POCKET MANUAL
OF
HOMOEOPATHIC MATERIA MEDICA
&
REPERTORY

COMPRISING OF
THE CHARACTERISTIC AND GUIDING SYMPTOMS OF ALL REMEDIES
(CLINICAL AND PATHOGENETIC)
INCLUDING INDIAN DRUGS

By

WILLIAM BOERICKE, M.D.

B. Jain Publishers (P) Ltd.
USA – EUROPE – INDIA

POCKET MANUAL OF HOMOEOPATHIC MATERIA MEDICA AND REPERTORY

58th impression, 2021

> **NOTE FROM THE PUBLISHERS**
> Any information given in this book is not intended to be taken as a replacement for medical advice. Any person with a condition requiring medical attention should consult a qualified practitioner or therapist.

All rights reserved. No part of this book may be reproduced, stored in a retrieval system or transmitted, in any form or by any means, mechanical, photocopying, recording or otherwise, without any prior written permission of the publisher.

© with the publisher

Published by Kuldeep Jain for
B. JAIN PUBLISHERS (P) LTD.
B. Jain House, D-157, Sector-63,
NOIDA-201307, U.P. (INDIA)
Tel.: +91-120-4933333 • Email: info@bjain.com
Website www.bjain.com

Printed in India

ISBN: 978-81-319-0128-1

PREFACE TO THE NINTH EDITION

In preparing the ninth edition of this work, I have followed the lines laid out for all the previous editions, namely, to present in a condensed form the homœopathic Materia Medica for practical use.

The book contains the well known verified characteristic symptoms of all our medicines besides other less important symptoms aiding the selection of the curative remedy. All the new medicines and essentials of the published clinical experience of the school have been added. In its present compact form it contains the maximum number of reliable Materia Medica facts in the minimum space.

I have tried to give a succinct resumé of the symptomatology of every medicine used in Homœopathy, including also clinical suggestions of many drugs so far not yet based on provings, thus offering the opportunity to experiment with these and by future provings discover their distinctive use and so enlarging our armamentarium.

I am aware that there is a difference of opinion about the advisability of further introduction of remedies, especially of such as seem obsolete or to some minds illusory. But it is not for the compiler to leave out information about any substance that has received the clinical endorsement from a reliable source.

Our Materia Medica must include all substances which have been proved and which have been used with apparent efficacy. It rests with the individual student to judge for himself the accuracy and reliability of such observation. In this connection, I cannot forego to avail myself of the high authority of that master of Homœopathy, Dr. Constantine Hering, favoring the introduction of all remedies capable of producing reactions in the body that may guide to their medicinal employment. "Homœopathy is essentially not only many-sided but all-sided. She investigates the action of all substances, whether articles of diet, beverages, condiments, drugs or poisons. She investigates their action on the healthy, the sick, animals and plants. She gives a new interpretation to that ancient, quoted saying of Paul, *Prove all things*—a new meaning, a new application that acts universally. Elimination of the useless may gradually take place with the growth of accurate physiological and pathological knowledge."

Again, imperfectly proved remedies necessitate the use of names of diseases at times instead of the component symptoms that alone are the legitimate guide to the choice of the curative remedy. Here, too, I have Hering as pioneer guide for the legitimacy of this method, which he also followed in his great work, the Guiding Symptoms. He said that he used the disease designations not for the purpose of recommending the particular remedy for that disease, but to show the great variety of remedies that may be used for any form of disease when otherwise indicated. For the same reason I have included nosological terms in the symptomatology and Therapeutic Index, as this is a practical handbook for every-day service, and any aid for finding the curative remedy ought to be utilized. As Dr. J. Compton Burnett expresses it:

"The fact is we need any and every way of finding the right remedy; the simple simile, the simple symptomatic similimum and the farthest reach of all—the pathologic similimum, and I maintain that we are still well within the lines of Homœopathy that is expansive, progressive, science fostered and science fostering."

The dosage needs some apology. It is, of course, suggestive only; more often to be wholly disregarded. I have followed the lines of the earlier Homœopathists in this regard, and given what was then considered the usual range of potency, to which I have added my own experience and that of many observing practitioners. Every teacher of Materia Medica is constantly importuned by students to suggest the potency—something to start with at least.

The book is in no sense a treatise, and must not be considered or judged as such. It is as accurate and reliable a compilation and the fullest collection of verified Materia Medica facts and clinical suggestions as it is possible to obtain within the compass of the volume. It supplements every other work on Materia Medica, and if used as a ready reminder of the essential facts of our vast symptomatology and as an introduction to the larger books of reference and record of provings, it will fulfill its purpose and prove a useful aid to the student and general practitioner. As such it is again offered with much appreciation of past endorsement to his professional brethren.

I have been aided in seeing this edition through the press by the efficient help of Mr. F. O. Ernesty, who has lightened the labor of making the manuscript more acceptable to the printers, and I desire to express my hearty appreciation of this kind and helpful service.

WILLIAM BOERICKE, M. D.

San Francisco, June, 1927.

PREFATORY NOTE TO THE REPERTORY

With the advent of the incomparable Ninth Edition of the progressive pocket Materia Medica, its modest companion, the Repertory, has been completely remodelled and brought up to date, by embodying much of the newly incorporated material. Many of the Sections have been carefully rewritten, and, with appropriate expansion, offer a more trustworthy guide for the selection of the homœopathic remedy. A few prefatory remarks, pertaining to the practical and expeditious use of the repertorial contents, may assist in clarifying a certain inevitable obscurity of plan.

Firstly, in conformity with established repertorial methods, the *division* of the *sections* in somewhat the old Hahnemannian order is adhered to, and may be stated as follows: Mind; Head; Eyes; Ears, etc.

Secondly, for the purpose of convenience, solely, *headings* and *sub-headings* and specific conditions or symptoms comprised under the latter are arranged in *alphabetical order*, and this is more or less consistently adhered to throughout the entire work. For example, under Mind the headings read, Awkward, brain-fag, catalepsy, etc.; likewise the heading Delirium embraces its various phases in alphabetical order.

Thirdly, all *headings* when *extensive in scope—e. g., Headache*, are presented under definite captions in the following order: Cause, Type, Location, Character of pain, Concomitants, Modalities—*i. e.*, Aggravations and Ameliorations. It is to be observed that some headings include only a few, whereas others include all of these divisions. This method has been resorted to simply to facilitate the task of the use of the repertory.

Fourth, to preserve uniformity, the *technical names of diseases* are bracketed, thereby assuming a subsidiary place, which is in strict accord with the homœopathic requirement, to prescribe for the symptoms of each specific case, and not for a mere name of a disease. Of course, being a clinical and not a truly symptomatological index (for which the practitioner and student are referred to the monumental works of Kent, Knerr and Clarke) technical terms are often selected as main headings, and when feasible, the more or less complete symptoms constitute the sub-headings.

Fifthly, the *remedies* are arranged in *alphabetical* order, and the *italics* indicate the more frequently verified *clinical* remedy. The abbreviations of the remedies are purely arbitrary and self-explanatory.

A complete alphabetical Index, newly added, will surely offer much assistance to the busy practitioner, in the ready reference to the specific information desired.

Lastly, it is only by the persistent use of *one* repertory, that its peculiar and intricate arrangements gradually crystallizes itself in definite outline, in the mind of the student of the same, and thus he attains the ready ease and practical insight of the collator, thereby rendering such a clinical bee-line well-nigh indispensable in our day of labor-saving devices.

OSCAR E. BOERICKE, M. D.

Philadelphia, Pa., June, 1927.

HOMŒOPATHIC MATERIA MEDICA

HOMŒOPATHIC MATERIA MEDICA

ABIES CANADENSIS—PINUS CANADENSIS
(Hemlock Spruce)

Mucous membranes are affected by Abies Can. and gastric symptoms are most marked, and a catarrhal condition of the stomach is produced. There are peculiar cravings and chilly sensations that are very characteristic, especially for women with uterine displacement, probably due to defective nutrition with debility. Respiration and heart action labored. Wants to lie down all the time; skin cold and clammy, hands cold; very faint. Right lung and liver feel small and hard. Gleet.

Head.—Feels light-headed, tipsy. Irritable.

Stomach.—Canine hunger with torpid liver. *Gnawing, hungry, faint feeling* at the epigastrium. Great appetite, craving for meat, pickles, radishes, turnips, artichokes, coarse food. *Tendency to eat far beyond capacity for digestion.* Burning and *distention of stomach and abdomen with palpitation.* Flatulence disturbs the heart's action. Pain in right shoulder-blade, and constipation, with burning in rectum.

Female.—Uterine displacements. Sore feeling at fundus of uterus, relieved by pressure. Prostration; wants to lie down all the time. Thinks womb is soft and feeble.

Fever.—Cold shiverings, as if blood were ice-water. [*Acon.*] Chills run down back. Cold-water feeling between shoulders. [*Ammon. mur.*] Skin clammy and sticky. Night-sweat [*China.*]

Dose.—First to third potency

ABIES NIGRA
(Black Spruce)

A powerful and long-acting remedy, in various forms of disease, whenever the characteristic stomach symptoms are present. Most of the symptoms are associated with the gastric disturbances. *In dyspeptic troubles of the aged*, with functional heart symptoms; also after tea or tobacco. *Constipation*. Pain in external meatus.

Head.—Hot, with flushed cheeks. Low-spirited. Dull during the day, wakeful at night. Unable to think.

Stomach.—*Pain in stomach always comes on after eating.* Sensation of a lump that hurts, *as if a hard-boiled egg had lodged in the cardiac end of stomach;* continual distressing constriction just above the pit of the stomach, as if everything were knotted up. Total loss of appetite in morning, but great craving for food at noon and night. Offensive breath. Eructations.

Chest.—Painful sensation, as if something were lodged in the chest and had to be coughed up; lungs feel compressed. Cannot be fully expanded. Worse coughing; waterbrash succeeds cough. Choking sensation in throat. Dyspnœa; worse lying down; Sharp, cutting pain in heart; *heart's action heavy and slow; tachycardia,* bradycardia.

Back.—Pain in small of back. Rheumatic pains and aching in bones.

Sleep.—Wakeful and restless at night, with hunger. Bad dreams.

Fever.—Alternate heat and cold; chronic intermittent fever, with pain in stomach.

Modalities.—*Worse* after eating.

Relationship.—Compare: (Lump in stomach—*China Bryon. Pulsat.*) also other Conifers—*Thuja, Sabina, Cupressus* (painful indigestion) also *Nux vom. Kali carb.*

Dose.—First to thirtieth potency.

ABROTANUM
(Southernwood)

A very useful remedy in *marasmus*, especially of lower extremities only, yet with good appetite. *Metastasis*. Rheumatism following checked diarrhœa. Ill effects of suppressed conditions especially in gouty subjects. *Tuberculous peritonitis. Exudative pleurisy* and other exudative processes. After operation upon the chest for hydrothorax or empyæmia, a pressing sensation remains. Aggravation of hæmorrhoids when rheumatism improves. Nosebleed and hydrocele in boys.

Great weakness after influenza. [*Kali phos.*]

Mind.—Cross, irritable, anxious, depressed.

Face.—Wrinkled, cold, dry, pale. Blue rings around dull-looking eyes. Comedones, with emaciation. Nosebleed. *Angioma of the face.*

Stomach.—Slimy taste. Appetite good, but emaciation progresses. Food passes undigested. Pain in stomach; worse at night; cutting, gnawing pain. *Stomach feels as if swimming in water;* feels cold. Gnawing hunger and whining. Indigestion, with vomiting of large quantities of offensive fluid.

Abdomen.—Hard lumps in abdomen. *Distended.* Alternate diarrhœa and constipation. Hæmorrhoids; frequent urging; bloody stools; worse as rheumatic pains abate. Ascarides. Oozing from umbilicus. Sensation as if bowels were sinking down.

Respiratory.—Raw feeling. Impeded respiration. Dry cough following diarrhœa. Pain across chest; severe in region of heart.

Back.—Neck so weak cannot hold head up. Back lame, weak, and painful. Pain in lumbar region extending along spermatic cord. Pain in sacrum, with hæmorrhoids.

Extremities.—Pain in shoulders, arms, *wrists*, and *ankles*. Pricking and coldness in fingers and feet. *Legs* greatly emaciated. Joints stiff and lame. Painful contraction of limbs. [*Amm. mur.*]

Skin.—Eruptions come out on face; are suppressed, and the skin becomes purplish. Skin flabby and loose. Furuncles. Falling out of hair. Itching chilblains.

Modalities.—*Worse*, cold air, checked secretions. *Better*, motion.

Relationship.—Compare: *Scrophularia; Bryonia; Stellaria; Benzoic acid*, in gout. *Iodine, Natr. mur.* in marasmus.

Dose.—Third to thirtieth potency.

ABSINTHIUM

(Common Wormwood)

A perfect picture of epileptiform seizure is produced by this drug. Nervous tremors precede attack. Sudden and severe giddiness, delirium with hallucinations and loss of consciousness. Nervous excitement and sleeplessness. Cerebral irritation, hysterical and infantile spasms come within range of this remedy. Poisoning by mushrooms. Chorea. *Tremor.* Nervousness, excitement, and sleeplessness in children.

Mind.—Hallucinations. Frightful visions. Kleptomania. Loss of memory. Forgets what has recently happened. Wants nothing to do with anybody. Brutal.

Head.—*Vertigo, with tendency to fall backward.* General confusion. Wants head low. Pupils dilated unequally. Face blue. *Spasmodic facial twitching.* Dull occipital headache. [*Gelsem. Picric ac.*]

Mouth.—Jaws fixed. Bites tongue; trembles; feels as if swollen and too large; protruding.

Throat.—Scalded sensation; as of a lump.

Stomach.—Nausea; retching; eructation. Bloated around waist and *abdomen.* Wind colic.

Urine.—Constant desire. Very strong odor; deep yellow color. [*Kali phos.*]

Sexual.—Darting pain in right ovary. Spermatorrhœa, with relaxed, enfeebled parts. Premature menopause.

Chest.—Sensation of weight on chest. Irregular, tumultuous action of heart can be heard in back.

Extremities.—Pain in limbs. Paralytic symptoms.

Relationship.—Compare: *Alcohol; Artemisia; Hydrocy. acid; Cina; Cicuta.*

Dose.—First to sixth potency.

ACALYPHA INDICA

(Indian Nettle)

A drug having a marked action on the alimentary canal and respiratory organs. It is indicated in incipient phthisis, with hard, racking cough, bloody expectoration, arterial hæmorrhage, but no febrile disturbance. Very weak in the morning, gains strength during day. Progressive emaciation. All pathological hæmorrhages having notably *a morning aggravation*.

Chest.—*Cough dry, hard, followed by hæmoptysis;* worse in morning and at night. Constant and severe pain in chest. Blood bright red and not profuse in morning; dark and clotted in afternoon. Pulse soft and compressible. Burning in pharynx, œsophagus, and stomach.

Abdomen.—Burning in intestines. *Spluttering diarrhœa with forcible expulsion of noisy flatus,* bearing down pains and tenesmus. Rumbling distention, and griping pain in abdomen. Rectal hæmorrhage; worse in morning.

Skin.—Jaundice. Itching and circumscribed furuncle-like swellings.

Modalities.—*Worse* in morning.

Relationship.—Compare: *Millefol.; Phosphor.; Acetic acid; Kali nit.*

Dose.—Third to sixth potency.

ACETANILIDUM
(Antifebrinum)

Depresses heart, respiration and blood pressure, lowers temperature. Cyanosis and collapse. Increased susceptibility to cold. Destroys red blood corpuscles; pallor.

Head.—Enlarged sensation. Fainting. Moral depravity.

Eyes.—Pallor of optic discs, contracted visual field and shrinking retinal vessel; mydriasis.

Heart.—Weak, irregular, with blue mucous membranes, albuminuria, œdema of feet and ankles.

Relationship.—Compare: *Antipyrin.*

Dose.—Used as a sedative and antipyretic for various forms of headache and neuralgia in doses of one to three grains. For the homœopathic indications use the third potency.

ACETIC ACID

(Glacial Acetic Acid)

This drug produces a condition of profound anæmia, with some dropsical symptoms, great debility, frequent fainting, dyspnœa. weak heart, vomiting, profuse urination and sweat. Hæmorrhage from any part. Especially indicated in pale, lean persons. with lax, flabby muscles. *Wasting and debility.* Acetic acid has the power to *liquify albuminous and fibrinous deposits.* Epithelial cancer, internally and locally (W. Owens). Sycosis with nodules and formations in the joints. Hard chancre. The 1x solution will soften and cause formation of pus.

Mind.—Irritable, worried about business affairs.

Head.—Nervous headache, from abuse of narcotics. Blood rushes to head with delirium. Temporal vessels distended. Pain across root of tongue.

Face.—*Pale, waxen, emaciated.* Eyes sunken, surrounded by dark rings. Bright red. Sweaty. Epithelioma of lip. Cheeks hot and flushed. Aching in left jaw-point.

Stomach.—*Salivation. Fermentation* in stomach. Intense burning thirst. Cold drinks distress. Vomits after every kind of food. Epigastric tenderness. Burning pain as of an ulcer. Cancer of stomach. Sour belching and vomiting. Burning waterbrash and profuse salivation. Hyperchlorhydria and gastralgia. *Violent burning pain in stomach and chest, followed by coldness of skin and cold sweat on forehead.* Stomach feels as if she had taken a lot of vinegar.

Abdomen.—Feels as if abdomen was sinking in. Frequent watery stools, worse in morning. *Tympanitic.* Ascites. Hæmorrhage from bowels.

Urine.—Large quantities of pale urine. Diabetes, with great thirst and debility. [*Phos. ac.*]

Female.—Excessive catamenia. *Hæmorrhages after labor.* Nausea of pregnancy. Breasts painfully enlarged, distended with milk. Milk impoverished, bluish, transparent, sour. Anæmia of nursing mothers.

Respiratory.—Hoarse, hissing respiration; *difficult breathing; cough when inhaling.* Membraneous croup. Irritation of trachea and bronchial tubes. False membrane in throat. Profuse bronchorrhœa, Putrid sore throat (gargle).

Back.—Pain in back, *relieved only by lying on abdomen.*

Extremities.—Emaciation. Œdema of feet and legs.

Skin.—Pale, waxen, œdematous. Burning, dry, hot skin, or bathed in profuse sweat. Dimished sensibility of the surface of body. Useful after stings, bites, etc. Varicose swellings. Scurvy; *anasarca.* Bruises; sprains.

Fever.—*Hectic, with drenching night-sweats. Red spot on left cheek. No thirst in fever.* Ebullitions. *Sweat profuse, cold.*

Relationship.—Acetic acid is antidotal to all anæsthetic vapors. Counteracts sausage poisoning.

Compare: *Ammon. acet.* (Profuse saccharine urine, patient is bathed in sweat.) *Benzoin oderiferum—Spice-wood (night sweats.) Ars.; China; Digitalis; Liatris. (General anasarca in heart and* kidney disease, *dropsy,* and chronic diarrhœa.)

Dose.—Third to thirtieth potency. Not to be repeated too often, except in croup.

ACONITUM NAPELLUS
(Monkshood)

A state of fear, anxiety; anguish of mind and body. *Physical and mental restlessness,* fright, is the most characteristic manifestation of *Aconite. Acute, sudden, and violent invasion, with fever,* call for it. Does not want to be touched. Sudden and great sinking of strength. *Complaints and tension* caused by exposure *to dry, cold weather,* draught of cold air, checked perspiration, also complaints from *very hot weather,* especially gastro-intestinal disturbances, etc. First remedy in inflammations, inflammatory fevers. Serous membranes and muscular tissues affected markedly. Burning in internal parts; *tingling, coldness and numbness.* Influenza. *Tension* of arteries; emotional and physical mental tension explain many symptoms. When prescribing Aconite remember Aconite causes only functional disturbance, no evidence that it can produce tissue change—its action is brief and *shows no periodicity.* Its sphere is in the beginning of an acute disease and not to be continued after pathological change comes. In Hyperæmia, congestion not after exudation has set in. *Influenza* [*Influenzin*]

Mind.—*Great fear, anxiety,* and worry accompany every ailment, however trivial. Delirium is characterized by unhappiness, worry, fear, raving, rarely unconsciousness. *Forebodings and fears.* Fears death but believes that he will soon die; predicts the day. *Fears the future,* a crowd, crossing the street. *Restlessness,* tossing about. Tendency to start. Imagination acute, clairvoyance. Pains are intolerable; they drive him crazy. Music is unbearable; makes her sad. [*Ambra.*] Thinks his thoughts come from the stomach—that parts of his body are abnormally thick. Feels as if what had just been done was a dream.

Head.—Fullness; *heavy,* pulsating, *hot, bursting,* burning, undulating sensation. Intercranial pressure. (*Hedera Helix.*) Burning headache, as if brain were moved by boiling water [*Indigo.*]. Vertigo; *worse on rising* [*Nux. Opium*] and shaking head. Sensation on vertex as if hair were pulled or stood on end. Nocturnal furious delirium.

Eyes.—Red, inflamed. Feel *dry and hot,* as if sand in them. *Lids swollen, hard and red.* Aversion to light. Profuse watering after exposure to dry, cold winds, *reflection from snow, after extraction of cinders* and other foreign bodies.

Ears.—Very *sensitive to noises;* music is unbearable. External ear hot, red, painful, swollen. Earache. [*Cham.*] Sensation as of drop of water in left ear.

Nose.—*Smell acutely sensitive. Pain at root of nose.* Coryza; much sneezing; throbbing in nostrils. Hæmorrhage of bright red blood. *Mucous membrane dry, nose stopped up; dry or with but scanty watery coryza.*

Face.—Red, hot, flushed, swollen. One cheek red, the other pale (*Cham., Ipec.*). *On rising the red face becomes deathly pale, or he becomes dizzy. Tingling* in cheeks and numbness. *Neuralgia, especially of left side, with restlessness, tingling, and numbness.* Pain in jaws.

Mouth.—Numb, *dry,* and tingling. Tongue swollen; *tip tingles.* Teeth sensitive to cold. Constantly moves lower jaw as if chewing. *Gums hot and inflamed. Tongue coated white.* [*Antim. crud.*]

Throat.—*Red, dry, constricted,* numb, prickling, burning, stinging. Tonsils swollen and dry.

ACONITUM NAPELLUS

Stomach.—*Vomiting, with fear, heat, profuse sweat and increased urination.* Thirst for cold water. *Bitter taste* of everything except water. *Intense thirst.* Drinks, vomits, and declares he will die. Vomiting, bilious, mucous and bloody, greenish. Pressure in stomach with dyspnœa. Hæmatemesis. Burning from stomach to œsophagus.

Abdomen.—Hot, tense, tympanitic. *Sensitive to touch. Colic, no position relieves.* Abdominal symptoms better after warm soup. Burning in umbilical region.

Rectum.—Pain with nightly itching and stitching in anus. Frequent, small stool with tenesmus; *green, like chopped herbs.* White with red urine. Choleraic discharge with collapse, anxiety, and restlessness. Bleeding hæmorrhoids. [*Hamam.*] Watery diarrhœa in children. They cry and complain much, are sleepless and restless.

Urine.—*Scanty, red, hot, painful.* Tenesmus and burning at neck of bladder. Burning in urethra. Urine suppressed, bloody. Anxiety always on beginning to urinate. *Retention, with screaming and restlessness,* and handling of genitals. Renal region sensitive. Profuse urination, with profuse perspiration and diarrhœa.

Male.—Crawling and stinging in glans. Bruised pain in testicles, swollen, hard. Frequent erections and emissions. Painful erections.

Female.—Vagina dry, hot, sensitive. Menses too profuse, with nosebleed, too protracted, late. Frenzy on appearance of menses. *Suppressed from fright, cold,* in plethoric subjects. Ovaries congested and painful. Sharp shooting pains in womb. *After-pains, with fear and restlessness.*

Respiratory.—Constant pressure in left chest; *oppressed breathing* on least motion. *Hoarse, dry, croupy cough;* loud, labored breathing. Child grasps at throat every time he coughs. Very sensitive to inspired air. *Shortness of breath.* Larynx sensitive. Stitches through chest. Cough, dry, short, hacking; *worse at night and after midnight.* Hot feeling in lungs. Blood comes up with hawking. Tingling in chest after cough.

Heart.—*Tachycardia.* Affections of the heart with pain in *left shoulder.* Stitching pain in chest. *Palpitation, with anxiety,* fainting, and *tingling* in fingers. *Pulse full, hard; tense and* *bounding;* sometimes intermits. Temporal and carotid arteries felt when sitting.

Back—Numb, stiff, painful. Crawling and tingling, as if bruised. Stiffness in nape of neck. Bruised pain between scapulæ.

Extremities.—*Numbness and tingling;* shooting pains; icy coldness and insensibility of hands and feet. Arms feel lame, bruised, heavy, numb. Pain down left arm [*Cact., Crotal., Kalmia, Tabac.*] *Hot hands and cold feet.* Rheumatic inflammation of joints; worse at night; red shining swelling, very sensitive. Hip-joint and thigh feel lame, especially after lying down. Knees unsteady; disposition of foot to turn. [*Æscul.*] Weak and lax ligaments of all joints. Painless cracking of all joints. *Bright red hypothenar eminences on both hands.* Sensation as if drops of water trickled down the thigh.

Sleep.—Nightmare. Nightly ravings. *Anxious dreams.* Sleeplessness, with restless and tossing about. [Use thirtieth potency.] Starts up in sleep. Long dreams, with anxiety in chest. Insomnia of the aged.

Skin.—Red, hot, swollen, dry, burning. *Purpura miliaris.* Rash like measles. Gooseflesh. Formication and numbness. Chilliness and formication down back. Pruritus *relieved* by stimulants.

Fever.—Cold stage most marked. Cold sweat and icy coldness of face. Coldness and heat alternate. Evening chilliness soon after going to bed. *Cold waves pass through him. Thirst and restlessness* always present. Chilly if uncovered or touched. Dry heat, red face. Most valuable febrifuge with mental anguish, restlessness, etc. Sweat drenching, on parts lain on; relieving all symptoms.

Modalities.—*Better* in open air; *worse* in warm room, in evening and *night; worse* lying on affected side, from music, from tobacco-smoke, dry, cold winds.

Vinegar in large doses is antidotal to poisonous effects.

Relationship.—Acids, wine and coffee, lemonade, and acid fruits modify its action.

Not indicated in malarial and low fevers or hectic and pyæmic conditions, and in inflammations when they localize themselves. *Sulphur* often follows it. Compare *Cham.* and *Coffea* in *intense pain* and sleeplessness.

Agrostis acts like Acon. in fever and inflammations, also *Spiranthes*.

Complementary: *Coffea; Sulph.* Sulphur may be considered a chronic Aconite. Often completes a cure begun with Aconite.

Compare: *Bellad.; Cham.; Coffea; Ferr. phos.*

Aconitine.—(Heavy feeling *as of lead;* pains in supraorbital nerve; ice-cold sensations creep up; hydrophobia symptoms. Tinnitus aurium 3x.) *Tingling* sensation.

Aconitum Lycotonum.—Great yellow wolfsbane.—(Swelling of glands; Hodgkin's disease. Diarrhœa after eating pork. Itching of nose, eyes, anus and vulva. Skin of nose cracked; taste of blood.)

Aconitum Cammarum.—(Headache with vertigo and tinnitus. Cataleptic symptoms. Formication of tongue, lips and face.)

Aconitum ferox.—Indian Aconite.—Rather more violent in its actions than *A. napellus*. It is more diuretic and less antipyretic. It has proved valuable in *cardiac dyspnœa*, neuralgia, and acute gout. *Dyspnœa. Must sit up. Rapid respiration.* Anxiety, with suffocation from feeling of paralysis in respiratory muscles. Cheynes-Stokes breathing. *Quebracho* (cardiac dyspnœa.) (*Achyranthes.*—A Mexican drug—very similar to Aconite in fevers, but of larger range, being also adapted to typhoidal states and intermittents. Muscular rheumatism. A great diaphoretic. Use 6x.) *Eranthis hymnalis*—(Winter Aconite—acts on solar plexus and works upwards causing dyspnœa. Pain in occiput and neck.)

Dose.—Sixth potency for sensory affections; first to third for congestive conditions. Must be repeated frequently in acute diseases. Acon. is a rapid worker. In Neuralgias tincture of the root often preferable, one drop doses (poisonous), or again, the 30th potency according to susceptibility of patient.

ACTEA SPICATA
(Baneberry)

Is a rheumatic remedy, especially of the *small joints;* tearing, tingling pains characterize it. *Wrist-rheumatism.* Pulsations over whole body, especially liver and renal region. Cardiovascular spasm. Pains worse from touch and motion.

Head.—Fearful, starts easily; confused. Ebullition of blood to head excited by drinking coffee. Vertigo, tearing headache, better in open air, throbbing in brain, pain from crown to between eyebrows; heat in forehead, pain in left frontal eminence as if bone were crushed. Itching of scalp alternating with heat; nose red at tip, fluent coryza.

Face.—Violent pain in upper jaw, running from teeth through malar bones to temples. Perspiration on face and head.

Stomach.—Tearing, darting pains in epigastric region, with vomiting. Cramp-like pains in stomach and epigastrium, with difficult breathing; sense of suffocation. Sudden lassitude after eating.

Abdomen.—Spasmodic retraction. Sticking pain and distension of hypogastrium.

Respiratory.—Short, irregular breathing at night, while lying. *Great oppression. Shortness of breath on exposure to cold air.*

Extremities.—Tearing pains in loins. *Rheumatic pains in small joints, wrist, [Ulmus] fingers, ankles, toes. Swelling of joints from slight fatigue. Wrist swollen,* red, worse any motion. Paralytic weakness in the hands. Lame feeling in arms. Pain in knee. Sudden lassitude after talking or eating.

Relationship.—Compare: *Cimicif.; Cauloph.; Led.*

Dose.—Third potency.

ADONIS VERNALIS
(Pheasant's Eye)

A heart medicine, after rheumatism or influenza, or Bright's disease, where the muscles of the heart are in stage of fatty degeneration, regulating the pulse and increasing the power of contractions of heart, with increased urinary secretions. Most valuable in cardiac dropsy. Low vitality, with weak heart and slow, weak pulse. Hydrothorax, ascites. Anasarca.

Head.—Feels light; aches across front, *from occiput around temples to eyes.* Vertigo on rising, turning head quickly or lying down. Tinnitus. Scalp feels tight. Eyes dilated.

Mouth.—Slimy. Tongue dirty yellow, sore, feels scalded.

Heart.—Mitral and aortic regurgitation. Chronic aortitis.

Fatty heart pericarditis. Rheumatic Endocarditis. [*Kalmia*].
Præcordial pain, palpitation, and dyspnœa. Marked venous engorgement. Cardiac asthma. [*Quebracho.*] Fatty heart.
Myocarditis, irregular cardiac action, constriction and vertigo.
Pulse rapid, irregular.

Stomach.—Heavy weight. Gnawing hunger. Faint feeling in epigastrium. Better out of doors.

Urine.—Oily pellicle on urine. Scanty, albuminous.

Respiratory.—Frequent desire to take a long breath. Feeling of weight on chest.

Sleep.—Restlesss, with horrible dreams.

Extremities.—Aching in nape. Spine stiff and aching. Œdema.

Relationship.—*Adonidin* is a cardiac tonic and diuretic. Quarter grain daily, or two to five grains of first decimal trit. increases arterial pressure and prolongs the diastole, favoring emptying engorged veins. Is an excellent substitute for Digitalis and is not cumulative in action.

Compare: *Digit.; Cratæg.; Conval.; Strophantus.*

Dose.—Five to ten drops of the tincture.

ADRENALIN
(An Internal Secretion of Suprarenal Glands)

Adrenalin or Epinephrin, the active principle of the medulla of the suprarenal gland, (cortical secretion not as yet isolated), is employed as a chemical messenger in the regulation of the activities of the body; in fact, its presence is essential to the activity of the sympathetic nerve. Adrenalin action on any part is the same as *stimulation of the sympathetic nerve endings* thereto. Local application [1: 1,000 solution] to mucous membranes promptly induces transient ischæmia, seen in a *blanching*, persisting several hours from conjunctival instillation. Its action is very prompt, efficient, *evanescent*, owing to rapid oxidation and therefore practically harmless, *unless* too frequently repeated, when atheroma and heart lesions—myocardial—in animals have been reported. Arteries, heart, supra-renal bodies and vaso-motor system are prominently affected.

The main action of Adrenalin is stimulation of the *sympa-*

thetic endings, notably the splanchnic area, causing *constriction of the peripheral arterioles*, with resulting *rise in blood pressure*. This is especially observed in stomach, intestines; less in uterus, skin; nil in brain and lungs. Furthermore, is noticed, *slowing of pulse*, (medullary vagus stimulation), and *strengthening of heart beat* (increased myocardial contractility), resembling Digitalis; increased glandular activity, glycosuria; depression of respiratory center; contraction of muscular tissue of eye, uterus, vagina; relaxation of muscular tissue of stomach, intestines, bladder.

Uses.—Its chief therapeutic use depends on its *vaso-constriction* action; therefore a most powerful and prompt *astringent* and *hæmostatic;* and invaluable in *checking* capillary hæmorrhages from *all* parts, where *local* or direct application is feasible: nose, ear, mouth, throat, larynx, stomach, rectum, uterus, bladder. Hemorrhagic condition not due to defective coagulation of the blood. Complete *bloodlessness*, ischæmia, may be induced with impunity.   Locally, solutions [1 : 10,000-1 : 1,000] sprayed or applied on cotton have been very efficient in bloodless operations about the eye, nose, throat, and larynx.

Congestions of the ethmoid and sphenoid sinuses, also hay fever, have been markedly alleviated by warm spray of Adrenalin chloride, 1 : 5,000. Here compare, Hepar 1x, which will start up secretions and so facilitate drainage. Werlhoff's disease, hypodermically, 1 : 1,000. Externally, it has been used in neuritis, neuralgia, reflex pains, gout, rheumatism, as an ointment, 1-2 m. of (1 : 1,000) solution, along the nerve trunk at point of skin nearest its origin which could be reached (H.G. Carlton).

Therapeutically, Adrenalin has been suggested in acute congestion of lungs, *Asthma*, Grave's and Addison's diseases, arterio-sclerosis, chronic aortitis, angina pectoris, hæmophilia, chlorosis, hay fever, serum rashes, acute urticaria, etc. Dr. P. Jousset reports success in treating, homœopathically, cases of angina and of aortitis, sub-acute and chronic, when Adrenalin has been prescribed *per os* and in infinitesimal dose. The symptom guiding to this is, *Sensation of thoracic constriction with anguish*. This, with vertigo, nausea and vomiting have been produced by the drug. *Abdominal pain. Shock* or heart failure during anesthesia, as it causes very prompt rise of blood pressure by its action on nerve endings in the vessel wall.

Dose.—Hypodermically, 1-5 m. [1 : 1,000 solution, as chloride] diluted in water. Internally, 5-30 m. of 1 : 1,000 solution.

Caution.—On account of its affinity for oxygen, the drug easily decomposes in watery and dilute acid solutions. The solution must be protected from air and light. It must not be too frequently repeated, owing to cardiac and arterial lesions. For homœopathic use 2x to 6x attenuation.

AESCULUS HIPPOCASTANUM
(Horse Chestnut)

The action of this drug is most marked on the lower bowel, producing engorged hæmorrhoidal veins, with characteristic backache, with absence of actual constipation. Much pain but little bleeding. Venous stasis general, varicose veins of purple color; everything is slowed down, digestion, heart, bowels, etc. Torpor and congestion of the liver and portal system, with constipation. The back aches and gives out and unfits the patient for business. Flying pains all over. *Fullness in various parts;* dry, swollen mucous membranes. Throat with hæmorrhoidal conditions.

Head.—Depressed and *irritable*. Head dull, confused, aching as from a cold. Pressure in forehead, with nausea, followed by stitches in right hypochondrium. Pain from occiput to frontal region, with bruised sensation of the scalp; worse in the morning. Neuralgic stitches from right to left through forehead, followed by flying pains in epigastrium. Vertigo when sitting and walking.

Eyes.—Heavy and hot, with lachrymation, *with enlarged blood vessels*. Eyeballs sore.

Nose.—Dry; inspired air feels cold, *nasal passages sensitive to it. Coryza,* sneezing. Pressure at root of nose. Membrane over turbinate bones distended and boggy, dependent upon hepatic disorders.

Mouth.—Scalded feeling. Metallic taste. Salivation. Tongue thickly coated, feels as if scalded.

Throat.—Hot, *dry,* raw, stitching pain into ears when swallowing. Follicular pharyngitis connected with hepatic congestion. *Veins in pharynx distended* and tortuous. Throat sensitive to inspired air; feels excoriated and constricted, burns like fire on swallowing, in afternoon. Early stages of atrophic pharyngitis in dried-up, bilious subjects. Hawking of ropy mucus of sweetish taste.

Stomach.—Weight of a stone, with gnawing, aching pain; most manifest about three hours after meals. Tenderness and fullness in region of liver.

Abdomen.—Dull aching in liver and epigastrium. Pain at umbilicus. Jaundice; throbbing in hypogastrium and pelvis.

Rectum.—Dry, aching. *Feels full of small sticks.* Anus raw, sore. Much pain after stool, with prolapse. *Hæmorrhoids,* with sharp shooting pains up the back; blind and bleeding; worse during climacteric. Large, hard, dry stools. Mucous membrane seems swollen and obstructs the passage. Irritation caused by ascarides and aids their expulsion. *Burning in anus with chills up and down back.*

Urinary.—Frequent, scant, dark, muddy, hot urine. Pain in kidneys, especially left and ureter.

Male.—Discharge of prostatic fluid at stool.

Female.—*Constant throbbing behind symphysis pubis.* Leucorrhea, with *lameness of back across the sacro-iliac articulation;* dark yellow, sticky corroding; worse after menses.

Chest.—Feels constricted. Heart's action full and heavy, can feel pulsations all over. Laryngitis; coughs *depending on hepatic disorders;* hot feeling in chest; pain around heart in hæmorrhoidal subjects.

Extremities.—Aching and soreness in limbs, in left acromion process with shooting down arms; finger tips numb.

Back.—Lameness in neck; aching between shoulder blades; region of *spine feels weak;* back and legs give out. *Backache affecting sacrum and hips; worse walking or stooping.* When walking feet turn under. Soles feel sore, tired, and swell. Hands and feet swell, and become red after washing, feel full.

Fever.—Chill at 4 p. m. Chilliness up and down back. Fever 7 to 12 p. m. Evening fever, skin hot and dry. Sweat profuse and hot with the fever.

Modalities.—*Worse*, in morning on awaking, and from any motion, *walking;* from moving bowels; after eating, afternoon, standing. *Better*, cool open air.

Relationship.—*Æsculus glabra* — Ohio-Buckeye Proctitis. Very painful, dark purple, external hæmorrhoids, with constipation and vertigo and portal congestion. Speech thick, tickling in throat, impaired vision, paresis. *Phytolacca* (throat dry, more often in acute cases.) *Negundium Americanum*—Boxelder—(Engorgements of rectum and piles with great pain, tendrop doses of tincture every two hours.) Compare also: *Aloe, Collinson. Nux. Sulphur.*

Dose.—Tincture, to third potency.

AETHIOPS MERCURIALIS-MINERALIS
(Sulph. and Quicksilver, or Black Sulphide Mercury)

This preparation is of use in *scrofulous* affections, ophthalmia, otorrhœa, painful, irritating, scabby eruptions, hereditary syphilis.

Skin.—Eruptions. Favus-like, scrofulous, herpetic and eczematous.

Dose.—The lower triturations, especially the second decimal.

Relationship.—*Æthiops Antimonalis* — (Hydrargyrum stibiato sulfuratum.)—(often more effective than the above in scrofulous eruptions, glandular swellings, otorrhœa and *scrofulous eye affections*, corneal ulcers. Third trituration.) Compare: *Calc.; Sil.; Psorin.*

AETHUSA CYNAPIUM
(Fool's Parsley)

The characteristic symptoms relate mainly to the brain and nervous system, connected with gastro-intestinal disturbance. Anguish, crying, and expression of uneasiness and discontent, lead to this remedy most frequently in disease in children, during dentition, summer complaint, when, with the diarrhœa, there is *marked inability to digest milk*, and poor circulation. Symptoms set in with *violence*.

Mind.—Restless, *anxious, crying*. Sees rats, cats, dogs, etc.

Unconscious, delirious. *Inability to think, to fix the attention.* Brain fag. Idiocy may alternate with furor and irritability.

Head.—Feels bound up, or in a vise. *Occipital pain extending down spine; better lying down and by pressure.* Head symptoms relieved by expelling flatus [*Sanguin.*] and by stool. Hair feels pulled. *Vertigo with drowsiness, with palpitation; head hot after vertigo ceases.*

Eyes.—Photophobia; *swelling of Meibomian glands.* Rolling of eyes on falling asleep. *Eyes drawn downward;* pupils dilated.

Ears.—*Feel obstructed.* Sense of something hot from ears. Hissing sound.

Nose.—Stopped up with much thick mucus. *Herpetic eruption* on tip of nose. Frequent ineffectual desire to sneeze.

Face.—*Puffed*, red-spotted, collapsed. Expression anxious, full of pain; *linea nasalis* marked.

Mouth.—Dry. Aphthæ. Tongue seems too long. Burning and pustules in throat, with difficult swallowing.

Stomach.—*Intolerance of milk;* vomiting as soon as swallowed or in large curds. Hungry after vomiting. *Regurgitation of food about an hour after eating.* Violent vomiting of a white frothy matter. Nausea at sight of food. Painful contraction of stomach. Vomiting, *with sweat and great weakness*, accompanied by anguish and distress, followed by sleepiness. Stomach feels turned upside down, with burning feeling up to the chest. Tearing pains in the stomach extending to œsophagus.

Abdomen.—Cold, internal and external, with aching pain in bowels. Colic, followed by vomiting, vertigo, and weakness. Tense, inflated, and sensitive. Bubbling sensation around navel.

Stool.—*Undigested, thin, greenish*, preceded by colic, with tenesmus, and followed by exhaustion and drowsiness. Cholera infantum; child cold, clammy, stupid, with staring eyes and dilated pupils. Obstinate constipation; feels as if all bowel action is lost. Choleraic affections in old age.

Urinary.—Cutting pain in bladder, with frequent urging. Pain in kidneys.

Female.—Lancinating pains in sexual organs. Pimples; itching when warm. Menses watery. Swelling of mammary glands, with lancinating pains.

Respiratory.—Difficult, oppressed, anxious respiration; crampy constriction. Sufferings render patient speechless.

Heart.—Violent palpitation, with vertigo, headache and restlessness. Pulse rapid, hard and small.

Back and Extremities.—Want of power to stand up or hold head up. Back feels as if in a vise. Aching in small of back. Weakness of lower extremities. Fingers and thumbs clenched. Numbness of hands and feet. Violent spasms. Squinting of eyes downward.

Skin.—Excoriation of thighs in walking. Easy perspiration. *Surface of body cold and covered with clammy sweat. Lymphatic glands swollen.* Itching *eruption around joints.* Skin of hands dry and shrunken. Ecchymosis. Anasarca.

Fever.—*Great heat; no thirst.* Profuse, cold sweat. *Must be covered during sweat.*

Sleep.—Disturbed by *violent startings;* cold perspiration. Dozing after vomiting or stool. *Child is so exhausted, it falls asleep at once.*

Modalities.—*Worse,* 3 to 4 a. m., and evenings; warmth, summer. *Better* in open air and company.

Compare: *Athamantha* (confused head, vertigo better lying down, *bitter* taste and saliva. Hands and feet icy cold); *Antimon.; Calc.; Ars.; Cicuta.* Complementary: *Calc.*

Dose.—Third to thirtieth potency.

AGARICUS MUSCARIUS—AMANITA
(Toad Stool—Bug Agaric)

This fungus contains several toxic compounds, the best known of which is *Muscarin.* The symptoms of poisoning do not develop at once, usuallly twelve to fourteen hours elapse before the initial attack. There is no antidote, treatment, entirely symptomatic (Schneider). Agaricus acts as an intoxicant to the brain, producing more vertigo and delirium than alcohol, followed by profound sopor with lowered reflexes.

Jerking, twitching, trembling, and itching are strong indications. Incipient phthisis; is related to the tubercular diathesis, anæmia, *chorea,* twitching ceases during sleep. Various forms of neuralgia and spasmodic affections, and neurotic skin troubles are pictured in the symptomatology of this remedy. It corresponds to various forms of cerebral excitement rather than congestion. Thus, in delirium of fevers, alcoholism, etc. General paralysis. *Sensation as if pierced by needles of ice.* Sensitive to pressure and cold air. *Violent bearing-down pains.* Symptoms appear diagonally as *right arm and left leg.* Pains are accompanied by sensation of cold, numbness and tingling.

Mind.—Sings, talks, but does not answer. *Loquacity.* Aversion to work. Indifference. *Fearlessness. Delirium* characterized by singing, shouting, and muttering; rhymes and prophesies. Begins with paroxysm of yawning.

The provings bring out four phases of cerebral excitement.

1. *Slight stimulation*—shown by increased cheerfulness, courage, loquacity, exalted fancy.

2. *More decided intoxication*—great mental excitement and incoherent talking, immoderate gaity alternates with melancholy. Perception of relative size of objects is lost, takes long steps and jumps over small objects as if they were trunks of trees—a small hole appears as a frightful chasm, a spoonful of water an immense lake. Physical strength is increased, can lift heavy loads. With it much twitching.

3. *Third stage* produces a condition of furious or raging delirium, screaming, raving, wants to injure himself, etc.

4. *Fourth stage*—mental depression, languor, indifference, confusion, disinclination to work, etc. We do not get the active cerebral congestion of Belladonna, but a general nervous excitement such as is found in delirium tremens, delirium of fevers, etc.

Head.—*Vertigo from sunlight,* and on walking. Head in constant motion. Falling backward, as if a weight in occiput. Lateral headache, as if from a nail. [*Coff.; Ignat.*] Dull headache from prolonged desk-work. Icy coldness, *like icy needles,* or splinters. Neuralgia with icy cold head. Desire to cover head warmly. [*Silica.*] Headache with *nose-bleed* or thick mucous discharge.

Eyes.—*Reading difficult, as type seems to move, to swim.* Vibrating specters. *Double vision* [*Gels.*], dim and flickering. Asthenopia from prolonged strain, *spasm* of accommodation. *Twitching of lids and eyeballs.* [*Codein.*] Margins of lids red; itch and burn and agglutinate. Inner angles very red.

Ears.—Burn and itch, as if frozen. Twitching of muscles about the ear and *noises*.

Nose.—*Nervous* nasal disturbances. *Itching* internally and externally. Spasmodic sneezing after coughing; sensitiveness; watery non-inflammatory discharge. Inner angles very red. Fetid, dark, bloody discharge. *Nosebleed in old people*. Sensation of soreness in nose and mouth.

Face.—*Facial* muscles feel stiff; *twitch;* face itches and burns. Lancinating, tearing pain in cheeks, as of splinters. Neuralgia, as if cold needles ran through nerves or sharp ice touched them.

Mouth.—Burning and smarting on lips. Herpes on lips. Twitching. Taste sweet. Aphthæ on roof of mouth. Splinter like pains in tongue. Thirsty all the time. Tremulous tongue. [*Lach.*] Tongue white.

Throat.—Stitches along eustachian tube to ear. Feels contracted. Small solid balls of phlegm thrown up. Dryness of pharynx, swallowing difficult. Scratching in throat; cannot sing a note.

Stomach.—Empty eructations, tasting of apples. Nervous disturbances, with spasmodic contractions, hiccough. Unnatural hunger. Flatulent distention of stomach and abdomen. Profuse inodorous flatus. Burning in stomach about three hours after a meal, changing into a dull pressure. *Gastric disturbance with sharp pains in liver region*.

Abdomen.—Stitching pains in liver, *spleen* [*Ceanothus*] and abdomen. Stitches under short ribs, left side. Diarrhœa with much fetid flatus. Fetid stools.

Urinary.—Stitches in urethra. Sudden and violent urging to urinate. Frequent urination.

Female.—Menses, increased, earlier. Itching and tearing, pressive pains of genitals and back. Spasmodic dysmenorrhœa. Severe *bearing-down pains, especially after menopause*. Sexual excitement. Nipples itch, burn. Complaints following parturition and coitus. Leucorrhœa, with much itching.

Respiratory Organs.—Violent attacks of coughing that can be suppressed by effort of will, worse eating, pain in head while cough lasts. Spasmodic cough at night after falling asleep, *with expectoration of little balls of mucus*. Labored, oppressed breathing. *Cough ends in a sneeze*.

Heart.—*Irregular, tumultuous palpitation,* after tobacco. Pulse intermittent and irregular. Cardiac region oppressed, as if thorax were narrowed. Palpitation with redness of face.

Back.—Pain, *with sensitiveness of spine to touch;* worse in dorsal region. Lumbago; worse in open air. Crick in back. *Twitching of cervical muscles.*

Extremities.—Stiff all over. Pain over hips. Rheumatism better motion. Weakness in loins. Uncertain gait. Trembling. *Itching of toes and feet as if frozen.* Cramp in soles of feet. Pain in shin-bone. Neuralgia in locomotor ataxia. Paralysis of lower limbs, with spasmodic condition of arms. Numbness of legs on crossing them. Paralytic pain in left arm followed by palpitation. Tearing painful contractions in the calves.

Skin.—*Burning, itching, redness, and swelling, as from frost-bites.* Pimples, hard, like flea-bites. Miliary eruption, with intolerable itching and burning. Chilblains. Angioneurotic œdema; rosacea. Swollen veins with cold skin. Circumscribed erythematous, papular and pustular and œdematous lesions.

Sleep.—*Paroxysms of yawning.* Restless from violent itching and burning. On falling asleep, *starts, twitches, and awakes often.* Vivid dreams. Drowsy in daytime. Yawning, followed by involuntary laughter.

Fever.—Very sensitive to cool air. Violent attacks of heat in evening. Copious sweat. Burning spots.

Modalities.—*Worse,* open cold air, after eating, after coitus. In cold weather, before a thunder-storm. Worse, pressure on dorsal spine, which causes involuntary laughter. *Better,* moving about slowly.

Relationship.—Compare: *Muscarine,* the alkaloid of Agaricus (has much power over secretions, increasing lachrymal, salivary, hepatic, etc., but diminishing renal; probably neurotic in origin, stimulating the terminal fibres of the secretory nerves of all these structures, hence *salivation, lachrymation and excessive perspiration.* Atropin exactly opposes *Muscarine.* Resembles *Pilocarpin in* action.) *Amanita vernus*—spring mushroom—a variety of *Agar Phalloides*—Death cup—active principle is *Phallin,* active like Muscarine. *Amanita phalloides* (Death Cup—Deadly Agaric.) The poison is a toxalbumin, resembling the poison in the rattle snake and the poison excreted by the cholera and diphtheria germs. It acts on the red blood corpuscles, dissolving them so that blood escapes into the alimentary canal and the whole system is drained. The amount of this toxic principle is small, even handling of specimens and breathing of spores affects some people unpleasantly. The poison is slow in development. Even 12 to 20 hours after taking it the patient feels all right, but vertigo violent choleraic symptoms with rapid loss of strength with death the second or third day, preceded by stupor and spasms. Fatty degeneration of liver, heart and kidneys, hemorrhages in lungs, pleura and skin (Dr. J. Schier) Vomiting and purging. Continuous urging to stool, but *no* gastric, abdominal or rectal *pain*. Intense thirst for cold water, dry skin. Lethargic but mentally clear. *Sharp changes* from rapid to slow and from slow to rapid breathing, extreme collapse, suppressed urine, but *no* cold extremities or cramps.) *Agaric. emet.* (severe vertigo; all symptoms *better, cold water; longing for ice-water;* gastritis cold sweat, vomiting sensation as if stomach was suspended on a string. *Tamus* (chilblains and freckles). *Cimicif.; Cann. ind.; Hyos.; Tarantula.*

Antidote: *Absinth.; Coffea; Camphor.*

Dose.—Third to thirtieth and two hundredth potency. In skin affections and brain exhaustions give the lower attenuations.

AGAVE AMERICANA
(Century Plant)

Indicated in stomacace, and painful erections in gonorrhœa, Strangury. Hydrophobia. Scurvy; countenance pale, gums swollen and bleeding, legs covered with dark purple blotches, swollen, painful and hard. Appetite poor; bowels constipated.

Relationship.—Compare: *Anhalonium; Lyssin; Lach.*

Dose.—Tincture.

AGNUS CASTUS
(The Chaste Tree)

The most effective point of attack of Agnus upon the organism is the sexual organism. It lowers sexual vitality, with corresponding mental depression and loss of nervous energy.

It shows this distinctive influence in both sexes, but is more pronounced in men. Premature old age from abuse of sexual power. History of repeated gonorrhœas. A prominent remedy for sprains and strains. *Gnawing itching in all parts, especially eyes.* Tachycardia caused by tobacco in neurotic young men.

Mind.—Sexual melancholy. Fear of death. *Sadness with impression of speedy death.* Absentminded, forgetful, lack of courage. Illusion of smell—herrings, musk. Nervous depression and mental forebodings.

Eyes.—*Pupils dilated.* [*Bell.*] Itching about eyes; photophobia.

Nose.—Odor of herring or musk. Aching in dorsum better pressure.

Abdomen.—Spleen swollen, sore. Stools soft, recede, difficult. Deep fissures in anus. Nausea with *sensation as if intestines were pressed downwards;* wants to support bowels.

Male.—Yellow discharge from urethra. No erections. *Impotence. Parts cold, relaxed. Desire gone.* [*Selen.; Con.; Sabal.*] Scanty emission without ejaculation. Loss of prostatic fluid on straining. Gleety discharge. Testicles, cold, swollen, hard, and painful.

Female.—Scanty menses. Abhorrence of sexual intercourse. Relaxation of genitals, with leucorrhœa. *Agalactia;* with sadness. Sterility. Leucorrhœa staining yellow; transparent. Hysterical palpitation with nose bleed.

Relationship.—Compare: *Selenium; Phosph. ac.; Camphor; Lycop.*

Dose.—First to sixth potency.

AGRAPHIS NUTANS
(Bluebell)

A relaxed condition of the system generally and a proneness to take cold on exposure to cold winds.

Catarrhal conditions; obstruction of nostrils. *Adenoids, throat deafness. Enlarged tonsils.* Mucous diarrhœa from cold. Chill from cold winds. Throat and ear troubles *with tendency to free discharge from mucous membranes.* Mutinism of childhood unconnected with deafness.

Relationship.—Compare: *Hydrast.; Cepa; Calc. phos.; Sulph. jod.; Calc. jod.*

Dose.—Third potency. Single doses of tincture. (Dr. Cooper).

AILANTHUS GLANDULOSA
(Chinese Sumach)

This remedy shows by its peculiar skin symptoms its pronounced power of disorganizing the blood, causing conditions we meet with in low fevers, low types of eruptive diseases, diphtheria, *follicular tonsillitis*, Streptococcus infection, Hemorrhagic diathesis, etc. *The skin appears livid or purplish;* face dark as mahogany, hot; sordes; throat swollen, purple, livid; semi-conscious, delirious; weak pulse, general torpor and prostration. Symptoms remarkably alike to malignant scarlatina. Diarrhœa, dysentery and *great weakness* are very marked. *Adynamia* characterizes all its conditions. Lividity, stupor and malignancy. Mucous membranes hemorrhagic and ulcerative [*Lach. Ars.*]

Head.—General stupor, with sighing. Confused mind, mental depression. *Headache, frontal,* with drowsiness. Passive congestion headaches. *Suffused, dilated eyes;* photophobia. Face dusky. Thin, *copious, ichorous,* bloody nasal discharge.

Throat.—Inflamed, œdematous, dusky red. *Much swelling, internal and external.* Dry, rough, scraping, choking feeling. *Neck tender and swollen.* Hoarse, croupy voice. *Tongue dry and brown. Teeth covered with sordes. Pain in swallowing* extends to the ears.

Respiratory.—Hurried breathing; irregular. Dry, hacking cough. Lungs sore and tired.

Sleep.—Drowsy, restless. Heavy, disturbed, unrefreshing.

Skin.—Miliary, livid rash, returns annually. Large blisters filled with dark serum. *Irregular, patchy, livid eruption,* disappearing on pressure. Cold. Raynaud's disease.

Relationship.—Antidotes: *Rhus; Nux.*

Compare: *Ammon. carb.; Bapt.; Arn.; Mur. ac.; Lach.; Rhus.*

Dose.—First to sixth potency.

ALETRIS FARINOSA
(Stargrass)

An anæmic, relaxed condition, especially of the female organism, is protrayed by this remedy. The patient *is tired all the time*, and suffers from prolapsus, leucorrhœa, rectal distress, etc. Marked anæmia. Chlorotic girls and pregnant women.

Mind.—Power and energy weakened. Confused feelings. Cannot concentrate mind. Fainting, with vertigo.

Mouth.—Much frothy saliva.

Stomach.—Disgust for food. Least food causes distress. Fainting spells, with vertigo. Vomiting during pregnancy. Nervous dyspepsia. Flatulent colic.

Rectum.—Loads up with fæces—paretic condition. Stool large, hard, difficult, great pain.

Female.—*Premature and profuse menses, with labor-like pains.* [*Bell.; Cham.; Kali c.; Plat.*] Retarded and scanty flow. (*Senecio.*) Uterus seems heavy. Prolapse, with pain in right inguinal region. Leucorrhœa due to weakness and anemia. Habitual tendency to abortion. Muscular pains during pregnancy.

Relationship.—Compare: *Helonias.; Hydrastis; Tanacet.; China.*

Dose.—Tincture to third potency.

ALFALFA
(Medicago Sativa. California Clover or Lucerne)

From its action on the sympathetic, Alfalfa favorably influences nutrition, evidenced in "toning up" the appetite and digestion resulting in greatly improved mental and physical vigor, with gain in weight. Disorders characterized by malnutrition are mainly within its therapeutic range, for example, neurasthenia, splanchnic blues, nervousness, insomnia, nervous indigestion, etc. Acts as a fat producer, corrects tissue waste. Deficient lactation. Increases quality and quantity of milk in nursing mothers. Its pronounced urinary action suggests it clinically in diabetes insipidus and phosphaturia; and it is claimed to allay vesical irritability of prostatic hypertrophy. The rheumatic diathesis seems especially amenable to its action.

Mind.—It induces mental exhilaration of buoyancy, *i. e.*, a general feeling of well being; clear and bright, so that all blues are dissipated. Dull, drowsy, stupid [*Gels.*]; gloomy and irritable, worse during evening.

Head.—Dull, heavy feeling in occiput, in and above the eyes, worse toward evening. Pain in left side of head. Violent headache.

Ears.—Stuffed feeling in eustachian tubes [*Kali mur.*] at night; patulous in morning.

Stomach.—Increased thirst. Appetite impaired, but chiefly increased even to bulimia. He must *eat* frequently, so that he cannot wait for regular meals; hungry in forenoon. [*Sul.*] Much nibbling of food and craving for sweets.

Abdomen.—Flatulence with distention. Shifting, flatulent pain along colon several hours after meals. Frequent, loose, yellow, painful stools, with burning of flatulence. Chronic appendicitis.

Urine.—Kidneys inactive; frequent urging to urinate. Polyuria. [*Phos. ac.*] Increased elimination of urea, indican and phosphates.

Sleep.—Slept better than usual, especially in early morning; it induces quiet, reposeful and refreshing sleep.

Relationship.—Compare: *Avena sat.; Dipodium punct.; Gels.; Hydr.; Kali phos.; Phos. ac.; Zinc.*

Dose.—The best results are elicited with material doses (5-10) drops of tincture, several times daily. Continue its use until tonic effects ensue.

ALLIUM CEPA
(Red Onion)

A picture of coryza, with *acrid nasal* discharge and laryngeal symptoms, eye secretion *bland;* singers' cold, *worse in warm room* and toward evening; better in open air is presented by this remedy. Specially adapted to phlegmatic patients; colds in *damp cold weather*. Neuralgic pains, *like a fine thread*, following amputations or injuries to nerves. Traumatic chronic

ALLIUM CEPA

neuritis. Burning in nose, mouth, throat, bladder and skin. Sensation of glowing heat on different parts of the body.

Head.—Catarrhal headache, mostly in forehead; *worse in warm room* towards evening. Thread-like pains in face. Headache ceases during menses; returns when flow disappears.

Eyes.—Red. Much *burning* and smarting lachrymation. *Sensitive to light.* Eyes suffused and watery; profuse, *bland* lachrymation, better in open air. Burning in eyelids.

Ears.—Earache, shooting in eustachian tube.

Nose.—Sneezing, especially when entering a warm room. *Copious, watery and extremely acrid discharge.* Feeling of a lump at root of nose. Hay-fever. [*Sabad.; Sil.; Psor.*] Fluent coryza with headache, cough, and hoarseness. Polypus.

Stomach.—Canine hunger. Pain in pyloric region. Thirst. Belching. Nausea.

Abdomen.—Rumbling, offensive flatus. Pains in left hypogastrium. Colic sitting, moving about.

Rectum.—Diarrhœa with very offensive flatus. Stitches in rectum; itching and rhagades in anus. Glowing heat in rectum.

Urinary—Sensation of weakness in bladder and urethra. Increased secretion of urine with coryza. Urine red with much pressure and burning in urethra.

Respiratory.—*Hoarseness. Hacking cough on inspiring cold air. Tickling in larynx. Sensation as if larynx is split or torn. Oppressed breathing* from pressure in middle of chest. Constricted feeling in region of epiglottis. Pain extending to ear.

Extremities.—Lame joints. Ulcers on heel. Painful affections of fingers about nails. Neuralgia of stump. Bad effects from getting feet wet. Limbs, especially arms, feel sore and tired.

Sleep.—Yawning with headache and drowsiness. Gaping in deep sleep. Dreams. Wakes at 2 a. m.

Modalities.—*Worse*, in the evening, in warm room. *Better*, in open air, and in cold room.

Relationship.—Compare: *Gels.; Euph.; Kali hyd.; Aconite, Ipecac.*

Complementary: *Phosphor.; Thuja; Puls.*

Antidotes: *Arn.; Cham.; Verat.*

Dose.—Third potency.

ALLIUM SATIVUM
(Garlic)

Acts directly on intestinal mucous membrane increasing peristalsis. Colitis, with pathological flora. Has vaso-dilatory properties. Arterial hypotension begins usually in 30 to 45 minutes after twenty to forty drop doses of the tincture.

Adapted to fleshy subjects with dyspepsia and catarrhal affections. High livers. Patients who eat a great deal more, *especially meat*, than they drink. *Pain in hip, pain in psoas and iliac muscles. Pulmonary tuberculosis.*

Cough and expectoration diminishes, temperature becomes normal, weight is gained, and sleep becomes regular. *Hæmoptysis.*

Head.—Heavy; pulsation in temples; catarrhal deafness.

Mouth.—Much sweetish saliva after meals and at night. Sensation of a hair on tongue or throat.

Stomach.—Voracious appetite. Burning eructations. Least change in diet causes trouble. Constipation, with constant dull pains in bowels. *Tongue pale, red papillæ.*

Respiratory.—Constant rattling of mucus in bronchi. Cough in the morning after leaving bedroom, with mucous expectoration, which is tenacious and difficult to raise. Sensitive to cold air. Dilated bronchi, with fetid expectoration. Darting pain in chest.

Female.—Pain in swelling of breasts. Eruption in vagina and on breasts and vulva during menses.

Relationship.—*Allium Sat.*, according to Dr. Teste, belongs to the Bryonia group, including Lycopod. Nux. Colocy, Digital, and Ignatia which affect deeply all flesh eating animals and hardly at all vegetarians. Hence their special applicability to meat eaters rather than to exclusive vegetarians.

Compare: *Capsicum; Arsenic; Senega; Kali nit.*

Complementary: *Arsenic.*

Antidote: *Lycopod.*

Dose.—Third to sixth potency. In tuberculosis, dose, four to six grammes in moderate state of dessication daily, in divided doses.

ALNUS

(Red Alder)

Has some reputation as a remedy for skin affections, glandular enlargements, and indigestion from imperfect secretion of gastric juice. It stimulates nutrition, and thus acts favorably upon strumous disorders, enlarged glands, etc. Ulcerated mucous membranes of mouth and throat. Fingers covered by crust caused by pustules, disagreeable odor. Indigestion from imperfect secretion of gastric juice.

Female.—Leucorrhœa, with erosions of cervix, bleeding easily. Amenorrhœa, with burning pains from back to pubis.

Skin.—Chronic herpes. Enlarged sub-maxiliary glands. Eczema, prurigo. Purpura hæmorrhagica. Poison-oak. Use locally.

Dose.—Tincture to third potency.

ALOE

(Socotrine Aloes)

An excellent remedy to aid in re-establishing physiological equilibrium after much dosing, where disease and drug symptoms are much mixed. There is no remedy richer in symptoms of portal congestion and none that has given better clinical results, both for the primary pathological condition and secondary phenomena. Bad effects from sedentary life or habits Especially suitable to lymphatic and hypochondriacal patients. The rectal symptoms usually determine the choice. Adapted to weary people, the aged, and phlegmatic, old beer-drinkers. Dissatisfied and angry about himself, alternating with lumbago. Heat internally and externally. Has been used successfully in the treatment of consumption by giving the pure juice.

Head.—Headache alternates with lumbago, with intestinal and uterine affections. Disinclination to mental labor. *Aches above forehead, with heaviness in eyes, must partially close them.* Headache after stool. Dull, pressive pain; worse from heat.

Eyes.—Compelled to make small during pain in forehead. Flickering before eyes. Redness of eyes with *yellow* vision. *Pain deep in orbits.*

Face.—Marked redness of lips.

Ears.—Cracking when chewing. Sudden explosion and clashing in left ear. Tinkling as of some thin, shivered, metallic globe in head.

Nose.—Coldness of tip. Bleeding in morning on awakening. Full of crusts.

Mouth.—Taste bitter and sour. Tasteless eructations. Lips cracked and dry.

Throat.—Thick lumps of tough mucus. Varicose condition of veins in pharynx. Dry, scrapy feeling.

Stomach.—Aversion to meat. Longing for juicy things. After eating, flatulence, *pulsation in rectum*, and sexual irritation. Nausea, with headache. Pain in pit when making false step.

Abdomen.—Pain around navel, worse pressure. Fullness in region of liver, pain under right ribs. *Abdomen feels full, heavy, hot, bloated*. Pulsating pain around navel. Weak feeling, as if diarrhœa would come on. Great accumulation of flatus, pressing downwards, causing distress in lower bowels. *Sensation of plug between symphysis pubis and os coccygis*, with urging to stool. Colic before and during stool. Burning, copious flatus.

Rectum.—Constant bearing down in rectum; bleeding, sore, and hot; relieved by cold water. Feeling of weakness and loss of power of sphincter ani. *Sense of insecurity in rectum*, when passing flatus. Uncertain whether gas or stool will come. Stool passes without effort, almost unnoticed. Lumpy, watery stool. Jelly-like stools, with soreness in rectum after stool. *A lot of mucus, with pain in rectum after stool*. Hæmorrhoids protrude like grapes; very sore and tender; better cold water application. *Burning in anus* and rectum. Constipation, with heavy pressure in lower part of abdomen. Diarrhœa from beer.

Urinary.—Incontinence in aged, bearing-down sensation and enlarged prostate. Scanty and high colored.

Female.—Bearing down in rectum, worse standing and during menses. Uterus feels heavy, cannot walk much on that account. Labor-like pains in loins; extend down legs. Climacteric hæmorrhage. Menses too early and too profuse.

Respiratory—Winter coughs, with itching. Difficult respiration, with stitches from liver to chest.

Back.—Pain in small of back; worse moving. Stitches through sacrum. *Lumbago alternating with headache and piles.*

Extremities.—Lameness in all limbs. *Drawing pains in joints.* Soles pain when walking.

Modalities.—*Worse*, early morning; summer; heat; in hot, dry weather; after eating or drinking. *Better*, from cold, open air.

Relationship.—Complementary: *Sulphur;* compare: *Kali bich.; Lycop.; Allium sat.*

Antidotes: *Opium; Sulph.*

Dose.—Sixth potency and higher. In rectal conditions, a few doses of the third, then wait.

ALSTONIA SCHOLARIS
(Dita Bark)

Malarial diseases, with diarrhœa, dysentery, anæmia, feeble digestion, are the general conditions suggesting this remedy. Characteristics are the gone sensation in stomach and sinking in abdomen, with debility. *A tonic after exhausting fevers.*

Abdomen.—Violent purging and cramp in bowels. Heat and irritation in lower bowels. Camp diarrhœa, bloody stool, *dysentery;* diarrhœa from bad water and malaria. *Painless watery stools.* [*Phosph. ac.*] Diarrhœa immediately after eating.

Relationship.—Compare: Similar in action to *Alstonia constricta*, the bitter bark or native quinine of Australia. *Ditain* (active principle, is anti-periodic, like quinine, but without unpleasant effects). *Cinchona* (similar in diarrhœa, chronic dyspepsia and debility) *Hydrastis; Fer. cit. et chin.*

Dose.—Tincture to third potency. Locally, for ulcers and rheumatic pains.

ALUMEN
(Common Potash Alum)

The clinical application of this remedy points to its bowel symptoms, both in obstinate constipation and in hæmorrhage from bowels in the course of typhoid—one phase of the *paralytic weakness* of the muscles in all parts of the body. Tendency to *induration* is also marked, a low form of tissue-making is favored. Hardening of tissues of tongue, rectum, uterus, etc.; ulcers with indurated base. Adapted to old people, especially bronchial catarrhs. *Sensation of dryness and constriction.* Mental paresis; dysphagia especially to *liquids*. Tendency to induration, Scirrhus of the tongue.

Head.—*Burning pain as of weight on top of head better by pressure* of hand. Vertigo, with weakness in pit of stomach. Alopecia.

Throat.—Throat relaxed. Mucous membrane red and swollen. Cough. Tickling in throat. Tendency to throat colds. *Enlarged and indurated tonsils.* Burning pain down the œsophagus. Complete aphonia. Every cold settles in throat. Constriction of œsophagus.

Heart.—Palpitation, *from lying down on right side.*

Rectum.—*Constipation of the most aggravated kind.* No desire for stool for days. Violent ineffectual urging to stool. No ability to expel stool. *Marble-like masses pass, but rectum still feels full.* Itching after stool. Itching in anus. Long lasting pain and smarting in rectum after stool; also hæmorrhoids. Yellow, like an infant's. Hæmorrhage from bowels.

Female.—Tendency to induration of neck of uterus and mammary glands. [*Carb. an.; Con.*] Chronic yellow vaginal discharge. Chronic gonorrhœa, yellow, with little lumps along urethra. Aphthous patches in vagina. [*Caul.*] Menses watery.

Resperitory.—Hæmoptysis, great weakness of chest; difficult to expel mucus. Copious, ropy morning expectoration in old people. Asthma.

Skin.—*Ulcers, with indurated base.* To be thought of in indurated glands, epithelioma, etc.; veins become varicose, and bleed. Indurations resulting from long-continued inflammatory irritations. Glands inflame and harden. Alopecia, Scrotal eczema and on back of penis.

Extremities.—*Weakness of all muscles*, especially arms and legs. Constricted feeling around limbs.

Modalities.—*Worse*, cold except headache, which is relieved by cold.

Dose.—First to thirtieth potency. The very highest potencies have proved efficacious. Powdered alum, 10 grains, placed on tongue, said to arrest an attack of asthma.

ALUMINA
(Oxide of Aluminum—Argilla)

A very general condition corresponding to this drug is *dryness* of mucous membranes and skin, and *tendency to paretic muscular states*. Old people, with lack of vital heat, or prematurely old, with debility. Sluggish functions, heaviness, numbness, and staggering, and the characteristic constipation find an excellent remedy in Alumina. Disposition to colds in the head, and eructations in spare, dry, thin subjects. Delicate children, products of artificial baby foods.

Mind.—Low-spirited; fears loss of reason. Confused as to personal identity. *Hasty, hurried.* Time passes slowly. *Variable mood.* Better as day advances. Suicidal tendency when seeing knife or blood.

Head.—Stitching, burning pain in head, with vertigo, worse in morning, but relieved by food. Pressure in forehead as from a tight hat. Inability to walk except with eyes open. Throbbing headache, with constipation. Vertigo, with nausea; better after breakfast. Falling out of hair; scalp itches and is numb.

Eyes.—Objects look yellow. Eyes feel cold. Lids dry, burn, smart, thickened, aggravated in morning; chronic conjunctivitis. Ptosis. Strabismus.

Ears.—Humming; roaring. Eustachian tube feels plugged.

Nose.—Pain at root of nose. Sense of smell diminished. Fluent coryza. Point of nose *cracked*, nostrils sore, *red;* worse touch. *Scabs with thick yellow mucus.* Tettery redness. *Ozæna atrophica sicca.* Membranes distended and boggy.

Face.—Feels as if albuminous substance had dried on it. Blood-boils and pimples. Twitching of lower jaw. Rush of blood to face after eating.

Mouth.—Sore. Bad odor from it. Teeth covered with sordes. Gums sore, bleeding. Tensive pain in articulation of jaw when opening mouth or chewing.

Throat.—*Dry*, sore; food cannot pass, œsophagus contracted. Feels as if splinter or plug were in throat. Irritable, and relaxed throat. Looks parched and glazed. Clergyman's sore throat in thin subjects. Thick, tenacious mucus drops from posterior nares. Constant inclination to clear the throat.

ALUMINA

Stomach.—Abnormal cravings—chalk, charcoal, dry food, tea-grounds. Heartburn; feels constricted. Aversion to meat. [*Graph.; Arn.; Puls.*] Potatoes disagree. No desire to eat. *Can swallow but small morsels at a time.* Constriction of œsophagus.

Abdomen.—Colic, like painter's colic. Pressing in both roins toward sexual organs. *Left-sided abdominal complaints.*

Stool.—*Hard, dry, knotty; no desire.* Rectum sore, dry, inflamed, bleeding. Itching and burning at anus. *Even a soft stool is passed with difficulty. Great straining.* Constipation of infants [*Collins.; Psor.; Paraf.*] and old people from inactive rectum, and in women of very sedentary habit. Diarrhœa on urinating. *Evacuation preceded by painful urging long before stool, and then straining at stool.*

Urine.—Muscles of bladder paretic, *must strain at stool in order to urinate.* Pain in kidneys, with mental confusion. Frequent desire to urinate in old people. Difficult starting.

Male.—Excessive desire. Involuntary emissions when straining at stool. Prostatic discharge.

Female.—Menses too early, short, *scanty, pale, followed by great exhaustion.* [*Carb. an.; Coccul.*] Leucorrhœa acrid, profuse, transparent, ropy, with-burning; worse during daytime, and after menses. Relieved by washing with cold water.

Respiratory.—Cough soon after waking in the morning. Hoarse, aphonia, tickling in larynx; wheezing, rattling respiration. Cough on talking or singing, *in the morning.* Chest feels constricted. Condiments produce cough. Talking aggravates soreness of chest.

Back.—Stitches. Gnawing pain, as if from hot iron. Pain along cord, with paralytic weakness.

Extremities.—Pain in arm and fingers, as if hot iron penetrated. Arms feel paralyzed. Legs feel asleep, *especially when sitting with legs crossed. Staggers on walking. Heels feel numb.* Soles tender; on stepping, feel soft and swollen. Pain in shoulder and upper arm. Gnawing beneath finger nails. *Brittle nails.* Inability to walk, except when eyes are open or in daytime. Spinal degenerations and paralysis of lower limbs.

Sleep.—Restless; anxious and confused dreams. Sleepy in morning.

Skin.—Chapped and dry tettery. Brittle nails. *Intolerable itching when getting warm in bed.* Must scratch until it bleeds; then becomes painful. Brittle skin on fingers.

Modalities.—*Worse*, periodically; in afternoon; from potatoes. *Worse*, in morning on awaking; warm room. *Better*, in open air; from cold washing; in evening and on alternate days. *Better*, damp weather.

Relationship.—Compare: *Aluminum chloridum* (Pains of loco-motor ataxia. Lower trits in water. *Slag Silico—Sulphocalcite of Alumina* 3x (anal itching, piles, constipation, flatulent distention); *Secale; Lathyr.; Plumb. Aluminum acetate* solution. (Externally a lotion for putrid wounds and skin infections. Arrests hæmorrhage from inertia of uterus. Parenchymatous hæmorrhage from various organs 2-3% solution. Hæmorrhage following tonsillectomy is controlled by rinsing out nasopharynx with a 10% sol.

Complementary: *Bryonia.*

Antidotes: *Ipecac.; Chamom.*

Dose.—Sixth to thirtieth and higher. Action slow in developing.

ALUMINA SILICATA
(Andalasite rock—Alumina 63, Silica 37 parts)

Deep acting remedy for chronic complaints of brain, spine and nerves. Constriction is a marked general symptom, also constriction of orifices. Venous distention. Weakness, especially spinal. Aching and burning in spine. Formication, numbness, pain in all limbs. Epileptiform convulsion. Coldness during pains.

Head.—Congestion of brain. Constriction of scalp. Pain in head, better heat, perspires. Pain in eyes, flickering. Frequent coryzas. Swelling and ulceration of nose.

Respiratory.—Catarrh of chest, pain, raw feeling. Feeling of great weakness in chest. Stitching pains. Spasmodic cough with purulent viscid expectoration.

Extremities.—Heaviness, jerking, numbness, aching and pains.

Skin.—Formication along course of nerves, veins feel full and distended. Sore to touch and pressure.

Modalities.—*Worse*, cold air, after eating, standing. *Better*, warmth, fasting, resting in bed.

Dose.—Higher potencies.

AMBRA GRISEA
(Ambergis—A Morbid Secretion of the Whale)

Suitable to excitable, nervous children and thin, nervous patients. Extreme *nervous hypersensitiveness*. External numbness of whole body in the morning and weakness. Nervous bilious temperament. Thin, scrawny women. Adapted to hysterical subjects, or those suffering from spinal irritation, with convulsive cough, eructation, etc. Also for patients *weakened by age* or overwork, who are anæmic and sleepless. Great remedy for the aged, with impairment of all functions, weakness, coldness and *numbness*, usually of single parts, fingers, arms, etc. One-sided complaints call for it. *Music aggravates symptoms.* Ebulitions and pulsations after walking in open air. One-sided complaints.

Mind.—Dread of people, and desire to be alone. Cannot do anything in presence of others. Intensely shy, blushes easily. *Music causes weeping.* Despair, loathing of life. Fantastic illusions. Bashful. Loss of love of life. Restless, excited, very loquacious. Time passes slowly. Thinking, difficult in the morning with old people. Dwells upon unpleasant things.

Head.—Slow comprehension. Vertigo, with weakness in head and stomach. Pressure on front part of head with mental depression. *Tearing pain in upper half of brain. Senile dizziness.* Rush of blood to head, when listening to music. *Hearing impaired.* Epistaxis, especially in the morning. Profuse bleeding from teeth. Hair falls out.

Stomach.—Eructations, with violent, convulsive cough Acid eructations, like heartburn. *Distention of stomach and abdomen* after midnight. Sensation of coldness in abdomen.

Urinary.—Pain in bladder and rectum at the same time. Burning in orifice of urethra and anus. *Feeling in urethra as if a few drops passed out.* Burning and itching in urethra while urinating. *Urine turbid, even during emission,* forming a brown sediment.

Female.—Nymphomania, *Itching of pudendum, with soreness and swelling.* Menses too early. Profuse, bluish leucorrhœa. Worse at night. *Discharge of blood between periods, at every little accident.*

Male.—Voluptuous itching of scrotum. Parts externally numb; burn internally. Violent erections without voluptuous sensations.

Respiratory.—Asthmatic breathing with eructation of gas. *Nervous, spasmodic cough,* with hoarseness and *eructation,* on waking in morning; worse in presence of people. Tickling in throat, larynx and trachea, chest oppressed, gets out of breath when coughing. *Hollow, spasmodic, barking cough, coming from deep in chest.* Choking when hawking up phlegm.

Heart.—*Palpitation, with pressure in chest as from a lump lodged there, or as if chest was obstructed.* Conscious of the pulse. Palpitation in open air with pale face.

Sleep.—*Cannot sleep from worry; must get up.* Anxious dreams. Coldness of body and twitching of limbs, during sleep.

Skin.—Itching and soreness, especially around genitals. Numbness of skin. Arms "go to sleep."

Extremities.—*Cramps in hands* and fingers, worse grasping anything. Cramps in legs.

Modalities.—*Worse,* music; presence of strangers; *from any unusual thing;* morning, warm room. *Better,* slow motion in open air; lying on painful part; cold drinks.

Relationship.—Do not confound with *Amber*—Succinum. q. v. *Moschus* frequently follows advantageously. Compare: *Oleum succinum* (hiccough). *Sumbul; Castor.; Asaf.; Crocus. Lilium.*

Dose.—Second and third potencies; may be repeated with advantage.

AMBROSIA
(Rag-Weed)

A remedy for hay-fever, *lachrymation* and *intolerable itching of the eye-lids.* Some forms of whooping-cough. Respiratory tract in its entire length stopped up. *Many forms of diarrhœa,* especially during summer months, also dysentery.

Nose.—Watery coryza; sneezing; watery discharge. *Nosebleed*. Stuffed up feeling of nose and head. Irritation of trachea and bronchial tubes, with asthmatic attacks. [*Aral.; Eucalypt.*] Wheezy cough.

Eyes.—Smart and burn. Lachrymation.

Relationship.—Compare in hay-fever: *Sabadilla, Wyethia; Succin. ac.; Ars. jod.; Arundo.*

Dose.—Tincture, to third potency; 10 drops in water during and after attack of epistaxis. In hay-fever high potencies.

AMMONIACUM-DOREMA
(Gum Ammoniac)

A remedy for the aged and feeble, especially in chronic bronchitis. Ill humor. Sensitive to cold. Sensation of burning and scratching in neck and œsophagus.

Head.—Catarrhal headache due to closure of frontal sinuses.

Eyes.—Dim sight. Stars and fiery points float before eyes. Easily fatigued from reading.

Throat.—Throat dry; worse inhaling fresh air. Full feeling, burning and scraping sensation. Immediately after eating, sensation as if something stuck in œsophagus, causing swallowing.

Respiratory.—*Difficult breathing*. Chronic bronchial catarrh. Large accumulation of purulent matter and feeble expectoration; worse cold weather. Mucus tough and hard. Heart beats stronger, extends to pit of stomach. Coarse rattling of chest in old people.

Relationship.—Antidotes: *Bry.; Arnica.*

Compare: *Senega; Tart. emet.; Balsam Peru.*

Dose.—Third trituration.

AMMONIUM BENZOICUM
(Benzoate of Ammonia)

One of the remedies for albuminuria, especially in the gouty Gout, with deposits in joints. Urinary incontinence in the aged.

Head.—Heavy, stupid.

Face.—Bloated, swollen eyelids. Swelling under tongue like ranula.

Urine.—Smoky, scanty. Albuminous and thick deposits.

Back.—Pain across sacrum, with urgency to stool. Soreness in region of right kidney.

Relationship.—Compare: *Terebinth.; Benz. ac.; Ammonia salts; Caust.*

In albuminuria compare: *Kalmia; Helon; Merc. cor.; Berb.; Canth.*

Dose.—Second trituration.

AMMONIUM BROMATUM
(Bromide of Ammonia)

Indicated in chronic laryngeal and pharyngeal catarrh, neuralgic headaches, and obesity. Constrictive pain in head, chest, legs, etc. Irritable feeling under finger nails; relieved only by biting them.

Head.—Cerebral congestion. Feeling of a band above ears. Sneezing; thick nasal discharge.

Eyes.—Edges of lids red and swollen, also Meibomian glands. Eyeballs feel large and pain around eyes into head.

Throat.—Smarting in mouth. Tickling in throat, *with inclination to dry, spasmodic cough, especially at night.* Burning in fauces. White, sticky, mucus. Chronic speakers' catarrh.

Respiratory.—Sudden, short cough, strangling. Tickling in trachea and bronchial tubes. Wakes at 3 a. m. with cough. Feels suffocated; continuous cough, when lying down at night; sharp pain in lungs. **Whooping Cough.**—Dry, spasmodic cough on lying down.

Relationship.—*Hyos.; Con.; Arg. nit.; Kali bich.*

Dose.—First potency.

AMMONIUM CARB
(Carbonate of Ammonia)

The diseased conditions met by this remedy are such as we find often in rather stout women who are always tired and weary, take cold easily, suffer from cholera-like symptoms before menses, lead a sedentary life, have a slow reaction generally, and are disposed to frequent use of the smelling-bottle. Too frequent and profuse menses. Mucous membranes of the respiratory organs are especially affected. Fat patients with weak heart, wheezing, feel suffocated. Very sensitive to cold air. Great aversion to water; cannot bear to touch it. Malignant scarlatina, with somnolence, swollen glands, dark red sore throat, faintly developed eruption. Uræmia. *Heaviness in all organs.* Uncleanness in bodily habits. Swelling of parts, glands, etc. Acid secretions. Prostration from trifles.

Mind.—Forgetful, ill-humored, gloomy during *stormy weather. Uncleanliness.* Talking and hearing others talk affects greatly. Sad, weepy, unreasonable.

Head.—Pulsating forehead; better, pressure and in warm room. Shocks through head.

Eyes.—Burning of eyes with aversion to light. Eye-strain. [*Nat. mur.*] Asthenopia. Sore canthi.

Ears.—Hardness of hearing. Shocks through ears, eyes, and nose, when gnashing teeth.

Nose.—Discharge of sharp, burning water. *Stoppage at night, with long-continued coryza. Cannot breathe through nose.* Snuffles of children. *Epistaxis after washing and after eating.* Ozæna, blows bloody mucus from nose. Tip of nose congested.

Face.—Tetters around mouth. Boils and pustules, during menses. Corners of mouth sore, cracked, and burn.

Mouth.—Great dryness of mouth and throat. Toothache. *Pressing teeth together sends shocks through head, eyes, and ears.* Vesicles on tongue. Taste sour; metallic. Cracking of jaw on chewing.

Throat.—Enlarged tonsils and glands of neck. Burning pain all down throat. Tendency to gangrenous ulceration of tonsils. Diphtheria *when nose is stopped up.*

Stomach.—Pain at pit of stomach, with heartburn, nausea, waterbrash, and chilliness. Great appetite, but easily satisfied. Flatulent dyspepsia.

Abdomen.—Noise and pain in abdomen. Flatulent hernia. Stools difficult, hard, and knotty. *Bleeding piles; worse during menses.* Itching at anus. Protruding piles, worse after stool, better lying down.

Urine.—Frequent desire; involuntary at night. Tenesmus of bladder. Urine white, sandy, bloody, copious, turbid and fetid.

Male.—Itching and pain of scrotum and spermatic cords. Erection without desire. Seminal emissions.

Female.—Itching, swelling and burning of pudendum. Leucorrhœa burning, acrid, watery. Aversion to the other sex. Menses too *frequent, profuse,* early, copious, clotted, black; colicky pains, and hard, difficult stool, with *fatigue,* especially of thighs; yawning and chilliness.

Respiratory.—Hoarseness. Cough every morning about three o'clock, with dyspnœa, palpitation, burning in chest; worse ascending. Chest feels tired. Emphysema. *Much oppression in breathing;* worse after any effort, and entering *warm room,* or ascending even a few steps. Asthenic *Pneumonia.* Slow labored, stertorous breathing; bubbling sound. Winter catarrh, with slimy sputum and specks of blood. Pulmonary œdema.

Heart.—Audible palpitation with fear, cold sweat, lachrymation, inability to speak, loud breathing and trembling hands. *Heart weak,* wakes with difficult breathing and palpitation.

Extremities.—Tearing in joints relieved by heat of bed; inclination to stretch limbs. Hands cold and blue; distended veins. Fingers swell when arm is hanging down. Panaritium, deep-seated periosteal pain. Cramps in calves and soles. Big toe painful and swollen. Felons in the beginning. Heel painful on standing. Tearing in ankle and bones of feet, better when warm in bed.

Sleep.—*Sleepiness* during the day. Starts from sleep strangling.

Skin.—Violent itching and burning blisters. Scarlet rash. Miliary rash. Malignant scarlatina. Faintly developed eruptions from defective vitality. Erysipelas in the aged, with brain symptoms. Eczema in the bends of extremities, between legs, about anus and genitals.

Modalities.—*Worse,* evenings, from cold, wet weather, wet applications, washing, and during 3 to 4 a. m., during menses. *Better,* lying on painful side and on stomach; in dry weather.

Relationship.—Inimical to *Lachesis.* Similar in action.

Antidotes: *Arnica; Camphor.*

Compare: *Rhus; Muriatic acid; Tartar emet.*

Of use in poisoning by charcoal fumes.

Dose.—Lower potencies deteriorate with age. Sixth potency best for general use.

AMMONIUM CAUSTICUM
(Hydrate of Ammonia—Ammonia Water)

This is a powerful cardiac stimulant. As such in *syncope*, thrombosis, hæmorrhage, snake-bites, chloroform narcosis, may be given by inhalation.

The œdema and ulceration of mucous membranes produced by this powerful drug have been utilized as guiding symptoms for its use; hence in membranous croup with burning in œsophagus. Aphonia. See *Causticum*.

Respiratory.—Difficult respiration. Accumulation of mucus with incessant coughing. *Loss of voice. Burning rawness in throat.* Spasm of the glottis with suffocation; patient gasps for breath. Pain in œsophagus on breathing deeply. Scraping and burning in throat and œsophagus. Uvula covered with white mucus. Nasal diphtheria, with burning excoriating discharge.

Extremities.—*Excessive exhaustion* and muscular debility. Rheumatism of shoulders. Skin hot and dry.

Dose.—First to third potency; also five to ten minims, well diluted with water.

AMMONIUM JODATUM
(Iodide of Ammonia)

Indicated when iodine has but partially relieved its cases of laryngitis and bronchitis, catarrhal pneumonia, œdema of lungs.

Head.—Dull headache, especially in young people, face stupid, heavy; vertigo, Meniere's disease.

Dose.—Second and third trit.

Compare: *Ammonium tartaricum* (Dry hacking cough after every cold).

AMMONIUM MURIATICUM
(Sal Ammoniac)

A state of prostration bordering on a typhoid state is produced by this remedy. All mucous secretions are increased and retained. It is especially adapted to fat and sluggish patients who have respiratory troubles. Coughs associated with catarrhs and affections of liver. A tendency to irregular circulation, blood seems to be in constant turmoil, pulsations, etc. Many groups of symptoms are accompanied by cough, *profuse glairy secretions*. Its periods of aggravations are peculiarly divided as to the bodily region affected; thus the head and chest symptoms are worse mornings, the abdominal in the afternoon, the pains in the limbs, the skin and febrile symptoms, in the evenings. "Boiling" sensation.

Mind.—Melancholy, apprehensive; like from internal grief. *Desire to cry*, but cannot. Consequences of grief.

Head.—Hair falls out, with itchings and dandruff. Feels full, compressed; worse mornings.

Eyes.—Mist before eyes, optical illusions in incipient cataract; capsular cataract.

Nose.—Free *acrid, hot watery discharge* corroding the lip. Sneezing. Nose sore to touch; ulcerative pain in nostrils. *Loss of smell. Obstructed, stuffy feeling;* constant and unavailing efforts to blow it out. Itching.

Face.—Inflammatory faceache. Mouth and lips sore and excoriated.

Throat.—Throbbing in, and swelling of tonsils, can scarcely swallow. Sore spot behind uvula, relieved by eating. Internal and external swelling of throat *with viscid phlegm*. So tough, it cannot be hawked up. Tonsillitis. Stricture of œsophagus.

Stomach.—Thirst for lemonade, regurgitation of food, bitter waterbrash. Nausea. Gnawing in stomach. Epigastric pain immediately after eating. Cancer of stomach.

Abdomen.—Splenic stitches, especially in the morning, with difficult breathing. Pain around navel. Abdominal symptoms appear during pregnancy. Chronic congestion of liver. Excessive fatty deposit around abdomen. Much flatus. Strained feeling in groin.

AMMONIUM MURIATICUM

Rectum.—Itching and hæmorrhoids, soreness with pustules. Hard, *crumbly* stool, or covered with glairy mucus. Stinging in perinæum. Green mucus stools alternate with constipation. During and after stool, burning and smarting in rectum. Hæmorrhoids after suppressed leucorrhœa.

Female.—Menses too early, too free, dark, clotted; *flow more at night.* Pain as if sprained in left side of abdomen during pregnancy. Diarrhœa, greenish mucous stools, and navel pain *during menses.* Leucorrhœa, like white of an egg [*Alum.; Bor.; Calc. p.*]; with pain about the navel; brown, slimy *after every urination.*

Respiratory.—*Hoarseness and burning in larynx.* Dry, hacking, scraping cough; worse lying on back or right side. Stitches in chest. Cough loose in afternoon, with profuse expectoration and rattling of mucus. Oppression of chest. Burning at small spots in chest. Scanty secretion. Cough with profuse salivation.

Back.—*Icy coldness between shoulders;* not relieved by warm covering, followed by itching. Bruised pain in coccyx when sitting. Backache, as if in a vise when sitting.

Extremities.—Pain as from ulceration in finger tips. Shooting and tearing *in tips of finger* and toes. Ulcerative pain in heels. *Contraction of hamstring tendons.* Sciatica, *worse sitting, better lying.* Neuralgic pain in amputated limbs. Offensive sweaty feet. Pain in feet during menses.

Skin.—Itching, generally evenings. Blisters on various parts. Intense burning better cold applications.

Fever.—*Chilliness evenings after lying down* and on awakening, without thirst. Heat in palms and soles. Sub acute, low fevers due to unhealthy climate. Lowest potencies.

Modalities.—*Better,* open air. *Worse,* head and chest symptoms in the morning; abdominal symptoms in the afternoon.

Relationship.—Antidotes: *Coffea; Nux; Caust.*

Compare: *Calcarea; Senega; Caustic.*

Dose.—Third to sixth potency.

AMMONIUM PHOSPHORICUM
(Phosphate of Ammonia)

A remedy for chronic gouty patients uric acid diathesis, indicated in bronchitis and *nodosities of the joints* of the fingers and backs of the hands. Facial paralysis. Pain in shoulder-joint. Tightness around chest. Heavienss of limbs, unsteady, tottering gait. Coldness from least draft of air.

Head.—Sneezing with excessive running from nose and eyes, *only in morning*.

Respiratory.—Deep rough cough with greenish expectoration.

Urine.—Rose-colored sediment.

Dose.—Third decimal trituration.

AMMONIUM PICRATUM
(Picrate of Ammonia)

A remedy for malarial fever and neuralgias and so-called bilious headaches. Pain in occiput and mastoid region. Whooping cough.

Head.—Periodical neuralgia *in right side of occiput;* boring extends to ear, orbit, and jaw. Vertigo on rising. Periodic bilious headaches. [*Sanguin.*]

Dose.—Third trituration.

AMMONIUM VALERIANICUM
(Valerianate of Ammonia)

A remedy for nervous, hysterical people, suffering with neuralgia headaches and insomnia. Great nervous erethism is always present.

Heart.—Pains in cardiac region. Functional disturbances, tachycardia.

Dose.—Lower triturations.

AMPELOPSIS
(Virginia Creeper)

Renal dropsies, hydrocele, and chronic hoarseness in scrofulous patients have been benefited by this drug. Choleric symptoms. Generally worse about 6 p. m. Dilated pupils.

Left costal region sore and sensitive. Elbow joints pain, back sore. Soreness of all limbs. Vomiting, purging with tenesmus. Rumbling in abdomen.

Dose.—Second to third potency.

AMYGDALUS PERSICA
(Peach Tree)

A most valuable remedy in vomiting of various kinds; *morning sickness*. Irritation of eyes. Ischuria and hæmaturia.

Hæmorrhage from the bladder.

Gastric irritation of children; no form of food tolerated. Loss of smell and taste. Gastric and intestinal irritation when the tongue is elongated and pointed, tip and edges red. Constant nausea and vomiting.

Relationship.—Compare: *Amygd. amara*—Bitter Almond. (Pains through tonsils, throat dark, difficult swallowing, vomiting, cough with sore chest.)

Dose.—Fresh infusion or mother tincture.

AMYL NITROSUM
(Amyl Nitrite)

On inhaling this drug, it rapidly dilates all arterioles and capillaries, producing flushings of face, heat, and throbbing in the head.—Superficial arterial hyperæmia. Palpitation of the heart and similar conditions are readily cured by it, especially the flushings and other discomforts at climacteric. *Hiccough and yawning.* Often relieves temporarily epileptic convulsions. Seasickness.

Head.—*Anxiety*, as if something might happen; *must have fresh air. Surging of blood to head and face;* sensation as if blood would start through skin. with heat and redness. *Flushings, followed by sweat at climacteric.* Ears hyperæmic. Throbbing.

Throat.—Constriction; collar seems too tight.

Chest.—Dyspnœa and asthmatic feelings. Great oppression and fullness of chest; spasmodic, suffocative cough. Præcordial anxiety. *Tumultuous action of heart.* Pain and constriction around heart. Fluttering at slightest excitement.

Female.—After-pains; hæmorrhage associated with facial flushing. *Climacteric headache and flushes of heat, with anxiety and palpitation.*

Fever.—Much flushing of heat; sometimes followed by cold and clammy skin and profuse sweat. Throbbing throughout whole body. *Abnormal sweat after influenza.*

Extremities.—*Constant stretching for hours.* Veins of hands dilated; pulsations felt in tips of fingers.

Relationship.—Compare: *Glonoine; Lachesis.*

Antidotes: *Cactus; Strychn.; Ergot.*

Dose.—Third potency.

For *palliations.* In all conditions where the blood-vessels are *spasmodically contracted,* as in angina pectoris, epileptic seizure, megrim, accompanied by cold, pallor, etc., also in paroxysms of asthma, chloroform asphyxia, inhalation of the *Amyl. nit.* will give immediate relief. For this non-homœopathic application, two to five minims (put up in pearls) dropped on a handkerchief and inhaled may be required.

ANACARDIUM
(Marking Nut)

The Anacardium patient is found mostly among the neurasthenics; such have a type of nervous dyspepsia, relieved by food; *impaired memory,* depression, and irritability; diminution of senses (smell, sight, hearing). Syphilitic patients often suffer with these conditions. Intermittency of symptoms. Fear of examination in students. Weakening of all senses, sight, hearing, etc. Aversion to work; lacks self-confidence; irresistible desire to swear and curse. *Sensation of a plug* in various parts— eyes, rectum, bladder, etc.; also *of a band.* Empty feeling in stomach; *eating temporarily relieves all discomfort.* This is a sure indication, often verified. Its skin symptoms are similar to Rhus, and it has proved a valuable antidote to Poison-Oak.

Mind.—Fixed ideas. Hallucinations; *thinks he is possessed of two persons or wills.* Anxiety when walking, as if pursued. Profound melancholy and hypochondriasis, with *tendency to use violent language. Brain-fag. Impaired memory. Absent mindedness. Very easily offended.* Malicious; seems bent on wickedness. Lack of confidence in himself or others. Suspicious [*Hyos.*]. Clairaudient, hears voices far away or of the dead. Senile dementia. Absence of all moral restraint.

Head.—Vertigo. Pressing pain, *as from a plug;* worse after mental exertion—in forehead; occiput, temples, vertex; *better during a meal.* Itching and little boils on scalp.

Eyes.—Pressure *like a plug* on upper orbit. Indistinct vision. *Objects appear too far off.*

Ears.—Pressing in the ears as from a plug. Hard of hearing.

Nose.—Frequent sneezing. *Sense of smell perverted.* Coryza with palpitation, especially in the aged.

Face.—Blue rings around eyes. Face pale.

Mouth.—Painful vesicles; fetid odor. Tongue feels swollen, impeding speech and motion, with saliva in mouth. Burning around lips as from pepper.

Stomach.—Weak digestion, with fullness and distention. *Empty feeling in stomach.* Eructation, nausea, vomiting. *Eating relieves the Anacardium dyspepsia.* Apt to choke when eating or drinking. Swallows food and drinks hastily.

Abdomen.—*Pain as if dull plug were pressed into intestines.* Rumbling, pinching, and griping.

Rectum.—Bowels inactive. *Ineffectual desire; rectum seems powerless, as if plugged up;* spasmodic constriction of sphincter ani; even soft stool passes with difficulty. *Itching at anus; moisture from rectum.* Hæmorrhage during stool. Painful hæmorrhoids.

Male.—Voluptuous itching; increased desire; seminal emissions without dreams. Prostatic discharge during stool.

Female.—Leucorrhœa, with soreness and itching. Menses scanty.

Respiratory.—Pressure in chest, as from a dull plug. Oppression of chest, with internal heat and anxiety, driving him into open air. Cough excited by talking, in children, after fit of temper. Cough after eating with vomiting of food and pain in occiput.

Heart.—Palpitation, with weak memory, with coryza in the aged; stitches in heart region. Rheumatic pericarditis with double stitches.

Back.—Dull pressure in the shoulders, as from a weight. Stiffness at nape of neck.

Extremities.—Neuralgia in thumb. Paralytic weakness. Knees feel paralyzed or bandaged. Cramps in calves. Pressure as from a plug in the glutei. Warts on palms of hands. Fingers swollen with vesicular eruption.

Sleep.—Spells of sleeplessness lasting for several nights. Anxious dreams.

Skin.—*Intense itching* eczema, with mental irritability; vesicular eruption; *swelling,* urticaria; eruption like that of Poison-Oak. [*Xerophyl.; Grindel.; Croton.*] Lichen planus; neurotic eczema. Warts on hands. Ulcer formation on forearm.

Modalities.—*Worse,* on application of hot water. *Better,* from eating. When lying on side, from rubbing.

Relationship.—Antidote: *Grindeleia; Coffea; Juglans; Rhus; Eucalyptus.*

Compare: *Anacard. occidentale* (cashew nut) (ersipelas, vesicular facial eruptions), anæsthetic variety of leprosy; warts, corns, ulcers, cracking of the skin on soles of feet). *Rhus; Cypriped.; Chelidon.; Xerophyl.*

Platina follows well. *Cereus serpentina* (swearing).

Dose.—Sixth to two hundredth potency.

ANAGALLIS
(Scarlet Pimpernel)

Marked action on skin, characterized by great itching and tingling everywhere. Favors expulsion of splinters. An old medicine for hydrophobia and dropsy. Possesses power of softening flesh and destroying warts.

Head.—Great hilarity; headache over supra-orbital ridges, with rumbling in bowels and eructations; better from coffee. Sick headache. Pain in facial muscles.

Extremities.—Rheumatic and gouty pains. Pain in shoulder and arm. Cramp in ball of thumbs and fingers.

Urine.—More or less irritation in urethra, inclining to coition. Burning pain on urinating, with agglutination of orifice. Urine passes in several streams; must press before it passes.

Skin.—*Itching;* dry, bran-like eruption, especially *on hands and fingers. Palms* especially affected. Vesicles in groups. Ulcers and swellings on joints.

Relationship.—Anagallis contains Saponin, *q. v.*

Compare: *Cyclamen; Primula obcon*

Dose.—First to third potency.

ANATHERUM
(Cuscus—An East Indian Grass)

A skin remedy of high order.
Painful swelling of various parts, going on to suppuration. Glandular inflammation.

Head.—Pains pierce brain like pointed arrows; worse in afternoon. Herpes, ulcers, and tumors on scalp. Wartlike growth on eyebrows. Boils and tumors on tip of nose. Tongue fissured, as if cut on edges; copious salivation.

Urine.—Turbid, thick, full of mucus. *Constant urging.* Bladder cannot hold smallest quantity. Involuntary. Cystitis.

Sexual.—Chancre-like sores. Scirrhus-like swelling of cervix. Breasts swollen, indurated, nipples excoriated.

Skin.—Diseased and deformed nails. Offensive foot-sweat. *Abscesses*, boils, *ulcers*. Erysipelas. Pruritus, herpes.

Relationship.—Compare: *Staphisag.; Mercur.; Thuja.*

Dose.—Third potency.

ANHALONIUM
(Mescal Button)

Mescal is a strong intoxicating spirit distilled from *Pulque fuerte.* Pulque is made from the Agave Americana of Mexico, locally known as Maguey and is the national beverage of Mexico. Indians call it Peyote. It weakens the heart, produces insanity. Its most striking effects appear in the *auditory nerve* for it makes "each note upon the piano a center of melody which seems to be surrounded by a halo of color pulsating to the rythm of the music." (Hom. World.)

Causes a form of intoxication accompanied by wonderful visions, remarkably beautiful and varied kaleidoscopic changes, and a sensation of increased physical ability. Also visions of monsters and various gruesome forms. A cardiac tonic and respiratory stimulant. Hysteria and insomnia. A remedy for brain-fag, delirium, megrim, hallucinations, with colored brilliant visions. Motor inco-ordination. Extreme muscular depression; increased patellar reflex. Paraplegia.

Mind.—Loss of conception of time. Difficult enunciation. Distrust and resentment. Lazy contentment.

Head.—Aches, with disturbed vision. Fantastic, brilliant, moving colored objects. Affected by beating time. Pupils dilated, vertigo, brain tired. *Polychrome spectra*. Exaggerated reverberation of ordinary sounds.

Dose.—Tincture.

Relationship.—Compare *Agave*. The intoxication of *Anhalonium* is similar to that of *Cannabis Indica* and *Oenanthe*.

ANEMOPSIS CALIFORNICA
(Yerba Mansa—Household Herb)

A mucous membrane medicine. Chronic forms of inflammation of the Schneiderian membrane with considerable relaxation and profuse discharge. Chief value in *catarrhal states*, with full stuffy sensation in head and throat. Useful in cuts, bruises and sprains; and as a diuretic and in malaria. Not yet proven, but found useful in profuse mucous or serous discharges; in nasal and pharyngeal catarrh, diarrhœa and urethritis. Recommended in heart disease, as a quieting agent when unduly excited. Flatulence; promotes digestion.

Relationship.—Compare *Piper meth*.

Dose.—The tincture internally and locally as a spray.

ANGUSTURA VERA
(Bark of Galipea Cusparia)

Rheumatic and paralytic complaints—great difficulty in walking. Crackling in all joints.

The greatest craving for coffee is a characteristic symptom. Caries of long bones. Paralysis. Tetanus. Stiffness of muscles and joints. *Oversensitive*.

Principal action on spinal motor nerves and mucous membranes.

Head.—Oversensitive. Headache, with heat of face. Acute pain in cheeks. Drawing in facial muscles. Pain in temporal muscles, when opening the jaws. Pain in articulation of jaw, in masseter muscles, as if fatigued by chewing too much. Cramp-pain on the zygomatic arch.

Stomach.—Bitter taste. *Irresistible desire for coffee.* Pain from navel into sternum. Atonic dyspepsia. Belching, with cough. [*Ambra.*]

Abdomen.—Diarrhœa and colic. Tenesmus with soft stool; chronic diarrhœa, with debility and loss of flesh. Burning in anus.

Back.—Itching along back. Pain in cervical vertebræ. Drawing in the neck. Pain in spine, at nape of neck and sacrum, worse on pressure. Twitching and jerking along back. Bends backward.

Extremities.—Stiffness and tension of muscles and joints. Pain in limbs on walking. Arms tired and heavy. Caries of long bones. Coldness of fingers. *Pain in knees.* Cracking in joints.

Skin.—Caries, very painful ulcers which affect the bone.

Relationship.—Compare: *Nux; Ruta; Mercur.; Brucea.*—Bark of Nux vomica or angustura falsa. (Tetanic spasms with undisturbed consciousness, worse noise, liquids, paralyzed lower extremities, worse least touch, *cries for fear of being touched.* Painful jerking of legs; cramp-like pain in knees; rigid and lame limbs of paralytics. For pain in the passing of calculus.)

Dose.—Sixth potency.

ANILINUM
(Coal Tar Product—Amidobenzene)

Marked giddiness and pain in head; *face has a purple hue.* Pain in penis and scrotum with swelling. *Tumors of the urinary passages.* Profound anæmia with discoloration of skin, blue lips, anorexia, gastric disturbances. Swelling of skin.

Relationship.—Compare: *Arsenic; Antipyrin.*

ANTHEMIS NOBILIS
(Roman Chamomile)

This remedy is akin to the ordinary Chamomilla. Gastric disturbance with coldness. Sensitive to cold air and cold things.

Respiration.—Coryza with much lachrymation, sneezing, and discharge of clear water from the nose. Symptoms worse indoors. Constriction and rawness of throat. Cough, tickling; worse in warm room.

Abdomen.—Aching in region of liver; griping and *chilliness inside of abdomen* and into legs. Itching of anus, with white putty-like stools.

Urinary.—Bladder feels distended. Pain along spermatic cord, which feels full, as if varicosed. Frequent urination.

Skin.—Itching of the soles, as if from chilblains. Gooseflesh.

Dose.—Use the third potency.

ANTHRACINUM
(Anthrax Poison)

This nosode has proven a great remedy in epidemic spleen-diseases of domestic animals, and in septic inflammation, *carbuncles*, and *malignant ulcers*. *In boils* and boil-like eruptions. ne. Terrible burning. Induration of cellular tissue, abscess, bo, and all inflammation of connective tissue in which there ists a purulent focus.

Tissues.—Hæmorrhages, black, thick, tar-like, rapidly decomposing, from any orifice. Glands swollen, *cellular tissues œdematous and indurated*. Septicemia. Ulceration, sloughing and *intolerable burning*. Erysipelas. Black and blue blisters Dissecting wounds. Insect stings. Bad effects from inhaling foul odors. Gangrenous parotitis. *Succession of boils*. Gangrene. Foul secretions.

Relationship.—Similar to Arsenic, which it often follows. Compare: *Pyrogen; Lachesis; Crotalus; Hippozœn; Echinac.; Silica* follows well. In the treatment of carbuncles, remember the prescription of the prophet Isaiah for King Hezekiah's carbuncle—*i. e.*, the pulp of a fig placed on a poultice and apply

Dose.—Thirtieth potency. *Tarani. Cubensis.*

ANTHRAKOKALI

(Anthracite Coal Dissolved in Boiling Caustic Potash)

Useful in skin affections, scabies, prurigo, chronic herpes, kracks and ulcerations. Papular-like eruption with a vesicular tendency, especially on scrotum, also on hands, tibia, shoulders and dorsum of feet. Intense thirst. Chronic rheumatism. Bilious attacks, vomiting of bile, tympanic distention of abdomen.

Dose.—Low triturations.

ANTIMONIUM ARSENICOSUM
(Arsenite of Antimony)

Found useful in *emphysema with excessive dyspnœa and cough*, much mucous secretion. Worse on eating and lying down. Catarrhal pneumonia associated with influenza. Myocarditis and cardiac weakness. Pleurisy, especially of left side, *with exudation*, and pericarditis, with effusion. Sense of weakness. Inflammation of eyes and œdema of face.

Dose.—Third trituration.

ANTIMONIUM CRUDUM
(Black Sulphide of Antimony)

For homœopathic employment, the mental symptoms, and those of the gastric sphere, determine its choice. *Excessive irritability and fretfulness*, together with a *thickly-coated white tongue*, are true guiding symptoms to many forms of disease calling for this remedy. All the conditions are aggravated by *heat and cold bathing*. Cannot bear heat of sun. Tendency to grow fat. An absence of pain, where it could be expected, is noticeable. Gout with gastric symptoms.

Mind.—Much concerned about his fate. Cross and contradictive; whatever is done fails to give satisfaction. Sulky; does not wish to speak. Peevish; vexed without cause. *Child cannot bear to be touched or looked at.* Angry at every little attention. Sentimental mood.

Head.—Aching, worse in vertex, on ascending, *from bathing, from disordered stomach*, especially from eating candy or drinking acid wines. Suppressed eruptions. Heaviness in forehead, with vertigo; nausea, and nosebleed. Headache with great loss of hair.

Eyes.—Dull, sunken, red, itch, inflamed, agglutinated. *Canthi raw and fissured.* Chronic *blepharitis.* Pustules on cornea and lids.

Ears.—Redness; swelling; pain in eustachian tube. Ringing and deafness. Moist eruption around ear.

Nose.—Nostrils *chapped and covered with crusts. Eczema of nostrils, sore, cracked and scurfy.*

Face.—Pimples, pustules, and boils on face. *Yellow crusted eruption on cheeks* and chin. Sallow and haggard.

Mouth.—*Cracks in corners of mouth.* Dry lips. Salti*** saliva. Much slimy mucus. *Tongue coated thick white, a   whitewashed.* Gums detach from teeth; bleed easily. Toothache in hollow teeth. Rawness of palate, with expectoration of much mucus. *Canker sores.* Pappy taste. No thirst. Subacute eczema about mouth.

Throat.—Much thick yellowish mucus from posterior nares. Hawking in open air. Laryngitis. Rough voice from over use.

Stomach.—*Loss of appetite. Desire for acids, pickles.* Thirst in evening and night. *Eructation tasting of the ingesta.* Heartburn, nausea, vomiting. After nursing, the child vomits its milk in curds, and refuses to nurse afterwards, and is very cross. Gastric and intestinal complaints from bread and pastry, acids, sour wine, cold bathing, overheating, hot weather. *Constant belching.* Gouty metastasis to stomach and bowels. Sweetish waterbrash. *Bloating after eating.*

Stool.—Anal itching. [*Sulpho-Calc. Alum.*] *Diarrhœa alternates with constipation,* especially in old people. Diarrhœa after acids, sour wine, baths, overeating; slimy, flatulent stools. Mucous piles; *continued oozing of mucus. Hard lumps mixed with watery discharge. Catarrhal proctitis.* Stools composed entirely of mucus.

Urine.—Frequent, with burning, and backache; turbid and foul odor.

Male.—Eruption on scrotum and about genitals. Impotence. Atrophy of penis and testicles.

Female.—Excited; parts itch. Before menses, toothache; menses too early and profuse. Menses suppressed from cold bathing, with feeling of pressure in pelvis and tenderness in ovarian region. Leucorrhœa watery; acrid, lumpy.

Respiratory.—Cough worse *coming into warm room*, with burning sensation in chest, *itching of chest*, oppression. Loss of voice from becoming overheated. *Voice harsh and badly pitched.*

Back.—Itching and pain of neck and back.

Extremities.—Twitching of muscles. Jerks in arms. *Arthritic pain in fingers.* Nails brittle; grow out of shape. Horny warts on hands and soles. Weakness and shaking of hands in writing followed by offensive flatulence. *Feet very tender;* covered with large horny places. Inflamed corns. Pain in heels.

Skin.—Eczema with gastric derangements. Pimples, vesicles, and pustules. Sensitive to cold bathing. Thick, hard, honey-colored scabs. *Urticaria*; measle-like eruption. Itching when warm in bed. Dry skin. *Warts.* [*Thuja; Sabina; Caust.*] Dry gangrene. Scaly, pustular eruption with burning and itching, worse at night.

Sleep.—*Continual drowsiness in old people.*

Fever.—Chilly even in warm room. Intermittent with disgust, nausea, vomiting, eructations, coated tongue, diarrhœa. Hot sweat.

Modalities.—*Worse* in evening, from heat, acids, wine, water, and washing. Wet poultices. *Better* in open air, during rest. Moist warmth.

Relationship.—Compare: *Antimonium Chloridum.* Butter of Antimony. (A remedy for cancer. Mucous membranes destroyed. Abrasions. Skin cold and clammy. Great prostration of strength. Dose—third trituration.)

Antimon. jodat. (Uterine hyperplasia; humid asthma. Pneumonia and bronchitis; loss of strength, and appetite, yellowish skin, sweaty, dull and drowsy.) In sub-acute and chronic colds in chest which have extended downwards from head and have fastened themselves upon the bronchial tubes in the form of hard, croupy cough with a decided wheeze and inability to raise the sputum, especially in the aged and weak patients (Bacmeister). Stage of resolution of pneumonia slow and delayed.

Compare: *Kermes mineral*—Stibiat sulph. rub. (Bronchitis.)
Also *Puls, Ipecac, Sulph*.
Complementary: *Sulph*.
Antidote: *Hepar*.
Dose.—Third to sixth potency.

ANTIMONIUM SULPHURATUM AURATUM
(Golden Sulphuret of Antimony)

A remarkable remedy for many forms of chronic nasal and bronchial catarrh. Acne. Amaurosis.

Nose and Throat.—*Nosebleed on washing*. Increased secretion in nose and throat. Rough and scrapy feeling. Loss of smell. Metallic styptic taste.

Respiratory.—Tickling in larynx. *Increased mucus* with fullness in bronchi. Respiration difficult, pressure in bronchi, with constriction. Tough mucus in bronchi and larynx. Dry hard cough. Congestion of upper lobe of left lung. Winter coughs, patient is sore all over. Pneumonia, when hepatization occurred and resolution failed to take place.

Skin.—Acne (pustular variety). Itching on hands and feet.
Dose.—Second or third trituration.

ANTIMONIUM TARTARICUM
(Tartar Emetic. Tartrate of Antimony and Potash)

Has many symptoms in common with Antimonium Crudum, but also many peculiar to itself. Clinically, its therapeutic application has been confined largely to the treatment of respiratory diseases, *rattling of mucus with little expectoration* has been a guiding symptom. There is much *drowsiness, debility and sweat* characteristic of the drug, which group should always be more or less present, when the drug is prescribed. Gastric affections of drunkards and gouty subjects. *Cholera morbus*. Sensation of coldness in blood-vessels. *Bilharziasis*. Antimonium tart is homœopathic to dysuria, strangury, hæmaturia, albuminuria, catarrh of bladder and urethra, burning in rectum, bloody mucous stools, etc. Antimon tart acts indirectly on the parasites by stimulating the oxidizing action of the protective substance. By-effects, following injection for Bilharziasis. *Chills and contractures* and pain in muscles.

Trembling of whole body, great prostration and faintness. Lumbago. Chills, contractures and muscular pains. Warts on glans penis.

Mind and Head.—Vertigo alternates with drowsiness. Great despondency. Fear of being alone. Muttering, delirium, and stupor. Vertigo, with dullness and confusion. Band-like feeling over forehead. Face pale and sunken. Child will not be touched without whining. Headache as from a band compressing. [*Nit. ac.*]

Tongue.—*Coated, pasty, thick white*, with red edges. Red and dry, especially in the center. Brown.

Face.—Cold, blue, *pale; covered with cold sweat. Incessant quivering of chin and lower jaw.* [*Gelsem.*]

Stomach.—Difficult deglutition of liquids. Vomiting in any position, excepting lying on right side. *Nausea, retching. and vomiting*, especially after food, with deathly faintness and prostration. *Thirst for cold water, little and often, and desire for apples, fruits, and acids generally.* Nausea produces fear; with pressure in præcordial region, followed by headache with yawning and lachrymation and vomiting.

Abdomen.—Spasmodic colic, much flatus. Pressure in abdomen, especially on stooping forward. Cholera morbus. Diarrhœa in eruptive diseases.

Urinary.—Burning in urethra during and after urinating. Last drops bloody with pain in bladder. Urging increased. Catarrh of bladder and urethra. Stricture. Orchitis.

Respiratory Organs.—Hoarseness. *Great rattling of mucus, but very little is expectorated.* Velvety feeling in chest. Burning sensation in chest, which ascends to throat. Rapid, short, difficult breathing; seems as if he would suffocate; must sit up. Emphysema of the aged. *Coughing and gaping consecutively.* Bronchial tubes overloaded with mucus. Cough excited by eating, with pain in chest and larynx. *Œdema and impending paralysis of lungs.* Much palpitation, with uncomfortable hot feeling. Pulse rapid, weak, trembling. Dizziness, with cough Dyspnœa relieved by eructaion. Cough and dyspnœa better lying on right side—(opposite *Badiaga*).

Back.—*Violent pain in sacro-lumbar region.* Slightest effort to move may cause retching and cold, clammy sweat. *Sensation of heavy weight at the coccyx, dragging downward all the time* Twitching of muscles; limbs tremulous.

Skin.—*Pustular eruption,* leaving a bluish-red mark. Smallpox. Warts.

Fever.—Coldness, trembling, and chilliness. Intense heat Copious perspiration. Cold, clammy sweat, with great faintness. Intermittent fever with lethargic condition.

Sleep.—*Great drowsiness.* On falling asleep electric-like shocks. Irresistible inclination to sleep with nearly all complaints.

Modalities.—*Worse,* in evening; from lying down at night; from warmth; in damp cold weather; from all sour things and milk. *Better,* from sitting erect; from eructation and expectoration.

Relationship.—Antidotes: *Puls.; Sepia.*

Compare: *Kali sulph.; Ipecac.*

Dose.—Second and sixth trituration. The lower potencies sometimes aggravate.

ANTIPYRINE

(Fhenazone—A Coal-tar Derivative)

Antipyrine is one of the drugs that induce leucocytosis, similar to ergotin, salicylates, and tuberculin. Acts especially on the vaso-motor centers, causing dilation of capillaries of skin and consequent circumscribed patches of hyperæmia and swelling. In large doses causes profuse perspiration, dizziness, cyanosis, and somnolence, albumen and blood in urine. Acute erythema multiforme.

Mind.—Fear of becoming insane: nervous anxiety; *hallucinations of sight and hearing.*

Head.—Throbbing headache; *sensation of constriction.* Flashes of heat. *Headache under ears with earache.*

Eyes.—Puffiness of lids. Conjunctiva red and œdematous, *with lachrymation.* Red spots. [*Apis.*]

Ears.—Pains and buzzing. *Tinnitus.*

Face.—Œdema and puffiness. Red and swollen.

Mouth.—Swelling of lips. Burning of mouth and gums.

Ulceration of lips and tongue; vesicles and bullæ. Small lump in cheek. Tongue swollen. Bloody saliva. Toothache along lower jaw.

Throat.—Pain on swallowing. Expectoration of fetid pus. Abscess, white false membrane. Sensation of burning.

Stomach.—Nausea and vomiting; burning and pain.

Urine.—Diminished. Penis black.

Female.—Itching and burning in vagina. Menses suppressed. Watery leucorrhœa.

Respiratory.—Fluent coryza. Nasal mucous membrane swollen. Dull pains in frontal sinus. Aphonia. Oppression and dyspnœa. Cheyne-Stokes repiration.

Heart.—Faintness, with sensation of stoppage of heart. Throbbing throughout the body. Rapid, weak, irregular pulse.

Nerves.—Epileptiform seizures. Contractures. Trembling and cramps. Crawling and numbness. *General prostration.*

Skin.—*Erythema*, eczema, pemphigus. *Intense pruritus. Urticaria*, appearing and disappearing suddenly, with internal coldness. Angioneurotic-œdema. Dark blotches on skin of penis, sometimes with œdema.

Dose.—Second decimal potency.

APIS MELLIFICA
(The Honey-Bee)

Acts on cellular tissues causing œdema of skin and mucous membranes.

The very characteristic effects of the sting of the bee furnish unerring indications for its employment in disease. Swelling or puffing up of various parts, *œdema*, red rosy hue, stinging pains, soreness, intolerance of heat, and slightest touch, and afternoon aggravation are some of the general guiding symptoms. Erysipelatous inflammations, dropsical effusions and anasarca, acute, inflammation of kidneys, and other parenchymatous tissues are characteristic pathological states corresponding to Apis. Apis acts especially on outer parts, skin, coatings of inner organs, serous membranes. It produces serous inflammation with effusion, membranes of brain, heart, pleuritic effusion, etc. Extreme sensitiveness to touch and general soreness is marked. *Constricted* sensations. Sensation of stiffness and as of something torn off in the interior of the body. Much prostration.

Mind.—Apathy, indifference, and unconsciousness. *Awkward; drops things readily.* Stupor, with sudden sharp cries and startings. Stupor alternating with erotic mania. Sensation of dying. Listless; cannot think clearly. Jealous, fidgety, hard to please. Sudden shrill, piercing screams. *Whining. Tearfulness.* Jealously, fright, rage, vexation, grief. Cannot concentrate mind when attempting to read or study.

Head.—Whole brain feels *very tired*. Vertigo with sneezing, worse on lying or closing eyes. Heat, throbbing, distensive pains, better on pressure, and worse on motion. Sudden stabbing pains. Dull, heavy sensation in occiput, as from a blow, extending to neck (better on pressure), accompanied with sexual excitement. Bores head into pillow and screams out.

Eyes.—Lids *swollen*, red, *œdematous*, everted, inflamed; burn and sting. Conjunctiva bright red, puffy. *Lachrymation hot.* Photophobia. *Sudden piercing pains.* Pain around orbits. *Serous exudation, œdema, and sharp pains. Suppurative inflammation of eyes.* Keratitis with *intense chemosis of ocular conjunctiva*. Staphyloma of cornea following suppurative inflammation. *Styes,* also prevents their recurrence.

Ears.—External ear red, inflamed, sore; stinging pains.

Nose—Coldness of tip of nose. *Red, swollen,* inflamed, with sharp pains.

Face.—Swollen, red, with piercing pain. Waxy, pale, œdematous. Erysipelas with stinging burning œdema. Extends from right to left.

Mouth.—Tongue fiery red, swollen, sore, and raw, with vesicles. Scalding in mouth and throat. Tongue feels scalded, red hot, trembling. Gums swollen. Lips swollen, especially upper. Membrane of mouth and throat glossy, as if varnished. *Red, shining, and puffy,* like erysipelas. Cancer of the tongue.

Throat.—Constricted, stinging pains. *Uvula swollen,* saclike. Throat swollen, inside and out; tonsils swollen, *puffy, fiery red.* Ulcers on tonsils. *Fiery red margin* around leathery membrane. Sensation of fishbone in throat.

Stomach.—Sore feeling. *Thirstless.* Vomiting of food. *Craving for milk.* [Rhus.]

Abdomen.—*Sore, bruised* on pressure, when sneezing. *Extremely tender*. Dropsy of abdomen. Peritonitis. Swelling in right groin.

Stool.—Involuntary on every motion; *anus seems open*. Bloody, painless. Anus feels raw. Hæmorrhoids, with stinging pain, after confinement. Diarrhœa watery, yellow; *cholera infantum type*. Cannot urinate without a stool. Dark, fetid, worse after eating. Constipation; feels as if something would break on straining.

Urine.—Burning and soreness when urinating. Suppressed, loaded with casts; frequent and involuntary; stinging pain and strangury; *scanty, high colored*. Incontinence. *Last drops* burn and smart.

Female.—Œdema of labia; relieved by cold water. Soreness and stinging pains; ovaritis; worse in *right* ovary. Menses suppressed, with cerebral and head symptoms, especially in young girls. Dysmenorrhœa, with severe ovarian pains. Metrorrhagia profuse, with heavy abdomen, faintness, stinging pain. Sense of tightness. Bearing-down, as if menses were to appear. Ovarian tumors, metritis with stinging pains. Great tenderness over abdomen and uterine region.

Respiratory.—Hoarseness; *dyspnœa*, breathing hurried and difficult. Œdema of larynx. Feels *as if he could not draw another breath*. Suffocation; short, dry cough, suprasternal. Hydrothorax.

Extremities.—Œdematous. Synovitis. Felon in beginning. Knee swollen, shiny, sensitive, sore, with stinging pain. Feet swollen and stiff. Feel too large. Rheumatic pain in back and limbs. Tired, bruised feeling. Numbness of hands and tips of fingers. Hives with intolerable itching. Œdematous swellings.

Skin.—Swellings after bites; *sore, sensitive*. Stinging. Erysipelas, with sensitiveness and swelling, rosy hue. Carbuncles, with burning, stinging pain. [*Ars.; Anthrac.*] Sudden puffing up of whole body.

Sleep.—Very *drowsy*. Dreams full of care and toil. Screams and *sudden starting during sleep*.

Fever.—*Afternoon chill, with thirst; worse on motion and heat*. External heat, with smothering feeling. Sweat slight, with sleepiness. Perspiration breaks out and dries up frequently.

Sleeps *after* the fever paroxysm. After perspiration, nettle rash, also with shuddering.

Modalities.—*Worse*, heat in any form; *touch;* pressure; late in afternoon; after sleeping; in closed and heated rooms. Right side. *Better*, in open air, uncovering, and cold bathing.

Relationship.—Complementary: *Nat. mur.* The "chronic," *Apis.;* also *Baryta carb.*, if lymphatics are involved. Inimical. *Rhus.*

Compare: *Apium virus* (auto-toxæmia, with pus products); *Zinc.; Canth.; Vespa; Lachesis.*

Dose.—Tincture to thirtieth potency. In œdematous conditions the *lower* potencies. Sometimes action is slow; so several days elapse before it is seen to act, and then urine is increased. *Apium virus*, sixth trituration.

APIUM GRAVEOLENS
(Common Celery)

Contains a soporific active principle. Obstinate retention of urine, throbbing headaches and heartburn, have been produced by celery. Swelling of throat, face, and hands. Rheumatic pain in muscles of neck also in sacrum. Growing pains. Hungry for apples. Dysmenorrhæa, with sharp, short pains, better flexing legs.

Head.—Depressed; energetic; feeling of fidgets; cannot sleep from thinking. Headache; better eating. Eyeballs feel sunken. Itching in eyes. Itching and smarting in inner canthus of left eye.

Abdomen.—Sore; sharp sticking pain as if stool was coming on; diarrhœa, sharp pain in left iliac region going over to right. Nausea increases with pains.

Female.—Sharp sticking pains in both ovarian regions, left, better bending over, by lying on left side, *with legs flexed;* nipples tender.

Respiratory.—Tickling, dry cough. *Intense constriction over sternum*, with drawing feeling through to back on lying down. Throat swollen, dyspnœa.

Skin.—Itching blotches; burning, creeping sensation. Profuse discharge from granulating ulcers. Urticaria with shuddering.

Sleep.—Unrefreshed; sleepless. Wakes from 1 to 3 a. m. Eating does not help sleep. Not fatigued from loss of sleep.

Dose.—First to thirtieth potency.

APOCYNUM ANDROSAEMIFOLIUM
(Dogbane)

The rheumatic symptoms of this remedy promise most curative results. Its pains are of a wandering nature, with much stiffness and drawing. Everything smells and tastes like honey. Worms. Trembling and prostration. Swollen sensations.

Extremities.—Pain in all joints. Pain in toes and soles. Swelling of hands and feet. Profuse sweat, with much heat in soles. Tingling pain in toes. Cramps in soles. Violent heat in soles. [*Sulph.*]

Dose.—Tincture and first potency.

APOCYNUM CANNABINUM
(Indian Hemp)

Increases secretions of mucous and serous membranes and acts on cellular tissue, producing œdema and dropsy and on skin causing diaphoresis. Acute hydrocephalus. A diminished frequency of the pulse is a prime indication. This is one of our most efficient remedies, in *dropsies*, ascites, anasarca and hydrothorax, and urinary troubles, especialy suppression and strangury In the digestive complaints of Bright's disease, with the nausea, vomiting, drowsiness, difficult breathing, it will be found of frequent service. The dropsy is characterized by great thirst and gastric irritability. Arhythmia. *Mitral and tricuspid regurgitation. Acute alcoholism.* Relaxation of sphincters.

Mind.—Bewildered. Low spirited.

Nose.—Long-continued sneezing. Snuffles of children. [*Sambucus.*] Chronic nasal catarrh with tendency to acute stuffiness with dull, sluggish memory. Dull headache. Takes cold easily, nostrils become congested and blocked up easily.

Stomach.—Nausea, with drowsiness. Thirst on walking. *Excessive vomiting.* Food or water is immediately ejected. Dull, heavy, sick feeling. Oppression in epigastrium and chest, impeding breathing. [*Lobelia infl.*] Sensation of sinking in stomach. Abdomen bloated. Ascites.

Stool.—*Watery*, flatulent, with soreness in anus; worse after eating. Feeling as if sphincter were open and stools ran right out.

Urine.—Bladder much distended. Turbid, hot urine, with thick mucus and burning in urethra, after urinating. Little expulsive power. Dribbling. Strangury. *Renal Dropsy.*

Female.—Amenorrhœa, with bloating; metrorrhagia with nausea; fainting, vital depression. Hæmorrhages at change of life. Blood expelled in large clots.

Respiratory.—Short, dry cough. *Respiration short and unsatisfactory.* Sighing. Oppression about epigastrium and chest.

Heart.—Tricuspid regurgitation; rapid and feeble, irregular cardiac action, low arterial tension, pulsating jugulars, general cyanosis and general dropsy.

Sleep.—Great restlessness and little sleep.

Modalities.—Worse, cold weather; cold drinks; uncovering.

Relationship.—*Cymarin* is the active principle of Apocyn., lowers pulse rate and increases blood-pressure. *Strophanthus* (extreme cardiac depression with intense gastric disturbance; dropsy). *Aralia hispida*—Wild Elder—a valuable diuretic. useful in dropsy of the cavities, either due to hepatic or renal disease with constipation. Urinary disorders, especially with dropsy. Scudder advises doses of five to thirty drops in sweetened cream of tartar, Solution). *Apis., Arsenic; Digital.; Helleb.*

Dose.—Tincture (ten drops three times daily) and in acute alcoholism 1 dram of decoction in 4 oz. water.

APOMORPHIA

(Alkaloid from Decomposition of Morphine by Hydrochloric Acid)

The chief power of this drug lies in the speedy and effective vomiting that it produces, which becomes a strong guiding symptom to its homœopathic use. The vomiting is preceded by nausea, lassitude and increased secretion of sweat, saliva, mucus and tears. Pneumonia with vomiting. *Combined alcoholism*, with constant nausea, constipation, insomnia.

Head and Stomach.—Vertigo. Dilated pupils. *Nausea and vomiting*. Violent inclination to vomit. Hot feeling all over body, especially head. Empty retching and headache; heartburn; pain between shoulder-blades. Reflex vomiting—pregnancy. *Seasickness*.

Non-Homœopathic Uses.—The hypodermic injection of one-sixteenth of a grain will cause full emesis within five to fifteen minutes in an adult without developing any other direct action apparently. Do not use in opium poisoning. *Apomorph.* hypodermically, one-thirtieth grain or less, acts as a safe and sure hypnotic. Acts well even in delirium. Sleep comes on in half an hour.

Dose.—Third to sixth potency.

AQUILEGIA
(Columbine)

A remedy for hysteria. Globus and clavus hystericus. Women at climaxis, with vomiting of green substance, especially in the morning. *Sleeplessness*. Nervous trembling of body; sensitive to light and noise. Dysmenorrhœa of young girls.

Female.—Menses scanty, with dull, painful, nightly increasing pressure in the right lumbar region.

Dose.—First potency.

ARAGALLUS LAMBERTI
(White Loco Weed—Rattle Weed)

Acts principally on nervous system, producing a bewildered, confused state. Symptoms of incoordination and paralysis. Locomotor ataxia. Tired in the morning.

Mind.—Great depression; worse in morning or evening. Cannot study. Cross, irritable, restless. *Bewildered*. Mental confusion and apathy. Desires to be alone. Difficulty in concentrating mind, absent-minded. Lack of ambition. Defective expression in writing. Restlessness and aimless wandering. Must concentrate his mind on walking.

Head.—Diplopia. Burning in eyes. Cracking of lower lip.

Throat.—Aches. Feels full. Sore with nausea. Pharynx dark, swollen, glazed.

Respiratory.— Weight on chest in region of ensiform cartilage. Constriction as of a wide band. Soreness of chest under sternum. Oppression.

Extremities.—Weakness of limbs. Pain in left sciatic nerve. Cramps of muscles on front of leg while walking.

Relationship.—Compare: *Astragallus* and *Oxytropis*, two varieties of Loco Weed; also *Baryta*.

Dose.—Sixth and two hundredth potencies.

ARALIA RACEMOSA
(American Spikenard)

This is a remedy for asthmatic conditions, with *cough aggravated on lying down*. Drenching sweat during sleep. Extreme sensitiveness to draughts. Diarrhœa, prolapse of rectum. Aching in rectum extending upwards; worse lying on side lain upon.

Respiratory.—*Dry cough coming on after first sleep*, about middle of night. *Asthma on lying down at night* with spasmodic cough; worse after first sleep, with tickling in throat. Constriction of chest; *feels as if a foreign body were in throat*. Obstruction worse in spring. Hay-fever; *frequent sneezing*. Rawness and burning behind sternum.

The least current of air causes sneezing, with *copious watery, excoriating nasal discharge*, of *salty acrid taste*.

Female.—Menses suppressed; leucorrhœa foul-smelling, acrid, with pressing-down pain. Lochia suppressed, with tympanites.

Modalities.—Worse about 11 p. m. (cough).

Relationship.—Compare: *Pecten—Scallop* (humid asthma. Quick, labored breathing. Constriction of chest, especially right side. Asthma preceded by coryza and burning in throat and chest. Attack ends with copious expectoration of tough, frothy mucus. Worse at night.) *Ars. iod.; Naphthaline; Cepa; Rosa; Sabad.; Sinapis.*

Dose.—Tincture, to third potency.

ARANEA DIADEMA
(Papal-Cross Spider)

All spider poisons powerfully affect the nervous system. (See tarentula, Mygale, etc.)

All symptoms of Aranea are characterized by *periodicity, and coldness*, and great susceptibility to dampness. It is the remedy for the constitution favorable to malarial poisoning, where every damp day or place favors chilliness. Patient feels cold to the very bones. Coldness not relieved by anything. *Feeling as if parts were enlarged and heavier.* Wake up at night with hands feeling twice their natural size. Spleen swollen. *Hydrogenoid* Constitution, *i. e.*, Abnormal sensitiveness to damp and cold, inability to live near fresh water, lakes, rivers, etc., or in damp, chilly places. [*Nat. Sulph. Thuja.*]

Head.—Pain in right trifacial nerve from periphery inwards. Confusion; *better by smoking in open air*. Heat and flickering in eyes; worse in damp weather. Sudden violent pain in teeth at night immediately after lying down.

Female.—*Menses too early, too copious*. Distention of abdomen. Lumbo-abdominal neuralgia.

Chest.—Pain in intercostal nerve from nerve endings to spine. Bright red hæmorrhage from lungs. [*Millefol.; Ferr. phos.*]

Stomach.—Cramps after eating a little; epigastrium painful to pressure.

Abdomen.—Enlarged spleen. Colic returns same hours. Heaviness in lower abdomen, as of a stone. Diarrhœa. Arms and legs feel as if asleep.

Extremities.—Bone-pains in extremities. Pain in *os calcis*. *Sensation of swelling*, and of parts going to sleep.

Sleep.—Restless and waking, as if hands and forearms were swollen and heavy.

Fever.—*Coldness, with pain in long bones*, and feeling of stone in abdomen at the same hour daily. *Chilly day and night;* always worse during rain.

Modalities.—*Worse*, damp weather; late in afternoon, and at midnight. *Better*, smoking tobacco.

Relationship.—*Tela aranearum*—Spider's web.—(Cardiac sleeplessness, increased muscular energy. Excitement and nervous agitation in febrile states. Dry asthma. harassing coughs; periodic headaches with *extreme nervous erethism*. *Obstinate intermittents*. Acts immediately on arterial system, pulse full, strong, compressible.

Lowers pulse rate frequency. Masked periodical diseases, hectic, broken down patients. Symptoms come on *suddenly* with cool, *clammy* skin. Numbness of hands and legs when at rest. *Continued chilliness*.

Aranea Scinencia—Grey Spider—(constant twitching of under eyelids. Sleepiness. Worse in warm room.)

Heloderma; Cedron; Arsenic.

Dose.—Tincture to thirtieth potency.

ARBUTUS ANDRACHNE
(Strawberry Tree)

A remedy for eczema associated with gouty and rheumatic symptoms. Arthritis; especially larger joints. Urine rendered more clear. Lumbago. Symptoms shift from skin to joints. Vesical symptoms.

Relationship.—*Arbutin; Ledum; Bryonia; Kalmia.*

Dose.—Tincture, to third potency.

ARECA
(Betel Nut)

Of use in Helminthiasis. Its alkaloid, *Areolin hydrobrom* contracts the pupil, acting more promptly and energetically but of shorter duration than *Eserine*. Serviceable in glaucoma. Acts also as a salivatory like *Pilocarpin*. Also increases the amplitude of pulsations of the heart and promotes the contractibility of the intestines.

ARGEMONE MEXICANA
(Prickly Poppy)

Colicky cramp and spasm of bowels. Painful neuro-muscular conditions, preventing sleep. Rheumatic disease associated with Bright's disease. (D. MacFarlan.)

Head.—Throbbing headache in eyes and temples. Head hot. Throat very dry, pain on swallowing.

Stomach.—Feels sick, like vomiting. Griping in pit of stomach. No appetite. Belching and passing gas.

Urinary.—Passes less urine. Changing color.

Female.—Menses suppressed. Diminished sexual desire with weakness.

Extremities.—Left knee stiff and painful. Feet swollen.

Modalities.—*Worse* at noon (weakness).

Dose.—Sixth potency. Fresh juice is applied to ulcers and warts.

ARGENTUM METALLICUM
(Silver)

Emaciation, a gradual drying up, desire for fresh air, dyspnœa, sensation of expansion and left-sided pains are characteristic. The chief action is centered on the articulations and their component elements, bones, cartilages, and ligaments. Here the small blood vessels become closed up or withered and carious affections result. They come on insidiously, lingering, but progress. The larynx is also a special center for this drug.

Mental.—Hurried feeling; time passes slowly; melancholy.

Head.—Dull paroxysmal neuralgia over left side, gradually increasing and ceasing suddenly. Scalp very tender to touch Vertigo, with intoxicated feeling, on looking at running water. *Head feels empty, hollow.* Eyelids red and thick. Exhausting coryza, with sneezing. Pain in facial bones. Pain between left eye and frontal eminence.

Throat.—Raw, hawking, gray, *jelly-like mucus*, and throat sore on coughing. *Profuse and easy* morning expectoration.

Respiratory.—*Hoarseness* Aphonia. Raw, sore feeling when coughing. Total loss of voice of professional singers. Larynx feels sore and raw. *Easy expectoration, looking like boiled starch. Feeling of raw spot near supra sternal fossa Worse from use of voice. Cough from laughing.* Hectic fever at noon. On reading aloud, must hem and hawk. *Great weakness of chest;* worse left side. Alteration in timbre of voice. Pain in left lower ribs.

Back.—Severe backache; must walk bent, with oppression of chest.

Urine.—Diuresis. Urine *profuse, turbid*, sweet odor. Frequent urination. Polyuria.

Extremities.—Rheumatic affections of joints, especially elbow and knee. Legs weak and trembling, worse descending stairs. Involuntary contractions of fingers, partial paralysis of forearm; writer's cramp. *Swelling of ankles.*

Male.—Crushed pain in testicles. *Seminal emissions, without sexual excitement.* Frequent micturation with burning.

Female.—Ovaries feel too large. Bearing-down pain. Prolapse of womb. *Eroded spongy cervix. Leucorrhœa* foul, excoriating. Palliative in scirrhus of uterus. Pain in left ovary. *Climacteric hæmorrhage.* Sore feeling throughout abdomen; worse by jarring. Uterine disease with pain in joints and limbs.

Modalities.—*Worse* from touch, toward noon. *Better* in open air; cough at night when lying down (opposite *Hyoscy*.)

Relationship.—Antidotes: *Mercur.; Puls.*

Compare: *Selen.; Alum.; Platina; Stannum; Ampelopsis.* (Chronic hoarseness in scrofulous patients.)

Dose.—Sixth trituration and higher. Not too frequent repetition.

ARGENTUM NITRICUM
(Nitrate of Silver)

In this drug the neurotic effects are very marked, many brain and spinal symptoms presenting themselves which give certain indications for its homœopathic employment. Symptoms of inco-ordination, loss of control and want of balance everywhere, mentally and physically; *trembling* in affected parts. Is an irritant of mucous membranes, producing violent inflammation of the throat, and a marked gastro-enteritis. Very characteristic is the great *desire for sweets*, the splinter-like pains, and free muco-purulent discharge in the inflamed and ulcerated mucous membranes. Sensation as if a part were expanding and other errors of perception are characteristic. Withered up and dried constitutions present a favorable field for its action, especially when associated with unusual or long continued mental exertion. Head symptoms often determine the choice of this remedy. Pains increase and decrease gradually. Flatulent state and prematurely aged look. Explosive belching, especially in neurotics. Upper abdominal affections brought on by undue mental exertion Paraplegia Myelitis and disseminated sclerosis of brain and cord. *Intolerance of heat.* Sensation of a sudden pinch. (Dudgeon). Destroys red blood corpuscles, producing anemia.

Mind.—Thinks his understanding will and must fail. Fearful and *nervous;* impulse to jump out of window. Faintish and tremulous. *Melancholic;* apprehensive of serious disease. *Time passes slowly.* [*Cann. ind.*] Memory weak. Errors of perception. *Impulsive; wants to do things in a hurry.* [*Lilium.*] *Peculiar mental impulses.* Fears and anxieties and hidden irrational motives for actions.

Head.—*Headache with coldness and trembling.* Emotional disturbances cause appearance of hemi-cranial attacks. Sense of *expansion.* Brain-fag, with general debility and trembling. Headache from mental exertion, from dancing. *Vertigo,* with buzzing in ears and with nervous affections. Aching in frontal eminence, with *enlarged feeling in corresponding eye.* Boring pain; *better on tight bandaging and pressure.* Itching of scalp. Hemi-crania; bones of head feel as if separated.

Eyes.—Inner canthi *swollen and red.* Spots before the vision. Blurred vision. Photophobia in warm room. *Purulent ophthalmia.* Great swelling of conjunctiva; *discharge abundant and purulent.* Chronic ulceration of margin of lids; sore, thick, swollen. Unable to keep eyes fixed steadily. Eye-strain from sewing; worse in warm room. Aching, tired feeling in eyes, better closing or pressing upon them. Useful in restoring power to the weakened ciliary muscles. Paretic condition of ciliary muscle. Acute granular conjunctivitis. Cornea opaque. Ulcer in cornea.

Nose.—Loss of smell. Itching. Ulcers in septum. **Coryza,** with chilliness, lachrymation, and headache.

Face.—Sunken, old, pale, and bluish. Old man's look; tight drawing of skin over bones.

Mouth.—Gums tender and bleed easily. Tongue has prominent papillæ; tip is red and painful. Pain in sound teeth. Taste coppery, like ink. Canker sores.

Throat.—Much *thick mucus* in throat and mouth causes hawking. Raw, rough and sore. *Sensation of a splinter in throat* on swallowing. Dark redness of throat. Catarrh of smokers, with tickling as of hair in throat. *Strangulated* feeling.

Stomach.—*Belching* accompanies most gastric ailments. Nausea, retching, vomiting of glairy mucus. Flatulence; *painful swelling of pit.* Painful spot over stomach that radiates to all parts of the abdomen. Gnawing ulcerating pain; burning and constriction. Ineffectual effort at eructation. *Great craving for sweets.* Gastritis of drunkards. Ulcerative pain in left side under ribs. Trembling and throbbing in stomach. Enormous distention. Ulceration of stomach, *with radiating pain.* Desire for cheese and salt.

Abdomen.—Colic, *with much flatulent distention.* Stitchy ulcerative pain on left side of stomach, below short ribs.

Stool.—Watery, noisy, flatulent; *green, like chopped spinach,* with shreddy mucus and enormous distention of abdomen; very offensive. Diarrhœa immediately after eating or drinking. *Fluids go right through him;* after sweets. After any emotion with flatulence. Itching of anus.

Urine.—Urine passes unconsciously, day and night. Urethra inflamed, with pain, burning, itching; pain as from a splinter. Urine scanty and dark. Emission of a few drops after having finished. Divided stream. Early stage of gonorrhœa; profuse discharge and terrible cutting pains; bloody urine.

Male.—Impotence. Erection fails when coition is attempted. Cancer-like ulcers. Desire wanting. Genitals shrivel. Coition painful.

Female.—Gastralgia at beginning of menses. Intense spasm of chest muscles. Orgasms at night. Nervous erethism at change of life. Leucorrhœa profuse, with erosion of cervix. bleeding easily. Uterine hæmorrhage, two weeks after menses; Painful affections of left ovary.

Respiratory.—*High notes cause cough.* Chronic hoarseness. Suffocative cough, as if from a hair in throat. Dyspnœa. Chest feels as if a bar were around it. Palpitation, pulse irregular and intermittent; worse lying on *right side;* [*Alumen.*] Painful spots in chest. Angina pectoris, nightly aggravation. Many people in a room seem to take away his breath.

Back.—Much pain. Spine sensitive with nocturnal pains, [*Oxal. acid.*] paraplegia; posterior spinal sclerosis.

Extremites.—Cannot walk with eyes closed. Trembling, with general debility. Paralysis, with mental and abdominal symptoms. Rigidity of *calves*. Debility in calves especially. Walks and stands unsteadily, especially when unobserved. Numbness of arms. Post-diphtheritic paralysis (after *Gelsem.*)

Skin.—Brown, tense, and hard. Drawing in skin, as from a spider-web, or dried albuminous substance, withered and dried up. Irregular blotches.

Sleep.—Sleepless, from fancies before his imagination; horrible dreams of snakes, and of sexual gratification. Drowsy stupor.

Fever.—Chills with nausea. Chilly when uncovered, yet feels smothered if wrapped up.

Modalities.—*Worse*, warmth in any form; at night; from cold food; *sweets;* after eating; at mentsrual period; from emotions, *left side*. *Better*, from eructation; fresh air; *cold;* pressure.

Relationship.—Antidote: *Nat. mur.*

Compare: *Ars.; Merc.; Phos.; Pulsat.; Argent. cyanatum* (angina pectoris, asthma, spasm of œsophagus); *Argent. iodat.* (throat disorders, hoarseness, gland affected.) *Protargol* (gonorrhœa after acute stage 2 per cent. solution; syphilitic mucous patches, chancres and chancroids, 10 per cent. solution applied twice a day; ophthalmia neonatorum, 2 drops of 10 per cent. solution).

Argent. phosph. (An excellent diuretic in dropsy.)

Argent. oxyd. (Chlorosis with menorrhagia and diarrhœa.)

Dose.—Third to thirtieth potency

Best form an aqueous solution 1 to 9, 2 or 3 drop doses. This solution in water preferable to lower triturations; unless fresh, these readily decompose into the oxide.

ARISTOLOCHIA MILHOMENS
(Brazilian Snake Root)

Stitching pains in various parts. Pain in heels, burning in anus and frequent irritation. Flatulence in stomach and abdomen. Pain in back and extremities. Stiffness of legs. Pain in tendo-Achillis. Itching and swelling around the malleoli.

Relationship.—Compare: *Aristolochia Serpentaria*—Virginia Snake Root—(Symptoms of intestinal tract; colliquative diarrhœa, meteorism. Flatulent dyspepsia. Brain congestion. Distention and cutting pains in abdomen. Symptoms like those of Poison-Oak.)

Dose.—Lower potencies.

ARNICA
(Leopard's Bane)

Produces conditions upon the system quite similar to those resulting from injuries, falls, blows, contusions. Tinnitus aurium. *Putrid phenomena*. Septic conditions; prophylactic of pus infection. Apoplexy, red, full face.

It is especially suited to cases when any injury, however remote, seems to have caused the present trouble. *After traumatic injuries*, overuse of any organ, strains. Arnica is disposed to cerebral congestion. Acts best in plethoric, feebly in debilitated with impoverished blood, cardiac dropsy with dyspnœa. A muscular tonic. Traumatism of grief, remorse or sudden realization of financial loss. Limbs and body ache as if beaten; joints as if sprained. Bed feels too hard. Marked effect on the blood. Affects the venous system inducing stasis. Echymosis and hæmorrhages. Relaxed blood vessels, black and blue spots. Tendency to hæmorrhage and low-fever states. Tendency to tissue degeneration, septic conditions, abscesses that do not mature. *Sore, lame, bruised feeling*. Neuralgias originating in disturbances of pneumo-gastric. Rheumatism of muscular and tendinous tissue, especially of back and shoulders. Aversion to tobacco. *Influenza*. Thrombosis. Hæmatocele.

Mind.—Fears touch, or the approach of anyone. Unconscious; when spoken to answers correctly, but relapses. Indifference; inability to perform continuous active work; morose, delirious. Nervous; cannot bear pain; whole body oversensitive. Says there is nothing the matter with him. Wants to be let alone. Agoraphobia (fear of space). After mental strain or shock.

Head.—*Hot, with cold body;* confused; sensitiveness of brain, with sharp, pinching pains. Scalp feels contracted. Cold spot on forehead. Chronic vertigo; objects whirl about especially when walking.

Eyes.—Diplopia from traumatism, muscular paralysis, retinal haemorrhage. Bruised, sore feeling in eyes after close work. Must keep eyes open. Dizzy on closing them. Feel tired and weary after sight-seeing, moving pictures, etc.

Ears.—Noises in ear caused by rush of blood to the head. Shooting in and around ears. Blood from ears. Dullness of hearing after concussion. Pain in cartilages of ears as if bruised.

Nose.—Bleeding after every fit of coughing, dark fluid blood. Nose feels sore; *cold.*

Mouth.—*Fetid breath.* Dry and thirsty. Bitter taste. [*Colocy.*] *Taste as from bad eggs.* Soreness of gums after teeth extraction. [*Sepia.*] Empyema of maxillary sinus.

Face.—*Sunken;* very red. Heat in lips. Herpes in face.

Stomach.—Longing for vinegar. Distaste for milk and meat. Canine hunger. Vomiting of blood. Pain in stomach during eating. Repletion with loathing. Oppressive gases pass upward and downward. Pressure as from a stone. *Feeling as if stomach were passing against spine.* Fetid vomiting.

Abdomen.—Stitches under false ribs. Distended; offensive flatus. Sharp thrusts through abdomen.

Stool.—*Straining of tenesmus in diarrhœa. Offensive,* brown, *bloody,* putrid, involuntary. Looks like brown yeast. Must lie down after every stool. Diarrhœa of consumption; worse lying on left side. Dysenteric stools with muscular pains.

Urine.—Retained from over-exertion. Dark brick-red sediment. Vesical tenesmus with very painful micturition.

Female.—Bruised parts after labor. Violent after-pains. Uterine hæmorrhage from mechanical injury after coition. Sore nipples. Mastitis from injury. Feeling as if fœtus were lying crosswise.

Respiratory.—Coughs depending on cardiac lesion, paroxysmal, at night, during sleep, worse exercise. Acute tonsillitis. swelling of soft palate and uvula. Pneumonia; approaching paralysis. Hoarseness from overuse of voice. Raw, sore feeling in morning. Cough produced by weeping and lamenting. Dry, from tickling low down in trachea. Bloody expectoration. Dyspnœa with hæmoptysis. All bones and cartilages of chest painful. *Violent spasmodic cough, with facial herpes.* Whooping cough, child cries before coughing. *Pleurodynia* [*Ranunc.; Cimicif.*]

Heart.—*Angina pectoris;* pain especially severe in elbow of left arm. Stitches in heart. Pulse feeble and irregular. Cardiac dropsy with distressing dyspnœa. Extremities distended, feel bruised and sore. Fatty heart and hypertrophy.

Extremities.—Gout. Great fear of being touched or approached. Pain in back and limbs, as if bruised or beaten. Sprained and dislocated feeling. Soreness after overexertion. Everything on which he lies seems too hard. Deathly coldness of forearm. Cannot walk erect, on account of bruised pain in pelvic region. Rheumatism begins low down and works up. [*Ledum.*]

Skin.—*Black and blue.* Itching, burning, eruption of small pimples. *Crops of small boils.* [*Ichthyol; Silica.*] Ecchymosis. Bed sores. [*Bovinine locally.*] Acne indurata, characterized by *symmetry in distribution.*

Sleep.—Sleepless and restless when overtired. Comatose drowsiness; awakens with hot head; dreams of death, mutilated bodies, anxious and terrible. Horrors in the night. Involuntary stools during sleep.

Fever.—Febrile symptoms closely related to typhoid. Shivering over whole body. Heat and redness of head, with coolness of rest of body. Internal heat; feet and hands cold. Nightly sour sweats.

Modalities.—*Worse,* least touch; motion; rest; wine; damp cold. *Better, lying down, or with head low.*

Relationship.—Antidotes: *Camph.*

Vitex trifolia.—Indian Arnica. (Sprains and pains, headache in temples, pain in joints; pain in abdomen; pain in testicles.)

Complementary: *Acon.; Ipec.*

Compare: *Acon.; Bapt.;Bellis; Hamam; Rhus.; Hyperic.*

Dose.—Third to thirtieth potency. Locally, the tincture, but should never be applied *hot* or at all when abrasions or cuts are present.

ARSENICUM ALBUM
(Arsenious Acid)—Arsenic Trioxide

A profoundly acting remedy on every organ and tissue. Its clear-cut characteristic symptoms and correspondence to many severe types of disease make its homœopathic employment constant and certain. Its general symptoms often alone lead to its successful application. Among these the all-prevailing debility, exhaustion, and *restlessness*, with *nightly aggravation*, are most important. *Great exhaustion after the slightest exertion.* This, with the peculiar irritability of fibre, gives the characteristic *irritable weakness*. *Burning pains.* Unquenchable thirst. Burning relieved by heat. *Seaside complaints* [*Nat. mur.; Aqua Marina*]. Injurious effects of fruits, especially more watery ones. Gives quiet and ease to the last moments of life when given in high potency. *Fear fright and worry.* Green discharges. Infantile Kala-azar. (Dr. Neatby).

Ars. should be thought of in ailments from alcoholism, *ptomaine poisoning*, stings, dissecting wounds, chewing tobacco; ill effects from decayed food or animal matter; odor of discharges is *putrid;* in complaints that return annually. Anæmia and chlorosis. Degenerative changes. Gradual loss of weight from impaired nutrition. Reduces the refractive index of blood serum (also *China* and *Ferr. phos.*). Maintains the system under the stress of malignancy regardless of location. Malarial cachexia. *Septic infections and low vitality.*

Mind.—*Great anguish and restlessness. Changes place continually. Fears*, of death, of being left alone. Great fear, with cold sweat. Thinks it useless to take medicine. Suicidal. Hallucinations of smell and sight. Despair drives him from place to place. Miserly, malicious, selfish, lacks courage. General sensibility increased [*Hep.*]. Sensitive to disorder and confusion.

Head.—Headaches relieved by cold, other symptoms worse. Periodical burning pains, with *restlessness;* with cold skin.

Hemicrania, with *icy feeling of scalp and great weakness*. Sensitive head in open air. Delirium tremens; cursing and raving; vicious. Head is in constant motion. Scalp *itches* intolerably; circular patches of bare spots; rough, dirty, sensitive, and covered with dry scales; nightly burning and itching; dandruff. Scalp very sensitive; cannot brush hair.

Eyes.—*Burning in eyes, with acrid lachrymation.* Lids red, ulcerated, scabby, scaly, granulated. Œdema *around* eyes. External inflammation, with extreme painfulness; *burning, hot*, and excoriating lachrymation. Corneal ulceration. *Intense photophobia;* better external warmth. Ciliary neuralgia, with fine burning pain.

Ears.—Skin within, raw and burning. *Thin, excoriating, offensive* otorrhœa. Roaring in ears, during a paroxysm of pain

Nose.—*Thin, watery, excoriating* discharge. Nose feels *stopped up.* Sneezing *without* relief. Hay-fever and coryza; worse in open air; better indoors. *Burning* and bleeding. Acne of nose. Lupus.

Face.—Swollen, pale, yellow, *cachectic*, sunken, cold, and covered with sweat. [*Acetic acid.*] Expression of agony. Tearing, *needle-like* pains; burning. Lips black, livid. Angry, circumscribed flush of cheeks.

Mouth.—Unhealthy, easily-bleeding gums. Ulceration of mouth with dryness and burning heat. Epithelioma of lips. Tongue dry, clean, and red; stitching and burning pain in tongue, ulcerated with blue color. Bloody saliva. Neuralgia of teeth; feel long and very sore; worse after midnight; better warmth. Metallic taste. *Gulping up of burning water.*

Throat.—Swollen, œdematous, constricted, *burning*, unable to swallow. Diphtheritic membrane, looks dry and wrinkled.

Stomach.—*Cannot bear the sight or smell of food. Great thirst; drinks much, but little at a time.* Nausea, retching, vomiting, after eating or drinking. Anxiety in pit of stomach. *Burning pain.* Craves acids and coffee. Heartburn; gulping up of acid and bitter substances which seem to excoriate the throat. Long-lasting eructations. Vomiting of blood, bile, green mucus, or brown-black mixed with blood. Stomach extremely irritable; seems raw, as if torn. Gastralgia from slightest food or drink. Dyspepsia from vinegar, acids, ice-

ARSENICUM ALBUM

cream, ice-water, tobacco. Terrible fear and dyspnœa, with gastralgia; also faintness, icy coldness, great exhaustion. Malignant symptoms. Everything swallowed seems to lodge in the œsophagus, which seems as if closed and nothing would pass. *Ill effects of vegetable diet, melons, and watery fruits generally.* Craves milk.

Abdomen.—Gnawing, burning pains like coals of fire; relieved by heat. *Liver and spleen enlarged and painful.* Ascites and anasarca. Abdomen swollen and painful. Pain as from a wound in abdomen on coughing.

Rectum.—Painful, spasmodic protrusion of rectum. Tenesmus. *Burning* pain and pressure in rectum and anus.

Stool.—*Small, offensive, dark, with much prostration.* Worse at night, and after eating and drinking; from chilling stomach, alcoholic abuse, spoiled meat. Dysentery dark, bloody, very offensive. Cholera, with intense agony, prostration, and burning thirst. Body cold as ice. [*Verat.*] Hæmorrhoids burn like fire; relieved by heat. Skin excoriated about anus.

Urine.—Scanty, burning, involuntary. Bladder as if paralyzed. *Albuminous.* Epithelial cells; cylindrical clots of fibrin and globules of pus and blood. After urinating, feeling of weakness in abdomen. Bright's disease. Diabetes.

Female.—Menses too profuse and too soon. Burning in ovarian region. Leucorrhœa, acrid, burning, offensive, thin. Pain as from red-hot wires; worse least exertion; causes great fatigue; better in warm room. *Menorrhagia.* Stitching pain in pelvis extending down the thigh.

Respiratory.—Unable to lie down; fears suffocation. Air-passages constricted. Asthma worse midnight. Burning in chest. Suffocative catarrh. Cough worse after midnight; worse lying on back. Expectoration scanty, frothy. *Darting pain through upper third of right lung.* Wheezing respiration. Hæmoptysis with pain between shoulders; burning heat all over. Cough dry, as from sulphur fumes; *after drinking.*

Heart.—Palpitation, pain, dyspnœa, faintness. Irritable heart in smokers and tobacco-chewers. *Pulse more rapid in morning.* [*Sulph.*] Dilatation. Cyanosis. Fatty degeneration. Angina pectoris, with pain in neck and occiput.

Back.—Weakness in small of back. Drawing in of shoulders. Pain and burning in back. [*Oxal. ac.*]

Extremities.—Trembling, twitching, spasms, weakness, heaviness, uneasiness. Cramps in calves. Swelling of feet. Sciatica. Burning pains. Peripheral neuritis. Diabetic gangrene. Ulcers on heel [*Cepa; Lamium*]. Paralysis of lower limbs with atrophy.

Skin.—Itching, burning, swellings; œdema, eruption, papular, *dry, rough, scaly; worse cold* and scratching. Malignant pustules. Ulcers with offensive discharge. Anthrax. Poisoned wounds. Urticaria, with burning and restlessness. *Psoriasis.* Scirrhus. Icy coldness of body. Epithelioma of the skin. Gangrenous inflammations.

Sleep.—Disturbed, anxious, restless. Must have head raised by pillows. Suffocative fits during sleep. Sleeps with hands over head. Dreams are full of care and fear. Drowsy, sleeping sickness.

Fever.—High temperature. *Periodicity marked with adynamia.* Septic fevers. *Intermittent. Paroxysms incomplete, with marked exhaustion. Hay-fever.* Cold sweats. Typhoid, not too early; often after Rhus. Complete exhaustion. Delirium; worse after midnight. Great restlessness. Great heat about 3 a. m. Sordes.

Modalities.—*Worse*, wet weather, after midnight; from cold, cold drinks, or food. Seashore. Right side. *Better* from heat; from head elevated; warm drinks.

Complementary: *Rhus; Carbo; Phos.; Thuja; Secale.* Antidotal to lead poison.

Antidotes: *Opium; Carbo; China; Hepar; Nux.* Chemical Antidotes: Charcoal; Hydrated Peroxide of Iron; Lime Water.

Compare: *Arsenic. stibiatum* 3x (Chest inflammations of children, restlessness with thirst and prostration, loose mucous cough, oppression, hurried respiration, crepitant rales). *Cenchris contortrix; Iod.; Phosph.; China; Verat. alb.; Carbo; Kali phos. Epilobium* (intractable diarrhœa of typhoid). *Hoang Nan. Atoxyl.*—Sodium arseniate 3x, sleeping sickness; commencing optic atrophy. *Levico Water*—(containing Ars., Iron and Copper of South Tyrol). (Chronic and dyscratic skin diseases, chorea minor and spasms in scrofulous and anæmic children. Favors assimilation and increases nutrition. Debility and skin diseases, especially after the use of higher potencies where progress seems suspended. Dose. Ten drops in wine glass of warm water 3 times a day after meals. (Burnett). *Sarcolactic acid* (influenza with violent vomiting).

Dose.—Third to thirtieth potency. The very highest potencies often yield brilliant results.

Low attenuations in gastric, intestinal, and kidney diseases; higher in neuralgias, nervous diseases, and skin. But if only surface conditions call for it, give the lowest potencies, 2x to 3x trit. Repeated doses advisable.

ARSENICUM BROMATUM
(Bromide of Arsenic)

Has proven a great anti-psoric and anti-syphilitic remedy. Herpetic eruptions, syphilitic excrescences, glandular tumors and indurations, carcinoma, locomotor ataxia, and obstinate intermittents, and *diabetes* are all greatly influenced by this preparation.

Face.—*Acne rosacea*, with violet papules on nose; worse in the spring. *Acne* in young people.

Dose.—Tincture, two to four drops daily in water. In diabetes, three drops three times a day in a glass of water.

ARSENICUM HYDROGENISATUM
(Arseniuretted Hydrogen)

The general action of Arsenic more accentuated. Anæmia. Anxiety; despair. *Hœmaturia*, with general blood disorganization. Hæmorrhages from mucous membranes. Urine suppressed, followed by vomiting. Prepuce and glans covered with pustules and round superficial ulcers. Collapse. Coldness; prostration. Sudden weakness and nausea. Skin becomes dark brown.

Head.—Violent vertigo on going upstairs. Eyes sunken; broad, blue circles around. Violent sneezing. Nose cold. Must be wrapped up with warm cloths.

Mouth.—Tongue enlarged; deep, irregular ulcer; nodular swelling. Mouth hot and dry; little thirst.

Dose.—Third potency.

ARSENICUM IODATUM
(Iodide of Arsenic)

Is to be preferred for persistently irritating, corrosive discharges. The discharge irritates the membrane *from* which it flows and *over* which it flows. The discharge may be fetid, watery, and the mucous membrane is always red, angry, swollen; itches and burns. Influenza, *hay-fever*, old nasal catarrhs, and catarrh of middle ear. Swelling of tissues within the nose. Hypertrophied condition of eustachian tube and deafness. Senile heart, myocarditis and fatty degeneration. Pulse shotty. Chronic aortitis. Epithelioma of the lip. Cancer of breast after ulceration has set in.

It seems probable that in Arsenic iod., we have a remedy most closely allied to manifestations of tuberculosis. In the early stages of tuberculosis, even though there is an afternoon rise in temperature, *Ars. jod.* is very effective. It will be indicated by a profound prostration, rapid, irritable pulse, recurring fever and sweats, emaciation; tendency to diarrhœa. Chronic pneumonia, with abscess in lung. Hectic; debility; night sweats.

This remedy is also to be remembered in phthisis with hoarse, racking cough and profuse expectoration of a purulent nature, and attended with cardiac weakness, emaciation and general debility; in chronic, watery diarrhœa in phthisical subjects; in cases of emaciation with good appetite; in amenorrhœa, with anæmic palpitation and dyspnœa. In chronic pneumonia, when abscess is about to form. Great emaciation. Arteriosclerosis, myocardial degeneration and senile heart. Threatened pyæmia. [*Pyrog.; Methyl. blue.*]

Head.—*Vertigo*, with tremulous feeling, especially in aged.

Nose.—*Thin, watery, irritating, excoriating discharge from anterior and posterior nares; sneezing.* Hay-fever. Irritation and tingling of nose constant desire to sneeze. [*Pollanin.*] *Chronic nasal catarrh;* swollen nose; profuse, thick, yellow discharge; ulcers; *membrane sore and excoriated.* Aggravation by sneezing.

Throat.—Burning in pharynx. Tonsils swollen. Thick membrane from fauces to lips. Breath fetid, glandular involvement. Diphtheria. Chronic follicular pharyngitis.

Eyes and Ears.—Scrofulous ophthalmia. Otitis, with fetid, corrosive discharge. Thickening of tympanum. *Burning, acrid coryza.*

Stomach.—Pain and pyrosis. Vomiting an hour after food. Nausea distressing. Pain in epigastrium. Intense thirst; water is immediately ejected.

Respiratory.—Slight hacking cough, with dry and stopped-up nostrils. Pleuritis exudativa. Chronic bronchitis. Pulmonary tuberculosis. Pneumonia that fails to clear up. Broncho-pneumonia after grippe. Cough dry, with little difficult expectoration. Aphonia.

Fever.—Recurrent fever and sweats. *Drenching night-sweats.* Pulse rapid, feeble, weak, irregular. Chilly, cannot endure cold.

Skin.—Dry, scaly, itching. *Marked exfoliation of skin in large scales,* leaving a raw exuding surface beneath. *Ichthyosis. Enlarged scrofulous glands. Venereal bubo.* Debilitating night-sweats. Eczema of the beard; watery, oozing, itching; worse, washing. Emaciation. Psoriasis. Acne hard, shotty, indurated base with pustule at apex.

Relationship.—Compare: *Tuberculinum; Antimon. iod.* In hay-fever, compare: *Aralia; Naphthalin; Rosa; Sang. nit.*

Dose.—Second and third trituration. Ought to be prepared fresh and protected from light. Continued for some time. Clinically, it has been found advisable in tuberculosis to begin with about the 4x and gradually go lower to the second x trit., 5 grains 3 times a day.

ARSENICUM METALLICUM
(Metallic Arsenic)

Arouses latent syphilis. Periodicity very marked; symptoms recur every two and three weeks. Weakness. Swollen feeling of parts.

Head.—Low spirited, memory weak. *Desire to be alone.* Annoyed by visions, causing her to cry. Head feels too large. Left-sided headache up to eyes and into ears. Headache worse stooping and lying down. Œdematous swelling of forehead.

Face.—Red, itching, burning and bloated. Eyes swelled and watery, burn with coryza. Eyes weak, day and gas light unpleasant.

Mouth.—The tongue coated white, and shows imprint of the teeth. Mouth sore and ulcerated.

Abdomen.—Sore pain in liver goes through to shoulders and spine. Pain in spleen down to groin. Pain in breast extends to hip and spleen. Diarrhœa, burning watery stools with relief of pain.

Dose.—Sixth potency.

ARSENICUM SULFURATUM FLAVUM—ARSENIC TRISULPH.

(Yellow Sulphuret of Arsenic. Orpiment)

Needle pricks from within outwards in chest; also on forehead, right side. Sticking behind ear. Difficult respiration. Skin chafed about genitals.

Leucoderma and squamous syphilides. Sciatica and pain around the knee.

Relationship.—*Arsenic sulph. rub.* (influenza with intense catarrhal symptoms, great prostration and high temperature, purulent discharges, psoriasis, acne, *and sciatica.* Chilly even before a fire. Itching in various parts. Pellagra.)

Dose.—Third trituration.

ARTEMISIA VULGARIS
(Mugwort)

Has some reputation as a remedy for epileptic conditions, and convulsive diseases of childhood and girls at puberty. Locally and internally is injurious to eyes. *Petit mal.* Epilepsy without aura; after fright and other violent emotions and after masturbation. Several convulsions close together. Somnambulism. Gets up at night and works, remembers nothing in the morning. [*Kali phos.*]

Head.—Drawn back by spasmodic twitchings. Mouth drawn to left. Congestion of brain.

Eyes.—*Colored light produces dizziness.* Pain and blurring of vision; better, rubbing; worse, using eyes.

Female.—Profuse menses. Violent uterine contractions. Spasms during menses.

Fever.—Profuse sweat, *smelling like garlic.*

Relationship.—Compare: *Absinth.; Cina; Cicuta.*

Dose.—First to third potency. Said to act better when given with wine.

ARUM DRACONTIUM
(Green Dragon)

A remedy for Pharyngitis with sore, raw and tender throat.

Head.—Heavy; shooting pain in ears, aching pain behind right ear.

Throat.—Dry, sore, worse swallowing. Raw and tender. Continued disposition to clear throat. Croupy, hoarse cough with sore throat.

Urinary.—Irresistible desire to pass urine, burns and smarts.

Respiratory.—Hoarseness; excess of mucus in larynx. Asthmatic at night. Expectoration thick, heavy.

Relationship.—*Arum Italicum.* (Brain-fag, with headache in occipital region.) *Arum maculatum* (inflammation and ulceration of mucous membranes. Nasal irritation with polypus).

Dose.—First potency.

ARUM TRIPHYLLUM
(Jack-in-the-Pulpit)

Arum maculatum, Italicum, Dracontium, have the same action as the Triphyllum. They all contain an irritant poison, causing inflammation of mucous surfaces and destruction of tissue. *Acridity* is the keynote of the kind of action characteristic of Arum.

Head.—Bores head in pillow. Headache from too warm clothing, from hot coffee.

Eyes.—Quivering of upper eyelids, especially left.

Nose.—Soreness of nostrils. *Acrid, excoriating discharge,* producing raw sores. *Nose obstructed; must breathe through mouth. Boring in the nose.* Coryza; discharge blood-streaked, watery. Nose completely stopped, with fluent, acrid discharge. Hay-fever, with pain over root of nose. Large scabs high up on right side of nose. Face feels chapped, as if from cold wind; feels hot. *Constant picking at nose until it bleeds.*

Mouth.—*Raw feeling at roof and palate.* Lips and soft palate sore and burning. Lips chapped and burning. *Corners of mouth sore and cracked.* Tongue red, sore; whole mouth raw. Picking lips until they bleed. Saliva profuse, acrid, corroding.

Throat.—Swelling of sub-maxillary glands. *Constricted and swollen; burns;* raw. Constant hawking. *Hoarseness.* Expectoration of much mucus. Lungs feel sore. Clergyman's sore throat. Voice uncertain, uncontrollable. Worse, talking, singing.

Skin.—Scarlet rash; *raw, bloody surfaces* anywhere. Impetigo contagiosa.

Modalities.—*Worse, northwest wind;* lying down.

Relationship.—Compare: *Ammon. carb.; Ailanthus; Cepa*
Antidotes: *Buttermilk; Acet. ac.; Puls.*

Dose.—Third to thirtieth potency.

ARUNDO
(Reed)

A remedy for catarrhal states. Hay-fever.

Head.—Itching; falling off of hair; roots of hair painful. Pustules. Pain in occiput, extends to right ciliary region. Deep seated pain in sides of head.

Ears.—Burning and itching in auditory canals. Eczema behind ears.

Nose.—Hay-fever begins with burning and *itching of palate* and conjunctiva. *Annoying itching in the nostrils and roof of the mouth.* [*Wyethia.*] Coryza; loss of smell. [*Nat. mur.*] Sneezing, *itching of nostrils.*

Mouth.—Burning and itching; bleeding of gums. Ulcers and exfoliations in the commissures. Fissures in tongue.

Stomach.—Coldness in stomach. Longing for acids.

Abdomen.—Movement as from something alive. Flatulence pain at pubic region.

Stool.—Greenish. Burning at anus. Diarrhœa of nursing children. [*Cham.; Calc. phos.*]

Urine.—Burning. Red sediment. [*Lyc.*]

Male.—Pain in spermatic cord after embrace.

Female.—Menses too early and profuse. Neuralgic pains from face to shoulders and pubis. Desire with vaginal pruritus.

Respiratory.—Dyspnœa; cough; bluish expectoration. Burning and pain in nipples.

Extremities.—Itching, burning; œdema of hands and feet. Burning and swelling of soles. Copious and offensive sweat of feet.

Skin.—Eczema; itching and crawling, especially of chest, upper extremities. Fissures in fingers and heels.

Relationship.—Compare: *Anthoxantum*—sweet vernal grass (a popular medicine for hay-fever and coryza). *Lolium; Cepa; Sabad.; Silica.*

Dose.—Third to sixth potency.

ASAFOETIDA
(Gum of the Stinkasand)

The flatulence and spasmodic contraction of stomach and œsophagus with reverse peristalsis are the most marked symptoms. In its selection, its relation to the hysterical and hypochondriacal patients, must be borne in mind. Besides these superficial symptoms, it has been found to affect favorably deep ulcerations, caries of bones, especially in the syphilitic organism; here the *extreme sensitiveness* and terrible throbbing, nightly pains, guiding to its use.

Head.—Irritable; complains of her troubles; sensitive. Boring above eyebrows. *Pressive pain from within outward.*

Eyes.—Orbital neuralgia; better, pressure and rest. Iritis and intraocular inflammations, with boring, throbbing pains at night. Stitches under left frontal eminences. Boring pains in and around eyes. Syphilitic iritis. Superficial corneal ulcer with digging pains; worse at night.

Ears.—Offensive otorrhœa, with boring pains in mastoid bone. Mastoid disease with pain in temporal region with *pushing out sensation*. Offensive, purulent discharge.

Nose.—Syphilitic ozæna, with very offensive purulent discharge. *Caries of nasal bones.* [*Aurum.*]

Throat.—*Globus hystericus.* Ball rises in throat. Sensation as if peristaltic motion were reversed, and œsophagus were driven from stomach to throat.

Stomach.—Great difficulty in bringing up wind. *Flatulence and regurgitation of liquid.* Hysterical flatulence. Great distention. Sensation of emptiness and weakness, with distention and beating in stomach and abdomen. Forcible eructation of gas. *Pulsation in pit of* stomach. Violent gastralgia; cutting and burning in stomach and region of diaphragm. Gurgling and rolling of wind, which escapes afterwards with loud and difficult eructation.

Female.—Mammæ turgid with milk in the unimpregnated. *Deficient milk*, with oversensitiveness.

Rectum.—Distended, griping, with hunger. Obstinate constipation. Pain in perineum, as if something dull pressed out. *Diarrhœa, extremely offensive, with meteorism*, and regurgitation of food.

Chest.—*Spasmodic tightness*, as if lungs could not be fully expanded. Palpitation more like a tremor.

Bones.—Darting pain and caries in bones. Periosteum painful, swollen, enlarged. Ulcers affecting bones; thin, ichorous pus.

Skin.—Itching, better scratching; ulcers painful on edges. Suppressed skin symptoms produce nervous disorders.

Modalities.—*Worse*, at night; from tough; left side, during rest, warm applications. *Better*, open air; from motion, pressure.

Relationship.—Antidotes: *China; Mercur.*
Compare: *Moschus; China; Mercur; Aurum.*
Dose.—Second to sixth potency.

ASARUM EUROPUM
(European Snake-root)

A remedy for nervous affections, loss of energy, with excessive *erethism. Scratching on silk or linen or paper unbearable.* Pains and spasmodic muscular actions. Nervous deafness and asthenopia. Cold shivers from any emotion. Feels as if parts were pressed together. Tension and contractive sensations. *Always feels cold.*

Mind.—Thoughts vanish, with drawing pressure in forehead. *Sensibility increased, even from mere imagination.*

Head.—Compressive pain. Tension of scalp; hair painful. [*China.*] Coryza, with sneezing.

Eyes.—Feel stiff; burn; feel cold. Better, in cold air or water; worse, sunlight and wind. Darting pains in eyes after operations. Asthenopia.

Ears.—Sensation as if plugged up. Catarrh with deafness. Heat of external ear. Noises.

Stomach.—Loss of appetite, flatulence, eructation, and vomiting. *Desire for alcoholic drinks.* Smoking tobacco tastes bitter. Nausea; worse after eating. Clean tongue. Great faintness. Accumulation of cold, watery saliva.

Rectum.—*Strings* of odorless, yellow mucus pass from bowels. Diarrhœa of tough mucus. *Undigested stools.* Prolapse.

Female.—Menses too early, long lasting, black. Violent pain in small of back. Tenacious, yellow leucorrhœa.

Respiratory.—Nervous, hacking cough. Short respiration.

Back.—Paralytic pain in muscles of nape of neck. Weakness, with staggering.

Fever.—Chilliness, single parts get icy cold. Easily excited perspiration.

Modalities.—*Worse,* in cold dry weather; penetrating sounds. *Better,* from washing; in damp and wet weather.

Relationship.—*Asarum Canadensa*—Wild Ginger. (Colds, followed by amenorrhœa and gastro-enteritis. Suppressed colds.) Compare: *Ipecac.*, especially in diarrhœa; *Silica; Nux; China.*

Dose.—Third to sixth potency.

ASCLEPIAS SYRIACA (CORNUTI)
(Silkweed)

Seems to act especially on nervous system and urinary organs. A remedy for dropsy, hepatic, renal or cardiac and post-scarlatinal; causes diaphoresis and augments the urinary secretion. Acute rheumatic inflammation of large joints. Intermittent, pressing-down uterine pains.

Head.—Feels as if *a sharp instrument were thrust through* *from temple to temple.* Constriction across forehead. Nervous headache, after suppressed perspiration, followed by *increased urine, with increase of specific gravity*. Headache from retention of effete matters in system.

Relationship.—Compare: *Asclepias Vincetoxicum.*—Swallow-wart—*Cynanchum*—(A gastro-intestinal irritant, producing vomiting and purgation.—(Useful in dropsy, diabetes, great thirst, profuse urination.)

Dose.—Tincture.

ASCLEPIAS TUBEROSA
(Pleurisy-root)

Its action on the chest muscles is most marked and has been verified. Sick headache, with flatulence in stomach and bowels. Dyspepsia. Bronchitis and pleurisy come within its range. Catarrhal states from cold and damp weather. Irritation of larynx with huskiness; grip, with pleuritic pain.

Respiratory.—Respiration painful, especially at base of left lung. Dry cough; throat constricted; causes pain in head and abdomen. Pain in chest; shooting downward from left nipple. A general eliminative remedy, acting specially on the sudoriparous glands. Chest pains are relieved by bending forward. Spaces between ribs close to sternum tender. Lancinating pain between shoulders. Catarrh, with frontal headache, and sticky yellow discharge.

Stomach.—Fullness, pressure, weight. Flatulence after meals. Sensitive to tobacco.

Rectum.—*Catarrhal dysentery, with rheumatic pains all over.* Stools smell like rotten eggs.

Extremities.—Rheumatic joints give sensation as if adhesions being broken up on bending.

Relationship.—Compare: *Asclepias Incarnata*—Swamp Milk Weed. (Chronic gastric Catarrh and leucorrhœa. (Dropsy with dyspnœa.) *Periploca græca*—One of the Asclepiades—(Cardiac tonic, acts on circulation and respiratory centre, accelerating respiration in a ratio disproportionate to pulse.) *Bryonia; Dulc.*

Dose.—Tincture and first potency.

ASIMINA TRILOBA
(American Papaw)

Produces a series of symptoms much like scarlet fever; sore throat, fever, vomiting, scarlet eruption; tonsils and submaxillary glands enlarged, with diarrhœa. Fauces red and swollen, face swollen. Desire for ice-cold things. *Hoarseness.* Languid, drowsy irritable.

Acne. Itching in evening on undressing.

Relationship.—Compare: *Capsic.; Bellad.*

ASPARAGUS OFFICINALIS
(Common Garden Asparagus)

Its marked and immediate action on the urinary secretion is well known. It causes weakness and cardiac depression with dropsy. Rheumatic pains. Especially about left shoulder and heart.

Head.—Confused. Coryza, with profuse, thin fluid. Aching in forehead and root of nose. Migrainous morning headache with scotoma. Throat feels rough, with hawking copious, tenacious mucus from throat.

Urine.—Frequent, with fine stitches in orifice of urethra; burning; of peculiar odor. Cystitis, with pus, mucus and tenesmus. Lithiasis.

Heart.—*Palpitation, with oppression of chest.* Pulse intermits, weak, pain about left shoulder and heart, associated with bladder disturbances. Great oppression in breathing. Hydrothorax.

Extremities.—Rheumatic pain in back, especially near shoulder and limbs. Pain at acromion process of left scapula under clavicle and down arm, with feeble pulse.

Relationship.—Antidote: *Acon.; Apis.*

Compare: *Althæa*—Marshmallow—(contains asparagin; irritable bladder, throat and bronchi.) *Physalis Alkekengi. Digital.; Sarsap.; Spigelia.*

Dose.—Sixth potency.

ASPIDOSPERMA
(Quebracho)

The digitalis of the lungs. (Hale.) Removes temporary obstruction to the oxidation of the blood by stimulating respiratory centres, increasing oxidation and excretion of carbonic acid. Pulmonary stenosis. Thrombosis of pulmonary artery. Uræmic dyspnœa. An effective remedy in many cases of asthma. It stimulates the respiratory centers and increases the oxygen in the blood. "Want of breath" during exertion is the guiding symptom. *Cardiac asthma.*

Relationship.—Compare: *Coca; Arsenic; Coffea.—Catalpa* (difficult respiration).

Dose.—First trituration or tincture, or Aspidospermin hydrochlorid 1 grain of 1x trit. Every hour for a few doses.

ASTACUS FLUVIATILIS—CANCER ASTACUS
(Crawfish)

Skin symptoms most important. *Urticaria.*

Skin.—Nettle-rash over whole body. Itching. Crusta lactea, with enlarged lymphatic glands. Erysipelas, and *liver affections with nettle-rash.* Swelling of cervical glands. Jaundice.

Fever.—Inward chilliness; very sensitive to air, worse uncovering; violent fever, with headache.

Relationship.—Compare: *Bombyx*—Caterpillar—Itching of whole body. (Urticaria.) *Apis; Rhus; Nat. m.; Homar.*

Dose.—Third to thirtieth potency.

ASTERIAS RUBENS
(Red Starfish)

A remedy for the sycotic diathesis; flabby, lymphatic constitution, flabby with *red* face. Lancinating pains. Nervous disturbances, neuralgias, chorea, and hysteria come within the range of this remedy. Has been used for cancer of the breast, and has an unquestioned influence over cancer disease. Excitement in both sexes.

Head.—Cannot bear contradiction. Shocks in brain; throbbing; *heat in head, as if surrounded by hot air*.

Face.—Red. Pimples on side of nose, chin and mouth. *Disposition to pimples at adolescence*.

Female.—Colic and other sufferings cease with appearance of flow. Breasts swell and pain in breasts; worse left. Ulceration with sharp pains, piercing to scapulæ. Pains down left arm to fingers, worse motion. Excitement of sexual instinct with nervous agitation.

Nodes and indurations of mammary gland, dull aching, neuralgic pain in this region. [*Conium.*]

Chest.—Breasts swollen, indurated. Neuralgia of left breast and arm. [*Brom.*] Pain under sternum and in muscles of præcordial region. *Left breast feels as if pulled inward*, and pain extends over inner arm to end of little finger. Numbness of hand and fingers of left side. *Cancer mammæ even in ulcerative stage. Acute, lancinating pain. Axillary glands swollen hard and knotted*.

Nervous System.—Gait unsteady; muscles refuse to obey the will. Epilepsy; preceded by twitching over whole body.

Stool.—Constipation. Ineffectual desire. Stool like olives. Diarrhœa, watery brown, gushing out in jet.

Skin.—Destitute of pliability and elasticity. Itching spots. Ulcers, with fetid ichor. Acne. Psoriasis and herpes zoster worse left arm and chest. Enlarged axillary glands, worse, at night and in damp weather.

Relationship.—Antidotes: *Plumb.; Zinc.*

Compare: *Conium; Carbo; Ars.; Condurango.*

Incompatible: *Nux; Coffea.*

Modalities.—*Worse*, coffee, night; cold damp weather, left side.

Dose.—Sixth potency.

ASTRAGALUS MOLLISSIMUS
(Purple or Woolly Loco-weed)

Affects animals like effects of alcohol, tobacco and morphine in man. First stage, period of hallucination or mania with defective eye sight during which the animal performs all sorts of antics. After acquiring a taste for the plant it refuses every other kind of food. Second stage brings emaciation, sunken eyeballs, lusterless hair and feeble movements—after a few months dies as from starvation. (U. S. Dept. Agriculture.) Irregularities in gait—paralytic affections. Loss of muscular co-ordination.

Head.—Fullness in right temple and upper jaw. Pain over left eyebrow. Painful facial bones. Dizzy. Pressive pain in temples. Pain and pressure in maxillæ.

Stomach.—Weakness and emptiness. Burning in œsophagus and stomach.

Extremities.—Purring sensation in right foot outer side from heel to toe. Icy coldness of left calf.

Relationship.—Compare: *Aragallus Lamberti*—White Loco-Weed—Rattleweed; *Baryta; Oxytropis*.

Dose.–Sixth potency.

AURUM METALLICUM
(Metallic Gold)

Given full play, Aurum develops in the organism, by attacking the blood, glands, and bone, conditions bearing striking resemblance to mercurial and syphilitic infections; and it is just for such deteriorations of the bodily fluids and alterations in the tissues, that Aurum assumes great importance as a remedy. Like the victim of syphilis, mental states of great depression are produced by it. Hopeless, despondent, and *great desire to commit suicide*. Every opportunity is sought for self-destruction. Exostosis, caries, nightly bone-pains, especially cranial, nasal, and palatine. Glands swollen in scrofulous subjects. Palpitation and congestions. Ascites often in conjunction with heart affections. Frequently indicated in secondary syphilis and effects of mercury. This use of gold as an anti-venereal and anti-scrofulous remedy is very old, but has been well-nigh forgotten by the old school until rediscovered and placed on its scientific basis by homœopathy, and now it can never be lost again. When syphilis is implanted on the scrofulous constitution, we have one of the most intractable

AURUM METALLICUM

morbid conditions, and gold seems to be especially suited to the vile combination. *Ennui.* Ozæna; sexual hyperæsthesia. *Arteriosclerosis*, high blood pressure; nightly paroxysms of pain behind sternum. Sclerosis of liver, arterial system, brain. Pining boys; low spirited, lifeless, weak memory.

Mind.—Feeling of self-condemnation and utter worthlessness. Profound despondency, with increased blood pressure, with thorough *disgust of life*, and thoughts of suicide. *Talks of commiting suicide.* Great fear of death. Peevish and vehement at least contradiction. Anthropophobia. Mental derangements. Constant rapid questioning without waiting for reply. Cannot do things fast enough. *Oversensitiveness;* [*Staph.*] *to noise*, excitement, confusion.

Head.—*Violent pain in head; worse at night*, outward pressure. Roaring in head. Vertigo. Tearing through brain to forehead. Pain in bones extending to face. Congestion to head. Boils on scalp.

Eyes.—*Extreme photophobia.* Great soreness all about the eyes and into eyeballs. Double vision; *upper half of objects invisible.* Feel tense. Sees fiery objects. Violent pains in bones around eye. [*Asaf.*] Interstitial keratitis. *Vascular cornea.* Pains from without inward. *Sticking pains inward.* Trachoma with pannus.

Ears.—Caries of ossicula and of mastoid. *Obstinate fetid otorrhœa* after scarlatina. External meatus bathed in pus. Chronic nerve deafness; Labyrinthine disease due to syphilis.

Nose.—*Ulcerated, painful*, swollen, obstructed. Inflammation of nose; caries; fetid discharge, purulent, bloody. Boring pains in nose; worse at night. *Putrid smell* from nose. Sensitive smell. [*Carbol. ac.*] Horrible odor from nose and mouth. Knobby tip of nose.

Mouth.—Foul breath in girls at puberty. Taste putrid or bitter. Ulceration of gums.

Face.—Tearing in zygoma. Mastoid and other facial bones inflamed.

Throat.—Stitches when swallowing; pain in glands. Caries of the palate.

Stomach.—Appetite and thirst increased, with qualmishness. Swelling of epigastrium. Burning at stomach and hot eructations.

Abdomen.—Right hypochondrium hot and painful. Incarcerated flatus. Swelling and suppuration of inguinal glands.

Urine.—Turbid, like buttermilk, with thick sediment. Painful retention.

Rectum.—Constipation, stools hard and knotty. Nocturnal diarrhœa, with burning in rectum.

Male.—Pain and *swelling of testicles*. Chronic induration of testicles. Violent erections. *Atrophy of testicles in boys*. Hydrocele.

Female.—Great sensitiveness of vagina. Uterus enlarged and prolapsed. Sterility; vaginismus.

Heart.—*Sensation as if the heart stopped beating* for two or three seconds, immediately followed by a tumultuous rebound, with sinking at the epigastrium. Palpitation. Pulse *rapid, feeble, irregular*. Hypertrophy. *High Blood Pressure*—Valvular lesions of arterio-sclerotic nature (Aurum 30).

Respiratory.—Dyspnœa at night. Frequent, deep breathing; stitches in sternum.

Bones.—Destruction of bones, like secondary syphilis. Pain in bones of head, lumps under scalp, exostosis with nightly pains in bones. Caries of nasal, palatine and mastoid bones. Soreness of affected bones, better in open air, worse at night.

Extremities.—All the blood seems to rush from head to lower limbs. Dropsy of lower limbs. Orgasm, as if blood were boiling in all veins. Paralytic, tearing pains in joints. Knees weak.

Sleep.—Sleepless. Sobs aloud in sleep. Frightful dreams.

Modalities.—*Worse*, in cold weather when getting cold. Many complaints come on only in winter; from sunset to sunrise.

Relationship.—Compare: *Aur. ars.* (chronic aortitis; lupus phthisis in syphilitic headaches; also in anæmia and chlorosis. It causes rapid increase of appetite.)

Aur. brom. (in headaches with neurasthenia, megrim, night terrors, valvular diseases.

Aur. mur. (Burning, yellow, acrid leucorrhœa; heart symptoms, glandular affections; warts on tongue and genitals; sclerotic and exudative degeneration of the nervous system. Multiple sclerosis. Morvan's disease. Second trituration. Aur. mur. is a sycotic remedy, causing suppressed discharges to reappear. Valuable in climacteric hæmorrhages from the womb. Diseases of frontal sinus. Stitching pain in left side of forehead. Weariness, aversion to all work. Drawing feeling in stomach. Cancer, tongue as hard as leather; induration after glossitis.)

Aur. mur. Kali.—Double chloride of Potassium and gold. (In uterine induration and hæmorrhage.)

Aur. iod. (Chronic pericarditis, valvular diseases, arteriosclerosis, ozæna, lupus, osteitis, ovarian cysts, myomata uteri, are pathological lesions, that offer favorable ground for the action of this powerful drug. *Senile paresis.*)

Aur. sulph. (Paralysis agitans; constant nodding of the head; affections of mammæ; swelling, pain, cracked nipples with lancinating pains.)

Also, *Asafæt.* (in caries of bones of ears and nose). *Syphilin: Kali iod.; Hep.; Merc.; Mez.; Nit. ac.; Phosph.*

Antidotes: *Bell.; Cinch.; Cupr ; Merc.*

Dose.—Third to thirtieth potency. Latter potency especially for increased blood pressure.

AURUM MURIATICUM NATRONATUM
(Sodium Chloroaurate)

This remedy has a most pronounced effect on the female organs, and most of its clinical application has been based thereon. Has more power over uterine tumors than any other remedy (Burnett). Psoriasis syphilitica. Periosteal swelling on lower jaw. Swelling of testicle. High blood pressure due to disturbed function of nervous mechanism. Arterio-sclerosis. Syphilitic ataxia.

Tongue.—Burning; stitches, and induration. Old cases of rheumatism and gouty pains. Hepatic cirrhosis. Interstitial nephritis.

Female.—Indurated cervix. Palpitation of young girls. Coldness in abdomen. Chronic metritis and prolapsus. Uterus fills up whole pelvis. Ulceration of neck of womb and vagina. Leucorrhœa, with spasmodic contraction of vagina. Ovaries indurated. Ovarian dropsy. Sub-involution. Ossified uterus.

Dose.—Second and third trituration.

AVENA SATIVA
(Common Oat)

Has a selective action on brain and nervous system, favorably influencing their nutritive function.

Nervous exhaustion, sexual debility, and the morphine habit call for this remedy in rather material dosage. Best tonic for debility after exhausting diseases. Nerve tremors of the aged; chorea, paralysis agitans, epilepsy. Post-diphtheritic paralysis. Rheumatism of heart. *Colds.* Acute coryza (20 drop doses in hot water hourly for a few doses). Alcoholism. Sleeplessness. especially of alcoholics. Bad effects of *Morphine* habit. Nervous states of many female troubles.

Mind.—Inability to keep mind on any one subject.

Head.—Nervous headache at menstrual period, with burning at top of head. Occipital headache, with phosphatic urine.

Female.—Amenorrhœa and dysmenorrhœa, with weak circulation.

Male.—Spermatorrhœa: impotency; after too much indulgence.

Extremities.—Numbness of limbs, as if paralyzed. Strength of hand diminished.

Relationship.—Compare: *Alfalfa.* (General tonic similar to avena—also in scanty and suppressed urine.)

Dose.—Tincture ten to twenty drop doses, preferably in hot water.

AZADIRACHTA INDICA
(Margosa Bark)

An afternoon fever and rheumatic pains in various parts are caused by this remedy. Pain in sternum and ribs, in back and shoulders and extremities; heat, pricking and aching in hands, especially palms, fingers, also toes.

Head.—Forgetful; giddy on rising; head aches, scalp sensitive; eyes burn, pain in right eyeball.

Fever.—Slight chill, afternoon fever, glowing heat in face, hands, and feet, copious sweat on upper part of body.

Relationship.—Compare: *Cedron; Natr. mur.; Arsenic.*

BACILLINUM

(A Maceration of a Typical Tuberculous Lung)
Introduced by Dr. Burnett

Has been employed successfully in the treatment of tuberculosis; its good effects seen in the change of the sputum, which becomes decreased and more aerated and less purulent. Many forms of chronic non-tubercular disease are influenced favorably by Bacillinum, especially when bronchorrhœa and dyspnœa are present. Respiratory pyorrhœa. *The patient expectorates less.*

Bacillinum is especially indicated for lungs of old people, with chronic catarrhal condition and enfeebled pulmonary circulation, attacks of suffocation at night with difficult cough. Suffucative catarrh. Tubercular meningitis. Favors falling off of tartar of teeth. Constant disposition to take cold.

Head.—Irritable, depressed. Severe, deep-in headache, also as of a tight hoop. Ringworm. Eczema of eyelids.

Abdomen.—Abdominal pains, enlarged lands in groins, tabes mesenterica. Sudden diarrhœa before breakfast. Obstinate constipation, with offensive flatus.

Respiratory.—*Oppression. Catarrhal dyspnœa. Humid asthma. Bubbling rales and muco-purulent expectoration.* Note. This muco-purulent expectoration of bronchitic patients is equally poly-bacillary; it is a mixture of diverse species and hence Bacillinum is truly indicated. (Cartier.) Often relieves congestion of the lungs, thus paving way for other remedies in Tuberculosis.

Skin.—*Ringworm;* pityriasis. Eczema of eyelids. Glands of neck enlarged and tender.

Modalities.—*Worse,* night and early morning; cold air.

Relationship.—*Antimon. iod.; Lach.; Arsenic. iod.; Myosotis. Levico,* 5-10 drops, follows as an intercurrent where much debility is present (Burnett).

Complementary: *Calc. phos.; Kali carb.*

Compare: Its effects seem to be identical to that of Koch's Tuberculinum. Both are useful in the tubercular diathesis before phthisis has developed. In the *early stages* of tubercular disease of glands, joints, skin and bones. *Psorinum.* Seem to be its chronic equivalent. *Bacillin. testium* (acts especially on lower half of the body.

Dose.—The dose is important. Should not be given below the thirtieth, and not repeated frequently. One dose a week often sufficient to bring about reaction. It is *rapid in action*, and good results ought to be seen soon, otherwise there is no need of repetition.

BADIAGA

(Fresh-water Sponge)

Soreness of muscles and integuments; worse motion and friction of clothes, with sensitiveness to cold. Glands swollen. General paresis. Basedow's disease. Lues, bubo, roseola.

Head.—Sensation of enlargement and fullness. Pain in forehead and temple, *extending to eyeballs*, worse in afternoon. Blueness under eyes. *Dandruff;* scalp sore, dry, tetter-like. Dull, dizzy feeling in head. *Coryza,* sneezing, watery discharge, with asthmatic breathing and suffocative cough. Influenza. Slight sounds are greatly accentuated.

Eyes.—Twitching of *left* upper lid; eyeballs tender; aching in eyeballs. Intermittent sore pain in eyeball, coming on at 3 p. m.

Respiratory.—Cough; worse in afternoon, better in warm room. The *mucus flies out of mouth and nostrils.* Whooping-cough, with thick yellow expectoration; flies out. Hay-fever, with asthmatic breathing. Pleuritic stitches in chest, neck, and back.

Stomach.—Mouth hot. Much thirst. Lancinating pain in pit of stomach extending to vertebra and scapula.

Female.—Metorrhagia; worse at night, with feeling of enlargement of head. [*Arg.*] Cancer of breast. [*Asterias; Con.; Carbo an.; Plumb. iod.*]

Heart.—Indescribable bad feeling about the heart with soreness and pain, flying stitches all over.

Skin.—Sore to touch. *Freckles. Rhagades.*

Back.—Stitches in nape, scapulæ. Pain in small of back, hips and lower limbs. Very stiff neck. *Muscles and skin sore, as if beaten.*

Modalities.—*Worse* by cold. *Better*, by heat.

Relationship.—Compare: *Merc.* similar but opposite modalities. *Spongia; Kali hyd.; Phytol.; Conium.*
Complementary: *Sulph.; Merc.; Iod.*

Dose.—First to sixth attenuation.

BALSAMUM PERUVIANUM
(Peruvian Balsam from Myroxylon Pereiræ)

Useful in bronchial catarrh, with copious, purulent expectoration. *Debility; hectic fever.*

Nose.—Profuse, thick discharge. Eczema, with ulceration. Chronic, fetid, nasal catarrh.

Stomach.—Vomiting of food and mucus. Catarrh of stomach.

Chest.—Bronchitis, and phthisis, *with muco-purulent, thick, creamy expectoration.* Loud rales in chest. [*Kali sulph.; Ant. tart.*] Very loose cough. Hectic fever and night-sweats, with irritating, short cough and scanty expectoration.

Urine.—Scanty; much mucus sediment. Catarrh of bladder. [*Chimaph.*]

Relationship.—*Balsamum Tolutanum*—the balsam of My roxylon toluifera—(chronic bronchitis with profuse expectoration). *Oleum caryophyllum*—oil of cloves—in *profuse* septic expectoration—3 to 5 minims in milk or capsules.)

Dose.—First attenuation: In hectic 6x.

Extra homœopathic uses locally:—As a stimulant to raw surfaces in indolent ulcers, scabies, cracked nipples, rhagades, itch. Promotes granulation, removes fetor. A one per cent. solution in alcohol or ether may be used with the atomizer in respiratory affections. Internally, as an expectorant, in chronic bronchitis. Dose, 5 to 15 M., made into an emulsion with mucilage or yolk of egg.

BAPTISIA
(Wild Indigo)

The symptoms of this drug are of an asthenic type, simulating low fevers, *septic conditions* of the blood, malarial poisoning, and extreme prostration. Indescribable sick feeling. *Great mus-*

cular soreness and putrid phenomena always are present. All the secretions are offensive—breath, stool, urine, sweat, etc. Epidemic influenza. Chronic intestinal toxæmias of children with fetid stools and eructations.

Baptisia in low dilutions produces a form of anti-bodies to the bac. typhosus, viz., the agglutinins. [*Mellon.*] Thus it raises the natural bodily resistance to the invasion of the bacillary intoxication, which produces the typhoid syndrome. Typhoid carriers. After inoculation with anti-typhoid serum. Intermittent pulse, especially in the aged.

Mind.—Wild, wandering feeling. Inability to think. Mental confusion. Ideas confused. Illusion of divided personalty. *Thinks he is broken or double, and tosses about the bed trying to get pieces together.* [*Cajeput.*] Delirium, wandering, muttering. Perfect indifference. Falls asleep while being spoken to. Melancholia, with stupor.

Head.—Confused, swimming feeling. Vertigo; pressure at root of nose. Skin of forehead feels tight; seems drawn to back of head. Feels too large, *heavy, numb.* Soreness of eyeballs. Brain feels sore. Stupor; falls asleep while spoken to. Early deafness in typhoid conditions. Eyelids heavy.

Face.—*Besotted look.* Dark red. Pain at root of nose. Muscles of jaw rigid.

Mouth.—Taste flat, bitter. Teeth and gums sore, ulcerated. *Breath fetid. Tongue feels burned;* yellowish-brown; edges red and shining. Dry and brown in center, with dry and glistening edges; surface cracked and sore. *Can swallow liquids only;* least solid food gags.

Throat.—Dark redness of tonsils and soft palate. *Constriction, contraction of œsophagus.* [*Cajeput.*] Great difficulty in swallowing solid food. *Painless sore throat,* and offensive discharge. *Contraction at cardiac orifice.*

Stomach.—Can swallow only liquids, vomiting due to spasm of œsophagus. Gastric fever. No appetite. Constant desire for water. *Sinking feeling at stomach.* Pain in episgastric region. Feeling of hard substance. [*Abies nig.*] All symptoms worse from beer. [*Kali bich.*] Cardiac orifice contracted convulsively and ulcerative inflammation of stomach and bowels.

Abdomen.—Right side markedly affected. Distended and rumbling. Soreness over region of gall-bladder, with diarrhœa. Stools very *offensive, thin, dark, bloody*. Soreness of abdomen in region of liver. Dysentery of old people.

Female.—Threatened miscarriage from mental depression, shock, watching, low fevers. Menses too early, too profuse. Lochia acrid, fetid. Puerperal fever.

Respiratory.—Lungs feel compressed, breathing difficult; seeks open window. Fears going to sleep on account of nightmare and *sense of suffocation*. Constriction of chest.

Back and Extremities.—Neck tired. Stiffness and pain, aching and drawing in arms and legs. Pain in sacrum, around hips and legs. *Sore and bruised*. Decubitus.

Sleep.—Sleepless and restless. Nightmare and frightful dreams. Cannot get herself together, feels scattered about bed. Falls asleep while answering a question.

Skin.—Livid spots all over body and limbs. Burning and heat in skin. [*Arsenic*.] Putrid ulcers with stupor, low delirium and prostration.

Fever.—Chill, with rheumatic pains and soreness all over body. Heat all over, with occasional chills. Chill about 11 a. m. *Adynamic fevers*. Typhus fever. Shipboard fever.

Modalities.—Worse; Humid heat; fog; indoors.

Relationship.—Compare: *Bryonia* and *Arsenic* may be needed to complete the favorable reaction. *Ailanthus* differs, being more painful. Baptisia more painless. *Rhus; Muriat. acid; Arsenic; Bryon.; Arnica; Echinac. Pyrogen.*

Baptisia confusia. (Pain in right jaw and oppression in left hypochondrium, producing dyspnœa and necessity to assume erect position.)

Dose.—Tincture, to twelfth attenuation. Has rather short action.

BAROSMA CRENATA
(Buchu)

Marked specific effects on genito-urinary system; *mucopurulent discharges*. Irritable bladder, with vesical catarrh; prostatic disorders. Gravel. Leucorrhœa.

Relationship.—Compare: *Copaiva; Thuja; Populus; Chimaph.* See Diosma.

Dose.—Tincture or tea from leaves.

BARYTA ACETICA
(Acetate of Barium)

Produces paralysis beginning at the extremities and spreading upward. Pruritus of aged.

Mind.—Forgetful; wavering long between opposite resolutions. Lack of self confidence.

Face.—Feeling of cobweb in face.

Extremities.—Drawing pain down whole left leg. Crawling, with burning stitches. *Paralysis.* Lumbago and rheumatic pain in muscles and joints.

Dose.—Second and third trituration in repeated dosage.

BARYTA CARB
(Carbonate of Baryta)

Specially indicated in *infancy* and *old age*. This remedy brings aid to scrofulous children, especially if they are backward mentally and physically, are dwarfish, do not grow and develop, have scrofulous ophthalmia, swollen abdomen, take cold easily, and then *always have swollen tonsils*. Persons subject to quinsy which is prone to suppurate; gums bleed easily. Diseases of old men when degenerative changes begin;—cardiac vascular and cerebral;—who have hypertrophied prostate or indurated testes, very sensitive to cold, offensive foot-sweats, very weak and weary, must sit or lie down or lean on something. Very averse to meeting strangers. Catarrh of posterior nares, with frequent epistaxis. Often useful in the dyspepsias of the young who have masturbated and who suffer from seminal emissions, together with cardiac irritability and palpitation. Affects glandular structures, and useful in general degenerative changes, especially in coats of arteries, *aneurism*, and senility. Baryta is a cardio-vascular poison acting on the muscular coats of heart and vessels. Arterial fibrosis. Blood-vessels soften and degenerate, become distended, and aneurisms, ruptures, and apoplexies result.

Mind.—Loss of memory, mental weakness. Irresolute. Lost confidence in himself. Senile dementia. Confusion. *Bashful.* Aversion to strangers. Childish; grief over trifles.

Head.—Vertigo; stitches, when standing in the sun, extending through head. Brain feels as if loose. Hair falls out. Confusion. *Wens.*

Eyes.—Alternate dilatation and contraction of pupils. Photophobia. Gauze before eyes. Cataracts. [*Calc.*; *Phos.*; *Sil.*]

Ears.—Hardness of hearing. *Crackling noise. Glands around ears painful and swollen.* Reverberation on blowing nose.

Nose.—Dry; sneezing; *coryza, with swelling of upper lip and nose.* Sensation of smoke in nose. Discharge of thick, yellow mucus. Frequent bleeding. Scabs around wings of nose.

Face.—Pale, puffed; sensation as of cobweb. [*Alumina.*] Upper lip swollen.

Mouth.—Awakes with dry mouth. Gums bleed and retract. Teeth ache before menses. Mouth filled with inflamed vesicles, foul taste. Paralysis of tongue. Smarting, burning pain in tip of tongue. Dribbling of saliva at dawn. Spasm of œsophagus when food enters.

Throat.—Submaxillary glands and tonsils swollen. *Takes cold easily, with stitches and smarting pain. Quinsy. Suppurating tonsils from every cold.* Tonsils inflamed, with swollen veins. Smarting pain when swallowing; worse empty swallowing. Feeling of a plug in pharynx. Can only swallow liquids. Spasm of œsophagus as soon as food enters œsophagus, causes gagging and choking. [*Merc. cor.*; *Graphit.*] Throat troubles from over use of voice. Stinging pain in tonsils, pharynx or larynx.

Stomach.—Waterbrash, hiccough, and eructation, which relieves pressure as of a stone. Hungry, but refuses food. Pain and weight immediately after a meal, with epigastric tenderness. [*Kali carb.*] Worse after warm food. Gastric weakness in the aged with possible malignancy present.

Abdomen.—*Hard and tense, distended.* Colicky. Enlarged mesenteric glands. Pain in abdomen swallowing food. Habitual colic, with hunger, but food is refused.

Rectum.—Constipation, with hard, knotty stools. Hæmorrhoids protrude on urinating. Crawling in rectum. Oozing at anus.

Urinary.—Every time patient urinates, his piles come down. Urging to urinate. Burning in urethra on urinating.

Male.—Diminished desire and premature impotence. Enlarged prostate. Testicles indurated.

Female.—Before menses, pain in stomach and small of back. Menses scanty.

Respiratory.—Dry, suffocative cough, especially in old people, full of mucus but lacking strength to expectorate, worse every change of weather. [*Senega.*] Larynx feels as if smoke were inhaled. Chronic aphonia. Stitches in chest; worse inspiration. Lungs feel full of smoke.

Heart.—Palpitation and distress in region of heart. Aneurism. [*Lycop.*] Accelerates the heart's action at first, blood pressure much increased, contraction of blood vessels. Palpitation when lying on left side, when thinking of it especially· pulse full and hard. Cardiac symptoms after suppressed foot-sweat.

Back.—*Swollen glands in nape of occiput.* Fatty tumors about neck. Bruised pain between scapulæ. Stiffness in sacrum. Weakness of spine.

Extremities.—Pain in axillary glands. Cold, clammy feet. [*Calc.*] *Fetid foot-sweats.* Numbness of limbs. Numb feeling from knees to scrotum; disappears when sitting down. Toes and soles sore; soles painful when walking. Pain in joints; burning pains in lower limbs.

Sleep.—Talking in sleep; awakens frequently; feels too hot. Twitching during sleep.

Modalities.—*Worse,* while thinking of symptoms; from washing; lying on painful side. *Better,* walking in open air.

Relationship.—Compare: *Digitalis; Radium; Aragallus; Oxytrop; Astrag.* Complementary: *Dulc.; Silica; Psorin.* Incompatible: *Calc.* Antidote for poisonous doses: *Epsom salts.*

Dose.—Third to thirtieth potency, the latter to remove the predisposition to quinsy. Baryta is slow in action, bears repetition.

BARYTA IODATA
(Iodide of Baryta)

Acts on the lymphatic system, *increased leucocytosis. Quinsy. Indurated glands, especially tonsils and breasts.* Strumous ophthalmia, with tumefaction of cervical glands and stunted growth. Tumors.

Relationship.—Compare: *Acon. lyccionum* (swelling of cervical, axillary, and mammary glands). *Lapis; Con. Merc. iod.; Carbo an.*

Dose.—Second and third trituration.

BARYTA MURIATICA
(Barium Chloride)

The different salts of Baryta are called for in organic lesions of the aged and dwarfish, both mentally and physically. Arterio-sclerosis and cerebral affections due to this condition. Headaches, but without acute crisis, occurring in old people; heaviness rather than pain. Vertigo, due to cerebral anæmia and noises in ears. Acts on lower alimentary canal, especially rectum; on muscles and joints, giving stiffness and weakness as from overwalking. The white blood corpuscles increased. Hypertension and vascular degeneration. Increased tension of pulse. Arterio-sclerosis [*Aurum; Secale*] where a high systolic pressure with a comparatively low diastolic tension is attended by cerebral and cardiac symptoms.

This remedy has indurated and *narrowing of the cardiac orifice with pain*, immediately after eating, and epigastric tenderness, which has been repeatedly verified, also its use in *aneurism* and chronic hypertrophy of the tonsils. Nymphomania and satyriasis. Convulsions. In every form of mania when the sexual desire is increased. *Icy coldness of body, with paralysis.* Multiple sclerosis of brain and cord. *Voluntary muscular power gone but perfectly sensible.* Paresis after influenza and diphtheria. General feeling of lassitude in the morning, especially weakness of the legs, with muscular stiffness. Children who go around with their mouth open and who talk through the nose. Stupid-appearing, hard of hearing.

Ears.—Whizzing and buzzing. Noises on chewing and swallowing, or sneezing. Earache; better sipping cold water. Parotids swollen. Offensive otorrhœa. Inflates middle ear on blowing nose.

Throat.—Difficult swallowing. *Tonsils enlarged.* Paresis of pharynx and eustachian tubes, with sneezing and noises. Tubes feel too wide open.

Respiratory.—*Bronchial affections of old people* with cardiac dilation. *Facilitates expectoration.* Great accumulation and rattling of mucus with difficult expectoration. Arterio-sclerosis of the lung, thus in senile asthma, modifies the arterial tension.

Stomach.—*Gone feeling at epigastrium* a good guiding symptom for it in chronic affections. Retching and vomiting. Sensation of heat ascending to head.

Urine.—*Great increase in uric acid*, diminution of chlorides.

Abdomen.—Throbbing [*Selen.*]; *induration of* pancreas; abdominal aneurism. Inguinal glands swollen. Spasmodic pain in rectum.

Relationship.—Compare in sclerotic degenerations, especially of spinal cord, liver, and heart. *Plumbum met.* and *Plumb. iod.* Also *Aurum mur.* (which will often accomplish more in sclerotic and exudative degenerations than other remedies. Multiple sclerosis, fulgurating pains, tremors, Morvan's disease, hypertrophy of fingers.)

Dose.—Third trituration. Bears repetition of dosage well.

BELLADONNA
(Deadly Nightshade)

Belladonna acts upon every part of the nervous system, producing active congestion, furious excitement, perverted special senses, twitching, convulsions and pain. It has a marked action on the vascular system, skin and glands. Belladonna always is associated with hot, red skin, flushed face, glaring eyes, throbbing carotids, excited mental state, hyperæsthesia of all senses, delirium, restless sleep, convulsive movements, dryness of mouth and throat with aversion to water, *neuralgic pains* that come and go suddenly. [*Oxytropis.*] *Heat, redness, throbbing and burning. Great children's remedy.* Epileptic spasms followed by nausea and vomiting. *Scarlet fever* and also prophylactic. Here use the thirtieth potency. *Exophthalmic goitre.* Corresponds to the symptoms of "air-sickness" in aviators. Give as preventive. *No thirst, anxiety or fear.* Belladonna stands for *violence* of attack and *suddenness* of onset. Bell. for the extreme of thyroid toxaemia. Use 1x (Beebe).

Mind.—Patient lives in a world of his own, engrossed by spectres and visions and oblivious to surrounding realities. While the retina is insensible to actual objects, a host of visual hallucinations throng about him and come to him from within. He is acutely alive and crazed by a flood of *subjective* visual impressions and fantastic illusions. Hallucinations; sees monsters, hideous faces. Delirium; frightful images; *furious;* rages, bites, strikes; *desire to escape.* Loss of consciousness. Disinclined to talk. Perversity, with tears. *Acuteness of all senses.* Changeableness.

Head.—Vertigo, with falling to left side or backwards. Sensitive to least contact. Much throbbing and heat. Palpitation reverberating in head with labored breathing. Pain; fullness, *especially in forehead,* also occiput, and temples. Headache from suppressed catarrhal flow. Sudden outcries. *Pain worse light, noise, jar, lying down and in afternoon;* better by pressure and semi-erect posture. Boring of head into pillow; drawn backward and rolls from side to side. Constant moaning. Hair splits; is dry and comes out. Headache worse on right side and when lying down; ill effects, colds, etc.; from having hair cut.

Face.—Red, *bluish-red,* hot, swollen, shining; convulsive motion of muscles of face. Swelling of upper lip. Facial neuralgia with twitching muscles and flushed face.

Eyes.—Throbbing deep in eyes on lying down. *Pupils dilated.* [*Agnus.*] Eyes feel swollen and protruding, *staring, brilliant;* conjunctiva red; *dry,* burn; photophobia; shooting in eyes. Exophthalmus. Ocular illusions; fiery appearance. *Diplopia,* squinting, spasms of lids. Sensation as if eyes were half closed. Eyelids swollen. Fundus congested.

Ears.—Tearing pain in middle and external ear. Humming noises. Membrana tympani bulges and injected. Parotid gland swollen. Sensitive to loud tones. Hearing very acute. *Otitis media. Pain causes delirium. Child cries out in sleep;*

throbbing and beating pain deep in ear, synchronous with heart beat. Hematoma auris. Acute and sub-acute conditions of Eustachian tube. Autophony—hearing one's voice in ear.

Nose.—Imaginary odors. Tingling in tip of nose. Red and swollen. *Bleeding of nose,* with red face. Coryza; mucus mixed with blood.

Mouth.—Dry. Throbbing pain in teeth. Gumboil. Tongue red on edges. Strawberry tongue. *Grinding of teeth.* Tongue swollen and painful. Stammering.

Throat.—Dry, as if glazed; angry-looking congestion [*Ginseng*]; *red, worse on right side.* Tonsils enlarged; *throat feels constricted; difficult deglutition;* worse, liquids. Sensation of a lump. Œsophagus dry; feels contracted. *Spasms* in throat. Continual inclination to swallow. Scraping sensation. Muscles of deglutition very sensitive. Hypertrophy of mucous membrane.

Stomach.—Loss of appetite. Averse to meat and milk. Spasmodic pain in epigastrium. Constriction; pain runs to spine. Nausea and vomiting. *Great thirst for cold water.* Spasms of stomach. Empty retching. Abhorrence of liquids. Spasmodic hiccough. *Dread of drinking.* Uncontrollable vomiting.

Abdomen.—Distended, hot. Transverse colon protrudes like a pad. Tender, swollen. Pain as if clutched by a hand; worse, jar, pressure. Cutting pain across; stitches in left side of abdomen, when coughing, sneezing, or touching it. Extreme sensitiveness to touch, bed-clothes, etc. [*Laches.*]

Stools.—Thin, green, dysenteric; in lumps like chalk. Shuddering during stool. Stinging pain in rectum; spasmodic stricture. Piles more sensitive with backache. Prolapsus ani. [*Ignatia; Podoph.*]

Urine.—*Retention.* Acute urinary infections. Sensation of motion in bladder as of a worm. Urine scanty, with tenesmus; *dark and turbid,* loaded with phosphates. Vesical region sensitive. Incontinence, continuous dropping. *Frequent and profuse.* Hæmaturia where no pathological condition can be found. Prostatic hypertrophy.

Male.—Testicles hard, drawn up, inflamed. Nocturnal sweat of genitals. Flow of prostatic fluid. Desire diminished.

Female.—Sensitive forcing downwards, *as if all the viscera would protrude at genitals*. Dryness and heat of vagina. Dragging around loins. Pain in sacrum. Menses increased; *bright red, too early, too profuse*. *Hæmorrhage hot*. Cutting pain from hip to hip. *Menses and lochia very offensive and hot*. Labor-pains come and go suddenly. *Mastitis* pain, throbbing, redness, streaks radiate from nipple. Breasts feel heavy; are hard and red. Tumors of breast, pain worse lying down. Badly smelling hæmorrhages, hot gushes of blood. Diminished lochia.

Respiratory.—Drying in nose, fauces, larynx, and trachea. *Tickling, short, dry cough; worse at night*. Larynx feels sore. Respiration oppressed, quick, unequal. Cheyne-Stokes respiration [*Cocain; Opium*.] *Hoarse;* loss of voice. Painless hoarseness. Cough with pain in left hip. Barking cough, whooping cough, with pain in stomach before attack, with expectoration of blood. Stitches in chest when coughing. *Larynx very painful;* feels as if a foreign body were in it, with cough. *High, piping voice. Moaning at every breath*.

Heart.—Violent palpitation, reverberating in head, with labored breathing. Palpitation from least exertion. Throbbing all through body. Dichrotism. Heart seemed too large. Rapid but weakened pulse.

Extremities.—Shooting pains along limbs. Joints swollen, red, shining, with red streaks radiating. Tottering gait. Shifting rheumatic pains. Phlegmasia alba dolens. Jerking limbs. Spasms. Involuntary limping. *Cold extremities*.

Back.—Stiff neck. *Swelling of glands of neck*. Pain in nape, as if it would break. Pressure on dorsal region most painful. Lumbago, with pain in hips and thighs.

Skin.—Dry and *hot;* swollen, sensitive; burns scarlet, smooth. Eruption like scarlatina, suddenly spreading. Erythema; pustules on face. *Glands swollen, tender,* red. *Boils*. Acne rosacea. Suppurative wounds. *Alternate redness and paleness of the skin*. Indurations after inflammations. Erysipelas.

Fever.—A high feverish state with comparative absense of toxæmia. *Burning, pungent, steaming, heat*. Feet icy cold. Superficial blood-vessels, distended. Perspiration dry only on head. *No thirst with fever*.

Sleep.—Restless, crying out, gritting of teeth. Kept awake by pulsation of blood-vessels. Screams out in sleep. Sleeplessness, with drowsiness. *Starting when closing the eyes or during sleep.* Sleeps with hands under head. [*Ars.; Plat.*]

Modalities.—*Worse*, touch, jar, noise, draught, after noon, lying down. *Better*, semi-erect.

Relationship.—Compare: *Sanguisorba officinalis* 2x-6x, a member of the Rosaceæ family, (*Profuse, long-lasting menses*, especially in nervous patients with congestive symptoms to head and limbs. Passive hemorrhages at climacteric. Chronic metritis. Hemorrhage from lungs. Varices and ulcers). *Mandragora*—(Mandrake). A narcotic of the ancients—Restless excitability and bodily weakness. Desire for sleep. Has antiperiodic properties like China and Aranea. Useful in epilepsy and hydrophobia, also *Cetonia* (A. E. Lavine). *Hyos.* (less fever, more agitation); *Stram.* (more sensorial excitement, frenzy); *Hoitzia*—A Mexican drug, similar in action to Bellad. (Useful in fever, scarlatinal eruption, measles, urticaria, etc. High fever with eruptive fevers. Dry mouth and throat, red face, injected eyes, delirium.) Calcar is often required after *Bell.; Atropia.* Alkaloid of Belladonna covers more the neurotic sphere of the Belladonna action. (Great *dryness of throat*, almost impossible to swallow. Chronic stomach affections, with great pain and vomiting of all food. Peritonitis. All kind of illusions of sight. Everything appears large. *Platina opposite.*) *Hypochlorhydria;* pyrosis. Motes over everything. On reading, *words run together;* double vision, *all objects seem to be elongated.* Eustachian tube and tympanic congestion. Affinity for the pancreas. Hyperacidity of stomach. Paroxysms of gastric pain; ovarian neuralgia.)

Non-Homoeopathic Uses.—*Atropia* and its salts are used for ophthalmic purposes, to dilate the pupil and paralyze the accommodation.

Given internally or hypodermically, it is antagonistic to Opium and Morphine. Physostigma and Prussic Acid. Narcotic poisons and mushroom poisoning. Renal colic 1-200 of a grain hypodermically.

Atropin injected subcutaneously in doses from a milligram upwards for intestinal obstruction threatening life.

Hypodermically 1-80 gr. night sweats in phthisis.

Atropia 1-20 gr. is antagonistic to 1 gr. Morphine.

Also used as a local anæsthetic, antispasmodic, and to dry up secretions, milk, etc. Hypodermically 1-80 gr. night sweats in phthisis.

Dose.—*Atropia Sulph.*, 1-120 to 1-60 grain.

Antidotes to Belladonna: *Camph.*; *Coff.*; *Opium*; *Acon.*

Complementary: *Calc.* Bellad. (contains lime). Especially in semi-chronic and constitutional diseases.

Incompatible: *Acet. ac.*

Dose.—First to thirtieth potency and higher. Must be repeated frequently in acute diseases.

BELLIS PERENNIS
(Daisy)

It acts upon the muscular fibers of the blood-vessels. Much muscular soreness. Lameness, as if sprained. Venous congestion, due to mechanical causes. First remedy in injuries to the deeper tissues, after major surgical work. Results of injuries to nerves with intense soreness and intolerance of cold bathing. After gout, debility of limbs.

Traumatism of the pelvic organs, auto-traumatism, expresses the condition calling for this remedy; ill effects from masturbation. Excellent remedy for sprains and bruises. Complaints due to cold food or drink when the body is heated, and in affections due to cold wind. Externally, in nævi. Acne. *Boils all over. Sore, bruised feeling in the pelvic region.* Exudations, stasis, swelling, come within the range of this remedy. Rheumatic symptoms. Does not vitiate the secretions. "It is a princely remedy for old laborers, especially gardeners." (Burnett.)

Head.—Vertigo in elderly people. Headache from occiput to top of head. Forehead feels contracted. *Bruised soreness.* Itching around scalp and over back, worse from hot bath and bed.

Female.—Breasts and uterus engorged. Varicose veins in pregnancy. *During pregnancy inability to walk.* Abdominal muscles lame. *Uterus feels sore, as if squeezed.*

Sleep.—Wakes early in morning and cannot get to sleep again.

Abdomen.—*Soreness of abdominal walls and of uterus.* Stitches in spleen, sore, enlarged. Yellow, painless diarrhœa, foul odor, worse at night. Bloated; rumbling in bowels.

Skin.—*Boils.* Ecchymosis, swelling, very sensitive to touch. Venous congestion due to mechanical causes. Varicose veins with bruised sore feeling. Exudations and swellings. Acne.

Extremities.—Joints sore, muscular soreness. Itching on back and flexor surfaces of thighs. Pain down anterior of thighs. Wrist feels contracted as from elastic band around joint. Sprains with great soreness. *Railway spine.*

Relationship.—Compare: *Arnica; Arsenic; Staphis.; Hamamelis; Bryonia; Vanadium* (degenerative states).

Modalities.—*Worse, left side;* hot bath and warmth of bed; before storms; cold bathing; cold wind.

Dose.—Tincture to third potency.

BENZENUM—COAL NAPHTHA
(Benzol, C_6, H_6)

The most striking fact in the proving of Benzol seems to be the influence it had on the circulatory system. It caused a slowing of the pulse stream which in the guinea-pigs brought about the formation of infarcts. In the human provers it resulted in a *decrease of the red and increase of white cells.* (R. F. Rabe, M.D.)

It ought to be of use in Leucæmia. Eye symptoms striking. Hallucinations—Epileptiform attacks, coma, and anasthesia.

Head.—Sense of falling through bed and floor. Pains from below upward. Tired and nervous.

Frontal headache to root of nose. Dizzy. Pressing feeling in head. Right sided headache.

Eyes.—Illusion of vision with wide open eyes. Twitching of lids. Photophobia, objects blurred. Aching in eyes and lids. Marked dilation of pupils. Failure to react to light, particularly daylight.

Nose.—Profuse fluent coryza. Especially in afternoon. Violent sneezing.

Male.—Swelling of right testicle. Severe pain in testicles. Itching of scrotum. Profuse urination.

Extremities.—Heavy limbs, cold legs, exaggerated knee-jerk. Pains from below upward.

Skin.—Eruption like measles. Perspiration on side not lain upon. Itching all over back.

Modalities.—Worse at night. Worse right side.

Dose.—Sixth potency.

Relationship.—Compare: *Benzin.*—Petroleum ether—not as pure a compound as Benzene (Benzol). It is the same, but with a mixture of hydrocarbons. It seems to exercise a special influence on the nervous system and on the blood. Oxyhaemoglobinæmia. Physical weakness, cramps, exaggeration of knee jerks, nausea, vomiting, dizziness, *heaviness* and coldness of limbs. Tremor of eyelids and tongue. *Benzin. dinitricum*—D. N. B.—(The most obvious results of poisoning by skin absorption are changes in the red blood corpuscles and liver degeneration in amblyopia, color-blindness, retinitis. Field of vision contracted. Black urine). *Benzin. nitricum. Mirbane.* (Dark, black blood, coagulates with difficulty; venous hyperæmia of the brain and general venous engorgement. Burning taste in mouth. Blue lips, tongue, skin, nails and conjunctivæ. Cold skin, pulse small, weak, breathing slow and irregular, unconsciousness, symptoms of apoplectic coma. *Rolling of eyeballs in their vertical axis; pupils dilated.* Nystagmus. Respiration very slow, difficult, sighing.) *Trinitrotoluene* (T. N. T.), Trotyl—is a high explosive, obtained by nitrating toluene—a product of coal tar distillation.

When the skin or hair is exposed to T. N. T. by contact a characteristic yellow or tawny-orange stain is produced, which lasts for some weeks. Indicated in graver forms of anemia (pernicious) and jaundice. Produces fatal toxic jaundice.

Dose.—Sixth potency.

BENZOICUM ACIDUM
(Benzoic Acid)

The most marked characteristic pertains to the odor and color of the urine. It has a marked action on metabolism. It produces and cures symptoms of a uric acid diathesis, with urine highly colored and very offensive, and gouty symptoms. Renal insufficiency. Child wants to be nursed in the arms, will not be laid down. Pains suddenly change their locality. Antisycotic. Gouty and asthmatic.

Mind.—Prone to dwell on unpleasant things in the past. Omits words in writing. Depression.

Head.—Vertigo inclination to fall sideways. Throbbing in temporal arteries, causes puffing around ears. Noises when swallowing. Ulceration of tongue. Swelling behind ears. [*Caps.*] Cold sweat on forehead. Pricking, puckered constriction of mouth, bluish and bleeding gums. Wens.

Nose.—Itching of septum. Pain in nasal bones.

Face.—Copper-colored spots. Red, with little blisters. Circumscribed redness of cheeks.

Stomach.—Sweat while eating; pressure in stomach, sensation of a lump.

Abdomen.—Cutting about navel. Stitching in liver region.

Rectum.—Stitches and *constricted* feeling. Puckering constriction of rectum. Itching and watery elevations around anus.

Stool.—Frothy, *offensive, liquid*, light-colored, like soapsuds, bowel movements mostly windy.

Urine.—*Repulsive odor;* changeable color; brown, acid. *Enuresis;* dribbling, *offensive urine of old men*. Excess of uric acid. Vesical catarrh from suppressed gonorrhœa. Cystitis.

Respiratory.—Hoarse in morning. Asthmatic cough; worse night; lying on right side. Chest very tender. Pain in region of heart. Expectoration, green mucus.

Back.—Pressure on spinal column. Coldness in sacrum. Dull pain in region of kidneys; worse, wine.

Extremities.—Joints crack on motion. Tearing with stitches. *Pain in tendo Achillis*. Rheumatic gout; nodes very painful. Gouty deposits. Ganglion; swelling of the wrist. Pain and swelling in knees. Bunion of great toe. Tearing pain in great toe.

Fever.—Cold hands, feet, back, knees. Chilliness; cold sweat. Internal heat on awakening.

Skin.—Red spots. Itching in spots.

Modalities.—*Worse*, in open air; by uncovering.

Relationship.—Useful after Colchic. fails in gout; after Copaiva in gonorrhœa.

Compare: *Nitric acid; Ammon. benz.; Sabina; Tropœolum*—Garden Nasturtium—(*fetid urine*).

Antidote: *Copaiva*.
Incompatible: *Wine*.
Dose.—Third to sixth potency

BERBERIS AQUIFOLIUM—MAHONIA
(Mountain Grape)

A remedy for the skin, chronic catarrhal affections, secondary syphilis. Hepatic torpor, lassitude and other evidences of incomplete metamorphosis; stimulates all glands and improves nutrition.

Head.—Sensation of a band just above ears. Bilious headache. "Scald head." Scaly eczema.

Face.—Acne. Blotches and pimples. Clears the complexion

Stomach.—Tongue thickly coated, yellowish-brown; feels blistered. Burning in stomach. Nausea and hunger after eating.

Urine.—Stitching, crampy pains; thick mucus, and brightred, mealy sediment.

Skin.—*Pimply, dry, rough, scaly*. Eruption on *scalp extending to face* and neck. Tumor of breast, with pain. Psoriasis. Acne. Dry Eczema. Pruritus. Glandular induration.

Relationship.—*Carbol. acid; Euonym.; Berb. vulg.; Hydr.*

Dose.—Tincture in rather material doses.

BERBERIS VULGARIS
(Barberry)

Rapid change of symptoms—pains change in regard to place and character—thirst alternates with thirstlessness, hunger, and loss of appetite, etc. Acts forcibly on the venous system, producing pelvic engorgements and hæmorrhoids.

Hepatic, and rheumatic affections, particularly with urinary, hæmorrhoidal and menstrual complaints.

Old gouty constitutions. Pain in region of kidneys is most marked; hence its use in renal and vesical troubles, gall-stones, and vesical catarrh. It causes inflammation of kidneys with hæmaturia. Pains may be felt all over body, emanating from small of back. It has also marked action on the liver, promoting the flow of bile. Often called for in arthritic affections with urinary disturbances. Wandering, *radiating* pains. Acts well in, fleshy persons, good livers, but with little endurance. Spinal irritation. All Berberis pains radiate, are not worse by pressure, but worse in various attitudes, especially standing and active exercise.

Head.—Listless, apathetic, indifferent. Puffy sensation, feeling as if becoming larger. Vertigo with attacks of fainting. Frontal headache. Chilliness in back and occiput. Tearing pain in auricle, and gouty concretions. *Sensation of a tight cap pressing upon the whole scalp.*

Nose.—Dry; obstinate catarrh of left nostril. Crawling in nostrils.

Face.—Pale, sickly. Sunken cheeks and eyes, with bluish circles.

Mouth.—Sticky sensation. /Diminished saliva. Sticky, frothy saliva, like cotton. [*Nux mosch.*] Tongue feels scalded; vesicles on tongue.

Stomach.—*Nausea before breakfast.* Heartburn.

Abdomen.—Stitches in region of gall-bladder; worse, pressure, extending to stomach. Catarrh of the gall-bladder with constipation and yellow complexion. Stitching pain in front of kidneys extending to liver, spleen, stomach, groins, Poupart's ligament. Sticking deep in ilium.

Stool.—Constant urging to stool. Diarrhœa painless, clay-colored, burning, and smarting in anus and perineum. Tearing around anus. *Fistula in ano.*

Urinary.—Burning pains. Sensation as if some urine remained after urinating. Urine with thick *mucus and bright-red*, mealy sediment. Bubbling, sore sensation in kidneys. Pain in bladder region. *Pain in the thighs and loins on urinating.* Frequent urination; urethra burns when not urinating.

Male.—Neuralgia of spermatic cord and testicles. Smarting, burning, stitching in testicles, in prepuce and scrotum.

Female.—Pinching constriction in mons veneris, vaginismus, contraction and tenderness of vagina. Burning and soreness in vagina. Desire diminished, cutting pain during coition. Menses scanty, gray mucus, with pain in kidneys and chilliness, pain down thighs. Leucorrhœa, grayish mucus, with painful urinary sumptoms. Neuralgia of ovaries and vagina.

Respiratory.—Hoarseness; polypus of larynx. Tearing stitches in chest and region of heart.

Back.—Stitches in neck and back; worse, respiration. Sticking pain in region of kidneys radiating thence around abdomen, to hips and groins. Numb, bruised sensation. Stitches from kidneys into bladder. Tearing, sticking with stiffness, making rising difficult, involving hips, nates, limbs, with numbness. Lumbago. [*Rhus; Tart. em.*] Metatarsus and metacarpus feel sprained. Post-operative pain in lumbar region; soreness with sharp pain following course of circumflex iliac nerve to bladder with frequent urination.

Extremities.—Rheumatic paralytic pain in shoulders, arms, hands and fingers, legs and feet. *Neuralgia under finger-nails*, with swelling of finger-joints. Sensation of cold on outside of thighs. Heels pain, as if ulcerated. Stitching between metatarsal bones as from a nail when standing. Pain in balls of feet on stepping. Intense weariness and lameness of legs after walking a short distance.

Skin.—Flat warts. *Itching*, burning and smarting; *worse, scratching;* better, cold applications. Small pustules over whole body. Eczema of *anus* and *hands*. *Circumscribed pigmentation* following eczematous inflammation.

Fever.—Cold sensation in various parts, as if spattered with cold water. Warmth in lower part of back, hips, and thighs.

Modalities.—*Worse*, motion, *standing*. It brings on, or increases, urinary complaints.

Relationship.—Compare: *Ipomea—Convolvulus Duartinus—Morning Glory.*—(Pain in left lumbar muscles on stooping. Kidney disorders with pain in back. Much abdominal flatulence. Aching in top of right shoulder renal colic; aching in small of back and extremities), *Aloe.; Lycopod.; Nux.; Sarsap. Xanthorrhœa arborea* (severe pain in kidneys, cystitis and gravel. Pain from ureter to bladder and testicles; pain in small of back returns from least chill or damp). *Xanthorrhiza apifolia*—Shrub Yellow Root—contains Berberine. Dilatation of stomach and intestines, atony, enlarged spleen.

Antidotes: *Camphor; Bell.*

Dose.—Tincture, to sixth potency.

BETA VULGARIS
(Beet-root)

Influences chronic catarrhal states and tuberculosis. The salt *Betainum hydrochloricum* obtained from the Beet root itself seems to be the best adapted to phthisical patients. Children yield very quickly to the action of the remedy. Use about the 2x Trit.

BETONICA
(Betony Wood)

Produces pains in various parts.

Head.—Stitches in right temple. Inability to concentrate mind.

Abdomen.—Pains in abdomen, hepatic region and of transverse colon, also in gall-bladder and right inguinal region and spermatic cords.

Extremities.—Shooting pain in back of both wrist joints. Wrist drops. Pain in right popliteal space down leg, which feels paralyzed.

BISMUTHUM
(Precipitated Sub-Nitrate of Bismuth)

Irritation and catarrhal inflammation of the alimentary canal, is the chief action of this drug.

Mind.—Solitude is unbearable. *Desire for company.* Complains about his condition. *Anguish.* Discontented.

Head.—Headache alternates with gastralgia. Neuralgic pain, as if torn by pincers; involves face and teeth; worse, eating; better, cold; alternate with gastralgia. Cutting or pressure above right orbit extending to occiput. Pressure in occiput; worse, motion; with heaviness.

Mouth.—*Gums swollen.* Toothache; better, cold water in mouth. [*Coff.*] Tongue white. Swollen. Black, gangrenous looking wedges on dorsum and sides of tongue. Profuse salivation, teeth loose. Thirst for cold drinks.

Stomach.—Vomits, with convulsive gagging and pain. *Water is vomited as soon as it reaches the stomach.* Eructation after drinking. Vomits all fluids. *Burning; feeling of a load.* Will eat for several days; then vomit. Slow digestion, with *fetid* eructations. Gastralgia; pain from stomach through to spine. Gastritis. *Better, cold drinks*, but vomiting when stomach becomes full.

Tongue coated white; sweetish, metallic taste. Inexpressible pain in stomach; must bend backwards. Pressure as from a load in one spot, alternating with burning, crampy pain and pyrosis.

Stool.—Painless diarrhœa, with great thirst, and frequent micturition and vomiting. Pinching in lower abdomen, with rumbling.

Respiratory.—Pinching in middle of diaphragm, extending transversely through chest. Angina pectoris; pain around heart, left arm to fingers.

Extremities.—Cramps in hands and feet. Tearing in wrist. Paralytic weakness, especially right arm. Tearing in tips of fingers under nails. [*Berb.*] Itching erosion near tibia and back of feet near joints. Cold limbs.

Sleep.—Restless on account of voluptuous dreams. Sleepy in morning, a few hours after eating.

Relationship.—Antidotes: *Nux; Capsic.; Calc.*

Compare: *Antimon.; Ars.; Bellad.; Kreosot.*

Dose.—First to sixth potency.

BLATTA AMERICANA
(Cockroach)

Ascites. Various forms of dropsy. Yellow complexion. Extreme weariness. Pain in urethra on urinating. Weariness on going upstairs.

Dose.—Sixth potency.

BLATTA ORIENTALIS
(Indian Cockroach)

A remedy for asthma. Especially when associated with bronchitis. Indicated after arsenic when this is insufficient.

Cough with *dyspnœa* in bronchitis and phthisis. Acts best in stout and corpulent patients. Much pus-like mucus.

Dose.—Lowest potencies during an attack. After the spasm, for the remaining cough, use the higher. Stop with improvement to prevent return of aggravation.

BOLETUS LARICIS—POLYPORUS OFFICINALE
(White Agaric)

Quotidian intermittent fever. Sweat is light, and without relief. Night-sweat in phthisis.

Head.—Feels light and hollow with deep frontal headache. Thick, yellow coating of tongue; teeth indented. Constant nausea.

Fever.—Chilliness along spine, with frequent, hot flashes. Yawns and stretches when chilly. Severe aching in shoulders and joints and small of back. *Profuse perspiration at night*, with hectic chills and fever.

Skin.—Hot and dry, especially in palms. Itching more between scapulæ and on forearms.

Relationship.—Compare: *Agaricin*, active constituent of Polyporus officinale (phthisical and other enervating night-sweats 1-4 to 1-2 gr. doses; also in chorea, in dilatation of heart with pulmonary Emphysema, fatty degeneration, profuse perspiration and erythema.) *Boletus luridus*. (Violent pain in epigastrium, urticaria tuberosa.) *Boletus satanus* (dysentery, vomiting, great debility, cold extremities, spasm of extremities and face).

Dose.—First attenuation.

BORICUM ACIDUM
(Boracic Acid)

Used as an antiseptic disinfectant, since it arrests fermentation and putrefaction.

Pain in region of ureters, with frequent urging to urinate. *Coldness.* [*Heloderm.*] *Diabetes*, tongue dry, red, and cracked. Cold saliva.

Skin.—Multiform erythema of trunk and upper extremities. Œdema around eyes. Exfoliating dermatitis. Oedema of tissues around eyes.

Female.—Climacteric flushings. [*Lach.; Amyl. nit.*] Vagina cold, as if packed with ice. Frequent urination with burning and tenesmus.

Dose.—Third trituration.

Non-Homoeopathic Uses.—When the diplococcus of Weichselbaum is present in the sputum of pharyngitis or bronchitis, pneumonia with tenacious sputum, hacking cough and pain, five-grain doses six times daily. A solution of Boracic Acid, as an injection, in chronic, cystitis, or, a teaspoonful to a glass of hot milk, taken internally. Boro-Glyceride in solution (1:40) is a powerful antiseptic. *Styes*, 15 gr. to 1 oz. water externally. As a dusting powder on ulcerated surfaces. In cystitis as an irrigating fluid.

BORAX
(Borate of Sodium)

Gastro-intestinal irritation. Salivation, nausea, vomiting, colic, diarrhœa, collapse, albuminuria, casts and vesical spasm. Delirium, visual changes, hæmaturia, and skin eruptions have all been observed from over-dosing.

Dread of downward motion in nearly all complaints. For homœopathic purposes, the peculiar nervous symptoms are very characteristic, and have frequently been verified, especially in the therapeutics of children. Of much value in epilepsy. Aphthous ulceration of mucous membranes.

Mind.—Extreme anxiety, especially from motions which have a downward direction, rocking, being carried downstairs, laid down. Anxious expression of face during the downward motions, starts and throws up hands on laying patient down, as if afraid of falling. Excessively nervous; easily frightened. *Sensitive to sudden noises*. Violent fright from report of a gun, even at a distance Fear of thunder.

Head.—Aches, with nausea and trembling of whole body. Hair tangled at tips, cannot be separated, as in Plica Polonica. [*Vinca min.*]

Eyes.—Lashes turn inward. Visions of bright waves. Eyelids inflamed, lids cut against eyeball. Entropium.

Ears.—*Very sensitive to slightest noise;* not so much disturbed by louder ones.

Nose.—Red nose, of young women. [*Nat. carb.*] Red and shining swelling, with throbbing and tensive sensation. Tip swollen and ulcerated. Dry crusts.

Face.—Pale, earthy, with suffering expression. Swollen, with pimples on nose and lips. Feeling of cobwebs.

Mouth.—*Aphthæ.* White fungous like growth. Mouth *hot* and tender; ulcers bleed on touch and eating. Painful gum-boil. Crying when nursing. Taste bitter. [*Bry.; Puls.; Cup.*] Taste of "cellar mould."

Stomach and Abdomen.—Distention after eating; vomiting. Gastralgia, depending upon uterine disturbance. Pain as if diarrhœa would result.

Stool.—*Loose, pappy, offensive stools in children.* Diarrhœa, offensive, preceded by colic; stools mucous, with aphthous sore mouth.

Urine.—Hot, smarting pain in orifice. Pungent smell. Child afraid to urinate, screams before urinating. [*Sarsap.*] Small red particles on diaper.

Female.—Labor pains with frequent eructations. *Galactorrhœa.* [*Cal.; Con.; Bell.*] In nursing, pain *in opposite breast.* Leucorrhœa like white of eggs, with sensation as if warm water was flowing. Menses *too soon, profuse,* with griping, nausea and pain in stomach extending into small of back. *Membranous dysmenorrhœa.* Sterility. Favors easy conception. Sensation of distention in clitoris with sticking. Pruritus of vulva and eczema.

Respiratory.—Hacking and violent cough; expectoration, mouldy taste and smell. *Stitches in chest,* with inspiration and cough. Cough with mouldy taste—breath smells mouldy. Pleurodynia; worse upper part of right chest. Arrest of breathing when lying; is obliged to jump and catch breath, which causes pain in right side. Out of breath on going up stairs.

Extremities.—Feeling as of cobwebs on hands. Itching on back of finger-joints and hands. Throbbing pain in tip of thumb. *Stitches in sole.* Pain in heel. Burning pain in great toe; inflammation of balls of toes. Eczema of toes and fingers with loss of nails.

Skin.—*Psoriasis.* Erysipelas in face. Itching on back of finger-joints. Unhealthy skin; slight injuries suppurate.

Herpes. [*Rhus.*] Erysipelatous inflammation with swelling and tension. Chilblains relieved in open air. Trade eruptions on fingers and hands, itching and stinging. Ends of hair become tangled.

Sleep.—Voluptuous dreams. Cannot sleep on account of heat, especially in head. Cries out of sleep as if frightened. [*Bell.*]

Modalities.—*Worse,* downward motion, noise, smoking, warm weather, after menses.

Better, pressure, evening, cold weather.

Relationship.—Acetic acid, vinegar, and wine are incompatible.

Antidoe: *Cham.; Coffea.*

Compare: *Calc.; Bryon.; Sanicula; Sulph, ac.*

Dose.—First to third trituration. In skin diseases continue its use for several weeks. Locally in pruritus pudendi. A piece of borax, the size of a pea, dissolved in the mouth, acts magically in restoring the voice, in cases of sudden hoarseness brought on by cold, and frequently for an hour or so, it renders the voice silvery and clear.

BOTHROPS LANCIOLATUS.—LACHESIS LANCIOLATUS
(Yellow Viper)

Its venom is most coagulating, (also *Lachesis*). We should expect to find under these remedies the symptomatology of thrombosis, also thrombotic phenomena, as hemiplegia, aphasia, inability to articulate. (Linn J. Boyd.)

Broken-down, hæmorrhagic constitutions; septic states. Great lassitude and sluggishness; hæmorrhages from every orifice of the body; black spots. Hemiplegia with aphasia. Inability to articulate, without any affection of the tongue. Nervous trembling. Pain in right big toe. Diagonal course of symptoms. Pulmonary congestion.

Eyes.—Amaurosis; blindness from hemorrhage into retina. Hemoralopia, day blindness, can hardly see her way after sunrise; conjunctivial hæmorrhage.

Face.—Swollen and puffy. Besotted expression.

Throat.—Red, dry, constricted; swallowing difficult, cannot pass liquids.

Stomach.—Epigastric distress. Black vomiting. Intense hæmatemesis. Tympanitis and bloody stools.

Skin.—Swollen, livid, cold with hæmorrhagic infiltration. Gangrene. Lymphatics swollen. Anthrax. Malignant erysipelas.

Modalities.—*Worse,* right side.

Relationship.—Compare: *Toxicophis.*—Moccasin Snake (pain and fever *recur* annually, after bite from this snake, and sometimes change location with disappearance of first symptoms. An unusual dryness of skin follows the bite. Œdematous swellings and periodical neuralgia. Pain travels from one part to another.) Other snake poisons, notably *Lachesis*.

Trachinus,—Stingfish (intolerable pains, swelling, acute blood poisoning, gangrene.)

Dose.—Sixth to thirtieth potency.

BOTULINUM
(Toxin of Bacillus Botulinum)

Food poisoning from canned spinach produced a clinical picture suggested in a bulbar paresis.

Eye symptoms, ptosis, double vision, blurred vision.

Difficulty in swallowing and breathing, choking sensation; weakness and uncertainty in walking, "blind staggers," dizziness, thickening of speech. Cramping pain in stomach.

Mask-like expression of face, due to weakness of facial muscles. Severe constipation.

Dose.—Higher potencies.

BOVISTA
(Puff-Ball)

Has a marked effect on the skin, producing eruption like eczema, also upon the circulation, predisposing to hæmorrhages; marked languor and lassitude. Adapted to stammering children, old maids with palpitation; and "tettery" patients. Stage of numbness and tingling in multiple neuritis. Asphyxia due to charcoal fumes.

Mind.—*Enlarged sensation.* [*Arg. n.*] Awkward; *everything falls from hands.* Sensitive.

Head.—Sensation *as if head were enlarging,* especially of occiput. Distensive headache; worse early morning, open air, lying. Discharge from nose *stringy,* tough. Dull, bruised pain in brain. *Stammering.* [*Stram.; Merc.*] Scalp itches; worse, warmth; sensitive; must scratch until sore.

Face.—Scurf and crusts about nostrils and corners of mouth. Lips chapped. Bleeding of nose and gums. Cheeks and lips feel swollen. *Acne* worse in summer; due to use of cosmetics.

Stomach.—Sensation as of a lump of ice. Intolerant of tight clothing around waist.

Female.—*Diarrhœa before and during menses.* Menses too early and profuse; *worse at night.* Voluptuous sensation. Leucorrhœa acrid, thick, tough, greenish, follows menses. *Cannot bear tight clothing around waist* [*Lach.*]. *Traces of menses between menstruation.* Soreness of pubes during menses. Metrorrhagia; Parovarian cysts.

Abdomen.—*Colic,* with red urine; *relieved by eating.* Must bend double. Pain around umbilicus. Stitches through perineum towards rectum and genitals.

Chronic diarrhœa of old people; worse at night and early morning.

Extremities.—Great weakness of all joints; clumsiness with her hands, drops things from hands. Weariness of hands and feet. Sweat in axillæ; *onion smell. Tip of coccyx itches intolerably.* Moist eczema on back of hand. Itching of feet and legs. Œdema in joints after fracture.

Skin.—Blunt instruments leave deep impression on the skin. *Urticaria on excitement,* with rheumatic lameness, palpitation and diarrhœa. [*Dulc.*] Itching on getting warm. Eczema, moist; formation of thick crusts. Pimples cover the entire body; scurvy; herpetic eruptions. Pruritus ani. Urticaria on waking in the morning, worse from bathing. Pellagra.

Relationship.—*Bovista* antidotes tar applications. Suffocation from gas. After *Rhus* in chronic urticaria.

Compare: *Calc.; Rhus; Sepia; Cicuta.*

Dose.—Third to sixth potency.

BRACHYGLOTTIS
(Puka-Puka)

Fluttering sensation. [*Caladium.*] Kidney and bladder symptoms predominate. Produces symptoms of albuminuria. Itching in ears and nostrils. *Bright's disease.* Oppression of chest. Writer's cramp.

Abdomen.—Feeling as if something rolling about. Fluttering in region of ovary.

Urinary.—Pressure in neck of bladder; urging to urinate. Sense of swashing in bladder. Soreness in urethra; feeling as if urine could not be retained. Urine contains mucous corpuscles and epithelium, albumen and casts.

Extremities.—Cramp in fingers, thumb, and wrist when writing—soreness extending along flexor carpi ulnaris.

Relationship.—Compare: *Apis; Helonias; Merc. cor.; Plumbum.*

Dose.—Third potency.

BROMUM
(Bromine)

Most marked effects are seen in the respiratory symptoms, especially in larynx and trachea. It seems to affect especially scrofulous children with enlarged glands. *Blond type.* Enlarged parotid and goitre. Tendency to spasmodic attacks. *Left-sided mumps.* Sense of suffocation; excoriating discharges, profuse sweats and great weakness. Complaints from being over-heated. *Tendency to infiltrate glands, become hard, but seldom suppurate.*

Mind.—Delusion that strange persons are looking over patient's shoulder and that she would see some one on turning. Quarrelsome.

Head.—Megrim of left side; worse stooping, especially after drinking milk. Headache; worse heat of sun and by rapid motion. Sharp pain through eyes. Dizzy when crossing stream of water.

Nose—Coryza, with corrosive soreness of nose. Stoppage of right nostril. Pressure at root of nose. *Tickling, smarting, as from cobwebs.* Fan-like motion of alæ. [*Lyc.*] Bleeding from nose relieving the chest.

Throat.—Throat feels raw, evening, with hoarseness. Tonsils pain on swallowing deep red, with network of dilated blood vessels. Tickling in trachea during inspiration. Hoarseness coming on from being overheated.

Stomach and Abdomen.—Sharp burning from tongue to stomach. Pressure as of stone. Gastralgia; better eating. Tympanitic distention of abdomen. Painful hæmorrhoids, with black stool.

Respiratory.—Whooping cough. (Use persistently for about ten days.) *Dry cough, with hoarseness* and burning pain *behind sternum. Spasmodic cough, with rattling of mucus* in the larynx; suffocative. *Hoarseness. Croup* after febrile symptoms have subsided. Difficult and painful breathing. Violent cramping of chest. Chest pains run upward. *Cold sensation when inspiring.* Every inspiration provokes cough. *Laryngeal diphtheria,* membrane begins in larynx and spreads upward. Spasmodic constriction. Asthma; difficulty in getting air *into* lung. (*Chlorum*, in expelling.) Better at sea, of seafaring men when they come on land. Hypertrophy of heart from gymnastics. [*Rhus.*] Fibrinous bronchitis, great dyspnœa. Bronchial tubes feel filled with smoke.

Male.—Swelling of testicles. Indurated, with pains worse slight jar.

Female.—Swelling of ovaries. Menses too early; too profuse, with membranous shreds. Low spirited before menses. Tumor in breasts, with stitching pains; worse left. Stitch pains from breast to axillæ. Sharp shooting pain in left breast, worse, pressure.

Sleep.—Full of dreams and anguish; jerking and starting during sleep, full of fantasy and illusions; difficult to go to sleep at night, cannot sleep enough in morning; trembling and weak on awaking.

Skin.—Acne, pimples and pustules. Boils on arms and face. *Glands stony, hard, especially on lower jaw* and throat. Hard goitre. [*Spong.*] Gangrene.

Modalities.—*Worse,* from evening, until midnight, and when sitting in warm room; warm damp weather when at rest and lying left side. *Better,* from any motion; exercise; at sea.

Relationship.—Antidotes: *Ammon. carb.*; *Camph.* Salt inhibits the action of Brom.

Compare: *Conium*; *Spongia*; *Iod.*; *Aster.*; *Arg. nit.* Avoid milk when taking Brom. *Hydrobromic acid.* (Throat dry and puckering; constriction in pharynx and chest; waves of heat over face and neck; pulsating tinnitus with great nervous irritability (Houghton); vertigo, palpitation; arms heavy; seemed as if parts did not belong to him. Seems to have a specific effect on the inferior cervical ganglion, increasing the tonic action of the sympathetic, thus promoting vaso-constriction. Relieves headache, tinnitus and vertigo, especially in vasomotor stomach disturbance. Dose, 20 minims.)

Dose.—First to third attenuation. Must be prepared fresh, as it is liable to rapid deterioration.

BRYONIA
(Wild Hops)

Acts on all serous membranes and the viscera they contain. Aching in every muscle. The general character *of the pain here produced is a stitching, tearing; worse by motion, better rest.* These characteristic stitching pains, greatly aggravated by any motion, are found everywhere, but especially in the chest; worse pressure. *Mucous membranes are all dry.* The Bryonia patient is irritable; has vertigo from raising the head, pressive headache; dry, parched lips, mouth; excessive thirst, bitter taste, sensitive epigastrium, and feeling of a stone in the stomach; stools large, dry, hard; dry cough; rheumatic pains and swellings; dropsical effusions into synovial and serous membranes.

Bryonia affects especially the constitution of a robust, firm fiber and dark complexion, with tendency to leanness and irritability. It prefers the right side, the evening, and open air. Warm weather after cold days, to manifest its action most markedly.

Children dislike to be carried or raised. *Physical weakness*, all-pervading apathy. Complaints apt to develop slowly.

Mind.—Exceedingly *irritable;* everything puts him out of humor. Delirium; wants to go home; *talks of business.*

Head.—Vertigo, nausea faintness on rising, confusion. *Bursting, splitting headache,* as if everything would be pressed out; as if hit by a hammer from within; worse from motion, stooping, opening eyes. Headache becomes seated in occiput. Drawing in bones towards zygoma. Headache; worse on motion, even of eyeballs. Frontal headache, frontal sinuses involved.

Nose.—*Frequent bleeding of nose when menses should appear.* Also in the morning, relieving the headache. Coryza with shooting and aching in the forehead. Swelling of tip of nose, feels as if it would ulcerate when touched.

Ears.—Aural vertigo. [*Aur.; Nat. sal.; Sil.; Chin.*] Roaring, buzzing.

Eyes.—Pressing, crushing, aching pain. Glaucoma. Sore to touch and when moving them.

Mouth.—*Lips parched, dry, cracked. Dryness of mouth, tongue, and throat, with excessive thirst.* Tongue coated yellowish, dark brown; heavily white in gastric derangement. Bitter taste. [*Nux; Col.*] Burning in lower lip in old smokers. Lip swollen, dry, black and cracked.

Throat.—Dryness, sticking on swallowing, scraped and constricted. [*Bell.*] Tough mucus in larynx and trachea, loosened only after much hawking; worse coming into warm room.

Stomach.—*Nausea and faintness when rising up.* Abnormal hunger, loss of taste. Thirst for large draughts. Vomiting of bile and water immediately after eating. Worse, warm drinks, which are vomited. *Stomach sensitive to touch. Pressure in stomach after eating, as of a stone.* Soreness in stomach when coughing. Dyspeptic ailments during summer heat. Sensitiveness of epigastrium to touch.

Abdomen.—Liver region swollen, sore, tensive. Burning pain, *stitches; worse, pressure, coughing, breathing.* Tenderness of abdominal walls.

Stool.—Constipation; stools hard, dry, as if burnt; seem too large. Stools brown, thick, bloody; *worse in morning, from moving,* in hot weather, after being heated, from cold drinks, every spell of hot weather.

Urine.—Red, brown, like beer; scanty, hot.

Female.—Menses too early, too profuse; worse from motion, with tearing pains in legs; *suppressed, with vicarious discharge or splitting headache.* Stitching pains in ovaries on taking a deep inspiration; very sensitive to touch. Pain in right ovary as if torn, extending to thigh. [*Lilium; Croc.*] Milk fever. Pain in breasts at menstrual period. *Breasts hot and painful, hard.* Abscess of mammæ. Frequent bleeding of nose at appearance of menses. Menstrual irregularities, with gastric symptoms. Ovaritis. *Intermenstrual pain, with great abdominal and pelvic soreness.* [*Ham.*]

Respiratory.—Soreness in larynx and trachea. Hoarseness; worse in open air. Dry, hacking cough from irritation in upper trachea. Cough, dry, at night; *must sit up; worse after eating or drinking,* with vomiting, *with stitches in chest,* and expectoration of rust-colored sputa. Frequent desire to take a long breath; *must* expand lungs. Difficult, quick respiration; worse every movement; caused by stitches in chest. Cough, with feeling as if chest would fly to pieces; presses his head on sternum; must support chest. Croupous and pleuro-pneumonia. Expectoration brick shade, tough, and falls like lumps of jelly. Tough mucus in trachea, loosened only with much hawking. *Coming into warm room excites cough.* [*Nat. carb.*] Heaviness beneath the sternum extending towards the right shoulder. Cough *worse* by going into warm *room.* Stitches in cardiac region. Angina pectoris (use tincture).

Back.—Painful stiffness in nape of neck. *Stitches and stiffness in small of back.* From hard water and sudden changes of weather.

Extremities.—Knees stiff and painful. Hot swelling of feet. *Joints red, swollen, hot,* with stitches and tearing; worse on least movement. Every spot is painful on pressure. Constant motion of left arm and leg. [*Helleb.*]

Skin.—Yellow; pale, swollen, dropsical; hot and painful. Seborrhœa. *Hair very greasy.*

Sleep.—Drowsy; starting when falling asleep. Delirium; busy with business matters and what he had read.

Fever.—Pulse full, hard, tense, and quick. Chill with external coldness, dry cough, stitches. Internal heat. Sour sweat after slight exertion. Easy, profuse perspiration. Rheumatic and typhoid marked by gastro-hepatic complications.

Modalities.—*Worse*, warmth, any motion, morning, eating, hot weather, exertion, touch. Cannot sit up; gets faint and sick. *Better*, lying on *painful side, pressure, rest, cold things*.

Relationship.—Complementary: *Upas* when Bryonia fails. *Rhus; Alumina. Illecebrum.*—A Mexican drug.—(Fever with catarrhal symptoms, gastric and typhoid fever symptoms.)

Antidotes: *Acon.; Cham.; Nux.*

Compare: *Asclep. tub.; Kali mur.; Ptelia.*

Dose.—First to twelfth attenuation.

BUFO

(Poison of the Toad)

Acts on the nervous system and skin. Uterine symptoms marked. Lymphangitis of septic origin. Symptoms of paralysis agitans. Striking rheumatic symptoms.

Arouses the lowest passions. Causes a desire for intoxicating drink, and produces impotence.

Of use in feeble-minded children. Prematurely senile. Epileptic symptoms. Convulsive seizures occur during sleep at night. More or less connected with derangements of the sexual sphere, seem to come within the range of this remedy. Injuries to fingers; pain runs in streaks up the arms.

Mind.—Anxious about health. Sad, restless. Propensity to bite. Howling; impatient; nervous; imbecile. *Desire for solitude. Feeble-minded.*

Head.—Sensation as if hot vapor rose to top of head. Numbness of brain. Face bathed in sweat. Epistaxis with flushed face and pain in forehead, better, nosebleed.

Eyes.—Cannot bear sight of brilliant objects. Little blisters form on eye.

Ears.—Music is unbearable. [*Ambra.*] Every little noise distresses.

Heart.—Feels too large. Palpitation. Constriction about heart. Sensation of heart swimming in water.

Female.—Menses too early and copious, clots and bloody discharge at other times; watery leucorrhœa. Excitement, with epileptic attacks. Epilepsy at time of menses. Induration in mammary glands. Pallative in cancer of the mammæ

Burning in ovaries and uterus. Ulceration of cervix. Offensive bloody discharge. Pains run into legs. Bloody milk. Milk-leg. Veins swollen. Tumors and polypi of womb.

Male.—Involuntary emissions; *impotence*, discharge too quick, spasms during coition. *Buboes*. Disposition to handle organs. [*Hyos.; Zinc.*] Effects of onanism.

Extremities.—Pains in loins, numbness of limbs, cramps, staggering gait, feeling as if a peg were driven in joints; swelling of bones.

Skin.—Panaritium; *pain runs up arm*. Patches of skin lose sensation. Pustules, suppuration from every slight injury. Pemphigus. Bullæ which open and leave a raw surface, exuding and ichorous fluid. Blisters on palms and soles. Itching and burning. Carbuncle.

Relationship.—Compare: *Baryt. carb.; Asterias; Salamand.* (Epilepsy and softening of brain.)

Antidotes: *Laches.; Seneg.*

Complementary: *Salamandra*

Modalities.—*Worse*, in warm room, on awakening. *Better*, from bathing or cold air; from putting feet in hot water.

Dose.—Sixth potency and higher.

BUTYRIC ACID
(A volatile acid obtained chiefly from butter)

Head.—Worries over trifles; impulsive thoughts of suicide; constant state of fear and nervousness. Headache makes him apprehensive about trifles; worse going upstairs or rapid motion. Dull, hazy ache of head.

Stomach.—Poor appetite. Much gas in stomach and bowels. Cramps in pit of stomach, worse at night. Stomach feels heavy and overloaded. Cramp in abdomen below umbilicus. Bowels irregular. Stool accompanied by pain and straining.

Back.—Tired feeling and dull pain in small of back, worse walking. Pain in ankles and up back of leg. Pain low down in back and extremities.

Sleep.—Pronounced sleeplessness; dreams of serious nature while asleep.

Skin.—Perspiration on slight exertion. *Profuse, offensive sweat of feet.* Crumbling away of finger-nails.

Modalities.—*Worse*, at night, fast walking, going upstairs.
Dose.—Third attenuation.

CACTUS GRANDIFLORUS—SELENICEREUS SPINULOSUS
(Night-blooming Cereus)

Acts on circular muscular fibers, hence constrictions. It is the heart and arteries especially that at once respond to the influence of Cactus, producing very characteristic *constrictions* as of an iron band. This sensation is found in various places, œsophagus, bladder, etc. The mental symptoms produced correspond to those found when there are heart affections, sadness, and melancholy. *Hemorrhage, constrictions, periodicity*, and *spasmodic pains*. Whole body feels as if caged, each wire being twisted tighter. Atheromatous arteries and weak heart. Congestions; irregular distribution of blood. *Favors formation of clots speedily*. Great periodicity. Toxic goitre with cardiac symptoms. Cactus is pulseless, panting and prostrated.

Mind.—Melancholy, taciturn, sad, ill-humored. Fear of death. Screams with pain. Anxiety.

Head.—Headache if obliged to pass dinner hour. [*Ars.; Lach.; Lyc.*] *Sensation as of a weight on vertex*. Right-sided pulsating pain. *Congestive headaches*, periodical, threatening apoplexy. Blood-vessels to the head distended. Feels as if head were compressed in a vise. Pulsation in ears. Dim sight. *Right-sided prosopalgia*, constricting pains, returns at same hour daily. [*Cedron.*]

Nose.—Profuse bleeding from nose. Fluent coryza.

Throat.—Constriction of œsophagus. Dryness of tongue, as if burnt; needs much liquid to get food down. Suffocative constriction at throat, with full, throbbing carotids in angina pectoris.

Stomach.—*Constriction*, pulsation, or heaviness in stomach. Vomiting of blood.

Stool.—Hard, black stools. Diarrhœa in morning. Hæmorrhoids swollen and painful. Sensation of great weight in anus. Hæmorrhage from bowels in malarial fevers and with heart symptoms.

Urine.—Constriction of neck of bladder, causing retention of urine. Hæmorrhage from bladder. Clots of blood in urethra. Constant urination.

Female.—Constriction in uterine region and ovaries. *Dysmenorrhœa;* pulsating pain in uterus and ovaries. Vaginismus. Menses early, dark, pitch-like. [*Cocc.; Mag. c.*]; cease on lying down, with heart symptoms.

Chest.—Oppressed breathing as from a weight on chest. *Constriction in chest, as if bound, hindering respiration.* Inflammation of diaphragm. *Heart-constriction, as from an iron band.* Angina pectoris. Palpitation; pain shooting down left arm. Hæmoptysis, with convulsive, spasmodic cough. Diaphragmitis, with great difficulty of breathing.

Heart.—*Endocarditis with mitral insufficiency together with violent and rapid action.* Acts best in the incipiency of cardiac incompetence. Heart weakness of arteriosclerosis. Tobacco heart. Violent palpitation; *worse lying on left side, at approach of menses.* Angina pectoris, with suffocation, cold sweat, and ever-present iron-band feeling. Pain in apex, shooting down left arm. Palpitation, with vertigo, dyspnœa, flatulence. *Constriction;* very acute pains and stitches in heart; pulse feeble, irregular, quick, without strength. Endocardial murmurs, excessive impulse, increased præcordial dullness, enlarged ventricle. Low blood pressure.

Extremities.—Œdema of hands and feet. Hands soft; feet enlarged. Numbness of left arm. Icy-cold hands. Restless legs.

Sleep.—Sleepless on account of pulsation in different parts of body. Frightful dreams.

Fever.—Fever every day at same hour. Coldness in back and icy-cold hands. Intermittent; paroxysms about midday (11 a. m.) incomplete in their stages, accompanied by hæmorrhages. Coldness predominates; cold sweat, with great anguish. Persistent *subnormal* temperature.

Modalities.—*Worse,* about noon, lying on left side; walking, going upstairs, 11 a. m. and 11 p. m. *Better,* open air.

Relationship.—Antidotes: *Acon.; Camph.; China.*

Compare: *Digital.; Spigel.; Convallar.; Kalmia; Naja; Magnol.*

Dose.—Tincture (best made from flowers), to third attenuation. Higher in nervous palpitation.

CADMIUM SULPH.
(Cadmic Sulphate)

Its pathogenesis gives symptoms corresponding to very low forms of disease, as in cholera, *yellow fever*, where, with exhaustion, vomiting, and *extreme prostration*, the disease runs deathward. Important gastric symptoms. Carcinoma ventriculi; persistent vomiting.

The attack is upon the stomach more especially. Patients must keep quiet. *Chilliness and coldness* even when near the fire.

Mind and Head.—Unconscious. Vertigo; room and bed seem to spin around. Hammering in head. Heat in head.

Nose.—*Ozæna*. Tightness at root. Nose obstructed; *polypus*. Caries of nasal bones. Boils on nose. Nostrils ulcerated.

Eyes.—*Opacity of cornea*. Blue circle around eyes. One pupil dilated. Night blindesss.

Face.—Distortion of mouth. Trembling of jaw. *Facial paralysis;* more left side.

Mouth.—Difficult swallowing. Œsophagus constricted. [*Bapt.*] Salty belching. Intense nausea, with pain and cold. Stringy, offensive exudation on mucous membrane. Salty taste.

Throat.—Sore throat, constant tickling; gagging and nausea, worse deep breathing; chilliness and aching.

Stomach.—Soreness in pit of stomach on pressure. Violent *nausea;* retching. *Black vomit*. Vomiting of mucus, green slime, blood, with great prostration, and great tenderness over the stomach. Burning and cutting pains in stomach. Carcinoma, helps the persistent vomiting. Coffee ground vomiting.

Abdomen.—Sore, tender, tympanitic. Region of liver sore. Coldness. Black, offensive clots of blood from bowels. Pain in abdomen, with vomiting. Tenderness and tympanites.

Stool.—Bloody, black, and offensive. Gelatinous, yellowish green; semi-fluid, with urinary suppression.

Urine.—Rawness and soreness in urethra, urine mixed with pus and blood.

Heart.—Palpitation, with constriction of chest.

Fever.—*Icy coldness.* [*Camph.; Verat.; Heloderm.*] *Yellow fever.* [*Crotalus; Carbo.*]

Skin.—Blue, yellow, sallow, scaly, cracking. Itching; better scratching. Chloasma, yellowish stains on nose and cheeks; worse exposure to sun and wind. Chilblains.

Sleep.—Stops breathing on going to sleep. Wakes up suffocating. Fears to go to sleep again. Protracted sleeplessness.

Modalities.—*Worse,* walking or carrying burdens; after sleep; from open air, stimulants. *Better,* eating and rest.

Relationship.—Compare: *Cadmium oxide; Cad. brom.* (pain and burning in stomach, and vomiting); *Cadmium jodat.* (Itching of anus and rectum felt during the day only; constipation, frequent desire, tenesmus, abdomen bloated); *Zinc.; Ars.; Carbo; Verat.*

Dose.—Third to thirtieth potency.

CAHINCA
(Brazilian Plant—Chiococca)

This remedy has been found of use in dropsical affections. Its urinary symptoms are well marked. Albuminuria, with dyspnœa on lying down at night. Ascites and anasarca, with dry skin.

Urinary.—Constant desire to urinate. Polyuria while traveling. Urine fiery. Burning pain in urethra, especially glandular portion.

Male.—Drawing in of testicles and spermatic cord. Pain worse during passage of pungent smelling urine.

Back.—Pain in region of kidneys; better lying bent backward. General fatigue.

Relationship.—Compare: *Apocyn.; Ars.; Coffea* (similar botanically and in relieving effects of fatigue).

Dose.—Third potency or lower.

CAJUPUTUM (OLEUM WITTNEBIANUM)
(Cajuput Oil)

Acts like Oil of Cloves. A remedy for *flatulence* and affections of the tongue. *Sense of enlargement.* Causes copious diaphoresis. Retrocedent gout. Neuralgic affections not inflammatory. Nervous dyspnœa.

Head.—Feels much enlarged. As if he could not get himself together. [*Baptisia.*]

Mouth.—Persistent sensation of choking. *Spasmodic stricture of œsophagus.* Constricted sensation on swallowing solid food. *Tongue feels swollen,* fills whole mouth.

Stomach.—*Hiccough,* on slightest provocation.

Abdomen.—*Flatulence colic;* tympanites. [*Tereb.*] Nervous distention of bowels. Urine smells like cat's urine. Spasmodic cholera.

Modalities.—*Worse,* about 5 a. m.; night.

Relationship.—Compare: Bovist.; Nux mosch.; Asaf.; Ign.; Bapt.

Dose.—First to third potency. (5 drops of oil.)

CALADIUM SEGUINUM
(American Arum)

This remedy has a marked action on the genital organs, and pruritus of this region. Coldness of single parts and inclination to lie down, with aggravation on lying on left side. Slightest noise startles from sleep. *Dread from motion.* Modifies craving for tobacco. Tobacco heart. Asthmatic complaints.

Head.—Headaches and mental states of smokers. Very forgetful, does not know about the occurrences of things. Confused headache with pain in shoulder, pressure in eyes and forehead; extremely sensitive to noise, throbbing in ear.

Stomach.—Gnawing in orifice of stomach, which prevents deep breathing, and eructations. Eructations. *Stomach feels full of dry food; sensation of fluttering.* Acrid vomiting, thirstless and tolerates only warm drinks. Sighing respiration.

Male.—*Pruritus.* Glans very red. Organs seem larger, puffed, relaxed, cold, sweating; skin of scrotum thick. Erections when half-asleep; cease when fully awake. *Impotency;*

relaxation of penis during excitement. No emission and no orgasm during embrace.

Female.—*Pruritus of vulva* [*Ambr.; Kreos.*] and vagina during pregnancy. (Hydrogen peroxyd 1 : 12 locally). Voluptuousness. Cramp pains in uterus at night.

Skin.—Sweet sweat—attracts flies. Insect bites burn and itch intensely. Itching rash alternates with asthma. *Burning sensation* and erysipelatous inflammation.

Respiratory.—Larynx seems constricted. Breathing impeded. Catarrhal asthma; mucus not readily raised. Patient afraid to go to sleep.

Modalities.—*Better*, after sweat, after sleeping in daytime. *Worse*, motion.

Relationship.—Incompatible: *Arum triph.*

Complementary: *Nitr. ac.*

Compare: *Capsic.; Phosph.; Caust.; Selen.; Lyc. Ikshugandha* (sexual weakness, emissions, prostatic enlargement).

Dose.—Third to sixth attenuation.

CALCAREA ACETICA
(Acetate of Lime)

Has had brilliant clinical results in inflammations of mucous membranes characterized by a *membranous exudation;* otherwise its action and application is like the carbonate. Cancer pains.

Head.—Vertigo in open air. *Senses obscure while reading. Megrim*, with great coldness in head and sour taste.

Female.—Membranous dysmenorrhœa [*Borax.*].

Respiratory.—Rattling expiration. *Cough loose, with expectoration of large pieces* like casts of bronchial tubes. Breathing difficult; better bending shoulders backward. Constrictive anxious sensation in chest.

Relationship.—Compare: *Brom.; Borax;* also *Calc. oxal.* in excruciating pains of open cancer.

Dose.—Third trituration.

CALCAREA ARSENICA
(Arsenite of Lime)

Epilepsy with rush of blood to the head before attack; aura felt in region of heart; flying sensation. Complaints in fat women around climacteric. Chronic malaria. Infantile enlarged liver and spleen. *Nephritis*, with great sensitivenss in kikney region. Complaints of drunkards after abstaining. [*Carbon. sulph.*] Fleshy women at climacteric, *slightest emotion causing palpitation*. Dyspnœa, with feeble heart. *Chilliness*. Albuminuria. Dropsy. Affections of spleen and mesenteric glands. Hæmoglobin and red corpuscles are low.

Mind.—Anger, anxiety. Desire for company. Confusion, delusions, illusions, Great depression.

Head.—Violent rush of blood to head with vertigo. Pain in head *better by lying on painful side*. Weekly headache. Benumbing headache mostly around ears.

Stomach.—Region of stomach distended. Enlarged liver and spleen in children. Pancreatic disease; relieves burning pain in cancer of pancreas. Belching with saliva and beating of heart.

Urinary.—*Kidney region sensitive to pressure*. Albuminuria, passes urine every hour.

Heart.—Constriction and pain in region of heart, suffocating feeling, *palpitation*, oppression and throbbing and pain in back extending to arms.

Female.—Offensive, bloody leucorrhœa. Cancer of uterus; burning pain in uterus and vagina.

Back.—Pain and stiffness near nape of neck. Violent backache, throbbing, drives out of bed.

Extremities.—Removes inflammatory products in veins of lower extremities. Weariness and lameness of lower limbs.

Modalities.—Worse from slight exertion.

Dose.—Third trituration.

CALCAREA CARBONICA—OSTREARUM
(Carbonate of Lime)

This great Hahnemannian anti-psoric is a constitutional remedy *par excellence*. Its chief action is centered in the vegetative sphere, impaired nutrition being the keynote of its action, the glands, skin, and bones, being instrumental in the changes wrought. Increased local and general perspiration, swelling of glands, scrofulous and rachitic conditions generally offer numerous opportunities for the exhibition of Calcarea. Incipient phthisis. [*Ars. jod.; Tuberculin.*] It covers the tickling cough, fleeting chest pains, nausea, acidity and dislike of fat. Gets out of breath easily. *A jaded state, mental or physical, due to overwork. Abscesses in deep muscles; polypi and exostoses.* Pituitary and thyroid disfunction.

Raised blood coagulability [*Strontium*]. Is a definite stimulant to the periosteum. Is a hæmostatic and gives this power probably to the gelatine injections.

Easy relapses, interrupted convalescence. Persons of scrofulous type, who take cold easily, with increased mucous secretions, children who grow fat, are large-bellied, with large head, pale skin, chalky look, the so-called leuco-phlegmatic temperament; affections caused by working in water. Great sensitiveness to cold; partial sweats. Children crave eggs and eat dirt and other indigestible things; are prone to diarrhœa. Calcarea patient is fat, fair, flabby and perspiring and cold, damp and sour.

Mind.—*Apprehensive;* worse towards evening; *fears loss of reason, misfortune,* contagious diseases. *Forgetful,* confused, low-spirited. Anxiety with palpitation. Obstinacy; slight mental effort produces hot head. Averse to work or exertion.

Head.—Sense of weight on top of head. Headache, with cold hands and feet. Vertigo on ascending, and when turning head. Headache from overlifting, from mental exertion, with nausea. Head feels hot and heavy, with pale face. *Icy coldness in, and on the head,* especially right side. Open fontanelles; head enlarged; *much perspiration, wets the pillow.* Itching of the scalp. Scratches head on waking.

Eyes.—Sensitive to light. Lachrymation in open air and early in morning. *Spots and ulcers on cornea.* Lachrymal ducts closed from exposure to cold. Easy fatigue of eyes. **Far-sighted.** Itching of lids, swollen, scurfy. *Chronic dilatation of pupils.* Cataract. Dimness of vision, as if looking through a mist. Lachrymal fistula; scrofulous ophthalmia.

Ears.—Throbbing; cracking in ears; stitches; pulsating pain as if something would press out. Deafness from working in water. Polypi which bleed easily. Scrofulous inflammation *with muco-purulent otorrhœa, and enlarged glands.* Perversions of hearing; hardness of hearing. Eruption on and behind ear [*Petrol.*] Cracking noises in ear. Sensitive to cold about ears and neck.

Nose.—Dry, *nostrils sore, ulcerated.* Stoppage of nose, also with fetid, yellow discharge. Offensive odor in nose. *Polypi;* swelling at root of nose. Epistaxis. Coryza. *Takes cold at every change of weather.* Catarrhal symptoms with hunger; coryza alternates with colic.

Face.—Swelling of upper lip. Pale, with deep-seated eyes, surrounded by dark rings. Crusta lactea; itching, burning after washing. Submaxillary glands swollen. Goitre. Itching of pimples in whiskers. Pain from right mental foramen along lower jaw to ear.

Mouth.—Persistent *sour taste.* Mouth fills with sour water. Dryness of tongue at night. Bleeding of gums. Difficult and delayed dentition. Teeth ache; excited by current of air, anything cold or hot. Offensive smell from mouth. Burning pain at tip of tongue; worse, anything warm taken into stomach.

Throat.—*Swelling of tonsils* and submaxillary glands; stitches on swallowing. Hawking-up of mucus. Difficult swallowing. *Goitre.* Parotid fistula.

Stomach.—Aversion to meat, boiled things; *craving for indigestible things—chalk, coal, pencils;* also for eggs, salt and sweets. Milk disagrees. *Frequent sour eructations; sour vomiting. Dislike of fat. Loss of appetite when overworked.* Heartburn and loud belching. Cramps in stomach; worse, pressure, cold water. Ravenous hunger. Swelling over pit of stomach, like a saucer turned bottom up. Repugnance to hot food. Pain in epigastric region to touch. Thirst; longing for *cold* drinks. Aggravation while eating. Hyperchlorhydria [*Phos.*].

Abdomen.—Sensitive to slightest pressure. Liver region painful when stooping. Cutting in abdomen; Swollen abdomen. Incarcerated flatulence. *Inguinal and mesenteric glands swollen* and painful. Cannot bear tight clothing around the waist. *Distention* with hardness. *Gall-stone colic.* Increase of fat in abdomen. Umbilical hernia. Trembling; weakness, as if sprained. Children are late in learning to walk.

Stool.—Crawling and constriction in rectum. Stool large and hard [*Bry.*]; whitish, watery, *sour*. Prolapse ani, and burning, stinging hæmorrhoids. Diarrhœa of undigested, food, fetid, with ravenous appeite. *Children's diarrhœa.* Constipation; stool at first hard, then pasty, then liquid.

Urine.—Dark, brown, sour, fetid, abundant, with white sediment, bloody. Irritable bladder. Enuresis. (Use 30th, also *Tuberculin.* 1 *m.*)

Male.—*Frequent emissions.* Increased desire. Semen emitted too soon. Coition followed by weakness and irritability.

Female.—Before menses, headache, colic, chilliness and leucorrhœa. Cutting pains in uterus during menstruation. Menses *too early, too profuse, too long,* with vertigo, toothache and *cold, damp feet;* the least excitement causes their return. Uterus easily displaced. Leucorrhœa, *milky* [*Sepia*]. Burning and itching of parts before and after menstruation; in little girls. Increased sexual desire; easy conception. Hot swelling breasts. Breasts tender and swollen before menses. Milk too abundant; disagreeable to child. Deficient lactation, with distended breasts in lymphatic women. Much sweat about external genitals. Sterility with copious menses. Uterine polypi.

Respiratory.—Tickling cough troublesome at night, dry and free expectoration in morning; cough when playing piano, or by eating. Persistent, irritating cough form arsenical wall paper. (Clarke.) Extreme dyspnœa. *Painless hoarseness;* worse in the morning. Expectoration only during the day; thick, yellow, sour mucus. Bloody expectoration; with sour sensation in chest. *Suffocating spells;* tightness, burning and soreness in chest; *worse going upstairs* or slightest ascent, must sit down. Sharp pains in chest from before backwards. *Chest very sensitive to touch, percussion, or pressure.* Longing for fresh air. Scanty, salty expectoration. [*Lyc.*]

Heart.—Palpitation at night and after eating. Palpitation with feeling of coldness, with restless oppression of chest; after suppressed eruption.

Back.—Pain as if sprained; can scarcely rise; from overlifting. Pain between shoulder-blades, impeding breathing. Rheumatism in lumbar region; weakness in small of back. Curvature of dorsal vertebræ. Nape of neck stiff and rigid. *Renal colic.*

Extremities.—Rheumatoid pains, as after exposure to wet. Sharp sticking, as if parts were wrenched or sprained. *Cold, damp* feet; feel as if damp stockings were worn. Cold knees. cramps in calves. Sour foot-sweat. Weakness of extremities. Swelling of joints, especially knee. Burning of soles of feet. Sweat of hands. Arthritic nodosities. *Soles of feet raw.* Feet feel cold and dead at night. Old sprains. Tearing in muscles.

Sleep.—Ideas crowding in her mind prevent sleep. Horrid visions when opening eyes. Starts at every noise; fears that she will go crazy. Drowsy in early part of evening. Frequent waking at night. *Same disagreeable idea always arouses from light slumber.* Night terrors [*Kali phos.*] Dreams of the dead.

Fever.—*Chill at 2 p. m. begins internally in stomach region. Fever with sweat.* Pulse full and frequent. Chilliness and heat. Partial sweats. *Night sweats, especially on head,* neck and chest. Hectic fever. Heat at night during menstruation, with restless sleep. *Sweat over head in children, so that pillow becomes wet.*

Skin.—Unhealthy; readily ulcerating; flacid. Small wounds do not heal readily. Glands swollen. Nettle rash; better in cold air. Warts on face and hands. *Petechial eruptions.* Chilblains. Boils.

Modalities.—*Worse,* from exertion, mental or physical; ascending; cold in every form; water, washing, moist air, wet weather; during full moon; standing. *Better,* dry climate and weather; lying on painful side. Sneezing (pain in head and nape).

Relationship.—Antidotes: *Camph.; Ipec.; Nit ac.; Nux.* Complementary: *Bell.; Rhus; Lycop.; Silica.*

Calcar. is useful after Sulphur where the pupils remain dilated. When Pulsatilla failed in school girls.

Incompatible: *Bry.;* Sulphur should not be given *after* Calc.

Compare: *Aqua calcar.*—Lime-water—(½ teaspoonful in

milk); (as injection for oxyuris vermicularis), and *Calc. caust.* —slaked lime—(pain in back and heels, jaws and malar bones; also symptoms of influenza). *Calc. brom.* (removes inflammatory products from uterus; children of lax fiber, nervous and irritable, with gastric and cerebral irritation. *Tendency to brain disease.* Insomnia and cerebral congestion. Give 1x trituration). *Sulph.* (differs in being worse by heat, hot feet, etc.).

Calcar. calcinata—Calcined oyster-shell—a remedy for warts. Use 3d trituration. *Calcarea ovorum. Ova tosta*—Toasted egg-shells—(*backache and leucorrhœa*. Feeling as if back were broken in two; tired feeling. Also effective in controlling suffering from cancer).

Calcar. lactic. (anemias, hæmophilia, urticaria, where the coagulability of the blood is diminished; nervous headache with œdema of eyelids, lips or hands; 15 grains three times a day, but low potencies often equally effective).

Calcar. lacto-phosph. (5 grains 3 times a day in cyclic vomiting and migraine).

Calc. mur.—*Calcium chloratum*—Rademacher's Liquor—(1 part to 2 of distilled water, of which take 15 drops in half a cup of water, five times daily. Boils. *Porrigo capitis. Vomiting of all food and drink*, with gastric pain. Impetigo, glandular swellings, angioneurotic œdema. Pleurisy with effusion. Eczema in infants).

Calcar. picrata, (peri-follicular inflammation; a remedy of prime importance in *recurring or chronic boils*, particularly when located on parts thinly covered with muscle tissue, as on shinbones, coccyx, *auditory canal*, dry, scurfy accumulation and exfoliation of epithelial scales, etc., styes, phlyctenules. Use 3x trit.)

Compare also with Calcarea: *Lycop.; Silica; Pulsat.; Chamom.*

Dose.—Sixth trit. Thirtieth and higher potencies. Should not be repeated too frequently in elderly people.

CALCAREA FLUORICA—FLUOR SPAR.
(Fluoride of Lime)

A powerful tissue remedy for hard, stony glands, varicose and enlarged veins, and malnutrition of bones. Hard knots in female breast. Goitre. Congenital hereditary syphilis. *Induration threatening suppuration.* Many cases of cataract have undoubtedly been influenced favorably by it. Congenital syphilis manifesting itself in ulceration of mouth and throat, caries and necrosis with boring pains and heat in parts. Arteriosclerosis; threatened apoplexy. Tuberculosis. Used after operations, the tendency to adhesions is reduced.

Mind.—Great depression; groundless fears of financial ruin.

Head.—Creaking noise in head. Blood-tumors of newborn infants. Hard excrescences on the scalp. Ulcers on the scalp with callous, hard edges.

Eyes.—Flickering and sparks before the eyes, spots on the cornea; conjunctivitis; cataract. *Strumous phlyctenular keratitis. Subcutaneous palpebral cysts.*

Ears.—Calcareous deposits on tympanum; sclerosis of ossicula and petrous portion of temporal bone, with deafness, ringing and roaring. *Chronic suppuration of middle ear.*

Nose.—Cold in the head; stuffy cold; dry coryza; ozæna. Copious, offensive, thick, greenish, lumpy, yellow nasal catarrh. Atrophic rhinitis, especially if crusts are prominent.

Face.—Hard swelling on the cheek, with pain or toothache, hard swelling on jaw-bone.

Mouth.—Gum-boil, with hard swelling on the jaw. Cracked appearance of the tongue, with or without pain. Induration of the tongue, hardening after inflammation. Unnatural looseness of the teeth, with or without pain; teeth become loose in their sockets. Toothache, with pain if any food touches the tooth.

Throat.—Follicular sore throat; plugs of mucus are continually forming in the crypts of the tonsils. Pain and burning in throat; better by warm drinks; worse, cold drinks. Hypertrophy of Luschka's tonsil. Relaxed uvula, tickling referred to larynx.

Stomach.—Vomiting of infants. Vomiting of undigested food. Hiccough [*Cajup.*; *Sulph.* ac.]. Flatulency. Weakness and daintiness of appetite, nausea and distress after eating in young children who are overtaxed by studies. *Acute indigestion from fatigue* and brain-fag; much flatulence.

Stool and Anus.—Diarrhœa in gouty subjects. Itching of anus. Fissure of the anus, and intensely sore crack near the lower end of the bowel. Bleeding hæmorrhoids. Itching of anus as from pin-worms. Internal or blind piles frequently, with pain in back, generally far down on the sacrum, and constipation. Much wind in lower bowels. Worse, pregnancy.

Male.—Hydrocele; indurations of the testicles.

Respiratory Organs.—Hoarseness. *Croup*. Cough with expectoration of tiny lumps of yellow mucus, with tickling sensation and irritation on lying down. Spasmodic cough. *Calc. Fluor.* removes fibroid deposits about the endocardium and restores normal endocardial structure. (Eli G. Jones, M. D.)

Circulatory Organs.—Chief remedy for vascular tumors with dilated blood-vessels, and for *varicose or enlarged veins*. Aneurism. Valvular disease. When the tuberculous toxins attack the heart and blood-vessels.

Neck and Back.—Chronic *lumbago;* aggravated on beginning to move, and ameliorated on continued motion. Osseous tumors. *Rachitic enlargement of femur in infants*. Pain lower part of back, with burning.

Extremities.—Ganglia or encysted tumors at the back of the wrist. Gouty enlargements of the joints of the fingers. Exostoses on fingers. Chronic synovitis of knee-joint.

Sleep.—Vivid dreams, with sense of impending danger. Unrefreshing sleep.

Skin.—Marked whiteness of skin. Scar tissue; adhesions after operations. Chaps and cracks. Fissures or cracks in the palms of the hands, or hard skin. Fissure of the anus. Suppurations with callous, hard edges. Whitlow. Indolent, fistulous ulcers, secreting thick, yellow pus. Hard, elevated edges of ulcer, surrounding skin purple and swollen. Knots, kernels, hardened glands in the female breast. *Swellings or indurated enlargements* having their seat in the fasciæ and capsular ligaments of joints, or in the tendons. *Indurations of stony hardness*.

Modalities.—*Worse*, during rest, changes of weather. *Better*, heat, warm applications.

Relationship.—Compare: *Con.; Lapis; Baryt. mur.; Hecla: Rhus; Cacodylate of Soda* (Tumors).

Calcar. sulph-stibiata (acts as an hæmostatic and absorptive in uterine myoma).

Mangifera indica (varicose veins).

Dose.—Third to twelfth trituration. A "chronic" remedy. Needs some time before manifesting its effects. Should not be repeated too frequently.

CALCAREA IODATA
(Iodide of Lime)

It is in the treatment of scrofulous affections, especially enlarged glands, tonsils, etc., that this remedy has gained marked beneficial results. Thyroid enlargements about time of puberty. Flabby children subject to colds. Secretions inclined to be profuse and yellow. Adenoids. Uterine fibroids. *Croup*.

Head.—Headache while riding against cold wind. Light-headed. Catarrh; worse at root of nose; sneezing; very little sensation. Polypi of nose and ear.

Throat.—Enlarged tonsils are filled with little crypts.

Respiratory.—Chronic cough; Pain in chest, difficulty breathing after syphilis and mercurialization (Grauvogl). Hectic fever; green, purulent expectoration. Croup. *Pneumonia*.

Skin.—*Indolent ulcers, accompanying varicose veins*. Easy perspiration. Copper-colored and papulous eruptions, tinea, favus, crusta lactea, swelling of the glands, skin cracked, falling out of hair.

Relationship.—Compare: *Agraphis*—Bluebell (adenoids with enlarged tonsils). Here *Sulph. iod.* follows both *Agraphis* and *Calc. iod. Acon. lycotonum* (swelling of glands, Hodgkin's disease).

Compare also: *Calc. fluor.; Sil.; Merc. iod.*

Dose.—Second and third trituration.

CALCAREA PHOSPHORICA
(Phosphate of Lime)

One of the most important tissue remedies, and while it has many symptoms in common with *Calcarea carb.*, there are some differences and characteristic features of its own. It is especially indicated in tardy dentition and troubles incident to that period, bone disease, non-union of fractured bones, and the anæmias after acute diseases and chronic wasting diseases. *Anæmic children who are peevish, flabby, have cold extremities and feeble digestion.* It has a special affinity where bones form sutures or symphyses, and all its symptoms are worse from any change of weather. *Numbness and crawling* are characteristic sensations, and tendency to perspiration and glandular enlargement are symptoms it shares with the carbonate. Scrophulosis, chlorosis and phthisis.

Mind.—Peevish, forgetful; after grief and vexation. [*Ignat.; Phos. ac.*] Always wants to go somewhere.

Head.—Headache, *worse near the region of sutures, from change of weather*, of school children about puberty. Fontanelles remain open too long. Cranial bones soft and thin. Defective hearing. Headache, with abdominal flatulence. Head hot, with smarting of roots of hair.

Eyes.—Diffused opacity in cornea following abscess.

Mouth.—Swollen tonsils; cannot open mouth without pain. Complaints during teething; teeth develop slowly; rapid decay of teeth. *Adenoid growths.*

Stomach.—Infant wants to nurse all the time and vomits easily. *Craving for bacon, ham, salted or smoked meats. Much flatulence.* Great hunger with thirst, flatulence temporarily relieved by sour eructations. Heartburn. Easy vomiting in children.

Abdomen.—*At every attempt* to eat, colicky pain in abdomen. *Sunken and flabby.* Colic, soreness and burning around navel.

Stool.—Bleeding after hard stool. Diarrhœa from juicy fruits or cider; during dentition. Green, slimy, *hot*, sputtering, undigested, *with fetid flatus*. Fistula in ano, alternating with chest symptoms.

Urine.—Increased, with sensation of weakness. Pain in region of kidneys when lifting or blowing the nose.

CALCAREA PHOSPHORICA

Female.—Menses too early, excessive, and bright in girls. If late, blood is dark; sometimes, first bright, then dark, with *violent backache*. During lactation with sexual excitement. Nymphomania, with aching, pressing, or weakness in uterine region. [*Plat.*] After prolonged nursing. Leucorrhœa, like *white of egg*. Worse morning. Child refuses breast; milk tastes salty. Prolapsus in debilitated persons.

Respiratory.—Involuntary sighing. Chest sore. Suffocative cough; better lying down. Hoarseness. Pain through lower left lung.

Neck and Back.—Rheumatic pain from draught of air, with stiffness and dullness of head. Soreness in sacro-iliac symphysis, as if broken. [*Æsc. hip.*]

Extremities.—Stiffness and pain, *with cold, numb* feeling, worse any change of weather. Crawling and coldness. Buttocks, back and limbs asleep. Pains in joints and bones. Weary when going upstairs.

Relationship.—Complementary: *Ruta; Hepar.*

Compare: *Calcar. hypophosporosa* (is to be preferred when it seems necessary to furnish the organism with liberal doses of phosphorus in consequence of continued abscesses having reduced the vitality. Give first and second decimal trits. Loss of appetite, rapid debility, night sweats; Acne pustulosa.— Pallor of skin, habitually *cold extremities*. Phthisis—diarrhœa and cough; acute pains in chest. Mesenteric tuberculosis. Bleeding from lungs; angina pectoris; asthma; affection of arteries. Veins stand out like whipcords. Attacks of pain occurring two hours after meals (relieved by a cup of milk or light food). *Cheiranthus* (effects of cutting wisdom teeth). *Calcarea renalis*—Lapis renalis—(arthritic nodosities. Rigg's disease; lessens tendency to accumulation of tartar on teeth; gravel and renal calculi). *Conchiolin.*—Mater perlarum.— Mother of pearl (Osteitis.—Has a wide range of action in bone affections, especially when the growing ends are affected. Petechiæ). *Silica; Psorin.; Sulph.*

Modalities.—*Worse*, exposure to damp, cold weather, melting snow. *Better, in summer;* warm, dry atmosphere.

Dose.—First to third trituration. Higher potencies often more effective.

CALCAREA SILICATA
(Silicate of Lime)

A deep, long acting medicine for complaints which come on slowly and reach their final development after long periods. Hydrogenoid constitution [*Nat. sulph.*]. Very sensitive to *cold*. *Patient is weak, emaciated, cold and chilly, but worse from being overheated;* sensitive generally. Atrophy of children.

Mind.—Absent-minded, irritable, irresolute, lacks self-confidence. *Fearful.*

Head.—Vertigo, head cold, especially at vertex; catarrh of nose and posterior nares, discharge thick, yellow, hard crusts. Corneal exudation.

Stomach.—Sensation of coldness, especially when empty. Sinking sensation at pit. Great thirst. Flatulence and distention after eating. Vomiting and eructations.

Female.—Uterus heavy, prolapsed. Leucorrhœa, painful and irregular menses. Flow between periods.

Respiratory.—Sensitive to cold air. Difficult respiration. Chronic irritation of air passages. Copious, yellow-green mucus. Coughs with coldness, weakness, emaciation, sensitiveness and peevishness, worse from cold air. Pain in chest walls.

Skin.—Itching, burning, cold and blue, very sensitive. Pimples, comedones, wens. Psoric eruptions.

Relationship.—Compare: *Arsenic; Tubercul.; Baryt. carb.; Iod.*

Dose.—All potencies from lowest to high.

CALCAREA SULPHURICA
(Sulphate of Lime—Plaster of Paris)

Eczema and torpid glandular swellings. Cystic tumors. Fibroids. Suppurative processes come within the range of this remedy, after pus has found a vent. *Mucous discharges are yellow, thick and lumpy.* Lupus vulgaris.

Head.—Scald-head of children, if there be purulent discharge, or yellow, purulent crusts.

Eyes.—*Inflammation of the eyes, with discharge of thick, yellow matter.* Sees only one-half an object. Cornea smoky. Ophthalmia neonatorum.

CALCAREA SULPHURICA

Ears.—Deafness, with discharge of matter from the middle ear, sometimes mixed with blood. Pimples around ear.

Nose.—Cold in the head, with thick, *yellowish, purulent secretion*, frequently tinged with blood. One-sided discharge from nose. *Yellowish discharge* from posterior nares. Edges of nostrils sore.

Face.—*Pimples and pustules on the face.* Herpes.

Mouth.—Inside of lips sore. Tongue flabby, resembling a layer of dried clay. Sour, soapy, acrid taste. Yellow coating at base.

Throat.—Last stage of ulcerated sore throat, with discharge of yellow matter. Suppurating stage of tonsillitis, when abscess is discharging.

Abdomen.—Pain in region of liver, in right side of pelvis, followed by weakness, nausea, and pain in stomach.

Stool.—Purulent diarrhœa mixed with blood. Diarrhœa after maple sugar and from change of weather. Pus-like, slimy discharge from the bowels. *Painful abscesses about the anus* in cases of fistula.

Female.—Menses late, long-lasting, with headache, twitching great weakness.

Respiratory.—Cough, with purulent and sanious sputa and hectic fever. Empyema, pus forming in the lungs or pleural cavities. Purulent, sanious expectoration. Catarrh, with thick, lumpy, white-yellow or pus-like secretion.

Extremities.—*Burning-itching of soles of feet.*

Fever.—Hectic fever, caused by formation of pus. With cough and burning in soles.

Skin.—Cuts, wounds, bruises, etc., unhealthy, discharging pus; they do not heal readily. Yellow, purulent crusts or discharge. Purulent exudations in or upon the skin. Skin affections with yellowish scabs. Many little matterless pimples under the hair, bleeding when scratched. Dry eczema in children.

Relationship.—Compare: *Hepar; Silica.*

Dose.—Second and third trituration. The twelfth potency has been found effective in Lupus.

CALENDULA OFFICINALIS
(Marigold)

A most remarkable healing agent, applied locally. Useful for open wounds, parts that will not heal, ulcers, etc. Promotes healthy granulations and rapid healing by first intention. Hæmostatic after tooth extraction. Deafness. Catarrhal conditions. Neuroma. Constitutional tendency to erysipelas. Pain is excessive and out of all proportion to injury. *Great disposition to take cold, especially in damp weather.* Paralysis after apoplexy. Cancer, as an intercurrent remedy. Has remarkable power to produce local exudation and helps to make acrid discharge healthy and free. Cold hands.

Head.—Extremely nervous; easily frightened; tearing headache; weight on brain. Submaxillary glands swollen, painful to touch. Pain in right side of neck. Lacerated *scalp* wounds.

Eyes.—Injuries to eyes which tend to suppuration; after operations; blenorrhœa of lachrymal sac.

Ears.—Deafness; worse in *damp* surroundings and with eczematous conditions. Hears best on a train, and distant sounds.

Nose.—Coryza in one nostril; with much green discharge.

Stomach.—Hunger immediately after nursing. Bulimia. *Heartburn with horripilations.* Nausea in *chest*. Vomiting. Sinking sensation. Epigastric *distention*.

Respiratory.—Cough, with green expectoration, hoarseness; with distention of inguinal ring.

Female.—*Warts at the os externum.* Menses suppressed, with cough. Chronic endocervicitis. Uterine hypertrophy, sensation of weight and fullness in pelvis; stretching and dragging in groin; pain on sudden movements. Os lower than natural. Menorrhagia.

Skin.— *Yellow;* goose-flesh. Promotes favorable cicatrization, with least amount of suppuration. Slough, proud flesh, and raised edges. Superficial burns and scalds. Erysipelas (use topically).

Fever.—*Coldness, great sensitiveness to open air;* shuddering in back, skin feels warm to touch. Heat in evening.

Modalities.—*Worse*, in damp, *heavy, cloudy* weather.

Relationship.—Compare: *Hamamel.; Hyperic.; Symph.; Arn.*

Compare in deafness: *Ferr. pic.; Kal. iod.; Calc.; Mag. .c; Graph.*

Antidote: *Chelidon.; Rheum*

Complementary: *Hepar.*

Dose.—Locally, Aqueous Calendula [*Marigoldin.*] for all wounds, the greatest healing agent. Also as an injection in leucorrhœa; internally, tincture, to third potency. For burns, sores, fissures, and abrasions, etc., use Calendula Cerate.

CALOTROPIS
(Madar Bark)

Has been used with marked success in the treatment of *syphilis* following Mercury; also, in elephantiasis, leprosy, and acute dysentery. Pneumonic phthisis. Tuberculosis.

Increases the circulation in the skin; has powerful effects as a sudorific. In the secondary symptoms of syphilis, where Mercury has been used but cannot be pushed safely any farther, it rapidly recruits the constitution, heals the ulcers and blotches from the skin, and perfects the cure. *Primary anæmia of syphilis. Heat in stomach* is a good guiding symptom. *Obesity*, while flesh decreases, muscles become harder and firmer.

Relationship.—Compare: *Merc.; Potass. iod.; Berb. aqui.; Sarsap; Ipecac.*

Dose.—Tincture, one to five drops; three times a day.

CALTHA PALUSTRIS
(Cowslip)

Pain in abdomen, vomiting, headache, singing in ears, dysuria and diarrhœa. Anasarca.

Skin.—Pemphigus. Bullæ are surrounded by a ring. Much itching. Face much swollen, especially around the eyes. Itching eruption on thighs. Pustules. *Uterine cancer.*

Dose.—Tincture.

CAMPHORA
(Camphor)

Hahnemann says: "The action of this substance is very puzzling and difficult of investigation, even in the healthy organism because its *primary action*, more frequently than with any other remedy, alternates and becomes intermixed with the vital reactions (after effects) of the organism. On this account it is often difficult to determine what belongs to the vital reactions of the body and *what to the alternating effects due to the primary action of the camphor.*"

Pictures a state of collapse. *Icy coldness* of the whole body; sudden sinking of strength; pulse small and weak. After operations, if temperature is subnormal, low blood pressure, 3 doses camph. 1x, 15-minute intervals. This condition is met with in cholera, and here it is that Camphor has achieved classical fame. *First stages of a cold, with chilliness and sneezing.* Subsultus and extreme restlessness. Cracking of joints. Epileptiform convulsions. Camphor has a direct relationship to muscles and fascia. In local rheumatic affections in cold climates necessary. Distention of veins. As a heart stimulant for emergency use of Camphor is the most satisfactory remedy. Drop doses on sugar as often as every five minutes.

It is characteristic of Camphor that the patient *will not be covered*, notwithstanding the icy coldness of the body. One of the main remedies in shock. *Pain better while thinking of it.* Very sensitive to cold and to touch. Sequelæ of measles. *Violent convulsion*, with wandering and hysterical excitement. Tetanic spasms. Scrofulous children and irritable, weakly blondes especially affected.

Head.—Vertigo, tendency to unconsciousness, feeling as if he would die. Influenza; headache, with catarrhal symptoms, sneezing, etc. Beating pain in cerebellum. Cold sweat. *Nose cold and pinched.* Tongue cold, flabby, trembling. *Fleeting stitches in temporal region and orbits.* Head sore. *Occipital throbbing, synchronous with the pulse.*

Eyes.—Fixed, staring; pupils dilated. Sensation as if all objects were too bright and glittering.

Nose.—Stopped; sneezing. Fluent coryza on sudden change

CAMPHORA

of weather. Cold and pinched. *Persistent epistaxis*, especially with goose-flesh state of skin.

Face.—Pale, haggard, *anxious*, distorted; *bluish*, cold. Cold sweat.

Stomach.—Pressive pain in pit of stomach. *Coldness*, followed by burning.

Stool.—Blackish; involuntary. *Asiatic cholera*, with cramps in calves, coldness of body, anguish, great weakness, *collapse*, tongue and mouth cold.

Urine.—Burning and *strangury*, with tenesmus of the neck of the bladder. Retention with full bladder.

Male.—Desire increased. Chordee. *Priapism*. Nightly emissions.

Respiratory.—Præcordial distress. Suffocative dyspnœa. Asthma. Violent, dry, hacking cough. Palpitation. *Breath cold*. Suspended respiration.

Sleep.—*Insomnia*, with cold limbs. Subsultus and extreme restlessness.

Extremities.—Rheumatic pain between shoulders. Difficult motion. Numbness, tingling and *coldness*. Cracking in joints. Cramps in calves. Icy cold feet, ache as if sprained.

Fever.—Pulse small, weak, slow. *Icy coldness of the whole body*. Cold perspiration. *Congestive chill*. *Tongue cold*, flabby, trembling.

Skin.—*Cold*, pale, blue, livid. Cannot bear to be covered. [*Secale*.]

Modalities.—*Worse*, motion, night, contact, cold air. *Better*, warmth.

Relationship.—Camphor antidotes or modifies the action of nearly every vegetable medicine—tobacco, opium, worm medicines, etc. *Laffa acutangula* (whole body ice-cold, with a restlessness and anxiety; burning thirst). *Camphoric acid*—(a prophylactic against catheter fever; cystitis 15 grains three times a day; also for prevention of night sweats).

Incompatible: *Kali nit.*

Complementary: *Canth.*

Antidotes: *Opium; Nitr sp. dulc.; Phos.*

Compare: *Carbo; Cuprum; Arsenic; Veratr*

Dose.—Tincture, in drop doses, repeated frequently, or smelling of Spirits of Camphor. Potencies are equally effective

CAMPHORA MONO-BROMATA
(Mono-bromide of Camphor)

Nervous excitability is the guiding condition. Suppression of milk. Nightly emissions. Painful erections. Paralysis agitans. Cholera infantum, and infantile convulsions. Intensifies the action of Quinine and renders it more permanent.

Mind.—Directions appear reversed, i. e., north seems south, and east seems west. Hysteria; weeping and laughing alternately. Trance-like state.

Dose.—Second trituration.

CANCHALAGUA
(Erythræa venusta—Centaury)

Used extensively as a fever remedy and bitter tonic [*Gentiana*], antimalarial and antiseptic. Of use in severe type of intermittent fever in hot countries; also, in influenza. Sore, as if bruised all over. Sensation of drops falling from and upon different spots.

Head.—Congested. Scalp feels tight; head feels as if bound; burning in eyes; buzzing in ears.

Fever.—Chill all over; worse in bed at night. Sensitive to cold trade-winds on Pacific Coast. General sore and bruised feeling; nausea and retching.

Skin.—Wrinkled like a washerwoman's. Scalp feels tight, as if drawn together by India-rubber.

Dose.—Tincture, in drop doses. Must be made from the fresh plant. Its medicinal properties are lost in the dry.

CANNABIS INDICA
(Hashish)

Inhibits the higher faculties and stimulates the imagination to a remarkable degree without any marked stimulation of the lower or animal instinct. A condition of *intense exaltation*. in which all perceptions and conceptions, all sensations and emotions are exaggerated to the utmost degree.

Subconscious or *dual nature state*. Apparently under the control of the second self, but, the original self, prevents the performance of acts which are under the domination of the second self. Apparently the two natures cannot act independently, one acting as a check upon the other. (Effects of one Dram doses by Dr. Albert Schneider.)

The experimenter feels ever and anon that he is distinct from the subject of the hashish dream and can think rationally.

Produces the most remarkable hallucinations and imaginations, *exaggeration of the duration of time and extent of space, being most characteristic*. Conception of time, space and place is gone. Extremely happy and contented, nothing troubles. Ideas crowd upon each other. Has great soothing influence in many nervous disorders, like epilepsy, mania, dementia, delirium tremens, and irritable reflexes. Exophthalmic goitre. Catalepsy.

Mind.—Excessive loquacity; *exuberance of spirits. Time seems too long; seconds seem ages; a few rods an immense distace*. Constantly theorizing. Anxious depression; constant fear of becoming insane. Mania, must constantly move. *Very forgetful; cannot finish sentence*. Is lost in delicious thought. *Uncontrollable laughter*. Delirium tremens. Clairvoyance. Emotional excitement; rapid change of mood. Cannot realize her identity, chronic vertigo as of floating off.

Head.—Feels *as if top of head were opening and shutting and as if calvarium were being lifted*. Shocks through brain. [*Aloe; Coca.*] Uræmic headache. Throbbing and weight at occiput. Headache with flatulence. *Involuntary shaking of head*. Migrain attack preceded by unusual excitement with loquacity.

Eyes.—Fixed. Letters run together when reading. Clairvoyance. Spectral illusions without terror.

Ears.—Throbbing, buzzing, and ringing. Noise like boiling water. Extreme sensitiveness to noise.

Face.—Expression drowsy and stupid. Lips glued together. *Grinding of teeth in sleep*. Mouth and lips dry. Saliva thick, frothy, and sticky.

Stomach.—Increased appetite. Pain at cardiac orifice; better, pressure. Distention. Pyloric spasm. Sensation of extreme tension in abdominal vessels—feel distended to bursting.

Rectum.—Sensation in anus as if sitting on a ball.

Urinary.—Urine loaded with slimy mucus. Must strain; *dribbling;* has to wait some time before the urine flows. Stitches and burning in urethra. Dull pain in region of right kidney.

Male.—After sexual intercourse, *backache.* Oozing of white, glairy mucus from glans. Satyriasis. Prolonged thrill. Chordee. Sensation of swelling in perineum or near anus, as if sitting on a ball.

Female.—Menses *profuse,* dark, painful, without clots. Backache during menses. Uterine colic, with great nervous agitation and sleeplessness. Sterility. [*Borax.*] Dysmenorrhœa with sexual desire.

Respiratory.—Humid asthma. Chest oppressed with deep, labored breathing.

Heart.—Palpitation awakes him. Piercing pain, with great oppression. *Pulse very slow.* [*Dig.; Kalmia; Apocyn.*]

Extremities.—*Pain across shoulders and spine; must stoop; cannot walk erect.* Thrilling through arms and hands, and from knees down. *Entire paralysis of the lower extremities.* Pain in soles and calves; sharp pains in knees and ankles; *very exhausted after a short walk.*

Sleep.—Very sleepy, but unable to do so. Obstinate and intractable forms of insomnia. Catalepsy. Dreams of dead bodies; prophetic. Nightmare.

Modalities.—*Worse,* morning; from coffee, liquor and tobacco; lying on right side. *Better* from fresh air, cold water, rest.

Relationship.—*Bellad.; Hyoscy.; Stram.; Laches.; Agaric.; Anhalon* (time sense disordered; time periods enormously overestimated, thus, minutes seem hours, etc.).

Dose.—Tincture and low attenuations.

CANNABIS SATIVA
(Hemp)

Seems to affect especially the urinary, sexual, and respiratory organs. It has characteristic sensations as of dropping water. Great fatigue, as from over-exertion; weary after meals. Choking in swallowing; things go down the wrong way. *Stuttering.* Confusion of thought and speech. Wavering speech. Wavering speech, hasty, incoherent.

Head.—Lectophobia. Vertigo; sensation of dropping water on head. Pressure on root of nose.

Eyes.—*Opacity of cornea.* Cataract from nervous disturbances, abuse of alcohol and tobacco; patient feels deeply approaching blindness. Misty sight. Pressure from back of eyes, forward. Gonorrhœal ophthalmia. Eyeballs ache. Scrofulous eye troubles. [*Sulph.; Calc.*]

Urine.—Retained, with obstinate constipation. Painful urging. Micturition in split stream. Stitches in urethra. Inflamed sensation, with soreness to touch. *Burning while urinating, extending to bladder.* Urine scalding, with spasmodic closure of sphincter. Gonorrhœa, acute stage; urethra very sensitive. Walks with legs apart. Dragging in testicles. Zigzag pain along urethra. Sexual overexcitement. Urethral caruncle [*Eucalypt.*], phimosis. Stoppage of urethra by mucus and pus.

Female.—Amenorrhœa when physical powers have been overtaxed, also with constipation.

Respiratory.—Oppression of breathing and palpitation; *must stand up.* Weight on chest; rattling wheezing breathing. Cough, with green viscid, also bloody, expectoration.

Heart.—Sensation as if drops were falling from the heart. Painful strokes and tension with palpitation. Pericarditis.

Sleep.—Frightful dreams. More tired in morning. Sleepy during day.

Extremities.—Contraction of fingers after a sprain. Dislocation of patella on going upstairs. Feet feel heavy on going upstairs. Paralytic tearing pains. Affections of the ball of the foot and under part of toes.

Modalities.—*Worse,* lying down; going upstairs.

Relationship.—Antidotes: *Camph.; Lemon juice.*

Compare: *Hedysarum*—Brazilian Burdock—(Gonorrhœa and inflammation of penis); *Canth.; Apis; Copaiva; Thuj.; Kal. nit.*

Dose.—Tincture to third attenuation. In stuttering the 30th.

CANTHARIS
(Spanish Fly)

This powerful drug produces a furious disturbance in the animal economy, attacking the urinary and sexual organs especially, perverting their function, and setting up violent inflammations, and causing a frenzied delirium, simulating hydrophobia symptoms. [*Anagallis.*] Puerperal convulsions. Produces most violent inflammation of the whole gastro-intestinal canal, especially lower bowel. Oversensitiveness of all parts. Irritation. *Raw, burning pains.* Hæmorrhages. *Intolerable, constant urging to urinate* is most characteristic. Gastric, hepatic and abdominal complaints *that are aggravated by drinking coffee.* Gastric derangements of pregnancy. *Dysuria*, with other complaints. Increases secretion of mucous membranes, tenacious mucus. The inflammations cantharis produces (bladder, kidneys, ovaries, meninges, pleuritic and pericardial membranes) are usually associated with bladder irritation.

Mind.—Furious delirium. Anxious restlessness, ending in rage. Crying, barking; worse touching larynx or drinking water. Constantly attempts to do something, but accomplishes nothing. *Acute mania,* generally of a sexual type; amorous frenzy; fiery sexual desire. Paroxysms of rage, crying, barking. *Sudden* loss of consciousness with red face.

Head.—Burning in brain. Sensation as if boiling water in brain. Vertigo; worse in open air.

Eyes.—Yellow vision. [*Santon.*] *Fiery, sparkling, staring look.* Burning in eyes.

Ears.—Sensation as if wind were coming from ear, or hot air. Bones about ear painful. [*Capsic.*]

Face.—Pale, wretched, death-like appearance. Itching vesicles on face, burning when touched. Erysipelas of face, with burning, biting heat with urinary symptoms. Hot and red.

Throat.—Tongue covered with vesicles; deeply furred; edges red. *Burning in mouth, pharynx, and throat;* vesicles in mouth. *Great difficulty in swallowing liquids.* Very *tenacious* mucus. [*Kal. bich.*] Violent spasms reproduced by touching larynx. Inflammation of throat; feels on fire. Constriction; aphthous ulceration. [*Hydr. mur.; Nit. ac.*] Scalding feeling. Burnt after taking too hot food.

Chest.—Pleurisy, as soon as effusion has taken place. Intense dyspnœa; palpitation; frequent, dry cough. *Tendency to syncope.* Short, hacking cough, blood-streaked *tenacious* mucus. Burning pains.

Stomach.—Burning sensation of œsophagus and stomach.

[*Carb.*] Disgust for everything—drink, food, **tobacco**. Burning thirst, with aversion to all fluids. Very sensitive, *violent burning*. Vomiting of blood-streaked membrane and violent retching. *Aggravation from drinking coffee;* drinking the smallest quantity increases pain in bladder, and is vomited. Thirst unquenchable.

Stool.—*Shivering with burning.* Dysentery; mucous stools, *like scrapings of intestines.* Bloody, with *burning* and *tenesmus and shuddering after stool.*

Urine.—*Intolerable urging* and tenesmus. Nephritis with bloody urine. Violent paroxysms of cutting and burning in whole renal region, with painful urging to urinate; bloody urine, by *drops*. Intolerable tenesmus; cutting before, during, and after urine. *Urine scalds him, and is passed drop by drop. Constant desire to urinate.* Membranous scales looking like bran in water. Urine jelly-like, shreddy.

Male.—*Strong desire;* painful erections. Pain in glans. [*Prunus; Pareira.*] Priapism in gonorrhœa.

Female.—Retained placenta [*Sep.*], with painful urination. Expels moles, dead fœtuses, membranes, etc. *Nymphomania.* [*Plat.; Hyos.; Lach.; Stram.*] Puerperal metritis, with inflammation of bladder. Menses too early and too profuse; black swelling of vulva with irritation. Constant discharge from uterus; worse false step. Burning pain in ovaries; extremely sensitive. Pain in os coccyx, lancinating and tearing.

Respiratory.—Voice low; weak feeling. Stitches in chest. [*Bry.; Kal. c.; Squilla.*] Pleurisy, *with exudation.*

Heart.—Palpitation; pulse feeble, irregular; tendency to syncope. *Pericarditis, with effusion.*

Back.—Pain in loins, with incessant desire to urinate.

Extremities.—Tearing in limbs. Ulcerative pain in soles; cannot step.

Skin.—Dermatitis venenata with bleb formation. Secondary eczema about scrotum and genitals, following excessive perspiration. Tendency to gangrene. Eruption with mealy scales. *Versicular eruptions*, with burning and itching. Sunburn. *Burns, scalds,* with rawness and smarting, relieved by cold applications, followed by undue inflammation. *Erysipelas,* vesicular type, with great restlessness. Burning in soles of feet at night.

Fever.—Cold hands and feet; cold sweat. Soles burn. Chill, as if water were poured over him.

Modalities.—*Worse*, from touch, or approach, urinating, drinking cold water or coffee. *Better*, rubbing.

Relationship.—Antidotes: *Acon.; Camph.; Puls.*

Compare: *Cantharidin*—(Glomerular nephritis). The immediate pharmacological action of Cantharidin is irritability of the capillaries, rendering the passage of nutritive fluids through them less difficult. This is most marked in the capillaries of the kidneys. The increase of blood sugar coincident with the glomular nephritis appears to be a valuable observation. *Vesicaria*—(Urinary and kidney remedy. Smarting, burning sensation along urethra and in bladder with frequent desire to void urine often with strangury. Cystitis irritable bladder. Tincture 5-10 drop doses). *Fuschina* coloring substance used in adulteration of wine. (Cortical nephritis with albuminuria, 6th-30th potency. Redness of ears, mouth, swollen gums; deep, red urine; red, profuse diarrhœa, with severe abdominal pains). *Androsace lactea* (urinary troubles, diuretic; dropsy) *Apis; Ars.; Merc. cor.*

Complementary: *Camph.*

Dose.—Sixth to thirtieth potency. Bears repeated doses well. Locally, in burns and eczema, 1x and 2x, in water, or as cerate.

CAPSICUM
(Cayenne Pepper)

Seems to suit especially persons of lax fiber, weak; diminished vital heat. A relaxed plethoric sluggish, cold remedy. Not much reactive force. Such persons are fat, indolent, opposed to physical exertion, averse to go outside of their routine, get homesick easily. *General uncleanliness of body*. Abstainers from accustomed alcoholics. It affects the mucous membranes, producing a sensation of *constriction*. Inflammation of petrous bone. Burning pains and general chilliness. Older people who have exhausted their vitality, especially by mental work, and poor living; blear-eyed appearance; who do not react. Fear of slightest draught. Marked tendency to suppuration in every inflammatory process. Prostration and

CAPSICUM

feeble digestion of alcoholics. Myalgia, aching and jerking of muscles.

Mind.—Excessive peevishness. *Homesickness*, with sleeplessness and disposition to suicide. Wants to be let alone. Peppery disposition. *Delirium tremens*.

Head.—Bursting headache; worse, coughing. Hot face. Red cheeks. Face red, though cold. [*Asafœt.*]

Ears.—Burning and stinging in ears. *Swelling and pain behind ears. Inflammation of mastoid. Tenderness over the petrous bone;* extremely sore and tender to touch. [*Onosmod.*] Otorrhœa and mastoid disease before suppuration.

Throat.—*Hot feeling in fauces.* Subacute inflammation of Eustachian tube with great pain. *Pain and dryness in throat* extending to the ears. *Sore throat of smokers and drinkers.* Smarting in; constriction. Burning constriction worse between acts of deglutition. Inflamed uvula and palate; swollen and relaxed.

Mouth.—Herpes labialis. (Apply one drop of the mother tincture.) *Stomatitis.* Disagreeable smell from mouth. *Fetid odor from mouth.*

Stomach.—Burning in tip of tongue. Atonic dyspepsia. Much flatulence, especially in debilitated subjects. Intense craving for stimulants. Vomiting, sinking at pit of stomach. *Much thirst; but drinking causes shuddering.*

Stool.—*Bloody mucus, with burning and tenesmus;* drawing pain in back after stool. *Thirsty after stool, with shivering.* Bleeding piles, with soreness of anus. Stinging pain during stool.

Urine.—Strangury, frequent, almost ineffectual urging *Burning in orifice.* Comes first in drops, then in spurts; neck of bladder spasmodically contracted. Ectropion of meatus.

Male.—*Coldness of scrotum*, with impotency, atrophied testicles, loss of sensibility in testicles, with softening and dwindling. Gonorrhœa, with chordee, excessive burning, pain in prostate.

Female.—Climacteric disturbances with burning of tip of tongue. [*Lathyrus.*] Uterine hæmorrhage near the menopause, with nausea. Sticking sensation in left ovarian region.

Respiratory.—*Constriction* of chest; arrests breathing

Hoarseness. Pain at apex of heart or in rib region, worse touch. Dry, hacking cough, expelling an offensive breath from lungs. Dyspnœa. Feels as if chest and head would fly to pieces. Explosive cough. Threatening gangrene of lung. *Pain in distant parts on coughing*—bladder, legs, ears, etc.

Extremities.—Pain from hips to feet. Sciatica, worse bending backward; *worse, coughing.* Tensive pain in the knee.

Fever.—Coldness, with ill-humor. *Shivering after drinking.* Chill begins in back; better, heat. Must have something hot to back. Thirst before chill.

Modalities.—*Better*, while eating, from heat. *Worse*, open air, uncovering, draughts.

Relationship.—Antidote: *Cina; Calad.*

Compare: *Pulsat.; Lycop.; Bell.; Centaurea* (surging of blood; homesickness; intermittent fever).

Dose.—Third to sixth attenuation. In delirium tremens, dram doses of tincture in milk or tincture of orange peel.

CARBO ANIMALIS
(Animal Charcoal)

Seems to be especially adapted to scrofulous and venous constitutions, old people, and after debilitating disease, with feeble circulation and lowered vitality. *Glands are indurated, veins distended, skin blue. Stitch remaining after pleurisy.* Easily strained from lifting. Weakness of nursing women. Ulceration and decomposition. All its secretions are offensive. Causes local congestions *without* heat.

Mind.—Desire to be alone, sad and reflective, *avoids conversation.* Anxiety at night, with orgasm of blood.

Head.—Headache, as if head had been blown to pieces. Rush of blood with confusion. Sensation as if something lay above eyes so that she could not look up. Bluish cheeks and lips. Vertigo followed by nose-bleed. Nose swollen, tip bluish small tumor on it. Hearing confused; *cannot tell direction of sound.*

Stomach.—Eating tires patient. Weak, empty feeling in stomach. Burning and griping. *Weak digestion. Flatulence.* Ptomaine poisoning. Repugnance to fat food. Sour water from mouth. Pyrosis.

Female.—Nausea of pregnancy; worse at night. Lochia offensive. [*Kreos.; Rhus; Secale.*] Menses too early, frequent long lasting, *followed by great exhaustion*, so weak, can hardly speak. [*Cocc.*], flow only in morning. [*Bor.; Sep.*] Burning in vagina and labia. Darting in breast; *painful indurations* in breast, especially right. Cancer of uterus, burning pain down thighs.

Respiratory.—Pleurisy, typhoid character, and remaining stitch. Ulceration of lung, with feeling of coldness of chest. Cough, with discharge of greenish pus.

Skin.—Spongy ulcers, copper-colored eruption. Acne rosacea. Chilblains, worse in evening, in bed and from cold. Verruca on hands and face of old people, with bluish color of extremities. *Glands indurated*, swollen, painful, in neck, axillæ, groin, mammæ; pains lancinating, cutting, burning. [*Con.; Merc. iod. flav.*] Burning, rawness and fissures; moisture. *Bubo.*

Extremities.—Pain in coccyx; burns when touched. Ankles turn easily. Straining and over-lifting produce great debility. Joints weak. Easy discoloration. Pain in hip joints at night. *Night sweat* fetid and profuse. Wrist pain.

Modalities.—*Worse*, after shaving, loss of animal fluids.

Relationship.—The Carbon group all have putrid discharges and exhalations. All act on the skin, causing interrigo and excoriations. Glandular enlargements and catarrhal states, flatulency and asphyxiation.

Carbon Tetrachlorid is said to cause fatty liver. [*Phosph.; Ars.; Chlorof.*] Paralysis of interosseus muscles of feet and hands. Wonderful clinical results in the treatment of Hook worm disease. See *Thymol* (Relationship).

Complementary: *Calc. phos.*

Antidotes: *Ars.; Nux.*

Compare: *Badiaga; Sepia; Sulph.; Plumb. ioa.*

Dose.—Third to thirtieth potency. The third trituration for insufflation in aural polypi.

CARBO VEGETABILIS
(Vegetable Charcoal)

Disintegration and *imperfect oxidation* is the keynote of this remedy. The typical Carbo patient is sluggish, fat and lazy and has a tendency to chronicity in his complaints. Blood seems to stagnate in the capillaries, causing blueness, coldness, and ecchymosis. Body becomes blue, icy-cold. Bacteria find a rich soil in the nearly lifeless blood stream and sepsis and typhoidal state ensues.

A lowered vital power from loss of fluids, after drugging; after other diseases; in old people with venous congestions; states of collapse in cholera, typhoid; these are some of the conditions offering special inducements to the action of Carbo veg. The patient may be almost lifeless, but the head is hot; coldness, breath cool, pulse imperceptible, oppressed and quickened respiration, and must have air, must be fanned hard, must have all the windows open. This is a typical state for Carbo veg. The patient faints easily, is worn out, and must have fresh air. Hæmorrhage from any mucous surface. Very debilitated. Patient seems to be too weak to hold out. *Persons who have never fully recovered from the effects of some previous illness*. Sense of weight, as in the head (occiput), eyes and eyelids, before the ears, in the stomach, and elsewhere in the body; putrid (septic) condition of all its affections, coupled with a burning sensation. General venous stasis, bluish skin, limbs cold.

Mind.—Aversion to darkness. Fear of ghosts. Sudden loss of memory.

Head.—*Aches from any over-indulgence*. Hair feels sore, *falls off easily;* scalp itches when getting warm in bed. Hat pressed upon head like a heavy weight. Head feels heavy, constricted. Vertigo with nausea and tinnitus. Pimples on forehead and face.

Face.—Puffy, cyanotic. Pale, hippocratic, cold with cold sweat; blue. [*Cup.; Opium.*] Mottled cheeks and red nose.

Eyes.—Vision of black floating spots. Asthenopia. Burning in eyes. Muscles pain.

Ears.—Otorrhœa following exanthematous diseases. Ears dry. Malformation of cerumen with exfoliation of dermoid layer of meatus.

Nose.—*Epistaxis in daily attacks, with pale face.* Bleeding after straining, with pale face; tip of nose red and scabby, itching around nostrils. Varicose veins on nose. Eruption in corner of alæ nasi. Coryza with cough, especially in moist, warm weather. Ineffectual efforts to sneeze.

Mouth.—Tongue coated white or yellow brown, *covered with aphthæ.* Teeth very sensitive where chewing; gums retracted and bleed easily. Blood oozing from gums when cleaning teeth. Pyorrhœa.

Stomach.—*Eructations, heaviness, fullness, and sleepiness;* tense from flatulence, with pain; worse lying down. Eructations after eating and drinking. Temporary relief from belching. Rancid, sour, or putrid eructations. Waterbrash, asthmatic breathing from flatulence. Nausea in the morning. Burning in stomach, extending to back and along spine. *Contractive pain extending to chest, with distention of abdomen.* Faint gone feeling in stomach, not relieved by eating Crampy pains forcing patient to bend double. Distress comes on a half-hour after eating. Sensitiveness of epigastric region. *Digestion slow; food putrefies* before it digests. Gastralgia of nursing women, with excessive flatulence, sour, rancid belching. Aversion to milk, meat, and *fat things. The simplest food distresses.* Epigastric region very sensitive.

Abdomen.—Pain as from lifting a weight; colic from riding in a carriage; excessive discharge of fetid flatus. Cannot bear tight clothing around waist and abdomen. Ailments accompanying intestinal fistulæ. *Abdomen greatly distended;* better, passing wind. *Flatulent colic.* Pain in liver.

Rectum and Stool.—Flatus hot, moist, offensive. Itching, gnawing and burning in rectum. *Acrid, corrosive moisture from rectum.* A musty, glutinous moisture exudes. Soreness, itching moisture of perineum at night. Discharge of blood from rectum. Burning at anus, burning varices. [*Mur. ac.*] Painful diarrhœa of old people. Frequent, involuntary cadaverous-smelling stools, followed by burning. White hæmorrhoids; excoriation of anus. *Bluish,* burning piles, *pain* after stool.

Male.—Discharge of prostatic fluid at stool. Itching and moisture at thigh near scrotum.

Female.—Premature and too copious menses; pale blood.

Vulva swollen; aphthæ; varices on pudenda. Leucorrhœa before menses, thick, greenish, milky, excoriating. [*Kreos.*] During menstruation, burning in hands and soles.

Respiratory.—Cough with itching in larynx; spasmodic with gagging and vomiting of mucus. Whooping cough, especially in beginning. Deep, rough voice, failing on slight exertion. *Hoarseness; worse, evenings,* talking; evening oppression of breathing, sore and raw chest. Wheezing and rattling of mucus in chest. Occasional spells of long coughing attacks. *Cough, with burning in chest;* worse in evening, in open air, after eating and talking. Spasmodic cough, bluish face, offensive expectoration, neglected pneumonia. Breath cold; *must be fanned.* Hæmorrhage from lungs. *Asthma in aged with blue skin.*

Extremities.—Heavy, stiff; feel paralyzed; *limbs, go to sleep;* want of muscular energy; joints weak. Pain in shins. Cramp in soles; feet numb and sweaty. *Cold from knees down.* Toes red, swollen. Burning pain in bones and limbs.

Fever.—Coldness, with thirst. Chill begins in forearm. Burning in various places. Perspiration on eating. Hectic fever, exhausting sweats.

Skin.—*Blue, cold ecchymosed.* Marbled with venous over distension. Itching; worse on evening, when warm in bed. Moist skin; *hot perspiration;* senile gangrene beginning in toes; bed sores; bleed easily. Falling out of hair, from a general weakened condition. Indolent ulcers, burning pain. Ichorous, offensive discharge; tendency to gangrene of the margins. Purpura. *Varicose ulcers,* carbuncles. [*Ars.; Anthrac.*]

Modalities.—*Worse,* evening; night and open air; cold; from fat food, butter, coffee, milk, warm damp weather; *wine. Better,* from eructation, *from fanning,* cold.

Relationship.—Antidotes: *Spirits Nitre; Camph.; Ambra; Arsenic.*

Compare: *Carboneum*—Lampblack. (Spasms commencing in tongue, down trachea and extremities. Tingling sensation.) *Lycop.; Ars.; China.*

Complementary: *Kali carb.; Dros.*

Dose.—First to third trituration in stomach disorders. Thirtieth potency and higher in chronic conditions, and in collapse.

CARBOLICUM ACIDUM
(Phenol—Carbolic Acid)

Carbolic Acid is a powerful irritant and anæsthetic. A languid, foul, painless destructive remedy. Stupor, paralysis of sensation and motion, feeble pulse and depressed breathing, death due to paralysis of respiratory centres. Acts primarily on the central nervous system. *Increased olfactory sensibility.*

Produces mental and bodily languor, disinclination to study, with headache like a band. Very marked *acuteness of smell* is a strong guiding symptom. Stomach symptoms are also important. Pains are terrible; come and go suddenly. Physical exertion brings on abscess somewhere. Putrid discharges. [*Bapt.*] Scarlet fever, with marked tendency to destruction of tissue internally, and fetid odor. Spasmodic coughs. Arthritis. (See Dose.)

Head.—Disinclined to mental work. Tight feeling, as if compressed by a rubber band. [*Gels.; Mahonia.*] Orbital neuralgia over right eye. Headache, better, by green tea, while smoking.

Nose.—*Smell very acute.* Putrid discharge. Ozæna, with fetor and ulceration. Influenza and resulting debility.

Throat.—Ulcerated patches on inside of lips and cheeks. *Burning in mouth to* stomach. Fauces red, and covered with exudation. Uvula whitened and shriveled. *Putrid discharge.* Almost impossible to swallow. *Diphtheria, fetid breath, regurgitation* on swallowing liquids, but little pain. [*Bapt.*] Face dusky red; white about mouth and nose. Rapid sinking of vital forces.

Stomach.—Appetite lost. *Desire for stimulants and tobacco.* Constant belching, nausea, *vomiting*, dark olive green. Heat rises up œsophagus. Flatulent distention of stomach and abdomen. Painful flatulence often marked in one part of the bowel. [*Sulpho-Carbolate of Soda.*] *Fermentative dyspepsia* with bad taste and breath.

Stool.—Constipation, with *very offensive breath*. Bloody, like scrapings of intestines. Great tenesmus. Diarrhœa; stools thin, black, putrid.

Urine.—Almost black. Diabetes. Irritable bladder in old

men with frequent urination at night, of probable prostatic nature. Use 1x).

Female.—Discharges always offensive. [*Nitr. ac.; Nux.; Sep.*] Pustules about vulva containing bloody pus. Agonizing backache across loins, with dragging-down thighs. Pain in left ovary; worse walking in open air. Erosions of cervix; fetid, acrid discharge. Leucorrhœa in children. [*Cann. s.; Merc.; Puls.; Sep.*] Puerperal fever, with offensive discharge. Irritating leucorrhœa, causing itching and burning. [*Kreos.*]

Extremities.—Cramps in fore part of leg, close to tibia *during walking*. Gnawing pains in shin bones. Arthritis.

Skin.—Itching vesicles, with burning pain. Burns tend to ulcerate.

Relationship.—Compare: *Chrysarobin* (locally *in ringworm* of the scalp 5-10 per cent. in glycerine and alcohol. Equal parts). *Ars.; Kreosot.; Carbo; Guano.* (Violent headache as from a band around head. Itching of nostrils, back, thighs, genitals. Symptoms like hay-fever.)

Antidote: *Alcohol; Vinegar; Chalk; Iod.* Glauber's Salt in watery solution.

Incompatible: *Glycerine* and *vegetable oils*.

Dose.—Third to thirtieth potency. Phenol in Arthritis, according to Goodno. Must be absolutely pure. Crystals Solution (25%) in equal parts of water and glycerine, dose 20 minims well diluted 3 times daily (Bartlett).

CARBONEUM HYDROGENISATUM
(Carburetted Hydrogen)

Symptoms resemble an apopletic attack. Spasm as in lockjaw. Trismus. Involuntary stools and urine.

Mind.—Stupefaction. Extraordinary sensation of contentment All thoughts appear in a moment as if seen in an inner mirror.

Eyes.—Lids half closed. Oscillation of eyeballs. Pupils insensible to light.

CARBONEUM OXYGENISATUM
(Carbonous Oxide)

Herpes zoster, pemphigus, and trismus are produced by this drug. Coldness, *sleepiness*, loss of consciousness are marked. Vertigo.

Head.—Cerebral congestion; hallucination of vision, hearing and touch. Inclination to turn in a circle. *Jaws firmly clenched.* Trismus. Heaviness of head. Sticking pain in temples. Roaring ears.

Eyes.—Ocular paralysis, hemianopsias, disturbed pupilary reaction, optic neuritis and atrophy, subconjunctival and retinal hemorrhages.

Skin.—Anæsthesia; vesication along course of nerves; *herpes zoster;* pemphigus, with large and small vesicles. Hand icy cold.

Sleep.—Deep. *Prolonged;* sleepiness for several days.

Dose.—First attenuation.

CARBONEUM SULPHURATUM
(Alcohol Sulphuris—Bisulphide of Carbon)

This drug has a deep and disorganizing action and an immense range of action judging from the symptomatology. Very useful in patients broken down by abuse of alcohol. Sensitive patients worse cold, wasted muscles, and skin and mucous membranes anæsthetic. Special affinity for eyes. Chronic rheumatism, sensitive and cold. Lack of vital heat. Diarrhœa every four to six weeks. Paralysis with intense congestion of nerve centres. Tabes. Sensory difficulties in limbs.

Impotence, sciatica, come within the therapeutic sphere of this remedy. Chronic plumbism. *Diminished sensibility* of arms, hands and feet. Peripheral neuritis.

Mind.—Irritable, anxious, intolerant; *stupor*. Sluggishness of mind. Hallucinations of sight and hearing. Changeable mood. Dementia alternating with excitement.

Head.—Headache and dizziness. Aches as from a tight cap. Ears feel obstructed. *Noises in head.* Ulceration of the lips, anæsthesia of mouth and tongue.

Eyes.—Myopia, asthenopia, and dis-chromotopsia, cloudiness and atrophy of optic disc and centrol scotoma for light and for red and green not for white. Optic neuritis advancing toward atrophy. Arteries and veins congested. Retinal congestion; optic disc pale. Everything seems in a fog. Vision greatly impaired. Color-blindness.

Ears.—Hearing impaired. Buzzing and singing noises like an æolian harp. *Tinnitus aurium. Meniere's disease.*

Abdomen.—Pain with *wandering swellings* as from flatus. Distention, with soreness and rumbling.

Male.—Desire lost, parts atrophied. Frequent profuse emissions.

Extremities.—Herpes on dorsal surface of hands. Sore, bruised limbs; anæsthesia of arms and hands. Cramps in limbs. Lightning-like pains, with cramps. Fingers swollen, *insensible*, rigid, stiff. Gait unsteady, tottering; worse in dark. Feet insensible. *Sciatica. Flying pains, returning regularly* for a long time. Pain in lower limbs, with cramps and formication. *Neuritis.*

Sleep.—Deep morning sleep with anxious, vexatious dreams.

Skin.—Anæsthesia; burning; itching; ulcers; small wounds fester. Useful to restrain the growth of cancer. Furunculosis. Chronic skin diseases with much itching.

Modalities.—*Better*, in open air. *Worse*, after breakfast; bathing. Sensitive to warm, damp, weather.

Relationship.—Compare: *Potass. Xantate*—(Similar in action. Acts on cortical substance; loss of memory, marked blood degeneration; impotence and senility. *Tuberculin; Radium; Carbo; Sulph.; Caust.; Salicyl. ac.; Cinch.* In eye symptoms compare: *Benzin. dinitric. Thyroidin* (progressive diminution of sight with central Scotoma).

Dose.—First attenuation. Locally in facial neuralgia and sciatica.

CARDUUS MARIANUS
(St. Mary's Thistle)

The action of this drug is centered in the liver, and portal system, causing soreness, pain, jaundice. Has specific relation to the vascular system. Abuse of alcoholic beverages, especially beer. *Varicose veins* and ulcers. Diseases of miners, associated with asthma. Dropsical conditions depending on liver disease, and when due to pelvic congestion and hepatic disease. Disturbs sugar metabolism. Influenza when liver is affected. Debility. Hæmorrhages, especially connected with hepatic disease.

Mind.—Despondency; forgetful, apathetic.

Head.—Contractive feeling above eyebrows. Dull heavy, stupid, with foul tongue. Vertigo, with tendency to fall forward. Burning and pressure in eyes. Nose-bleed.

Stomach.—Taste bitter. Aversion to salt meat. Appetite small; tongue furred; *nausea; retching; vomiting of green, acid fluid*. Stitches in left side of stomach, near spleen. [*Ceanoth.*] Gallstone disease with enlarged liver.

Abdomen.—Pain in region of liver. Left lobe very sensitive. Fullness and soreness, with moist skin. Constipation; *stools hard, difficult, knotty;* alternates with diarrhœa. Stools bright yellow. Swelling of gall bladder with painful tenderness. Hyperæmia of liver, with jaundice. Cirrhosis, with dropsy.

Rectum.—Hæmorrhagic piles, prolapse or rectum, burning pain in anus and rectum, hard and knotting, clayey stools. Profuse diarrhœa due to rectal cancer. 10 drop doses (Wapler).

Urine.—Cloudy; golden-colored.

Chest.—Stitching pains in lower right ribs and front; worse, moving, walking, etc. *Asthmatic respiration*. Pain in chest, going to shoulders, back, loins and abdomen, with urging to urinate.

Skin.—Itching on lying down at night. *Varicose ulcers.* [*Clematis vitalba.*] Eruption on lower part of sternum.

Extremities.—Pain in hip-joint, spreading through buttocks and down thigh; *worse from stooping*. Difficult rising. Weakness felt in feet, especially after sitting.

Relationship.—Compare: *Card. benedictus* (strong action on eyes, and sensation of contraction in many parts; stomach symptoms similar); *Chelidon.; Chionanthes; Merc.; Podophyl.; Bry.; Aloe.*

Dose.—Tincture and lower potencies.

CARLSBAD
(The Waters of the Sprudel Springs)

Famous for its action on the liver and in the treatment of obesity, diabetes, and gout. In homœopathic potencies useful in weakness of all organs, constipation, great liability to take cold. Periodicity, effects repeated after from two to four weeks. [*Oxal. ac.; Sulph.*] *Flashes of heat all over.* Itching on various parts.

Mind.—Discouraged and anxious about domestic duties.

Head.—Aches, with swollen temporal veins [*Sang.*]; better, motion, in open air.

Face.—Yellow; sallow; red and hot; pain in zygomatic process; feels as if cobwebs were on it.

Stomach.—Tongue coated white. Offensive smell from mouth. Furry sensation. Sour or salty taste. Hiccough and yawning. Heartburn. [*Carbo.*]

Urine.—Stream *weak and slow;* only passed by pressing abdominal muscles.

Rectum.—*Fæces held back.* Stool slow, and only passed by much abdominal pressure. Burning in rectum and anus. Bleeding piles.

Relationship.—Compare: *Nat. sulph.; Nux.*

Dose.—Lower potencies.

CASCARA SAGRADA—RHAMNUS PURSHIANA
(Sacred Bark)

Introduced as a palliative for constipation (non-homœopathic), fifteen drops of fluid extract here it restores normal function by its tonic effects, but it has a wider sphere of action, as careful provings will show. Chronic indigestion, cirrhosis and jaundice. Hæmorrhoids and constipation. Gastric headache. Broad, flabby tongue; foul breath.

Urine.—Must wait for minute before flow starts then first in drops.

Extremities.—*Rheumatism of muscles and joints, with obstinate constipation.*

Relationship.—Compare: *Hyd.; Nux.; Rhamnus Californica* (tincture for constipation; tympanites and appendicitis and especially *rheumatism*).

Dose.—Tincture to sixth potency.

CASCARILLA
(Sweet Bark)

Acts on the digestive tract; constipation. Aversion to smell of tobacco. *Inclination to vomit* very marked.

Stomach.—Hunger after meals. Desire for hot drinks. *Nausea and vomiting*. Pain in stomach as from a shock. Pressing colic.

Rectum.—Constipation; stools hard, covered with mucus. [*Graph.*] Bright blood with stool. Diarrhœa alternating with hard, lumpy stool, with backache and lassitude, preceded by griping. Gnawing pain high up in rectum.

Dose.—First to third potency.

CARCINOSIN
(A Nosode from Carcinoma)

It is claimed the Carcinosin acts favorably and modifies all cases in which either a history of carcinoma can be elicited, or symptoms of the disease itself exist. (J. H. Clarke, M. D.)

Carcinoma of the mammary glands with great pain and induration of glands; of uterus, the offensive discharge, hæmorrhage and pain are greatly relieved.

Indigestion, accumulation of gas in stomach and bowels; rheumatism—Cancerous cachexia.

Relationship.—Compare: *Bufo; Conium; Phytolacca, Asterias*.

Dose.—Thirtieth and 200th potency, a dose at night or less frequently.

CASTANEA VESCA
(Chestnut Leaves)

A useful remedy in *whooping-cough*, especially in the early stage, with dry, ringing, violent, spasmodic cough. Desire for warm drinks. Very thirsty. Loss of appetite. Diarrhœa. Thick urine.

Lumbago, weak back, can hardly straighten up.

Relationship.—Compare: *Pertussin*—Whooping-cough (when symptoms return again after being allayed. *Dros.; Mephitis; Naphthal.; Ammon. brom.*

Dose.—Tincture.

CASTOR EQUI
(Rudimentary Thumb-nail of the Horse)

General action on thickening of the skin and epithelium. *Psoriasis linguæ*. The clinical experience of Hering and his fellow-provers has shown this to be highly useful remedy in *cracked and ulcerated nipples*. Affects principally female organs. Acts on the nails and bones; pain in right tibia and coccyx. Warts on forehead. Warts on breast. Chapped hands.

Chest.—Cracked, sore nipples, excessively tender. Swelling of mammæ. Violent itching in breasts; areola reddened.

Relationship.—Compare: *Graphites; Hippomanes; Calc.Oxal.*

Dose—Sixth and twelfth potency.

CASTOREUM
(The Beaver)

A great remedy for hysteria. Prostration marked.

Hysterical symptoms. Day-blindness; cannot endure the light. Nervous women who do not recover fully, but are continually irritable, and suffer from debilitating sweats. Spasmodic affections after debilitating diseases. Constant yawning. Restless sleep with frightful dreams and starts.

Tongue.—Swollen. Rounded elevation size of a pea in center, with drawing sensation from center to hyoid bone.

Female.—Dysmenorrhœa; blood discharged in drops with tenesmus. Pain commences in middle of thighs. Amenorrhœa, with painful tympanites.

Fever.—Predominant chilliness. Attacks of chilliness with ice-coldness in back.

Relationship.—Compare: *Ambra; Moschus; Mur. acid; Valeriana*.

Antidote: *Colch*.

Dose.—Tincture, and lower potencies.

CATARIA NEPETA
(Catnip)

Children's remedy for *Colic*, also for nervous headache and hysteria, abdominal complaints, pain, flexing of thighs, twisting of body, crying. Similar to chamomilla and magnes. phosph.

Dose.—5 to 10 drops of the tincture.

CAULOPHYLLUM
(Blue Cohosh)

This is a woman's remedy. Want of tonicity of the womb. During labor, when the pains are deficient and the patient is exhausted and fretful. Besides, it has a special affinity for the smaller joints. *Thrush*, locally and internally.

Stomach.—*Cardialgia, spasms of stomach.* Dyspepsia with spasmodic symptoms.

Female.—Extraordinary rigidity of os. [*Bell.; Gels.; Ver. v.*] Spasmodic and severe pains, which fly in all directions; shivering, without progress; false pains. Revives labor pains and furthers progress of labor. After pains. Leucorrhœa, with moth-spots on forehead. Habitual abortion from uterine debility. [*Helon.; Puls.; Sab.*] Needle-like pains in cervix. Dysmenorrhœa, with pains flying to other parts of body. Lochia protracted; great atony. Menses and leucorrhœa profuse.

Skin.—Discoloration of skin in women with menstrual and uterine disorder.

Extremities.—Severe drawing, erratic pain and stiffness in small joints, fingers, toes, ankles, etc. Aching in wrists. Cutting pains on closing hands. Erratic pains, changing place every few minutes.

Relationship.—Incompatible: *Coffea.*

Compare: *Viol. Odor.* (rheumatic carpal and metacarpal joints); *Cimicif.; Sepia; Pulsat.; Gels.*

Dose.—Tincture to third attenuation.

CAUSTICUM
(Hahnemann's Tinctura acris sine Kali)

Manifests its action mainly in chronic rheumatic, arthritic and paralytic affections, indicated by the tearing, drawing pains in the muscular and fibrous tissues, with deformities about the joints; progressive loss of muscular strength, tendinous contractures. Broken down seniles. In catarrhal affections of the air passages, and seems to choose preferably dark-complexioned and rigid-fibered persons. Restlessness at night, with tearing pains in joints and bones, and faint-like sinking of strength. This weakness progresses until we have gradually appearing paralysis. Local paralysis, vocal cords, muscles of deglutition, of tongue, eyelids, face, bladder and extremities. Children are slow to walk. The skin of a Causticum person is of a *dirty white* sallow, with warts, especially on the face. Emaciation due to disease, worry, etc., and of long standing. *Burning, rawness, and soreness* are characteristic.

Mind.—Child does not want to go to bed alone. Least thing makes it cry. Sad, hopeless. *Intensely sympathetic.* Ailments from long-lasting grief, sudden emotions. Thinking of complaints, aggravates, especially hæmorrhoids.

Head.—Sensation of empty space between forehead and brain. Pain in right frontal eminence.

Face.—Paralysis of right side. Warts. Pain in facial bones. Dental fistula. Pain in jaws, with difficulty in opening mouth.

Eyes.—Cataract with motor disturbances. Inflammation of eyelids; ulceration. Sparks and dark spots before eyes. *Ptosis.* [*Gels.*] Vision impaired, as if film were before eyes. Paralysis of ocular muscles after exposure to cold.

Ears.—Ringing, roaring, pulsating, with deafness; words and steps re-echo; chronic middle-ear catarrh; accumulation of ear-wax.

Nose.—*Coryza, with hoarseness.* Scaly nose. Nostrils ulcerated. *Pimples and warts.*

Mouth.—Bites inside of cheek from chewing. Paralysis of tongue, with indistinct speech. Rheumatism of articulation of lower jaw. Gums bleed easily.

Stomach.—Greasy taste. Aversion to sweets. Feels as if lime were burned in stomach. Worse after eating fresh meat; smoked meat agrees. Sensation of ball rising in throat. *Acid dyspepsia.*

Stool.—Soft and small, size of goose-quill. [*Phos.*] Hard, tough, covered with mucus; shines like grease; small-shaped; expelled with much straining, or only on standing up. Pruritus. Partial paralysis of rectum. Rectum sore and burns. Fistula and large piles.

Urine.—Involuntary when coughing, sneezing. [*Puls.*] Expelled very slowly, and sometimes retained. Involuntary during first sleep at night; also from slightest excitement. *Reten-*

tion after surgical operations. Loss of sensibility on passing urine.

Female.—*Uterine inertia during labor.* Menses cease at night; *flow only during day.* [*Cycl.; Puls.*] Leucorrhœa at night, with great weakness. [*Nat. mur.*] Menses delay, late. [*Con.; Graph.; Puls.*]

Respiratory.—*Hoarseness* with pain in chest; *aphonia.* Larynx sore. *Cough, with raw soreness of chest.* Expectoration scanty; *must be swallowed.* Cough *with pain in hip,* especially left worse in evening; *better, drinking cold water;* worse, warmth of bed. Sore streak down trachea. Mucus under sternum, which he cannot *quite reach.* Pain in chest, with palpitation. Cannot lie down at night. Voice re-echoes. Own voice roars in ears and distresses. Difficulty of voice of singers and public speakers (Royal).

Back.—Stiffness between shoulders. Dull pain in nape of neck.

Extremities.—Left-sided sciatica, with numbness. Paralysis of single parts. Dull, tearing pain in hands and arms. Heaviness and weakness. Tearing joints. Unsteadiness of *muscles of forearm* and hand. Numbness; loss of sensation in hands. *Contracted tendons.* Weak ankles. Cannot walk without suffering. *Rheumatic tearing in limbs; better by warmth, especially heat of bed.* Burning in joints. Slow in learning to walk. Unsteady walking and easily falling. *Restless legs at night.* Cracking and tension in knees; stiffness in hollow of knee. Itching on dorsum of feet.

Skin.—Soreness in folds of skin, back of ears, between thighs. *Warts* large, jagged, bleeding easily, on tips of fingers and nose. Old burns that do not get well, and ill effects from burns. Pains of burns. Cicatrices freshen up; old injuries reopen. Skin prone to intertrigo during dentition.

Sleep.—Very drowsy; can hardly keep awake. Nocturnal sleeplessness, with dry heat, inquietude.

Relationship.—According to the careful investigations of Dr. Wagner of Basel, Causticum corresponds to Ammon. causticum 4x. *Causticum* does not agree with *Phosphorus;* the remedies should not be used after each other. *Diphtherotoxin* follows, causticum in chronic bronchitis.

Antidote: Paralysis from lead-poisoning.

Complementary: *Carbo; Petrosel.*

Compare: *Rhus; Arsenic; Amm. phos.* (facial paralysis).

Modalities.—*Worse*, dry, cold winds, in *clear fine* weather, *cold* air; from motion of carriage. *Better*, in *damp, wet weather; warmth.* Heat of bed.

Dose.—Third to thirtieth attenuation. In chronic ailments and especially in paralytic states, the higher potencies once or twice a week.

CEANOTHUS

(New Jersey Tea)

This remedy seems to possess a specific relation to the spleen. Ague cake of malaria. A left-sided remedy generally. Anæmic patients where liver and spleen are at fault. Chronic bronchitis with profuse secretion. Marked blood pressure, reducing powers. Active hemastatic, materially reducing the clotting of blood.

Abdomen.—Enormous enlargement of the spleen. *Splenitis; pain all up the left side.* Deep-seated pain in left hypochondrium, hypertrophy of spleen. Leucæmia. Violent dyspnœa. Menses profuse, and yellow weakening leucorrhœa. Unable to lie on left side. Pain in liver and back.

Rectum.—Diarrhœa; bearing down in abdomen and rectum.

Urine.—Constant urging to urinate. Green; frothy; contains bile, sugar.

Relationship.—Compare: *Tinospora cordifolia* (a Hindoo medicine for chronic cases of fever with enlarged spleen). *Polymnia uvedalia*—Bearsfoot—(acute splenitis with tenderness over left hypochondriac region; spleen enlarged, ague cake. Vascular atony, tissues sodden, flabby and non-elastic. Enlarged glands; influences all ductless glands). *Ceanothus thrysiflorus*—California Lilac—(Pharyngitis, tonsillitis, nasal catarrh, diphtheria. Tincture internally and as a gargle.)

Compare: *Berberis; Myrica; Cedron; Agaricus* (spleen).

Modalities.—*Worse*, motion, lying on left side.

Dose.—First attenuation. Locally as hair tonic.

CEDRON-SIMARUBA FERROGINEA
(Rattlesnake Bean)

Periodicity is the most marked characteristic of this drug. Is particularly useful in tropical or in damp, warm, marshy countries. It has been found curative in malarial affections, especially neuralgia. Adapted to persons of a voluptuous disposition, excitable, nervous temperament. Has powers of antidoting snake-bites and stings of insects. Tincture of pure bean scraped on wound. Mania.

Head.—Pain from temple to temple across eyes. Pain over whole right side of face, coming on about 9 a. m. Crazy feeling from pain across forehead; worse, working on black. Roaring in ears produced by Cinchona. Whole body seems numb with headache.

Eyes.—Shooting over left eye. Severe *pain in eyeball, with radiating pains around eye,* shooting into nose. Scalding lachrymation. *Supra-orbital neuralgia periodic.* Iritis, choroiditis.

Extremities.—Lancinating pain in joints; worse, feet and hands. Sudden pain in ball of right thumb, extending up arm to shoulder. Pain in ball of right foot, extending to knee. Shingles, with radiating pain. Dropsy of knee-joint.

Fever.—Chilliness towards evening; then frontal headache extending into parietal region. Red eyes. Heat, with itching of eyes, tearing pain in limbs, *numbness of limbs.*

Relationship.—Antidote: *Lach.*

Compare: *Ars.; China.*

Dose.—Tincture to third attenuation.

CENCHRIS CONTORTRIX—ANCISTRODON
(Copperhead Snake)

Like the other snake poisons, it affects the system profoundly. Like arsenic, it has dyspnœa, mental and physical restlessness, thirst for small quantities of water, necessity for having clothing loose, like Laches. Marked alternation of moods; vivid dreams. Is a wonderful restorative and deep acting remedy. Increased sexual desire in both sexes. Ineffectual attempts to recline. Right ovarian region painful.

Head.—Forgetful, absent-minded, alternating moods. Aching pain in left frontal eminence and left side of teeth. Swelling around eyes, aching and itching in eyes.

Heart.—Feels distended, fills whole chest, as if it fell down in abdomen; sharp stitches, fluttering under left scapula.

Sleep.—Dreams horrible and vivid; lascivious.

Modalities.—*Worse*, pressure; lying down; afternoon and night.

Relationship.—Compare: *Ars.; Laches. Clotho Arictans*—Puff Adder.—Should have a great sphere of usefulness in many conditions where excessive swelling is a leading feature. (John H. Clarke, M. D.)

Dose.—Sixth potency.

CEREUS BONPLANDII
(A Night-blooming Cereus)

Mind.—Great desire to work and to be doing something useful.

Head.—Occipital headache and *pain through the globe of the eyes* and orbits. [*Cedron; Onos.*] Pain across the brain from left to right. Pain along right malar bone running to temple.

Chest.—Convulsive pains at the heart; feels as if transfixed. Pain in chest through heart, with pain running toward spleen. Pain in left pectoral muscle and cartilages of left lower ribs. Sensation of a great weight on heart, and pricking pain. Hypertrophy of heart. Difficult, sighing respiration, as from some compression of chest.

Skin.—Itching of skin. [*Dolich.; Sulph.*]

Extremities.—Pain in neck, back, shoulders, down arms, hands and fingers. Pain in knees and joints of lower extremities.

Relationship.—Compare: *Cactus; Spigel.; Kalmia; Cereus serpentinus.* (Very irritable with tendency to swear; wild anger and low morals. Disturbance in speech; in writing leaves off the last syllable. Paralyzed feeling. Pains in heart, and dwindling of sexual organs. Emissions, followed by pain in testicles.)

Dose.—Third to sixth attenuation.

CERIUM OXALICUM
(Oxalate of Cerium)

Spasmodic reflex vomiting and spasmodic cough are within the sphere of this remedy. *Vomiting of pregnancy*, and of half-digested food. Whooping cough, with vomiting and hæmorrhage. Dysmenorrhæa in fleshy, robust women. Better when flow is established.

Relationship.—Compare: *Ingluvin*—(made from gizzard of a fowl). Vomiting of pregnancy; gastric neurasthenia. Infantile vomiting and diarrhœa. 3x Trit. *Amygdal.; Lactic ac.; Ipecac.*

Dose.—First trituration.

CHAMOMILLA
(German Chamomile)

The chief guiding symptoms belong to the mental and emotion group, which lead to this remedy in many forms of disease. Especially of frequent employment in diseases of children, where peevishness, restlessness, and colic give the needful indications. A disposition that is mild, calm and gentle; sluggish and constipated bowels contra-indicate chamomilla.

Chamomilla is *sensitive, irritable, thirsty, hot, and numb.* Oversensitiveness from abuse of coffee and narcotics. *Pains unendurable*, associated with numbness. Night-sweats.

Mind.—*Whining restlessness.* Child wants many things which he refuses again. Piteous moaning because he cannot have what he wants. Child can only be quieted when carried about and petted constantly. *Impatient*, intolerant of being spoken to or interrupted; extremely sensitive to every pain; always complaining. Spiteful, *snappish.* Complaints from *anger* and vexation. *Mental calmness contraindicates Chamom.*

Head.—Throbbing headache in one-half of the brain. Inclined to bend head backward. Hot, clammy sweat on forehead and scalp.

Ears.—Ringing in ears. *Earache*, with soreness; *swelling and heat driving patient frantic.* Stitching pain. Ears feel stopped.

Eyes.—Lids smart. Yellow sclerotic. Spasmodic closing of lids.

Nose.—Sensitive to all smells. Coryza, with inability to sleep.

Face.—*One cheek red* and hot; the other pale and cold. Stitches in jaw extending to inner ear and teeth. *Teeth ache worse after warm drink;* worse, coffee, at night. Drives to distraction. Jerking of tongue and facial muscles. Distress of teething children. [*Calc. phos.; Terebinth.*]

Throat.—Parotid and submaxillary glands swollen. Constriction and pain as from a plug.

Mouth.—Toothache, if anything warm is taken, from coffee, during pregnancy. Nightly salivation.

Stomach.—Eructations, foul. Nausea after coffee. Sweats after eating or drinking. Aversion to warm drinks. Tongue yellow; taste bitter. Bilious vomiting. Acid rising; regurgitation of food. Bitter, bilious vomiting. Pressive gastralgia, as from a stone. [*Bry.; Abies n.*]

Abdomen.—Distended. Griping in region of navel, and pain in small of back. Flatulent colic, after anger, *with red cheeks and hot perspiration.* Hepatic colic. Acute duodenitis. [*Kali bich.* (chronic).]

Stool.—Hot, *green,* watery, fetid, *slimy,* with colic. Chopped white and yellow mucus like chopped eggs and spinach. Soreness of anus. Diarrhœa during dentition. Hæmorrhoids, with painful fissures.

Female.—Uterine hæmorrhages. Profuse discharge of clotted, *dark blood, with labor-like pains.* Labor pains spasmodic; press upward. [*Gels.*] Patient intolerant of pain. [*Caul.; Caust.; Gels.; Hyos.; Puls.*] Nipples inflamed; tender to touch. Infants' breasts tender. Yellow, acrid leucorrhœa. [*Ars.; Sep.; Sulph.*]

Respiratory.—Hoarseness, hawking, *rawness* of *larynx. Irritable, dry, tickling cough;* suffocative tightness of chest, with bitter expectoration in daytime. Rattling of mucus in child's chest.

Back.—Insupportable pain in loins and hips. *Lumbago.* Stiffness of neck muscles.

Extremities.—Violent rheumatic pains drive him out of bed at night; compelled to walk about. Burning of soles at night.

[*Sulph.*] *Ankles give way in the afternoon.* Nightly paralytic loss of power in the feet, unable to step on them.

Sleep.—Drowsiness with moaning, weeping and wailing during sleep; anxious, frightened dreams, with half-open eyes.

Modalities.—*Worse*, by *heat*, anger, open air, wind, *night*. *Better*, from being carried, warm wet weather.

Relationship.—Compare: *Cypriped; Anthemis; Aconite; Puls.; Coffea; Bellad.; Staphis.; Ignat.* Follows Belladonna in diseases of children and abuse of opium. *Rubus villosus*—Blackberry—(diarrhœa of infancy; stools watery and clay colored).

Antidotes: *Camph.; Nux; Puls.*

Complementary: *Bell.; Mag. c.*

Dose.—Third to thirtieth attenuation.

CHAPARRO AMARGOSO
(Goat-bush)

Chronic diarrhœa. Tenderness over liver. Stools little pain, but with much mucus. Dysentery. Acts as a tonic and antiperiodic.

Compare: *Kali carb.; Cup, ars.; Caps.*

Dose.—Third attenuation.

CHELIDONIUM MAJUS
(Celandine)

A prominent liver remedy, covering many of the direct reflex symptoms of diseased conditions of that organ. The jaundiced skin, and especially the *constant pain under inferior angle of right scapula*, are certain indications. Paralytic drawing and lameness in single parts. The great general lethargy and indisposition to make any effort is also marked. Ailments brought on or renewed by change of weather. *Serous effusions. Hydrocele. Bilious complications during gestation.*

Head.—Icy coldness of occiput from the nape of neck; *feels heavy as lead.* Heavy, lethargic; drowsiness very marked, with general numbness; vertigo, associated with heptic disturbance. Inclination to fall forward. Right-sided headache down behind ears and shoulder-blade. *Neuralgia over right eye*, right cheek-bone and right ear, with excessive lachrymation, preceded by pain in liver.

Nose.—Flapping of alæ nasi. [*Lyc.*]

Eyes.—Dirty yellow color of whites. Sore sensation on looking up. Tears fairly gush out. Orbital neuralgia of right eye, with profuse lachrymation; pupils contracted, relieved by pressure.

Face.—*Yellow;* worse nose and cheeks. Wilted skin.

Stomach.—Tongue yellow, with imprint of teeth; large and flabby. [*Merc.; Hyd.*] Taste bitter, pasty. Bad odor from mouth. *Prefers hot food and drink.* Nausea, vomiting; *better, very hot water.* Pain through stomach to back and right shoulder-blade. Gastralgia. *Eating relieves temporarily,* especially when accompanied with hepatic symptoms.

Abdomen.—Jaundice due to hepatic and gall-bladder obstruction. Gall-colic. Distention. Fermentation and sluggish bowels. Constriction across, as by a string. Liver enlarged. Gallstones. [*Berberis.*]

Urine.—Profuse, foaming, yellow urine, like beer. [*Chenop.*] dark, turbid.

Stool.—Constipation; stools hard, round balls, like sheep's dung, bright yellow, pasty; clay-colored, stools float in water; *alternation of diarrhœa and constipation.* Burning and itching of anus. [*Ratanh.; Sulph.*]

Female.—Menses too late and too profuse.

Respiratory.—Very quick and short inspirations; pain on deep inspiration. Dyspnœa. Short, exhausting cough; sensation of dust not relieved by cough. Whooping-cough; spasmodic cough; loose, rattling; expectoration difficult. Pain in *right* side of chest and shoulder, with embarrased respiration. Small lumps of mucus fly from mouth when coughing. Hoarse in afternoon. Constriction of chest.

Back.—Pain in nape. Stiff neck, head drawn to left. *Fixed pain under inner and lower angle of right scapula.* Pain at lower angle of left scapula.

Extremities.—Pain in arms, shoulders, hands, tips of fingers. *Icy coldness of tips of fingers;* wrists sore, tearing in metacarpal bones. Whole flesh sore to touch. Rheumatic pain in hips and thighs; intolerable pains in heels, as if pinched by too narrow a shoe; worse, right. Feels paralyzed. Paresis of the lower limbs with rigidity of muscles.

Skin.—Dry heat of skin; itches, *yellow.* Painful red pimples and pustules. Old, spreading, offensive ulcers. Wilted skin. Sallow, cold, clammy.

Modalities.—Worse, right side, motion, touch, change of weather, very early in morning. *Better*, after dinner, from pressure.

Relationship.—*Chelidonin.*—(Spasm of smooth muscle everywhere, intestinal colic, uterine colic, bronchial spasm, tachycardia, etc.) *Boldo*—Boldoa fragrans—(Bladder atony; cholecystitis and biliary calculus. Bitter taste, no appetite; constipation, hypochondriasis languor, congestion of liver; burning weight in liver and stomach. Painful hepatic diseases. Disturbed liver following malaria.) *Elemuy Gauteria*—(Stones in kidneys and bladder; grain doses of powdered bark in water or 5 drops of tincture. Pellagra).

Sulph. often completes its work.

Complementary: *Lycop.; Bryon.*

Antidote: *Chamom.*

Compare: *Nux; Sulph.; Bry.; Lyc.; Opium; Podophyl.; Sanguin.; Ars.*

Dose.—Tincture and lower attenuations.

CHENOPODIUM ANTHELMINTICUM
(Jerusalem Oak)

Characteristic pain in scapula very marked. Symptoms of apoplexy, right hemiplegia, and aphasia. Stertorous breathing. [*Opium.*] Sudden *vertigo*. Meniere's disease. Affections of auditory nerves. [*Nat. salicyl.*] Oil of Chenopodium for hookworm and roundworm.

Ears.—Torpor of auditory nerve. Hearing better for *high-pitched* sounds. Comparative deafness to sound of voice, but *great sensitiveness to sound, as of passing vehicles* and also a shrinking from low tones. Buzzing in ears. Enlargement of tonsils. *Aural vertigo.*

Back.—*Intense pain between angle of right shoulder-blade near spine*, and through the chest.

Urine.—Copious, yellow, foaming urine, with acrid sensation in urethra. Yellowish sediment. [*Chel.*]

Relationship.—Compare: *Opium; China; Chelid.*

Dose.—Third potency. Oil of Chenopodium for hookworm, 10 minim doses every 2 hours for 3 doses; also *Carbon tetrachloride.*

CHENOPODI GLAUCI APHIS
(Plant-lice from Chenopodium)

Partakes largely of the properties of the plant upon which the insect lives.

Head.—Sad; aching, worse from motion. Brain seems swashed hither and thither. Coryza, with burning or biting in nostrils. Noise in ears, as of cannon. Yellow face. Orbital right neuralgia, with profuse lachrymation. *Toothache, relieved by general warm sweat.* [*Cham.*] Toothache extends to ear, temple, and cheek-bone. [*Plantago.*]

Stomach.—No appetite for meat and bread. Vesicles at end of tongue. Much mucus. Colic with much rumbling and ineffectual urging to stool.

Stools.—Hard and knotty. Diarrhœa in morning, with painful urging and burning in anus, and pressure in rectum and bladder.

Urine.—Voluptuous feeling in glans. Burning in urethra. Urination frequent, copious, frothy.

Back.—Severe pains in region of *lower inner angle of left shoulder-blade,* running into chest.

Fever.—Shuddering all over; burning in palms; hot sweat in bed.

Relationship.—Compare: *Nat. sulph.; Nux.*

Dose.—Sixth to thirtieth potency.

CHELONE
(Snakehead)

A remedy in liver affections with pain or soreness of the left lobe of the liver and extending downwards. Dumb ague. Soreness of external parts, as if skin were off; debility. Malaise, following intermittents. Dyspepsia with hepatic torpor. Jaundice. *Round and thread worms.* It is an enemy to every kind of worm infesting the human body.

Dose.—Tincture, in one to five drop doses.

CHIMAPHILA UMBELLATA
(Pipsissewa)

Acts principally on kidneys, and genito-urinary tract; affects also lymphatic and mesenteric glands and female mammæ. Plethoric young women with dysuria. Women with large breasts. Hepatic and renal dropsies; chronic alcoholics. Incipient and progressive cataracts.

One of the remedies whose symptoms point to its employment in bladder affections, notably catarrh, acute and chronic. *Scanty urine, and loaded with ropy, muco-purulent sediment. Prostatic enlargement.*

Head.—Pain in left frontal protuberance. Halo about the light. Itching of eyelids. Stabbing pain in left eye with lachrymation.

Mouth.—Toothache, worse after eating and exertion, better cool water. Pain as if tooth was being gently pulled.

Urinary.—Urging to urinate. Urine turbid, offensive, containing ropy or bloody mucus, and depositing a copious sediment. Burning and scalding during micturition, and straining afterwards. *Must strain* before flow comes. Scanty urine. Acute prostatitis, retention, and *feeling of a ball in perineum.* [*Cann. ind.*] Fluttering in region of kidney. *Sugar in urine.* Unable to urinate without standing with feet wide apart and body inclined forward.

Female.—Labia inflamed, swollen. Pain in vagina. Hot flashes. Painful *tumor of mammæ*, not ulcerated, with undue secretion of milk. Rapid atrophy of breasts. Women with *very large breasts* and tumor in the mammary gland with *sharp* pain through it.

Male.—Smarting in urethra from neck of bladder to meatus. Gleet. Loss of prostatic fluid. Prostatic enlargement and irritation.

Skin.—Scrofulous ulcers. Glandular enlargements.

Extremities.—Feeling of a band above left knee.

Modalities.—*Worse*, in damp weather; from sitting on cold stones or pavements: left side.

Relationship.—Compare: *Chimaph. maculata* (intense gnawing hunger; burning fever; sensation of swelling in arm pits); *Uva.; Ledum; Epigœa.*

Dose.—Tincture, to third attenuation.

CHININUM ARSENICOSUM
(Arsenite of Quinine)

The symptoms of general *weariness and prostration* produced by the drug have been utilized in prescribing it homœopathically as a general tonic, often with very marked beneficial and prompt effect. In diphtheria with great prostration, cases that are prolonged, especially, and in malarial affections, neuralgia, etc., it has been found curative. Asthmatic attacks which recur periodically, with great prostration. Icy skin. Pressure in the solar plexus, with tender spine back of it.

Head.—Tired feeling. Head feels too full. Throbbing. Great anxiety. Great irritability. Vertigo; worse looking up. Dull, heavy headache, frontal and occipital. Darting pains running up into head.

Eyes.—Intense photophobia and orbicular spasm; gushing hot tears. Flickering with pain and lachrymation.

Mouth.—Tongue thickly furred; yellow, slimy coating. Bitter taste. No appetite.

Stomach.—Alternation of hyperacidity and decrease of acid. Hyperchlorhydria. [*Robinia; Arg. nit.; Orexine tannate*]. Thirst for water, yet it disturbs. *Anorexia. Eggs produce diarrhœa.*

Heart—Palpitation. Sensation as if heart stopped. Suffocative attacks, occurrng in periodical paroxysms. Must have open air. Short of breath on ascending; cardiac dyspnœa; circulatory weakness after acute infections; early myocardial degeneration.

Sleep.—Sleeplessness due to nervous causes. (Single dose of 5th or 6th potency.)

Extremities.—Weak limbs. *Coldness of hands and feet, knees and limbs.* Tearing pains.

Fever.—Continuous, with weakness. System depleted.

Relationship.—Compare: *Chininum;* also *Ferrum Citricum* (in nephritis with great anæmia; acid dyspepsia in chloros's

Morbus maculosus Werlhoffii); *Chinin. mur.* (in severe neuralgic pains around eyes, with chills; exaggerated sensitiveness to alcohol and tobacco; prostration and restlessness). *Œnothera* (effortless diarrhœa with nervous exhaustion; incipient hydrocephaloid). *Macrozamia spiralis* (extreme debility after illness; collapse).

Dose.—Second and third trituration.

CHININUM SULPHURICUM
(Sulphite of Quinine)

A dose of Chinin, sulph. in high potency sometimes arouses suppressed malaria, and brings back the paroxysm. Aside from its undoubted influence over malaria, it is indicated homœopathically whenever there is marked periodicity and spinal sensitiveness. *Acute articular rheumatism.* Polyarticular gout. Pruritus and congested conditions of the rectum. Symptoms of *chronic interstitial nephritis*. Retro-bulbar neuritis with sudden loss of sight. Thready vessels. Hiccough.

Blood.—An immediate and rapid decrease in red blood cells and reduction in hæmoglobin with increase in elimination of chlorides. Tendency to polynucleated leucocytosis.

Head.—Pain in forehead and temples, increasing gradually at noon, of malarial origin, with vertigo and pulsation. Worse left side. Falling in street. Inability to remain standing. Amaurosis.

Ears.—Violent ringing, buzzing, *and roaring in ears, with deafness.*

Face.—Neuralgia commences under eye; extends into and around it. Pains return with great regularity; *relieved by pressure.*

Spine.—*Great sensitiveness of the dorsal vertebræ;* pain on pressure. Last cervical sensitive. Pain extends to head and neck.

Urine.—Bloody. Turbid, slimy, clay-colored, greasy sediment. Small amount of urea and phosphoric acid with excess of uric acid and abundance of chlorides, accompanied by subnormal temperature. Excessive flow. Albuminuria.

Skin.—Itching; erythema, urticaria, icterus, vesication, pustules, purpura. Great sensitiveness. Shriveled skin.

Fever.—Chill daily at 3 p. m. Painful swelling of various veins during a chill. Shivering even in a warm room. Anguish. Subnormal temperature.

Relationship.—Compare: *Chin. salicyl.* (Deafness, tinnitus, and Meniere's disease.) *Ars.; Eupat.; Methyl. blue. Camphor mono-bromide* (is said to intensify the action of Quinine and render it more permanent.) *Baja*, an East Indian drug, (said to be almost infallible in intermittent fever, quartan type; pulsating headache injected eyes, flushed face. Liver and spleen enlarged. Œdema.) Also *Pambotano*, Mexican remedy for intermittent and tropical fevers.

Antidotes: *Parthenum; Natr. mur.; Lach.; Arn.; Puls.*

Dose.—First to third triturations; also thirtieth potency and higher.

CHIONANTHUS
(Fringe-tree)

This remedy is often of service in many types of headaches, neurasthenic, *periodical sick*, menstrual and bilious. Taken for several weeks, drop doses, will often break up the sick headache habit. The pain in the forehead, chiefly over eyes. Eyeballs very painful, with pressure over root of nose. Hepatic derangements. *Jaundice*. Enlarged spleen. [*Ceanoth.*] Jaundice, with arrest of menses. A prominent liver remedy. *Gallstones*. [*Berberis; Cholest.; Calc.*] Diabetes mellitus. Paroxysmal, abdominal pain.

Head.—Listless, apathetic. Dull frontal headache, over root of nose, over eyes, through temples, worse stooping, motion, jar. *Yellow conjunctiva*.

Tongue.—Broad with thick yellow fur.

Mouth.—Dry sensation not relieved by water, also profuse saliva.

Abdomen and Liver.—Aching in umbilical region, griping. Feels as if a string were tied in a "slip-knot" around intestines which was suddenly drawn tight and then gradually loosened. Sore; *enlarged, with jaundice* and constipation. Clay-colored stool, also soft, yellow and pasty. Tongue heavily coated. No appetite. Bilious colic. Hepatic region tender. Pancreatic disease and other glandular disorders.

Urine.—Large amount of high specific gravity; frequent urination; bile and sugar in urine. Urine very dark.

Skin.—Yellow; marked moisture of skin. Sallow, greenish, itching.

Relationship.—Compare: *Cinchona; Ceanoth.; Chelidon.; Carduus; Podophyl.; Lept.*

Dose.—Tincture and first attenuation.

CHLORALUM
(Chloral Hydrate)

This drug, used in physiological doses, is a powerful hypnotic and cardiac depressant. It has a marked effect on the skin, producing erythema, ecchymosis, etc., which symptoms have been utilized homœopathically with much success, especially in the treatment of hives. Emotional excitability, hallucinations. Night terrors in children. Muscular prostration.

Head.—Morning headache; worse in forehead, also in occiput, on motion; better in open air. Passive cerebral hyperæmia (use 30th). Feeling as if hot band were drawn from temple to temple. Hears voices.

Eyes.—Eyes blood-shot and watery. Circles of light, black spots. Illusions of sight where eyes are closed or at night. Dim vision. Conjunctivitis, burning in eye and lids; eyeball feels too large; everything looks *white*.

Skin.—Red blotches, like measles. *Urticaria, worse, spirituous liquors*, hot drinks. Erythema aggravated by alcoholic drinks, with palpitation; causes pain in tendons and extensors. Intense itching. Surface of body *stone-cold*. Wheals come on from a chill; better, warmth. Purpura. [*Phos.; Crotal.*]

Respiratory.—Extreme dyspnœa, with sensation of weight and constriction of chest. Asthma, with sleeplessness.

Sleep.—Insomnia, hallucinations, horrid dreams. Somnolence.

Modalities.—*Worse*, after hot drinks, stimulants, eating, night.

Relationship.—Antidotes: *Ammon.; Atrop.; Dig.; Mosch.*
Compare: *Bell.; Opium; Apis; Veronal*—(a dangerous drug made by the action of alcohol upon urea and contains the same radical that alcohol does. Makes a man just as drunk as pure alcohol. Staggers, cannot stand up. (Dr. Varney.) (Confluent, reddish spots; dermatitis, itching of glans and prepuce; circumscribed dermatitis patch on first metacarpal phalangeal joint.) *Luminal*—(Sleeplessness with skin symptoms in migraine; lethargy like epidemic encephalitis). (Dr. Royal.)

Dose.—First trituration in hives, otherwise, higher potencies. Locally, in offensive foot-sweat, bathe with one per cent. solution. For its physiological effects, five to twenty grains. Use cautiously.

CHLOROFORMUM
(Chloroform)

General anæsthetic, antispasmodic. Complete muscular relaxation. Weak and quick pulse, shallow or stertorous breathing. Convulsions, nephritic or biliary colic, gastralgia.

Symptoms obtained by Dr. D. Macfarlan with the 6th potency.

Great weakness, especially on right side. Limbs very tired from knees down. Much perspiration all over face and chest; drowsy and dizzy; dry lips and throat; dry tickling cough at night. Flatulence; food regurgitates; sore and bruised feeling in stomach; catching pain around heart. Sharp pain in right chest when he takes long breath; shortness of breath on exertion.

Head.—Delirium where excitement and violence predominate. Head drawn down upon the shoulders, eyes opened and closed rapidly, pupils contracted; rapid convulsive movements of face, of muscles, of extremities.

Relationship.—*Ether* Post-operative Bronchitis (Prof. Bier). *Spiritus Aetheris Compositus.*—(Hoffman's Anodyne)—(Flatulence; angina pectoris. Dose 5m to 1 dram in water.)

Dose.—Higher attenuations, or sixth. *Phosphorus* is the remedy to give in narcosis of chloroform.

CHLORUM
(Chlorine Gas in Water)

The marked effect on the respiratory organs, producing spasm of the glottis, is the chief symptom of the drug. Asthma to relieve the spasm of glottis. Useful externally and internally in gangrene.

Mind.—Fear of becoming crazy. Marked loss of memory, *especially for names*.

Respiratory.—Sooty, smoky nostrils. Coryza with sudden gushes of sharp, corroding fluid, making nose sore inside and about the alæ. *Constriction, with suffocation. Spasm of the glottis.* Irritation of epiglottis, larynx, and bronchi. Loss of voice from damp air. *Sudden dyspnœa from spasm of the vocal cords*, with staring protruding eyes, blue face, cold sweat, pulse small. *Inspiration free, with obstructed expiration.* [*Mephit.*] Livid face. Prolonged, loud, whistling rales. Extreme dryness of tongue.

Dose.—Chlorine water, when required of full strength, must be freshly prepared. Fourth to sixth potency.

CHOLESTERINUM
(Cholesterine — The proximate principle. Furnished by the epithelium lining of gall bladder and the larger ducts)

For cancer of the liver. *Obstinate hepatic engorgements.* Burning pain in side; on walking holds his hand on side, hurts him so. Opacities of the vitreous. Jaundice; gallstones. Cholesterine is the physiological opponent of Lecithin. Both seem to play some unknown part in the growth of tumors. Gallstones and insomnia.

Relationship.—Compare: *Taurocholate of soda* in Homœopathy.—Dr. I. P. Tessier, in an interesting study of the action of bile and its salts, in hepatic affections, analyzes a number of experiments by leading authorities, with the object of determining this action, and concludes that in the *Taurocholate of Soda,* homœopathy has a useful remedy against certain forms of hypoglobular anæmia. The claim that its pathogenesis and toxicology clearly indicate its value, and that it should also serve us as a remedy in cases of hypertrophy of the spleen and ganglia. He calls our attention to the fact, that it produces dyspnœa, the Cheyne-Stokes rhythm, acute pulmonary œdema, and intense exaggeration of the cardiac pulsations, offering a good field for clinical studies and experimentation of great interest, which may give fruitful and important results.

Dose.—Third trituration.

CHROMICUM ACIDUM
(Chromic Acid)

Diphtheria, post-nasal tumors, and epithelioma of the tongue have been benefited by this drug. Bloody, foul-smelling lochia. Symptoms come and go *suddenly*, and return periodically; offensive discharges.

Nose.—Ulcer and scabs in nose. Offensive smell. Corrosive pain. Ozæna. [*Aur.*]

Throat.—Diphtheria; sore throat. Tough mucus, with inclination to swallow it; worse, causing hawking. Post-nasal tumors.

Extremities.—Uneasiness in limbs. Pain in shoulder-blades and back of neck. Pain in knees and balls of feet. Drawing pain in soles while walking.

Stool.—Watery, frequent, copious, with nausea and vertigo. Hæmorrhoids, internal and bleeding. Weakness in small of back.

Relationship.—Compare: *Kali bich.; Rhus; Chromium Sulphate* (in locomotor ataxia, goitre, *prostatic hypertrophy*. Herpes preputialis. Wry neck. Also exophthalmic, inhibits the vagus, relieving tachycardia. Acts like a nerve tonic where there is lack of nervous tone. Fibroid tumors. Infantile paralysis. Dose for adults, 3 to 5 grains after meals and at bedtime).

Dose.—Homœopathically, third to sixth trituration.

CHRYSAROBINUM
(Goa Powder—Andira araroba)

Acts as a powerful irritant of the skin and used successfully in skin diseases especially in *ringworm, psoriasis,* herpes tonsurans, acne rosacea. Vesicular or squamous lesions, associated with foul smelling discharge and crust formation, tending to become confluent and to give the appearance of a single crust covering the entire area. (Bernstein.) *Violent itching,* thighs, legs and *ears.* Dry, scaly eruption, especially around eyes and ears, scabs with pus underneath. [*Mezer.*]

Eyes.—Blepharitis, conjunctivitis keratitis. Intense photophobia. Optical hyperaesthesia.

Ears.—Eczema behind ears. Filthy, scabby condition with tendency to form thick crust. Whole ear and surrounding tissue appears to be one scab.

Relationship.—Chrysarobinum contains chrysophan, which is rapidly oxydized into chrysophanic acid. This is also contained in Rhubarb and Senna.

Dose.—Locally, as a cerate, 4-8 grains to the ounce, of vaseline. Internally, third to sixth potency. Used externally; should be used with caution on account of its ability to produce inflammation.

CICUTA VIROSA
(Water Hemlock)

The action on the nervous system, producing spasmodic affections, viz., hiccough, trismus, tetanus, and convulsions, give the pathological picture calling especially for this remedy, whenever this is further characterized, by the more individual symptoms of the drug. Among these, are the *bending of the head, neck, and spine backwards,* and the general action of the patient is *violent,* with frightful distortions. Violent, strange desires. Sensation of internal chill. Moaning and howling. Does absurd things. Marked action on the skin.

Mind.—Delirium, with singing, dancing and funny gestures. Everything appears strange and terrible. Confounds present with the past; feels like a child. Stupid feeling. Melancholy, with indifference. Mistrustful. Epilepsy; moaning and whining. Vivid dreams.

Head.—*Head turned or twisted to one side. Cerebro-spinal meningitis. Cervical muscles contracted.* Vertigo, with gastralgia, and muscular spasms. Sudden, violent shocks through head. Stares persistently at objects. *Convulsions* from concussion of brain. Thick, yellow scabs on head. Head symptoms relieved by emission of flatus.

Eyes.—When reading, letters disappear. *Pupils dilated, insensible strabismus.* Objects recede, approach, and seem double. Eyes stare. Pupils get behind upper lids as head inclines. Effects of exposure to snow. Spasmodic affections of eyes and its appendages. Strabismus; periodic, spasmodic after a fall or a blow.

Ears.—Difficult hearing. Sudden detonations especially on swallowing. *Hæmorrhage from ears.*

Face.—Pustules which run together forming thick, yellow scabs on face and head, corners of mouth and chin, with burning pain. *Red face.* Trismus; disposition to grind teeth.

Throat.—Dry. Feels as if grown together. Spasms of œsophagus; cannot swallow. Effects on œsophagus from swallowing sharp piece of bone.

Stomach.—Thirst; burning pressure; *hiccough.* Throbbing in pit of stomach, which has become raised to size of fist. Desire for unnatural things, *like coal.* [*Alum.; Calc.*] Indigestion, with insensibilty, frothing at mouth.

Abdomen.—Flatulence with anxiety and crossness. Rumbling in. Distended and painful. Colic, with convulsions.

Rectum.—Diarrhœa in morning, with irresistible desire to urinate. Itching in rectum.

Respiratory.—Chest feels tight; can hardly breathe. Tonic spasm in pectoral muscles. Heat in chest.

Back and Extremities.—Spasms and cramps in muscles of nape of neck, and spasmodic drawing backward of head. Curved limbs cannot be straightened nor straight ones bent. *Back bent backward like an arch.* Jerking, tearing in coccyx, especially during menses.

Skin.—Eczema; no itching; exudation forms into a *hard,* *lemon-colored crust.* Suppressed eruption causes brain disease. Elevated eruptions, as large as peas. Chronic impetigo.

Modalities.—*Worse,* from touch, draughts, concussion, tobacco smoke.

Relationship.—Antidotes: *Opium; Arn.*

Compare: *Cicuta Maculata*—Water Hemlock—(Effects very similar; the most prominent symptoms being: Falls unconscious, tetanic or clonic convulsions. Body covered with sweat. Consider in epilepsy and tetanus. Tincture and lower potencies.) *Hydrocy. acid; Con.; Œnanth.; Strychnia; Bellad.*

Dose.—Sixth to two hundredth attenuation.

CIMEX — ACANTHIA
(Bedbug)

Of use in intermittent fever, with weariness and inclination to stretch. Hamstrings feel too short. [*Ammon mur.*] Flexors mostly affected. Sensation of retraction of arm tendons. Stretching.

Head.—Violent headache, caused by drinking. Great rage; vehement at beginning of chilly stage. Would like to tear everything to pieces. Pain under right frontal bone.

Female.—Shooting pain from vagina up towards left ovary.

Fever.—Chilliness of whole body. Sensation as of wind blowing on knees. *Pains in all joints, as if tendons were too short,* especially knee-joints. Chill; worse lying down. Thirst during apyrexia, but little during chilly stage; still less during hot stage, and none during sweating. Musty, offensive sweat.

Bowels.—Constipation, fæces dry and in small balls [*Op.; Plumb.; Thuj.*] and hard. Ulcer of rectum.

Dose.—Sixth to two hundredth attenuation.

CIMICIFUGA RACEMOSA — (ACTAEA RACEMOSA) (MACROTYS)
(Black Snake-root)

Has a wide action upon the cerebrospinal and muscular system, as well as upon the uterus and ovaries. Especially useful in rheumatic, nervous subjects with ovarian irritation, uterine cramps and heavy limbs. Its muscular and crampy pains, primarily of neurotic origin, occurring in nearly every part of the body, are characteristic. *Agitation and pain* indicate it. Pains like electric shocks here and there. Migraine. Symptoms referable to the pelvic organs prominent. "It lessens the frequency and force of the pulse soothes pain and allays irritability."

Mental.—Sensation of a cloud enveloping her. Great depression, with *dream of impending evil*. Fears riding in a closed carriage, of being obliged to jump out. Incessant talking. Visions of rats, mice, etc. Delirium tremens; tries to injure himself. Mania following disappearance of neuralgia.

Head.—Wild feeling in brain. Shooting and throbbing pains in head after mental worry, over-study, or reflex of uterine disease. Waving sensation or *opening and shutting sensation in brain*. Brain feels too large. *Pressing-outward* pain. Tinnitus. Ears sensitive to least noise.

Eyes.—Asthenopia associated with pelvic trouble. Deep-seated throbbing and *shooting pains* in eyes, with photophobia from artificial light. *Intense aching of eyeball. Pain from eyes to top of head.*

Stomach.—Nausea and vomiting caused by pressure on spine and cervical region. Sinking in epigastrium. [*Sep.; Sulph.*] *Gnawing pain.* Tongue pointed and trembling.

Female.—Amenorrhœa (use Macrotin preferably(. Pain in ovarian region; shoots upward and down anterior surface of thighs. Pain immediately before menses. Menses profuse, dark, *coagulated*, offensive with backache, nervousness; always irregular. Ovarian neuralgia. *Pain across pelvis, from hip to hip.* After-pains, with great sensitiveness and *intolerance to pain*. Infra-mammary pains worse, left side. Facial blemishes in young women.

Respiratory.—Tickling in throat. Dry, short cough, *worse speaking* and at night. Cough when secretion is scanty—spasmodic, dry with muscular soreness and nervous irritation.

Heart.—Irregular, slow, trembling pulse. Tremulous action. Angina pectoris. Numbness of left arm; feels as if bound to side. Heart's action ceases suddenly, impending suffocation. Left-sided infra-mammary pain.

Back.—Spine very sensitive, especially upper part. *Stiffness and contraction in neck and back.* Intercostal rheumatism.

Rheumatic pains in muscles of back and neck. Pain in lumbar and sacral region, down thighs, and through hips. Crick in back.

Extremities.—Uneasy, restless feeling in limbs. Aching in limbs and *muscular soreness*. Rheumatism affecting the belly of muscles, especially large muscles. Choreic movements, accompanied by rheumatism. Jerking of limbs. Stiffness in tendo-Achilles. Heaviness in lower extremities. Heavy, aching, tensive pain.

Sleep.—Sleeplessnes. Brain irritation of children during dentition.

Skin.—Locally and internally for ivy poisoning.

Modalities.—*Worse*, morning, cold (except headache), during menses; the more profuse the flow, the greater the suffering. *Better*, warmth, eating.

Relationship.—Compare: *Rhamnus Californica (muscular pains*, lumbago, pleurodynia, acute rheumatism). *Derris pinnata* (Neuralgic headaches of rheumatic origin). *Aristolochia milhomens* (pain in tendo-Achilles; diabetes). *Caulophyl.; Pulsat.; Lilium; Agar.; Macrotin* (especially for lumbago).

Dose.—First to thirtieth attenuation, third most frequently used.

CINA
(Worm-seed)

This is a children's remedy,—big, fat, rosy, scrofulous, corresponding to many conditions that may be referred to intestinal irritation, such as worms and accompanying complaints. An irritability of temper, variable appetite, grinding of teeth, and even convulsions, with screams and violent jerkings of the hands and feet, are all within its range of action. The Cina patient is hungry, cross, ugly, and wants to be rocked. *Pain in shocks*. Skin sensitive to touch.

Mind.—Ill-humor. Child *very cross;* does not want to be touched, or crossed, or carried. Desires many things, but rejects everything offered. Abnormal consciousness, as if having committed some evil deed.

Head.—Headache, alternating with pain in abdomen. Relieved by stooping. [*Mezer.*] Pain in head when using eyes.

Eyes.—Dilated pupils; yellow vision. Weak sight from masturbation. Strabismus from abdominal irritation. Eye-strain, especially when presbyopia sets in. *Pulsation of superciliary muscle.*

Ears.—Digging and scratching in ears.

Nose.—Itching of nose all the time. *Wants to rub it* and pick at it. *Bores at nose* till it bleeds.

Face.—Intense, circumscribed redness of cheeks. *Pale, hot, with dark rings around eyes.* Cold perspiration. *White and bluish about the mouth.* Grits teeth during sleep. *Choreic movements of face* and hands.

Stomach.—Gets hungry soon after a meal. *Hungry, digging, gnawing sensation.* Epigastric pain; worse, first waking in morning and before meals. Vomiting and diarrhœa immediately after eating or drinking. Vomiting with a clean tongue. Desires many and different things. Craving for sweets.

Abdomen.—*Twisting pain about navel.* [*Spig.*] Bloated and hard abdomen.

Stool.—White mucus, like small pieces of popped corn, preceded by pinching colic. *Itching of anus.* [*Teuc.*] Worms. [*Sabad.; Naphth.; Nat. phos.*]

Urine.—Turbid, white; turns milky on standing. Involuntary at night.

Female.—Uterine hæmorrhage before puberty.

Respiratory.—Gagging cough in the morning. Whooping-cough. Violent recurring paroxysms, as of down in throat. Cough ends in a spasm. Cough so violent as to bring tears and sternal pains; feels as if something had been torn off. Periodic; returning spring and fall. Swallows after coughing. *Gurgling from throat to stomach after coughing.* Child is afraid to speak or move for fear of bringing on paroxysm of coughing. After coughing, moaning, anxious, gasps for air and turns pale.

Extremities.—*Twitching* and jerking distortion of limbs, trembling. Paralyzed shocks; patient will jump suddenly, as though in pain. Child throws arms from side to side. Nocturnal convulsions. *Sudden inward jerking of fingers of right* *hand. Child stretches out feet spasmodically.* Left foot in constant spasmodic motion.

Sleep.—Child gets on hands and knees in sleep; on abdomen. Night terrors of children; cries out, screams, wakes frightened. *Troubles while yawning.* Screams and talks in sleep. Grits teeth.

Fever.—Light chill. Much fever, associated with clean tongue. Much hunger; colicky pains; chilliness, with thirst. Cold sweat on forehead, nose, and hands. In Cina fever, face is cold and hands warm.

Modalities.—*Worse*, looking fixedly at an object, from worms, at night, in sun, in summer.

Relationship.—Compare: *Santonin*—(often preferable in worm affections; same symptoms as Cina; corresponding to the "pain in shocks" produced by Cina. Visual illusions, *yellow* sight; violet light not recognized, colors not distinguishable. Urine deep saffron color. Spasms and twitchings, chronic gastric and intestinal troubles sometimes removed by a single dose (physiological) of Santonin. Dahlke.) *Helmintochortos*—Worm-moss (acts very powerfully on intestinal worms, especially the lumbricoid.) *Teucrium; Ignat.; Cham.; Spig.*

Antidote: *Camph.; Caps.*

Dose.—Third attenuation. For nervous irritable children, thirtieth and two-hundredth preferable. *Santonin* in first (with care) and third trituration.

CINCHONA OFFICINALIS
(Peruvian Bark — China)

Debility from exhausting discharges, from loss of vital fluids, together with a *nervous erethism*, calls for this remedy. Periodicity is most marked. Sensitive to draughts. Seldom indicated in the earlier stages of acute disease. Chronic gout. Chronic suppurative pyelitis. Post operative gas pains, no relief from passing it.

Mind.—Apathetic, indifferent, disobedient, taciturn, despondent. Ideas crowd in mind; prevent sleep. Disposition to hurt other people's feelings. Sudden crying and tossing about.

Head.—As if skull would burst. Sensation as if brain were balancing to and fro, and striking against skull, receiving great pain. [*Sulph.; Sulph. ac.*] Intense *throbbing* of head and carotids. Spasmodic headache in vertex, with subesquent pain, as if bruised in sides of head. Face flushed after hæmorrhages, or sexual excesses, or loss of vital fluids. Relieved from pressure and warm room. Scalp sensitive; worse combing hair. Aches worse in open air, from temple to temple. Worse by contact, current of air, stepping. Dizzy when walking.

Eyes.—Blue color around eyes. Hollow eyes. Yellowish sclerotica. Black specks, bright dazzling illusions; night blindness in anæmic retina. Spots before eyes. Photophobia. Distortion of eyeballs. Intermittent ciliary neuralgia. *Pressure in eyes*. Amaurosis; scalding lachrymation.

Ears.—*Ringing* in ears. External ear sensitive to touch. Hearing sensitive to noise. Lobules red and swollen.

Nose.—Checked catarrh. Easily bleeding from nose, especially on rising. Coryza, sneezing, watery discharge. Violent *dry* sneezing. Cold sweat about nose.

Face.—Sallow complexion. Face bloated; red.

Mouth.—Toothache; better pressing teeth firmly together, and by warmth. Tongue coated thick, dirty; tip burns, succeeded by ptyalism. Bitter taste. Food tastes too salty.

Stomach.—Tender, cold. Vomiting of undigested food. Slow digestion. Weight after eating. Ill effects of tea. Hungry without appetite. Flat taste. Darting pain crosswise in hypogastric region. Milk disagrees. Hungry longing for food, which lies undigested. *Flatulence; belching* of bitter fluid or regurgitation of food *gives no relief;* worse eating fruit. *Hiccough*. Bloatedness better by movement.

Abdomen.—Much flatulent colic; better bending double. *Tympanitic abdomen*. Pain in right hypochondrium. *Gallstone colic*. [*Triumfetta semitriloba*.] Liver and spleen swollen and enlarged. Jaundice. Internal coldness of stomach and abdomen. Gastro-duodenal catarrh.

Stool.—Undigested, frothy, yellow; *painless;* worse at night, after meals, during hot weather, from *fruit*, milk, beer. Very weakening, with much flatulence. Difficult even when soft. [*Alum.; Plat.*]

Male.—Excited lascivious fancy. Frequent emissions, followed by great weakness. Orchitis.

Female.—Menses too early. *Dark clots and abdominal distention.* Profuse menses with pain. Desire too strong. Bloody leucorrhœa. Seems to take the place of the usual menstrual discharge. Painful heaviness in pelvis.

Respiratory.—Influenza, with debility. Cannot breathe with head low. Labored, slow respiration; constant choking. *Suffocative catarrh; rattling in chest;* violent, hacking cough *after every meal.* Hæmorrhage from lungs. Dyspnœa, sharp pain in left lung. Asthma; worse damp weather.

Heart.—Irregular with weak rapid beats followed by strong, hard beats. Suffocative attacks, syncope; anæmia and dropsy.

Back.—Sharp pains across kidneys, worse movement and at night. Knife-like pains around back. (D. MacFarlan.)

Extremities.—*Pains in limbs and joints,* as if sprained; *worse, slight touch;* hard pressure relieves. Sensation as of a string around limb. Joints swollen; very sensitive, with dread of open air. Great debility, trembling, with numb sensation. Averse to exercise; sensitive to touch. Weariness of joints; worse, mornings and when sitting.

Skin.—*Extreme sensitiveness to touch,* but hard pressure *relieves. Coldness;* much sweat. One hand ice cold, the other warm. Anasarca. [*Ars.; Apis.*] *Dermatitis;* erysipelas. Indurated glands; scrofulous ulcers and caries.

Sleep.—Drowsiness. Unrefreshing or constant stupor. Wakens early. Protracted sleepiessness. Anxious, frightful dreams with confused consciousness on waking, so that the dream cannot be rid of and fear of dream remains. Snoring, especially with children.

Fever.—Intermittent, paroxysms anticipate; return every week. All stages well marked. Chill generally in forenoon, commencing in breast; thirst before chill, and little and often. Debilitating night-sweats. Free perspiration caused by every little exertion, especially on single parts. Hay fever, watery coryza, pain in temples.

Modalities.—*Worse, slightest touch.* Draught of air; every other day; loss of vital fluids; at night; *after eating;* bending over. *Better,* bending double; hard pressure; open air; warmth.

Relationship.—Antidotes: *Arn.; Ars.; Nux; Ipec.*

Compare: *Quinidin*—(Paroxysmal tachycardia and *auricular fibrillation*. Heart is slowed, and the auriculo-ventricular conduction time is lengthened. Dose ½ grain t. i. d.) *Cephalanthus*—Button Bush—Intermittent fever, sore throat, rheumatic symptoms, vivid dreams). *Ars.; Cedron; Nat. sulph. Cydonia vulgaris*—Quince (supposed to be of use to strengthen the sexual organs and stomach).

Complementary: *Ferrum; Calc. phos.*

Dose.—Tincture, to thirtieth potency.

CINERARIA
(Dusty Miller)

Has some reputation in the cure of cataract and corneal opacities. Is used externally, by instilling into the eye one drop four or five times a day. This must be kept up for several months. Most effective in traumatic cases. Compare in cataract *Phosph.; Platanus; Cannabis; Causticum; Naphthalin; Ledum; Nat. mur.; Silica.*

CINNABARIS — MERCURIUS SULPHURATUS RUBER
(Mercuric Sulphide)

For certain forms of ciliary neuralgia and ulceration upon a syphilitic base, this remedy is most effective. Sleepless during night.

Head.—Congestion to head; face purple red.

Eyes.—*Pains from lachrymal duct around eye to temple, from inner canthus across brows to ear. Severe shooting pain in bones of orbit, especially running from inner to outer canthus in the bone. Redness of whole eye.* Lids granulated; canthi and lids red.

Nose.—Pressive sensation, as from heavy spectacles. Pain about root, extending into bones on each side. [*Aur.; Kal. hyd.*]

Throat.—Stringy mucus passed through posterior nares into throat. Dryness of mouth and throat; must rinse the mouth. Fiery-looking ulcers in mouth and throat.

Male.—Prepuce swollen; *warts on it which bleed easily;*

testicles enlarged; buboes; angry-looking chancres. Syphilides, squamous and vesicular.

Female.—Leucorrhœa. Feeling of pressure in vagina.

Extremities.—Pain in forearm from elbow down, including hands. Pain in long bones when barometer lowers; coldness of joints.

Skin.—*Very fiery-red* looking ulcers. Nodes on shin-bones. Buboes. Condyloma, easily bleeding.

Modalities.—*Worse,* lying on right side (feels as if contents of body were being dragged over to that side).

Relationship.—Compare: *Hepar; Nitr. ac.; Thuja; Sep.* Antidotes: *Hepar; Sulph.*

Dose.—First to third trituration.

CINNAMONUM
(Cinnamon)

Cancer where pain and fetor are present. Best when skin is intact. Its use in hæmorrhages has abundant clinical verification. Nosebleed. Hæmorrhages from bowels, hæmotysis, etc. A strain in loins or false step brings on a profuse flow of bright blood. *Post-partum hæmorrhage.* Flatulency and diarrhœa. Feeble patients with languid circulation.

Female.—Bearing-down sensation. Menses *early, profuse, prolonged, bright red.* Sleepy. No desire for anything. Fingers seem swollen. Uterine hæmorrhages caused by overlifting, during puerperal state; menorrhagia.

Relationship.—Compare: *Ipec.; Sil.; Trill.*

Antidote: *Acon.*

Dose.—Tincture to third potency. For cancer, strong decoction, one-half pint in a day. *Oil of cinnamon* in aqueous solution best local disinfectant. 3-4 drops in two quarts of water as a douche, wherever a germicide and disinfectant is needed. Three drops on sugar for hiccough.

CISTUS CANADENSIS
(Rock Rose)

A deep-acting anti-psoric remedy, with marked action in glandular affections, herpetic eruptions, chronic swellings, when patient is *extremely sensitive to cold. Sensation of coldness in various parts.* Scrofulous ophthalmia. Poisoned wounds, bites, phagedenic ulcers. *Malignant disease of the glands of the neck.* Cistus has affinity for naso-pharynx; aborts colds that center in posterior nose. Sniffling.

Face.—Itching, burning, and crusts on right zygoma. Lupus, caries; open, bleeding cancer. Tip of nose painful.

Mouth.—Scorbutic swollen gums. *Mouth feels cold;* putrid, impure breath. *Pyorrhœa.* [*Merc. cor.; Caust.; Staph.; Kreos.*] *Hurts to protrude the tongue.*

Ears.—Watery discharge; also fetid pus. Tetter on and around ears, extending to external meatus.

Throat.—Spongy feeling; *very dry* and *cold air passing over parts causes pain*. Breath, tongue, and throat feel cold. Uvula and tonsils swollen. A small, dry spot in throat; must sip water frequently. Hawking of mucus. Swelling and suppuration of glands of throat. Head drawn to one side by swellings in neck. Sore throat from inhaling the least *cold air*. Heat and itching in throat.

Stomach.—*Cool feeling* in stomach before and after eating. *Cool feeling* in whole abdomen. Desire for cheese.

Stool.—Diarrhœa from coffee and fruit, thin, yellow, urgent; worse in morning.

Chest.—Coldness in chest. The neck is studded with tumors. Induration of mammæ. Hæmorrhage from lungs.

Extremities.—Sprained pain in wrist. Tips of fingers sensitive to cold. Tetter on hands. Cold feet. Syphilitic ulcers on lower limbs, with hard swelling around. White swelling.

Sleep.—Cannot sleep from coldness in throat.

Female.—Induration and inflammation of mammæ. Sensitive to cold air. Bad smelling leucorrhœa.

Respiratory.—Asthmatic after lying down (trachea feels narrow), preceded by formication.

Skin.—Itching all over. Small, painful pimples; lupus. *Glands inflamed and indurated.* Mercurio-syphilitic ulcers. Skin of hands hard, thick, dry, fissured; deep cracks. Itching of swollen hands and arms; general itching which prevents sleep. Hemicrania.

Modalities.—*Worse*, slightest exposure to cold air; mental exertion, excitement. *Better* after eating.

Relationship.—Antidotes: *Rhus; Sepia.*
Compare: *Conium; Carbo; Calc; Arg. n.*
Dose.—First to thirtieth attenuation. Locally as a wash to arrest fetid discharges.

CITRUS VULGARIS
(Bitter Orange)

Headache with nausea, vomiting and vertigo. Facial neuralgias mostly right-sided. Thoracic oppression. Frequent and irresistible yawning. Disturbed sleep.

Relationship.—*Citrus decumana*—Grape-fruit. (Tinnitus, *head noises* and ringing in ears. Sensation of pressure in the temporal region.) *Aurantium*-Orange (neuralgic and skin symptoms. Itching, redness and swelling of hands. Diseases of the aged with coldness and chilliness. Boiled dried *orange peel* excites the intestine in a manner similar to other forms of cellulose or agar. There is an increased flow of bile which continues for hours. It unites both a cholagogue action with a mechanical stimulus to peristalsis.) Compare: *Citrus Limonum* (scorbutus, sore throat and cancer pains; checks excessive menstruation.) (*Citric Acid.*—Useful in *scurvy* and chronic rheumatism and hæmorrhages. All forms of *Dropsy* are benefitted with Citric acid and lemon juice, tablespoonful every 3-4 hours. Pain from cancer of tongue. Used as a local application and mouth wash, one dram to 8 ozs. of water. For cancer pains generally, often effective.)

CLEMATIS ERECTA
(Virgin's Bower)

Scrofulous, rheumatic, gonorrhœal, and syphilitic patients. Acts especially on skin, *glands* and genito-urinary organs, especially testicles. A remedy of much importance in disturbances of sleep, and neuralgic *pains* in various parts. Many of these pains are relieved by perspiration. Muscles relaxed or twitching. Great emaciation. *Great sleepiness.* Distant pulsation in whole body.

Head.—Boring pain in temples. *Confused feeling; better in open air.* Eruption on occiput at base of hair, moist, pustular, sensitive, itching.

Eyes.—Heat in eyes and *sensitive to air;* must close them. Chronic blepharitis, with sore and swollen meibomian glands. Iritis, great *sensitiveness to cold.* Flickering before eyes. Pustular conjunctivitis, with tinea capitis; eyes inflamed and protruding.

Face.—White blisters on face and nose, as if burned by sun. Swelling of submaxillary glands, with hard tubercles; throbbing, aggravated on being touched. Pain in right side of face to eye, ear and temple; better, holding cold water in mouth.

Teeth.—*Ache; worse, at night and from tobacco.* Teeth feel too long.

Stomach.—After eating, weakness in all limbs and pulsation in arteries.

Male.—Ilio-scrotal neuralgia. *Testicles indurated with bruised feeling.* Swelling of scrotum. [*Orchitis.*] Right-half only. Troubles from suppressed gonorrhœa. Violent erections with stitches in urethra. Testicles hang heavy or retracted, with pain along spermatic cord; worse, right side.

Urinary.—Tingling in urethra lasting some time after urinating. Frequent, scanty urination; burning at orifice. *Interrupted flow.* Urethra feels constricted. Urine emitted drop by drop. Inability to pass all the urine; dribbling after urinating. Pain worse at night, pain along the spermatic cord. Commencing stricture.

Skin.—Red, burning, vesicular, scaly, scabby. Itches terribly; worse, washing in cold water; worse face and hands and *scalp around occiput. Glands* hot, painful, *swollen;* worse inguinal glands. Glandular indurations and tumors of breast. Varicose ulcers.

Modalities.—*Better,* in open air. *Worse,* at night and warmth of bed (washing in cold water; new moon—(monthly aggravation).

Relationship.—Compare: *Clematis vitalba* (varicose and other ulcers); *Sil.; Staph.; Petrol.; Oleand.; Sarsap.; Canth.; Phos. ac.; Pulsat.*

Antidotes: *Bryon.; Camph.*

Dose.—Third to thirtieth potency.

COBALTUM
(The Metal Cobalt)

Adapted to neurasthenic spinal states. Sexual disturbances. Fatigue, agitation, and bone pains, worse in morning.

Mind.—All mental excitement increases suffering. Constant interchange of mental moods.

Head.—Aches; worse, bending head *forward*. Itching of hairy scalp and beard.

Teeth.—Feel too long. Pain in teeth. Cracks across tongue. Coated white. [*Ant. cr.*]

Abdomen.—Shooting in liver. Pain in spleen.

Rectum.—Constant dropping of blood from the anus, no blood from the stools.

Male.—Pain in right testicle; better, urinating. *Emissions* without erection. Impotence. Backache in lumbar region and weak legs. Lewd dreams. Pain in end of urethra; greenish discharge; brown spots on genitals and abdomen.

Back.—*Pain in back and sacrum; worse while sitting;* better, walking or lying. Weakness in legs and backache after emissions.

Extremities.—Aching in wrist-joints. Shooting into thighs from liver. *Weak knees.* Trembling in limbs. Tingling in feet. Foot-sweat, mostly between toes.

Sleep.—Unrefreshing; *disturbed by lewd dreams.*

Skin.—Dry and pimply. Pimples about nates, chin, hairy scalp.

Relationship.—Compare: *Cannab. Ind.; Sepia; Zinc.; Agnus; Selen.*

Dose.—Sixth to thirtieth potency.

COCA—ERYTHROXYLON COCA
(The Divine Plant of the Incas—but the Spanish priests denounced it as "un delusio del demonio")

The mountaineer's remedy. Useful in a variety of complaints incidental to mountain climbing, such as palpitation, dyspnœa, anxiety and insomnia. Exhausted nervous system from physical and mental strain. Caries of teeth. *Loss of voice.*—Give 5-6 drops, every half hour, two hours before expected demand on voice. Nocturnal enuresis. Emphysema [*Quebracho*].

Mind.—Melancholy; bashful, ill at ease in society, irritable, delights in solitude and obscurity. Sense of right and wrong abolished.

Head.—Fainting fit from climbing mountains. Shocks coming from occiput with vertigo. *Noises in ear.* Headache with vertigo, preceded by flashes of light. Like a band across forehead. Diplopia. Tongue furred. *Headaches of high altitudes.* Tinnitus.

Stomach.—Peppery sensation in mouth.[11] Longing for alcoholic liquors and tobacco. Great satiety for a long time. Incarcerated flatus; rises with noise and violence, as if it would split the œsophagus. Tympanitic distention of abdomen. No appetite but for sweets.

Heart.—*Palpitation*, with weak heart and dyspnœa.

Male.—Diabetes, with impotency. [*Phos. ac.*]

Respiratory.—Hawking of small, transparent pieces of mucus. Weak vocal cords. *Hoarseness;* worse after talking. *Want of breath, short breath*, especially in aged athletes, and alcoholic users. Hæmoptysis. *Asthma*, spasmodic variety.

Sleep.—Can find no rest anywhere, but sleepy. Nervousness and nightly restlessness during teething.

Modalities.—*Better*, from wine; riding, quick motion in open air. *Worse*, ascending, high altitudes.

Relationship.—Compare: *Ars.; Paulin.; Cyp.; Chamom.* Antidote: *Gels.*

Dose.—Tincture to third attenuation.

COCAINA

(An Alkaloid from Erythroxylon Coca)

Besides the great usefulness of Cocaine as a local anæsthetic, it has specific homœopathic uses, though the symptoms are mainly clinical only.

Sensation *as if small foreign bodies or worms were under the skin.*

Mind.—Talkative. Constant desire to do something great, *to undertake vast feats of strength.* Cerebral activity. Frightful persecutory hallucinations; *sees and feels bugs and worms. Moral sense blunted.* Personal appearance neglected. Thinks he hears unpleasant remarks about himself. Hallucinations of hearing. Irrational *jealousy*. Insomnia.

Head.—Throbbing and bursting sensation. *Pupils dilated.* Hearing greatly increased. Roaring and noises in head.

Eyes.—Glaucoma, increased tension, decreased corneal sensibility. Eyes staring, expressionless.

Throat.—Dry, burning, tickling, constricted, paralysis of muscles of deglutition. Speech difficult.

Stomach.—Loss of appetite for solid food. *Likes sweets. Hæmorrhages* from bowels, stomach.

Nervous System.—Chorea; paralysis agitans; alcoholic tremors and senile trembling. Local sensory paralysis. Formication and numbness in hands and forearms.

Sleep.—Restless, cannot sleep for hours after retiring.

Fever.—Coldness with intense pallor.

Relationship.—Compare: *Stovain* (an analgesic, a vasomotor dilator). Antidote to disagreeable effects occasionally resulting from injection of cocaine into skin or gums, drop doses of nitro-glycer. 1% sol.

Dose.—Lower potencies. As a local application to mucous membranes, 2-4%.

COCCINELLA SEPTEMPUNCTATA
(Lady Bug)

This remedy ought to be remembered in neuralgias, teeth, gums, mouth, etc. Is awakened by profuse accumulation of saliva. Uvula feels too long. Symptoms of hydrophobia; worse, by any bright object.

Head.—Pain in forehead over right eye, sensitive to touch; from superior molars to forehead. Aching in temples and occiput. Rush of blood to face. *Throbbing toothache. Cold sensation in teeth* and mouth. [*Cistus.*] Periodical attacks of frontal neuralgia. Cannot open eyes during paroxysm. Pain worse from any bright object; better, sleep.

Stomach.—Hiccough and burning in stomach.

Back.—*Pain in region of kidneys and loins.* Icy cold extremities.

Relationship.—Compare: *Canth.; Mayn. c.*

Dose.—Third potency.

COCCULUS
(Indian Cockle)

Within the sphere of action of Cocculus are many spasmodic and paretic affections, notably those affecting one-half of the body. Affects the cerebrum, will not cure convulsive seizures proceeding from the spinal cord. (A. E. Hinsdale.) *Painful contracture* of limbs and trunk; tetanus. Many of the evil *effects of night-watching* are relieved by it. It shows a special attraction *for light-haired females*, especially during pregnancy, causing much nausea and backache. Unmarried and childless women, sensitive and romantic girls, etc. All its symptoms are worse riding in a carriage or on shipboard; hence its use in seasickness. Sensation of *hollowness*, or emptiness, as if parts had gone to sleep. Feels too weak to talk loud.

Mind.—Capricious. Heavy and stupid. *Time passes too quickly;* absorbed in reveries. Inclination to sing irresistible. Slow of comprehension. Mind benumbed. *Profound sadness.* Cannot bear contradiction. Speaks hastily. Very anxious about the health of others.

Head.—Vertigo, nausea, *especially when riding* or sitting up. Sense of emptiness in head. Headache *in occiput* and nape; worse, lying on back of head. Sick headache from carriage-riding, cannot lie on back part of head. Pupils contracted. Opening and shutting sensation, especially in occiput. Trembling of head. Pain in eyes as if torn out of head.

Face.—Paralysis of facial nerve. Cramp-like pain in masseter muscle; *worse, opening mouth.* Prosopalgia in afternoon, with wide radiations of pain.

Stomach.—Nausea from riding in cars, boat, etc., or looking at boat in motion; worse on becoming cold or taking cold. Nausea, with faintness and vomiting. *Aversion to food*, drink, tobacco. *Metallic taste.* Paralysis of muscles preventing deglutition. Dryness of œsophagus. Seasickness. [*Resorcin.* 1x.] Cramp, in stomach during and after meal. Hiccough and spasmodic yawning. Loss of appetite. Desire for cold drinks, especially beer. Sensation in stomach as if one had been a long time without food until hunger was gone. Smell of food disgusts. [*Colch.*]

Abdomen.—Distended, with wind, and feeling as *if full of sharp stones when moving;* better, lying on one side or the other. Pain in abdominal ring, as if something were forced through. Abdominal muscles weak; it seems as if a hernia would take place.

Female.—Dysmenorrhœa, with profuse dark menses. Too early menses, clotted, with spasmodic colic. Painful pressing in uterine region, followed by hæmorrhoids. Purulent, gushing leucorrhœa between menses; *very weakening*, can scarcely speak. So weak during menstruation, scarcely able to stand.

Respiratory.—Sensation of emptiness and cramp in chest. Dyspnœa as from constriction of trachea, as if irritated by smoke. Choking constriction in upper part of œsophagus, oppressing breathing and inducing cough.

Back.—Cracking of cervical vertebræ when moving head. *Paralytic pain in small of the back.* Pain *in shoulder and arms as if bruised.* Pressure in scapula and nape. Stiffness on moving shoulders.

Extremities.—Lameness; worse by bending. *Trembling* and pain in limbs. Arms go to sleep. One-sided paralysis; worse after sleep. Hands are alternately hot and cold; numbness and cold sweat now of one, now of the other hand. Numb and unsteady. *Knees crack on motion.* Lower limbs very weak. Inflammatory swelling of knee. Intensely painful, paralytic drawing. Limbs straightened out, painful when flexed.

Sleep.—Spasmodic yawning. Coma vigil. Constant drowsiness. After loss of sleep, night-watching, nursing.

Fever.—Chill, with flatulent colic, nausea, vertigo, coldness of lower extremities, and heat of head. Sweat general. Nervous form of low fever. *Chilliness, with perspiration, and heat of skin.*

Modalities.—*Worse*, eating, after loss of sleep, open air, smoking, riding, swimming, touch, noise, jar; afternoon. Menstrual period. After emotional disturbance.

Relationship.—Antidotes: *Coffee; Nux.*

Compare: *Picrotoxin*—alkaloid of Cocculus—(epilepsy, attacks in the morning on leaving horizontal position, hernia, locomotor ataxia, night-sweats); *Symphoricarpus* (morning sickness); *Petrol.; Puls.; Ignat.*

Dose.—Third to thirtieth potency.

COCCUS CACTI
(Cochineal)

The clinical application of the symptoms of this remedy, place it among the medicines for spasmodic and whooping coughs, and catarrhal conditions of the bladder; spasmodic pains in kidneys, with visceral tenesmus. Anuria, anasarca, ascites.

Mind.—Early morning or afternoon sadness.

Head.—Suboccipital soreness; worse after sleep and exertion. Headache, worse from lying on back, better with the head high. Dull pain over right eye in morning. *Sensation of a foreign body between upper lid and eyeball.* Distress from cinders lodged in eye.

Respiratory.—Constant hawking from enlarged uvula; coryza, with inflamed fauces; *accumulation of thick viscid mucus*, which is expectorated with great difficulty. *Tickling in lárynx.* Sensation of a crumb behind larynx, must swallow continually: brushing teeth causes cough. Fauces very sensitive. Suffocative cough; worse, first waking, with tough, white mucus, which strangles. Spasmodic morning cough. *Whooping cough attacks end with vomiting of this tough mucus.* Chronic bronchitis complicated with gravel; large quantities of albuminous, tenacious mucus, are expectorated. Walking against wind takes breath away.

Heart.—Sensation as if everything were pressed toward the heart.

Urinary.—Urging to urinate; *brick-red sediment.* Urinary calculi, hæmaturia, urates, and uric acid; lancinating pains from kidney to bladder. Deep-colored, thick urine. Dysuria.

Female.—Menses too early, profuse, *black* and thick; *dark clots*, with dysuria. Intermittent menstruation; flow only in evening and at night. *Large clots* escape when passing water. *Labia* inflamed.

Modalities.—*Worse*, left side, after sleep, touch, pressure of clothing, brushing teeth, slightest exertion. *Better*, walking.

Relationship.—Compare: *Canth.; Cact.; Sars.*

Dose.—Lower triturations.

COCHLEARIA ARMORACIA—ARMORACIA SATIVA
(Horse-radish)

Frontal bone and sinus, antrum and salivary glands are specifically affected by this drug. Bloated sensation. Raises vital forces. Used as a gargle in scorbutic gums and sore throat. Hoarseness and in relaxed conditions of the fauces. Internally in gonorrhœa. Useful as a condiment in enfeebled states of the stomach. An infusion of the root in cider, for dropsy, causes copious diuresis. Locally cures dandruff.

Head.—Thinking is difficult. Anxiety, driven to despair by pain. Pressing, boring pain as if frontal bone would fall out. Violent headache with vomiting. Impaired hearing.

Eyes.—*Sore and scrofulous;* traumatic inflammation of eyes, blearedness and cataract. Copious running from eyes.

Stomach.—Pain towards back; worse, pressure on dorsal vertebræ. Belching and cramps. Colic with backache. *Violent cramp from stomach through both sides around to back.* Griping around navel.

Back.—Pain in back as from incarcerated flatulence *from abdomen through to back and down into sacrum.*

Respiratory.—Dry, hacking, laryngeal cough, also post-influenzal cough, dry or loose, worse lying down. Chest painful to touch. Coryza, with hoarseness. Mucous asthma. Œdema of lungs. Throat feels rough and hoarse.

Urinary.—Burning and cutting at glans penis before, during, and after urination. Frequent urination.

Modalities.—Worse evening and at night.

Relationship.—Compare: *Cannab; Sinapis; Caps.*

Dose.—First to third attenuation.

CODEINUM
(An Alkaloid from Opium)

Trembling of whole body. Involuntary twitching of muscles of arms and lower limbs. *Itching*, with feeling of warmth, numbness and prickling. Diabetes.

Head.—Pain from occiput to back of neck. Skin of face and scalp sore after neuralgia.

Eyes.—Involuntary twitching of lids. [*Agar.*]

Stomach.—Spasmodic pain at pit of stomach. Eructations. Great thirst, with desire for bitter substances.

Respiratory.—Short and irritating cough; worse, at night. Copious, purulent expectoration. Night cough of phthisis.

Relationship.—Compare: *Opium; Agaricus; Hyoscy.; Ammon. brom.*

Dose.—One-quarter of a grain doses to third trituration.

COFFEA CRUDA
(Unroasted Coffee)

Stimulates the functional activity of all organs, increasing the nervous and vascular activity. The drinking of coffee by the aged is likely to increase production of uric acid, causing irritation of kidneys; muscle and joint pains, and with the increased susceptibility of old people to the stimulating action of coffee and tea, their use should be curtailed or carefully watched. Great nervous agitation and restlessness. Extreme sensitiveness characterizes this remedy. Neuralgia in various parts; always with great nervous excitability and *intolerance of pain*, driving to despair. *Unusual activity of mind and body.* Bad effects of sudden emotions, surprises, joy, etc. Nervous palpitation. Coffea is specially suited to tall, lean, stooping persons with dark complexions, temperament choleric and sanguine. Skin hypersensitive.

Mind.—Gaiety, easy comprehension, irritability, excited; senses acute. Impressionable, especially to pleasurable impressions. Full of ideas, quick to act. Tossing about in anguish. [*Acon.*]

Head.—Tight pain, worse from noise, smell, narcotics. Seems as if brain were torn to pieces, *as if nail were driven in head.* Worse in open air. *Sensitive hearing.*

Face.—Dry heat, with red cheeks. Prosopalgia extending to molar teeth, ears, forehead, and scalp.

Mouth.—Toothache; temporarily relieved by holding ice-water in the mouth. [*Mangan. opposite.*] Hasty eating and drinking. Delicate taste.

Stomach.—Excessive hunger. Intolerance of tight clothing. After wine and liquor.

Female.—Menses too early and long lasting. Dysmenorrhœa, large clots of black blood. *Hypersensitive vulva and vagina.* Voluptuous itching.

Sleep.—Wakeful; on a constant move. Sleeps till 3 a. m., after which only dozing. Wakes with a start, sleep disturbed by dreams. *Sleepless, on account mental activity;* flow of ideas, with nervous excitability. Disturbed by itching of anus.

Respiratory.—Short, dry cough of measles in nervous, delicate children.

Heart.—Violent irregular palpitation especially after excessive joy or surprise. Rapid high tension pulse and urinary suppression.

Extremities.—Crural neuralgia; worse, motion, afternoon and night; better, by pressure.

Modalities.—*Worse,* excessive emotions (joy), narcotics. strong odors, noise, open air, cold, night. *Better,* warmth, from lying down; holding ice in mouth.

Relationship.—Incompatible: *Camph.; Coccul.* Complementary: *Acon.*

Compare: *Coffea tosta.* (Roasting develops certain vitaminlike substances (P. T. Mattei). Pigeons which have developed "deficiency" neuritis and paralysis on diet of polished rice lost their disabilities on the addition of 8cc to a 5% infusion of coffee to their food. Unroasted coffee was useless.) *Caffein.*—(A crystalline alkaloid—is a direct heart stimulant and diuretic. Dropsy depending on cardiac insufficiency. Myocardial degeneration. Cardiac insufficiency in pneumonia and other infectious diseases. Raises the blood pressure, increases pulse rate and stimulates the heart muscle; hence, a support in extreme feebleness or threatened failure. Stimulates the respiratory centre, nerve centres and *increases diuresis.* One of the best stimulants of the vaso-motor centres. Acute pulmonary edema. Brachialgia and other neuralgias characterized by *nocturnal exacerbations.* Jousset uses equal parts of caffein and sachar. lac. 3 grains taken in divided doses every other day. Hypodermically, ¼ grain. Excruciating facial neuralgia from decayed teeth); *Acon.; Cham.; Nux; Cyp.; Caffein* and plants containing it, as *Kola, Thea,* etc.

Strong black coffee, drunk as hot as possible, is indispensable as an antidote in a large number of poisons, especially narcotics. Hot coffee by rectum in cases of extreme collapse.

Antidotes: *Nux; Tabac.*

Dose.—Third to two hundredth potency.

COLCHICUM
(Meadow Saffron)

Affects markedly the muscular tissues, periosteum, and synovial membranes of joints. Has specific power of relieving the gouty paroxysms. It seems to be more beneficial in chronic affections of these parts. The parts are red, hot, swollen. Tearing pains; worse, in the evening and at night and from touch; stubbing the toes hurts exceedingly. *There is always great prostration,* internal *coldness,* and tendency to collpase. Effects of night watching and hard study. Shocks as from electricity through one half of body. Bad effects from suppressed sweat. Dreams of mice.

Head.—Headache chiefly frontal and temporal, but also occipital and in nape of neck, worse afternoon and evening.

Eyes.—Pupils unequal; left pupil contracted. Variations in visual acuity. Lachrymation worse in open air; violent tearing pain in eyes. Dim vision after reading. Spots before eyes.

Ears.—Itching in ears; sharp, shooting pains below right tragus.

Face.—Pain in facial muscles, moving about. Tingling and œdematous swelling; cheeks red, hot, sweaty. Very irritable with the pains. [*Cham.*] Pain behind angle of right lower jaw.

Stomach.—Dry mouth, tongue burns, gums and teeth pain. *Thirst;* pain in stomach and flatulence. The *smell of food causes nausea even to fainting,* especially fish. Profuse salivary secretion. Vomiting of mucus, bile and food; worse, any motion; *great coldness in stomach. Craving for various things,* but is averse to them when smelling them, seized then with nausea. Gouty gastralgia. Burning or *icy coldness in stomach* and abdomen. Thirst for effervescent, alcoholic beverages. Pain in transverse colon.

Abdomen.—*Distention* of abdomen, with gas, inability to stretch out legs. Borborygmi. Pain over liver. Cæcum and ascending colon much distended. Fullness and continuous rumbling. Ascites.

Stool.—Painful, scanty, transparent, jelly-like mucus; pain, as if anus were torn open, with prolapse. Autumnal dysentery; stools contain *white shreddy particles* in large quantities. Ineffectual pressing; feels fæces in rectum, but cannot expel them.

Female.—Pruritus of genitals. Cold feeling in thigh after period. Sensation of swelling in vulva and clitoris.

Urine.—Dark, scanty or suppressed; bloody, brown, black, inky; contains clots of putrid decomposed blood, albumin, sugar.

Heart.—Anxiety in region of heart. Impulse not felt. Pericarditis, with severe pain, oppression and dyspnœa, pulse threadlike. Sound of heart become weaker, pulse of low tension.

Extremities.—Sharp pain down left arm. Tearing in limbs during warm weather, stinging during cold. Pins and needles in hands and wrists, fingertips numb. Pain in front of thigh. Right plantar reflex abolished. Limbs, lame, weak, tingling. Pain worse in evening and warm weather. Joints stiff and feverish; shifting rheumatism; pains worse at night. Inflammation of great toe, gout in heel, *cannot bear to have it touched or moved*. Tingling in the finger nails. Knees strike together, can hardly walk. Œdematous swelling and coldness of legs and feet.

Back.—Aching in lumbar and lumbo-sacral region. Dull pain across loins. Backache, better, rest and pressure.

Skin.—Blotchy papular rash on face. Pink spots on back, chest and abdomen. Urticaria.

Modalities.—*Worse*, sundown to sunrise; motion, loss of sleep, smell of food in evening, mental exertion. *Better*, stooping.

Relationship.—Antidotes: *Thuja; Camph.; Coccul.; Nux; Puls.*

Compare: *Colchicine* (intestinal catarrh with shreddy membranes; convulsive jerkings of right hand; rheumatic fever, gout, endo and pericarditis, pleurisy, arthritis, deformans in early stages; *intense pain of rheumatism* 3x trit.). Also, *Carbo; Arnica; Lilium; Arsen.; Verat.*

Dose.—Third to thirtieth attenuation.

COLLINSONIA CANADENSIS
(Stone-Root)

Pelvic and portal congestion, resulting hæmorrhoids and constipation, especially in females. Depressed arterial tension, general atony of muscular fiber. *Chronic nasal, gastric, and pharyngeal catarrh,* due to portal obstruction. Dropsy from cardiac disease. Pruritus in pregnancy, with piles. *Constipation of children from intestinal atony.* Said to be of special value when given before operations, for rectal diseases. Sense of weight and constriction. Venous engorgement.

Head.—Dull frontal headache; from suppressed hæmorrhoids. Chronic catarrh. Yellow-coated tongue. Bitter taste. [*Colocy.; Bry.*]

Rectum.—*Sensation of sharp sticks in rectum. Sense of constriction.* Vascular engorgement of rectum. Dry fæces. *Most obstinate constipation,* with protruding hæmorrhoids. Aching in anus and hypogastrium. Constipation during pregnancy; with membranous dysmenorrhœa, following labor. [*Nux.*] Painful bleeding piles. Dysentery, with tenesmus. *Alternate constipation and diarrhœa,* and great flatulence. *Itching of anus.* [*Teucrium; Ratanh.*]

Female.—Dysmenorrhœa; *pruritus of vulva;* prolapse of womb; swelling and dark redness of genitals; pain on sitting down. Membranous dysmenorrhœa, with constipation. Pruritus. Cold feeling in thighs after menstruation. Sensation of swelling of labia and of clitoris.

Respiratory.—*Cough from excessive use of voice;* "minister's sore throat;" sharp pain in larynx. Hoarseness. Harassing, dry cough.

Heart.—Palpitation; rapid but weak. Dropsy. After heart symptoms relieved, piles or menses return. Chest-pains alternate with hæmorrhoids. Oppression, faintness, and dyspnœa. [*Acon. ferox.*]

Modalities.—*Worse,* from the slightest mental emotion or excitement; cold. *Better,* heat.

Relationship.—Antidote: *Nux.*

Compare: *Æscul.; Aloes; Hamam.; Lycopus; Negundo; Sulph.; Nux.*

Dose.—Tincture, to third attenuation. Higher potencies where there is organic heart affection.

COLOCYNTHIS
(Bitter Cucumber)

Often indicated in the transition season when the air is cold, but the sun is still powerful enough to heat the blood.

Develops most of its symptoms in the abdomen and head, causing intense neuralgias. It is especially suitable for irritable persons easily angered, and ill effects therefrom. Women with copious menstruation, and of sedentary habits. Persons with a tendency to corpulency. The neuralgic pains are nearly always relieved by pressure. Cramps and twitching and shortening of muscles. Constrictions and contractions. Cystospasm following operations on orifices. [*Hyper.*] Urinous odor of perspiration. [*Berb.; Nitr. ac.*] *Agonizing pain in abdomen*, causing patient to bend double, is most characteristic. Sensations: Cutting, twisting, grinding, contracting and bruised; *as if clamped with iron bands.*

Mind.—Extremely irritable. Becomes angry when questioned. Mortification caused by offense. Anger, with indignation. [*Cham.; Bry.; Nux.*]

Head.—Vertigo when turning head *to the left.* Lateral cutting headache, with nausea, vomiting. Pains (better pressure and heat), with soreness of *scalp.* Burning pains, digging, rending, and tearing. Frontal headache; worse, stooping, lying on back, and moving eyelids.

Eyes.—Pains sharp, boring, *better pressure.* Sensation on stooping, as if eye would fall out. Gouty affections of eyes. Violent pain in eyeballs which precede the development of glaucoma.

Face.—Tearing, shooting, and swelling of face; left side great soreness. Get relief from pressure. [*China.*] Neuralgia, *with chilliness;* teeth seems too long. *Sounds re-echo in ears.* Pain in stomach, always with pain of teeth or head.

Stomach.—Very *bitter* taste. Tongue rough, as from sand, and feels scalded. Canine hunger. Feeling in stomach as if something would not yield; drawing pain.

Abdomen.—Agonizing cutting pain in abdomen *causing patient to bend over double*, and pressing on the abdomen. Sensation as if stones were being ground together in the abdomen, and would burst. Intestines feel as if bruised. Colic with cramps in calves. Cutting in abdomen, especially after anger. Each paroxysm is attended with general agitation and a chill over the cheeks, ascending from the hypogastrium. Pain in small spot below navel. *Dysenteric stool renewed each time by the least food or drink. Jelly-like* stools. Musty odor. Distention.

Female.—*Boring pain in ovary. Must draw up double, with great restlessness.* Round, small cystic tumors in ovaries or broad ligaments. Wants abdomen supported by pressure. Bearing-down cramps, causing her to bend double. [*Opium.*]

Urine.—Intense burning along urethra during stool. Vesical catarrh, discharge like fresh white of egg. *Viscid.* [*Phos. acid*] fetid; small quantities, with frequent urging. Itching at orifice. Red, hard crystals, adhering firmly to vessel. Tenesmus of bladder. Pains on urinating *over whole abdomen*.

Extremities.—*Contraction of muscles.* All the limbs are drawn together. Pain in right deltoid. [*Guaco.*] *Cramp-like pain in hip;* lies on affected side; pain from hip to knee. Spontaneous luxation of the hip-joints. Stiffness of joints and shortening of tendons. Sciatic pain, left side, drawing, tearing; better, *pressure and heat;* worse, gentle touch. Contraction of the muscles. Pain down right thigh; muscles and tendons feel too short; numbness with pains. [*Gnaphal.*] Pain in left knee joint.

Modalities.—*Worse*, from anger and indignation. *Better*, doubling up, hard pressure, warmth, lying with head bent forward.

Relationship.—Antidote: *Coffea; Staphis.; Cham. Colocynth* is the best antidote to lead poisoning. (Royal).

Compare: *Lobelia erinus* (violent cork-screw-like pains in abdomen). *Dipodium punctatum* (*Writhing.* Twisting like a dying snake. Intractable insomnia.) *Dioscor.; Chamom.; Coccul.; Merc.; Plum.; Magn. phos.*

Dose.—Sixth to thirtieth potency.

COMOCLADIA DENTATA
(Guao)

Important eye and skin symptoms. Affections of antrum. Sacro-iliac and abdominal pain. *Throbbing pains worse by heat.* Pain in joints and ankles.

Eyes.—Ciliary neuralgia with eyes feeling large and protruded, especially *right*. Worse, *near warm stove;* feels as if pressed outward. Sees only glimmer of light with left eye. Glaucoma, sense of fullness; *eyeball feels too large.* Motion of eyes aggravates.

Face.—Swollen, with eyes projecting.

Skin.—Itches, red and pimples. *Redness all over, like scarlatina.* Erysipelas. Deep ulcers, with hard edges. Leprosy. Red stripes on skin. [*Euphorb.*] Eczema (papular) of the trunk and extremities; also pustular type.

Chest.—Acute pain in left mammary gland. Pain from right side of chest down arm to fingers. Cough with pain under left breast, going through to left scapula.

Modalities.—*Better*, open air, scratching; by motion. *Worse,* touch, warmth, rest; night.

Relationship.—Compare: *Rhus; Anacard.; Euphorb.*

Dose.—First to thirtieth potency.

CONDURANGO
(Condor Plant)

Stimulates the digestive functions and thus improves the general health. Allays the pain in gastralgia accompanying cancer of stomach. Modifies secretions of digestive glands. Varicose ulcers. Lupus.

Painful cracks in corner of mouth is a guiding symptom of this drug. Chronic gastric catarrh, syphilis, and cancer. Tumors; stricture of œsophagus. The active principle [*Condurangin*] produces locomotor ataxia.

Stomach.—Painful affections of the stomach; ulceration. Vomiting of food and indurations, constant burning pain. Stricture of œsophagus, with burning pains behind sternum, where food seems to stick. Vomiting of food, and indurations in left hypochondrium with constant burning pain.

Skin.—Fissures form about the muco-cutaneous outlets. Epithelioma of lips or anus. Ulcerative stage of carcinoma cutis when fissures form.

Relationship.—Compare: *Asterias; Conium; Hydrast.; Arsenic.*

Dose.—Tincture, or bark, 5-grain doses before meals in water. Also the thirtieth potency, in tumors.

CONIUM
(Poison Hemlock)

An old remedy, rendered classical by Plato's graphic description of its employment in the death of Socrates. The *ascending paralysis* it produces, ending in death by failure of respiration, shows the ultimate tendency of many symptoms produced in the provings, for which Conium is an excellent remedy, such as difficult gait, trembling, sudden loss of strength while walking, painful stiffness of legs, etc. Such a condition is often found in old age, a time of weakness, languor, local congestions, and sluggishness. This is the special environment that Conium chooses to manifest its action. It corresponds to the debility, hypochondriasis, urinary troubles, weakened memory, sexual debility found here. Troubles at the change of life, old maids and bachelors. Growth of tumors invite it also. General feeling as if bruised by blows. Great debility in the morning in bed. *Weakness of body and mind, trembling,* and palpitation. Cancerous diathesis. Arterio-sclerosis. Caries of sternum. Enlarged glands. Acts on the glandular system, engorging and indurating it, altering its structure like scrofulous and cancerous conditions. Tonic after grippe. Insomnia of multiple neuritis.

Mind.—Excitement causes mental depression. Depressed, timid, averse to society, and afraid of being alone. No inclination for business or study; takes no interest in anything. Memory weak; unable to sustain any mental effort.

Head.—*Vertigo, when lying down, and when turning over in bed,* when turning head *sidewise,* or turning eyes; worse, shaking head, slight noise or conversation of others, especially towards the left. Headache, stupefying, with nausea and vomiting of mucus, with a feeling as of foreign body under the skull. Scorched feeling on top. Tightness as if both temples were compressed; worse *after a meal*. [*Gels.; Atropine.*] Bruised, semilateral pains. Dull occipital pain on rising in morning.

Eyes.—*Photophobia and excessive lachrymation.* Corneal pustules. Dim-sighted; worse, artificial light. On closing eyes, he sweats. Paralysis of ocular muscles. [*Caust.*] In superficial inflammations, as in phlyctenular conjunctivitis and keratitis. *The slightest ulceration or abrasion will cause the intensest photophobia.*

Ears.—Defective hearing; discharge from ear blood colored.

Nose.—Bleeds easily—becomes sore. Polypus.

Stomach.—Soreness about the root of tongue. Terrible nausea, acrid *heartburn*. and acid eructations; *worse on going to bed.* Painful spasms of the stomach. Amelioration from eating and aggravation a few hours after meals; acidity and burning; painful spot the level of the sternum.

Abdomen.—Severe aching in and around the liver. Chronic jaundice, and pains in right hypochondrium. Sensitive, bruised, swollen, knife-like pains. Painful tightness.

Stool.—Frequent urging; hard, with tenesmus. *Tremulous weakness after every stool.* [*Verat.; Ars.; Arg. n.*] Heat and burning in rectum during stool.

Urine.—Much difficulty in voiding. *It flows and stops again.* [*Ledum.*] *Interrupted discharge.* [*Clematis.*] Dribbling in old men. [*Copaiva.*]

Male.—Desire increased; power decreased. Sexual nervousness, with feeble erection. *Effects of suppressed sexual appetite.* Testicles hard and enlarged.

Female.—Dysmenorrhœa, with drawing-down thighs. Mammæ lax and shrunken, *hard*, painful to touch. *Stitches in nipples.* Wants to press breast hard with hand. Menses delayed and scanty; parts sensitive. *Breasts enlarge and become painful* before and during menses. [*Calc. c.; Lac can.*] Rash before menses. Itching around pudenda. Unready conception. Induration of os and cervix. Ovaritis; ovary enlarged, indurated; lancinating pain. Ill effects of *repressed sexual* desire or suppressed menses, or from excessive indulgence. Leucorrhœa after micturition.

Respiratory.—Dry cough, almost continuous, hacking; worse, evening and at night; *caused by dry spot in larynx* with *itching* in chest and throat, *when lying down*, talking or laughing, and during pregnancy. Expectoration only after long coughing. Want of breath on taking the least exercise; oppressed breathing, constriction of chest; pains in chest.

Back.—Dorsal pain between shoulders. Ill effects of bruises and shocks to spine. Coccyodynia. Dull aching in lumbar and sacral region.

Extremities.—Heavy, weary, paralyzed; trembling; hands unsteady; fingers and toes numb. *Muscular weakness*, especially of lower extremities. *Perspiration of hands*. *Putting feet on chair relieves pain.*

Skin.—*Axillary glands pain, with numb feeling down arm.* Induration after contusions. Yellow skin, with papular eruption; yellow finger-nails. *Glands enlarged and indurated*, also mesenteric. Flying stitches through the glands. Tumors; piercing pains; worse, at night. Chronic ulcers with fetid discharge. *Sweat as soon as one sleeps*, or even when closing eyes. Night and morning sweat, with offensive odor, and smarting in skin.

Modalities.—*Worse*, lying down, *turning* or rising in bed; *celibacy;* before and during menses, from taking cold, bodily or mental exertion. *Better*, while fasting, in the dark, from letting limbs hang down, motion and pressure.

Relationship.—Compare: *Scirrhinum*—Cancer nosode—(cancerous diathesis; enlarged glands; cancer of breast; worms); *Baryt.; Hydrast.; Iod.; Kali phos.; Hyos.; Curare.*

Dose.—Best in higher potencies given infrequently, especially for growths, paretic states, etc. Otherwise sixth to thirtieth.

CONVALLARIA MAJALIS
(Lily of the Valley)

A heart remedy. Increases energy of hearts' action, renders it more regular. Of use when the ventricles are overdistended and dilatation begins, and when there is an absence of compensatory hypertrophy, and when venous stasis is marked. Dyspnœa, dropsy, aneuric tendency. *Anasarca.*

Mind and Head.—Dull intellect. Grieves easily. Dull headache; worse, ascending, hawking. Scalp sensitive. Irritability. Hysterical manifestations.

Face.—Hydroa in nose and lips; raw and sore. Epistaxis. Sees imaginary gray spot about three inches square.

Mouth.—Grating of teeth in the morning. Coppery taste. Tongue feels sore and scalded; broad and thick with heavy, dirty coating.

Throat.—Raw feeling in back of throat when inspiring.

Abdomen.—Sensitive. Clothes feel too tight. Gurgling and pain on taking deep breath. Movement in abdomen like fist of a child. Colicky pains.

Urinary Organs.—Aching in bladder; feels distended. Frequent urination; offensive; scanty urine.

Female.—Great *soreness in uterine region, with sympathetic palpitation of heart.* Pain in sacro-iliac joints, running down leg. Itching at urinary meatus and vaginal orifice.

Respiratory.—Pulmonary congestion. Orthopnœa. *Dyspnœa while walking.* Hot feeling in throat.

Heart.—Feeling as if heart beat throughout the chest. Endocarditis, with extreme orthopnœa. *Sensation as if heart ceased beating, then starting very suddenly.* Palpitation from the least exertion. Tobacco heart, especially when due to cigarettes. Angina pectoris. Extremely rapid and irregular pulse.

Back and Extremities.—Pain and aching in lumbar region; aching of legs; in big toe. Trembling of hands. Aching in wrists and ankles.

Fever.—Chilly in back and down spine, followed by fever, little sweat. Thirst and headache during chill. Dyspnœa during fever.

Relationship.—Compare: *Digit.; Cratæg.; Lilium; Adonis* (feeble heart action due only to functional disturbance).

Modalities.—*Better,* in open air. *Worse,* in warm room.

Dose.—Third attenuation, and for symptoms of heart failure, tincture, one to fifteen drops.

COPAIVA
(Balsam of Copaiva)

Acts powerfully on mucous membranes, especially that of the urinary tract, the respiratory organs, and the skin, here producing a well-marked nettle-rash. Colds and catarrhs.

Head.—Excessive sensitiveness; pain in occiput. Dull, frontal headache, passes to occiput and back again, with throbbing, worse right side and motion. Scalp sensitive. Sensitive to sharp sounds.

Nose.—Rawness and soreness of nostrils with stopped-up feeling; dryness of posterior nares. Profuse, thick, fetid discharge from nasal passages, running down throat at night. *Burning and dryness*, crusts on turbinated bones. Marked catarrhal condition in upper respiratory tract.

Stomach.—Food seems too salty. Gastric troubles during menstruation or following urticaria. Gas and intestinal flatulence, urging to stool and difficult passage with pain.

Urinary.—Burning pressure; painful micturition by drops. Retention, with pain in bladder, anus, and rectum. *Catarrh of bladder;* dysuria. Swelling of orifice. Constant desire to urinate. Urine smells of violets. Greenish, turbid color; peculiar pungent odor.

Rectum.—*Mucous Colitis*. Stools covered with mucus, with colic and chilliness. Burning and itching of anus, caused by piles.

Male.—Testicles sensitive and swollen.

Female.—Itching of vulva and anus, with bloody purulent discharge. Profuse, strong-smelling menstrual discharge, with pains radiating to hip bones, with nausea.

Respiratory.—Cough, with profuse, gray, purulent expectoration. Tickling in larynx, trachea, and bronchi. Bronchial catarrh, with profuse greenish, offensive discharge.

Skin.—*Hives*, with fever and constipation. Roseola. Erysipelatous inflammation, especially around abdomen. Circumscribed, lenticular patches, with itching; mottled appearance. Chronic urticaria in children. Bullous eruptions.

Relationship.—Antidotes: *Bell.; Merc.*

Compare: *Santalum*—(aching in kidneys); *Cannab.; Canth.; Barosma; Cubeb; Apis; Vespa; Erig.; Senecio; Sepia.*

Dose.—First to third attenuation.

CORALLIUM
(Red Coral)

The provings of coral develop much coryza and epistaxis, and even ulceration within the nostrils. It is to be thought of for whooping and spasmodic coughs, especially when the attack comes on with a *very rapid* cough, and the attacks follow so closely as to almost run into each other. Often preceded by sensation of smothering, followed by exhaustion. Congestion of face after dinner. Patient becomes purple in face. *Violence of paroxysm*, even with *expectoration* of blood. Feeling as if cold air were streaming through skull and air-passages. One is too cold when uncovered and too hot when covered; relieved by artificial heat.

Head.—Feels very large; violent pain as if parietal bones were forced apart; worse stooping. Eyes hot and painful. Deep-seated frontal headache with severe pain back of eyeballs. Pain aggravated by breathing cold air through nose.

Nose.—Odors of smoke, onions, etc. Painful ulcer in nostrils. *Post-nasal catarrh. Profuse secretion of mucus dropping through posterior nares;* air feels cold. Dry coryza; nose stopped up and ulcerated. Epistaxis.

Mouth.—Food tastes like sawdust. Bread tastes like straw. Beer tastes sweet. Pain in articulation of left lower jaw. Craves salt.

Respiratory.—Hawking of profuse mucus. Throat very sensitive, *especially to air*. Profuse, nasal catarrh. Inspired air feels cold. [*Cistus.*] *Profuse secretion of mucus dropping through posterior nares.* Dry, *spasmodic*, suffocative cough; very rapid cough, short, barking. Cough with great sensitiveness of air-passages; *feel cold on deep inspiration.* Continuous hysterical cough. Feels suffocated and greatly exhausted after whooping-cough.

Male.—Ulcers on glans and inner prepuce, with yellow ichor. Emissions and weakened sexual power. Profuse perspiration of genitals.

Skin.—Red, flat ulcers. Coral-colored, then dark red spots, changing to copper-colored spots. Psoriasis of palms and soles.

Modalities.—Worse in open air, changing from a warm to cold room.

Relationship.—Complementary: *Sulph.*
Compare: *Bellad.; Droser.; Mephit.; Caust.*
Dose.—Third to thirtieth attenuation.

CORALLORHIZA
(Crawley Root)

Hectic fever, coming on 9 to 10 a. m., and lasting till midnight. Intensely nervous and restless, burning of palms and soles; no thirst, chill or perspiration. Can bear only slightest covering.

CORNUS CIRCINATA
(Round-leaved Dogwood)

Chronic malaria, hepatitis, jaundice. Weakness in morning. Pain in pit of stomach, with distended abdomen. Vesicular eruption associated with chronic liver disease or aphthous stomatitis.

Mouth.—Ulceration of tongue, gums and mouth; aphthæ. Burning in mouth, throat and stomach.

Stool.—Loose, windy, dark stool, immediately after dinner. Burning in anus. Dark, bilious, offensive diarrhœa, with sallow complexion.

Skin.—Vesicular eczema of face in infants, with nursing sore mouth.

Relationship.—Compare: *Cornus alternifolia*—Swamp Walnut—(Weak and tired; disturbed sleep, fever, restlessness, eczema; *skin cracked;* chest feels cold, as if full of ice); *Cornus florida* (chronic malaria; indigestion and distressing acid heartburn; general debility from loss of fluids and night sweats; neuralgic pains in arms, chest, and trunk, and sensation as if broken in two; intermittent fever, *with drowsiness;* feels cold, but is warm to touch; great exhaustion in intervals; general clammy sweat. Chill is preceded by drowsiness, heat is associated with drowsiness. Headache after quinine.)

Dose.—Tincture to sixth attenuation.

CORYDALIS (DICENTRA CANADENSIS)
(Turkey-pea)

Syphilitic affections. Ulcers of mouth and fauces. Cancer cachexia pronounced. Gummata and night-pains. Chronic diseases, with atony. Tongue clean, broad, and full. Tissues flabby, doughy, cold. Gastric catarrh. [*Hydrast.*]

Skin.—Dry, scaly scabs on face of old people. Lymphatic glands swollen.

Relationship.—*Nit. ac.; Kali iod.; Fluor. ac.*

Dose.—Tincture, twenty drops three times a day.

COTYLEDON
(Pennywort)

Marked action on heart; oppression of chest; fulness in throat. Epilepsy. Numb aching in muscular and fibrous tissue. Sciatica. Well-marked pains through the breast to scapula. Catarrh of larynx and trachea. Hysterical joint.

Mind.—Lost, confused feeling. Could not articulate for some time on awaking. Pressing vertex headache. Ailments from suppressed emotion. *Feeling as if a part of the body were absent.*

Breast.—Pain under left nipple, and aching in right breast. Pain through to scapula from region of left breast. Pain at angles of scapulæ. Full, bursting feeling, as if from obstruction at heart. Choking fulness in throat. Breathing oppressed.

Extremities.—Aching in back and thighs. Aching in all joints. Skin sensitive, rubbing of trousers causes an acute sting. Legs and arms feel heavy and sore.

Relationship.—Compare: *Ambra; Asafæt.; Hepatica; Ignatia; Laches.*

Dose.—Tincture to third potency.

CRATAEGUS
(Hawthorn Berries)

Produces giddiness, lowered pulse, and air hunger and reduction in blood-pressure. Acts on muscle of heart, and *is a heart tonic*. No influence on the endocardium.

Myocarditis. Failing compensation. *Irregularity of heart.* Insomnia of aortic sufferers; anæmia; œdema; cutaneous chilliness. High arterial tension. Is a sedative in cross, irritable patients with cardiac symptoms.

Chronic heart disease, with extreme weakness. Very feeble and irregular heart action. General anasarca. Very nervous, with pain in back of head and neck. Collapse of typhoid. Hæmorrhage from bowels. Cold extremities, pallor; irregular pulse and breathing. Painful sensation of pressure in left side of chest below the clavicle. Dyspepsia and nervous prostration, with heart failure. In the beginning of heart mischief after rheumatism. *Arteriosclerosis.* Said to have a solvent power upon crustaceous and calcareous deposits in arteries.

Head.—Apprehensive, despondent. Very nervous and irritable, with pain in back of head and neck. Mental dullness conjunctival irritation nasal discharges.

Urinary.—*Diabetes,* especially in children.

Heart.—*Cardiac dropsy.* Fatty degeneration. Aortic disease. *Extreme dyspnœa on least exertion,* without much increase of pulse. Pain in region of heart *and under left clavicle.* Heart muscles seem flabby, worn out. Cough. *Heart dilated; first sound weak.* Pulse accelerated, *irregular, feeble, intermittent.* Valvular murmurs, angina pectoris. Cutaneous chilliness, blueness of fingers and toes; all aggravated by exertion or excitement. Sustains heart in infectious diseases.

Skin.—Excessive perspiration. Skin eruptions.

Sleep.—Insomnia of aortic patients.

Modalities.—*Worse,* in warm room. *Better,* fresh air, quiet and rest.

Relationship.—*Strophantus; Digit.; Iberis; Naja; Cactus.*

Dose.—Fluid extract or tincture, one to fifteen drops. Must be used for some time in order to obtain good results.

CROCUS SATIVA
(Saffron)

Is a remedy often useful in hæmorrhages that are black and stringy. Tingling in various parts. Chorea and hysterical affections. Frequent and extreme changes in sensations and mental conditions. Anger with violence followed by repentance. *Laughing* mania. Drowsiness and *lassitude;* better by literary labor.

Mind.—*Vacillating;* pleasant mania; sings and laughs. Happy and affectionate; then angry. Sudden changes from hilarity to melancholy. Vivid recollection from music heard. [*Lyc.*]

Head.—Throbs, pulsates, during climacteric; worse during menses.

Eyes.—Appearance as of electric sparks. Must wipe eyes as if mucus or water were in them. *Feeling in eyes as after violent weeping.* Sensation as if she had been looking through too sharp spectacles. *Eyes feel as if in smoke.* Pupils enlarged and react slowly. Lids heavy. Ciliary neuralgia, pain from eyes to top of head. *Sensation as if cold air was rushing through eye.* [*Fluor. ac.; Syph.*] Asthenopia with extreme photophobia. Threatened glaucoma; embolism of arteria centralis retinal.

Nose.—Epistaxis. *Dark, stringy, clotted. Strings of dark blood* hanging down the nose.

Abdomen.—*Obstinate constipation* due to portal stagnation. Constipation in infants. Crawling and stitches in anus. *Sensation of something alive in abdomen, stomach, etc.*, especially on left side. [*Calend.*] Abdomen swollen, feeling of something heavy.

Female.—Threatened abortion, especially when hæmorrhage is *dark and stringy.* Urging of blood to genitals. Menses dark, viscid, too frequent and copious, *black and slimy.* Uterine hæmorrhage; *clots with long strings;* worse from least movement. Jerking pain in interior of left breast, as if drawn toward back by means of thread. [*Crot. tig.*] A bounding feeling, as if something alive in right breast.

Respiratory.—Wheezy cough, with frothy expectoration, containing threads like fine twine; worse, lying down. Breath has offensive, sickly smell. Feeling as if the uvula is elongated in hysterical patients.

Back.—Sudden feeling of coldness in back as if cold water were thrown over him; icy-cold extremities.

Extremities.—Spasmodic contractions and twitchings of single set of muscles. Chorea and hysteria, with great alterations of feeling. Whole upper extremity falls asleep. Cracking in hip-joint and *knees.* Weakness in knees and legs. Pain in ankles and soles.

Modalities.—*Worse*, lying down, hot weather, warm room, in morning, fasting, before breakfast, looking fixedly at an object. *Better*, in open air.

Relationship.—Antidote: *Opium; Bell.*
Compare: *Ipec.; Trillium; Plat.; China; Sabina.*

Dose.—Tincture, to thirtieth attenuation.

CROTALUS HORRIDUS
(Rattlesnake)

Snake poisons are supposed to be chemically *Cyan. hydrates* of Soda and other salts. Alcohol is the natural solvent of these salts and is an antidote. Has a profound trophic action. Old age nutritional troubles.

Low septic states. General disorganization of the blood, hæmorrhages and jaundice. A crotalin injection decreases the rate of coagulation of the blood. In epilepsy the average rate is far greater than in normal conditions. Blood decomposition, *hæmorrhages* (dark fluid that forms no clots), tendency to carbuncles, malignant scarlatina, *yellow fever*, the plague, cholera, give opportunity to use this remedy. *Hæmorrhagic diathesis*. Acts as a sedative. Sleeps into his symptoms. More right-sided in its action.

Mind.—Weeping mood; clouded perception and memory; impatient. Loquacious, with desire to escape. Sadness. Delusions of cerebral decay.

Head.—Vertigo, with weakness and trembling. Dull heavy occipital pain, on right side and right eye. Headache with pain in heart on lying on left side. Headache; must walk on tip-toe to avoid jarring.

Eyes.—Very sensitive to light, especially *lamp light*. Yellow color of eyes. Illusions; blue colors. *Ciliary neuralgia;* tearing, boring pain, as if a cut had been made around eye. *For absorption of intra-ocular hæmorrhages*, into the vitreous, but particularly for non-inflammatory retinal hæmorrhages. Diplobia

Ears.—Auditory vertigo Blood oozes from ears. Feeling of stoppage in right ear.

Nose.—Epistaxis, *blood black and stringy*, ozæna, after exanthemata or syphilis.

CROTALUS HORRIDUS

Face.—Acne. Lips swollen and numb. Leaden-colored and yellow face. Lockjaw.

Mouth.—Tongue red and small, but feels swollen. Tongue fiery red, dry in center, smooth and polished. Mouldy smell of breath. Fills up with saliva. Tongue when protruding, goes to right. Spasmodic grinding of teeth at night. Cancer of tongue with hæmorrhage.

Throat.—Dry, swollen, dark red. Spasm of ophagus; cannot swallow any solid substance. Tight constriction. Gangrenous, with much swelling.

Stomach.—Intolerance of clothing around stomach. Unable to retain anything; violent vomiting of food; bilious vomiting, vomiting of blood. Constant nausea and vomiting every month, after menstruation. Cannot lie on right side, without vomiting dark-green matter. Black or coffee-grounds vomiting. Cancer of stomach with vomiting of bloody, slimy mucus. Trembling, fluttering feeling below the epigastrium. Intolerance of clothing about epigastrium. Faintness and sinking at stomach. Ulceration of the stomach. Atonic dyspepsia. Gastritis in chronic alcoholism. Hungry, craves stimulants, sugar; averse to meat.

Abdomen.—Distended, hot, and tender. Pain in region of liver.

Stool.—Black, thin, offensive, like coffee-grounds. Intestinal hæmorrhage; blood dark, fluid, non-coagulable. Blood oozes from rectum when standing or walking.

Female.—Prolonged menses. Dysmenorrhœa; pain extends down thighs, with aching in region of heart. Uterine hæmorrhage with faintness at stomach. Puerperal fever; offensive lochia. Phlegmasia alba dolens. Sensation as though uterus would drop out. Painful drawing in uterine ligaments. Cannot keep legs still.

Urinary.—Dark, bloody urine. Casts. Inflamed kidney. Albuminous, dark, scanty. [*Merc. cor.*]

Heart.—Action feeble, pulse tremulous. Palpitation, especially at menstrual period. Trembling feeling of heart.

Respiratory.—Cough, with bloody expectoration. Tickling from a dry spot in larynx.

Extremities.—Hands tremble, swollen. Lower extremities go to sleep easily. *Right-sided paralysis.*

Fever.—Malignant fevers of a *hæmorrhagic or putrescent character.* Low bilious remittents. Yellow fever. Bloody sweat. Cerebro-spinal meningitis. [*Cicuta; Cup. acet.*] Cold sweats.

Skin.—Swelling and discoloration, skin tense and shows every tint of color, with excruciating pain. Vesication. *Sallow.* Yellow color of the whole body. Great sensitiveness of skin of *right half* of body. *Purpura hæmorrhagica.* Hæmorrhage from every part of body. Bloody sweat. Chilblains, felons. Dissecting wounds. Pustular eruptions. Insect stings. Post-vaccination eruptions. Bad effects of vaccination. Lymphangitis and septicæmia. Boils, carbuncles, and eruptions are surrounded by purplish, mottled skin and œdema. Anthrax. Sore sensation relieved by pressure.

Sleep.—Dreams of the dead. Starting in sleep. Yawning. Smothering sensation when awaking.

Modalities.—*Worse,* right side; open air; evening and morning; in spring, coming on of warm weather; yearly; on awaking; damp and wet; *jar.*

Relationship.—Compare: *Bothrops; Naja* (more nervous phenomena); *Lachesis* (more markedly worse on left side); *Elaps* (preferable in otorrhœa and affections of right lung); *Crotalus cascavella* (thoughts and dreams of death. Paralysis of articulation, embarrassed stertorous breathing and semi-consciousness. A magnetic state is produced; cutting sensation all around eyeball.) *Bungarus-Krait*—(poliomyelitis).

Antidote: *Lach.; Alcohol.* Radiant heat; camphor.

Dose.—Third to sixth potency.

CROTON TIGLIUM
(Croton-oil Seed)

Is a valuable remedy in diarrhœa, summer complaint, and *skin affections.* These may alternate with each other. Feels tight all over. It is one of the antidotes to Rhus poisoning, as is evident from its wide and intense action upon skin and mucous surface, causing both irritation and inflammation, with formation of vesicles and mucous discharges. Has elective affinity for skin of face and external genitals. *Burning in the œsophagus.*

Head.—Pressing pain in forehead, especially orbits.

Eyes.—Granular lids; pustules of cornea. Red and raw appearance. *Feel drawn backward.* Eruptions around eyes. *Tensive pain above right orbit.*

Stool.—Copious watery stools, with much urging; *always forcibly shot out*, with gurgling in intestines; worse, drinking the least quantity, or even while eating. Constant urging to stool, followed by sudden evacuation. Swashing sensation in intestines.

Urine.—Night urine foaming; dark orange color; turbid on standing; greasy particles floating on top. Day urine is pale, with white sediment.

Chest.—*Drawing-pain through the left chest into the back.* *Asthma*, with cough; cannot expand the chest. Nursing women; every suck the child gives produces *pain from nipple back.* Inflamed breasts. Cough; as soon as he touches the pillow must get up. Sensitive to deep breathing.

Skin.—*Feels hide-bound. Intense itching; but scratching is painful.* Pustular eruption, especially on face and *genitals*, with fearful itching, followed by painful burning. Vesicles; confluent oozing. Vesicular erysipelas, itching exceedingly. Herpes zoster; stinging, smarting pains of the eruption.

Modalities.—*Worse*, least food or drink; during summer; *touch*, night and morning, washing.

Relationship.—Compare: *Momordica charantia*—Hairy Mordica—(has marked drastic properties, producing colic, nausea, vomiting, cholera-like symptoms, abdomen seems full of fluid discharged explosively, thin, watery, yellow. Great thirst). *Rhus; Anagallis; Anacard.; Sepia.*

Antidoe: *Ant. tart.*

Dose.—Sixth to thirtieth potency.

CUBEBA
(Cubebs)

Mucous membranes generally, but especially that of the urinary tract, are chiefly affected by this remedy. Frequent urination of a nervous origin. Leucorrhœa in little girls.

Urine.—Urethritis, with much mucus, especially *in women*. Cutting after urination, with constriction. Hæmaturia. Prostatitis, with thick yellow discharge. Cystitis.

Respiratory.—Catarrh of nose and throat, with fetid odor and expectoration. Mucus trickles from posterior nares. Rawness of throat and hoarseness.

Relationship.—Compare: *Cucurbita; Copaiva; Piper meth.; Sandal*.

Dose.—Second and third attenuation.

CUCURBITA PEPO
(Pumpkin Seed)

Intense nausea immediately after eating. Vomiting of pregnancy. Seasickness. One of the most efficient and least harmful of teniafuges.

Relationship.—Compare: *Filix; Cuprum oxid. nig.*

Dose.—Tincture. The seeds are a valuable remedy for tape-worm. Scald the seeds and peel off the outer skins when softened, the green inner pulp being the part used. Dose: two ounces of seed, yielding one of pulp. May be mixed with cream and taken like porridge. Take in morning after twelve hours' fasting, and follow in two hours by castor oil.

CUCURBITA CITRULLUS
(Seeds of Watermelon)

Infusion for painful urination with sense of constriction and backache.

CUPHEA
(Flux-weed)

Vomiting of undigested food. *Cholera infantum*, much acidity; frequent green, watery, acid stools. Tenesmus and great pain. High fever; restlessness, and sleeplessness. Obstinate constipation.

Relationship.—Compare: *Æthusa; Coto*—Para-coto Bark—(intestinal catarrh, chronic, copious, exhausting diarrhœa and dysentery; colliquitine sweats of phthisis and chronic diarrhœa.)

Typha latifolia—Cat-tail flag (diarrhœa, dysentery, summer complaint of children. Tincture and first attenuation.)

Dose.—Tincture.

CUPRUM ACETICUM
(Acetate of Copper)

Hay-fever, with burning excoriation, paroxysmal cough; tough, tenacious mucus, and fear of suffocation. *Protracted labor.* Chronic psoriasis and lepra.

Head.—Violent throbbing and lancinating pains in forehead. Left-sided brow ague. Brain seems void. Inclined to gape and cry. Loses consciousness; *head reels when in high-ceiled room.* Constant protrusion and retraction of tongue. [*Laches.*] Neuralgia with heaviness of head, burning, stinging and stitching in temples and forehead.

Face.—Collapsed, hippocratic. Facial neuralgia in cheekbone, upper jaw, and behind right ear. Better by chewing, pressure, and external warmth.

Stomach.—Violent spasmodic pains in stomach and abdomen. Vomiting. Slimy brown diarrhœa. Violent tenesmus. Cholera.

Respiratory.—Attacks of angina pectoris coming on when excited. Violent spasmodic cough. Short, difficult respiration. Spasmodic constriction of chest. Dyspnœa.

Skin.—Leprous-like eruption, without itching, over whole body, in spots of various sizes.

Modalities.—*Worse*, mental emotions, touch. *Better*, chewing, pressure, night, lying on affected side, and warmth.

Relationship.—Acts similarly to *Cuprum met.* but is more violent in action.

Dose.—Third to sixth trituration.

CUPRUM ARSENITUM
(Arsenite of Copper — Scheele's Green)

A remedy for symptoms depending on deficient kidney action, various intestinal affections, cholera morbus and infantum; entero-colitis, diarrhœa, and dysentery. Gastro-intestinal disturbances of influenza and typhoid. *Uræmic convulsions*, headache, vertigo and unconscious conditions resulting from brain œdema. Nephritis of pregnancy. Convulsions preceded by gastro-intestinal symptoms. Chlorosis. Bronchial asthma and with emphysema. Purulent endocarditis (Royal). Painful neuroses, enteroptosis. Delirium and tremor cordis.

Mouth.—Tongue thickly coated, dirty brown, white, metallic taste; thirst. Dry mouth.

Heart.—Cardiac rhythm and force altered due to defective elimination.

Abdomen.—Gastro-enteritis. Violent abdominal pain. Diarrhœa in phthisis. Cholera. [*Ars.; Verat.; Camph.*] Rumbling and sharp cutting pain. Dark liquid stools.

Back.—Persistent lameness. Pain in lumbar region and in lower left shoulder-blade; chest feels tight.

Urinary.—Renal inefficiency and uræmia. *Garlicky odor*. Diabetes. Urine of high specific gravity; increased, acetones and diacetic acid.

Male.—Perspiration of scrotum; is constantly damp and moist. Boils on scrotum. Purulent discharge of a *white* color from urethra; tingling and burning in urethra; pain in prostate; pains in penis.

Extremities.—*Cramps in calves of legs*, worse after midnight, only relieved by getting out of bed and standing. Ulcers; gangrene.

Skin.—Icy cold. Sweat, and skin even when dry. Cold, clammy perspiration of an intermittent nature. Acne, pustules on face and in the cruro-genital region; ulcers look like chancre. Gangrene; carbuncles.

Dose.—Third trituration.

CUPRUM METALLICUM
(Copper)

Spasmodic affections, *cramps*, convulsions, beginning in fingers and toes, violent, contractive, and intermitting pain, are some of the more marked expressions of the action of Cuprum; and its curative range therefore includes tonic and clonic spasms, convulsions, and epileptic attacks. Chorea brought on by fright. Nausea greater than in any other remedy. In epilepsy, aura begins at knees, ascends to hypogastrium; then unconsciousness, foaming, and falling. Symptoms disposed to appear periodically and in groups. Complaints begin in left side. [*Laches.*] Tape worm (colloidal Cuprum 3x).

Where eruptions trike in, as in scarlet fever, complaints may result, such as excessive vomiting, stupor, convulsions, which come within the sphere of this remedy. The pains are increased by movement and touch.

Head.—Fixed ideas, malicious and morose. Uses words not intended. Fearful. Empty feeling. Purple, red swelling of head, with convulsions. Bruised pain in brain and eyes on turning them. Meningitis. Sensation as if water were poured over head. Giddiness accompanies many ailments, head falls forward on chest.

Eyes.—Aching over eyes. Fixed, stary, sunken, glistening, turned upward. Crossed. Quick rolling of eyeballs, with closed eyes.

Face.—Distorted, pale *bluish,* with blue lips. *Contraction of jaws,* with foam at mouth.

Nose.—Sensation of violent congestion of blood to nose. [*Melilot.*]

Mouth.—*Strong metallic, slimy taste,* with flow of saliva. Constant protrusion and retraction of the tongue, like a snake. [*Lach.*] Paralysis of tongue. Stammering speech.

Stomach.—Hiccough preceding the spasms. *Nausea.* Vomiting, relieved by drinking cold water; with colic, diarrhœa, spasms. Strong metallic taste. [*Rhus.*] *When drinking, the fluid descends with gurgling sound.* [*Laur.*] Craves cool drink.

Abdomen.—Tense, hot and tender to touch; *contracted.* Neuralgia of abdominal viscera. *Colic,* violent and intermittent. Intussusception.

Stool.—Black, painful, bloody, with tenesmus and weakness. Cholera; with cramps in abdomen and calves.

Female.—Menses too late, protracted. Cramps, extending into chest, before, during, or after suppression of menses. Also, from suppressed foot sweats. [*Sil.*] Ebullition of blood; palpitation. Chlorosis. *After-pains.*

Heart.—Angina pectoris. Slow pulse; or hard, full and quick. Palpitation, præcordial anxiety and pain. Fatty degeneration. [*Phytol.*]

Respiratory.—Cough has a gurgling sound, better by drinking cold water. Suffocative attacks, worse 3 a. m. [*Am. c.*] *Spasm and constriction* of chest; spasmodic asthma, alternating with spasmodic vomiting. Whooping-cough, better, swallow water, with vomiting and spasms and purple face. Spasm of the glottis. Dyspnœa with epigastric uneasiness. Spasmodic dyspnœa before menstruation. Angina with asthmatic symptoms and cramps (Clarke).

Extremities.—Jerking, twitching of muscles. Coldness of hands. Cramps in palms. Great weariness of limbs. *Cramps in calves and soles.* Epilepsy; aura begins in knees. Clenched thumbs. Clonic spasms, beginning in fingers and toes.

Skin.—*Bluish*, marbled. Ulcers, itching spots, and pimples at the folds of joints. Chronic psoriasis and lepra (Hughes).

Sleep.—Profound, with shocks in body. During sleep constant rumbling in abdomen.

Modalities.—*Worse*, before menses; from vomiting, contact. *Better*, during perspiration, drinking cold water.

Relationship.—Antidotes: *Bell.; Hepar; Camph.* Copper is found in *Dulcam., Staphisag., Conium* and some other plants. Also in *King-crab* [Limulus].

Complementary: *Calc.*

Compare: *Cupr. sulph. (burning at vertex;* incessant, spasmodic cough; worse at night; tongue and lips bluish; locally, *Cupr. sulph.* in 1-3 per cent. sol. in inoperable sarcoma). *Cupr. cyan.* (meningitis basilaris); *Cholas terrapina* (cramps in calves and feet; rheumatism, with cramp-like pains); *Plumb.; Nux; Veratr. Cuprum oxydatum nigrum* 1x (all kinds of worms, including tape-worms and trichinosis according to Zopfy's 60 years' experience).

Dose.—Sixth to thirtieth potency.

CURARE — WOORARI
(Arrow-poison)

Muscular paralysis without impairing sensation and consciousness. Paralysis of respiratory muscles. *Reflex action diminished.* Debility of the aged [*Baryta*] and from loss of fluids. Catalepsy. Nervous debility. Trismus. Glycosuria with motor paralysis. Curare decreases the output of adrenalin. Vomiting of bile in cirrhosis of liver. Diabetes mellitus, 4th dilution (Dr. Barkhard).

Mind.—Indecision; no longer wishes to think, or act for herself.

Head.—Lancinating pains all over head. Head drawn backward. Falling out of hair. Brain feels full of fluid.

Eyes.—Sharp, stitching pains over right eye. Black spots before vision. Ptosis of right side.

Ears.—Noises; unbearable earache. Lancinating pains start from ears; extending down to legs. Swelling of lobes of ear.

Nose.—Ozæna. Tubercles on nose; fetid lumps of pus.

Face.—Facial and buccal paralysis. Tongue and mouth drawn. Red face. Tongue and mouth drawn to right.

Female.—Dysmenorrhœa. Menses too early, during menses, colic, headache, kidney pain. Leucorrhœa, thick, purulent, offensive.

Respiratory.—*Threatened paralysis of respiration* on falling asleep. Short breath. Short dry cough; provokes vomiting, followed by fainting. *Chest sore to pressure. Very distressing dyspnœa.*

Extremities.—Tired pain up and down spine. *Arms weak, heavy.* Cannot lift the fingers. Weakness of hands and fingers in pianists. Legs tremble; give way in walking. Debility; paralysis. Catalepsy. Favors development of corns. Reflexes lessened or abolished.

Skin.—Leprosy. Dirty-looking skin. Boils. Tubercles on nose. Liver spots. Blood oozes through. Itching.

Modalities.—*Worse,* dampness, cold weather, cold wind; 2 a. m.; right side.

Relationship.—Compare: *Cystisin* (motor paralysis); *Conium; Causticum; Crotalus; Nux.* Curare antidotes *Strychnin.*

Dose.—Sixth to thirtieth potency.

CYCLAMEN
(Sow-bread)

Large doses produce violent purging and vomiting; disturbed digestion with very salty saliva. Anæmic and chlorotic conditions. Affections of uterus. Gastro-intestinal and genito-urinary tracts affected, inducing secondary anæmia and various reflexes. *Sleepiness, moroseness, and lassitude.* Cough at night while asleep without waking, especially in children. [*Cham.; Nitr. ac.*]

Head.—Terrors of conscience. Grieves over duty neglected. Depression, with weeping desire to be alone. Aching in morning, with *flickering before eyes;* sneezing with itching in ear. Vertigo; things turn in a circle; better in the room; worse, open air. One-sided headache. Frequent sneezing with itching in ears.

Eyes.—Dim vision, worse on waking, with spots before eyes. *Flickering of various colors.* Convergent strabismus. *Sees countless stars.* Diplopia. Disturbance of vision, associated with gastric disturbances.

Stomach.—*Salty taste;* hiccough-like eructation worse, fat food. Diarrhœa after every cup of coffee; *hiccough.* Satiety after a few mouthfuls. Disgust for meat, especially pork. Desire for lemonade. No thirst all day.

Rectum.—*Pain about anus and perineum,* as if a spot were suppurating, when walking or sitting.

Female.—Menses *profuse, black,* membranous, *clotted, too early, with labor-like pains* from back to pubes. Flow less when moving about. Menstrual irregularities with megrim and blindness, or fiery spots before eyes. *Hiccough during pregnancy.* Post-partum hæmorrhage, with colicky bearing-down pains, with relief after gush of blood. After menses, swelling of breasts, with milky secretion.

Extremities.—Pains in parts where bones lie near surface. Burning, *sore pain in heels.* Cramp-like contraction of right thumb and index finger. Pains in periosteum. Chilblains.

Skin.—Acne in young women, pruritus better scratching and appearance of menses.

Modalities.—*Worse,* open air, evenings, sitting, standing, and cold water. *Better,* during menstrual flow, by moving about, rubbing parts; in warm room, lemonade.

Relationship.—Compare: *Ambra; Pulsat.; Cinchona; Fer. cit. et Chin.*

Dose.—Third attenuation.

CYPRIPEDIUM
(Yellow Lady's Slipper)

The skin symptoms correspond to those of poisoning by Rhus, for which it has been found an efficient antidote. Nervousness in children; from teething and intestinal troubles. Debility after gout. *Hydrocephaloid* symptoms, result of long, exhausting diarrhœa. *Sleeplessness.* Cerebral hyperasthesia in young children often the result of overstimulation of brain.

Head.—Child cries out at night; is wakeful and begins to laugh and play. Headaches of elderly people and during climacteric.

Relationship.—Compare: *Ambra; Kali brom.; Scutellar.; Valerian; Ignat.* Skin relatives: *Grindelia; Anacard.*

Dose.—Tincture, to sixth attenuation. For Poison Oak, 5 drops of tincture per dose, also locally.

DAPHNE INDICA
(Spurge Laurel)

Acts on lower tissues, muscles, bones and skin. Sudden, lightning jerks in different parts of the body. *Craving for tobacco.* Burning in stomach. Parts of the body feel separated. [*Bapt.*] Fetid breath, urine, sweat.

Head.—Feels as if skull would burst; *as if head were separated from body.* Heat in head, especially in vertex. *Tongue coated on one side only.* [*Rhus.*] Foul-smelling, ptyalism hot.

Urine.—Thick, turbid, yellowish, like rotten eggs.

Extremities.—Right toe swollen, painful. Pain shoots upward into abdomen and heart. Rheumatic pains in thighs and knees. Cold feeling on buttocks. Shooting pains, shift rapidly; worse, cold air.

Sleep.—Entire inability to sleep; sometimes caused by aching in bones. Dreams, with nightmare. Dreams of cats, black cats. Starting on falling to sleep with chilliness and clamminess.

Relationship.—Antidotes: *Bry.; Rhus.*
Compare: *Fluor. ac.; Aur.; Mez.; Staph.*

Dose.—First to sixth attenuation.

DIGITALIS

(Foxglove)

Comes into play in all diseases where the heart is primarily involved, where the pulse is *weak, irregular, intermittent, abnormally slow*, and dropsy of external and internal parts. *Weakness and dilatation of the myocardium.* Its greatest indication is in failure of compensation and especially when *auricular fibrillation has set in.* Slow pulse in recumbent posture, but irregular and dicrotic on sitting up. Auricular flutter and fibrillation especially when subsequent to rheumatic fever. Heart block, very slow pulse. Other symptoms of organic heart disease, such as great weakness and sinking of strength, faintness, coldness of skin, and irregular respiration; cardiac irritability and ocular troubles after tobacco; jaundice from induration and *hypertrophy of the liver*, frequently call for Digitalis. Jaundice with heart disease. Faint, as if dying. *Bluish* appearance of face. *Cardiac muscular failure* when asystole is present. Stimulates the heart's muscles, increases force of systole, increases length. Prostration from slight exertion. Collapse.

Mind.—Despondency; fearful; *anxious* about the future. Dullness of sense. Every shock strikes in epigastrium. Melancholia, dull lethargic with *slow* pulse.

Head.—Vertigo, when walking and on rising, in cardiac and hepatic affections. Sharp, shooting frontal pain, extending into nose, after drinking cold water or eating ice-cream. Heaviness of head, with sensation as if it would fall backward. Face bluish. Confusion, fullness and noise in head. Cracking sounds during a nap. Blue tongue and lips.

Eyes.—Blueness of eyelids. Dark bodies, like flies, before eyes. *Change in acuteness of perception of shades of green.* Objects appear green and yellow. Mydriasis; lid margins red, swollen, agglutinated in morning. Detachment of retina. Dim vision, irregular pupils, diplopia.

Stomach.—Sweet taste with constant ptyalism. *Excessive nausea*, not relieved by vomiting. Faintness, *great weakness in stomach*. Burning in stomach extending to œsophagus. After cold water or ice-cream, sharp pain in forehead, extending to nose. *Faintness* and vomiting from motion. Discomfort, even after a small quantity of food, or from mere sight or smell. *Tenderness of epigastrium.* Copious salivation. *Neuralgic pain in stomach,* unconnected with taking food.

Abdomen.—Pain in left side apparently in descending colon and under false ribs. Severe abdominal pains, pulsation in abdominal aorta, and epigastric constriction. *Enlarged, sore, painful liver.*

Stool.—*White, chalk-like, ashy, pasty stools.* Diarrhœa during jaundice.

Urine.—Continued urging, in drops, dark, hot, burning, with sharp cutting or *throbbing* pain at neck of bladder, *as if a straw was being thrust back and forth;* worse at night. Suppressed. Ammoniacal, and turbid. *Urethritis,* phimosis, strangury. Full feeling after urination. Constriction and burning, as if urethra was too small. Brick-dust sediment.

Female.—Labor-like pains in abdomen and back before menses. Uterine hæmorrhage.

Male.—Nightly emission [*Digitalin*], with great weakness of genitals after coitus. Hydrocele; scrotum enlarged like a bladder. Gonorrhœa, balanitis [*Merc.*], with œdema of prepuce. Dropsical swelling of genitals. [*Sulph.*] Enlarged prostate.

Respiratory.—Desire to take a deep breath. Breathing irregular, difficult; deep sighing. Cough, with raw, sore feeling in chest. Expectoration sweetish. Senile pneumonia. Great weakness in chest. *Dyspnœa,* constant desire to breathe deeply, lungs feel compressed. Chronic bronchitis; passive congestion of the lungs, giving bloody sputum due to failing myocardium. *Cannot bear to talk.* Hæmoptysis with weak heart.

Heart.—The least movement causes violent palpitation, and sensation as if it would cease beating, if he moves. [Opposite: *Gels.*] Frequent stitches in heart. *Irregular heart especially of mitral disease. Very slow pulse. Intermits; weak.* Cyanosis. Inequality of pulse; it varies. *Sudden sensation as if heart stood still. Pulse weak, and quickened by least movement.* Pericarditis, copious serous exudation. Dilated heart, tired, irregular, with slow and feeble pulse. Hypertrophy with dilatation. Cardiac failure following fevers. Cardiac dropsy.

Extremities.—Swelling of the feet. Fingers go to sleep easily.

Coldness of hands and feet. Rheumatic pain in joints. Shining, white swelling of joints. Muscular debility. Nocturnal swelling of fingers. Sensation in legs as *if a red hot wire* suddenly darted through them (Dudgeon).

Sleep.—*Starts from sleep in alarm* that he is falling from a height. Continuous sleepiness.

Fever.—Sudden flushes of heat, followed by great nervous weakness.

Skin.—Erythema, deep red, worse on back, like measles. Blue distended veins on lids, ears, lips and tongue. *Dropsical*. Itching and jaundiced.

Modalities.—*Worse*, when sitting erect, after meals and music. *Better*, when stomach is empty; in open air.

Relationship.—Antidotes: *Camph.; Serpentaria*. Incompatible: *China*. Compare: *Nerium odorum* (resembles in heart effects Digitalis, but also has an action like Strychnia on spinal cord. Spasms appear more in upper part of body. Palpitation; weak heart will be strengthened by it. Lock-jaw). *Adonia; Cratægus* (a true heart tonic); *Kalmia; Spigel.; Liatris;* Compare also: *Digitoxinum* (Digitalis dissolved in Chloroform; which has yellow vision very marked, and distressing nausea, *aggravated by champagne and aerated waters.*) *Nitri. spir. dulc.* increases action of Digit. *Ichthyotoxin*. Eel Serum. (Experiments show great analogy between the serum and the venom of vipera. Indicated whenever the systole of the heart is insufficient, decompensated valvular disease, irregular pulse due to fibrillation of the auricle. Assytole, feeble, frequent, irregular pulse, dyspnœa and scanty urine. Liver enlarged, dyspnœa, albuminuria. No œdema.) *Convallaria* (heart disease with vertigo and digestive disturbances). *Quinidin*—Isomeric methoxyl compound.—(Restores normal rhythm in auricular fibrillation, often supplements the action of Digitalis. Two doses of 3 grains each, three hours apart—if no symptoms of cinchonism develop, 4 doses 6 grs. each daily. (C. Harlan Wells.) Paroxysmal tachycardia. Establishes normal heart rhythm at least temporarily, less in valvular lesions.)

Dose.—The third to thirtieth attenuation will bring about reaction when the drug is homœopathically indicated; but for palliative purposes the physiological dosage is required. For this purpose, the tincture made from the *fresh* plant, in doses of five to twenty drops, when the cardiac stimulation is desired, or the infusion of 1½ per cent. Dose, one-half to one ounce if the diuretic action is wanted. The tincture may be given on sugar or bread, and nothing liquid be taken for twenty minutes before or after its administration. Of the powdered leaves, ½ to 2 grains in capsules. Digitoxin 1-250 grain. No matter what form of digitalis is given the dose should be reduced as soon as the pulse rate has been lowered to 80 beats a minute and the normal rhythm has been partially or completely restored. Under such conditions a good rule is to cut the dose in half and still more if there be a sudden falling off of the urinary output.

DIOSCOREA VILLOSA
(Wild Yam)

As a remedy for many kinds of *pain*, especially colic, and in severe, painful affections of abdominal and pelvic viscera; it ranks with the polychrests of the Materia Medica. Persons of feeble digestive powers; tea-drinkers, with much flatulence. *Gall stone colic.*

Mind.—Calls things by the wrong name.

Head.—Dull pain in both temples; better pressure, but worse afterwards. Buzzing in head.

Stomach.—Mouth dry and bitter in morning, tongue coated, no thirst. Belching of large quantities of offensive gas. Neuralgia of stomach. *Sinking at the pit of the* stomach; pyrosis. *Pain along sternum and extending into arms.* Eructations of sour, bitter wind, *with hiccough.* Sharp pain in epigastrium, relieved by standing erect.

Abdomen.—Pains suddenly shift to different parts; *appear in remote localities, as fingers and toes.* Rumbling, with emission of much flatus. Griping, cutting in hypogastric region, with intermittent cutting in stomach and small intestines. Colic; better walking about; pains radiate from abdomen to back, chest, arms; worse, bending forwards and while lying. *Sharp pains from liver, shooting upward to right nipple.* Pain from gall-bladder to chest, back, and arms. Renal colic, with pain in extremities. Hurried desire for stool.

Heart.—Angina pectoris; pain back of sternum into arms;

labored breathing; *feeble action of heart.* Especially with flatulence and pain through chest and tightness across.

Rectum.—Hæmorrhoids, with darting pains to liver; look like bunches of grapes or red cherries; protrude after stool, with pain in anus. Diarrhœa (worse in morning), yellowish, followed by exhaustion, as if flatus and feces were hot.

Male.—*Relaxation and coldness of organs.* Pains shoot into testicles from region of kidneys. *Strong-smelling sweat* on scrotum and pubes. *Emissions* in sleep, or from sexual atony, *with weak knees.*

Female.—Uterine colic; pains radiate from uterus. Vivid dreams.

Respiratory.—Tight feeling all along sternum. Chest does not seem to expand on breathing. Short-winded.

Extremities.—Lameness in back; worse, stooping. Aching and stiffness in joints. Sciatica; pains shoot down thigh; worse, right side; better, when perfectly still. *Felons* in beginning, when pricking is first felt. Nails brittle. Cramps in flexors of fingers and toes.

Modalities.—*Worse,* evening and night, *lying down,* and *doubling up. Better,* standing erect, motion in open air; pressure.

Relationship.—Antidotes: *Chamom.; Camph.*

Compare: *Colocy.* (differs in modalities); *Nux; Cham.; Bry.*

Dose.—Tincture, to third potency.

DIOSMA LINCARIS
(Buku — from Cape of Good Hope)

Pathogenically it produces: Somnolence; nervous insomnia; night sweats. Erratic pains, with bad humor, desire to weep or fear of sickness. Violent vertigo. Cephalalgia, chiefly frontal, radiating to the occiput. Eyes brilliant, with lachrymation or itching, the conditions accompanied by a species of stupefaction, with hardness of hearing or noises from aural pressure. Earthy face with disseminated rosaceous eruption . Nausea, fetid breath, with sensation of emptiness. *Sensation of meteorism, with stinging pains in the spleen.* Painful sensation in the abdomen, with pubic pressure—the pressure of the clothing becomes insupportable, with emission of high-colored, bloody urine. Frequent yellow diarrhœa, worse at night. Catamenia abundant, anticipating, sometimes metrorrhagic in type; crampy pains on ingesting food. Sensation of heat or of cold in the hands, with convulsive movements of the fingers. Weakness of the legs, aggravated by sitting down.

Clinically, this pathogeny should be useful in cerebral affections with dullness or stupefaction; in convulsive or epileptiform attacks; in *hysteria;* in *hepatitis* (cirrhosis or atrophy); in hematuria with ovarian or uterine lesions.

In splenitis, where it should surpass Ceanothus. Mental disorders in nervous or ascetic individuals, particularly where there is constant fear of death, or erotic or maniacal attacks. *Gastralgia. Gastro-enteritis.* Sudden fright, with trembling and weakness of the legs. (Dr. C. Leal La Rota.)

DIPHTHERINUM
(Potentized Diphtheritic Virus)

Adapted to patients prone to catarrhal affections of respiratory organs, scrofulous individuals. Diphtheria, laryngeal diphtheria, *post-diphtheritic paralysis.* Malignancy from the start. Glands swollen; tongue red, swollen; breath and discharge very offensive. Diphtheritic membrane thick, dark. Epistaxis; profound prostration. Swallows without pain, but fluids are vomited or returned by the nose.

Relationship.—Compare: *Diphtherotoxin* (Cahis) (Chronic bronchitis with rales. Cartier suggests it in the vago-paralytic forms of Bronchitis of the aged or in toxic bronchitis after grip.)

Dose.—Thirtieth, two-hundredth or C. M. potency. Must not be repeated too frequently.

DOLICHOS PURIENS — MUCUNA
(Cowhage)

A right-sided medicine, with pronounced liver and skin symptoms. A general *intense itching* without eruption. Exalted nervous sensibility. Senile pruritus. Hæmorrhoidal diathesis.

Throat.—*Pain in throat, worse swallowing, below right angle of jaw, as if splinter were imbedded vertically.* Pain in gums prevents sleep.

Abdomen.—Colic from getting feet wet. *Constipation, with intense itching; bloated abdomen.* White stools. Swelling of liver. Hæmorrhoids, with burning sensation.

Skin.—*Intense itching*, with no swelling or rash; worse across shoulders, also about elbows and knees and hairy parts. Jaundice. Yellow in spots; itching excessively at night. Herpes zoster. [*Ars.*]

Modalities.—*Worse*, at night, scratching, right side.

Relationship.—Compare: *Rhus; Bell.; Hep.; Nit. ac.; Fagopyr.*

Dose.—Sixth potency. Tincture, drop doses, in hæmorrhoids.

DORYPHORA
(Colorado Potato-bug)

The center of this drug's action seems to be in the urinary organs, and hence its employment in gonorrhœa and gleet. Urethritis in children from local irritation and gleet. Great trembling in extremities. Prostration. Swelling of body. *Burning sensation.*

Urinary.—Difficult micturition. Urethra inflamed, with excruciating pain when urinating. Pain in back and loins. Severe trembling in limbs.

Relationship.—Antidote: *Stram.*

Compare: *Agar.; Apis; Canth.; Lach.; Coccion.*

Dose.—Sixth to thirtieth potency.

DROSERA
(Sundew)

Affects markedly the respiratory organs and was pointed out by Hahnémann as the principal remedy for whooping-cough. Drosera can break down resistance to tubercle and should therefore be capable of raising it (Dr. Tyler). Laryngeal phthisis is benefited by it. Phthisis pulmonum; vomiting of food from coughing with gastric irritation and profuse expectoration. Pains about hip-joint. Tubercular glands.

Head.—Vertigo when walking in open air, with inclination to fall to the *left side.* Coldness of left half of face, with stinging pains and dry heat of *right half.*

Stomach.—Nausea. Aversion to and bad effects from acids.

Respiratory Organs.—Spasmodic, dry irritative cough, like whooping-cough, the *paroxysms following each other very rapidly;* can scarcely breathe; chokes. Cough very deep and hoarse; worse, after midnight; yellow expectoration, *with bleeding from nose* and mouth; *retching. Deep, hoarse voice; hoarseness;* laryngitis. Rough, scraping sensation deep in the fauces and soft palate. Sensation as if crumbs were in the throat, of feather in larynx. Laryngeal phthisis, with rapid emaciation. Harassing and titillating cough in children—not at all through the day, but commences as soon as the head touches the pillow at night. Clergyman's sore throat, with rough, scraping, dry sensation deep in the fauces; voice hoarse, deep, toneless, cracked, requires exertion to speak. *Asthma when talking,* with contraction of the throat at every word uttered.

Extremities.—Paralytic pains in the coxo-femoral joint and thighs. Stiffness in joints of feet. All limbs feel lame. Bed feels too hard.

Fever.—Internal chilliness; shivering, with hot face, cold hands, no thirst. Is always too cold, even in bed.

Modalities.—*Worse,* after midnight, lying down, on getting warm in bed, drinking, singing, laughing.

Relationship.—Antidote: *Camph.*

Compare: *Fluoroform* (2 per cent. watery solution, 2-4 drops, after paroxysms, considered specific for whooping-cough.) *Ouabain* from leaves of Carissa schimperi—arrow poison. (Respiratory spasm—Whooping cough is cut short in first stage and reduced in frequency of attacks and hastens convalescence.) *Chelid.; Corall.; Cupr.; Castanea; Argent.; Menyanth.*

Dose.—First to twelfth attenuation.

DUBOISIA
(Corkwood Elm)

Acts chiefly on the nervous system, eyes, upper respiratory tract. Recommended in pharyngitis sicca, with black, stringy mucus. It dilates the pupil, dries the mouth, checks perspiration, causes headache and drowsiness. On the eye it acts more promptly than Atropia, much stronger as a mydriatic. *Red spot floats in the field of vision.* Sensation as if stepping on empty space. *Vertigo with pale face;* not gastric in origin. Scarlet fever; locomotor ataxia. Palliative in exophthalmic goitre.

Mind.—Absent-minded, incoherent, *silly and nonsensical*, memory impaired.

Head.—Impossible to stand with eyes shut, tendency to fall backwards.

Eyes.—*Conjunctivitis*, acute and chronic. *Mydriasis.* Paralysis of accommodation. Hyperæmia of retina with weakness of accommodation, fundus red, blood-vessels full and tortuous; pupils dilated, with dim vision. *Pain over eye*, between it and brow.

Respiratory.—Larynx dry, voice hoarse, phonation difficult. Dry cough with oppressed breathing.

Extremities.—Loss of power in limbs, staggers; feels as if he stepped on empty space. Trembling, numbness and weakness.

Relationship.—It antagonizes *Muscarine. Duboisin sulphate* 1-100 gr. *sedative in mania.* 2-4 millegrams a day. Hysteroepilepsy. Motor restlessness of insane. *Has been used as a substitute for Atropia* in doses of 1-20 of a grain hypodermically.) Antidotes: *Morphia; Pilocarp.* Compare: *Bellad.; Stram.; Hyos.*

Dose.—Third to twelfth potency.

DULCAMARA
(Bitter-sweet)

Hot days and cold nights towards the close of summer are especially favorable to the action of Dulcamara, and is one of the remedies that correspond in their symptoms to the conditions found as effects of damp weather, colds after exposure to wet, especially diarrhœa. It has a specific relation also to the *skin, glands*, and digestive organs, *mucous membranes* secreting more profusely while the skin is inactive. The *rheumatic troubles* induced by damp cold are aggravated by every cold change and somewhat relieved by moving about. Results from sitting on cold, damp ground. Icy coldness. One-sided spasms with speechlessness. Paralysis of single parts. Congestive headache, with neuralgia and dry nose. Patients living or working in damp, cold basements. [*Nat. sulph.*] Eruptions on hands, arms or face around the menstrual period.

Head.—Mental confusion. Occipital pain ascending from nape of neck. Headache relieved by conversation. Rejects things asked for. Back part of head chilly, heavy, aching, during cold weather. Ringworm of scalp. *Scaldhead, thick brown crusts*, bleeding when scratched. Buzzing in head.

Nose.—Dry coryza. Complete stoppage of nose. *Stuffs up when there is a cold rain.* Thick, yellow mucus, bloody crusts. Profuse coryza. Wants nose kept warm, least cold air stops the nose. Coryza of the new born.

Eyes.—Every time he takes cold it settles in eyes. Thick, yellow discharge; granular lids. Hay-fever; profuse, watery discharge, worse in open air.

Ears.—Earache, buzzing, stitches, and swelling of parotids. Middle-ear catarrh [*Merc. dulc.; Kal. mur.*]

Face.—Tearing in cheek extending to ear, orbit, and jaw, *preceded by coldness of parts, and attended by canine hunger.* Humid eruption on cheeks and face generally.

Mouth.—Saliva tenacious, soapy. Dry, rough tongue, rough scraping in throat, after taking cold in damp weather. Cold-sores on lips. Facial neuralgia; worse, *slightest exposure to cold.*

Stomach.—Vomiting of white, tenacious mucus. *Aversion to food. Burning thirst for cold drinks.* Heartburn. Nausea accompanies the desire for stool. Chilliness during vomiting

Abdomen.—Colic from cold. Acts prominently on umbilical region. *Cutting pain about navel.* Swelling of inguinal glands [*Merc.*]

Stool.—Green, watery, slimy, bloody, *mucus*, especially in summer, when the weather suddenly becomes cold; *from damp, cold weather* and repelled eruptions.

Urine.—Must urinate *when getting chilled.* Strangury, painful micturition. Catarrh of bladder from taking cold. Urine has thick, *mucous*, purulent sediment. Ischuria from wading with bare feet in cold water.

Female.—Suppression of menses from cold or dampness. Before appearance of menses, *a rash appears on skin*, or sexual excitement. Dysmenorrhœa, with blotches all over; mammæ engorged and sore, delicate, sensitive to cold.

Respiratory.—Cough worse cold, wet weather, with free expectoration, tickling in larynx. Cough, hoarse, spasmodic. Whooping-cough, with excessive secretion of mucus. Winter coughs, dry, teasing. Asthma with dyspnœa. Loose, rattling cough; worse wet weather. Must cough a long time to expel phlegm. Cough *after physical exertion*.

Back.—Stiff neck. *Pain in small of back*, as after long stooping. Stiffness and lameness across neck and shoulders, after getting cold and wet.

Extremities.—Paralysis: paralyzed limbs, *feet icy cold*. Warts on hands. Perspiration on palms of hands. Pain in shin-bones. Rheumatism alternates with diarrhœa. Rheumatic symptoms after acute skin eruptions.

Skin.—*Adenitis. Pruritus, always worse in cold, wet weather.* Herpes zoster, pemphigus. Swelling and indurated glands from cold. Vesicular eruptions. Sensitive bleeding ulcers. Little boils. Red spots, *urticaria*, brought on by exposure, or sour stomach. Humid eruptions on face, genitals, hands etc. *Warts*, large, smooth, on face and palmar surface of hands. Anasarca. Thick, brown-yellow crusts, bleeding when scratched.

Fever.—Dry burning heat all over. Chilliness towards evening, mostly in back. Icy coldness, with pains. Dry heat and burning of skin. Chilliness with thirst.

Modalities.—*Worse*, at night; from *cold* in general, *damp, rainy weather. Better*, from moving about, external warmth.

Relationship.—Antidotes: *Camph.; Cupr.*

Complementary: *Baryta carb.*

Incompatible: *Bellad.; Laches.*

Compare: *Pimpinello*—(Bibernell).—Respiratory mucous membrane sensitive to draughts, pain and coldness in occiput and nape. Whole body weak; heavy head and drowsiness; lumbago and stiff neck; pain from nape to shoulder; chilliness. *Rhus; Cimicif.; Calc.; Puls.; Bry.; Nat. sulph.*

Dose.—Second to thirtieth potency.

ECHINACEA—RUDBECKIA
(Purple Cone-flower)

We are indebted to the Eclectic school for this remarkable medicine as a "corrector of blood dyscrasia." Acute autoinfection. Symptoms of *blood poisoning, septic conditions generally*. Diarrhœa in typhoid. Gonorrhœa. Boils. *Erysipelas* and foul ulcers. *Gangrene.* Goitre with exophthalmic symptoms; full doses, also injecting 5-10 drops into thyroid gland. Tendency to malignancy in acute and subacute disorders. Last stages of cancer to ease pain. *Venom infection.* Cerebro-spinal meningitis. Puerperal infections. *Tired feeling.* Piles. Pustules. Acts on vermiform appendix thus has been used for appendicitis, but remember it promotes suppuration and a neglected appendicitis with pus formation would probably rupture sooner under its use. Lymphatic inflammation; crushing injuries. *Snake bites* and bites and stings generally. Foul discharges with emaciation and great debility.

Head.—Confused, depressed. Aches with a peculiar periodical flushing of the face, even to the neck; dizziness and profound prostration.

Nose.—Foul-smelling discharge, membranous formations protruding. Post-nasal catarrh with ulceration and fetor. Nose feels stuffed up. Right nostril raw, bleeding.

Mouth.—Canker; gums recede and bleed easily; corners of mouth and lips crack; tongue dry and swollen; sores; dirty brownish. Tongue, lips, and fauces *tingle*, with sense of fear about heart. [*Acon.*] White coating of tongue, with red edges. Promotes the flow of saliva.

Throat.—Tonsils purple or black, gray exudation extending to posterior nares and air-passages. Ulcerated sore throat.

Stomach.—Sour belching and heartburn. Nausea; better lying down.

Chest.—Pain as of a lump in chest and under sternum. Pain in pectoral muscles. [*Aristolochia.*]

Urine.—Albuminous, scanty, frequent, and involuntary.

Female.—*Puerperal septicæmia;* discharges suppressed; abdomen sensitive and tympanitic; offensive, excoriating leucorrhœa.

Extremities.—*Aching in limbs* and general lassitude.

Skin.—Recurring boils. Carbuncles. Irritations from insect bites and poisonous plants. Lymphatics enlarged. Old tibial ulcers. Gangrene.

Fever.—*Chilliness, with nausea.* Cold flashes all over back. *Malarial fever.*

Relationship.—Compare: *Cenchris contortrix; Bothrops; Ars.; Laches.; Baptis.; Rhus; Cistus; Hepar; Calendula.*

Dose.—Tincture, one to ten drops, every two hours, and larger doses.

Locally, as a cleansing and antiseptic wash.

ELAPS CORALLINUS
(Coral-snake)

Similar to snake-poisons generally. Has very marked *black discharges*. *Cold things disagree.* Desire for sweetened buttermilk. Nausea and vomiting. Prostrating diarrhœa of consumption. Acidity of stomach, with faint feeling. Sudden pain in stomach. Spasm of œsophagus; pharynx constricted; food and liquids suddenly arrested, and then fall heavily into stomach. Spasms followed by paresis. *Cold feeling in stomach.* Fruits and ice-water lie very cold. *Right-sided paralysis.* Must have oscillatory motion. Rheumatic constitutions. Ear, nose and throat symptoms important.

Mind.—Depressed; imagines he hears someone talking; dreads to be left alone. *Fear of rain.* Can speak, but cannot understand speech. Fears apoplexy.

Head.—Violent headache, extending from forehead *to occiput;* first one eye, then the other. Pain in ears. Vertigo with tendency to fall forward. Weight and pain in forehead. Fulness in head.

Eyes.—Aversion to light; letters run together when reading. Veil before eyes. Burning in lids. Bloated around the eyes in the morning. Large red fiery spot before eyes.

Ears.—Cerumen *black* and hard, with difficult hearing, or serous *greenish* discharge, offensive; buzzing, and illusion of hearing. Sudden attack of nightly deafness, with roaring and crackling in ears, cracking in ears on swallowing. Intolerable itching in ear.

Nose.—*Chronic nasal catarrh, with fetid odor and greenish crusts.* Ozæna; yellowish-green discharge. Mucous membrane wrinkled; nostrils plugged up with dry mucus. Pains from nose to ears on swallowing. *Nostrils stopped up.* Nasal bleeding. Pain at root of nose. Eruption about nose.

Throat.—Thick, very offensive, dry, greenish-yellow crusts upon the posterior pharyngeal wall and extremely foul breath. Spasmodic contraction of œsophagus; passage of fluids arrested.

Chest.—*Coldness in chest after drinking.* Hæmorrhage from lungs black as ink and watery; stitches *in apex of right lung.* Fainting caused by stooping. Oppression in going upstairs. Peeling off of skin from palms and fingers. *Cough,* with terrible pain through lungs. Worse right and expectoration of black blood. Sensation of a sponge in œsophagus.

Stomach.—*Feels cold.* Sensation as if food turned like a corkscrew on swallowing; desire for sweetened buttermilk. Acidity after every mouthful.

Female.—Dysmenorrhœa, with black blood. Discharge of black blood between menses. Itching of vulva and vagina.

Sleep.—Dreams about dead persons.

Skin.—Glands and skin of axillæ affected; itching with tetter. Tips of fingers peel off. Itching eruption in axillæ.

Extremities.—Icy cold feet. Vesicular eruptions on feet. Arms and hands swollen bluish. Knee-joints feel sprained. Pricking under the nails.

Fever.—Cold perspiration all over. Typhoid when ulcers have eaten into tissues, and black blood is discharged.

Modalities.—*Worse* eating fruit; cold drinks; *wet weather.*

Relationship.—Compare: *Kino*—from *Pterocarpus* (Hæmoptysis and hemorrhage from intestines). *Eucalyptus rostrata* (offensive dark discharge from right ear). *Crotalus; Alumen; Carbo; Ars.; Lach.*

Dose.—Sixth to thirtieth potency.

ELATERIUM—ECBALIUM
(Squirting Cucumber)

This is an invaluable remedy in violent vomiting and purging, especially if the evacuations are copious and watery. It is a very efficient remedy in certain forms of dropsy. Much yawning and stretching. *Beriberi;* choleraic conditions; urticaria and mental disorders coming on as a consequence of suppressed malaria. Irresistible desire to wander from home at night. Effects of damp weather.

Stomach.—Nausea and vomiting, with great weakness. Griping pains in bowels.

Stool.—*Watery, copious, forceful. Squirting diarrhœa;* frothy, olive green, with cutting in abdomen.

Extremities.—Sharp pains in fingers and thumbs, knees, toes, and instep. Gouty pain in great toes. Pain extends down extremities; pain in hip-joints with diarrhœa. Arthritic nodules.

Skin.—Smarts, stings, and burns. Dropsical. Urticaria from suppressed intermittent. Skin, orange color.

Fever.—Chill comes on with much *yawning and stretching*, lasting all through chill. Pain in extremities, darting into fingers and toes. Chills and fever, with spurting diarrhœa.

Modalities.—Worse, from exposure on damp ground.

Relationship.—Compare: Bry.; Croton; Gambogia.

Dose.—Third to thirtieth potency. As a hydragogue cathartic to produce free discharge in dropsies, Elaterin 1-20 of a grain. Palliative only.

EOSIN

A remedy for cancer, polyarthritis. Proved in potencies by Dr. B. C. Woodbury.

Summary of symptoms:

Burning under finger nails and toe nails, on soles.

Itching and redness of knee-caps.

Redness of palms.

Redness, burning and *numbness* of tongue.

Peculiar sensation of being very tall with tendency to vertigo.

Burning in various parts on skin.

Shifting location after scratching which relieves.

Dose.—Second decimal (1% sol.).

EPIGEA REPENS
(Trailing Arbutus)

Chronic cystitis, with *dysuria;* tenesmus after micturition; *muco-pus and uric-acid deposit,* gravel, renal calculi. Fine sand in urine of a *brown color.* Burning in neck of bladder whilst urinating and tenesmus afterward. Pyelitis, incontinence of urine. Croaking noise and rumbling in bowels.

Relationship.—Compare: *Uva; Chimaph.; Lyc.; Pareira.* Epigea contains Arbutin, also Formic acid.

Dose.—Tincture in 5-drop doses every three hours.

EPIPHEGUS—OROBANCHE
(Beechdrop)

A remedy for sick, neurasthenic, and nervous headaches, especially in women, brought on or made worse by exertion, shopping, etc. Tongue coated yellow; bitter taste. Drowsy after meals. Loose stools. *Subinvolution,* with painful menstruation and congestion.

Head.—Pressing pain in temples *from without inwards; worse, left side. Viscid salivation;* constant inclination to spit. Sick headache coming on when deviating from ordinary pursuits. Headaches from nerve tire caused by mental or physical exhaustion, *preceded by hunger.*

Modalities.—*Worse,* from working in open air. *Better,* from sleep.

Relationship.—Compare: *Iris; Melilot.; Sanguinar. Fagus —Beech-nuts—*(headache and salivation); swelling of mouth; dread of water).

Dose.—First to thirtieth potency.

EQUISETUM
(Scouring-rush)

Principal action on the bladder. A remedy for enuresis and dysuria.

Urinary.—Severe, dull pain and feeling of fullness in bladder, not relieved by urinating. Frequent urging with severe pain *at the close of urination.* Urine flows only drop by drop. Sharp, *burning,* cutting pain in urethra while urinating.

Incontinence in children, with dreams or night-mares when passing urine. Incontinence in old women, also with involuntary stools. Retention and dysuria during pregnancy and after delivery. Much mucus in urine. Albuminuria. Involuntary urination.

Kidney.—Deep pain in region of right kidney, extending to lower abdomen, with urgent desire to micturate. Right lumbar region painful.

Modalities.—*Worse,* right side; movement, pressure, touch, sitting down; *better,* in afternoon from lying down.

Relationship.—Compare: *Hydrangea; Ferr. phos.; Apis; Canth.; Linaria; Chimaph.* Equisitum contains silica in appreciable quantity.

Dose.—Tincture, to sixth potency. A decoction, teaspoonful doses, or the tincture in hot water, is found useful to allay irritability of urinary tract, calculus, dysuria, etc.; also for pleuritic effusion and dropsy.

ERECHTHITES
(Fire-weed)

A hæmorrhagic remedy. Epistaxis of bright blood. Hæmorrhage from any part, especially lungs; always attended by excitement of the circulation. Flashes of heat and coldness. Scanty urine, œdema of the extremities.

Skin.—*Symptoms like Rhus poisoning.*

Relationship.—Compare: *Erig.; Millef.; Hamam.; Rhus.*

Dose.—Tincture. Locally for Poison Oak.

ERIGERON—LEPTILON CANADENSE
(Fleabane)

Hæmorrhages are caused and cured by this remedy. Persistent hæmorrhage from the bladder. Hæmorrhage from the uterus, with painful micturition. *Profuse bright-red blood.* Pain in left ovary and hip. Chronic gonorrhœa, with burning micturition; continual dribbling. *Dysentery,* with soreness and burning in bladder. *Tympanites.*

Female.—Metrorrhagia, with violent irritation of rectum and bladder, and prolapsus uteri. Bright-red flow. Menorrhagia; profuse leucorrhœa; *bloody lochia returns after least motion,* comes in gushes; between periods, *leucorrhœa with urinary irritation;* pregnant women with "weak uterus;" a bloody discharge on slight exertion. Bleeding hæmorrhoids; nosebleed instead of menses. [*Bry.*]

Modalities.—*Worse,* left side.

Relationship.—Terebinthina similar.

Dose.—Tincture, to third potency. Oil of Erigeron 1x internally for *tympanites.* An enema of one dram of the oil with the yolk of an egg and pint of milk will reduce the most enormous tympanites.

ERIODICTYON
(Yerba Santa)

A remedy for asthmatic and bronchial affections. Bronchial phthisis, with night-sweats and emaciation. Asthma relieved by expectoration. *Cough after influenza.* Furthers absorption of effusion in plural cavity. Appetite poor and impaired digestion. Whooping cough.

Head.—Dizzy, feels intoxicated. Pressure outwards; worse, occiput. Pain in ears. Coryza. Burning in throat. Foul mouth in morning. Coryza with dizziness and sneezing.

Respiratory.—Wheezing; asthma, with coryza and *mucous secretions.* Dull pain in right lung. Burning in fauces. Chronic bronchitis, bronchial tuberculosis, with profuse, easily raised bronchial secretion, giving relief.

Male.—Sore, dragging in testicle, could not bear any pressure; better gentle support.

Relationship.—Compare: *Grind.; Aral.; Eucalyp.; Ipec.*

Dose.—Tincture in doses of 2 to 20 drops and attenuations.

ERYNGIUM AQUATICUM
(Button Snake-root)

A remedy for urinary disorders. Strangury, etc., with nervous erethism. *Thick, yellow mucous discharges.* Influenza. Uridrosis, sweat of urinous odor in evening.

Respiratory.—Cough, with sense of constriction. Smarting in throat and larynx.

Urinary.—Tenesmus of bladder and urethra. Difficult and frequent micturition. Pain behind pubes. Spasmodic stricture. *Renal colic.* [*Pareira; Calc.*] Congestion of kidneys with dull pain in back, running down the ureters and limbs. Irritable bladder from enlarged prostate gland, or from pressure of uterus.

Male.—Discharge of prostatic fluid from slight causes. Seminal emissions without erections, with lassitude. [*Dioscor.; Phos. ac.*]

Relationship.—Compare: *Conium; Cannab.: Dios.; Ocim.; Clemat.*

Dose.—Tincture, to third potency.

ESCHSCHOLTZIA CALIFORNICA
(California Poppy)

Experiments upon animals showed it to act more powerfully than morphine which is contained in the plant. It causes general weakness, torpor, accelerated respiration, complete paralysis of the limbs. Slowing of circulation.

A soporic remedy which is harmless. Use the tincture.

EUCALYPTUS GLOBULUS
(Blue Gum-tree)

Eucalyptus is a powerful antiseptic and destructive to low forms of life, a stimulating expectorant and an efficient diaphoretic. Atonic dyspepsia, gastric and intestinal catarrh. A remedy with marked effects on catarrhal processes, malaria, and intestinal disturbance. *Influenza.* Fevers of a *relapsing* character. Produces diuresis and great increase of urea. Hæmorrhages internally and locally. [*Hamam.*] *Typhoid.* Symptoms of exhaustion and toxæmia. Conditions of the mucous surfaces of the air passages, genito-urinary organs and gastro-intestinal tract. A gastro-intestinal irritant with pain in stomach and upper intestines several hours after eating.

Head—Exhilaration. Desire for exercise. Dull congestive headache. *Coryza;* sore throat. Eyes smart and burn.

Nose.—*Stuffed-up sensation;* thin, watery coryza; nose does not stop running; tightness across bridge. *Chronic catarrhal, purulent and fetid discharge.* Ethmoid and frontal sinus involved.

Throat.—Relaxed, aphthous condition of mouth and throat. Excessive secretion of saliva. Burns, feels full. Constant sensation of phlegm in throat. Enlarged, ulcerated tonsils and inflamed throat. (Use tincture locally.)

Stomach.—*Slow digestion.* Much fetid gas. Beating and goneness with pulsation in epigastric arteries. Spleen hard and contracted. Pain in epigastrium and upper abdomen ameliorated by food. Malignant disease of stomach with vomiting of blood and sour fluid.

Abdomen.—*Acute diarrhœa.* Aching pains in bowels with feeling of impending diarrhœa. *Dysentery*, with rectal heat; tenesmus; hæmorrhage. Diarrhœa; stools thin, watery, preceded by sharp pains. Typhoid diarrhœa.

Urinary.—*Acute nephritis complicating influenza.* Hæmaturia. Suppurative inflammation of kidneys. Urine contains pus and is deficient in urea. Bladder feels loss of expulsive force. Burning and tenesmus; *catarrh of bladder;* diuresis; *urethral caruncle.* Spasmodic stricture; gonorrhœa.

Respiratory.—*Asthma,* with great dyspnœa and palpitation. Moist asthma. Expectoration white, thick mucus. Bronchitis in the aged. Bronchorrhœa. [*Bals. Peru.*] Profuse expectoration of offensive muco-pus. Irritative cough. Whooping-cough in rachitic children. Fetid form of bronchitis, bronchial dilatation and emphysema.

Female.—Leucorrhœa, acrid, fetid. Ulcer around orifice of urethra.

Extremities.—Rheumatic pains; worse at night, walking or carrying anything. Stiff, weary sensation. *Pricking sensation, followed by painful aching.* Nodular swellings over metacarpal and metatarsal joints.

Skin.—Glandular enlargements and nodular swelling over joints. Foul and indolent ulcers. Herpetic eruptions.

Fever.—Elevation of temperature. Continued and typhoid fevers. Scarlet fever (protective and curative). Discharges show a tendency to foulness, high temperature, accelerated but not strong pulse. Use the tincture.

Relationship.—Compare: *Oil of Eucalyptus.*—(Produces remarkable bodily exhaustion, no desire for any motion, unable to do any real mental work, study, etc. The volatile oil possesses, in common with other terpenes, the property of converting water, in presence of air and sunlight, into hydrogen peroxide, or to convert oxygen into ozone, which is the explanation usually given of its deodorizing and antiseptic properties. (Merrel.) Locally, in catarrhal affections, especially when of a suppurating or putrid nature.) *Eucalyptus tereticoris* (menstrual cough and *prostration*). *Eucalyptol* (depresses temperature of healthy body more than *Quinine;* acts on kidneys like *Terebinth.*); *Anacard.; Hydrast.; Kali sulph. Eucalyptus* neutralizes ill effects of *Strychnin. Angophora*—Red Gum— (dysentery, pains, tenesmus; better lying flat on face; obstinate constipation). *Eucalyptus rostrata; Kino.*

Dose.—Tincture in one to 20 drop doses, and lower potencies. Also Oil of Eucalyptus in five-drop doses.

EUGENIA JAMBOS—JAMBOSA VULGARIS
(Rose-apple)

Eugenia produces a state of intoxication like alcohol. Everything appears beautiful and larger; excitement soon changing to depression. Acne, simple and indurated. The pimples are painful for some distance around. Acne rosacea. *Nausea. better smoking. Comedones.*

Head.—Headache as if a board were lying on right side. Talkative. *Hot lachrymation.*

Extremities.—*Nightly cramp in soles of feet.* [*Cupr.; Zing* | Skin cracks about toes. Fissures between toes. Skin recedes from the nails, forming pus.

Relationship.—Compare: Eugenia chekun—Myrtus chekan (chronic Bronchitis); *Antim.; Berb. aquif.*

EUONYMUS ATROPURPUREA
(Wahoo. Burning Bush)

Brunettes more easily affected, producing headache, mental disturbances and much distress in hepatic and renal region; albuminuria. Migraine. Passive Congestion and torpor of liver; chronic catarrhal affections of stomach and intestines. Weak heart. Chronic rheumatism and gout.

Mind.—Mental confusion, despondent, irritable; loss of memory, unable to recall familiar names.

Head.—Heavy frontal headache. Sore, tired feeling; bruised feeling of scalp. Pain over right eye extending back through the head. Bilious headache; coated tongue, bad taste, constipation. Vertigo, obscure vision and gastric derangement, associated with albuminuria. Headache over eyebrows.

Stomach.—Mouth dry, pasty taste; thirsty, stomach full and uncomfortable.

Abdomen.—Flatus and pain. Anus very sore and burning. Constipation with hæmorrhoids and severe backache. Diarrhœa; stools variable and profuse, bloody. Pain about umbilical region.

Urinary.—Urine scanty, high-colored; acidity increased, poured out rapidly.

Back.—Dull pain between shoulders and about renal and splenic region; pain in lumbar region better lying down.

Extremities.—Aching in all joints, especially ankles. Feet feel swollen and tired.

Modalities.—Better cool draught, pressure. Worse evening.

Relationship.—*Euonymus Europœa*—Spindle-tree (Liver disorders, biliousness, lumbago, gastric derangements with albuminuria. Cutting pains in malar bones, tongue, penis up to bladder); *Podophyl; Ammon. pic.; Chel.; Euonymin* 1x trit. (albuminuria).

Dose.—Tincture and lower attenuations.

EUPATORIUM AROMATICUM
(Pool-root)

Nervous erethism; restlessness and morbid watchfulness. Hysteria and chorea. Low fevers, with extreme restlessness. Aphthous disease. *Sore nipples.* Sore mouth in infants. Vomiting of bile, pain in stomach, headache, and fever.

Relationship.—*Lapsana communis*—Nipple-wort—useful in sore nipples and piles. *Hyosc.; Passiflor.; Hydr. mur.*

Dose.—Tincture, locally, in sore mouth and sore nipples. Internally, tincture to third attenuation.

EUPATORIUM PERFOLIATUM
(Thoroughwort)

Known as "Bone-set," from the prompt manner in which it relieves pain in limbs and muscles that accompanies some forms of febrile disease, like malaria and influenza. Eupatorium acts principally upon the gastro-hepatic organs and bronchial mucous membrane. It is a boon in miasmatic districts, along rivers, marshes, etc., and in all conditions where there is a great deal of *bone-pain*. Cachexia from old chronic, bilious intermittents. Worn-out constitutions from inebriety. Sluggishness of all organs and functions. Bone-pains, general and severe. Soreness. Marked periodicity. [*Ars.; China; Cedron.*]

Head.—Throbbing pain. Pressure as if a cap of lead pressed over the whole skull. Vertigo; sensation of falling to *left*. Vomiting of bile. Top and back of head with pain *and soreness of eyeballs*. Periodical headache, every third and seventh day. *Occipital pain after lying down, with sense of weight.*

Mouth.—Cracks in corners of mouth, yellow coated tongue, thirst.

Stomach.—Tongue yellow. Taste bitter. Hepatic region sore. Great thirst. Vomiting and purging of bile, of green liquid several quarts at a time. Vomiting preceded by thirst. Hiccough. [*Sulph. ac.; Hydrocy. ac.*] Avoids tight clothing.

Stool.—Frequent, **green,** watery. Cramps. Constipated, with sore liver.

Respiratory.—Coryza, with sneezing. *Hoarseness and cough, with soreness in chest;* must support it. *Influenza,* with great soreness of muscles and bones. *Chronic* loose cough, chest sore; *worse at night.* Cough relieved by getting on hands and knees.

Fever.—Perspiration relieves all symptoms except headache. Chill between 7 and 9 a. m., *preceded by thirst with great soreness and aching of bones.* Nausea, vomiting of bile at close of chill or hot stage; throbbing headache. Knows chill is coming on because he cannot drink enough.

Extremities.—*Aching pain in back. Aching in bones of extremities with soreness of flesh. Aching in arms and wrists.* Swelling of left great toe. Gouty soreness and inflamed nodosities of joints, associated with headache. Dropsical swelling.

Modalities.—*Worse,* periodically. *Better,* by conversation, by getting on hands and knees.

Relationship.—Compare: *Bryon.; Sepia.; Natr. mur.; Chelidon. Nyctanthes arbor-tristis* (bilious fever; insatiable thirst; bitter vomiting at close of chill; also constipation of children).

Dose.—Tincture, to third attenuation.

EUPATORIUM PURPUREUM
(Queen of the Meadow)

Albuminuria, diabetes, strangury, *irritable bladder,* enlarged prostate are a special field for this remedy. Excellent in renal dropsy. Chills and pains run upwards. Impotency and sterility. Homesickness.

Head.—*Left-sided headache with vertigo.* Pain from left shoulder to occiput. Sick headache beginning in morning, worse afternoon and evening, worse in cold air.

Urinary. Deep, dull pain in kidneys. Burning in bladder and urethra on urinating. Insufficient flow; milky. Strangury. Hæmaturia. Constant desire; bladder feels dull. Dysuria. *Vesical irritability in women. Diabetes insipidus.*

Back.—Weight and heaviness in loins and back.

Female.—Pain around left ovary. Threatened abortion. External genitals feel as though wet.

Fever.—*No thirst during* chill, but much frontal ache. *Chill commences in back.* Violent shaking, with comparatively little coldness. Bone-pains.

Relationship.—Compare: *Senecio; Cannab. sat.; Helon.; Phos. ac.; Triticum; Epigea.*

Dose.—First potency.

EUPHORBIA LATHYRIS
(Gopher-Plant, Caper Spurge)

The fresh milky juice is exceedingly acrid when applied to the skin and the fruit is highly purgative and poisonous. The juice causes redness, itching, pimples, sometimes gangrene. The symptoms point to its use in erysipelas, Poison Oak, etc. Rheumatic pains during rest. Paralytic, weakness in joints.

Mind.—Delirium and hallucinations. Stupor, coma.

Eyes.—Almost closed from *œdema of lids*.

Nose.—End of nose very much inflamed externally. Very *sensitive and œdematous* mucous membranes with ulceration

Face.—At first ruddy glow on cheeks, afterwards death-like pallor. Cold perspiration in beads on forehead. Red, puffed, and in spots suppurating. Erythema, beginning on face, gradually extending into the hair parts, and then spreading over whole body, taking eight days to do so; eruption glossy, rough œdematous, with burning and smarting; aggravated by touch and cold air; ameliorated by close room and sweet-oil applications. Fine bran-like desquamation. Sensation of cobwebs. Stinging, smarting, and burning of face when touched.

Mouth.—Tongue coated, slimy; acrid taste. Breath cold, musty odor.

Stomach.—Nausea and vomiting of copious clear water, intermingled with white, gelatinous lumps.

Stool.—Drastic purgation from large doses; mild laxative condition from smaller doses; followed several weeks afterwards by obstinate constipation. Stools of white, transparent, gelatinous mucus; later mingled with blood.

Urine.—Copious flow of urine.

Male.—Inflammation of scrotum, resulting in deep acrid ulcers, with intense itching and burning; worse, touching the parts from washing.

Respiratory.—Labored breathing. Breath cold, musty odor. Cough; first, a hacking, as from inhalation of sulphur; later on, paroxysmal, like whooping-cough, in regular parosysms, ending in diarrhœa and vomiting, with sleepiness between each paroxysm.

Heart.—Weak and fluttering heart-action. Pulse 120, full, bounding, somewhat irregular.

Sleep.—Restlesness at night. Sleep disturbed, anxious dreams.

Fever.—Temperature increased. Body bathed in profuse perspiration, standing out like beads on forehead; later, cold, clammy perspiration on forehead.

Skin.—Erythema, beginning on uncovered parts, on face, and spreading over whole body; glossy, rough, œdematous, with burning and smarting. Fine bran-like desquamation following in the wake of the erythema. Eruption rough, scaly, smarting, and burning; when scratched forms deep, ragged ulcers; skin where ulcerated remains red.

Modalities.—*Worse*, touch and cold air; *better*, close room and sweet-oil application.

Relationship.—Antidoted by *Rhus tox.* (skin symptoms); *Veratr. alb.* (vomiting, purging, cough and coma).

Dose.—Third to thirtieth potency.

EUPHORBIUM

(Spurge—The Resinous Juice of Euphorbia Resinifera)

An irritant to the skin and mucous membranes. Burning pain in bones. Pains in limbs and paralytic weakness in the joints. Important respiratory and skin symptoms. Terrible burning pains. *Pains of cancer.* Everything appears larger than it really is.

Head.—Acute mania. Violent, pressive headache.

Face.—Erysipelas; yellow blisters. Burning in cheek; worse, left. Eyes inflamed and agglutinated in morning. Red swelling of cheeks. Nasal pruritus with mucous secretions from naso-pharynx.

Stomach.—Great hunger. Sialorrhœa (**profuse salty saliva**). Waterbrash. Thirst for cold drinks.

Abdomen.—Sunken; spasmodic, flatulent colic. Stools fermented, profuse, clayey. Feels hollow.

Respiratory.—Breathing oppressed, as if chest were not wide enough Spasmodic, dry cough, day and night, with asthma. Violent, fluent coryza, with burning and cough. Constant cough, with stitches from pit of stomach to sides of chest. Croup, dry, hollow, cough. Warm feeling in chest, as if hot food had been swallowed.

Extremities.—Paralytic pains. Pain in hip-joint and coccyx.

Skin.—Erysipelatous inflammation, especially of the cheek. Biting and stinging, red, swollen. *Vesicular erysipelas.* Carbuncle; old, torpid, indolent ulcers with biting, lancinating pain. Old torpid ulcer, pustules; *gangrene.* [*Echinac.; Secale.*] Ulcerating carcinoma and epithelioma of the skin.

Relationship.—Compare: *Euphorbia amygdaloides*—Wood Spurge (in pain in antrum, illusion of smell, *odor of mice.* Sense of taste blunted. Diarrhœa; stools difficult, with painful anal spasm).

Euphorbia corollata—Large Flowering Spurge—(a diaphoretic expectorant and cathartic of the old school in gastro-enteric disturbance, with deathly nausea. Vomiting of food, water, and mucus, and copious evacuations. Attacks recur after short intermissions. Feeling of clawing in stomach; cold sweat). (*Verat. alb.*)

Euphorbia marginata—Snow on the mountain—(Honey from the flowers is poisonous, detected by the hot, acrid taste. The milky juice produces skin symptoms like *Rhus*).

Euphorbia pilulifera—Pillbearing Spurge—(Humid asthma, cardiac dyspnœa, hay-fever, and bronchitis. Urethritis, with intense pain on urinating, and much urging. Acrid leucorrhœa; worse least movement. Hæmorrhages from sunstroke and traumatism).

Compare, also: *Psoralea*—A Columbian plant—(Pain of cancer, ulcers. Leucorrhœa fetid. Pruritus. Uterine tumors.) *Croton; Jatropha; Colchic.*

Antidotes: *Camph.; Opium.*

Dose.—Third to sixth potency.

EUPHRASIA

(Eyebright)

Manifests itself in inflaming the conjunctival membrane especially, producing profuse lachrymation. Patient is better in open air. Catarrhal affections of mucous membranes especially of eyes and nose. Profuse *acrid* lachrymation and bland coryza; worse, evening. Hawking up of offensive mucus.

Head.—Bursting headache with dazzling of eyes. *Catarrhal headache,* with profuse discharge from eyes and nose.

Nose.—*Profuse, fluent coryza,* with violent cough and abundant expectoration.

Eyes.—*Catarrhal* conjunctivitis; discharge of acrid matter. *The eyes water all the time.* Acrid lachrymation; bland coryza. [Opposite: *Cepa.*] Discharge thick and exoriating. [*Mercur.* thin and acrid.] Burning and swelling of the lids. Frequent inclination to blink. Free discharge of acrid matter. Sticky mucus on cornea; must wink to remove it. Pressure in eyes. Little blisters on cornea. Opacities. Rheumatic iritis. Ptosis. [*Gels.; Caust.*]

Face.—Redness and heat of cheeks. Stiffness of upper lip.

Stomach.—Vomiting from hawking mucus. Nausea and bitterness after smoking.

Rectum.—Dysentery. Prolapse ani. Pressure down in anus when sitting. *Constipation.*

Female.—Menses *painful; flow lasts only an hour or day;* late, scanty, short. *Amenorrhœa, with ophthalmia.*

Male.—Spasmodic retraction of genitals, with pressure above pubic bone. Condyloma and sycotic excrescences. *Prostatitis.* Nocturnal irritability of bladder; dribbling urine.

Respiratory.—Frequent yawning when walking in open air. Profuse, fluent coryza in morning, with much cough and expectoration. Influenza. Gags when clearing the throat in morning. Whooping-cough only in day-time, with profuse lachrymation.

Skin.—First stage of measles; eye symptoms marked. Consequence of external injuries.

Sleep.—Yawning when walking in open air. Sleepy during day

Fever.—Chilly and cold. Sweat mostly on chest, at night during sleep.

Modalities.—*Worse*, in evening, indoors, warmth; south winds; from light. *Better*, from coffee, in dark.

Relationship.—Antidotes: *Camph.; Puls.* Compare: *Hydrophyllum*—Burr-flower—(catarrhal inflammation of eyes; hot lachrymation with itching, swollen lids, dull headache; also for effects of Poison-Oak); *Cepa; Ars.; Gels.; Kali hyd.; Sabadilla.*

Dose.—Third to sixth potency.

EUPION

(Wood-tar distillation)

Marked female symptoms, and backache. A remedy for *uterine displacements*. Pain in back, followed by a bland leucorrhœa. Menses too early and copious; flow thin. *Intense sweat from slightest exertion*. Disgusting dreams. Sensation as if whole body were made of jelly.

Head.—Vertigo; everything turns round on sitting up in bed. Heat at vertex; stitches from vertex down limbs into abdomen and genitals. Sore painful spots on head. Painful pulsation in forehead.

Female.—*Burning in right ovary. Gushing leucorrhœa.* Chronic tubal disease. Uterine flexions. Menses too early and copious. During menses, irritable and disinclined to talk; burning and stitches in chest and heart. After menses, yellow *leucorrhœa, with severe backache.* When pain in back ceases, the discharge gushes out. Sore pain between labia during urination. Pruritus pudendi; labia swollen.

Extremities.—*Cramps in the calves;* worse at night.

Back.—Sacrum pains, as if broken. Severe backache; must lean against something for support. Pains extended into pelvis.

Relationship.—*Kreosot.; Graph.; Lach.*

Dose—Third potency.

FABIANA IMBRICATA
(Pichi)

A South American shrub cultivated in Southern California. It is a terebrinthine diuretic. It has also tonic and chologogue properties, used in the treatment of nasal catarrh, jaundice, dyspepsia and to increase the secretion of bile (Albert Schneider). Useful in the uric acid diathesis, cystitis, gonorrhœa, *prostatitis*, dysuria, vesical catarrh with suppurative prostatic conditions; post-gonorrhœal urinary conditions; cholethiasis and liver affections. Vesical tenesmus and burning after urination. Excoriating urine and calculi.

Dose.—Ten to twenty drops of the tincture.

FAGOPYRUM
(Buckwheat)

Its action on the skin, producing pruritus, is very marked. Visible pulsation of arteries. Fluent coryza. Offensive excretions. Itching erythema. *Pruritus senilis*. Post-nasal catarrh; dry crusts, granular appearance of posterior nares with itching.

Head.—Inability to study or remember. Depressed and irritable. Itching of eyes and ears. Pains deep in head, *with upward pressure*. Itching in and around eyes and ears. Head hot, better bending backward, with tired neck. Occipital headache. Bursting pains. Cerebral hyperæmia.

Nose.—Sore, red, inflamed. Fluent coryza, with sneezing, followed by dryness and crust formation.

Eyes.—*Itching* and smarting, swelling, heat and soreness.

Throat.—Soreness and feeling of excoriation, deep down pharynx. Uvula elongated, tonsils swollen.

Stomach.—Eructations of *scalding, hot,* acid, watery substance; better, coffee. Bad taste in the morning. Persistent, morning nausea. Drooling.

Heart.—Pain around heart, better lying on back, extending to left shoulder and arm. *Throbbing in all arteries* after retiring. Palpitation with oppression. Pulse irregular, intermittent, rapid. Light feeling in chest.

Female.—*Pruritus vulvæ, with yellow leucorrhœa,* worse, rest. Burning in right ovary.

Extremities.—Stiffness and bruised sensation in the muscles of the neck, with sensation as if nape of neck could not support head. Pain in shoulder, with pain along fingers. *Vehement itching in arms and legs;* worse towards evening. Feet numb and pricking. Streaking pains in arms and legs.

Skin.—*Itching;* better by bathing in cold water; worse scratching, touch and retiring. Sore red blotches. Blind boils. Itching of knees and elbows and hairy portions. *Itching of hands, deep in.* Vesicular, pustular; phlegmonous dermatitis. Skin hot, swollen.

Modalities.—*Better,* cold water, coffee; *worse,* in afternoon; from sunlight, scratching.

Relationship.—Compare: *Dolichos; Bovista; Urtica.*

Dose.—Third potency and 12x.

FEL TAURI
(Ox-gall)

Increases the duodenal secretion, emulsifies fats and increases the peristaltic action of the intestines. Liquifies bile and acts as a purgative and chologogue Disordered digestion, diarrhœa. and pain in nape of neck are among its chief symptoms. Obstruction of gall ducts. Biliary calculi. Jaundice.

Stomach.—Eructations, gurgling in stomach and epigastric region. Violent peristaltic movements. *Tendency to sleep after eating.*

Relationship.—Compare: *Merc. dulc.; Cholesterin.* In Biliary Lithiasis, *China. Calculobili*—Triturate Gall stones— 10-12x (Gall stones).

Dose.—Lower triturations. Purified oxgall 1 to 10 gr.

FERRUM IODATUM
(Iodide of Iron)

Scrofulous affections, glandular enlargements, and tumors call for this remedy. Crops of boils. Acute nephritis following eruptive diseases. Uterine displacements. Body emaciated Anemia Exophthalmic goitre following suppression of menses. Debility following drain upon vital forces. Impetigo of the cheek.

Stomach.—Food seems to push up into throat, as if it had not been swallowed.

Abdomen.—Fullness, even after a little food; stuffed feeling, as if she could not lean forward.

Throat.—Sore, as if of a splinter, shooting in different directions. Hoarse.

Respiratory.—Coryza; discharge of mucus from nose, trachea, and larynx. Pressure beneath sternum. Scrofulous swelling of nose. Chest feels oppressed. Hæmoptysis.

Urinary.—Urine dark. Sweet smelling. *Crawling sensation in urethra and rectum.* Sensation as if urine were stopped at fossa navicularis. Difficulty in retaining urine. Incontinence in anemic children.

Female.—On sitting, *feeling as if something pressed upward in vagina.* Much bearing down. Retroversion and prolapse of uterus. Leucorrhœa like boiled starch. Menses suppressed or scanty. Itching and soreness of vulva and vagina.

Dose.—Third trituration. Does not keep long.

FERRUM MAGNETICUM
(Loadstone)

Marked symptoms in intestinal tract. Pain in nape of neck. Paralytic weakness. Small warts on hands.

Stomach.—During a meal, flatulence; afterwards lassitude taciturn and hot, pain in epigastrium, especially on breathing.

Abdomen.—Movements and grumbling in abdomen. Loose evacuations with much flatulency, especially left side with pullings in legs. Abundant and frequent emission of fetid flatus.

Dose.—Third potency.

FERRUM METALLICUM
(Iron)

Best adapted to young weakly persons, anæmic and chlorotic, with pseudo-plethora, who flush easily; cold extremities; *oversensitiveness;* worse after any active effort. *Weakness* from mere speaking or walking though *looking* strong. *Pallor* of skin, mucous membranes, face, alternating with flushes. Orgasms of blood to face, chest, head, lungs, etc. Irregular distribution of blood. Pseudo-plethora. Muscles flabby and relaxed.

Mind.—Irritability. *Slight noises unbearable.* Excited from slightest opposition. Sanguine temperament.

Head.—Vertigo on seeing flowing water. Stinging headache. Ringing in ears before menses. *Hammering,* pulsating, congestive headache; pain extends to teeth, with cold extremities. Pain in *back of head,* with roaring in neck. Scalp painful. Must take down the hair.

Eyes.—Watery, dull red; photophobia; letters run together.

Face.—Fiery-red and *flushed from least pain, emotion, or exertion. Red parts become white,* bloodless and puffy.

Nose.—Mucous membrane relaxed, boggy, anæmic, pale.

Mouth.—*Pain in teeth; relieved by icy-cold water.* Earthy, pasty taste, like rotten eggs.

Stomach.—*Voracious* appetite, or absolute loss of appetite. Loathing of sour things. Attempts to eat bring on diarrhœa. *Spits up food by the mouthful.* [*Phos.*] Eructations of food after eating, without nausea. Nausea and vomiting after eating. *Vomiting immediately after eating. Vomiting after midnight. Intolerance of eggs.* Distention and pressure in the stomach after eating. Heat and burning in stomach. Soreness of abdominal walls. Flatulent dyspepsia.

Stool.—Undigested, at night, while eating or drinking, painless. Ineffectual urging; stool hard, followed by backache or cramping pain in rectum; prolapsus recti; itching of anus, especially young children.

Urine.—Involuntary; worse daytime. Tickling in urethra extending to bladder.

Female.—Menses remit a day or two, and then return. Discharge of long pieces from uterus. Women who are weak, delicate, chlorotic, yet have a fiery-red face. Menses too early, too profuse, last too long; pale, watery. Sensitive vagina. Tendency to abortion. Prolapse of vagina.

Respiratory.—Chest *oppressed;* breathing difficult. Surging of blood to chest. Hoarseness. Cough dry, spasmodic. Hæmoptysis. [*Millefol.*] With the cough pain in occiput.

Heart.—Palpitation; worse, movement. Sense of oppression.

Anæmic murmur. *Pulse full, but soft and yielding; also, small and weak.* Heart suddenly bleeds into the blood vessels, and as suddenly draws a reflux, leaving pallor of surface.

Extremities.—Rheumatism of the shoulder. Dropsy after loss of vital fluids. Lumbago; better, slow walking. Pain in hip-joint, tibia, soles, and heel.

Skin.—Pale; flushes readily; pits on pressure.

Fever.—General coldness of extremities; head and face hot. *Chill at 4 a. m.* Heat in palms and soles. Profuse, debilitating sweat.

Modalities.—*Better*, walking slowly about. Better after rising. *Worse*, while sweating; while sitting still. After cold washing and overheating. *Midnight aggravation.*

Relationship.—Antidotes: *Ars.; Hep.*

Complementary: *Chin.; Alum.; Hamamel.*

Compare: *Rumex* (similar in respiratory and digestive sphere and contains organic iron.)

Ferrum aceticum (alkaline urine in acute diseases. Pain in right deltoid. Epistaxis; especially adapted to thin, pale, weak children who grow rapidly and are easily exhausted; *varices of the feet;* copious expectoration of greenish pus; asthma; worse, sitting still and lying; phthisis, constant cough, vomiting of food after eating, hæmoptysis).

Ferrum arsenicum (enlarged liver and spleen, with fever; undigested stool; albuminuria). Simple and pernicious anæmia and chlorosis. Skin dry. Eczema, psoriasis, impetigo. Use 3x trituration.)

Ferrum bromatum (sticky, excoriating leucorrhœa; uterus heavy and prolapsed, scalp feels numb).

Ferrum cyanatum (neuroses with irritable weakness and hypersensitiveness, especially of a periodical character; *epilepsy;* cardialgia, with nausea, flatulence, constipation, alternating with diarrhœa; chorea).

Ferrum magneticum (small warts on hands).

Ferrum muriaticum. (Arrested menstruation; tendency to seminal emissions or copious urination at puberty; very dark, watery stools; diphtheria; phlegmonous erysipelas; pyelitis; hæmoptysis of dark, clotty blood; dyspareunia; pain in *right shoulder*, right elbow, and marked tendency to cramps and round red spots on cheeks; bright crystals in urine. Anæmia, 3x, after meals. Tincture 1-5 drops 3 times daily for chronic interstitial nephritis.)

Ferrum sulphuricum. (Watery and painless stools; menorrhagia, pressing, throbbing between periods with rush of blood to head. Basedow's disease. Erethism. (Pain in gall-bladder; toothache; acidity; eructation of food in mouthfuls); *Ferrum pernitricum* (cough, with florid complexion); *Ferrum tartaricum* (cardialgia; heat at cardiac orifice of stomach).

Ferrum protoxalatum (Anæmia). Use 1x trit. Compare also: *Graph.; Mangan.; Cupr.*

Dose.—States of debility where the blood is poor in hematin require material doses; plethoric, hæmorrhagic conditions call for small doses. from the second to the sixth potency.

FERRUM PHOSPHORICUM
(Phosphate of Iron)

In the early stages of febrile conditions, it stands midway between sthenic activity of Aconite and Bell, and the asthenic sluggishness and torpidith of *Gels.* The typical *Ferr. phos.* subject is not full blooded and robust, but nervous, sensitive, anæmic with the false plethora and easy flushing of Ferrum. Prostration marked; face more active than *Gels.* The superficial redness never assumes the dusky hue of *Gels.* Pulse soft and flowing; no anxious restlessness of *Acon.* Susceptibility to chest troubles. Bronchitis of young children. In acute exacerbation of tuberculosis, a fine palliative of wonderful power. Corresponds to Grauvogl's Oxygenoid Constitution, the inflammatory, febrile, emaciating, wasting consumptive.

The remedy for first stage of all febrile disturbances and inflammations before exudation sets in; especially for catarrhal affections of the respiratory tract. *Ferr. phos.* 3x increases hæmoglobin. In pale, anæmic subjects, with violent local congestions. Hæmorrhages, bright from any orifice.

Head.—Soreness to touch, cold, noise, jar. Rush of blood to head. Ill effects of sun-heat. Throbbing sensation. Vertigo. Headache *better cold applications.*

Eyes.—Red, inflamed, with burning sensation. Feeling as

of sand under lids. Hyperæmia of optic disc and retina, with blurred vision.

Ears.—Noises. Throbbing. First stage of otitis. Membrana tympani red and bulging. Acute otitis; when Bellad. fails, prevents suppuration.

Nose.—First stage of colds in the head. Predisposition to colds. *Epistaxis;* bright red blood.

Face.—Flushed; cheeks sore and hot. Florid complexion. Facial neuralgia; worse, shaking head and stooping.

Throat.—Mouth hot; fauces red, inflamed. Ulcerated sore throat. Tonsils red and swollen. Eustachian tubes inflamed. Sore throat of singers. Subacute laryngitis with fauces inflamed and red (2x). After operations on throat and nose to control bleeding and relieve soreness. First stage of diphtheria. Ranula in vascular, sanguine constitutions.

Stomach.—Aversion to meat and milk. Desire for stimulants. *Vomiting of undigested food.* Vomiting of bright red blood. *Sour eructations.*

Abdomen.—First stage of peritonitis. Hæmorrhoids. Stools watery, bloody, undigested. First stage of dysentery, with much blood in discharges.

Urinary.—Urine spurts with every cough. Incontinence. Irritation at neck of bladder. Polyuria. *Diurnal enuresis.*

Female.—Menses every three weeks, with bearing-down sensation and pain on top of head. Vaginismus. Vagina dry and hot.

Respiratory.—*First stage of all inflammatory affections.* Congestions of lungs. Hæmoptysis. Short, painful tickling cough Croup. Hard, dry cough, with sore chest. Hoarseness. *Expectoration of pure blood in pneumonia.* [*Millefol.*] Cough better at night.

Heart.—Palpitation; pulse rapid. First stage of cardiac diseases. *Short, quick, soft pulse.*

Extremities.—Stiff neck. Articular rheumatism. Crick in back. Rheumatic pain in shoulder; pains extend to chest and wrist. Whitlow. Palms hot. Hands swollen and painful.

Sleep.—Restless and sleepless. Anxious dreams. Night sweats of anæmia.

Fever.—Chill daily at 1 p. m. All catarrhal and inflammatory fevers; first stage.

Modalities.—*Worse*, at night and 4 to 6 a. m.; touch, jar, motion, right side. *Better*, cold applications.

Relationship.—Compare: (Oxygenoid Constitution. *Acon.; China; Arsenic; Graphit.; Petrol.*) Ferrum pyrophosph. (congestion of brain and headache following great loss of blood; tarsal cysts); *Acon.; Gelsen.; China.*

Dose.—Third to twelfth potency.

FERRUM PICRICUM
(Picrate of Iron)

Is considered a great remedy to complete the action of other medicines. The symptom that specially calls for it is failure of the function of an organ under exertion: e. g., the voice fails after public speaking. Acts best in dark-haired patients, plethoric, with sensitive livers. Warts and epithelial growths; corns with yellowish discoloration. *Senile hypertrophy of the prostate. Epistaxis.* Chronic deafness and tinnitus due to gout. Meatus dry. Pseudo-leucæmia.

Ears.—Deafness before menses. Crackling in ears and low-pitched voice. Vascular deafness. Dental neuralgia, radiating towards ears and eyes. Humming in ears as from telegraph wires. Tinnitus.

Stomach.—Indigestion, furred tongue, headache after meals, especially in bilious, dark-haired persons.

Urinary.—Pain along entire urethra. *Frequent micturition at night, with full feeling and pressure in rectum.* Smarting at neck of bladder and penis. [*Barosma.*] Retention of urine.

Extremities.—Pain in right side of neck and down right arm. Locomotor ataxia, ocular stage. Hands covered with warts.

Dose.—Second and third trituration.

FICUS RELIGIOSA
(Ashwathya)

This East Indian drug causes and cures hæmorrhages of many kinds. Hæmatemesis, menorrhagia, hæmoptysis, etc. Bloody urine.

Head.—Melancholic—quiet: burning at vertex; vertigo and slight headache.

Stomach.—Nausea, vomiting of bright red blood; pain and sick feeling in stomach.

Respiratory.—Difficult breathing; cough with vomiting of blood; pulse very weak.

Relationship.—Compare: *Acalypha; Millefol.; Thlaspi; Ipecac.*

Dose.—First potency.

FILIX MAS—ASPIDIUM
(Male Fern)

A remedy for worm symptoms, especially with constipation. Tapeworm. Soporific conditions. *Torpid inflammations of lymphatic glands.* (Maceration of fresh root.) Pulmonary tuberculosis in young patients, no fever, with limited, ulcerated lesions, formerly classified as scrofula.

Eyes.—Blindness, monocular amblyopia.

Abdomen.—Bloated. Gnawing-pain; worse eating sweets. Diarrhœa and vomiting. Worm colic, with itching of nose, pale face, blue rings around eyes. Painless hiccough.

Relationship.—Compare: *Aspidium Alhamanticum.*—Panna —3 doses, 2 grammes each, all in half hour, fasting in a glass of milk. Tasteless and will remove tape worm. *Cina; Granat.; Kousso.*

Dose.—First to third potency. For the expulsion of tapeworm, a full dose of ½ to 1 dram of the Oleoresin, fasting.

FLUORICUM ACIDUM
(Hydrofluoric Acid)

Especially adapted to chronic diseases with syphilitic and mercurical history. *Glabella region bloated.* Acts especially upon lower tissues, and indicated in deep, destructive processes, bedsores, ulcerations, varicose veins, and ulcers. Patient is compelled to move about energetically. Complaints of old age, or the prematurely aged, with weak, distended blood vessels. Hob-nailed liver of alcoholics. *Goitre* (Dr. Woakes) (Kali fluoride produced bronchocele in dogs). Early decay of teeth. Old cases of nightly fevers, coming on periodically.

Mind.—Indifference towards those loved best; inability to realize responsibility; buoyancy. Mentally elated and gay.

Head.—Alopecia. Caries of skin. Pressure on sides of head from within outward. Caries of ossicles and mastoid, with copious discharge; worse warmth. [*Silica;* worse cold.] Exostosis.

Eyes.—*Sensation as of wind blowing through eyes.* Lachrymal fistula. Violent itching of inner canthus.

Nose.—Chronic nasal catarrh with ulceration of the septum; nose obstructed and dull heavy pain in forehead.

Mouth.—Dental fistula, with persistent bloody, salty discharge. Syphilitic ulceration of throat, which is very sensitive to cold. Teeth feel warm. Affects teeth and bones of upper jaw.

Stomach.—Heaviness and weight in stomach. Heat in stomach before meals. Sour eructations. Averse to coffee, wants fancy dishes. Stomach symptoms relieved by tight clothes. Desire for highly seasoned food. Craves cold water, hungry. Warm drinks produce diarrhœa.

Abdomen.—Soreness over liver. Flatus and eructations.

Stool.—Bilious diarrhœa, with aversion to coffee.

Male.—Burning in urethra. Sexual passion and desire increased, with erections at night, during sleep. *Swollen scrotum.*

Urine.—Scanty, dark. In dropsy, produces frequent and free discharge, with great relief.

Female.—Menses copious, frequent, too long. Ulceration of uterus and os. Copious and excoriating leucorrhœa. Nymphomania.

Respiratory.—Oppression of chest, difficult breathing, great dyspnœa. Hydrothorax.

Extremities.—Inflammation of joints of fingers. Feeling as of a splinter under nail. Nails crumble. Caries and necrosis, especially of long bones. Coccygodynia. Ulcer over tibia.

Skin.—*Varicose veins.* Nævi. Ulcers; red edges and vesicles. Decubitus; worse, warmth. Syphilitic rupia. Itching of cicatrices. Feels as if burning vapor were emitted from pores. *Itching especially of the orifices*, and in spots, worse warmth. Nails grow rapidly. Periosteal abscess. Profuse, sour, offensive perspiration. Syphilitic tubercles. *Dropsy of limbs* in old, feeble constitutions. Atony of capillary and venous system. **Tissues bloated.**

Modalities.—*Worse,* warmth, morning, warm drinks. *Better,* cold, while walking.

Relationship.—Compare: *Thiosinaminum* (action on cicatricial tissues; adhesions, strictures, tumors); *Calc. fluor.; Silica.*
Complementary: *Silica.*

Dose.—Sixth to thirtieth potency.

FORMALIN
(Aqueous Solution (35 per cent) of Formaldehyde Gas)

Is a powerful disinfectant and deodorant; a potent poison. Prevents growth and kills almost any pathogenic micro-organism. It seems to have the peculiar property of eating into malignant tumors, leaving the surrounding healthy tissue uncharred and unchanged. A plug of cotton wool soaked in a 20 per cent. solution of Formaldehyde, and applied for a few hours, will produce a necrotic slough, which must be scraped away before the next application, otherwise it hardens.

Formalin in hot water as vapor most valuable therapeutic agent in pertussis, phthisis, in catarrhal affections of upper air-passages.

Mind.—*Forgetfulness.* Anxiety. Unconscious.

Head.—Coryza; eyes water; *vertigo.*

Mouth.—Ptyalism, thick saliva; loss of taste.

Stomach.—Food feels as if it were a ball in stomach. Burning in mouth and stomach.

Abdomen.—Intense urging to stool, watery stools.

Urinary.—Anuria; albuminous urine.

Respiratory.—*Dyspnœa. Laryngismus stridulus. Whooping-cough.*

Fever.—Chills in forenoon, followed by long fever. Bones ache during whole paroxysm. During fever forgets where he was.

Skin.—Puckers skin like leather; wrinkles; scales off. Eczema in neighborhood of wound. Damp sweat most marked on right upper extremity.

Relationship.—Antidote: *Ammonia water.* Compare: *Ammonium formaldehyde,* known commercially as *Cystogen.* (Dose, five to seven grains two to four times daily, dissolved in hot water, after meals. Prevents the decomposition of urine in the bladder, kidneys, and ureters. Turbid urine rendered clear and non-irritating; phosphatic deposits dissolved, and growth of pyogenic bacteria arrested). Also, *Urotropin*. (A diuretic and solvent of uric acid concretions; relieves cystitis associated with putrefaction. Three to five grains well diluted. When administered invariably appears in the cerebro-spinal fluid and therefore advised in threatened meningeal infection.)

Dose.—As vapor in hot water in respiratory affections; 1 per cent. spray, otherwise 3x potency.

FORMICA RUFA (MYRMEXINE)
(Crushed Live Ants)

An *arthritic* medicine. Gout and articular rheumatism; pains worse, motion; better, pressure. Right side most affected. Chronic gout and stiffness in joints. Acute outbursts of gouty poisons, especially when assuming the neuralgic forms. Tuberculosis, carcinoma, and lupus; chronic nephritis. Complaints from overlifting. Apoplectic diseases. *Has a marked deterrent influence on the formation of polypi.*

Head.—Vertigo. Headache with cracking in left ear. Brain feels too heavy and large. Sensation as if a bubble burst in forehead. Forgetful in the evening. *Exhilarated.* Coryza and *stopped-up* feeling in nose. Rheumatic iritis. *Nasal polypi.*

Ears.—Ringing and buzzing. Cracking in left ear with headache. Parts around ear feel swollen. Polypi.

Stomach.—Constant pressure at the cardiac end of the stomach, and a burning pain there. Nausea, with headache, and vomiting of yellowish bitter mucus. Pain shift from stomach to vertex. Gas cannot be passed.

Abdomen and Stool.—In the morning, difficult passages of small quantities of flatus; afterwards diarrhœa-like urging in the rectum. Pain in bowels before stool, with shuddering chilliness. Constriction in the anus. Drawing pain *around navel* before stool.

Urine.—Bloody, albuminous, with much urging; quantities of urates.

Respiratory.—Hoarseness, with dry, sore throat; cough worse at night, with aching in forehead and constrictive pain in chest; pleuritic pains.

Sexual.—Seminal emissions; weakness. "Slothful to venery."

Extremities.—Rheumatic pains; stiff and contracted joints. Muscles feel strained and torn from their attachment. *Weakness of lower extremities.* Paraplegia. Pain in hips. *Rheumatism comes on with suddenness and restlessness. Sweat does not relieve.* Relief after midnight and from rubbing.

Skin.—*Red, itching and burning.* Nettle-rash. Nodes around joints. [*Ammon. phos.*] Profuse sweat without relief.

Modalities.—*Worse,* cold and cold washing, dampness, before a snowstorm. *Better,* warmth, *pressure,* rubbing. Combing hair.

Relationship.—Compare: *Formic acid.* (Chronic myalgia. Muscular pains and soreness. Gout and articular rheumatism, which appear suddenly. Pains usually worse on right side, motion and better from pressure. *Failing vision.* Increases muscular strength and resistance to fatigue. Feels stronger and more "fit" in ordinary walking. Marked diuretic effect, greater elimination of products of disassimilation, particularly urea. *Tremor.* Tuberculosis, chronic nephritis and carcinoma, lupus, etc., have been treated successfully with injections of Formic acid of a dilution corresponding to the 3d and 4th centesimal. In prescribing it for varicose veins, polypi, catarrh, Dr. J. H. Clarke orders an ounce or two of a solution of Formic acid in the proportion of one part of the acid to eleven of distilled water. Of this one teaspoonful is taken in a tablespoonful of water after food once or twice daily. Pain in aponeurosis and muscles of head, neck and shoulders before a snowstorm.) *Rhus; (Dulcam, Urtica* and *Juniperus* contain *Formic acid), Wood alcohol,* when taken as a constituent of a beverage so common in these prohibition days, is not eliminated easily and is slowly converted into *Formic acid,* attacking the brain and causes death or blindness.

Dr. Sylwestrowicz of the Hering Research Laboratory of Hahnemann College, Philadelphia contributes his experience with *Formic Acid,* as follows:

"The best field for the formic acid treatment are cases of

atypical gout. Under this classification are to be mentioned disturbances in the muscles such as myositis, periostitic processes of the bones in form of doughy swellings, changes of the fascias such as Dupyutren's contraction, skin troubles such as chronic eczema, psoriasis and loss of hair, kidney disturbances such as subacute and chronic nephritis. In these cases *formic acid* in 12x and 30x, hypodermically 1 cc. is indicated at intervals of 2-4 weeks. Eight till twelve days after the first injection an aggravation is often noticed.

In acute rheumatic fever and acute gonorrhœic arthritis *formic acid* 6x, every six days 1 cc., sometimes 12x in sensitive patients shows often splendid results abolishing the pains and preventing reoccurrence.

Chronic arthritis needs a special discussion. Clinical experiments of the Hering research Laboratory of the Hahnemann Medical College of Philadelphia on a great number of cases of arthritis with *formic acid* showed that it preferrably acts on the ligaments, capsula and bursa of the joints. Such kind of cases respond very readily to treatment.

The prognosis depends to a large extent upon the etiology of the case. The most satisfactory cases are chronic arthritis in connection with gouty diathesis. Chronic arthritis following an attack of acute rheumatic fever shows also remarkable results although often pains of a neuralgic character persisting in certain spots are very stubborn. Finally chronic arthritis of traumatic nature can be cured by formic acid. In the latter case *formic acid* 6x showed quicker and better results than 12x or 30x which are indicated in the previous cases. In general the disappearance of the stiffness of the joint is the first sign of improvement. Then the pain and swelling cease gradually in 1-6 months time.

The prognosis of the formic acid treatment is not so favorably in chronic arthritis in which deformans processes have already taken place on the articular surfaces. Such processes in the beginning can be checked completely, advanced cases frequently show an improvement. But there is always the possibility that this improvement is only temporary. This is particularly to be expected in the cases of the so-called arthritis deformans in which even the inflammations on the ligaments and capsula are of a very progressive character."

Dose.—Sixth to thirtieth attenuation.

FRAGARIA
(Wood-strawberry)

Acts on digestion and mesenteric glands. Prevents formation of calculi, removes tartar from teeth and prevents attacks of gout. The fruit has refrigerant properties. Strawberries produce symptoms of poisoning in certain susceptible individuals, such as urticarial rashes (strawberry anaphylaxis). Here give Fragaria high potency.

Chilblains; worse during hot weather. Lack of mammary secretion. *Psilosis.* (Spruce.)

Mouth.—Tongue *swollen; strawberry* tongue.

Skin.—*Urticaria;* petechial and erysipelatous eruptions. Swelling of whole body.

Relationship.—Compare: *Apis. Calcarea.*

FRANCISCEA
(Manaca)

Chronic stiffnes of the muscles. Gonorrhœal rheumatism. Syphilis and rheumatism, great heat over body, much aching, better sweat. Pain in back of head and spine; band-like feeling around head. Pericarditis with rheumatism. Rheumatic pains in feet and lower part of legs. Urine contains uric acid.

Dose.—Tincture or Fluid Extract 10 to 60 minims.

FRAXINUS AMERICANA
(White Ash)

Enlargement of the uterus. Fibrous growths, subinvolution, and prolapse. Uterine tumors, with bearing-down sensations. Fever sores on lips. Cramps in feet. Cold creeping and hot flashes. Infantile eczema.

Head.—Throbbing pain in back of head. Depression, with nervous restlessness, anxiety. *Hot spot on top of head.*

Female.—*Uterus enlarged,* and patulous. Watery, unirritating leucorrhœa. Fibroids with bearing-down sensation, cramping in feet. worse in afternoon and night. Dysmenorrhœa.

Abdomen.—Tenderness in left inguinal region; bearing-down pain, extending down thigh.

Relationship.—Compare: *Fraxinus excelsior*—European Ash —(*Gout;* rheumatism. Infusion of ash-leaves. Rademacher). *Galega*—Goat's Rue—Backache; debility; anæmia and impaired nutrition. Increases the quantity and quality of the milk in nursing women, also the appetite). *Epiphegus; Sepia; Lilium.*

Dose.—Ten to fifteen drops of tincture, three times a day.

FULIGO LIGNI
(Soot)

Acts on glandular system, mucous membranes and obstinate ulcers, epidermis, tetters, eczema. Chronic irritations of mucous membranes of mouth; pruritus-vulvæ; uterine hæmorrhage; cancer, especially of scrotum—chimney sweeper's cancer; epithelial cancers; cancer of womb with metorrhagia; sadness, thoughts of suicide.

Relationship.—Compare: *Kreosot.*

Dose.—Sixth trituration.

FUCUS VESICULOSUS
(Sea Kelp)

A remedy for obesity and *non-toxic goitre;* also exophthalmic. Digestion is furthered and flatulence diminished. Obstinate constipation; forehead feels as if compressed by an iron ring. Thyroid enlargement in obese subjects.

Relationship.—Compare: *Phytol.; Thyroidine; Badiaga; Iodum.*

Dose.—Tincture, five to sixty drops three times a day before meals.

FUCHSINA—MAGENTA
(A Coloring Substance Used in Adulteration of Wine)

Produces redness of ears, deep red discoloration of mouth, swollen gums, with burning and tendency to salivation; deep red urine, albuminous, and light red, profuse diarrhœa with abdominal pains. Cortical substance of kidneys degenerated. Useful in cortical nephritis with albuminuria.

Dose.—6x to 30th potency.

GALANTHUS NIVALIS
(Snow-drop)

Proving by Dr. A. Whiting Vancouver.

Faintness, sinking sensations. Sore dry throat with dull headache. Half conscious and worried feeling during sleep. Heart weak with sensation of collapse as if she must fall. Pulse very irregular, rapid and uneven, violent palpitation. Systolic murmur at apex. Therapeutically—decided benefit in cases of Mitral Regurgitation with broken down compensation. *Myocarditis* with some degree of mitral insufficiency.

Dose.—First potency to fifth.

GALIUM APARINE
(Goose-Grass)

Galium acts on the urinary organs, is a diuretic and of use in dropsies, gravel and calculi. Dysuria and cystitis. Has power of suspending or modifying cancerous action. Has clinical confirmation of its use in cancerous ulcers and nodulated tumors of the tongue. Inveterate skin affections and scurvy. Favors healthy granulations on ulcerated surfaces.

Dose.—Fluid extract; half-dram doses, in cup of water or milk, three times a day.

GALLICUM ACIDUM
(Gallic Acid)

Should be remembered as a remedy in *phthisis*. It checks the morbid secretions, gives tone to the stomach, and increases the appetite. Passive hæmorrhages when pulse is feeble and capillaries relaxed, cold skin. Hæmaturia. Hæmophilia. Itching of skin. *Pyrosis.*

Mind.—Wild delirium at night; very restless, jumps out of bed; sweats; is afraid to be alone; is rude and abuses every one.

Head.—Pain in back of head and neck. Thick, stringy discharge from nose; photophobia with burning of lids.

Respiratory.—Pain in lungs; *pulmonary hæmorrhage;* excessive expectoration. Much mucus in throat in the morning. Dry at night.

Urinary.—Kidneys painful, distress along ureters into bladder. Dull heavy pain in bladder, directly over pubis. Urine loaded with thick, cream-colored mucus.

Rectum.—Copious stool; anus feels constricted. Faint feeling after stool. Chronic mucous discharges.

Relationship.—Compare: *Ars.; Iod.; Phos.*

Dose.—First trituration and pure acid 2 to 5 grain doses.

GAMBOGIA—GARCINIA MORELLA
(Gummi Gutti)

The use of this drug in Homœopathy has been confined to its action on the alimentary tract. It produces a diarrhœa very similar to Croton. From its pathogenesis, it is very evident that it has very intense and definite action especially on the gastro-enteric tract.

Head.—Heavy, with inertia, and drowsiness. Itching and burning in eyes; lids stick together, with *sneezing*.

Gastro-enteric Symptoms.—Feeling of coldness at edge of teeth. Great irritability of the stomach; burning, smarting, and dryness of the tongue and throat. Pain in the stomach after food. Tenderness in epigastrium. Pain and distention of abdomen from flatulence, after stool. *Rumbling and rolling.* Dysentery, with retained scybala, with pain in sacral region. Diarrhœa, with *sudden and forcible ejection of* bilious stools. *Tenesmus after, with burning at anus.* Ileo-cæcal region sensitive to pressure. Profuse, watery diarrhœa in hot weather, particularly old people. Pain in coccyx.

Modalities.—Worse, towards evening and at night.

Relationship.—Compare: *Croton; Aloes; Pod.*

Dose.—Third to thirtieth potency. Gamboge painted on the chest in lung tuberculosis is considered by Abrams specific and incipient cases are symptomatically cured in several weeks.

GAULTHERIA
(Wintergreen)

Inflammatory rheumatism, pleurodynia, *sciatica*, and other neuralgias, come within, the spere of this remedy. Cystic and prostatic irritation, undue sexual excitement, and renal inflammation.

Head.—Neuralgia of head and face.

Stomach.—Acute gastritis, severe pain in epigastrium; *prolonged vomiting*. Uncontrollable appetite, notwithstanding irritable stomach. Gastralgia from nervous depression. (Give five drops of 1x of Oil.)

Skin.—Smarting and burning. Intense erythema, worse, cold bathing; better, olive oil and cool air blowing on part.

Relationship.—Compare: *Spiræa*. Gaultheria contains Arbutin. *Salycyl. acid. Methylium salicylicum* (an artificial Gaultheria oil for rheumatism, especially when the salicylates cannot be used. Pruritus and epididymitis, locally). After *Cantharis* in burns.

Dose.—Tincture and lower potencies.

GELSEMIUM
(Yellow Jasmine)

Centers its action upon the nervous system, causing various degrees of *motor paralysis*. General prostration. *Dizziness, drowsiness, dullness, and trembling*. Slow pulse, tired feeling mental apathy. *Paralysis* of various groups of muscles about the eyes, throat, chest, larynx, sphincter, extremities, etc. Post-diphtheritic paralysis. *Muscular weakness*. Complete relaxation and prostration. Lack of muscular co-ordination. General depression from heat of sun. Sensitive to a falling barometer; cold and dampness brings on many complaints. Children fear falling, grab nurse or crib. Sluggish circulation. Nervous affections of cigarmakers. *Influenza*. Measles. Pellagra.

Mind.—Desire to be quiet, to be left alone. *Dullness, languor, listless*. "Discernings are lethargied." *Apathy regarding his illness*. Absolute lack of fear. Delirious on falling to sleep. Emotional excitement, fear, etc., lead to bodily ailments. Bad effects from fright, fear, exciting news. Stage fright. Child starts and grasps the nurse, and screams as if afraid of falling. [*Bor.*]

Head.—*Vertigo*, spreading from occiput. Heaviness of head; *band-feeling* around and *occipital* headache. *Dull, heavy ache*, with heaviness of eyelids; bruised sensation; better, compression and lying with head high. *Pain in temple, extending into* *ear* and wing of nose, chin. Headache, with muscular soreness of neck and shoulders. Headache preceded by blindness; better, profuse urination. Scalp sore to touch . Delirious on falling asleep. Wants to have head raised on pillow.

Eyes.—Ptosis; *eyelids* heavy; patient can hardly open them. Double vision. Disturbed muscular apparatus. Corrects blurring and discomfort in eyes even after accurately adjusted glasses. Vision blurred, smoky. [*Cycl.; Phos.*] *Dim-sighted;* pupils dilated and insensible to light. *Orbital neuralgia, with contraction and twitching of muscles.* Bruised pain back of the orbits. One pupil dilated, the other contracted. Deep inflammations, with haziness of vitreous. *Serous inflammations.* Albuminuric retinitis. Detached retina, glaucoma and descemetitis. *Hysterical amblyopia.*

Nose.—Sneezing; fullness at root of nose. Dryness of nasal fossæ. Swelling of turbinates. Watery, excoriating discharge. Acute coryza, with dull headache and fever.

Face.—*Hot heavy, flushed, besotted-looking.* [*Bapt.; Op.*] Neuralgia of face. Dusky hue of face, with vertigo and dim vision. Facial muscles contracted, especially around the mouth. Chin quivers. Lower jaw dropped.

Mouth.—Putrid taste and breath. Tongue numb, thick, coated, yellowish, *tremble,* paralyzed.

Throat.—Difficult swallowing, especially of warm food. Itching and tickling in soft palate and naso-pharynx. Pain in sterno-cleido-mastoid, back of parotid. Tonsils swollen. Throat feels rough, burning. *Post-diphtheritic paralysis.* Tonsillitis; shooting pain into ears. *Feeling of a lump in throat that cannot be swallowed.* Aphonia. Swallowing causes pain in ear. [*Hep.; Nux.*] Difficult swallowing. *Pain from throat to ear.*

Stomach.—As a rule, the Gelsemium patient has no thirst. Hiccough; worse in the evening. Sensation of emptiness and weakness at the pit of the stomach, or of an oppression, like a heavy load.

Stool.—Diarrhœa *from emotional excitement,* fright, bad news. [*Phos. ac.*] Stool painless or involuntary. *Cream-colored* [*Calc.*], *tea-green.* Partial paralysis of rectum and sphincter.

Urine.—*Profuse, clear, watery,* with chilliness and tremulousness. Dysuria. Partial paralysis of bladder; flow intermittent. [*Clematis*.] Retention.

Female.—Rigid os. [*Bell*.] Vaginismus. False labor-pains; pains pass up back. *Dysmenorrhœa*, with scanty flow; menses retarded. Pain extends to back and hips. Aphonia and sore throat during menses. Sensation as if uterus were squeezed. [*Cham.; Nux v.; Ustilago*.]

Male.—Spermatorrhœa, *without erections*. Genitals cold and relaxed. [*Phos. ac*.] Scrotum continually sweating. Gonorrhœa, first stage; discharge scanty; tendency to corrode; little pain, but much heat; smarting at meatus.

Respiratory.—Slowness of breathing, with great prostration. Oppression about chest. Dry cough, with sore chest and fluent coryza. *Spasm of the glottis*. Aphonia; acute bronchitis, respiration quickened, spasmodic affections of lungs and diaphragm.

Heart.—*A feeling as if it were necessary to keep in motion, or else heart's action would cease*. Slow pulse. [*Dig.; Kalm.; Apoc. can*.] Palpitation; pulse soft, weak, full and flowing. Pulse slow when quiet, but greatly accelerated on motion. *Weak, slow pulse of old age*.

Back.—Dull, heavy pain. Complete relaxation of the whole muscular system. Languor; muscles feel bruised. Every little exertion causes fatigue. Pain in neck, especially upper sternocleido muscles. Dull aching in lumbar and sacral region, passing upward. Pain in muscles of back, hips, and lower extremities, mostly deep-seated.

Extremities.—Loss of power of muscular control. Cramp in muscles of forearm. Professional neuroses. Writer's cramp. Excessive *trembling* and weakness of all limbs. Hysteric convulsions. Fatigue after slight exercise.

Sleep.—Cannot get fully to sleep. Delirious on falling asleep. Insomnia from exhaustion; from uncontrollable thinking; tobacco. Yawning. Sleepless from nervous irritation. [*Coffea*.]

Fever.—*Wants to be held, because he shakes so*. Pulse slow, full, soft, compressible. Chilliness up and down back. Heat and sweat stages, long and exhausting. Dumb-ague, with much muscular soreness, great prostration, and violent headache. *Nervous chills*. Bilious remittent fever, with stupor, dizziness, faintness; thirstless, prostrated. Chill, without thirst, along spine; wave-like, extending upward from sacrum to occiput.

Skin.—Hot, dry, itching, measle-like eruption. Erysipelas. *Measles, catarrhal symptoms; aids in bringing out eruption.* Retrocedent, with livid spots. Scarlet fever with stupor and flushed face.

Modalities.—*Worse*, damp weather, fog, before a thunderstorm, emotion, or excitement, *bad news*, tobacco-smoking, when thinking of his ailments; at 10 a. m. *Better*, bending forward, by profuse urination, open air, continued motion, stimulants.

Relationship.—Compare: *Ignatia* (gastric affections of cigarmakers); *Baptisa; Ipecac.; Acon.; Bell.; Cimicif.; Magnes. phos.* (Gelsem. contains some Magnes. phos.) *Culex*— (vertigo on blowing the nose with fulness of the ears.)

Antidotes: China; Coffea; Dig. Alcoholic stimulants relieve all complaints where *Gelsem.* is useful.

Dose.—Tincture, to thirtieth attenuation; first to third most often used.

GENTIANA LUTEA
(Yellow Gentian)

Stomach symptoms marked. Acts as a tonic, increasing appetite.

Head.—Vertigo, worse, rising or motion; better open air Frontal headache, better eating and open air. Brain feels loose, head tender. Aching in eyes.

Throat.—Dry. Thick saliva.

Stomach.—Acid risings, ravenous hunger, nausea, weight and aching in stomach. Inflation and tension of stomach and abdomen. [*Pothos.*] Colic, umbilical region sensitive to touch. Flatulence.

Relationship.—Compare: *Gentiana quinque flora* (intermittent fever; dyspepsia, cholera infantum, weakness); *Gentiana cruciata* (throat symptoms in addition to similar stomach symptoms; dysphagia; vertigo with headache; pressing inward sensation in eyes; constricted throat and head and abdomen. Distention, fulness and tightness in abdomen. Creeping over body as from fleas. *Hydrast.; Nux.*

Dose.—First to third attenuation.

GERANIUM MACULATUM

(Crane's-bill)

Habitual sick headaches. *Profuse, hæmorrhages*, pulmonary and from different organs. Vomiting of blood. *Ulceration of stomach. Atonic and foul ulcers.* Summer complaint.

Head.—Giddiness, with diplopia; better, closing eyes. Ptosis and dilated pupils. Sick headache.

Mouth.—Dry; tip of tongue burning. Pharyngitis.

Stomach.—Catarrhal gastritis with profuse secretion, tendency to ulceration and passive hæmorrhage. *Lessens the vomiting in gastric ulcer.*

Stool.—Constant desire to go to stool, with inability to pass anything for some time. Chronic diarrhœa, with offensive mucus. Constipation.

Female.—Menses too profuse. Post-partum hæmorrhage. Sore nipples. [*Eup. arom.*]

Relationship.—Compare: *Geranin.* 1x. Constant hawking and spitting in elderly people. *Erodium*—Hemlock—Stork's bill—(a popular hæmostatic in Russia, and especially used for metrorrhagia and menorrhagia); *Hydrastinin; Cinch.; Sabin.*

Dose.—Tincture, half-dram doses in gastric ulcer. Tincture, to third attenuation, as a general rule. Locally, in ulcers, it will destroy the pyogenic membrane.

GETTYSBURG WATER

Stringy mucus from throat and posterior nares. *Rawness.* Neck muscles rigid. Joints weak. Cannot lift things. *Ligaments rigid.* Subacute gouty state. Evaporated and residium triturated to 6x. Of use in sub-acute and chronic rheumatism. White coated tongue. High colored urine with red sandy sediment. Sensation of rigidity *worse moving*. Especially in lumbar region and joints of hips, shoulders and wrists. *Not perceived when quiet.* More in morning. Cannot remain long in one position. Stiffness of muscles on moving. Pain in ligaments relieved by rest.

Relationship.—*Lycopodium*, Phosphor. Rhus Pulsat., but modalities differ.

Modalities.—*Worse*, stiffness of muscles on moving. *Better*, rest (ligaments and stiffness of muscles).

Dose.—Lower triturations. Also thirtieth potency.

GINSENG
(Aralia Quinquefolia—Wild Ginseng—Panax)

Said to be a stimulant to the secretory glands, especially salivary. Acts on the lower part of the spinal cord. *Lumbago, sciatica, and rheumatism.* Paralytic weakness. *Hiccough.* Skin symptoms, itching pimples on neck and chest.

Head.—Vertigo, with gray spots before eyes; semi-lateral headache; occipital; difficult opening of eyelids; objects appear double.

Throat.—Tonsillitis, just like Bellad, but in dark-complexioned people.

Abdomen.—Tense, painful, rumbling. Pain in right side. Loud gurgling in ileo-cæcal region. Perityphlitis.

Male.—Rheumatic pains after frequent emissions. Weakness of genital organs. Voluptuous tickling at end of urethra. Sexual excitement. Pressure in testicles.

Extremities.—Hands feel swollen. Skin feels tight. Contraction. Coldness in back and spine. Bruised pain in small of back and thighs; nightly digging in right lower limb to toes. Burning heat in tips of fingers. Eruption on upper inner thighs. *Stiff, contracted joints,* heaviness of lower limbs. Crackling in joints. Stiffness in back.

Relationship.—Compare: *Aral.; Coca. Hedera*—Ivy—mental depression and skin irritation antidoted by Gunpowder.

Dose.—Tincture, to third potency.

GLONOINE = GL. = Glycerine
O = Oxygen
N = Nitrogen
(Nitro-glycerine) (Spirits Glycerinus Nitrate)

Recent German provings of Glonoine confirm the original American provings and clinical indications and bring out very marked nerve disturbances. Great lassitude, no inclination to work; extreme irritability, easily excited by the slightest opposition, ending in congestive head symptoms. The sixth potency alone produced itching all over body with later acne and furuncle formation, also bulimy.

Great remedy for congestive headaches, hyperæmia of the brain from excess of heat or cold. Excellent for the intercranial, climacteric disturbances, or due to menstrual suppression. Children get sick when sitting before an open fire. *Surging of blood to head and heart.* Tendency to sudden and violent irregularities of the circulation. Violent convulsions, associated with cerebral congestion. *Sensation of pulsation throughout body. Pulsating pains.* Cannot recognize localities. Sciatica in otheromatous subjects, with cold shriveled limb; seasickness.

Head.—*Confusion*, with dizziness. Effects of sunstroke; heat on head, as in type-setters and workers under gas and electric light. *Head heavy, but cannot lay it on pillow. Cannot bear any heat about head.* Better from uncovering head. *Throbbing* headache. Angio-spastic neuralgia of head and face. Very irritable. Vertigo on assuming upright position. Cerebral congestion. Head feels enormously large, as if skull were too small for brain. Sun headaches; increases and decreases with the sun. Shocks in head, synchronous with pulse. Headache in place of menses. Rush of blood to head in pregnant women. Threatened apoplexy. Meningitis.

Eyes.—See everything half light, half dark. Letters appear smaller. Sparks before eyes.

Mouth.—Pulsating toothache.

Ears.—Throbbing; each beat of heart is heard in ears; full feeling.

Face.—Flushed, hot, livid, pale; sweaty; pains in root of nose; faceache. Dusky face.

Throat.—Neck feels full. Collars must be opened. Chokes and swells up under ears.

Stomach.—Gastrlagia in anæmic patients with feeble circulation. Nausea and vomiting. Faint, gnawing, and empty feeling at pit of stomach. Abnormal hunger.

Abdomen.—Constipation, with itching, painful hæmorrhoids, with pinching in abdomen before and after stool. Diarrhœa; copious blackish, lumpy stools.

Female.—Menses delayed, or sudden cessation with congestion to head. Climacteric flushing.

Heart.—Laborious action. Fluttering. Palpitation with dyspnœa. Cannot go uphill. Any exertion brings on rush of blood to heart and fainting spells. Throbbing in the whole body to finger-tips.

Extremities.—Itching all over, worse extremities. Pain in left biceps. Drawing pain in all limbs. Backache.

Modalities.—*Better*, brandy. *Worse*, in sun; exposure to sun-rays, gas, open fire; jar, stooping, having hair cut; peaches, stimulants; lying down; from 6 a. m. to noon; left side.

Relationship.—Antidote: *Acon.*

Compare: *Amyl. nit.; Bellad.; Opium; Stram.; Verat. vir.*

Dose.—Sixth to thirtieth potency

For palliative (non-homœopathic) purposes, in angina pectoris, asthma, heart-failure. etc., physiological doses—i. e., 1-100 of drop—must be given. Here it is the great emergency remedy. The conditions calling for it are small, wiry pulse, pallor, arterial spasm, anæmia of brain, *collapse*, feeble heart, syncope, dicrotic pulse, vertigo,—the opposite of those indicating a homœopathic dosage. Often thus used to lower the arterial tension in chronic interstitial nephritis.

GLYCERINUM
(Glycerine)

Used homœopathically, dynamized Glycerine seems to act deeply and long, building up tissue, hence of great use in marasmus, debility, mental and physical, diabetes, etc. It disturbs nutrition in its primary action, and, secondarily, seems to improve the general state of nutrition. (Dr. Wm. B. Griggs.)

Head.—Feels full, throbs; mentally confused. Severe headache two days before menstruation. Occiput feels full.

Nose.—Stopped up, sneezing, irritating coryza. Sensation of crawling on mucous membrane. Post-nasal dripping.

Chest.—Hacking cough with sense of weakness. Chest seems full. Influenzal pneumonia.

Stomach.—Fermentation, burning in stomach and œsophagus.

Urinary.—Profuse and frequent urination. Increased specific gravity and sugar. Diabetes.

Female.—Profuse, long-lasting flow with bearing down heaviness in uterus. General sense of exhaustion.

Extremities.—Rheumatic pains of a remittent type. Feet painful and hot, feel enlarged.

Relationship.—Compare: *Lactic acid; Gelsemium; Calc.*

Dose.—Thirtieth and higher potencies. Pure Glycerine in teaspoonful doses, t. i. d., with lemon juice for pernicious anæmia.

GNAPHALIUM
(Cud-weed)—Old Balsam

A remedy of unquestioned benefit in sciatica, when pain is associated with *numbness* of the part affected. Rheumatism and morning diarrhœa. Polyuria.

Face.—Intermittent pains of superior maxillary of both sides.

Abdomen.—Borborygmus. Colic; pain in various parts of the abdomen. Irritated prostate. First stage of cholera infantum; vomiting and purging.

Female.—Weight and fullness in pelvis. *Dysmenorrhœa*, with scanty and painful menses.

Back.—Chronic backache in lumbar region; better resting on back. Lumbago with numbness in lower part of back and weight in pelvis.

Extremities.— Cramps in calves of legs and feet when in bed. Rheumatic pain in ankle joints and legs. *Intense pain along the sciatic nerve; numbness alternates with pain.* Frequent pains in calves and feet. Gouty pains in big toes. Better, drawing limbs up, flexing thigh on abdomen. Gouty concretions. [*Ammon. benz.*] Anterior crural neuralgia. [*Staph.*] Pain in joints as if they lacked oil. Chronic muscular rheumatism of back and neck.

Relationship.—Compare: *Xanthoxyl.; Chamom.; Pulsat.*

Dose.—Third to thirtieth potency.

GOLONDRINA
(Euphorbia Polycarpa)

An antidote to snake-poison. Its use also renders the body immune to the influence of the snake venom, and thus as a prophylactic. [*Indigo.*]

Relationship.—Compare: *The Euphorbias. Euphobia Prostata*—(Used by Indians as an infallible remedy against bites of poisonous insects and snakes, especially the rattle-snake). *Plumeria cellinus* Tincture internally and locally every 15 minutes for snake poisoning (Dr. Correa). *Cedron. Micania guacho*, a Brazilian snake cure. *Selaginella*—(Macerate in milk, locally and internally for bites of snakes and spiders.) *Iodium*, tincture for rattle snake bites externally and one drop doses every 10 minutes. *Gymnema sylvestre* (will abolish the taste of bitter things; *sense of taste altered;* powdered root for snakebite); *Sisyrinchium*—Blue-eyed grass—Ten to fifteen drop doses of tincture (rattlesnake bites).

GOSSYPIUM
(Cotton-plant)

A powerful emmenagogue, used in physiological doses. Homœopathically, it corresponds to many reflex conditions, depending on disturbed uterine function and pregnancy. Gossypium will relieve tardy menses, especially with sensation that the flow is about to start and yet does not do so. Tall, bloodless patients, with nervous chills.

Head.—Pain in cervical region with tendency for head to draw backward with nervousness.

Stomach.—Nausea, with inclination to vomit before breakfast. Anorexia, with uneasy feeling at scrobiculum at time of menses.

Female.—Labia swollen and itching. *Intermittent pain in ovaries.* Retained placenta. Tumor of the breast with swelling of axillary glands. Morning sickness, with sensitive uterine region. Suppressed menstruation. Menses too watery. Backache, weight and dragging in pelvis. Uterine sub-involution and fibroids, with gastric pain and debility.

Relationship.—Compare: Action similar to Ergot when made from fresh green root. *Lilium; Cimicif.; Sabina.*

Dose.—Tincture, to sixth attenuation.

GRANATUM
(Pomegranate)

As a vermifuge for the expulsion of tapeworm, and homœopathically for the following symptomatic indications. *Salivation,* with nausea, and vertigo. Spasm of the glottis.

Head.—Feels empty. Sunken eyes; pupils dilated; weak sight. *Vertigo very persistent.*

Stomach.—*Constant hunger.* Poor digestion. Loses flesh. Vomiting at night.

Abdomen.—Pain in stomach and abdomen; worse *about umbilicus* [*Cocc.; Nux m.; Plumb.*]; ineffectual urging. Itching at anus. Dragging in vaginal region, as if hernia would protrude. Swelling resembling umbilical hernia.

Chest.—Oppressed, with sighing. Pain between shoulders; even clothing is oppressive.

Skin.—*Itching in palms.* Sensation as if pimples would break out. Jaundiced complexion.

Extremities.—Pain around shoulders, as if heavy load had been carried. Pain in all finger-joints. Tearing in knee-joint. Convulsive movements.

Relationship.—Compare: *Pelletierine* (one of its constituents—an anthelminitic, especially for tapeworm); *Cina; Kousso.*

Dose.—First to third potency.

GRAPHITES
(Black Lead)—Plumbago

Like all the carbons, this remedy is an anti-psoric of great power, but especially active in patients who are rather stout, of fair complexion, with tendency to skin affections and constipation, *fat, chilly, and costive,* with delayed menstrual history. take cold easily. Children impudent, teasing, laugh at reprimands. Has a particular tendency to develop the skin phase of internal disorders. *Eradicates tendency to erysipelas.* Anæmia with redness of face. Tendency to obesity. Swollen genitals. Gushing leucorrhœa. Aids absorption of cicatricial tissue. Induration of tissue. Cancer of pylorus. Duodenal ulcer.

Mind.—Great tendency to start. Timid. Unable to decide. Want of disposition to work. Fidgety while sitting at work. *Music makes her weep.* Apprehensive, despondency, indecision.

Head.—Rush of blood to head with flushed face also with nose bleed and distension and flatulence. Headache in morning on waking, mostly on one side, with inclination to vomit. Sensation of cobweb on forehead. Feels numb and pithy. Rheumatic pains on one side of head, extending to teeth and neck. *Burning on vertex.* Humid, itching eruption on hairy scalp, emitting a fetid odor. Cataleptic condition.

Eyes.—Ophthalmia, with intolerance of artificial light. *Eyelids red and swollen.* Blepharitis. Dryness of the lids. *Eczema of lids; fissured.*

Ears.—*Dryness of inner ear.* Cracking in ears when eating. *Moisture and eruptions behind the ears. Hears better in noise.* Hardness of hearing. Hissing in the ears. Detonation in ear like report of a gun. Thin, white, scaly membrane covering membrana tympani, like exfoliated epithelium. Fissures in and behind the ear.

Nose.—Sore on blowing it; is painful internally. Smell abnormally acute; cannot tolerate flowers. Scabs and fissures in nostrils.

Face.—Feels as if cobwebs were on it. Eczema of nose. Itching pimples. Moist eczema around mouth and chin. Erysipelas, burning and stinging.

Mouth.—Rotten odor from mouth. Breath smells like urine. Burning blisters on tongue, salivation. Sour eructations.

Stomach.—Aversion to meat. Sweets nauseate. *Hot drinks disagree.* Nausea and vomiting after each meal. Morning sickness during menstruation. Pressure in stomach. Burning in stomach, causing *hunger.* Eructation difficult. *Constrictive pain in stomach.* Recurrent gastralgia. Flatulence. Stomach pain is temporarily relieved by eating, hot drinks especially milk and lying down.

Abdomen.—Nauseous feeling in abdomen. Fullness and hardness in abdomen, as from incarcerated flatulence; *must loosen clothing;* presses painfully at abdominal ring. Croaking in abdomen. Inguinal region sensitive, swollen. Pain of gas opposite the side on which he lies. Chronic diarrhœa, stools brownish, liquid, undigested, *offensive.* Very fetid gas preceded by colic.

Stool.—Constipation; large, difficult, knotty stools united by mucus threads. Burning hæmorrhoids. Prolapse, diarrhœa; stools of brown fluid, mixed with undigested substance, *very fetid,* sour odor. Smarting, sore anus, itching. Lump stool, conjoined with threads of mucus. Varices of the rectum. Fissure of anus. [*Ratanhia; Paeonia.*]

Urine.—Turbid, with sediment. Sour smelling.

Female.—Menses *too late,* with constipation; pale and scanty, with tearing pain in epigastrium, and itching *before.* Hoarseness, coryza, cough, sweats and morning sickness during menstruation. Leucorrhœa, *pale,* thin, *profuse, white, excoriating,* with great weakness in back. Mammæ swollen and hard. Induration of ovaries and uterus and mammæ. Nipples sore, cracked, and blistered. Decided aversion to coitus.

Male.—Sexual debility, with increased desire; aversion to coition; too early or no ejaculation; herpetic eruption on organs.

Respiratory.—Constriction of chest; spasmodic asthma, suffocative attacks wakes from sleep; must eat something. Pain in middle of chest, with cough, scraping and soreness. Chronic hoarseness with skin affections. Inability to control the vocal chords; hoarseness on beginning to sing and for breaking voice.

Extremities.—Pain in nape of neck, shoulders and back and limbs. Spinal pains. Pain in small of back with great weakness. Excoriation between thighs. Left hand numb; arms feel asleep; finger-nails *thick,* black, and rough. matrix inflamed. [*Psor.; Fluor. ac.*] Œdema of lower limbs. Toe-nails crippled. Stiffness and contraction of toes. **Nails brittle and crumbling. Nails deformed, painful, sore, thick, and crippled. Cracks or fissures in ends of fingers. Offensive perspiration of feet.**

Skin.—Rough, hard, persistent dryness of portions of skin unaffected by eczema. Early stage of keloid and fibroma. Pimples and acne. *Eruptions, oozing out a sticky exudation. Rawness in bends of limbs, groins, neck, behind ears. Unhealthy skin; every little injury suppurates.* Ulcers discharging a *glutinous* fluid, thin and sticky. Swelling and induration of glands. Gouty nodosities. Cracks in nipples, mouth, between toes, anus. Phlegmonous erysipelas of face; burning and stinging pain. Swelling of feet. *Wens.* Chronic Poison Oak.

Modalities.—*Worse*, warmth, at night, during and after menstruation. *Better*, in the dark, from wrapping up.

Relationship.—Complementary: *Argent. nit.* (follows well in gastric derangements); *Caustic.; Hep.; Lycop.: Ars.; Tuberc.*

Compare: *Petrol.; Sep.; Sulph.; Fluor. ac.* The associated constipation with mucus-covered stools and gastric flatulency should be taken into consideration and differentiate it from such remedies as *Petrol.* and *Lycop.* (Raue.)

Antidote: *Nux.; Acon.; Ars.*

Dose.—Sixth to thirtieth potency. Locally as a cerate, in sore nipples.

GRATIOLA
(Hedge Hyssop)

Acts especially on gastro-intestinal tract. Chronic catarrhal conditions, leucorrhœa and gonorrhœa. Obstinate ulcers. Useful in mental troubles from overweening pride. Especially useful in females. Nux symptoms in females often met by Gratiola.

Head.—Sick headache. *Rush of blood* with vanishing of sight. Sensation as if brain was contracting and head became smaller. Tightness in forehead, with wrinkles in skin. Eyes dry, burn. Myopia.

Stomach.—Vertigo during and after meals; hunger and feeling of emptiness after meals. Dyspepsia, with much distention of the stomach. Cramps and colic after supper and during night, with swelling of abdomen and constipation. Dysphagia for liquids.

Stool.—Diarrhœa; *green, frothy water,* followed by anal burning, *forcibly evacuated without pain.* Constipation, with gouty acidity. Hæmorrhoids, with hypochondriasis. Rectum constricted.

Sleep.—Insomnia.

Female.—*Nymphomania.* Menses too profuse, premature, and too long. Leucorrhœa.

Modalities.—*Worse,* drinking too much water.

Relationship.—Compare: Dig.; Euph.; Tab.; Cham.; Ammon. pic.; Nux vom.

Dose.—Second to third potency.

GRINDELIA
(Rosin-wood)

Both Grindelia robusta and Grindelia squarrosa have been used for the symptoms here recorded. There is practically no difference in their action, although the G. Squarrosa is credited with more *splenic* symptoms, dull pains and fullness in left hypochondrium; chronic malaria; gastric pains associated with splenic congestion. Induces paralysis, beginning in extremities. Its action is shown on the heart first quickening, then retarding it.

Acts on the cardio-pulmonary distribution of the pneumo gastric in dry catarrh (Tart Emetic in muco-purulent). Produces a paresis of the pneumo-gastric, interfering with respiration. *Smothering after falling asleep.* Asthmatic conditions, chronic bronchitis. Bronchorrhœa with tough mucus, difficult to detach. Raises the blood pressure. Nausea and retching of gastric ulcer. Sugar in urine. An effective antidote to Rhus-poisoning, locally and internally; also for burns, blisters, vaginal catarrh and herpes zoster. Hyperchlorhydria when attended with asthmatic and other neurotic symptoms. Hyperæmia of gastric mucous membrane with difficult respiration.

Head.—Feels full, as from quinine. *Pain in eyeballs,* running back to brain; worse, moving eyes. Pupils dilated. Purulent ophthalmia and iritis.

Respiratory.—An efficacious remedy for wheezing and oppression in bronchitic patients. The sibilant rales are disseminated with foamy mucus, very difficult to detach. Acts on the pulmonary circulation. Asthma, with profuse tenacious expectoration, which relieves. *Stops breathing when falling asleep;* wakes *with a start,* and gasps for breath. Must sit up to breathe. *Cannot breathe when lying down.* Pertussis, with profuse mucous secretion. [*Coccus.*] Bronchorrhœa, with tough, whitish, mucous expectoration. Sibilant rales. Weak heart and respiration. Cannot breathe lying down. Cheyne-Stokes respiration.

Spleen.—Cutting pain in region of spleen, extending to hips. Spleen enlarged. [*Ceanoth., Carduus.*]

Skin.—Rash, like roseola, with severe burning and itching. Vesicular and papular eruptions. Herpes zoster. Itching and burning. *Poison oak* (locally as a wash). Ulcers, with swollen, purplish skin.

Relationship.—Compare: *Tart-emet. Eriodictyon; Lach.; Sanguinar.*

Dose.—Tincture in 1 to 15 drop doses, also lower potencies.

GUACO
(Mikania, Climbing Hemp Weed)

Acts on nervous system and female organs. Antidote to bites of scorpions and serpents. [*Golondrina.*] Cholera. *Bulbar paralysis. Syphilis.* Cancer. Deafness—tongue heavy and difficult to move. *Spinal irritation.* Spinal symptoms most marked and verified. Beer drinkers threatened with apoplexy. *Diarrhœa and dysentery with aching in sacrum and loins.*

Headache, red face. Heaviness and difficulty in moving tongue.

Throat.—Larynx and trachea constricted; difficult deglutition. Tongue feels heavy, difficult to move.

Female.—Leucorrhœa copious, corroding, putrid, debilitating. Itching and smarting at night, as if fire were running out of parts.

Urine.—Increased, cloudy, phosphatic. Pain over region of bladder.

Back.—Pain between scapulæ, extending to forearm. Burning in nape of shoulders. *Pain along spine; worse,* bending. Weariness through hips and lumbar region.

Extremities.—Pain in deltoid, shoulders, elbows, arms, and fingers. Pain about hip-joint. Legs heavy. Pain in ankle-joints and soles. *Paralysis of lower extremities.*

Modalities.—*Worse,* from motion.

Relationship.—Compare: *Oxal. ac.; Lathyr.; Caust.*

Dose.—Third to sixth potency.

GUAIACUM
(Resin of Lignum Vitæ)

Chief action on fibrous tissue, and is especially adapted to the arthritic diathesis, rheumatism, and tonsillitis. Secondary syphilis. Very valuable in acute rheumatism. *Free foul secretions. Unclean odor from whole body.* Promotes suppuration of abscesses. Sensitiveness and aggravation from local heat. Contraction of limbs, stiffness and immobility. Feeling that he must stretch.

Mind.—Forgetful; thoughtless; staring. Slow to comprehend.

Head.—*Gouty and rheumatic pain in head* and face, *extending to neck.* Tearing pain in skull; worse, cold, wet weather. Feels swollen, and blood-vessels distended. Aching in left ear. *Pains often end in a stitch,* especially in head.

Eyes.—Pupils dilated. Eyelids appear too short. Pimples around eyes.

Throat.—Rheumatic sore throat with weak throat muscles. Throat dry, burns, swollen, stitches toward ear. *Acute tonsillitis.* Syphilitic sore throat.

Stomach.—Tongue furred. *Desire for apples* and other fruits. Aversion to milk. Burning in stomach. Constricted epigastric region.

Abdomen.—Intestinal fermentation. Much wind in bowels. Diarrhœa, cholera infantum.

Urinary.—Sharp stitches after urinating. Constant desire.

Respiratory.—*Feels suffocated.* Dry, tight cough. Fetid breath after coughing. *Pleuritic stitches.* Chest pains in articulations of ribs, with shortness of breathing till expectoration sets in.

Female.—Ovaritis in rheumatic patients, with irregular menstruation and dysmenorrhœa, and irritable bladder.

Back.—Pain from head to neck. *Aching in nape. Stiff neck and sore shoulders.* Stitches between scapulæ to occiput. Contractive pain between scapulæ.

Extremities.—Rheumatic pain in shoulders, arms and hands. *Growing pains.* [*Phos. ac.*] Pricking in nates. Sciatica and lumbago. Gouty tearing, with contractions. Immovable stiffness. Ankle pain extending up the leg, causing lameness. Joints swollen, painful, and intolerant of pressure; can bear no heat. Stinging pain in limbs. Arthritic lancinations followed by contraction of limbs. *A feeling of heat* in the affected limbs.

Modalities.—*Worse*, from motion, heat, cold wet weather; pressure, touch, from 6 p. m. to 4 a. m. *Better*, external pressure.

Relationship.—*Guaiacol* (in the treatment of gonorrhœal epididymitis, 2 parts to 30 vaselin, locally).

Antidote: *Nux.* Follows Sepia.

Compare: *Merc.; Caust.; Rhus; Mezer.; Rhodod.*

Dose.—Tincture, to sixth attenuation.

GUAREA
(Ballwood)

Eye symptoms have been verified. Chemosis and pterygium have been cured with it. Lupus of an ochre-red color.

Eyes.—Conjunctiva inflamed, swollen. Tearing pain in eyeballs; tension, forced-out feeling. Objects appear gray, upside down. Eye symptoms alternate with diminished hearing. Epiphora.

Head.—Sensation as if brain were falling forwards; as from a blow on head.

Respiratory.—Cough with sweat, pain and tightness of chest; larynx irritated.

Dose.—Tincture.

GYMNOCLADUS
(American Coffee-tree)

Sore throat, dark livid redness of **fauces**, and erysipelatous swelling of face are most marked. Hives. Desire for heat and quiet. Headache, throbbing in forehead and temples and over eyes, with *bluish-white coating of tongue*. Burning in eyes.

Face.—Sensation as of flies crawling over face. Erysipelas. Great sensibility of teeth.

Throat.—Sore: dark livid redness of fauces and tonsils. Sticking pain. Mucus in throat and hawking. Tickling, with dry cough.

Relationship.—Compare: *Lachnant.; Laches.; Ailanth.; Rhus.*

Dose.—Lower attenuations.

HAEMATOXYLON
(Logwood)

Sense of constriction is characteristic. *Sensation as if a bar lay across chest*. Angina pectoris.

Head.—Feels constricted; heavy, hot. Eyelids heavy.

Stomach.—Painful digging from abdomen to throat, causing pain in region of heart with oppression. Colic, tympanitis. Borborygmi and diarrhœa. Swollen, painful.

Chest.—Constriction, extending to epigastrium. Sensation of a bar across chest. Convulsive pain in heart region with oppression. Great soreness in region of heart. Palpitation.

Female.—Pain in hypogastrium, attended with slimy, whitish leucorrhœa. *Weak feeling, with painful bearing down sensation at menstrual period*.

Relationship.—Compare: *Cactus; Colocy.; Naja.*

Dose.—Third potency.

HAMAMELIS VIRGINICA
(Witch-hazel)

Venous congestion, hæmorrhages, varicose veins, and hæmorrhoids, with *bruised soreness of affected parts*, seem to be the special sphere of this remedy. Acts upon the coats of the veins causing relaxation with consequent engorgement. Passive venous hæmorrhages from any part. Great value in open, painful wounds, with weakness from loss of blood. After operations, supercedes the use of morphia (Helmuth).

Head.—Wants "the respect due to me" shown. Feeling as of a bolt from temple to temple. Fullness, followed by epistaxis. Numbness over frontal bone.

Eyes.—Painful weakness; *sore pain* in eyes; bloodshot appearance; inflamed vessels greatly injected. Hastens absorption of intraocular hæmorrhage. Eyes feel forced out.

Nose.—Bleeding from nose profuse; flow passive, non-coagulable, with tightness in bridge of nose. Bad odor from nose.

Throat.—Mucous membrane distended and bluish; varicosis of throat.

Stomach.—Tongue feels burnt. Thirst. Blisters on side. Hæmatemesis of black blood. Throbbing and pain in stomach.

Stool.—Anus feels sore and raw. *Hæmorrhoids, bleeding profusely, with soreness*. Dysentery. Pulsation in rectum.

Urine.—Hæmaturia, with increased desire.

Female.—Ovarian congestion and neuralgia; feel very sore. Vicarious menstruation. Uterine hæmorrhage, bearing-down pain in back. Menses *dark, profuse, with soreness in abdomen. Metrorrhagia, occurring midway between menstrual periods.* Intermenstrual pain (Jas. W. Ward). Vagina very tender. Profuse leucorrhœa. Vulva itches. Milk-leg, hæmorrhoids, and sore nipples, after confinement. Metrorrhagia; passive flow. Vaginismus, ovaritis, soreness over whole abdomen. Phlegmasia alba.

Male.—Pain in spermatic cord, running into testes. Varicocele. Pain in testicles. Orchitis. Testicles enlarged, hot, and painful. Epididymitis.

Respiratory.—Hæmoptysis: tickling cough. Chest feels sore and constricted.

Back.—Sore pain down cervical vertebræ. Severe pain in lumbar and hypogastric region, extending down legs.

Extremities.—Tired feeling in arms and legs. Very sore muscles and joints. Varicose veins. Chilliness in back and hips, extending down legs. Neuralgia of internal saphenous nerve.

Skin.—Bluish chilblains. Phlebitis. Purpura. Varicose veins and ulcers; very sore. Burns. Ecchymosis. Traumatic inflammations. [*Arnica.*]

Modalities.—*Worse*, warm, moist air.

Relationship.—Compare in hæmorrhoids: *Calc. fluor.; Aloe; Mur. ac.* in varicose veins. *Mangifera indica.*

Compare: *Arnica; Calend.; Trillium; Bellis; Sulph. ac.; Pulsatilla.*

Antidote: *Arnica.*

Complementary: *Ferrum.*

Dose.—Tincture, to sixth attenuation. Distilled extract locally.

HEDEOMA
(Pennyroyal)

Female symptoms are most marked; usually associated with nervous disturbances. Red sand in urine. *Pain along ureter.* Flatulent colic. Antidotes effects of Poison-oak. [*Grindelia.*]

Head.—Dull, heavy feeling in morning. Sore pain, as from a cut. Weak, faint; better, lying down.

Stomach.—Gastritis. *Everything taken into stomach causes pain.* Tongue coated thin white. Nausea.

Abdomen.—Distended, sore, and sensitive.

Urine.—Frequent urging, cutting pains. Pain along left ureter. Dragging pain from kidney to bladder. Dull burning pain over left kidney. Burning irritation at neck of bladder causing frequent intense desire to urinate and inability to retain urine for more than few minutes, better urinating.

Female.—Bearing-down pains, with much backache; worse, least movement. Leucorrhœa, with itching and burning Ovaries congested and painful; bearing-down spasmodic contractions.

Extremities.—*Pain in thumb-joint.* Pain, coldness, and paretic condition. Twitchings, jerkings, soreness. Tendo-Achilles painful, as if sprained and swollen; walking painful.

Relationship.—Compare: *Mentha; Sepia; Lilium; Ocimum* (uric acid diathesis, pain in ureters). *Hedera Helix*—Common Ivy—(Delirium and chronic convulsions. Chronic hydrocephalus Rhinorrhœa, cerebro-spinalis. Cataract. Acts on blood vessels, menorrhagia.) *Glechoma Hederacea*—Ground Ivy—(Hæmorrhoids with *rectal irritation* and bleeding. Diarrhœa. Anus feels raw and sore. Cough with laryngeal and tracheal irritation. Glandula sub-mentalis inflamed.)

Dose.—First potency.

HEKLA LAVA
(Lava Scoriæ from Mt. Hecla)

Marked action upon *the jaws*. Of great use in exostosis, gum abscess, difficult teething. Nodosities, caries of bone, etc. Osteitis, periostitis, osteosarcoma; rachitis. *Tumors* in general. Bone necrosis. Necrosis and sinus after mastoid operation.

Face.—Ulceration of nasal bones. *Facial neuralgia from carious teeth* and after extraction. Toothache, with swelling about jaws. Abscess of gums. *Enlargement of maxillary bone.* Cervical glands enlarged and indurated.

Relationship.—Compare: *Silica; Mercur.; Phos.; Conchiolinum*—Mother of pearl (diaphysis of bone affected; parts extremely sensitive to touch).

Amphisbæna—Snail-like lizard (great affinity for the jaw bones, worse by air and dampness.

Slag—(Great itching of parts).

Dose.—Lower triturations.

HELLEBORUS
(Snow-rose)

Produces a condition of *sensorial depression*. Sees, hears, tastes imperfectly, and general *muscular weakness*, which may go on to complete paralysis, accompanied by dropsical effusions. Hence, a remedy in low states of vitality and serious disease. Characteristic aggravation from 4 to 8 p. m. [*Lycop.*] *Sinking sensation*. State of effusion in hydrocephalus. Mania of a melancholy type.

Mind.—Slow in answering. Thoughtless; staring. *Involuntary sighing. Complete unconsciousness. Picks lips and clothes*.

Head.—Forehead wrinkled in folds. Cold sweat. Stupefying headache. *Rolls head* day and night; moaning, sudden screams. *Bores head into pillow;* beats it with hands. Dull pain in occiput, with sensation of water swashing inside. Headache culminates in vomiting.

Eyes.—Eyeballs turn upwards; squinting, vacant look. Pupils dilated. Eyes wide open, sunken. Night-blindness.

Nose.—Dirty, dry nostrils. Rubs nose. Smell diminished. Nose pointed.

Face.—Pale, sunken. Cold sweat. Wrinkled. Neuralgia on left side; parts so tender he cannot chew.

Mouth.—*Horrible smell from mouth*. Lips dry and cracked. Tongue red and dry. *Falling of lower jaw*. Meaningless picking of lips. Grinding of teeth. *Chewing motion*. Greedily swallows cold water, though unconscious. Child nurses greedily, with disgust for food. Ptyalism, with sore corners of mouth.

Abdomen.—Gurgling, as if bowels were full of water. Swollen, painful to touch.

Stool.—Jelly-like, white mucus; involuntary.

Urine.—Suppressed; scanty, dark; coffee-grounds sediment. Frequent urging. Child cannot urinate. Bladder overdistended.

Respiratory.—Frequent sighing. Respiration irregular. Chest constricted; **gasps for breath**. Hydrothorax. [*Merc. sulph.*]

Extremities.—*Automatic motion of one arm and leg.* Limbs heavy and painful. Stretching of limbs. Thumb drawn into palm. [*Cupr.*] Vesicular eruption between fingers and toes.

Sleep.—Sudden screams in sleep. Soporous sleep. *Cri encephalique.* Cannot be fully aroused.

Skin.—*Pale, dropsical,* itching. Livid spots on skin. Sudden, watery, swelling of skin. Falling off of hair and nails. Angio-neurotic œdema.

Modalities.—*Worse,* from evening until morning, from uncovering.

Relationship.—(*Hellebor. fætidus* or, *Polymnia*—Bear's foot—Acts especially on spleen [*Ceanothus*[; also rectum and sciatic nerve. Splenic pains extend to scapula, neck and head, worse left side and evening; chronic ague cake; hypertrophied uterus; glandular enlargements; hair and nails falling off; skin peeling.) *Hellebor. orientalis* (salivation).

Antidote: *Camphor; Cinch.*

Compare: Threatening effusion; *Tuberc.; Apis; Zinc.; Opium; Cinch.; Cicuta; Iodoform.*

Dose.—Tincture, to third potency.

HELIANTHUS
(Sunflower)

Old cases of intermittent fever. Coryza, catarrh, nasal hæmorrhage and thick scabs in nose. Rheumatic pain in left knee. Vomiting, black stools, congestion and dryness of mouth and pharynx, redness and heat of skin. Symptoms aggravated by heat and relieved by vomiting. Spleen remedy. Marked effects on stomach, with nausea and vomiting. Stools black. [*Leptandra.*] Dry mouth. Externally, as a vulnerary like Arnica and Calendula.

HELODERMA
(Gila Monster)

The result of the bite is a benumbing paralysis like paralysis agitans or locomotor ataxia. There is no tetanic phase—a condition almost reverse in objective symptoms to Hydrocy. acid or Strychnia. The most unusual action of the drug is noted upon the eye of the mouse. *The eyeball becomes more prominent and the cornea shows opacities.* The exophthalmus is due to the pressure of the blood behind the eyeball (Boyd). Homœopathically, it is indicated in many forms of disease characterized by *great coldness*—"arctic" coldness. Cold waves from occiput to feet or ascending.

Head.—Very depressed. Sensation as if would fall to right side. *Cold* band around head; cold pressure within the skull. Eyelids heavy. Pain beginning in right ear, extending round back of head to left ear.

Face.—Cold crawling feeling, as if facial muscles were tight.

Mouth.—Tongue cold, tender, and dry. Very thirsty. Swallowing difficult. Breath cold.

Chest.—Cold feeling in lungs and in heart. Slow labored thumping of heart.

Back.—Coldness across scapulæ. Burning along spine.

Extremities.—Numbness and trembling. Cyanosis of hands. Coldness. Sensation as if walking on sponge, and as if feet were swollen. Staggering gait. Cock's gait. When walking, lifts feet higher than usual, and puts down heel hard. Feet cold as ice or burn. Stretching relieves pains in muscles and limbs.

Fever.—*Internal coldness*, as if frozen to death. Cold rings around body. Cold waves. [*Abies c.; Acon.*] *Cold spots.* Arctic coldness. Temperature subnormal—96°. [*Camph.*]

Relationship.—Compare: *Lacerta*—Green Lizard (skin eruptions. Vesicles under tongue. Increased mental acumen. Difficult swallowing. Constant accumulation of saliva in the mouth. *Nausea;* violent pressure in stomach). *Camphor; Lachesis.*

Dose.—Thirtieth potency.

HELONIAS—CHAMAELIRIUM
(Unicorn-root)

Sensation of weakness, dragging and weight in the sacrum and pelvis, with great languor and prostration, are excellent indications for this remedy. There is a sensitiveness expressed as a consciousness of a womb. Tired, backachy females. The weakness shows itself also in a tendency to prolapse and other malposition of the womb. The menses are often suppressed and the kidneys congested. It seems as if the monthly congestion, instead of venting itself as it should through the uterine vessels, had extended to the kidneys. With it all, there is a profound melancholia. Patient must be doing something to engage the mind. Remember it, for women with prolapsus from atony, enervated by indolence and luxury (better when attention is engaged—hence when the doctor comes), or for those worn out with hard work; tired, strained muscles burn and ache; sleepless. Diabetes mellitus, and insipidus. Constant aching and tenderness over kidneys.

Mind.—Profound melancholy. *Patient is better when kept busy,* with mind engaged, when doing something. Irritable; cannot endure the least contradiction.

Head.—Burning sensation on top. Headache, better mental exertion.

Back.—*Pain and weight in back;* tired and weak. Aching and burning across the lumbar region; *can trace outlines of kidneys by constant burning.* Boring pain in lumbar region, extending down legs. Great languor, better exercising.

Female.—Dragging in sacral region, with prolapse, especially after a miscarriage. *Pruritus vulvæ.* Backache after miscarriage. [*Kali c.*] Weight and soreness in womb; *conscious of womb. Menses too frequent, too profuse.* Leucorrhœa. Breasts swollen, nipples painful and tender. Parts hot, red, swollen; burn and itch terribly. Albuminuria during pregnancy. Debility attending the menopause.

Urine.—*Albuminous,* phosphatic; profuse and clear, saccharine. Diabetes.

Extremities.—Sensation as if a cool wind streamed up calves of legs. Feet feel numb when sitting.

Modalities.—*Better,* when doing something (mental diversion). *Worse,* motion, touch.

Relationship.—Compare: *Agrimonia*—Cockleburr—(painful kidneys, impaired digestion and menstrual difficulties; Bronchorrhœa and catarrh of bladder. Cough with profuse expectoration attended with expulsion of urine. Tincture 1-10 gtt). *Aletris; Lilium; Puls.; Senecio; Stannum.*

Dose.—Tincture, to sixth attenuation.

HEPAR SULPHURIS CALCAREUM
(Hahnemann's Calcium Sulphide)

Suits especially scrofulous and lymphatic constitutions who are inclined to have eruptions and glandular swellings. Unhealthy skin. Blondes with sluggish character and weak muscles. *Great sensitiveness to all impressions.* Sweating patient pulling blanket around him. Locally, it has special affinity to the respiratory mucous membrane, producing croupous catarrhal inflammation, profuse secretion; also easy perspiration. After abuse of Mercury. Infected sinus with pus forming. *The tendency to suppuration* is most marked, and has been a strong guiding symptom in practice. The lesions spread by the formation of small papules around the side of the old lesion. Chilliness, hypersensitiveness, splinter-like pains, craving for sour and strong things are very characteristic. *Feeling as if wind were blowing on some part.* The side of the body on which he lies at night becomes gradually insufferably painful; he must turn. *Pellagra* (material doses required). Syphilis after antispecific gross medication.

Mind.—Anguish in the evening and night, with thoughts of suicide. *The slightest cause irritates him.* Dejected and sad. Ferocious. Hasty speech.

Head.—Vertigo and headache, when shaking the head or riding. Boring pain in the right temple and in root of nose every morning. Scalp sensitive and sore. Humid scald-head itching and burning. Cold sweat on head.

Eyes.—*Ulcers on cornea.* Iritis, with pus in anterior chamber; purulent conjunctivitis, with marked chemosis, profuse discharge, great sensitiveness to touch and air. Eyes and lids red and inflamed. Pain in the eyes, as if pulled back into the head. Boring pain in upper bones of the orbits. Eyeballs sore to touch. Objects appear red and too large. Vision obscured by reading; field reduced one-half. Bright circles before eyes. *Hypopion.*

Ears.—Scurfs on and behind the ears. Discharge of fetid pus from the ears. Whizzing and throbbing in ears, with hardness of hearing. Deafness after scarlet fever. Pustules in auditory canal and auricle. Mastoiditis.

Nose.—Sore, ulcerated. Soreness of nostrils, with catarrhal troubles. Sneezes every time he goes into a cold, dry wind, with running from nose, later, thick, offensive discharge. Stopped up every time he goes out into cold air. *Smell like old cheese. Hay-fever.* (Hepar 1x will often start secretions and profuse drainage in stuffy colds.)

Face.—Yellowish complexion. Middle of lower lip cracked. Vesicular erysipelas, with pricking in parts. Neuralgia of right side, extending in streak into temple, ear, alæ, and lip. Pains in bones of face, especially when being touched. Ulcers in corners of mouth. Shooting in jaw on opening mouth.

Mouth.—Ptyalism. Gums and mouth painful to touch and bleed readily.

Throat.—When swallowing, sensation as if a plug and *of a splinter in throat.* Quinsy, *with impending suppuration.* Stitches in throat extending to the ear when swallowing. Hawking up of mucus.

Stomach.—Longing for acids, wine, and strong-tasting food. Aversion to fat food. Frequent eructations, without taste or smell. Distention of stomach, compelling one to loosen the clothing. Burning in stomach. Heaviness and pressure in stomach after a slight meal.

Abdomen.—Stitching in region of liver when walking, coughing, breathing, or touching it. [*Bry.; Merc.*] Hepatitis, hepatic abscess; abdomen distended, tense; chronic abdominal affections.

Stool.—Clay-colored and soft. *Sour,* white, undigested, *fetid.* Loss of power to expel even a soft stool.

Urine.—Voided slowly, without force—drops vertically bladder weak. Seems as if some always remained. Greasy pellicle on urine. Bladder difficulties of old men. [*Phos.; Sulph. Copaiva.*]

Male.—Herpes, sensitive, bleed easily. Ulcers externally on prepuce similar to chancre. [*Nitr. acid.*] Excitement and emission without amorous fancies. Itching of glans, frænum, and scrotum. Suppurating inguinal glands. Figwarts of offensive odor. Humid soreness on genitals and between scrotum and thigh. Obstinate gonorrhœa "does not get well."

HEPAR SULPHURIS CALCAREUM

Female.—Discharge of blood from uterus. Itching of pudenda and nipples, worse during menses. Menses late and scanty. *Abscesses of labiæ with great sensitiveness.* Extremely offensive leucorrhœa. Smells like old cheese. [*Sanicula.*] Profuse perspiration at the climacteric. [*Tilia; Jaborandi.*]

Respiratory.—Loses voice and coughs when exposed to dry, cold wind. Hoarseness, with loss of voice. Cough troublesome when walking. Dry, hoarse cough. Cough excited *whenever any part of the body gets cold or uncovered*, or from eating anything cold. Croup with loose, rattling cough; worse in morning. *Choking cough.* Rattling, croaking cough; suffocative attacks; has to rise up and bend head backwards. Anxious, wheezing, moist breathing, asthma worse in dry cold air; better in damp. Palpitation of heart.

Extremities.—Finger-joints swollen; tendency to easy dislocation. Nail of great toe painful on slight pressure.

Skin.—Abscesses; suppurating glands are very sensitive. *Papules* prone to suppurate and extend. Acne in youth. Suppurate with prickly pain. Easily bleed. Angio-neurotic œdema. *Unhealthy skin; every little injury suppurates.* Chapped skin, with *deep cracks on hands and feet*. Ulcers, with bloody suppuration, smelling like old cheese. *Ulcers very sensitive* to contact, burning, stinging, easily bleeding. Sweats day and night without relief. *"Cola-sores" very sensitive.* Cannot bear to be uncovered; *wants to be wrapped up warmly.* Sticking or pricking in afflicted parts. Putrid ulcers, *surrounded by little pimples.* Great sensitiveness to slightest touch. *Chronic and recurring urticaria.* Small-pox. Herpes circinatus. Constant offensive exhalation from the body.

Fever.—Chilly in open air or from *slightest draught*. Dry heat at night. *Profuse sweat;* sour, sticky, offensive.

Modalities.—*Worse*, from dry cold winds; cool air; slightest draught; from Mercury, touch; lying on painful side. *Better*, in damp weather, from wrapping head up, from warmth, after eating.

Relationship.—Antidotes: *Bellad.; Cham.; Sil.*

Compare: *Acon.; Spongia; Staphis.; Silica; Sulph.; Calc. sulph.; Myristica. Hepar* antidotes bad effects from *Mercury,*

Iodine, Potash, Cod-liver Oil. Removes the weakening effects of ether.

Dose.—First to 200th. The higher potencies may abort suppuration, the lower promote it. If it is necessary to hasten it, give 2x.

HEPATICA
(Liver-Wort)

Pharyngeal catarrh, with profuse, serous sputa and hoarseness. Tickling and irritation of the throat. *Scraping and rough sensation.* Induces free and easy expectoration. Viscid, thick, tenacious phlegm causes continued hawking. Soreness at the nostrils. Sensation about epiglottis *as if particles of food remained.* Sputa sweet, profuse, creamy.

Dose.—Second potency.

HERACLEUM—BRANCA URSINA
(Hogweed)

Recommended as a spinal stimulant; in epilepsy with flatulency, gouty and skin symptoms.

Head.—Aches, with drowsiness, worse moving in open air, better tying up head with cloth. *Much fatty perspiration on head* and violent itching. Seborrhœa capitis. Sick headache.

Stomach.—Pain with inclination to vomit. Bitter risings and taste. Hungry but unable to eat. Abdominal and spleenic pain.

Dose.—Third potency.

HIPPOMANES
(A Meconium Deposit out of the Amniotic Fluid taken from the Colt)

The old famous Aphrodisiacum of the Greek authors.

Stomach.—*Icy coldness* in stomach.

Male.—Sexual desire increased. Prostatitis. Drawing pain in testicles.

Extremities.—Violent pain in wrist. Paralysis of wrists. *Sprained sensation in wrist.* Great weakness of hands and fingers. Weakness in joints of feet, knee, and soles. *Chorea.* Much weakness after growing too fast.

Relationship.—Compare: *Caustic.*

Dose.—Sixth to thirtieth potency.

HIPPOZAENIUM
(Gladerine-mallein—Farcine)

This powerful nosode introduced by Dr. J. J. Garth Wilkinson, covers symptoms which suggest integral parts of consumption, cancer, syphilis, etc., and promises useful service in the treatment of ozæna, scrofulous swellings, pyæmia, erysipelas. Chronic rhinitis; saneous secretion.

Nose.—Red, swollen. *Catarrh, ozæna,* ulceration. Discharge acrid, corroding, bloody, offensive. Tubercles on alæ nasi. Papules and ulceration in frontal sinus and pharynx.

Face.—All glands swollen; painful; form abscesses.

Respiratory.—Hoarseness. Bronchial asthma. Noisy breathing; short, irregular. Cough, with dyspepsia. Excessive secretion. Suffocation imminent. *Bronchitis in the aged,* where suffocation from excessive secretion is imminent. Tuberculosis.

Skin.—Lymphatic swellings. Articular non-fluctuating swellings. Nodules in arm. Malignant erysipelas. Pustules and abscesses. Ulcers. Rupia. Eczema.

Relationship.—Compare: *Muco-toxin* (Cahis' preparation with the micrococcus catarrhalis. Friedlander's Bacillus of Pneumonia and the micrococcus tetragenius—for acute and chronic mucous catarrhs in children and old people.); *Aur.; Kali bich.; Psor.; Bacill.*

Dose.—Thirtieth potency.

HIPPURIC ACID
(Proved by Dr. Wm. B. Griggs)

Its chief action is on the external tissues of the eyes and nasopharynx, joint surfaces, liver and mucous membranes. Right side especially affected, general muscular soreness.

Head.—Pain over right eye, dull, constant, worse in warm room. Eyelids inflamed and swollen.

Throat.—Sore, raw, dry, swallowing difficult, foul odor, gummy exudate; thickness and infiltration of all tissues around throat.

Stomach.—Acid rising. Lump in pit of stomach. Soreness and pressure over liver.

Female.—Menstrual flow for three weeks with complete relief of muscular and joint pains.

Extremities.—Backache extending down hips. Pain in shoulders and extremities and sore swollen joints. Pain in middle of thigh posteriorly shooting down right leg. Tired, grating sensation in the joints.

Skin.—Itching, burning. Papules looking like goose flesh on chest.

Relationship.—Benzoic acid seems to be an analogue.

Dose.—Lower potencies.

HOANG NAN—STRYCHNOS GAULTHERIANA
(Tropical Bind-weed)

Exhaustion with vertigo; numbness and tingling in hands and feet; involuntary action of lower jaw. Pustules and boils; tertiary syphilis and Paralysis, Eczema, prurigo, old ulcers, leprosy, cancer of glandular structures and bites of serpents. Removes fetor and hæmorrhage in cancer, revives the healing process. Follows Arsenic.

Dose.—Five drops of the tincture. May be increased to twenty.

HOMARUS
(Digestive Fluid of Live Lobster)

Dyspepsia, sore throat, and headache seems to be a combination that may be controlled by this remedy. Frontal and temporal pain chiefly, with soreness in eyes. Throat sore, *raw*, burns, with tough mucus. Pain in stomach and abdomen, better after eating. Belching. Chilliness and pain all over. Itching of skin.

Modalities.—*Worse*, from milk, after sleep. *Better*, from motion, after eating.

Relationship.—Compare: *Sepia; Asterias; Astacus; Æthusa.*

Dose.—Sixth potency.

HURA BRAZILIENSIS
(Assacu)

Used in leprosy, when skin feels as if it were hide bound. Tense vesicles; sensation of splinter under thumb-nails. Skin of forehead feels drawn tight. Stiff neck, pain in back. Throbbing in finger tips. Itching, pimples on all projecting portions of bone, malar bones, etc.

Dose.—Sixth potency.

Relationship.—Compare Calotropis or *Madura album*—(Leprosy; livid and gangrenous tubercles; thickening of the skin).

HYDRANGEA
(Seven-barks)

A remedy for gravel, profuse deposit of white amorphous salts in urine. Calculus, renal colic, bloody urine. Acts on ureter. Pain in lumbar region. Dizziness. Oppression of chest.

Urine.—Burning in urethra and frequent desire. Urine hard to start. Heavy deposit of mucus. *Sharp pain in loins*, especially left. Great thirst, with abdominal symptoms and *enlarged prostate*. [*Ferr. pic.; Sabal.*] Gravelly deposits. Spasmodic stricture. Profuse deposit of white amorphous salts.

Relationship.—Compare: *Lycopod.; Chimaphil.; Berberis; Pareira; Uva; Sabal; Oxydendron; Geum*—Water-Avens—(Severe jerking pains from deep in the abdomen to end of urethra; affections of bladder, with pains in penis; worse, eating; relaxed mucous membranes, with excessive and depraved secretions; imperfect digestion and assimilation.) *Polyctrichum*—Haircap moss—(according to Dr. A. M. Cushing in mother tincture or infusion for enlarged prostate—prostatitis.)

Dose.—Tincture.

HYDRASTIS
(Golden Seal)

Acts especially on mucous membranes, **relaxing them and** producing a *thick, yellowish, ropy* secretion. The catarrh may be anywhere,—throat, stomach, uterus, urethra,—it is always characterized by this peculiar mucous discharge. Hydrastis is especially active in old, easily-tired people, cachectic individuals, with great debility. Cerebral effects prominent, feels his wits sharpened, head cleared, facile expression. Weak muscular power, poor digestion and obstinate constipation. Lumbago. Emaciation and prostration. Its action on the liver is marked. Cancer and cancerous state, before ulceration, when pain is principal symptom. *Goitre* of puberty and pregnancy. *Smallpox* internally and locally. The power of Hydrastis over smallpox seen in modifying the disease, abolishing its distressing symptoms, shortening its course, lessening its danger and greatly mitigating its consequences. (J. J. Garth Wilkinson.)

Mind.—Depressed; sure of death, and desires it.

Head.—Dull, pressing frontal pain, especially connected with constipation. Myalgic pain in scalp and muscles of neck. [*Cimicif.*] Eczema on forehead along line of hair. *Sinusitis,* after coryza.

Ears.—Roaring. Muco-purulent discharge. Deafness. *Eustachian catarrh*, with high-pitched voice.

Nose.—*Thick, tenacious secretion from posterior nares* to throat. Watery, *excoriating* discharge. Ozæna, with ulceration of septum. Tends to blow nose all the time.

Mouth.—Peppery taste. Tongue white, swollen, large, flabby, slimy; *shows imprint of teeth* [*Merc.*]; as if scalded; stomatitis. Ulceration of tongue, fissures toward the edges.

Throat.—Follicular pharyngitis. Raw, smarting, excoriating sensation. Hawking of yellow, tenacious mucus. [*Kali bich.*] Child is aroused suddenly from sleep by this tenacious postnasal dropping. Goitre of puberty and pregnancy.

Stomach.—Sore feeling in stomach more or less constant. Weak digestion. *Bitter taste.* Pain as from a hard-cornered substance. Gone feeling. Pulsation in epigastrium. Cannot eat bread or vegetables. Atonic dyspepsia. Ulcers and cancer. Gastritis.

Abdomen.—Gastro-duodenal catarrh. Liver torpid, tender. Jaundice. Gallstones. Dull dragging in right groin with cutting sensation into right testicle.

Back.—Dull, heavy, dragging pain and stiffness, particularly across lumbar region, *must use arms in raising himself from seat.*

Rectum.—Prolapsed; anus fissured. *Constipation*, with sinking feeling in stomach, and dull headache. During stool, smarting pain in rectum. After stool, long-lasting pain. [*Nit. ac.*] Hæmorrhaids; even a light flow exhausts. Contraction and spasm.

Urine.—*Gleety discharge.* Urine smells decomposed.

Male.—Gonorrhœa, second stage; discharge thick and yellow.

Female.—Erosion and excoriation of cervix. Leucorrhœa, worse after menses [*Bov.; Calc. c.*]; acrid and corroding, shreddy, tenacious. Menorrhagia. Pruritus vulvæ, with profuse leucorrhœa. [*Calc. c.; Kreos.; Sep.*] Sexual excitement. Tumor of breast; nipple retracted.

Respiratory.—Chest raw, sore, burning. Dry, harsh cough. Bronchial catarrh, later stages. Bronchitis in old, exhausted persons, *with thick, yellow, tenacious expectoration.* Frequent fainty spells, with cold sweat all over. Feels suffocating when lying on left side. Pain from chest to left shoulder.

Skin.—Eruption like variola. Lupus; *ulcers,* cancerous formations. General tendency to profuse perspiration and unhealthy skin. [*Hepar.*]

Relationship.—Antidote: *Sulph.*

Useful after too much Chlorate of Potash for sore throat.

Compare: *Xanthorrhiza apifolia; Kali bich.; Conium; Ars. iod.; Phytol.; Galium* (cancer—nodulated tumor of the tongue); *Asterias; Stann.; Puls.* Also *Manzanita* (diarrhœa, gonorrhœa, gleet, leucorrhœa, catarrhal conditions). *Hydrastinum muriaticum*—Muriate of Hydrastia. (Locally, in aphthous sore mouth, ulcers, ulcerated sore throat, ozæna, etc. Internally, third dec. trit. Is a uterine hæmostatic and vasoconstrictor; metrorrhagia, especially from fibroid tumors; hæmorrhages; *in dilatation of the stomach,* and chronic digestive disorders). *Hydrastin sulph* 1x (hæmorrhage of bowels in typhoid).

Marrubium—Hoarhound—(a stimulant to mucous membranes, especially laryngeal and bronchial; chronic bronchitis, dyspepsia, and hepatic disorders; colds and coughs).

Dose.—Tincture, to thirtieth attenuation. Locally colorless Hydrastis, mother tincture, or fluid extract.

HYDROCOTYLE
(Indian Pennywort)

Curative in disorders that exhibit interstitial inflammation and cellular proliferation in any part. Hypertrophy and induration of connective tissue. Has considerable reputation in *leprosy* and *lupus*, when there is no ulceration. The skin symptoms are very important. Of great use in ulceration of womb. Difficulty in maintaining the upright posture. Very copious perspiration. Pains of cervical cancer.

Face.—Pain in left cheek-bones and about orbits.

Female.—Pruritus of vagina. Inflammation of neck of bladder. *Heat within vagina. Granular ulceration of womb.* Profuse leucorrhœa. Dull pain in ovarian region. Cervical redness.

Skin.—Dry eruptions. *Great thickening of epidermoid layer and exfoliation of scales.* Psoriasis *gyrate*, on trunk and extremities, palms and soles. Pustules on chest. Circular spots, with scaly edges. *Intolerable itching, especially of soles.* Profuse sweat. Syphilitic affections. *Acne.* Leprosy. *Elephantiasis* [*Ars.*] Lupus non-exedens.

Relationship.—Compare: *Elæis*—South American Palm—(scleroderma, elephantiasis, leprosy, skin thickened, itching and hardened. Anæsthesia). *Hura; Trychnos Gaultheriana* (bites of serpents, ulcers and cutaneous affections generally); *Hoang-Nan. Chaulomoogra oil* from seeds of *Taraktogenos; Hydrast.; Arsenic; Aurum; Sepia.*

Dose.—First to sixth potency.

HYDROCYANIC ACID
(Prussic Acid)

One of the most toxic agents known. Convulsions and paralysis express the action of this remedy. Spasmodic constriction in larynx, feeling of suffocation, pain and tightness in chest, palpitation; pulse weak, irregular. *Singing sensation at the epigastrium.* Hysterical and epileptic convulsions. Cyanosis. Collapse, due to some pulmonary condition not a cardiac collapse. Catalepsy. Cholera. Stage of collapse. [*Ars.; Verat.*] Coldness. Tetanus narcolepsy.

Mind.—Unconscious. Wild delirium. Fear of imaginary troubles. *Fears* everything—horses, wagons, houses falling, etc.

Head.—Violent stypefying headache. Brain feels on fire. Pupils motionless or dilated. Supra-orbital neuralgia, with flushing on same side of face.

Face.—Jaws clenched in rigid spasm. Froths at mouth. Pale, bluish lips.

Stomach.—Tongue cold. *Drink rumbles through throat and stomach.* Gastralgia; worse when stomach is empty. *Great sinking at pit of stomach.* Pulsative pain in præcordial region.

Respiratory.—Noisy and agitated breathing. Dry, spasmodic, suffocative cough. Asthma, with contraction of throat. Whooping-cough. Paralysis of lungs. [*Aspidos.*] Marked cyanosis; venously congested lung.

Heart.—Violent palpitation. Pulse, *weak, irregular.* Cold extremities. Torturing pain in chest. Angina pectoris. [*Spigel.; Oxal. ac.*]

Sleep.—Yawning, with shivering. Irresistible drowsiness. Vivid, incoherent dreams.

Relationship.—Antidotes: *Ammon.; Camph.; Opium.* Compare: *Cicuta; Œnanthe; Camph.; Lauroc.*

Dose.—Sixth and higher potencies.

HYDROPHOBINUM
(Lyssin—Saliva of Rabid Dog)

Affects principally the nervous system; aching in bones. Complaints from abnormal sexual desire. Convulsions brought on by dazzling light or sight of running water.

Head.—Lyssophobia; fear of becoming made. Emotion and bad news aggravate; also, thinking of fluids. *Hypersensitiveness of all senses.* Chronic headache. Boring pain in forehead.

Mouth.—Constant spitting; saliva tough, viscid. Sore throat; constant desire to swallow, which is difficult; gagging when swallowing water. Froths at mouth.

Male.—Lascivious; priapism, with frequent emissions. No emission during coition. Atrophy of testicles. Complaints from abnormal sexual desire.

Female.—Uterine sensitiveness; conscious of womb [*Helon.*] Feels prolapsed. Vagina sensitive, rendering coition painful. [*Berberis.*] Uterine displacements.

Respiratory.—Voice altered in tone. Breathing held for a time. Spasmodic contraction of respiratory muscles.

Stool.—Desire for stool on hearing or seeing running water. Profuse, watery stools, with pain in bowels; worse, evening. Constant desire to urinate on seeing running water.

Modalities.—*Worse*, sight or sound of running water or pouring water, or even thinking of fluids; dazzling or reflected light; heat of sun; stooping.

Relationship.—Compare: *Xanthium spinosum*—Cockle—(said to be specific for hydrophobia and is recommended for chronic cystitis in women). *Canth.; Bell.; Stram.; Lach.; Nat. mur.*

Dose.—Thirtieth potency.

HYOSCYAMUS
(Henbane)

Disturbs the nervous system profoundly. It is as if some diabolical force took possession of the brain and prevented its functions. It causes a perfect picture of *mania of a quarrelsome and obscene character*. Inclined to be unseemly and immodest in acts, gestures and expressions. Very talkative, and persists in stripping herself, or uncovering genitals. Is jealous, afraid of being poisoned, etc. Its symptoms also point to weakness and *nervous agitation;* hence typhoid and other infections with *coma vigil. Tremulous weakness and twitching of tendons.*

Subsultus tendinum. Muscular twitchings, spasmodic affections, generally with delirium. Non-inflammatory cerebral activity. *Toxic gastritis.*

Mind.—*Very suspicious.* Talkative, obscene, lascivious mania, uncovers body; jealous, *foolish.* Great hilarity; *inclined to laugh at everything.* Delirium, with attempt to run away. Low, muttering speech; *constant carphologia, deep stupor.*

Head.—Feels light and confused. Vertigo as if intoxicated. Brain feels loose, fluctuating. Inflammation of brain, with unconsciousness; head is shaken to and fro.

Eyes.—Pupils dilated, sparkling, fixed. Eyes open, but does not pay attention; downcast and dull, fixed. Strabismus. Spasmodic closing of lids. Diplopia. Objects have colored borders.

Mouth.—Tongue dry, red, cracked, stiff and immovable, protruded with difficulty; speech impaired. Foams at mouth. Teeth covered with sordes. Lower jaw drops.

Throat.—Stinging dryness. Constriction. Cannot swallow liquids. *Uvula elongated.*

Stomach.—Hiccough, eructations empty, bitter. Nausea, with vertigo. Vomiting, with convulsions; hæmatemesis; violent cramps, relieved by vomiting; burning in stomach; epigastrium tender. *After irritating food.*

Abdomen.—Colic, as if abdomen would burst. Distention. Colic, with vomiting, belching, hiccough screaming. Tympanites. Red spots on abdomen.

Stool.—Diarrhœa, colicky, pains; *involuntary,* aggravated by mental excitement or during sleep. Diarrhœa during the lying-in period. Involuntary defecation.

Urine.—*Involuntary* micturition. Bladder paralyzed. Has no will to urinate. [*Caust.*]

Male.—Impotence. Lascivious; exposes his person; plays with genitals during fever.

Female.—Before menses, hysterical spasms. Excited sexual desire. During menses, convulsive movements, urinary flux and sweat. Lochia suppressed. Spasms of pregnant women. Puerperal mania.

Chest.—Suffocating fits. Spasm, forcing bending forward. *Dry, spasmodic cough at night (worse lying down;* better sitting up), from itching in the throat, as if uvula were too long. Hæmoptysis.

Extremities.—*Picking at bed-clothes;* plays with hands; reaches out for things. Epileptic attacks ending in deep sleep. Spasms and convulsions. Cramps in calves and toes. Child sobs and cries without waking.

Sleep.—Intense sleeplessness. Sopor, with convulsions. *Starts up frightened.* Coma vigil.

Nerves.—Great restlessness; *every muscle twitches.* Will not be covered.

Modalities.—*Worse,* at night, during menses, after eating, when lying down. *Better,* stooping.

Relationship.—Antidotes: *Bell.; Camph.*

Compare: *Bellad.; Stram.; Agaric.; Gels.;*

Hyosc. hydrobrom.—Scopolamine hydrobromide. (Paralysis agitans; *tremors of disseminated sclerosis.* Sleeplessness and nervous agitation. Dry cough in phthisis. Similar in its effects to alcohol, both recent and remote. Corresponds to the effects of strong poisons introduced into or generated within the body. Symptoms of uræmia and acute nervous exhaustion. A remedy for shock. Third and fourth dec. trituration. In physiological dosage (1-200 gr.) mania and chorea; insomnia. *Scopola* (Japanese Belladonna)—chemically identical with Hyoscine. (Joyous delirium, licking of lips and smacking of mouth; sleepless; tries to get out of bed; sees cats, picks imaginary hairs, warms hands before imaginary fire, etc.)

Dose.—Sixth, to 200th potency.

HYPERICUM
(St. John's-wort)

The great remedy for injuries to nerves, especially of fingers, toes and nails. Crushed fingers, especially tips. Excessive painfulness is a guiding symptom to its use. Prevents lockjaw. *Punctured* wounds. Relieves pain after operations. Quite supersedes the use of Morphia after operations. (Helmuth.)

HYPERICUM

Spasms after every injury. Has an important action on the rectum; hæmorrhoids. *Coccydynia.* Spasmodic asthmatic attacks with changes of weather or before storms, better by copious expectoration. Injured nerves from bites of animals. Tetanus. Neuritis, tingling, burning and numbness. Constant drowsiness.

Mind.—Feels as if lifted high in air, or anxiety lest he fall from heights. Mistakes in writing. Effects of shock. Melancholy.

Head.—Heavy; feels as if touched by *an icy cold hand. Throbbing in vertex;* worse in close room. Brain seems compressed. Right side of face aches. Brain-fag and neurasthenia. Facial neuralgia and toothache of a pulling, tearing character, with sadness. *Head feels longer*—elongated to a point. In fractured skull, bone splinters. Brain feels alive. Pains in eyes and ears. Falling out of hair.

Stomach.—Craving for wine. Thirst; *nausea.* Tongue coated white at base, tip clean. Feeling of lump in stomach. [*Abies nig.; Bry.*]

Rectum.—Urging, dry, dull, pressing pain. *Hæmorrhoids,* with pain, bleeding, and tenderness.

Back.—Pain in nape of neck. *Pressure over sacrum.* Spinal concussion. Coccyx injury from fall, with pain radiating up spine and down limbs. Jerking and twitching of muscles.

Extremities.—Darting pain in shoulders. Pressure along ulnar side of arm. Cramp in calves. Pain in toes and fingers, especially in tips. *Crawling in hand and feet.* Lancinating pain in upper and lower limbs. *Neuritis,* with tingling, burning pain, numbness and flossy skin. Joints feel bruised. Hysterical joints. Tetanus. [*Physost.; Kali brom.*] Traumatric neuralgia and neuritis.

Respiratory.—Asthma *worse* foggy weather and relieved by profuse perspiration.

Skin.—Hyperidrosis, sweating of scalp, worse in morning after sleep; falling of hair from injury; eczema of hands and face, intense itching, eruption seems to be under the skin. Herpes zoster. Old ulcers or sores in mouth when very sensitive. Lacerated wounds with much prostration from loss of blood.

Modalities.—*Worse*, in cold; dampness; in a *fog;* in close room; least exposure; touch. *Better*, bending head backward.

Relationship.—Compare: *Ledum* (punched wounds and bites of animals); *Arnica; Staphis.; Calend.; Ruta; Coff.*

Antidotes: *Ars.; Cham.*

Dose.—Tincture, to third potency.

IBERIS
(Bitter Candytuft)

State of nervous excitement. Has marked action upon the heart. Possesses great efficacy in cardiac diseases. Controls vascular excitement in hypertrophy with thickening of the heart's walls. Cardiac debility after influenza. Liver region full and painful. White stools.

Mind.—Sad and sighing; fearful and trembling. Irritable.

Head.—Vertigo and pains around heart. Constant hawking of thick, stringy mucus until after a meal. Hot, flushed face. Vertigo, *as if occiput were turning around;* eyes feel forced outwards.

Heart.—Conscious of heart's action. On turning on left side, stitching pain as of needles through ventricles felt at each systole. Palpitation, *with vertigo and choking in throat.* Stitching pains in cardiac region. *Pulse full, irregular, intermittent.* Worse, least motion and in warm room. Sensation of weight and pressure, with occasional sharp, stinging pains. Dropsy, with enlarged heart. Violent palpitation *induced by slightest exertion, or by laughing, or coughing. Darting pains through heart.* Cardiac dyspnœ. Dilation of heart. Wakes with palpitation about 2 a. m. Throat and trachea fills up with mucus. Cough causes redness of face. *Tachycardia.*

Extremities.—Numbness and tingling in left hand and arm. Whole body sore, lame and trembling.

Modalities.—*Worse,* lying down; on left side; motion, exertion; warm room.

Relationship.—Compare: *Cact.; Dig.; Amyl.; Bell.*

Dose.—Tincture and first potency.

ICHTHYOLUM

(A Combination of Sulphonated Hydrocarbons; a Fossil Product of Complex Structure found in Tyrol, supposed to be Fish Deposits, contains 10% Sulphur.)

Its action on skin, mucous membranes, and kidneys is prompt and useful. It is strongly antiparasitic; redness, pain and inflammation; decreases tension. Excellent in winter coughs of old people. Polyarthritis. Chronic rheumatism. *Uric acid diathesis.* Hay-fever. *Chronic hives. Tuberculosis, aids nutrition.* Alcoholism when nothing will stay on stomach.

Mind.—Irritable and depressed. Forgetful, lack of concentration.

Head.—Dull, aching; better cold, pressure. Dull frontal and supra-orbital headache; worse moving eyes, cold air; better, warmth.

Face.—Skin feels dry and itches. Acne on chin.

Throat.—Irritated; pain to ears; sore, dry, with hawking and expectoration.

Eyes.—Burn, red; worse, any change of temperature.

Nose.—Bland coryza; stuffed feeling; feels sore inside. Irresistible desire to sneeze.

Stomach.—Disagreeable taste, burning sensation, very thirsty. *Nausea. Increased appetite.*

Abdomen.—Disposition to soft, shapeless stools. Griping in umbilical and left hypogastric region. Early morning diarrhœa.

Urine.—Increased in quantity and frequency. Burning pain in meatus. Uric acid deposits.

Female.—Fullness in lower abdomen. Nausea at time of menses.

Respiratory.—Coryza; *dry, teasing cough.* Bronchiectasis and phthisis. Bronchitis, especially of the aged.

Skin.—Heat and irritation; *itching.* Scaly and itching eczema. *Crops of boils.* Pruritus of pregnancy. Psorisis, Acne, rosacea, erysipelas.

Extremities.—Lameness in right shoulder and right lower extremity.

Relationship.—Compare: *Hepar; Calc.; Silica; Sulph.; Ars.; Petrol.*

Dose.—Lower potencies.

Externally, it is used as an ointment, with Lanoline 20 to 50 per cent.; for chronic eczema and psoriasis, also acne rosacea and gouty joints. Chilblains, scabies. Rectal suppositories for senile prostate.

IGNATIA

(St. Ignatius Bean)

Produces a marked hyperæsthesia of all the senses, and a tendency to clonic spasms. Mentally, *the emotional element is uppermost, and co-ordination of function is interfered with.* Hence, it is one of the chief remedies for hysteria. It is especially adapted to the nervous temperament—women of sensitive, easily excited nature, dark, mild disposition, quick to perceive, rapid in execution. Rapid change of mental and physical condition, opposite to each other. Great contradictions. Alert, nervous, apprehensive, rigid, trembling patients who suffer acutely in mind or body, at the same time made worse by drinking coffee. The *superficial* and *erratic character* of its symptoms is most characteristic. *Effects of grief* and worry. Cannot bear tobacco. Pain is small, circumscribed spots. [*Oxal. ac.*] *The plague.* Hiccough and hysterical vomiting.

Mind.—Changeable mood; introspective; silently brooding. Melancholic, sad, tearful. Not communicative. *Sighing and sobbing.* After shocks, grief, disappointment.

Head.—Feels hollow, heavy; *worse, stooping.* Headache as if a nail were driven out through the side. Cramp-like pain over root of nose. Congestive headaches following anger or grief; *worse, smoking or smelling tobacco*, inclines head forward.

Eyes.—*Asthenopia*, with spasms of lids and neuralgic pain about eyes. [*Nat. m.*] Flickering zigzags.

Face.—*Twitching of muscles* of face and lips. Changes color when at rest.

Mouth.—*Sour taste.* Easily bites inside of cheeks. Constantly full of saliva. Toothache; worse after drinking coffee and smoking.

Throat.—Feeling of a lump in throat that cannot be swallowed. Tendency to choke, globus hystericus. Sore throat; stitches when not swallowing; better, eating something solid. Stitches between acts of swallowing. Stitches extend to ear. [*Hep.*] Tonsils inflamed, swollen, *with small ulcers*. *Follicular tonsillitus*.

Stomach.—Sour eructation. All-gone feeling in stomach; *much flatulence;* hiccough. Cramps in stomach; worse slightest contact. Averse to ordinary diet; longs for great variety of indigestible articles. Craving for acid things. *Sinking in stomach, relieved by taking a deep breath*.

Abdomen.—Rumbling in bowels. Weak feeling in upper abdomen. Throbbing in abdomen. [*Aloe; Sang.*] Colicky, griping pains in one or both sides of abdomen.

Rectum.—Itching and stitching up the rectum. *Prolapse*. Stools pass with difficulty; *painful constriction of anus after stool*. Stitches in hæmorrhoids during cough. Diarrhœa from fright. Stitches from anus deep into rectum. Hæmorrhage and pain; worse when stool is loose. *Pressure as of a sharp instrument from within outward*.

Urine.—Profuse, watery. [*Phos. ac.*]

Respiratory.—Dry, spasmodic cough in quick successive shocks. Spasm of glottis [*Calc.*] Reflex coughs. Coughing increases the desire to cough. *Much sighing*. Hollow spasmodic cough, worse in the evening, little expectoration, leaving pain in trachea.

Female.—Menses, *black*, too early, too profuse, or scanty. During menses great languor, with spasmodic pains in stomach and abdomen. Feminine sexual frigidity. Suppression from grief.

Extremities.—Jerking of limbs. Pain in tendo-Achilles and calf. Ulcerative pain in soles.

Sleep.—Very light. Jerking of limbs on going to sleep. Insomnia from grief, cares, with itching of arms and violent yawning. Dreams continuing a long time; troubling him.

Fever.—Chill, with thirst; not relieved by external heat. During fever, itching; nettle-rash all over body.

Skin.—Itching, nettle-rash. Very sensitive to draught of air. Excoriation, especially around vagina and mouth.

Modalities.—*Worse*, in the morning, open air, after meals, *coffee*, smoking, liquids, external warmth. *Better*, while eating, change of position.

Relationship.—Compare: *Zinc.; Kali phos.; Sep.; Cimicif. Panacea arvensis*—Poor man's Mercury—(Sensitiveness over gastric region with hunger but an aversion to food).

Complementary: *Nat. mur.*

Incompatible: *Coffea; Nux; Tabac.*

Antidotes: *Puls.; Cham.; Cocc.*

Dose.—Sixth, to 200th potency.

ILLICIUM
(Anise)

Should be remembered in the treatment of flatulent conditions. So-called three-months' colic, especially if it recurs at regular hours; much rumbling in abdomen. One symptom is worthy of special remembrance—*pain in region of third rib*, about an inch or two from the sternum, generally on right side, but occasionally on left. Frequent cough with this pain. Purulent tracheal and gastric catarrh of old drunkards. Old asthmatics. Vomiting, epileptiform convulsions with biting of tongue.

Nose.—Sharp stitches beneath lip. Acute catarrh. Burning and numbness of inner lower lip.

Respiratory.—Dyspnœa. Pain near third intercostal cartilage. Cough, with pus-like phlegm. Palpitation, with aphthæ. Hæmoptysis.

Dose.—Third potency.

ILEX AQUIFOLIUM
(American Holly)

Intermittent fever. Marked eye symptoms, spleen pain. All symptoms better in winter.

Eye.—Infiltration of cornea; staphyloma; nightly burning in orbits, rheumatic inflammation of eye; psilosis.

Relationship.—*Ilex Paraguayensis*—Yerba Mate—(Persistent epigastric pain; sense of dryness of mouth and pharynx, anorexia, pyrosis, nervous depression, neurasthenia. Somnolence; incapacity for work, diminution of urinary secretion, headache and pruritus. Hemicrania. Renal colic. Is said to be of use as a prophylactic against sunstroke, being a safe stimulant to the circulation, to diaphoresis and diuresis.) *Ilex vomitoria*—Yaupon—(Emetic properties—Possesses also tonic and digestive qualities, free from sleepless effects. Has an active principle said to act as a powerful diuretic—employed in nephritis and gout). *Ilex Cassine*—(Christmas berry Tea)—Excellent diuretic and substitute for tea.

INDIGO

(Indigo—Dye-stuff)

Marked action on the nervous system, and of undoubted benefit in the treatment of epilepsy with great sadness. Excited mood and desire to be busy. Neurasthenia and hysteria. Pure powdered Indigo placed on the wound cures snake and spider poison. [*Kali permang.; Golondrina; Cedron.*] Stricture of œsophagus; blue color. [*Cupr.*]

Head.—Vertigo with nausea. Convulsions. Sensation of a band around forehead. Undulating sensation through whole head. Sensation as if brain were frozen. Gloomy; cries at night. Hair feels pulled from vertex. Head feels frozen.

Nose.—Excessive sneezing and bleeding from nose.

Ears.—Pressure and roaring.

Stomach.—Metallic taste. *Eructations.* Bloating. Anorexia. Flushes of heat rising from stomach to head.

Rectum.—Falling of rectum. Aroused at night with horrible itching at anus.

Urinary.—Constant desire to urinate. Urine turbid. Catarrh of bladder.

Extremities.—*Sciatica.* Pain from middle of thigh to knee. Boring pain in knee-joint; better, walking. *Pain in limbs worse after every meal.*

Nerves.—Hysterical symptoms where pain predominates. Excessive nervous irritation. Epilepsy; flashes of heat from abdomen to head; fit begins with dizziness. Aura from a painful spot between shoulders. Reflex spasms from worms.

Modalities.—*Worse*, during rest and sitting. *Better*, pressure, rubbing, motion.

Relationship.—Compare: *Cuprum; Œstrus cameli*, an Indian medicine for epilepsy.

Dose.—Third to thirtieth potency.

INDIUM
(The Metal Indium)

Headaches and migraine. Seminal emissions. *Backache.*

Head.—Pain in head when straining at stool. Bursting in head during stool. Dull pains in temples and forehead, *with nausea*, weakness, *sleepiness.* Gone feeling in stomach about 11 a. m. Violent attack of sneezing. Sexual psychopathy.

Face.—Painful suppurating pimples. Corners of mouth cracked and sore. [*Condur.*]

Male.—Horribly offensive smell of urine after standing a short time. Emissions too frequent. Diminished power. Testicles tender; drawing pains along spermatic cord.

Throat.—Uvula enlarged, ulcerated; thick, tough mucus in back part of pharynx. Worse evening.

Extremities.—Stiffness in neck and shoulders. Pain, especially in left arm. Legs restless and weary. Toes itch. [*Agar.*

Dose.—Sixth to 200th potency.

Relationship.—Compare: *Selenium; Titanium* (male sexual organs).

INDOL
(A Crystalline Compound Derivable from Indigo, but also a product of Putrefaction of Proteids)

Primary action is to increase the elimination of Indican. Auto-intoxication. Compare: *Skatol.*

Persistent desire to sleep, dull, discontented mental state, hideous delusions and nervousness, constant motion of fingers and feet. Intestinal putrefaction.

Head.—Dull occipital and frontal headache in afternoon. Dull sensation over eyes. Eyeballs hot and hurt when moved. Pupils dilated with headache.

Stomach.—Bloated feeling. Hungry sensation after full meal. Great thirst. Constipation.

Extremities.—Very tired and sore in lower limbs. Feet burn. Knee-joints sore.

Sleep.—*Sleepiness.* Continuous dreaming.

Dose.—Sixth attenuation.

INSULIN

(An active principle from the pancreas which affects sugar metabolism.)

Besides the use of Insulin in the treatment of diabetes, restoring the lost ability to oxidize carbohydrate and again storing glycogen in the liver, some use of it homœopathically has been made by Dr. Wm. F. Baker, showing its applicability in acne, carbuncles, erythema with itching eczema. In the gouty, transitory glycosuria when skin manifestations are persistent give three times daily after eating. Given a persistent case of skin irritation, boils or varicose ulceration with polyuria, it is indicated.

Dose.—3x to 30x.

INULA
(Scabwort)

A mucous membrane medicine. Bearing-down sensations in pelvic organs and bronchial symptoms are most marked. Substernal pain. Diabetes.

Head.—Vertigo on stooping; throbbing after eating, pressure in temples and forehead.

Respiratory.—Dry cough; worse at night and lying down; larynx painful. Chronic bronchitis; cough, with much thick expectoration, with languor and weak digestion. Stitches behind sternum. Teasing cough with much and free expectoration. Palliative in tubercular laryngitis.

Female.—Menses too early and painful. Labor-like pains; urging to stool; dragging in genitals, with violent backache. Itching of legs during menses, chattering of teeth from cold during menstruation. Moving about in abdomen, stitches in genitals. Chronic metritis.

Rectum.—Pressing toward rectum as of something extruding.

Urinary.—Frequent urging to urinate; passes only in drops. Violet odor. [*Tereb.*]

Extremities.—Pain in right shoulder and wrist; tearing in left palm, unable to double fingers; pain in lower limbs, feet and ankles.

Relationship.—Compare: *Crocus; Ignatia; Arum dracontium* (loose cough worse at night on lying down).

Dose.—First to third potency.

IODOFORMUM
(Iodoform)

Should not be forgotten in the treatment of tubercular meningitis, both as a local application to the head and internally. [*Bacil.*] *Tuberculous conditions.* Subacute and chronic diarrhœa of children.

Head.—Sharp, neuralgic pain. Head feels heavy, as if it could not be lifted from pillow. Itching of occiput. *Meningitis.* Sleep interrupted by sighing and cries. Very drowsy.

Eyes.—Pupils, *dilated;* contract unequally, react poorly. Diplopia. Failing sight due to retro-bulbar neuritis, central scotoma—partial atrophy of optic disc.

Chest.—Sore pain in apex of right lung. Feeling of a weight on chest, as if smothering. Cough and wheezing on going to bed. Pain in left breast, like a hand grasping at the base of the heart. Hæmoptysis. Asthmatic breathing.

Abdomen.—Scaphoid abdomen. Chronic diarrhœa with suspected tuberculosis. Abdomen distended; mesenteric glands enlarged. *Cholera infantum. Chronic diarrhœa; stools greenish, watery, undigested, with irritable temper.*

Extremities.—Legs weak; cannot stand and walk with eyes closed. Weakness of knees when going upstairs.

Dose.—Second trituration. Three grains on the back of the tongue will relieve attack of asthmatic breathing.

IODUM
(Iodine)

Rapid metabolism: *Loss of flesh* with great appetite. Hungry with much thirst. Better after eating. *Great debility, the slightest effort induces perspiration.* Iod. individual is exceedingly thin, dark complexioned, with enlarged lymphatic glands, has voracious appetite but gets thin. Tubercular type.

All glandular structures, respiratory organs, circulatory system are especially affected; they atrophy. Iodine arouses the defensive apparatus of the system by assembling the mononuclear leucocytes whose phagocytic action is marked, at a given point. Lead poisoning. Tremor. Iodine craves cold air.

Acute exacerbation of chronic inflammation. Arthritis deformans. *Acts prominently on connective tissue. The plague. Goitre.* Abnormal vaso-constriction; capillary congestion followed by œdema, ecchymosis, hæmorrhages, and nutritive disturbances are the pathological conditions at the basis of its symptomatology. Sluggish vital reaction, hence chronicity in many of its aspects. Acute catarrh of all mucous membranes, rapid emaciation, notwithstanding good appetite, and glandular atrophy call for this remedy, in numerous wasting diseases and in scrofulous patients. Acute affections of the respiratory organs. *Pneumonia,* rapid extension. Iodine is warm, and wants cool surroundings. Weakness and loss of breath going upstairs. *Adenoid vegetations.* Tincture internally and locally to swollen glands and rattlesnake bites.

Mind.—Anxiety *when quiet. Present* anxiety and depression, no reference to the future. Sudden impulse to run and do violence. Forgetful. Must be busy. Fear of people, shuns every one. Melancholy. Suicidal tendency.

Head.—Throbbing; *rush of blood,* and feeling of a tight band. Vertigo; worse from stooping, worse in warm room. Chronic, congestive headache of old people. [*Phos.*]

Eyes.—Violent lachrymation. Pain in eyes. Pupil dilated. Constant motion of eyeballs. *Acute dacryocystitis.*

Nose.—Sneezing. Sudden violent influenza. Dry coryza becomes fluent in open air, also a *fluent hot coryza* with general heat of skin. Pain at root of nose and frontal sinus. Nose stopped up. Tendency to ulceration. Loss of smell. *Acute nasal engorgement* associated with high blood pressure.

Mouth.—Gums loose and bleed easily. Foul ulcers and salivation. Profuse, fetid ptyalism. Tongue thickly coated. Offensive odor from mouth.

Throat.—Larynx feels constricted. *Eustachian deafness.* Thyroid enlarged. Goitre, with sensation of constriction. Swollen submaxillary glands. Uvula swollen.

Stomach.—Throbbing at pit of stomach. *Ravenous hunger* and much thirst. Empty eructations, as if every particle of food were turned into gas. Anxious and worried if he does not eat. [*Cina; Sulph.*] Loses flesh, yet hungry and eating well. [*Abrot.*]

Abdomen.—Liver and spleen sore and enlarged. Jaundice. Mesenteric glands enlarged. Pancreatic disease. Cutting pain in abdomen.

Stool.—Hæmorrhage at every stool. Diarrhœa, whitish, frothy, fatty. Constipation, with ineffectual urging; better by drinking cold milk. Constipation alternating with diarrhœa. [*Ant. cr.*]

Urine.—Frequent and copious, *dark yellow-green (Bovista)*, thick, acrid with cuticle on surface.

Male.—Testicles swollen and indurated. Hydrocele. Loss of sexual power, with atrophied testes.

Female.—Great weakness during menses. [*Alum.; Carbo an.; Coccul.; Hæmatox.*] Menstruation irregular. Uterine hæmorrhage. Ovaritis. [*Apis; Bell.; Lach.*] *Wedge-like pain from ovary to uterus. Dwindling of mammary glands.* Nodosities in skin of mammæ. Acrid leucorrhœa, thick, slimy, corroding the linen. *Wedge-like pain in the right ovarian region.*

Respiratory.—Hoarse. *Raw* and tickling feeling provoking a dry cough. *Pain in larynx.* Laryngitis, with painful roughness; worse during cough. Child grasps throat when coughing. Right-sided pneumonia with high temperature. Difficult expansion of chest, blood-streaked sputum; internal dry heat, external coldness. Violent heart action. Pneumonia. Hepatization spreads rapidly with persistent high temperature; absence of pain in spite of great involvement, worse warmth; craves cool air Croup in scrofulous children with dark hair and eyes. [*Brom.* opposite.] Inspiration difficult. Dry, morning cough, from tickling in larynx. *Croupy cough*, with difficult respiration; wheezy. *Cold extends downwards* from head to throat and bronchi. Great weakness about chest. Palpitation from least exertion. Pleuritic effusion. Tickling all over chest. Iod. cough is worse indoors, in warm, wet weather, and when lying on back.

Heart.—Heart feels squeezed. Myocarditis, painful compression around heart. Feels as if squeezed by an iron hand [*Cactus*] followed by great weakness and faintness. Palpitation from least exertion. Tachycardia.

Extremities.—Joints inflamed and painful. Pain in bones at night. White swelling. Gonorrhœal rheumatism. Rheumatism of nape and upper extremities. Cold hands and feet. Acrid sweat of feet. Pulsation in large arterial trunks. Rheumatic pains, nightly pains in joints; constrictive sensations.

Skin.—Hot, dry, yellow and withered. Glands enlarged. Nodosities. Anasarca of cardiac disease.

Fever.—Flushes of heat all over body. Marked fever, restlessness, red cheeks, apathetic. Profuse sweat.

Modalities.—*Worse*, when quiet, in warm room, right side. *Better*, walking about, in open air.

Relationship.—Yatren. Iod. pathogenesis is similar to that of *Carbol. acid.* Antidotes: *Hepar; Sulph.; Gratiola.*

Complementary: *Lycopod.; Badiaga.*

Compare: *Brom.; Hepar; Mercur.; Phosph.; Abrot; Nat. mur.; Sanic.; Tuber.*

Dose.—The crude drug in saturated solution may be required. Third to thirtieth potency. Ioduretted solution of Potass. iod. (35 grains Potassa and 4 grains Iodine to 1 oz. of water, 10 drops three times a day) expels tapeworms dead.

Locally the most powerful, least harmful and easily managed microbicide. Ideal agent to keep wounds clean and disinfected. Bites of insects, reptiles, etc. Gunshot wounds and compound fractures, excellent. Great skin disinfectant.

IPECACUANHA
(Ipecac-root)

The chief action is on the ramifications of the pneumogastric nerve, producing spasmodic irritation in chest and stomach. Morphia habit. The principal feature of Ipecacuanha is its *persistent nausea* and vomiting, which form the chief guiding symptoms. Indicated after indigestible food, raisins, cakes, etc. Especially indicated in fat children and adults, who are feeble and catch cold in relaxing atmosphere; warm, moist weather. Spasmodic affections. Hæmorrhages *bright-red* and *profuse*.

Mind.—Irritable; holds everything in contempt. Full of desires, for what they know not.

Head.—Bones of skull feel crushed or bruised. Pain extends to teeth and root of tongue.

Eyes.—Inflamed, red. Pain through eyeballs. Profuse lachrymation. Cornea dim. Eyes tire from near vision. State of vision constantly changing. Spasm of accommodation from irritable weakness of the ciliary muscle. Nausea from looking on moving objects.

Face.—Blue rings around eyes. Periodical orbital neuralgia, with lachrymation, photophobia, and smarting eyelids.

Nose.—Coryza, with stoppage of nose and nausea. Epistaxis.

Stomach.—*Tongue usually clean.* Mouth, moist; *much saliva. Constant nausea* and vomiting, with pale, twitching of face. Vomits food, bile, blood, mucus. Stomach feels relaxed, as if hanging down. Hiccough.

Abdomen.—Amebic dysentery with tenesmus; while straining pain so great that it nauseates; little thirst. Cutting, clutching; *worse, around the navel* Body rigid; stretched out stiff.

Stools.—Pitch-like, green as grass, *like frothy molasses*, with griping at navel. Dysenteric, slimy.

Female.—Uterine hæmorrhage, *profuse, bright, gushing, with nausea.* Vomiting during pregnancy Pain from navel to *uterus.* Menses too early and too profuse.

Respiratory.—Dyspnœa; constant *constriction in chest.* Asthma. Yearly attacks of difficult shortness of breathing. Continued sneezing; coryza; wheezing cough. *Cough incessant and violent, with every breath.* Chest seems full of phlegm, but does not yield to coughing. Bubbling rales. Suffocative cough; child becomes stiff, and blue in the face. Whooping-cough, with nosebleed, and from mouth. Bleeding from lungs, *with nausea;* feeling of constriction; rattling cough. Croup. Hæmoptysis from slightest exertion. [*Millef.*] *Hoarseness,* especially at end of a cold. Complete aphonia.

Fever.—Intermittent fever, irregular cases, after Quinine. *Slightest chill* with *much* heat, *nausea,* vomiting, and dyspnœa. Relapses from improper diet.

Sleep.—With eyes half open. Shocks in all limbs on going to sleep. [*Ign.*]

Extremities.—Body stretched stiff, followed by spasmodic jerking of arms towards each other.

Skin.—Pale, lax. Blue around eyes. Miliary rash.

Modalities.—*Worse,* periodically; from veal, moist warm wind, lying down.

Relationship.—Compare: *Emetine*—principal alkaloid of Ipecac. (A powerful amebicide, but is not a bactericide. Specific for amæbiasis; of remarkable value in treatment of amæbic dysentery; also as a remedy in pyorrhœa, ½ gr. daily for three days, then less. Emetin, ½ gr. hypodermically, in Psoriasis. Emetin hydroch. 2x, diarrhœa with colicky, abdominal pains and nausea. Emetin for endamœbic dysentery. In physiological doses must be carefully watched. May produce hepatization of lungs, rapid heart action, tendency for the head to fall forward and lobar pneumonia. In hæmetemesis and other hæmorrhages, compare: *Gelatin* (which has a marked effect on the coagulability of the blood. Hypodermically; or if by mouth, a 10 per cent. jelly, about 4 oz., three times a day). *Arsenic; Cham.; Puls.; Tart. em.; Squill. Convolvulus* (colic and diarrhœa). *Typha latifolia*—Cat-tail flag (dysentery, diarrhœa) and summer complaint. *Euphorbia hypericifolia*—Garden Spurge—(Very similar to Ipecac. Irritation of the respiratory and gastro-intestinal tracts and female organs).

Lippia mexicana—(Persistent dry, hard, bronchial cough—asthma and chronic bronchitis).

In Asthma, compare: *Blatta orientalis*.

Antidotes: *Arsenic; China; Tabac*.

Complementary: *Cuprum; Arn*.

Dose.—Third to 200th potency.

IRIDIUM
(The Metal)

Intestinal putrefaction and septicæmia. *Anæmia*, increases red corpuscles. Epilepsy; lupus. Rheumatism and gout. Uterine tumors. Spinal paresis. *Exhaustion after disease*. Children who are puny, weak-limbed, and grow too fast. Nephritis of pregnancy.

Head.—Difficult concentration of thought. Sensation as if mind were void. Though confused. "Woodeny" feeling in right side of head. Right side of scalp sensitive. Profuse, watery coryza, better indoors. Ozæna.

Respiratory.—Hoarse cough, worse talking; posterior nares feel raw, inflamed, profuse, thick, yellowish discharge. Chronic laryngeal catarrh.

Back and Extremities.—Weakness in the kidney region. Spinal paresis, especially for the aged and after disease. Pressing in groin and left thigh. Tension in both thighs, especially left. Dislocated feeling in left hip-joint and dull pain toward left gluteal region.

Relationship.—Compare: *Iridium chloride*. (Produces salivation and stiffness of jaws followed by head and nervous symptoms. Congestion of nares and bronchi. Dragging pain in lower back. Headache worse right side, heavy feeling as of liquid lead.)

Compare: *Platina; Palladium; Osmium*.

Dose.—Sixth and higher.

IRIS VERSICOLOR
(Blue Flag)

Thyroid, *pancreas*, salivary, intestinal glands, and **gastro** intestinal mucous membrane, are especially affected. **Increases** the flow of bile. Sick headaches and cholera morbus are a special therapeutic field for its action.

Head.—Frontal headache, with nausea. Scalp feels constricted. Right temples especially affected. Sick headache, worse rest; begins with a blur before eyes, after relaxing from a mental strain. Pustular eruption on scalp.

Ears.—Roaring, buzzing, *ringing* in ears, with deafness. Aural vertigo, with intense noises in ears.

Face.—Neuralgia after breakfast, beginning in infra-orbital nerve, and involving whole face.

Throat.—Mouth and tongue feel scalded. Heat and smarting in throat. *Burning.* Profuse flow of saliva; ropy. *Goitre.*

Stomach.—*Burning of whole alimentary canal. Vomiting,* sour, bloody, biliary. Nausea. Profuse flow of saliva. [*Merc.; Ipec.; Kali iod.*] *Deficient appetite.*

Abdomen.—Liver sore. Cutting pain. Flatulent **colic.** Diarrhœa; stools watery, with *burning at anus* and through intestinal canal. Periodical night diarrhœa, with pain and green discharges. *Constipation* (give 30th).

Extremities.—Shifting pains. Sciatica, as if left hip-joint were wrenched. Pain extends to popliteal space. Gonorrhœal rheumatism (use *Irisin*).

Skin.—Herpes zoster, associated with gastric derangements. Pustular eruptions. Psoriasis; irregular patches with shining scales. Eczema, with nightly itching.

Modalities.—*Worse*, in evening and at night, from rest. *Better*, from continued motion.

Relationship.—Antidote: *Nux.*

Compare: *Iris florentina*—Orris-root—(delirium, convulsions, and paralysis); *Iris factissima* (headache and hernia); *Iris germanica*—Blue Garden Iris—(dropsy and freckles); *Iris tenax*—*I. minor*—(dry mouth; deathly sensation at point of stomach, *pain in ileo-cæcal region;* appendicitis. Pain from adhesions after). *Pancreatinum*—a combination of several enzymes—(Indicated in intestinal indigestion; pain an hour or more after eating. Lienteric diarrhœa. Dose.—3-5 grains, better not given during the active period of stomachic digestion). *Pepsinum*—(Imperfect digestion with pain in gastric region. Marasmus of children who are fed on artificial foods. Diarrhœa due to indigestion. Dose.—3-4 grains). (Diseases of pancreas, gout, diabetes); *Ipec.; Podoph.; Sanguin.; Ars.; Ant. cr.*

Dose.—Tincture to thirtieth potency. Favorable reports from the very highest potencies.

JACARANDA
(Brazilian Caroba-tree)

Has reputation as a remedy in venereal diseases and rheumatism. Morning sickness. The urinary and sexual symptoms are important. Rheumatic symptoms.

Head.—Vertigo on rising, with heavy forehead. Eyes pain; are inflamed and watery. Coryza with heavy head.

Throat.—Sore, dry, constricted. Vesicles in pharynx.

Urinary.—Urethra inflamed; discharge of yellow matter.

Male.—Heat and pain in penis; painful erections; phimosis. Prepuce painful and swollen. Chancroid. Chordee. Itching pimples on glans and prepuce.

Extremities.—Rheumatic pain in right knee. Weakness of lumbar region. Morning soreness and stiffness of muscles. Gonorrhœal rheumatism. Itching pimples on hands. Gonorrhœal and syphilitic arthritis.

Relationship.—Compare: *Thuja; Corallium; Jacaranda Gualandai* (in syphilitic symptoms, especially of eye and throat. Chancroids; *atonic ulcers*. Dark, painless diarrhœa).

Dose.—Tincture, to third potency.

JALAPA—EXOGONIUM PURGA
(Jalap)

Causes and cures colic and diarrhœa. The child is good all day, but screams and is restless and troublesome at night.

Gastro-intestinal.—Tongue, smooth, glazed, dry, smarting.— Pain in right hypochondrium. Flatulence and nausea. Pinching and griping. Watery diarrhœa; thin, muddy stools. Abdomen distended. Face cold and blue. Anus sore.

Extremities.—Aching in arms and legs. Pain in large joint of great toe. Smarting at root of nail. Burning of soles.

Relationship.—Antidotes: *Elater.; Cann. sat.*

Compare: *Camph.; Colocy.*

Dose.—Third to twelfth potency.

JATROPHA
(Purging Nut)

Of value in cholera and diarrhœa. The abdominal symptoms are most important. Suppressed measles (H. Farrington).

Stomach.—Hiccough, followed by copious vomiting. Nausea and vomiting, brought on by drinking, with acrid feeling from throat. Great thirst. *Very easy vomiting.* Heat and burning in stomach, with crampy, constrictive pain in epigastrium.

Abdomen.—Distended, with gurgling noises. Pain in hypochondria. Pain in region of liver and under right scapula to shoulder. Violent urging to urinate.

Stool.—Sudden, profuse, watery, like rice-water. *Diarrhœa; forced discharge; loud noise in abdomen like gurgling of water coming out of a bung-hole,* associated with coldness, cramps, nausea, and vomiting.

Extremities.—Cramps in muscles, especially calves, legs, and feet. *Coldness* of whole body. Pain in ankles, feet and toes. Heels sensitive.

Modalities.—*Better,* by placing hands in cold water.

Relationship.—Compare: *Camph.; Verat.; Gambog.; Croton.; Jatropha urens*—Sponge-nettle—(œdema and cardiac paresis).

Dose.—Third to thirtieth potency.

JEQUIRITY—ARBRUS PRECATORIUS
(Crab's Eye Vine)

Epithelioma, lupus, ulcers, granular lids.

Eyes.—Purulent conjunctivitis; inflammation spreads to face and neck. Granular ophthalmia. Keratitis.

Relationship.—Compare: *Jequiritol* (in cases of trachoma and pannus to engraft a new purulent inflammation. The proteid poisons contained in Jequirity seeds are almost identical in their physiological and toxic properties with the similar principles found in snake venom).

Dose.—Mother tincture diluted locally and 3x internally.

JONOSIA ASOCA
(Bark of an Indian Tree, introduced by
Dr. N. D. Ray, Calcutta)

Has extensive sphere of action on female organs. Amenorrhœa and metrorrhagia.

Head.—Unilateral headache; reflex uterine, congestive headache, better open air and by free flow. Pain in eyeballs; supraorbital pains, photophobia. Nasal catarrh, profuse, watery discharge. Loss of sense of smell.

Gastric.—Desire for sweets, also acid things. Thirsty, excessive nausea; obstinate constipation, hæmorrhoids.

Female.—Delayed and irregular menses; menstrual colic; amenorrhœa, pain in ovaries before flow; menorrhagia, irritable bladder; leucorrhœa.

Sleep.—Disturbed. Dreams of traveling.

Back.—Pain along spine radiating to abdomen and thighs.

Dose.—Tincture.

JUGLANS CINEREA
(Butternut)

A faulty elimination that produces jaundice and various skin eruptions, is pictured by this drug. The sharp, *occipital headache*, usually associated with liver disturbances, is very characteristic. Pain in chest, axilla and scapula, with suffocative sensation. Feeling as if all internal organs were too large, especially those of left side. Cholelithiasis.

Head.—Dull, full head. Eruption on scalp. *Sharp, occipital headache.* Head feels enlarged. Pustules on lids and around eyes.

Nose.—Tingling in nose; sneezing. Coryza, preceded by *pain under sternum*, with threatening suffocation. Later, copious, bland, thick mucous discharge.

Mouth.—Acrid feeling in mouth and throat. Soreness in region of tonsils externally. Dryness of root of tongue and fauces.

Stomach.—Atonic dyspepsia with much eructation and flatulent distention. Soreness in region of liver.

Back.—Muscles of neck rigid, lame. Pain between scapula and under right. Pain in lumbar vertebræ.

Skin.—Red, like flush of scarlatina. Jaundice, with pain about liver and right scapula. *Itching* and pricking when heated. *Pustules.* Eczema, especially on lower extremities, sacrum and hands. Erythema and erysipelatous redness.

Stool.—Yellowish-green, with tenesmus and burning at anus. Camp diarrhœa.

Modalities.—*Better*, getting heated, exercise, scratching, on rising in morning. *Worse*, walking.

Relationship.—Compare: *Juglandin* (duodenal catarrh; bilious diarrhœa); *Chelidon.; Bryon.; Iris.*

Dose.—Tincture, to third potency.

JUGLANS REGIA
(Walnut)

Skin eruptions are prominent.

Head.—Confused; feels as if head were floating in air. *Occipital sharp pain.* Styes.

Female.—Menses early, black, pitch-like coagula. Abdomen distended.

Skin.—Comedones and acne of the face. Crusta lactea, with soreness around ears. Itching and eruptions of small red pustules. Scalp red, and itches violently at night. Chancre-like ulcer. Axillary glands suppurate.

Relationship.—Compare: *Juglans cinerea.*

Dose.—Tincture, and lower potencies.

JUNCUS EFFUSUS
(Common Rush)

A diuretic. Urinary affections. Dysuria, strangury, and ischuria. *Asthmatic symptoms in hæmorrhoidal subjects.* Bubbling sensations. Abdominal flatulence. Arthritis and Lithiasis.

Dose.—Tincture, and first potency.

JUNIPERUS COMMUNIS
(Juniper Berries)

Catarrhal inflammation of kidneys. Dropsy, with suppression of urine. Old persons, with poor digestion and scanty secretion of urine. Chronic pyelitis.

Urinary.—Strangury; bloody, scanty urine, violet odor. [*Tereb.*] Weight in kidney region. Prostatic discharge. Renal hyperæmia. [*Eucalyptol.*]

Respiratory.—Cough with scanty, loaded urine.

Relationship.—Compare: *Sabina; Juniperus Virginianus*—Red Cedar—(Violent tenesmus vesical. Persistent dragging in back; hyperæmia of the kidneys; pyelitis and cystitis; dropsy of the aged with suppressed urine. Dysuria, burning, cutting pain in urethra when urinating. Constant urging apoplexy, convulsions, strangury, uterine hæmorrhage). *Terebinthina.*

Dose.—Best form is the infusion. One ounce to a pint of boiling water. Dose, one-half to two ounces, or tincture, one to ten drops.

JUSTICIA ADHATODA BASAKA
(An Indian Shrub, Singhee)

Highly efficacious medicine for acute catarrhal conditions of the respiratory tract (used in the beginning).

Head.—Irritable, sensitive to external impressions; hot, full and heavy head; lachrymation, with *coryza, profuse,* fluent, with constant sneezing; loss of smell and taste; *coryza with cough.*

Throat.—Dry, pain during empty swallowing, tenacious mucus. Mouth dry.

Respiratory.—Dry cough from sternal region all over chest. Hoarseness, larynx painful. *Paroxysmal cough*, with suffocative obstruction of respiration. *Cough with sneezing.* Severe dyspnœa with cough. *Tightness across chest.* Asthmatic attacks, cannot endure a close, warm room. *Whooping-cough.*

Relationship.—Seems to come between *Cepa* and *Euphrasia*, which compare.

Dose.—Third potency and higher. Severe aggravation have been noticed from lower potencies.

KALI ARSENICUM
(Fowler's Solution)

The *Kali ars.* patient tends towards malignancy, and inveterate skin diseases. He is restless, nervous and anemic.

Skin.—Intolerable itching, worse undressing. *Dry, scaly, wilted.* Acne; pustules worse during menses. Chronic eczema; itching worse *from warmth*, walking, undressing. *Psoriasis*, lichen. Phagedænic ulcers. Fissures in bends of arms and knees. Gouty nodosities; worse, change of weather. Skin cancer, where suddenly an alarming malignancy without any external signs sets in. Numerous small nodules under skin.

Female.—Cauliflower excrescences of os uteri, with flying pains, foul smelling discharge, and pressure below pubis.

Relationship.—*Radium.*

Dose.—Third to thirtieth potency.

KALI BICHROMICUM
(Bichromate of Potash)

The special affinities of this drug are the mucous membrane of stomach, bowels, and air-passages; bones and fibrous tissues. Kidneys, heart, and liver are also affected. Incipient parenchrymatous; nephritis. Nephritis with gastric disturbances. Cirrhosis of liver. Anæmia and absence of fever are characteristic. General weakness bordering on paralysis. It is especially indicated for fleshy, fat, light complexioned persons subject to catarrhs or with syphilitic or scrofulous history. Symptoms are worse in the morning; *pains migrate quickly,* rheumatic and gastric symptoms alternate. More adapted to subacute rather than the violent acute stage. Mucous membranes everywhere are affected. Catarrh of pharynx, larynx, bronchi and nose. and a *tough, stringy, viscid secretion* is produced, which condition is a very strong guiding symptom for this drug. *Perforation of the septum.* Chronic atonic catarrh. Polypus. Dilatation of stomach and heart.

Head.—Vertigo with nausea when rising from seat. Headache over *eyebrows,* preceded by blurred vision. *Aching and fullness in glabella.* Semilateral headache in small spots, and from suppressed catarrh. Frontal pain; usually over one eye. *Bones and scalp feel sore.*

Eyes.—Supra-orbital neuralgia, right side. Eyelids burn, swollen, œdematous. Discharge *ropy* and yellow. Ulcers on cornea; no pain or photophobia. *Descemetitis,* with only moderate irritation of eye. Croupous conjunctivitis; granular lids, with pannus. Iritis, with punctate deposits on inner surface of cornea. Slight pain, with severe ulceration or inflammation. [*Conium* opposite.]

Ears.—Swollen, with tearing pains. Thick, yellow, stringy, fetid discharge. Sharp stitches in left ear.

Nose.—Snuffles of children, *especially fat, chubby babies. Pressure and pain at root of nose,* and sticking pain in nose. *Septum ulcerated;* round ulcer. *Fetid smell. Discharge thick, ropy, greenish-yellow.* Tough, elastic plugs from nose; leave a raw surface. Inflammation extends to frontal sinuses, with distress and fullness at root of nose. Dropping from posterior nares. [*Hydr.*] *Loss of smell.* Much hawking. Inability to breathe through nose. Dryness. *Coryza, with obstruction* of nose. *Violent sneezing.* Profuse, watery nasal discharge. Chronic inflammation of frontal sinus with stopped-up sensation.

Face.—Florid complexion. Blotchy, red appearance. Acne. [*Juglans; Kal. ars.*] Bones sensitive, especially beneath orbits.

Mouth.—Dry; viscid saliva. Tongue mapped, *red, shining, smooth, and dry*, with dysentery; broad, flat, indented, thickly coated. Feeling of a hair on tongue.

Throat.—Fauces red and inflamed. Dry and rough. Parotid glands swollen. Uvula relaxed, *œdematous, bladder-like*. Pseudo-membranous deposit on tonsils and soft palate. Burning extending to stomach. Aphthæ. Diphtheria, with profound prostration and soft pulse. Discharge from mouth and throat, tough and stringy.

Stomach.—Nausea and vomiting after beer. Load immediately after eating. Feels as if digestion had stopped. Dilatation of stomach. Gastritis. *Round ulcer of stomach.* Stitches in region of liver and spleen and through to spine. Dislikes water. Cannot digest meat. Desire for beer and acids. Gastric symptoms are relieved after eating, and the rheumatic symptoms reappear. Vomiting of bright yellow water.

Abdomen.—Cutting pain in abdomen, soon after eating. Chronic intestinal ulceration. Soreness in right hypochondrium. fatty infiltration of liver and increase in soft fibrous tissue. Painful retraction, soreness and burning.

Stool.—Jelly-like, gelatinous; *worse, mornings*. Dysentery; tenesmus, stools brown, frothy. Sensation of a plug in anus. Periodic constipation, with pain across the loins, and brown urine.

Urinary.—Burning in urethra. *After urinating a drop seems to remain which cannot be expelled.* Ropy mucus in urine. Urethra becomes clogged up. Congestion of kidneys; nephritis, with scanty, albuminous urine and casts. Pyelitis; urine mixed with epithelial cells, mucus, pus, or blood. *Hæmatochyluria.*

Male.—Itching and pain of penis, with pustules. Ulcers, with paroxysmal stitches; aggravated at night. Constriction at root of penis, at night on awakening. Syphilitic ulcers, with cheesy, tenacious exudation. Erections. [*Picric. ac.*]

Female.—Yellow, tenacious leucorrhœa. Pruritus of vulva, with great burning and excitement. Prolapsus uteri; *worse in hot weather.*

Respiratory.—Voice hoarse; worse, evening. Metallic, hacking cough. *Profuse, yellow expectoration, very glutinous and sticky, coming out in long, stringy, and very tenacious mass.* Tickling in larynx. Catarrhal laryngitis cough has a brassy sound. True membranous croup, extending to larynx and nares. Cough, with pain in sternum, extending to shoulders; worse when undressing. Pain at bifurcation of trachea on coughing; from mid-sternum to back.

Heart.—Dilatation, especially from coexisting kidney lesion. Cold feeling around heart. [*Kali nit.*]

Back.—*Cutting through loins;* cannot walk; extends to groins. Pain in coccyx and sacrum extending up and down.

Extremities.—Pains fly rapidly from one place to another. [*Kali sulph.; Puls.*] Wandering pains, along the bones; worse cold. Left-sided sciatica; better, motion. Bones feel sore and bruised. *Very weak.* Tearing pains in tibia; syphilitic rheumatism. [*Mez.*] Pain, swelling and stiffness and crackling of all joints. Soreness of heels when walking. Tendo Achilles swollen and painful. Pains in small spots. [*Oxalic ac.*]

Skin.—Acne. Papular eruptions. *Ulcer with punched-out edges*, with tendency to penetrate and tenacious exudation. Pustular eruption, resembling small-pox, with burning pains. Itching with vesicular eruption.

Modalities.—*Better,* from heat. *Worse,* beer, morning, hot weather, undressing.

Relationship.—Compare: *Tari. emet.; Brom.; Hepar; Ind.; Calc.; Ant. cr.* In the production of false membranes compare: *Brom.; Ammon. caust.; Sulph. ac.; Ipecac*

Antidotes: *Ars.; Lach.*

Dose.—Third trituration, also thirtieth attenuation and higher.

The lower preparations of this salt should not be kept too long.

KALI BROMATUM
(Bromide of Potash)

Like all Potash Salts, this weakens the heart and lowers temperature. Brominism is caused by it. General failure of mental power, loss of memory, melancholia, anæsthesia of the

KALI BROMATUM

mucous membranes, especially of eyes, throat, and skin; acne; loss of sexual desire, paralysis. Leading remedy in psoriasis. Nodular form of chronic gout. *Symptoms of apoplectic attacks*, uræmic or otherwise; somnolence and stertor, convulsions, aphasia, albuminaria. Epilepsy (with salt-free diet).

Mind.—Profound, melancholic delusion; feeling of moral deficiency; religious depression; delusions of conspiracies against him. Imagines he is singled out as an object of divine wrath. Loss of memory. Must do something—move about; gets fidgety. [*Tarant.*] Fear of being poisoned. [*Hyos.*] Amnesic aphasia; can pronounce any word told, but cannot speak otherwise. *Night terrors.* Horrid illusions. Active delirium.

Head.—Suicidal mania with tremulousness. Face flushed. *Numb feeling in head.* Brain-fag. Coryza with tendency to extension into throat.

Throat.—Congestion of uvula and fauces. *Anæsthesia* of fauces, pharynx, and larynx. Dysphagia, especially of liquids. [*Hyos.*]

Stomach.—Vomiting, with *intense thirst*, after each meal. *Persistent hiccough.* [*Sulph. ac.*]

Abdomen.—Sensation as if bowels were falling out. *Cholera infantum*, with reflex cerebral irritation, jerking and twitching of muscles. Green, watery stools with intense thirst, vomiting, eyes sunken. Prostration. *Internal coldness* of abdomen. Diarrhœa, with much blood. Green, watery stools. *Retraction* of abdomen.

Urinary.—Sensibility of urethra diminished. Urine profuse, with thirst. Diabetes. [*Phos. ac.*]

Male.—Debility and impotence. Effects of sexual excesses, especially loss of memory, impaired co-ordination, numbness and tingling in limbs. Sexual excitement during partial slumber.

Female.—Pruritus. Ovarian neuralgia with great nervous uneasiness. *Exaggerated sexual* desire. Cystic tumors of ovaries.

Respiratory.—Spasmodic croup. Reflex cough during pregnancy. Dry, fatiguing, hacking cough at night.

Extremities.—*Fidgety hands;* busy twitching of fingers. Jerking and twitching of muscles.

Skin.—*Acne* of face, pustules. Itching; worse on chest, shoulders, and face. Anæsthesia of skin. *Psoriasis.*

Sleep.—Restless sleep. Extreme drowsiness. Sleeplessness due to worry and grief and sexual excess. Night terrors. Grinding teeth in sleep. Horrible dreams. Somnambulism.

Modalities.—*Better,* when occupied mentally or physically.

Dose.—A few grains of the crude salt to the third trituration. Remember the unstable character of this salt. Said to be much more active if salt is eliminated from the diet.

KALI CARBONICUM
(Carbonate of Potassium)

The weakness characteristic of all Potassium Salts is seen especially in this, with soft pulse, coldness, general depression, and very characteristic *stitches,* which may be felt in any part of the body, or in connection with any affection. All Kali pains are *sharp and cutting;* nearly all better by motion. Never use any Salts of Potash where there is fever (T. F. Allen). Sensitive to every atmospheric change, and *intolerance of cold weather.* One of the best remedies following labor. Miscarriage, for consequent debilitated states. Early morning aggravation is very characteristic. Fleshy aged people, with dropsical and paretic tendencies. *Sweat, backache, and weakness.* Throbbing pains. Tendency to dropsy. Tubercular diathesis. Pains from within out, and of stinging character. "Giving-out" sensation. Fatty degenerations. Stinging pains in muscles and internal parts. Twitching of muscles. Pain in small spot on left side Hypothyroidism. Coxitis.

Mind.—Despondent. Alternating moods. *Very irritable.* Full of fear and imaginations. Anxiety felt in stomach. Sensation as if bed were sinking. Never wants to be left alone. Never quiet or contented. Obstinate and *hypersensitive* to pain, noise, touch.

Head.—Vertigo on turning. Headache *from riding in cold wind.* Headache comes on with yawning. Stitches in temples; aching in occiput, one-sided, with nausea, on riding in carriage. Loose feeling in head. Great *dryness of hair;* falls out. [*Fluor ac.*

KALI CARBONICUM

Eyes.—Stitches in eyes. Spots, gauze, and black points before eyes. Lids stick together in morning. *Swelling over upper lid, like little bags.* Swelling of glabella between brows. Asthenopia. Weak sight from excessive sexual indulgence. On shutting eyes, painful sensation of light penetrating the brain.

Ears.—Stitches in ears. Itching, cracking, ringing and roaring.

Nose.—Nose *stuffs up in warm room.* Thick, fluent, yellow discharge. Post-nasal dropping. [*Spigel.*] Sore, scurfy nostrils; bloody nasal mucus. Crusty nasal openings. Nosebleed on washing face in morning. *Ulcerated nostrils.*

Mouth.—Gums separate from teeth; pus oozes out. Pyorrhœa. Aphthæ. Tongue white. Much saliva constantly in mouth. Bad, slimy taste.

Throat.—Dry, parched, rough. Sticking pain, as from a fish-bone. Swallowing difficult; food goes down œsophagus slowly. Mucous accumulation in the morning.

Stomach.—Flatulence. Desire for sweets. Feeling of lump in pit of stomach. Gagging. Dyspepsia of old people; burning acidity, bloating. Gastric disorders from ice-water. *Sour eructations. Nausea;* better lying down. Constant feeling as *if stomach were full of water.* Sour vomiting; throbbing and cutting in stomach. Disgust for food. *Anxiety felt in stomach.* Epigastrium sensitive externally. Easy choking when eating. Epigastric pain to back.

Abdomen.—Stitches in region of liver. Old chronic liver troubles, with soreness. Jaundice and dropsy. Distention and coldness of abdomen. Pain from left hypochondrium through abdomen; must turn on right side before he can rise.

Rectum.—*Large,* difficult stools, with stitching pain an hour before. Hæmorrhoids, large, swollen, painful. Itching, ulcerated pimples around anus. Large discharge of blood with natural stool. Pain in hæmorrhoids when coughing. Burning in rectum and anus. Easy prolapsus. [*Graph.; Pod.*] Itching. [*Ignat.*]

Urine.—Obliged to rise several times at night to urinate. Pressure on bladder long before urine comes. Involuntary urination when coughing, sneezing, etc.

Male.—Complaints from coition. Deficient sexual instinct. Excessive emissions, *followed by weakness*.

Female.—Menses early, profuse [*Calc. c.*] or *too late, pale and scanty*, with soreness about genitals; pains from back pass down through gluteal muscles, with cutting in abdomen. Pain through left labium, extending through abdomen to chest. Delayed menses in young girls, with chest symptoms or ascites. Difficult, first menses. *Complaints after parturition.* Uterine hæmorrhage; constant oozing after copious flow, with violent backache, relieved by sitting and pressure.

Respiratory.—Cutting pain in chest; worse lying on right side. Hoarseness and loss of voice. Dry, hard cough about 3 a. m., with *stitching pains* and dryness of pharynx. Bronchitis, *whole chest is very sensitive*. Expectoration scanty and tenacious, but *increasing* in morning and after eating; aggravated right lower chest and lying on painful side. *Hydrothorax.* Leaning forward relieves chest symptoms. Expectoration must be swallowed; cheesy taste; copious, offensive, lump. *Coldness of chest.* *Wheezing.* Cough *with relaxed uvula.* Tendency to tuberculosis; constant cold taking; *better in warm climate.*

Heart.—Sensation as if heart were suspended. Palpitation and *burning in heart region.* *Weak, rapid pulse; intermits,* due to digestive disturbance. Threatened heart failure.

Back.—Great exhaustion. Stitches in region of kidneys and right scapula. *Small of back feels weak.* Stiffness and paralytic feeling in back. Burning in spine. [*Guaco.*] Severe backache during pregnancy, and after miscarriage. Hip-disease. Pain in nates and thighs and hip-joint. Lumbago with sudden sharp pains extending up and down back and to thighs.

Extremities.—*Backs and legs give out.* Uneasiness, heaviness, and tearing in limbs and jerking. Tearing pain in limbs with swelling. Limbs sensitive to pressure. White swelling of knee. Tearing in arms from shoulder to wrist. Lacerating in wrist-joint. Paralysis of old people, and dropsical affections. Limbs go to sleep easily. Tips of toes and fingers painful. *Soles very sensitive.* Itching of great toe, with pain. *Pain from hip to knee. Pain in knees.*

Skin.—Burning as from a mustard plaster.

Sleep.—Drowsy after eating. Wakes about two o'clock and cannot sleep again.

Modalities.—*Worse*, after coition; in cold weather; from soup and coffee; in morning about three o'clock; lying on left and painful side. *Better*, in warm weather, though moist; during day, while moving about.

Relationship.—Complementary: *Carbo;* (Lowness of vitality may suggest a preliminary course of Carbo to nurse up recuperation to the point that Kali carb. would come in helpfully.) Follows *Nux* often in stomach and bladder troubles.

Compare: *Kali salicylicum* (vomiting, especially of pregnancy; arteriosclerosis, with chronic rheumatism); *Kali silicum* (gouty nodosities); *Kali aceticum* (diabetes, diarrhœa, dropsy, alkaline urine, very much increased in quantity); *Kali citricum* (Bright's disease—1 gr. to wine-glass of water); *Kali ferrocyanatum*—Prussian blue—(physical and mental prostration following infection. Inability to sustained routine work. Neuralgic affections depending on impoverished blood and exhausted nerve centers, especially spinal. Fatty and functional heart troubles. Pulse weak, small, irregular. Uterine symptoms, like Sepia, bearing-down sensation and gastric sinking; profuse, pus-like leucorrhœa and passive hæmorrhage); use 6x); *Kali oxalicum* (lumbago, convulsions); *Kali picro-nitricum* and *Kali picricum* (jaundice, violent eructations); *Kali tartaricum* (paraplegia); *Kali telluricum* (garlicky odor of breath, salivation, swollen tongue). Also compare: *Calc.; Ammon. phos.; Phos.; Lycop.; Bry.; Natrum; Stann.; Sepia.*

Antidotes: *Camph.; Coffea.*

Dose.—Thirtieth and higher. Sixth trit. Do not repeat too often. Use cautiously in old gouty cases, advanced Bright's and tuberculosis.

KALI CHLORICUM
(Chlorate of Potassium—K clo. 3)

Acts very destructively upon the kidneys, producing a croupous nephritis, hæmoglobinuria, etc. Parenchymatous nephritis with stomatitis. Produces most acute ulcerative and follicular stomatitis. *Noma. Toxæmic conditions of pregnancy* (urinary symptoms). *Chronic nephritis;* hepatitis. Septicæmia. Anemia.

Mouth.—Profuse secretion of acid saliva. Whole mucous surface red, tumid, with gray-based ulcers. Tongue swollen. *Stomatitis*—aphthous and *gangrenous.* Fetor. Mercurial stomatitis (as a mouth wash).

Stomach.—Feeling of weight in epigastric and umbilical region. Flatulence. Vomiting of greenish-black matter.

Stool.—Diarrhœa; profuse, greenish mucus.

Urine.—Albuminous, scanty, suppressed. Hæmaturia: diuresis. Nucleo-albumin and bile, high Phosphoric acid, with low total solids.

Skin.—Jaundice. Itching miliary or papular eruptions. Discolored; chocolate tint.

Dose.—Second to sixth potency. Use cautiously locally as it is poisonous.

KALI CYANATUM
(Potassium Cyanide)

Sudden sinking sensation. Cancer of tongue and agonizing neuralgia have been benefitted by this drug. Sick headache; sciatica; epilepsy.

Tongue.—Ulcer of tongue, with indurated edges. Speech difficult. Power of speech lost but intelligence intact.

Face.—Severe neuralgia in temporal region, recurring daily at same hour. Pain in orbital and supra-maxillary region, with screaming and loss of consciousness.

Respiratory.—Cough prevents sleep; respiration weak; cannot take deep breath.

Modalities.—*Worse,* from 4 a. m. to 4 p. m.

Relationship.—Compare: *Platin.; Stann.; Cedron; Mezer.; Mur. ac.*

Dose.—Sixth potency and 200th.

KALI HYDRIODICUM
(Iodide of Potassium)

The profuse, watery, acrid coryza that the drug produces serves as a sure guiding symptom, especially when associated with pain in frontal sinus. It acts prominently on fibrous and connective tissues, producing infiltration, œdema, etc. *Glandular swellings.* Purpura and hæmorrhagic diathesis. *Syphilis* may be indicated in all stages: 1. In acute form with evening remitting fever, going off in nightly perspiration. 2. Second stage, mucous membranes and skin ulcerations. 3. Tertiary symptoms; nodes. Give material doses. *Diffused sensitiveness*—(glands, scalp, etc. Rheumatism in *neck, back*, feet, especially heels and soles; worse, cold and wet. Iodide of Potass. in material doses acts in the different forms of Fungoid disease. (thrush, ringworm, etc.), offer simulating syphilis and bacterial diseases like tuberculosis. Symptoms like loss of weight, spitting of blood, etc. Tea-taster's cough due to inhaling the fungus; also brings about often favorable reaction in many chronic ailments even when not clearly symptomatically indicated.

Mind.—Sad, anxious; harsh temper. Irritable; congestion to head, heat and throbbing.

Head.—Pain through *sides* of head. Violent headache. Cranium swells up in hard lump. Pain intense over eyes and *root of nose*. Brain feels enlarged. Hard nodes, with severe pain. *Facial neuralgia.* Lancinating pain in upper jaw.

Nose.—Red, swollen. Tip of nose red; *profuse, acrid, hot, watery, thin discharge. Ozæna, with perforated septum.* Sneezing. Nasal catarrh, involving frontal sinus. Stuffiness and dryness of nose, without discharge. Profuse, *cool,* greenish, unirritating discharges.

Eyes.—Conjunctiva red, injected; profuse lachrymation. *Syphilitic iritis.* Pustular keratitis and chemosis. Bony tumors of the orbit.

Ear.—Noises in ear. Boring pain in ears.

Stomach.—Saliva increased. Faintness at epigastrium. Cold food and drink, especially milk, aggravate. Much thirst. Throbbing, painful burning. Flatulence.

Female.—Menses late, profuse. During menses uterus feels as if squeezed. Corrosive leucorrhœa, with subacute inflammatory conditions of the womb in young married women. Fibroid tumors, metritis, sub-involution, hypertrophy, 1x or 1 gr. crude, 3 times a day.

Respiratory.—Violent cough; worse in morning. Pulmonary

œdema. *Larynx feels raw.* Laryngeal œdema. Awakes choking. *Expectoration like soap-suds, greenish.* Pneumonia, when hepatization commences. *Pneumococcic meningitis.* Stitching pains through lungs to back. Asthma. Dyspnœa on ascending, with pain in heart. Hydrothorax. [*Merc. sulph.*] *Pleuritic effusion. Cold travels downward to chest.*

Extremities.—Severe bone-pains. Periosteum thickened, especially tibia; sensitive to touch. [*Kali b.; Asaf.*] Rheumatism; pains at night and in damp weather. Contraction of joints. *Rheumatism of knees with effusion.* Pain in small of back and coccyx. Pain in hip, forcing limping. *Sciatica;* cannot stay in bed; worse at night and lying on affected side. Formication of lower extremities when sitting, better lying down.

Skin.—Purple spots; worse on legs. Acne, hydroa. Small boils. *Glands* enlarged, indurated. Hives. *Rough nodules all over,* worse any covering; heat of body intense. Fissured anus of infants. Tendency to œdematous swellings, eyelids, mouth, uvula, etc. *Acne rosacea.*

Modalities.—*Worse,* warm clothing, warm room, at night, damp weather. *Better,* motion, open air.

Relationship.—Antidote: *Hepar.*

Compare: *Iod.; Mercur.; Sulph.; Mezer. Chopheenee,* a Hindoo remedy for syphilitic eruptions, ulcerations and bone-pains. Used in tincture.

Dose.—Crude drug, in material officinal dosage, but remember Dr. Meyhoffer's statements in his chronic diseases of organs of respiration: "From the moment the drug produces pathogenetic symptoms, it exaggerates the function of the tissue, exhausts the already diminished vitality, and thence, instead of stimulating the organic cell in the direction of life, impairs or abolishes its power of contraction. We use, as a rule, the first dilution from 6 to 20 drops a day; if after a week no decided progress is visible, one drop of the tincture of Iodine is added to each hundred of the first dilution. In this way, the mucous tubercles, gummy deposits and ulcerations resulting therefrom in the larynx undergo a favorable termination in laryngeal syphilis." When strictly homœopathically indicated, as in acute respiratory affections the third potency.

KALI MURIATICUM
Chloride of Potassium—(K. Cl.)

Although not proven, this remedy has a wide clinical use, through its introduction by Schuessler. It certainly is of great value in catarrhal affections, in sub-acute inflammatory states, fibrinous exudations, and glandular swellings. *White or gray coating of base of tongue*, and expectoration of thick, white phlegm, seem to be special guiding symptoms. Bursitis præpatellaris.

Head.—Imagines he must starve. Headache, with vomiting. Crusta lactea. Dandruff.

Eyes.—White mucus, purulent scabs. Superficial ulcer. Trachoma. Corneal opacities.

Ears.—*Chronic, catarrhal conditions of the middle ear*. Glands about the ear swollen. *Snapping and noises in the ear*. Threatened mastoid. Great effusion about the auricle.

Nose.—Catarrh; phlegm white, thick. Vault of pharynx covered with adherent crusts. Stuffy cold. Nosebleed. [*Arn.; Bry.*]

Face.—Cheek swollen and painful.

Mouth.—Aphthæ; thrush; white ulcers in mouth. Swollen glands about jaw and neck. Coating of tongue *grayish-white*, dryish, or slimy.

Throat.—*Follicular tonsillitis*. Tonsils inflamed; enlarged so much, can hardly breathe. Grayish patches or spots in the throat and tonsils. Adherent crusts in vault of pharynx. "Hospital" sore throat. Eustachian catarrh.

Stomach.—*Fatty or rich food causes indigestion*. Vomiting of white, opaque mucus; water gathers in the mouth. Pain in the stomach, with constipation. Bulimia; hunger disappears by drinking water.

Abdomen.—Abdominal tenderness and swelling. Flatulence. Thread-worms, causing itching at the anus.

Stool.—Constipation; light-colored stools. Diarrhœa, after fatty food; clay-colored, white, or slimy stools. Dysentery; purging, with slimy stools. *Hæmorrhoids;* bleeding; blood dark and thick; fibrinous, clotted.

Female.—Menstruation too late or suppressed, checked or too early; excessive discharge; *dark-clotted*, or tough, black blood, like tar. [*Plat.*] Leucorrhœa; discharge of milky-white mucus, thick, non-irritating, bland. Morning sickness, with vomiting of white phlegm. Bunches in breast feel quite soft and are *tender*.

Respiratory Organs.—Loss of voice; hoarseness. Asthma, with gastric-derangements; mucus white and hard to cough up. Loud, noisy stomach cough; cough short, acute, and spasmodic, like whooping-cough; expectoration thick and white. Rattling sounds of air passing through thick, tenacious mucus in the bronchi; difficult to cough up.

Back and Extremities.—Rheumatic fever; exudation and *swelling around the joints*. Rheumatic pains felt only during motion, or increased by it. Nightly rheumatic pains; worse from warmth of bed; lightning-like from small of back to feet; must get out of bed and sit up. Hands get stiff while writing.

Skin.—Acne, erythema, and eczema, with *vesicles* containing thick, white contents. Dry, flour-like scales on the skin. [*Arsenic.*] Bursitis.

Modalities.—*Worse*, rich food, fats, motion.

Relationship.—Compare: *Bellad.* which Kali mur. follows well in catarrhal and hypertrophic conditions. *Kino* (otorrhœa, with stitches in right ear); *Bry.; Mercur.; Puls.; Sulph.*

Dose.—Third to twelfth potency.

External use in skin affections with burning sensation.

KALI NITRICUM—NITRUM
(Nitrate of Potassium—Saltpeter)

Often indicated in asthma, also valuable in cardiac asthma; of great value in *sudden dropsical swellings over the whole body*. Gastro-intestinal inflammation, with much debility, and relapse in phthisis, call for this remedy. Suppurative nephritis.

Head.—Scalp very sensitive. Headache, with vertigo, as if falling to right side and backwards; worse, stooping. Ennui.

Eyes.—Vision becomes clouded. Turbid corpus vitreum. [*Arn.; Ham.; Solan. n.; Phos.*] Variegated-colored rings before eyes. Burning and lachrymation.

KALI NITRICUM

Nose.—Sneezing. Swollen feeling; *worse, right nostril.* Point red and itching. Polypus. [*Sang. nit.*]

Mouth.—Tongue red, with burning pimples; burns at tip. Throat constricted and sore.

Stool.—Thin, watery, bloody. Membranous shreds, with tenesmus. *Diarrhœa from eating veal.*

Female.—Menses too early, profuse, *black;* preceded and with violent backache. Leucorrhœa. Burning pains in the ovarian region only during menses. [*Zinc.* after.]

Respiratory.—Hoarseness. Dry, morning cough, with pain in chest and bloody expectoration. Bronchitis, with sharp, short, dry, hacking cough. *Asthma,* with excessive dyspnœa, nausea, dull stitches, and burning in chest. Dyspnœa so great that breath cannot be held long enough to drink, though thirsty. Chest feels constricted. Oppression worse in morning. Sour-smelling expectoration. Expectoration of clotted blood, after hawking mucus. Acute exacerbations in phthisis; congestion of lungs. *Spasmodic croup;* paroxysm of crowing. Laryngeal diphtheria.

Heart.—Pulse weak, *small,* thready. Violent stitch in præcordia, and beating of heart.

Extremities.—Stitches between shoulder-blades. Tearing and sticking in shoulders and joints. Hands and fingers seem swollen.

Modalities.—*Worse,* eating veal; towards morning and in afternoon. *Better,* drinking sips of water.

Relationship.—Antidotes: *Opium; Nitr. sp. dulc.*

Antidote to Opium and Morphine poisoning, 8-10 grains to glass of water.

Compare: *Gun-powder* (Nitre with sulphur and charcoal—2x trit. "Blood poisoning." Septic suppuration. Protractive against wound infection. Antidote to Ivy and Primula rash [Clarke]. *Herpes facialis;* crops of boils. Carbuncles. Osteo-myelitis. *Cannab. sat.* (which contains a large amount of *Kali nit.*). *Lycop.; Sanguin.; Allium sat.; Antimon. iod.*

Dose.—Third to thirtieth potency.

KALI PERMANGANICUM
(Permanganate of Potassium)

Intense irritation of nose, throat, and larynx. Diphtheria. Dysmenorrhœa. Bites of serpents and for other animal poisons. Septic conditions; tissues infiltrated with tendency to sloughing.

Respiratory.—Bleeding from nose. Nasal discharge. Smarts and irritates. Constrictive, smarting sensation in throat. Larynx feels raw. Short, hacking cough.

Throat.—Swollen and painful. Everything hawked up streaked with blood. Posterior nares painful. Muscles of neck feel sore. Swollen uvula. Fetor of breath.

Dose.—Locally, 1 dram to a quart of water, to correct fetor in cancer, ulcer, ozæna, and other foul odors. Also as an injection in leucorrhœa and gonorrhœa. Internally, 2x dilution in water. Saturated solution locally in eruption of small-pox.

Potassium Permanganate for Morphine Poisoning.—Potassium permanganate is recognized as being the most effective chemical antidote in cases of morphine or opium poisoning, acting directly on the morphine and oxidizing it to less toxic substances. To be effective the permanganate must come in direct contact with the opium or morphine in the stomach; hypodermatic or intravenous injections are absolutely useless, as the salt would be decomposed by the blood serum at once. The approved treatment is administration of two to five grains of potassium permanganate in dilute aqueous solution as soon as possible after the poison is taken, this amount to be increased if very large doses of the poison have been taken. Washing out the stomach with a quantity of 1 to 500 solution of permanganate is also recommended, using at least a pint of this solution either by a stomach pump or by enforced vomiting. *Permang. of Potash* counteracts effects of alkaloids of many poisonous plants. Owing to its oxidizing powers if given before the alkaloid has been absorbed. (Dr. Chestnut in Dept. of Agriculture.)

KALI PHOSPHORICUM
(Phosphate of Potassium)

One of the greatest nerve remedies. *Prostration.* Weak and tired. Especially adapted to the young. Marked disturbance of the sympathetic nervous system. Conditions arising from *want of nerve power*, neurasthenia, mental and physical depression, are wonderfully improved by this remedy. The causes are usually excitement, overwork and worry. Besides, *it corresponds to states of adynamia and decay*, gangrenous conditions. In these two directions it has won many clinical laurels. Remember it in the treatment of suspected malignant tumors. After removal of cancer when in nealing process skin is drawn *tight* over the wound. Delayed labor.

Mind.—Anxiety, *nervous dread*, lethargy. Indisposition to meet people. Extreme lassitude and depression. Very nervous, starts easily, *irritable.* Brain-fag; hysteria; *night terrors.* Somnambulance. Loss of memory. *Slightest labor seems a heavy task.* Great despondency about business. Shyness; disinclined to converse.

Head.—Occipital headache; better, after rising. Vertigo, from lying, on standing up, from sitting, and when looking upward. [*Granat.*] *Cerebral anæmia.* Headache of students, and those worn out by fatigue. Headaches are relieved by gentle motion. Headache, with weary, empty, gone feeling at stomach. [*Ign.; Sep.*]

Eyes.—Weakness of sight; loss of perceptive power; after diphtheria; from exhaustion. Drooping of eyelids. [*Caust.*]

Ears.—*Humming and buzzing in the ears.*

Nose.—Nasal disease, with offensive odor; fetid discharge.

Face.—Livid and sunken, with hollow eyes. Right-sided neuralgia, relieved by cold applications.

Mouth.—*Breath offensive, fetid.* Tongue coated brownish, like mustard. *Excessively dry*, in the morning. Toothache, with easily-bleeding gums; they have a bright-red seam on them. Gums spongy and receding. [*Caps.; Hamam.; Lach.*]

Throat.—Gangrenous sore throat. Paralysis of the vocal cords.

Stomach.—A nervous "gone" sensation at the pit of the stomach. [*Ign.; Sep.; Sulph.*] Feels seasick without nausea.

Abdomen.—Diarrhœa; foul, *putrid odor;* occasioned by fright, with depression and exhaustion. Diarrhœa while eating. Dysentery; stools consist of pure blood; patient becomes delirious; abdomen swells. Cholera; stools have the appearance of rice water. [*Verat.; Ars.; Jatrop.*] Prolapsus recti. [*Ign.; Pod.*]

Female.—Menstruation *too late or too scanty* in pale, irritable, sensitive, lachrymose females. Too profuse discharge, deep-red or blackish-red, thin and not coagulating; sometimes with offensive odor. Feeble and ineffectual labor pains.

Male.—Nocturnal emissions; sexual power diminished; utter prostration after coitus. [*Kali carb.*]

Urinary Organs.—Enuresis. Incontinence of urine. Bleeding from the urethra. *Very yellow urine.*

Respiratory.—Asthma; least food aggravates. Short breath on going upstairs. Cough; *yellow* expectoration.

Extremities.—Paralytic lameness in back and extremities. Exertion aggravates. Pains, with depression, and subsequent exhaustion.

Fever.—Subnormal temperature.

Modalities.—*Worse*, excitement, worry, mental and physical exertion; eating, cold, early morning. *Better*, warmth, rest, nourishment.

Relationship.—Compare: *Kali hypophosph.* (Debility with *wasting of muscular tissue.* Phosphaturia with general anemia or leucocythemia. Effects of excessive tea drinking. Chronic bronchitis where the expectoration is *thick* and *fetid,* sometimes *scanty* and *tough.* Dose.—5 grains of crude to 3x.) *Genista*— Dyer's Weed—(contains scopolamin; frontal headache and vertigo, worse motion, better open air and eating. Dry throat, awakes with waterbrash. Itching eruption on elbows, knees and ankles. Promotes diuresis in dropsical conditions.) *Macrozamia Spiralis.* (Extreme debility after severe illness; collapse. Weariness from no assignable cause, no pains. Boring pain at vertex; vomiting and retching all night; impossible to open eyes, giddiness and cold.) *Zinc.; Gels.; Cimicif.; Laches.; Mur. ac.*

Dose.—Third to twelfth trituration. The highest potencies seem to be indicated in certain cases.

KALI SILICATUM
(Silicate of Potash)

A deep-acting remedy. Lassitude is very marked. Desire to lie down all the time. Emaciation.

Head.—Absent-minded, anxious, indolent, timid. Feeble will power. Head congested, blood surges from body to head. Vertigo, coldness of head; photophobia. Nasal catarrh, discharge *bloody*, excoriating, offensive nose, swollen, ulcerated.

Gastric.—Weight in stomach after eating, nausea, pain, flatulence. Pain in liver region. Constipation. Construction of anus during stool.

Extremities.—Stiffness over body and limbs. Creeping sensation over limbs. Twitching of muscles. Weak and weary.

Modalities.—*Worse*, open air, drafts, cold, exertion, motion uncovering, bathing.

Dose.—Higher potencies.

KALI SULPHURICUM
(Potassium Sulphate)

Ailments accompanied by profuse desquamation. Applicable to the later stages of inflammation. *Yellow*, mucous and serous discharges, profuse and intermittent. Has been found of much use in oxaluria.

Head.—Rheumatic headache, beginning in evening. Bald spots. Dandruff and scaldhead.

Ears.—Eustachian deafness. Discharge of *yellow* matter. [*Hydr.*]

Nose.—Colds, *with yellow*, slimy expectoration. Nose obstructed. Smell lost. [*Nat. mur.*] *Engorgement of the nasal pharyngeal mucous membrane*, mouth breathing, snoring, etc., remaining after removal of adenoids.

Face.—Aches in heated room. Epithelioma.

Stomach.—Tongue coated yellow and slimy. Insipid, pappy taste. Gums painful. Burning thirst, nausea, and vomiting. Load feeling. Dread of hot drinks.

Abdomen.—Colicky pains; abdomen feels cold to touch; tympanitic, tense. Yellow, slimy diarrhœa. Constipation, with hæmorrhoids. [*Sulph.*]

Male.—Gonorrhœa; discharge slimy, yellowish-green. Orchitis. Gleet.

Female.—Menses too late, scanty, with feeling of weight in abdomen. Metrorrhagia.

Respiratory.—Coarse rales. *Rattling of mucus in chest.* [*Tart. em.*] Post-grippal cough, especially in children. Bronchial asthma, with yellow expectoration. Cough; worse in evening and in hot atsmosphere. Croupy hoarseness. [*Hep.; Spong.*]

Extremities.—Pain in nape, back and limbs, worse in warm room. *Shifting, wandering pains.*

Fever.—Rise of temperature at night. Intermittent fever, with yellow, slimy tongue.

Skin.—Psoriasis. [*Ars.; Thyroid.*] Eczema; burning, itching, papular eruption. Nettle-rash. Polypi. Epithelioma. Seborrhœa. Favus. Ring-worm of scalp or beard with abundant scales.

Modalities.—*Worse*, in evening, heated room. *Better*, cool, open air.

Relationship.—Compare: *Kali sulph. chromico.*—*Alum of chrome*—3x. (Produces in the nasal passages very fine threads from the septum to external wall; affections of nasal fossæ and hay-fever. Chronic colds. Sneezing, red, watery eyes, irritation of mucous membrane). *Pulsat.; Kali bich.; Nat. m.*

Dose.—Third to twelfth potency.

KALI LATIFOLIA
(Mountain Laurel)

A rheumatic remedy. Pains shift rapidly. Nausea and slow pulse frequently accompanying. Has also a prominent action on the heart. In small doses, it accelerates the heart's action; in larger it moderates it greatly. Neuralgia; *pains shoot downwards, with numbness. Fulgurating pains of locomotor ataxia.* Protracted and continuous *fevers*, with tympanites. Paralytic

KALMIA LATIFOLIA

sensations; pains and achings in limbs accompany nearly every group of symptoms. *Albuminuria.*

Head.—*Vertigo;* worse stooping. Confusion of brain. Pain in front and temporal region from head to nape and to teeth; from cardiac origin.

Eyes.—Vision impaired. *Stiff, drawing sensation when moving eyes.* Rheumatic iritis. Scleritis, *pain increased by moving the eye.*

Face.—Neuralgia; worse *right side.* Stitches in tongue. Stitches and tearing in bones of jaw and face.

Stomach.—Warm, glowing sensation in epigastrium. *Nausea;* vomiting. *Pain in pit of stomach; worse by bending forward; relieved by sitting erect.* Bilious attacks, with nausea, vertigo, and headache. Sensation of something being pressed under the epigastrium.

Urinary.—Frequent, with sharp pains in lumbar region. Post-scarlatinal nephritis.

Heart.—Weak, *slow* pulse. [*Dig.; Apoc. can.*] Fluttering of heart, with anxiety. *Palpitation; worse leaning forward.* Gouty and rheumatic metastasis of heart. Tachycardia, with pain. [*Thyroid.*] Tobacco heart. Dyspnœa and pressure from epigastrium toward the heart. *Sharp pains take away the breath.* Shooting through chest above heart into shoulder-blades. Frequent pulse. Heart's action tumultuous, rapid and visible. Paroxysms of anguish around heart.

Female.—Menses too early, or suppressed, with pain in limbs and back and inside of thighs. Leucorrhœa follows menses.

Back.—Pain from neck down arm; in upper three dorsal vertebræ extending to shoulder-blade. Pain down back, as if it would break; in localized regions of spine: through shoulders. *Lumbar pains, of nervous origin.*

Extremities.—Deltoid rheumatism especially right. Pains from hips to knees and feet. *Pains affect a large part of a limb,* or several joints, and pass through quickly. Weakness, numbness, pricking, and sense of coldness in limbs. *Pains along ulnar nerve,* index finger. Joints red, hot, swollen. Tingling and numbness of left arm.

Sleep.—Sleepless, *wakes very early in morning.*

Modalities.—*Worse*, leaning forward [*opposite*, *Kali carb.*]; looking down; motion, open air.

Relationship.—Compare: Kalmia contains Arbutin g. v. *Derris pinuta* (of great service in neuralgic headaches of rheumatic origin).

Compare: *Spigelia; Pulsat.*

Complementary: *Benz. acid.*

Dose.—Tincture, to sixth potency.

KAOLIN
Bolus alba (China Clay) Alumina Silicate

A remedy for croup and bonchitis.

Nose.—Itching and burning. Discharge *yellow. Sore, scabby,* stopped up.

Respiratory.—*Soreness of chest* along trachea; cannot stand percussion. Gray sputa. Capillary bronchitis. Larynx and chest sore. Membranous croup—extends down trachea.

Dose.—Lower triturations.

KOUSSO—BRAYERA
(Hagenia Abyssinica)

A *Vermifuge*—Nausea and vomiting, vertigo, precordial anxiety slowing and irregular pulse, subdelirium and collapse. Rapid and extreme prostration. To expel tape-worm.

Dose.—½ oz. Mix with warm water and let stand 15 minutes; stir well and administer. May be preceded by a little lemon juice (Merrell).

Relationship.—Compare: *Mallotus*—Kamala—An efficient remedy for tape-worm in 30-60 minims of tincture taken in cinnamon water.

KREOSOTUM
(Beechwood Kreosote)

Kreosotum is a mixture of phenols obtained from this distillation.

Pulsations all over the body, and profuse bleeding from small wounds. Very severe, old neuralgic affections; pains rather aggravated by rest. *Excoriating*, burning, and offensive discharges. Hæmorrhages, ulcerations, cancerous affections. Rapid decomposition of fluids and secretions, and burning pains. Overgrown, poorly developed children. Post-climacteric diseases. Tumefaction, puffiness, gangrene. Ailings of teething children.

Mental.—Music causes weeping and palpitation. Vanishing of thought; stupid, forgetful, peevish, irritable. Child wants everything but throws it away when given.

Head.—Dull pain, as from a board pressing against forehead. Menstrual headache. Occipital pain. [*Gels.*; *Zinc. pic.*]

Eyes.—Salty lachrymation. Lids red and swollen.

Ears.—Eruption around and pimples within. Difficult hearing and buzzing.

Face.—Sick, suffering expression; hot, cheeks red.

Mouth.—Lips red, bleeding. *Very painful dentition;* child will not sleep. *Very rapid decay of teeth, with spongy, bleeding gums;* teeth dark and crumbly. [*Staph.; Ant. c.*] Putrid odor and bitter taste.

Nose.—Offensive smell and discharge. Chronic catarrh of old people. Acrid rawness. Lupus. [*Ars.*]

Throat.—Burning, choking sensation. *Putrid odor.*

Stomach.—Nausea; vomiting of food several hours after eating; of sweetish water in the morning. Feeling of coldness, as of ice water in stomach. Soreness; better eating. Painful hard spot. Hæmatemesis. Bitter taste after a swallow of water.

Abdomen.—Distended. Burning hæmorrhoids. Diarrhœa; very offensive; dark brown. Bloody, fetid stools. *Cholera infantum* in connection with painful dentition, green stools, nausea, dry skin, exhaustion, etc.

Urine.—*Offensive.* Violent itching of vulva and vagina, worse when urinating. Can urinate only when lying; cannot get out of bed quick enough during first sleep. Dreams of urinating. Enuresis in the first part of night. *Must hurry when desire comes to urinate.*

Female.—Corrosive itching within vulva, burning and swelling of labia; violent itching between labia and thighs. During menses, *difficult hearing;* buzzing and roaring; eruption after. Burning and soreness in external and internal parts. Leucorrhœa, yellow, acrid; odor of green corn; worse between periods. Hæmorrhage after coition. Menses too early, prolonged. Vomiting of pregnancy, with ptyalism. *Menstrual flow intermits* [*Puls.*]; ceases on sitting or walking; reappears on lying down. Pain worse after menses. Lochia offensive; *intermits*.

Respiratory.—*Hoarse, with pain in larynx.* Cough; worse evening, with efforts to vomit, with pain in chest. Raw burning in chest; pains and oppression. Cough after influenza. [*Eriodyction.*] Winter coughs of old people, *with heavy pressure on sternum.* Gangrene of lungs. After every cough, *copious, purulent expectoration.* Hæmoptysis; periodic attacks. Sternum feels pressed in.

Back.—Dragging backache, extending to genitals and down thighs. Great debility.

Extremities.—Pain in joints, hip and knee. Boring pain in hip-joints. Scapulæ sore.

Skin.—Itching, worse towards evening. Burning in soles. Senile gangrene. Small wounds bleed freely. [*Crot.; Lach.; Phos.*] Pustules and herpes. Ecchymosis; dorsal surface of fingers and hands eczematous.

Sleep.—Disturbed with tossing. Paralytic sensation in limbs on waking. Anxious dreams of pursuit, fire, erections, etc.

Modalities.—*Worse*, in open air, cold, rest, when lying; after menstruation. *Better*, from warmth, motion, warm diet.

Relationship.—Antidote: *Nux.* Inimical: *Carbo.*

Complementary in malignant diseases: *Ars.; Phos.; Sulph.*

Guaiacol (is the principal constituent of Kreosote, and similar in action. Used in pulmonary tuberculosis. Dose 1 to 5 m.)

Matico—Artanthe or Piper augustifolia, (Gonorrhœa, hemorrhage from lungs; catarrhal conditions of genito-urinary organs and gastro-intestinal tract. Topically a hæmostatic. Difficult, dry, deep, winter cough. Use tincture.)

Compare also: *Fuligo ligni; Carbol. ac.; Iod.; Laches.*

Dose.—Third to thirtieth potency. The 200th in sensitive patients.

LABURNUM
(Cystisus Laburnum)

All parts of this shrub are poisonous, producing inflammation of stomach and intestines, with vomiting, diarrhœa, headache, paleness of face and cold skin. Widespread anæsthesia, and convulsions are some of the chief effects of this drug. Cerebrospinal meningitis. Great prostration, sense of contriction in throat, stiffness of nape, tearing from nape into occiput, lustreless eyes.

Head.—Stupefaction; indifference. [*Phos ac.*] Unequally dilated pupils; *giddiness;* twitching of facial muscles. [*Agaric.*] Hydrocephalus. Constant vertigo, intense sleepiness.

Stomach.—Excessive thirst. Constant nausea, vomiting; burning pain in epigastrium.

Tenesmus and erections. Grass-green urine.

Extremities.—Numbness and pain in hands. Difficulty in moving them.

Compare: *Nux; Gels. Cystine* (produces motor paralysis resembling that of curare and death through respiratory paralysis).

Dose.—Third potency.

LAC CANINUM
(Dog's Milk)

This remedy is of undoubted value in certain forms of sore throat and diphtheria, and rheumatism. Corresponds to a low-vitiated, non-feverish type of sickness. The keynote symptom is, *erratic pains, alternating sides.* Feels as if walking on air, or of not touching the bed when lying down. Great lassitude. Ozæna. Decided effect in drying up milk in women who cannot nurse the baby. *Great weakness and prostration.* Sinking spells every morning. Mastitis.

Mind.—Very forgetful; in writing, makes mistakes. *Despondent;* thinks her disease incurable. Attacks of rage. *Visions of snakes.* Thinks himself of little consequence.

Head.—Sensation of walking or floating in the air. [*Sticta.*] Pain first one side, then the other. Blurred vision, nausea and vomiting at height of attack of headache. Occipital pain, with shooting extending to forehead. Sensation as if brain were alternately contracted and relaxed. Noises in ears. Reverberation of voice.

Nose.—Coryza; one nostril stuffed up, the other free; alternate. Alæ nasi and corners of mouth cracked. Bones of nose sore to pressure. Bloody pus discharged.

Mouth.—Tongue coated white with bright red edges; profuse salivation. Drooling in diphtheria. *Cracking of jaw while eating.* [*Nit. ac.; Rhus.*] Putrid taste increased by sweets.

Throat.—Sensitive to touch. Painful swallowing; pain extends to ears. Sore throat and cough with menstruation. *Tonsillitis and diphtheria symptoms change repeatedly from side to side. Shining glazed* appearance of deposit, *pearly-white* or like pure white porcelain. *Stiffness of neck* and tongue. Throat feels burned raw. Tickling sensation causes constant cough. Sore throat beginning and ending with menses.

Female.—Menses too early, profuse, *flow in gushes. Breasts swollen; painful before* [*Calc. c.; Con.; Puls.*] and better on appearance of menses. Mastitis; *worse, least jar. Helps to dry up milk.* Sinking at epigastrium. Sexual organs easily excited. Backache; spine very sensitive to touch or pressure. *Galactorrhœa.*

Extremities.—Sciatica, right-side. Legs feel numb and stiff, cramps in feet. Rheumatic pains in extremities and back, from one side to the other. Pain in arms to fingers. Burning in palms and soles.

Sleep.—Dreams of snakes.

Modalities.—*Worse*, morning of one day and in the evening of next. *Better*, cold, cold drinks.

Relationship.—Compare: *Lach.; Con.; Lac felinum*—Cat's Milk—(ciliary neuralgia; eye symptoms, photophobia; *asthenopia;* dysmenorrhœa); *Lac vaccinum*—Cows' Milk—(headache, rheumatic pains, constipation); *Lac vaccinum coagulatum*—Curds—(nausea of pregnancy); *Lactis vaccini floc*—Cream—(diphtheria, leucorrhœa, menorrhagia, dysphagia); *Lactic ac.*

Dose.—Thirtieth and the highest potencies.

LAC DEFLORATUM
(Skimmed Milk)

A remedy for diseases with faulty nutrition; sick headaches, with profuse flow of urine *during* pain. *Car sickness*.

Head.—Despondent. Pain begins in forehead to occiput, in morning on rising. *Intense throbbing*, with nausea, vomiting, blindness, and obstinate constipation; worse, noise, light, motion, during menses, with great prostration, and better by pressure and bandaging head tightly.

Stool.—*Constipation*. Stools hard, large, with great straining; painful, lacerating anus.

Relationship.—Compare: *Colostrum*. (Diarrhœa in infants. Whole body smells sour. Colic.) *Nat. mur*.

Dose.—Sixth, to thiritieth potency and higher.

LACHESIS
(Bushmaster or Surucucu)

Like all snake poisons, Lachesis decomposes the blood, rendering it more fluid; hence a hæmorrhagic tendency is marked. Purpura, septic states, diphtheria, and other low forms of disease, when the system is thoroughly poisoned and the prostration is profound. The modalities are most important in guiding to the remedy. Delirium tremens with much trembling and confusion. Very important during the climacteric and for patients of a melancholic disposition. Ill effects of suppressed discharges. Diphtheritic paralysis. [*Botulinum*.] Diphtheria carriers. Sensation of tension in various parts. Cannot bear anything tight anywhere.

Mind.—Great *loquacity*. Amative. Sad in the morning; no desire to mix with the world. Restless and uneasy; does not wish to attend to business; wants to be off somewhere all the time. Jealous. [*Hyos*.] Mental labor best performed at night. Euthanasia. Suspicious; nightly delusion of fire. Religious insanity. [*Verat*.; *Stram*.] Derangement of the *time sense*.

Head.—Pain through head on awaking. Pain at root of nose. Pressure and burning on vertex. Waves of pain; worse after moving. Sun headaches. With headache, flickerings, dim vision, very pale face. Vertigo. Relieved by onset of a discharge (menses or nasal catarrh).

Eyes.—Defective vision after diphtheria, extrinsic muscles too weak to maintain focus. Sensation as if eyes were drawn together by cords which were tied in a knot at root of nose.

Ears.—Tearing pain from zygoma into ear; also with sore throat. Ear-wax hard, dry.

Nose.—Bleeding, nostrils sensitive. Coryza, preceded by headache. Hay asthma; paroxysms of sneezing. [*Silica.; Sabad.*]

Face.—Pale. Trifacial neuralgia, left side, heat running up into head. [*Phos.*] Tearing pain in jaw-bones. [*Amphisbæna; Phos.*] Purple, mottled, puffed; looks swollen, bloated, jaundiced, chlorotic.

Mouth.—Gums swollen, spongy, bleed. Tongue swollen, burns, trembles, red, dry and cracked at tip, catches on teeth. *Aphthous and denuded spots* with burning and rawness. Nauseous taste. *Teeth ache, pain extends to ears.* Pain in facial bones.

Throat.—Sore, *worse left side, swallowing liquids. Quinsy.* Septic parotiditis. Dry, intensely swollen, externally and internally. Diphtheria; membrane dusky, blackish; *pain aggravated by hot drinks;* chronic sore throat, with much hawking; mucus sticks, *and cannot be forced up or down. Very painful; worse slightest pressure, touch is even more annoying.* In diphtheria, etc., the trouble *began* on the left side. Tonsils purplish. Purple, livid color of throat. Feeling as if something was swollen which must be swallowed; *worse, swallowing saliva or liquids. Pain into ear. Collar and neck-band must be very loose.*

Stomach.—Craving for alcohol, oysters. Any food causes distress. Pit of stomach painful to touch. Hungry, cannot wait for food. Gnawing pressure *made better by eating,* but returning in a few hours. Perceptible trembling movement in the epigastric region. Empty swallowing more painful than swallowing solids.

Abdomen.—Liver region sensitive, *cannot bear anything around waist.* Especially suitable to drunkards. Abdomen tympanitic, sensitive, painful. [*Bell.*]

Stool.—Constipated, *offensive stool*. Anus *feels tight*, as if nothing could go through it. Pain darting up the rectum every time he sneezes or coughs. Hæmorrhage from bowels like charred straw, *black particles*. Hæmorrhoids protrude, become *constricted, purplish*. Stitches in them on sneezing or coughing. Constant urging in rectum, not for stool.

Female.—Climacteric troubles, palpitation, flashes of heat, hæmorrhages, vertex headache, fainting spells; worse, pressure of clothes. Menses too short, too feeble; *pains all relieved by the flow*. [*Eupion.*] Left ovary very painful and swollen, indurated. Mammæ inflamed, bluish. Coccyx and sacrum pain, especially on *rising* from sitting posture. Acts especially well at beginning and close of menstruation.

Male.—Intense excitement of sexual organs.

Respiratory.—Upper part of windpipe very susceptible to touch. Sensation of suffocation and strangulation on lying down, particularly *when anything is around throat;* compels patient to spring from bed and rush for open window. Spasm of glottis; feels as if something ran from neck to larynx. Feels *he must take a deep breath*. Cramp-like distress in præcordial region. Cough; dry, suffocative fits, tickling. Little secretion and much sensitiveness; worse, pressure on larynx, *after sleep*, open air. *Breathing almost stops on falling asleep*. [*Grind.*] Larynx painful to touch. Sensation as of a plug [*Anac.*] which moves up and down, with a short cough.

Heart.—Palpitation, with fainting spells, especially during climacteric. Constricted feeling causing palpitation, with anxiety. Cyanosis. Irregular beats.

Back.—Neuralgia of coccyx, *worse rising from sitting posture;* must sit perfectly still. Pain in neck, worse cervical region. Sensation of threads stretched from back to arms, legs, eyes, etc.

Extremities.—Sciatica, right side, better lying down. *Pain in tibia* (may follow sore throat.) Shortening of tendons.

Sleep.—Patient *sleeps into an aggravation*. Sudden starting when falling asleep. Sleepiness, yet cannot sleep. [*Bell.; Op.*] Wide-awake in evening.

Fever.—Chilly in back; feet icy cold; hot flushes and hot perspiration. Paroxysm returns after acids. Intermittent fever every spring.

Skin.—Hot perspiration, *bluish, purplish appearance*. Boils, carbuncles, ulcers, with bluish, purple surroundings. Dark blisters. Bed-sores, with black edges. Blue-black swellings. Pyæmia; dissecting wounds. Purpura, with intense prostration. *Senile erysipelas*. Wens. Cellulitis. Varicose ulcers.

Modalities.—*Worse*, after sleep, (*Kali bich.*) Lachesis sleeps *into* aggravation; ailments that come on during sleep [*Calc.*]; left side, in the spring, warm bath, pressure or constriction, hot drinks. Closing eyes. *Better*, appearance of discharges, warm applications.

Relationship.—Antidotes: *Ars.; Merc.; Heat; Alcohol; Salt*.

Complementary: *Crotalus cascavella* often completes curative work of Lachesis. [*Mure.*] *Lycop.; Hep.; Salamandra.*

Incompatible: *Acet. ac.; Carb. ac.*

Compare: *Cotyledon* (climacteric troubles); *Nat. m.; Nit. ac.; Crotal.; Amphisbœna*—snake lizard—(right jaw swollen and painful, lancinating pains; headaches, lancinating pains. Eruption of vesicles and pimples); *Naja; Lepidium.*

Dose.—Eighth to 200th potency. Doses ought not be repeated too frequently. If well indicated, a single dose should be allowed to exhaust its action.

LACHNANTES
(Spirit-weed)

Head, chest and circulation are affected. Bridge of nose as if pinched. A remedy for torticollis, rheumatic symptoms about neck. *Tuberculosis*—light-complexioned people. Early stages, and established chest cases, with much coldness. Produces a desire to talk—a flow of language and the courage to make a speech.

Head.—Right-sided pain, extending down to jaw; *head feels enlarged;* worse, least noise. Scalp painful. Sleepless. Circumscribed red cheeks; scalp feels sore, as if hair was standing on end; burning in palms and soles. Bridge of nose feels as if pinched.

Chest.—Sensation of heat—bubbling and boiling around heart region rising to head.

Back.—*Chilliness between the shoulder-blades;* pain and stiffness in back.

Neck.—*Drawn over to one side* in sore throat. Rheumatism of the neck. Stiffness of neck. Pain in nape, as if dislocated.

Skin.—Body icy cold; face yellow, tendency to sweat.

Relationship.—Compare: *Dulc.; Bry.; Puls.;* also *Fel tauri* (nape of neck pains, and great tension there).

Dose.—Third potency. Tincture in phthisis, unit doses, once or twice a week, or three drops every four hours.

LACTICUM ACIDUM
(Lactic Acid)

Morning sickness, *diabetes*, and rheumatism offer a field for this remedy. *Troubles in the breasts.* Locally, in the tuberculous ulceration of vocal cords.

Stomach.—Tongue dry, parched. Thirst; voracious hunger. Canker, *copious salivation and water-brash. Nausea;* morning sickness, especially *in pale anæmic* women. Hot, acrid eructation. *Nausea;* better, *eating.* Burning, hot gas from stomach to throat, causing profuse secretion of tenacious mucus, *worse smoking.*

Throat.—Fullness or lump like a puff ball. Keeps swallowing. Constricted low down.

Chest.—Pain in breasts, *with enlargement of axillary glands, and pain extends into hand.*

Extremities.—Rheumatic pain in joints and shoulders, wrists, knees, with much weakness. Trembling of whole body while walking. Limbs feel chilly.

Urine.—Large quantities passed, frequently. Saccharine.

Relationship.—Compare: *Sarcolactic acid q. v. Lithia; Phos. ac.*

Dose.—Third to thirtieth potency. Six to ten drops in a small glass of water in acute gastro-enteritis (Cartier.).

LACTUCA VIROSA
(Acrid Lettuce)

This remedy acts principally upon the brain and circulatory system. Delirium tremens with sleeplessness, coldness, and tremor. Hydrothorax and ascites. Impotence. Sense of lightness and *tightness* affecting whole body, especially chest. Seems to be *a true galactogogue*. Marked action on extremities.

Mind.—Stupefaction of sense. Great restlessness.

Head.—Dull, heavy, confused, dizzy. Heat of face and headache, with general coldness. Headache, with affections of respiratory organs.

Abdomen.—Sensation of weight, of fullness; borborygmi; abundant emission of wind. Colic in early morning, abdomen tense, relieved somewhat by evacuation and passing of wind.

Chest.—Difficult breathing. Suffocative breathing from dropsy of the chest. Constant tickling cough. Incessant, spasmodic cough, as if chest would fly to pieces. Squeezing sensation in lower chest.

Female.—Promotes catamenia. *Increase of milk* in breasts. [*Asafoet.*]

Sleep.—Restless; impossible to get to sleep. Deep, comatose sleep.

Extremities.—Lame hip down left side; worse walking. Coldness and numbness of feet and legs. Tremor of hands and arms. Cramps in shin bones, extending to toes and side of leg involving calves.

Relationship.—Antidotes: *Acet. ac.; Coff.*

Compare: *Nabalus*—Prenanthes Serpentaria—Rattlesnake root—White Lettuce, similar to Lactuca, (chronic diarrhœa, worse after eating, nights and towards morning. Pain in abdomen and rectum; emaciation. Constipation and somnolence; susceptible to aura of others. Dyspepsia, with acid burning eructation. *Craving for acid food.* Leucorrhœa with throbbing in uterus); *Lach.; Kali carb.; Spiranthes* (galactagogue).

Dose.—Tincture.

LAMIUM
(White Nettle)

Has a special affinity for female and urinary organs.

Headache, *with backward and forward motion of head*. Leucorrhœa and menses too early and scanty. Hæmorrhoids; hard stool, with blood. Sensation in urethra as though a drop of water were flowing through it. Tearing in the extremities. Hæmoptysis. Blisters on heel from slight rubbing. Ulcers on heel. [*Cepa.*]

Dose.—Third potency.

LAPIS ALBUS
(Silico-fluoride of Calcium)

Affections of glands, *goitre*, pre-ulcerative stage of carcinoma. Burning, stinging pain in breast, stomach, and uterus. Connective tissue about glands specially affected. Fat anæmic babies with Iodine appetite. Ravenous appetite. Remarkably successful in scrofulous affections, except in malarial cases. *Uterine carcinoma.* Fibroid tumors with *intense burning* pains through the part with *profuse hæmorrhage*. Glands have a certain elasticity and pliability about them rather than the stony hardness of *Calc. fluor.* and *Cistus.*

Ears.—Otitis media suppurativa. Where Silica is indicated progress is hastened by *Lapis* (Bellows).

Chest.—Persistent pains in mammary region. Glandular hardening.

Skin.—Scrofulous abscesses and sores. Enlargement and induration of glands, *especially cervical.* Lipoma, sarcoma, carcinoma. Pruritus

Relationship.—Compare: *Silica.; Badiaga; Ars. iod.; Calc. iod.; Con.; Kal. iod.; Asterias.*

Dose.—First to sixth potency.

LAPPA—ARCTIUM
(Burdock)

Very important in skin therapeutics. Eruptions on the head, face, and neck; pimples; acne. Styes and ulcerations on the edge of the eyelids. Profuse and frequent urination. Crops of boils and styes. [*Anthracin.*]

Extremities.—Pain in hands, knees, and ankles extending downward to fingers and toes. Pain in all joints. Eruption on extremities.

Female.—Uterine displacements. An exceedingly sore, bruised feeling in uterus, with great relaxation of the vaginal tissues; apparently entire lack of tonicity of pelvic contents. These symptoms all aggravated by standing, walking, a misstep, or sudden jar.

Dose.—Tincture, to third potency.

LATHYRUS
(Chick-pea)

Affects the lateral and anterior columns of the cord. Does not produce pain. *Reflexes always increased.* Paralytic affections of lower extremities; spastic paralysis; lateral sclerosis; Beri-beri. Athetosis. Infantile paralysis. After influenza and wasting, exhaustive diseases where there is much weakness and heaviness, slow recovery of nerve power. Sleepy, constant yawning.

Mind.—Depressed; hypochrondriacal. Vertigo when standing with eyes closed.

Mouth.—Burning pain in *tip of tongue;* with tingling and numbness of tongue and lips, as if scalded.

Extremities.—Tips of fingers numb. Tremulous, tottering gait. Excessive rigidity of legs; spastic gait. Knees knock against each other when walking. Cramps in legs worse cold, and cold feet. Cannot extend or cross legs when sitting. Myelitis, with marked spastic symptoms. Rheumatic paralysis. Gluteal muscles and lower limbs emaciated. Legs blue; swollen, if hanging down. Stiffness and lameness of ankles and knees, toes do not leave the floor, heels do not touch floor.

Muscles of calves very tense. Patient sits bent forward, straightens up with difficulty.

Urine.—Increased bladder reflex. Frequent, must hurry, else voided involuntarily.

Relationship.—Compare: *Oxytrop.*; *Secale*; *Petiveria*, a South American plant. (Paralysis; paraplegia with numbness. Sensation of internal coldness.) *Agrostema githago*—Corncockle—(Burning sensations, in stomach, through œsophagus into throat, in lower abdomen and anus; nausea, bitter vomiting, impaired locomotion; difficulty in remaining erect; vertigo and *headache, burning from lower jaw to vertex*).

Dose.—Third potency.

LATRODECTUS MACTANS
(Spider)

The bite produces tetanic effects that last several days. A picture of *angina pectoris* is presented by the action of the drug. The præcordial region seems to be the center of attack. Constriction of chest muscles, with radiation to shoulders and back. Lowered coagulability.

Head.—Anxiety. Screams with pain. Pain in neck to back of head. Occipital pain.

Respiratory.—Extreme apnœa. Gasping respiration. Fears losing breath.

Chest.—Violent, præcordial pain extending to the axilla and down the arm and forearm to fingers, with numbness of the extremity. Pulse feeble and rapid. Sinking sensation at the Cramping pain from chest to abdomen.

Extremities.—Pain in left arm, feels paralyzed. Weakness of legs followed by cramps in the abdominal muscles. Paræsthesia of lower limbs.

Skin.—Coldness of whole surface. Skin cold as marble.

Relationship.—Compare: *Latrodectus Hasselti*— New South Wales Black Spider—(Long lasting effects seem to indicate it as a *"chronic"* blood poisoning. Arrests intense pain in pyæmia. Great œdema in neighborhood of wound; paralysis of limbs, with great wasting of muscles. Violent, darting, burning pains.

preceding paralysis; vertigo, tendency to fall forward; septicæmic conditions; constant delusion of *flying*. Loss of memory. Roaring noises.) *Aranea; Mygale; Theridion; Latrodectus Kalipo*—New Zealand spider— (lymphangitis and nervous twitchings, scarlet burning eruption.) *Triatema*—Kissing bug —(Swelling with violent itching of fingers and toes. Smothering sensation and difficult breathing succeeded by fainting and rapid pulse.)

Dose.—Sixth potency.

LAUROCERASUS
(Cherry-laurel)

Spasmodic tickling cough, especially in cardiac patients, is often magically influenced by this drug. *Lack of reaction*, especially in chest and heart affections. *Drink rolls audibly through œsophagus and intestines.* General coldness, not ameliorated by warmth. Violent pain in stomach with loss of speech. Spasm of facial muscles and œsophagus. Asphyxia neonatorum.

Fever.—Coldness; chills and heat alternate. Thirst, with dry mouth in afternoon.

Respiratory.—Cyanosis and dyspnœa; worse, sitting up. Patient puts hands on heart. Cough, with valvular disease. Exercise causes pain around heart. Tickling, *dry cough.* Dyspnœa. Constriction of chest. Cough, with copious, jelly-like, or bloody expectoration. Small and feeble pulse. Threatening paralysis of lungs. *Gasping for breath;* clutches at heart.

Heart.—Mitral regurgitation. Clutching at heart and palpitation. Cyanosis neanotorum.

Sleep.—Spells of deep sleep, with snoring and stertorous breathing.

Extremities.—Toe and finger nails become knotty. Skin blue. Sprained pains in hips, thighs and heels. Cold, clammy feet and legs. Clubbing of fingers. Veins of hands distended.

Relationship.—Compare: *Hydrocy. ac.; Camphor; Secale; Ammon. carb.; Ambra.*

Dose.—Tincture, to third potency. Cherry-laurel water, two to five drop doses.

LECITHIN

(A Phosphorus-containing Complex Organic Body prepared from the yolk of egg and animal brains)

Lecithin is important in the vital processes of plant and animal organisms. Lecithin has a favorable influence upon the nutritive condition and especially upon the blood hence its use in anæmia and convalescence, neurasthenia and insomnia. Increasing the number of red corpuscles and amount of hemoglobin. Excellent galactagog, renders milk more nourishing and increases quantity.

Causes an immediate decrease in the excretion of the phosphates. Mental exhaustion and impotency. Tuberculosis, causing marked improvement in nutrition and general improvement. Tired, weak, short breath, loss of flesh; symptoms of general break-down. Sexually weak.

Mind.—Forgetful, dull, confused.

Head.—Aching, especially in occiput—pulsating and ringing in ears. Pain in zygoma; face pale.

Stomach.—Loss of appetite, thirsty, craves wine and coffee, bloated, sore pain in stomach rising toward throat.

Urine.—Scanty, with phosphates, sugar or albumen.

Sexual.—Male power lost or enfeebled. Anaphrodisia and ovarian insufficiency.

Extremities.—Soreness, aching, lack of energy. Tired and weak.

Relationship.—Compare: *Phosphor*.

Dose.—One-half to 2 grains of crude and potencies. Twelfth potency.

LEDUM

(Marsh-Tea)

Affects especially the rheumatic diathesis, going through all the changes, from functional pain to altered secretions and deposits of solid, earthy matter in the tissues. The Ledum rheumatism begins in feet, and travels upward. It affects also the skin, producing an eruption like Poison-oak, and is antidotal thereto, as well as to stings of insects. *There is a general lack of animal heat*, and yet heat of bed is intolerable. For punctured wounds, produced by sharp-pointed intruments or bites, particularly if the *wounded parts are cold*, this is the remedy. Tetanus with twitching of muscles near wound.

Head.—Vertigo when walking, with tendency to fall to one side. Distress when head is covered. Nosebleed. [*Mellilot.; Bry.*]

Eyes.—Aching in eyes. Extravasation of blood in lids, conjunctiva, aqueous or vitreous. Contused wounds. Cataract with gout.

Face.—*Red pimples on forehead and cheeks;* stinging when touched. Crusty eruption around nose and mouth.

Mouth.—Dry, retching with eructation. Musty taste with catarrhal affection.

Respiratory.—Burning in nose. Cough, with bloody expectoration. Dyspnœa; chest feels constricted. Suffocative arrest of breathing. Pain along trachea. Bronchitis with emphysema of aged. Oppressive constriction of chest. Tickling in larynx; spasmodic cough. Hæmoptysis, alternating with rheumatism. Chest hurts when touched. Whooping-cough; spasmodic, *double inspiration* with sobbing.

Rectum.—*Anal fissures.* Hæmorrhoidal pain.

Extremities.—Gouty pains shoot all through the foot and limb, and in joints, but especially small joints. Swollen, hot, pale. Throbbing in right shoulder. Pressure in shoulder, worse motion. Cracking in joints; worse, warmth of bed. Gouty nodosities. Ball of great toe swollen. [*Bothrops.*] Rheumatism begins in lower limbs and *ascends*. [*Kalmia* opposite.] Ankles swollen. *Soles painful,* can hardly step on them. [*Ant. c.; Lyc.*] Easy spraining of ankle.

Fever.—Coldness, want of animal heat. Sensation as of cold water over parts; general coldness with heat of face.

Skin.—Acne on forehead, sticking pain therein. Eczema (facial). Itching of feet and ankles; worse, scratching and warmth of bed. Ecchymosis. Long discoloration after injuries. *Carbuncles.* [*Anthracin. Tarant. cuben.*] *Antidote to Rhus poisoning.* [*Grindel.; Cyprip.; Anac.*]

Modalities.—*Better*, from cold, putting feet in cold water. *Worse*, at night, and from heat of bed.

Relationship.—Compare: Ledum antidotes spider poisons. *Ruta; Ham.; Bellis; Arnica.*

Dose.—Third to thirtieth potency.

LEMNA MINOR
(Duckweed)

A catarrhal remedy. Acts especially upon the nostrils. *Nasal polypi; swollen turbinates. Atrophic rhinitis.* Asthma from nasal obstruction; worse in wet weather.

Nose.—*Putrid smell;* loss of smell. Crusts and mucopurulent discharge very abundant. Post-nasal dropping. Pain like a string from nostrils to ear. Reduces nasal obstruction when it is an œdematous condition. Dryness of naso-pharynx.

Mouth.—*Putrid taste* on rising in the morning. Dry pharynx and larynx.

Abdomen.—Disposition to noisy diarrhœa.

Modalities.—*Worse*, in damp, rainy weather, especially *heavy rains*.

Relationship.—Compare: *Dulc.* (damp surroundings and foggy weather). *Calc.; Teucr.; Calend.; Nat. sulph.*

Dose.—Third to thirtieth potency.

LEPIDIUM BONARIENSE
(Cress—Brazilian Cress)

Affections of breast, heart, lancinating pains.

With heart symptoms, numbness and pain in left arm, sensation of sinking in pit of stomach.

Left side of head, face, chest, hip to knee, all have lancinating pain.

A streak of pain from the temple to the chin, as if the face were cut with a razor. Burning in throat, roaring in ears. Sensation of a tight girdle around chest, as of a knife piercing the heart. Pain in neck, back, and extremities. Compare: *Arnica; Lachesis.*

LEPTANDRA
(Culver's Root)

A liver remedy, with jaundice and *black, tarry stools*. Bilious states. Enfeebled portal circulation. Malarial conditions.

Head.—Dull frontal pain; vertigo, drowsiness, and depression. Smarting and aching in eyes.

Stomach.—Tongue coated *yellow*. Great distress in stomach and intestines, with desire for stool. Aching in region of liver extending to spine, which feels chilly.

Stool.—Profuse *black, fetid stools*, with pain at umbilicus. Bleeding piles. Typhoid stools turn black and look like tar. Clay-colored stools with jaundice. Prolapse of rectum with hæmorrhoids. Rectal hæmorrhage.

Relationship.—Compare: *Podop.; Iris; Bry.; Merc.; Ptel.; Myrica.*

Dose.—Tincture, to third potency.

LIATRIS SPICATA—SERRATULA
(Colic Root)

A vascular stimulant. Increases functional activity of the skin, mucous membranes.

Of use in dropsy due to liver and spleen diseases, also renal dropsy. Here the suppressed urination is most favorably influenced. *General anasarca* due to heart and kidney disease. *Diarrhœa*, with violent urging and pain in lower part of back. Colic. Locally, applied to ulcers and unhealthy wounds.

A prompt diuretic.

Dose.—1 to 4 drams of tincture or infusion.

LILIUM TIGRINUM
(Tiger-lily)

Manifests powerful influence over the pelvic organs, and is adapted to many reflex states dependent on some pathological condition of uterus and ovaries. More often indicated in unmarried women. The action on the heart is very marked. Pain in small spots. [*Oxal. ac.*] Rheumatic arthritis.

LILIUM TIGRINUM

Mind.—Tormented about her salvation. Consolation aggravates. *Profound depression of spirits.* Constant inclination to weep. Anxious; *fears some organic and incurable disease.* Disposed to curse, strike, think obscene things. *Aimless, hurried manner;* must keep busy.

Head.—Hot, dull, heavy. Faint in warm room. Wild feeling in head.

Eyes.—Hyperæsthesia of retina. Pain, extending back into head; lachrymation; and impaired vision. *Myopic astigmia.* Useful in restoring power to the weakened ciliary muscle. [*Arg. nit.*]

Stomach.—Flatulent; nausea, with sensation of lump in stomach. Hungry; longs for meat. Thirsty, drinks often and much, and before severe symptoms.

Abdomen.—Abdomen sore, distended; trembling sensation in abdomen. Pressure downwards and backwards against rectum and anus; worse, standing; better, walking in open air. Bearing down in lower part of abdomen.

Urinary.—Frequent urging. Urine milky, scanty, *hot.*

Stool.—Constant desire to defecate, *from pressure in rectum,* worse standing. Pressure down the anus. Early-morning urgent stool. Dysentery; mucus and blood, with tenesmus, especially in plethoric and nervous women at change of life.

Heart.—Sensation as if heart were grasped in a vise. [*Cact.*] Feels full to bursting. Pulsations over whole body. Palpitation; irregular pulse; very rapid. Pain in cardiac region, with feeling of a load on chest. Cold feeling about heart. Suffocating feeling in a crowded and warm room. Angina pectoris with pain in right arm.

Female.—Menses early, scanty, *dark, clotted, offensive; flow only when moving about. Bearing-down sensation with urgent desire for stool, as though all organs would escape. Ceases when resting.* [*Sep.; Lac. c.; Bell.*] *Congestion of uterus,* prolapse, and anteversion. Constant desire to support parts externally. Pain in ovaries and down thighs. Acrid, brown leucorrhœa; smarting in labia. Sexual instinct awakened. Bloated feeling in uterine region. Sub-involution. Pruritus pudendi.

Extremities.—Cannot walk on uneven ground. Pain in back and spine, with trembling, but oftener in front of a pressing-down character. Pricking in fingers. Pain in right arm and hip. Legs ache; cannot keep them still. Pain in ankle joint. Burning palms and soles.

Sleep.—Unrefreshing, with disagreeable dreams. Unable to sleep, with wild feeling in head.

Fever.—Great heat and lassitude in afternoon, with throbbing throughout body.

Modalities.—*Worse*, consolation, warm room. *Better*, fresh air.

Relationship.—Compare: *Cact.; Helon.; Murex; Sep.; Plat.; Pallad.*

Antidote: *Helon.*

Dose.—The middle and higher potencies seem to have done best. Its curative action sometimes is slow in developing itself.

LIMULUS. (XIPHOSURA)
(Horse-foot—King-crab)

Limulus was introduced by C. Hering and partially proved by him and Lippe. Hering was surprised to see the blood of the Kingcrab that he dissected, blue, which on investigation, was found to contain copper as he had surmised and which he thought would prove to be another medicine for Cholera. Further provings are necessary to establish this, though symptoms so far observed make this probable. Hering's fertile mind always lead him to pioneer paths into practical therapeutics.

Bodily and mental exhaustion; drowsiness *after sea bathing*. Gastro-enteric symptoms. Painful fulness of whole right side of body.

Head.—Mental depression. Difficult to remember names, confused with heat of face, rush of blood to face, worse when meditating. Pain behind left eye-ball.

Nose.—Fluent coryza. Sneezing worse drinking water. Constant nasal dropping. Pressure above nose and behind eyes.

Abdomen.—Colic with heat. Cramp-like pain with watery stools. Abdomen hot and constricted. Piles, constriction of anus.

Respiratory.—Husky voice. Dyspnœa after drinking water. Oppression of chest.

Extremities.—Crural neuralgia. Soles of feet ache, feel numb. Pain in right hip-joint. Heels sore.

Skin.—*Itching spots and vesicles* on face and *hands*. Burning in palms.

Relationship.—Compare: *Asterias; Homarus; Cuprum.*

Dose.—Sixth potency.

LINARIA
(Toad-flax—Snap Dragon)

Acts prominently within the domain of the pneumogastrics. Eructations, nausea, salivation, pressure on stomach. Jaundice, splenic and hepatic hypertrophy. Enteric symptoms and *great drowsiness* very marked. Cardiac *fainting*. Enuresis. Rectal symptoms. Tongue rough, dry; throat constricted. Coldness. Confusion in head. Irresistible sleepiness. Symptoms worse walking in open air.

Dose.—Third potency.

LINUM USITATISSIMUM
(Common Flax)

The application of Linseed poultice has produced in sensitive subjects severe respiratory disturbances, as asthma, hives, etc. Its action in such cases is marked by *intense irritation*. It has been found to contain small quantity of Hydrocyanic acid, which may account for this intensity. The decoction is of service in inflammation of the urinary passages, cystitis, strangury, etc. Also in diseases of the intestinal tract. It has a place in the treatment of asthma, hay-fever and urticaria. Trismus and paralysis of the tongue.

Relationship.—Compare: *Linum Catharticum*—Purging flax —(Similar respiratory symptoms, but also colic and diarrhœa).

Dose.—Lower potencies.

LITHIUM CARBONICUM
(Carbonate of Lithium)

Chronic *rheumatism connected with heart lesions* and asthenopia offer a field for this remedy. Rheumatic nodes. Uric acid diathesis. Whole body is *sore*. Gout and tophi.

LITHIUM CARBONICUM

Head.—Tension, as if bound; better, sitting and going out. Externally sensitive. *Headache ceases while eating.* Trembling and throbbing. Pain in heart; extends to head. Dizzy states with ringing in ears. Both cheeks covered with dry, bran-like scales.

Eyes.—Half vision; invisible right half. Photophobia. Pain over eyes. Dry lids. Eyes pain after reading.

Stomach.—Acidity, nausea, *gnawing, relieved by eating*. [*Anacard.*] Cannot endure slightest pressure of clothes. [*Laches.*]

Urine.—Tenesmus. Turbid urine, with mucus and red deposit. Pain in region of right kidney. Free and colorless. While urinating, pressure in heart. Cystitis, subacute and chronic.

Respiratory.—Constriction of chest. Violent cough when lying down. Air feels cold when inspired. Pain in mammary glands, *which extend into the arms and fingers*.

Heart.—Rheumatic soreness in cardiac region. Sudden shock in heart. Throbbing, dull stitch in cardiac region. Pains in heart before menses, and associated with pains in bladder, and before urinating; better, after. Trembling and fluttering in heart, extending to back.

Urinary.—Soreness of bladder; pain in right kidney and ureter. Turbid urine with mucus, scanty and dark, acrid; sandy deposit.

Extremities.—Paralytic stiffness all over. Itching about joints. Rheumatic pains throughout shoulder-joint, arm, and fingers and small joints generally. Pain in hollow of foot, extending to knee. Swelling and tenderness of finger and toe joints; better, hot water. Nodular swellings in joints. Ankles pain when walking.

Skin.—Scabby, tettery eruption on hands, head, and cheeks, preceded by red, raw skin. Dull stitch, ending in itching. *Barber's itch* (use high). Rough rash all over body, much loose epithelium, tough, dry, itchy skin.

Modalities.—Worse, in morning, right side. *Better*, rising and moving about.

Relationship.—Compare: *Lyc.*; *Ammon. phos.*; *Benz. ac.*; *Calc.*; *Lithium chlor.* (symptoms of cinchonism, viz.: *Dizzy* head, full, *blurring of vision.* Ringing in ears; marked tremors; *general weakness;* marked muscular and general prostration; no gastro-intestinal effects. Nose sore, heartburn, pain in teeth). *Lithium lacticum* (rheumatism of shoulder, and small joints relieved by moving about; worse, resting). *Lithium benzoicum* (deep-seated pains in loins; in small of back; uneasiness in bladder. Cystic irritation. Gallstones. Frequent desire. Diminishing uric acid deposit). *Lithium bromatum* (cerebral congestion, threatened apoplexy, insomnia and epilepsy).

Dose.—First to third trituration.

LOBELIA INFLATA
(Indian Tobacco)

Is a vaso-motor stimulant; increases the activity of all vegetative processes; spends its force mainly upon the pneumogastric nerve, producing a depressed relaxed condition with oppression of the chest and episgastrium, impeded respiration, nausea and vomiting.

Languor, relaxation of muscles, *nausea, vomiting and dyspepsia* are the general indications that point to the use of this remedy, in asthma and gastric affections. Best adapted to light-complexioned fleshy people. Bad effects of drunkenness. *Suppressed discharges.* [*Sulph.*] Diphtheria. *Catarrhal jaundice.* [*Chionanth.*]

Head.—Vertigo, and fear of death. Gastric headache, with nausea, vomiting, and great prostration; worse, afternoon until midnight; tobacco. Dull, heavy pain.

Face.—Bathed in cold sweat. Sudden pallor.

Ears.—*Deafness due to suppressed discharges* or eczema. Shooting pain from throat.

Mouth.—Profuse flow of saliva; acrid burning taste; *mercurial taste;* tenacious mucus, tongue coated white.

Stomach.—Acidity, flatulence, shortness of breath after eating. Heartburn with profuse flow of saliva. *Extreme nausea and vomiting.* Morning sickness. *Faintness and weakness at epigastrium. Profuse salivation, with good appetite.* Profuse sweat and prostration. Cannot bear smell or taste of tobacco. Acrid, burning taste; acidity, with contractive feeling in pit of stomach. Flatulence, shortness of breath after eating. Heartburn.

Respiratory.—*Dyspnœa from constriction of chest;* worse, any exertion. Sensation of pressure or weight in chest; *better by rapid walking.* Feels as if heart would stop. Asthma; attacks, with weakness, felt in pit of stomach and preceded by *prickling all over.* Cramp, ringing cough, short breath, catching at throat. Senile emphysema.

Back.—Pain in sacrum; cannot bear slightest touch. Sits leaning forward.

Urinary.—Deep red color and copious red sediment.

Skin.—Prickling, itching with intense nausea.

Modalities.—*Worse,* tobacco, afternoon, slightest motion, cold, especially cold washing. *Better,* by rapid walking; (chest pain), toward evening, and from warmth.

Relationship.—Antidote: *Ipec.*

Compare: *Tabac.; Ars.; Tart. e.; Verat.; Rosa.*

Lobelia syphilitica or cerulea (gives a perfect picture of sneezing influenza, involving the posterior nares, palate, and fauces. Very depressed. Pain in forehead over eyes; pain and gas in bowels, followed by copious watery stools with tenesmus and soreness of anus. Pain in knees. Prickling in soles. *Great oppression in lower part of chest,* as if air could not reach there. *Pain in chest under short ribs of left side.* Dry, hacking cough. Breathing difficult. Dull, aching pain over root of nose. Eustachian catarrh. Pain in posterior part of spleen.) *Lobelia erinus* (*malignant growths,* extremely rapid development; colloid cancer of the omentum; cork-screw-like pains in abdomen; great dryness of skin, nasal and buccal mucous membranes; distaste for brandy; dry, eczematous patches covering points of first fingers. Malignant disease of the face. Epithelioma).

Dose.—Tincture, to thirtieth potency. Locally the tincture is antidotal to Poison-oak. Often the *Acetum Lobelia* acts better than any other preparation. Lobelia hypodermically acts clinically almost precisely as the antitoxin of diphtheria does upon the infection and renders the system stronger to resist future infections (F. Ellingwood).

LOBELIA PURPURASCENS
(Purple Lobelia)

Profound prostration of all the vital forces and of the nervous system; *respiratory paralysis. Nervous prostration of influenza.* Coma. Tongue white and paralyzed.

Head.—Confused and depressed. Headache with nausea, vertigo; especially between eyebrows. Cannot keep eyes open; spasmodic closure of lids.

Chest.—Superficial respiration; heart and lungs feel paralyzed; respiration slow. Heart beats sound to him like boom of a drum.

Eyes.—Impossible to keep open. Drowsy.

Relationship.—Compare: *Baptisia; Lobelia cardinalis* (debility, especially of lower extremities; oppressed breathing, pleurisy, *sticking* pain in chest on taking a long breath. Pain in *left* lung, intermitting pricking during the day).

Dose.—Third potency.

LOLIUM TEMULENTUM
(Darnel)

Has been made use of in cephalalgia, sciatica, paralysis. Prostration and restlessness.

Head.—Anxious and depressed, confused. Vertigo; must close eyes. Head heavy. Noises in ears.

Stomach.—Nausea, vomiting. Pain in pit of stomach and abdomen. Severe purging.

Extremities.—Gait unsteady. *Trembling of all limbs.* Loss of power in extremities. *Violent pain in calves, as if bound with cords.* Cold extremities. Spasmodic motions of arms and legs. Cannot write; cannot hold a glass of water. Trembling of hands in paralysis.

Relationship.—Compare: *Secale; Lathyr; Astrag.*

Dose.—Sixth potency.

LONICERA XYLOSTEUM
(Fly-woodbine)

Convulsive symptoms. Uræmic convulsions. Albuminuria. Syphilis.

Head.—Congestion of head and chest; coma. Contraction of one pupil and dilatation of the other. Sopor, eyes half open, red face.

Extremities.—Jerking of limbs. Trembling of whole body. Violent convulsions. Limbs and head fall over as if paralyzed. Extremities cold. Cold perspiration.

Relationship.—Compare: *Lonicera pericylmenum*—Honeysuckle—(irritability of temper, with violent outburst [*Crocus.*])

Dose.—Third to sixth potency.

LUPULUS—HUMULUS
(Hops)

Is a good remedy in unstrung conditions of the nervous system attended with nausea, dizziness, headache following a night's debauch. *Infantile jaundice*. Urethral burning. Drawing and twitching in almost every muscle. Nervous tremors; wakefulness and delirium of drunkards. *Giddiness* and *stupefaction*. *Slow* pulse. Perspiration profuse, clammy, greasy.

Head.—Morbid vigilance. Highly excited. Dull, heavy headache with dizziness. Drawing and twitching in every muscle.

Sleep.—*Drowsy* during the day. Sopor.

Male.—Painful erections. Emissions, *depending on sexual weakness and after onanism*. Spermatorrhœa.

Skin—Scarlatina-like eruption on face. Feels like insects crawling under skin; feels chapped, skin peels.

Relationship.—Antidotes: *Coffea; Vinegar.*

Compare: *Nux; Urtica; Cannab.*

Dose.—Tincture, to third potency. *Lupulin* 1x trit. (Best in seminal emissions. Locally in painful cancers.)

LYCOPODIUM
(Club Moss)

This drug is inert until the spores are crushed. Its wonderful medicinal properties are only disclosed by trituration and succussion.

In nearly all cases where Lycopodium is the remedy, some evidence of urinary or digestive disturbance will be found. Corresponds to Grauvogle's carbo-nitrogenoid constitution, the non-eliminative lithæmic. Lycopodium is adapted more especially to ailments gradually developing, functional power weakening, with failures of the digestive powers, where the function of the liver is seriously disturbed. *Atony. Malnutrition.* Mild temperaments of lymphatic constitution, with catarrhal tendencies; older persons, where the skin shows yellowish spots, earthy complexion, uric acid diathesis, etc.; also precocious, weakly children. Symptoms characteristically run from right to left, acts especially on *right* side of body, and are worse from about 4 to 8 p. m. In kidney affections, *red sand in urine,* backache, in renal region; worse before urination. Intolerant of cold drinks; *craves everything warm.* Best adapted to persons intellectually keen, but of weak, muscular power. Deep-seated, progressive, chronic diseases. Carcinoma. *Emaciation.* Debility in morning. Marked regulating influence upon the glandular (sebaceous) secretions. *Pre-senility.* Ascites, in liver disease. Lycop. patient is thin, withered, full of gas and dry. Lacks vital heat; has poor circulation, cold extremities. Pains come and go suddenly. Sensitive to noise and odors.

Mind.—*Melancholy; afraid to be alone.* Little things annoy. Extremely sensitive. Averse to undertaking new things. Headstrong and haughty when sick. Loss of self-confidence. Hurried when eating. Constant fear of breaking down under stress. *Apprehensive.* Weak memory, confused thoughts; *spells or writes wrong words* and syllables. Failing brain-power. [*Anac.; Phos.; Baryt.*] Cannot bear to see anything new. Cannot read what he writes. Sadness in morning on awaking.

Head.—Shakes head without apparent cause. Twists face and mouth. Pressing headache on vertex; worse from 4 to 8 p. m., and from lying down or stooping, if not eating regularly. [*Cact.*] Throbbing headache after every paroxysm of coughing. Headaches over eyes in severe colds; *better, uncovering.* [*Sulph.*] Vertigo in morning on rising. Pain in temples, as if they were screwed toward each other. Tearing pain in occiput; better, fresh air. Great falling out of hair. Eczema; moist oozing behind ears. Deep furrows on forehead. Premature baldness and gray hair.

Eyes.—Styes on lids near internal canthus. Day—blindness. [*Bothrops.*] Night-blindness more characteristic. Sees only one-half of an object. Ulceration and redness of lids. Eyes half open during sleep.

Ears.—Thick, yellow, offensive discharge. Eczema about and behind ears. Otorrhœa and deafness with or without tinnitus; after scarlatina. *Humming and roaring with hardness of hearing;* every noise causes peculiar echo in ear.

Nose.—Sense of smell very acute. Feeling of dryness posteriorly. Scanty excoriating, discharge anteriorly. Ulcerated nostrils. Crusts and elastic plugs. [*Kal. b.; Teuc.*] Fluent coryza. *Nose stopped up.* Snuffles; child starts from sleep rubbing nose. *Fan-like motion of alæ nasi.* [*Kali. brom.; Phos.*]

Face.—Grayish-yellow color of face, with blue circles around eyes. Withered, shriveled, and emaciated; copper-colored eruption. *Dropping of lower jaw,* in typhoid fever. [*Lach.; Opium.*] Itching; scaly herpes in face and corner of mouth.

Mouth.—Teeth excessively painful to touch. Toothache, with swelling of cheeks; relieved by warm application. Dryness of mouth and tongue, without thirst. Tongue dry, black, cracked, swollen; oscillates to and fro. Mouth waters. *Blisters on tongue.* Bad odor from mouth.

Throat.—Dryness of throat, without thirst. Food and drink regurgitates through nose. Inflammation of throat, with stitches on swallowing; *better, warm drinks.* Swelling and suppuration of tonsils. Ulceration of tonsils, *beginning on right side.* Diphtheria; *deposits spread from right to left; worse, cold drinks.* Ulceration of vocal bands. Tubercular laryngitis, especially when ulceration commences.

LYCOPODIUM

Stomach.—Dyspepsia due to farinaceous and fermentable food, cabbage, beans, etc. Excessive hunger. Aversion to bread, etc. Desire for sweet things. *Food tastes sour*. Sour eructations. Great weakness of digestion. Bulimia, with much bloating. After eating, pressure in stomach, with bitter taste in mouth. *Eating ever so little creates fullness*. Cannot eat oysters. Rolling of flatulence. [*Chin.; Carb.*] Wakes at night feeling hungry. Hiccough. *Incomplete burning eructations rise only to pharynx, there burn for hours*. Likes to take food and drink hot. Sinking sensation; worse night.

Abdomen.—Immediately after a light meal, abdomen is *bloated, full*. Constant sense of fermentation in abdomen, like yeast working; upper left side. Hernia, right side. Liver sensitive. Brown spots on abdomen. Dropsy, due to hepatic disease. Hepatitis, atrophic form of nutmeg liver. Pain shooting across lower abdomen from right to left.

Stool.—Diarrhœa. Inactive intestinal canal. Ineffectual urging. Stool *hard, difficult, small*, incomplete. *Hæmorrhoids; very painful to touch, aching*. [*Mur. ac.*]

Urine.—Pain in back before urinating; ceases after flow; *slow in coming*, must strain. Retention. *Polyuria during the night*. Heavy red sediment. Child cries before urinating. [*Bor.*]

Male.—No erectile power; *impotence*. Premature emission. [*Calad.; Sel.; Agn.*] Enlarge prostate. Condylomata.

Female.—Menses too late; last too long, too profuse. Vagina dry. Coition painful. Right ovarian pain. Varicose veins of pudenda. Leucorrhœa, acrid, with burning in vagina. Discharge of blood from genitals during stool.

Respiratory.—Tickling cough. Dyspnœa. Tensive, constrictive, burning pain in chest. Cough worse going down hill. Cough deep, hollow. Expectorations gray, thick, bloody, purulent, *salty*. [*Ars.; Phos.; Puls.*] Night cough, tickling as from Sulphur fumes. Catarrh of the chest in infants, seems full of mucus rattling. Neglected pneumonia, with great dyspnœa, flaying of alæ nasae and presence of mucous rales.

Heart.—*Aneurism*. [*Baryta carb.*] Aortic disease. Palpitation at night. Cannot lie on left side.

Back.—*Burning* between scapulæ as of hot coals. Pain in small of back.

Extremities.—Numbness, also drawing and tearing in limbs, especially while at rest or at night. Heaviness of arms. Tearing in shoulder and elbow joints. One foot hot, the other cold. Chronic gout, with chalky deposits in joints. Profuse sweat of the feet. Pain in heel on treading as from a pebble. Painful callosities on soles; toes and fingers contracted. *Sciatica, worse right side. Cannot lie on painful side.* Hands and feet numb. Right foot hot, left cold. Cramps in calves and toes at night in bed. Limbs go to sleep. Twitching and jerking.

Fever.—Chill between 3 and 4 p. m., followed by sweat. Icy coldness. Feels as if lying on ice. One chill is followed by another. [*Calc.*; *Sil.*; *Hep.*]

Sleep.—Drowsy during day. Starting in sleep. Dreams of accidents.

Skin.—Ulcerates. Abscesses beneath skin; worse warm applications. Hives; worse, warmth. Violent itching; fissured eruptions. *Acne.* Chronic eczema associated with urinary, gastric and hepatic disorders; bleeds easily. Skin becomes thick and indurated. Varicose veins, nævi, erectile tumors. Brown spots, freckles worse on left side of face and nose. *Dry,* shrunken, especially palms; hair becomes prematurely gray. Dropsies. Offensive secretions; *viscid and offensive perspiration,* especially of feet and axilla. Psoriasis.

Modalities.—*Worse,* right side, from right to left, from above downward, 4 to 8 p. m.; from heat or warm room, hot air, bed. Warm applications, except throat and stomach which are better from warm drinks. *Better,* by *motion,* after midnight, from warm food and drink, on getting cold, from being uncovered.

Relationship.—Complementary: *Lycop.* acts with special benefit *after Calcar.* and *Sulphur. Iod.*; *Graphites*; *Lach.*; *Chelidon.*

Antidotes: *Camph.*; *Puls.*; *Caust.*

Compare: Carbo-Nitrogenoid Constitution: *Sulphur*; *Rhus*; *Urtica*; *Mercur.*; *Hepar. Alumina.* (Lycop. is the only vegetable that takes up aluminum. T. F. Allen.) *Ant. c.*; *Nat. m.*; *Bry.*; *Nux*; *Bothrops* (day-blindness; can scarcely see after sunrise; pain in right great toe). *Plumbago littoralis*—A Brazilian plant—(Costive with red urine, pain in kidneys and joints and body generally; milky saliva, ulcerated mouth). *Hydrast.* follows *Lycop.* in indigestion.

Dose.—Both the lower and the highest potencies are credited with excellent results. For purposes of aiding elimination the second and third attenuation of the *Tincture*, a few drops, 3 times a day, have proved efficacious, otherwise the 6th to 200th potency, and higher, in not too frequent doses.

LYCOPUS VIRGINICUS
(Bugle-weed)

Lowers the blood pressure, reduces the rate of the heart and increases the length of systole to a great degree. Passive hæmorrhages. [*Adrenalin* 6x.]

A heart remedy, and of use in exophthalmic goitre and hæmorrhoidal bleeding. Indicated in diseases with tumultuous action of the heart and more or less pain. *Hæmoptysis due to valvular heart disease*. Beneficial in toxic goitre used in the pre-operative stage. Dose, 5 drops of tincture (Beebe).

Head.—Frontal headache; worse, frontal eminences; often succeeded by labored heart. Nosebleed.

Eyes.—Protrusion, pressing, outward, with tumultuous action of heart. Supraorbital pain, with aching in testicles.

Mouth.—Toothache in lower molars.

Heart.—Rapid heart action of smokers. Precordial pain; constriction, tenderness, pulse, weak, irregular, intermittent, tremulous, rapid. Cyanosis. Heart's action tumultuous and forcible. Palpitation from nervous irritation, with oppression around heart. Rheumatoid, flying pains, associated with heart disease. Cardiac asthma [*Sumbul*].

Respiratory.—Wheezing. Cough, with *hæmoptysis*, bleeding small but frequent.

Urine.—Profuse flow of limpid, watery urine, especially when the heart is most irritable; also scanty urine. Bladder feels distended when empty. Diabetes. *Pain in testicles*.

Rectum.—Bleeding from rectum. Hæmorrhoids.

Sleep.—Wakefulness and morbid vigilance with inordinately active, but weak circulation.

Relationship.—Compare: *Ephedra*—Teamster's Tea—(in exophthalmic goitre; eyes feel pushed out with *tumultuous* action of heart); *Fucus; Spartein; Cratægus. Adrenalin* 6x.

Dose.—First to thirtieth potency.

MAGNESIA CARBONICA
(Carbonate of Magnesia)

Gastro-intestinal catarrh, with marked acidity. Often used with advantage for complaints arising in people who have been taking this drug to sweeten the stomach. Is frequently indicated in children; whole body smells sour, and disposed to boils. Broken-down, "worn-out" women, with uterine and climacteric disorders. With numbness and distention in various parts and nerve prostration. Sensitive to the least start, noise, touch, etc. Affections of the antrum of Highmore. Effects of shock, blows, mental distress. Sense of numbness; nerve prostration; tendency to constipation after nervous strain; *sensitive to least touch*, it causes starting, or cold winds or weather or from excess of care and worry with constipation and heaviness. Intense neuralgic pains.

Head.—Sticking pain in the side of the head on which he lies, as if the hair was pulled; worse, mental exertion. Itching of scalp worse in damp weather. Pain above margin of right orbit. Black motes before eyes.

Ears.—Diminished hearing. Deafness; comes suddenly and varies. Numbness of outer ear. Feeling of distention of middle ear. Subdued tinnitus.

Face.—Tearing pain in one side; worse, quiet; must move about. Toothache, especially during pregnancy; worse at night; worse, cold and quiet. Teeth feel too long. Ailments from cutting wisdom teeth. [*Cheiranthus.*] Pain in malar bone, worse during rest, night. Swelling of malar bone with pulsating pain, worse exposure to cold wind.

Mouth.—Dry at night. Sour taste. Vesicular eruption; bloody saliva. Sticking pain in throat; hawking up fetid, pea-colored particles.

Stomach.—Desire for fruit, acids, and vegetables. Eructations *sour, and vomiting of bitter water*. Craving for meat.

Abdomen.—Rumbling, gurgling. Dragging towards pelvis. *Very heavy;* contractive, pinching pain in right iliac region.

Stool.—Preceded by griping, colicy pain. *Green, watery, frothy, like a frog-pond's scum.* Bloody mucous stools. *Milk passes undigested in nursing children. Sour,* with tenesmus

[*Rheum.*] Constipation after mental shock or severe nervous strain.

Female.—*Sore throat before menses appear.* Before menses, coryza and nasal stoppage. Menses too *late and scanty*, thick, dark, like pitch; mucous leucorrhœa. Menses flow only in sleep; more profuse at night [*Amm. m.*], or when lying down; cease when walking.

Respiratory.—Tickling cough, with *salty*, bloody expectoration. Constrictive pains in chest, with dyspnœa. Soreness in chest during motion.

Extremities.—Tearing in shoulders as if dislocated. Right shoulder painful, cannot raise it. [*Sang.*] Whole body feels tired and painful, especially legs and feet. Swelling in bend of knee.

Skin.—Earthy, sallow and parchment-like; emaciation. Itching vesicles on hands and fingers. Nodosities under skin. Sore; sensitive to cold.

Fever.—Chilly in evening. Fever at night. Sour, greasy perspiration.

Sleep.—Unrefreshing; more tired on rising than on retiring.

Modalities.—*Worse*, warmth of bed; change of temperature; cold wind or weather; every *three weeks*; rest. *Better*, warm air; walking in open air.

Relationship.—Antidotes: *Ars.; Merc.*

Complementary: *Cham.*

Compare: *Rheum; Kreos.; Aloes; Cheiranthus*—Wall flower—(deafness, otorrhœa, nose stopped up at night *from irritation of cutting wisdom-teeth.*

Dose.—Third to thirtieth potency.

MAGNESIA MURIATICA
(Muriate of Magnesia)

A liver remedy with pronounced characteristic constipation. Chronic liver affections with tenderness and pain, extending to spine and epigastrium, worse after food. Especially adapted to diseases of women, with a long history of indigestion and uterine disease; children who cannot digest milk. Evil effects of sea bathing.

Head.—Sensitive to noise; bursting headache; worse, motion, open air; better, pressure, and wrapping up warmly. [*Sil.; Stront.*] Much sweating of head. [*Calc.; Sil.*] Facial neuralgia pains, dull, aching, worse damp weather, slightest draft, better pressure heat.

Nose.—Nostrils ulcerated. Coryza. Nose stopped and fluent. *Loss of smell and taste*, following catarrh. Cannot lie down. Must breathe through mouth.

Mouth.—Blisters on lips. Gums swollen, bleed easily. Tongue feels burnt and scalded. Throat dry, with hoarseness.

Stomach.—Appetite poor, bad taste in mouth. Eructations like rotten eggs. Continued rising of white froth into mouth. *Cannot digest milk.* Urine can be passed only by pressing abdominal muscles.

Abdomen.—Pressing pain in liver; worse lying on right side. *Liver enlarged with bloating of abdomen;* yellow tongue. Congenital scrotal hernia. Must use abdominal muscles to enable him to urinate.

Urinary.—Urine difficult to void. Bladder can only be emptied by straining and pressure.

Bowels.—Constipation of infants during dentition; only passing small quantity; *stools knotty*, like sheep's dung, *crumbling at verge of anus*. Painful smarting hæmorrhoids.

Female.—Menses black, clotted. Pain in back and thighs. Metrorrhagia; worse at night. Great excitement at every period. Leucorrhœa with every stool and after exercise. Tinea ciliaris, eruptions in face and forehead worse before menses.

Heart.—Palpitation and cardiac pain *while sitting; better by moving about*. [*Gels.*] Functional cardiac affections *with liver enlargement*.

Respiratory.—Spasmodic dry cough; worse forepart of night, with burning and sore chest.

Extremities.—Pain in back and hips; in arms and legs. Arms "go to sleep" when waking in morning.

Sleep.—Sleep during day; restless at night on account of heat and shock; anxious dreams.

Modalities.—*Worse*, immediately after eating, lying on right side; *from sea bathing. Better*, from pressure, motion; open air, except headache.

Relationship.—Antidotes: *Camph.; Cham.*

Compare: *Nat. m.; Puls.; Sep.; Amm. m.; Nasturtium aquaticum*—Water-cress—(useful in scorbutic affections and constipation, related to strictures of urinary apparatus; supposed to be aphrodisiacal in its action. Is also antidotal to *tobacco* narcosis and sedative in neurotic affections, neurasthenia, hysteria. Cirrhosis of liver and dropsy.

Dose.—5 drops of tincture. Third to 200th potency.

MAGNESIA PHOSPHORICA
(Phosphate of Magnesia)

The great anti-spasmodic remedy. Cramping of muscles with radiating pains. Neuralgic pains *relieved by warmth*. Especially suited to tired, languid, exhausted subjects. Indisposition for mental exertion. Goitre.

Mind.—Laments all the time about the pain. Inability to think clearly. Sleepless on account of indigestion.

Head.—Vertigo on moving, falls forward on closing eyes, better walking in open air. Aches after mental labor, with chilliness; always better warmth. [*Sil.*] Sensation as if contents were liquid, as if parts of brain were changing places, as of a cap on head.

Eyes.—Supraorbital pains; worse, right side; relieved by warmth applied externally. Increased lachrymation. Twitching of lids. Nystagmus, strabismus, ptosis. Eyes hot, tired, vision blurred, colored lights before eyes.

Ears.—*Severe neuralgic pain;* worse behind right ear; worse, by going into cold air, and *washing face and neck with cold water.*

Mouth.—*Toothache; better by heat and hot liquids.* Ulceration of teeth, with swelling of glands of face, throat and neck, and *swelling* of tongue. *Complaints of teething children.* Spasms without febrile symptoms.

Throat.—Soreness and stiffness, especially right side; parts seem puffy, *with chilliness*, and aching all over.

Stomach.—Hiccough, with retching day and night. Thirst for very cold drinks.

Abdomen.—*Enteralgia*, relieved by pressure. *Flatulent colic, forcing patient to bend double; relieved by rubbing, warmth, pressure; accompanied with belching of gas, which gives no relief.*

Bloated, full sensation in abdomen; must loosen clothing, walk about, and constantly pass flatus. Constipation in rheumatic subjects due to flatulence and indigestion.

Female.—*Menstrual colic. Membranous dysmenorrhœa.* Menses too early, dark, stringy. Swelling of external parts. Ovarian neuralgia. Vaginismus.

Respiratory.—Asthmatic oppression of chest. Dry, tickling cough. *Spasmodic cough,* with difficulty in lying down. *Whooping-cough.* [*Corall.*] Voice hoarse, larynx sore and raw. Intercostal neuralgia.

Heart.—*Angina pectoris.* Nervous spasmodic palpitation. Constricting pains around heart.

Fever.—*Chilliness* after dinner, in evening. *Chills run up and down the back, with shivering,* followed by a suffocating sensation.

Extremities.—Involuntary shaking of hands. Paralysis agitans. Cramps in calves. Sciatica; feet very tender. Darting pains. Twitchings. *Chorea.* Writers' and players' cramp. Tetanic spasms. Weakness in arms and hands, finger-tips stiff and numb. General muscular weakness.

Modalities.—*Worse,* right side, *cold,* touch, night. *Better,* warmth, bending double, pressure, friction.

Relationship.—Compare: *Kali phos.; Colocy.; Silica; Zinc.; Diosc.*

Antidotes: *Bell.; Gels.; Lach.*

Dose.—First to twelfth potency. Sometimes the highest potencies are preferable. Acts especially well, given in hot water.

MAGNESIA SULPHURICA
(Epsom Salt)

The skin, *urinary*, and female symptoms are most marked. The purgative action of Sulphate of Magnesia is not a quality of the drug, but a quality of its physical state, which renders its absorption impossible. The properties inherent in the substance itself can only be discovered by attenuation. (Percy Wilde.)

Head.—Apprehensive; vertigo; head heavy during menses. Eyes burn, noises in ears.

Stomach.—Frequent eructations, tasting like bad eggs. Rising of water in mouth.

Urinary.—Stitches and burning the orifice of the urethra after urinating. Stream intermits and dribbles. The urine passed in the morning copious, bright yellow, soon becomes turbid, and deposits a copious red sediment. The urine is greenish as passed; is of a clear color, and in a large quantity. Diabetes. [*Phos. ac.; Lact. ac.; Ars. brom.*]

Female.—Thick leucorrhœa, as profuse as the menses, with weary pain in the small of the back and thighs, on moving about. Some blood from the vagina between the menses. Menstruation returned after fourteen days; the discharge was thick, black, and profuse. Menses too early, intermit.

Neck and Back.—Bruised and ulcerative pain between the shoulders, with a feeling as of a lump as large as the fist, on which account she could not lie upon her back or side; relieved by rubbing. Violent pain in the small of the back, as if bruised, and as before menstruation.

Extremities.—The left arm and foot fall asleep in bed, in the morning after waking.

Skin.—Small pimples over the whole body, that itch violently. Suppressed itch. [*Sulph.*] Crawling in the tips of the fingers of the left hand; better on rubbing. *Warts.* Eyrsipelas (applied locally as a saturated solution). Dropsy (physiological doses).

Fever.—Chill from 9 to 10 a. m. Shuddering in back; heat in one part and chill in another.

Relationship.—It is claimed that the addition of a small amount of *Magnes. Sulph.* to the usual hypodermic of Morphine increases the value of the hypodermic from 50 to 100%.

Physiologic Dosage.—Magnes. Sulph. is of diagnostic and therapeutic value in Gallstone colic. From 2 to 4 teaspoonfuls in glass hot water taken at onset of a colicky attack may abort or stop the colic.

Epsom salt is one of the most active saline cathartics, operating with little pain or nausea, especially if pure. It has but little if any effect on intestinal peristalsis, its action causing a rush of fluid into the intestine, which by producing a distention of the bowel produces evacuation. It causes little or no irritation in the intestine. In common with the other salines, it is the classical evacuant to be employed in connection with mercurials and anthelmintics and in cases of poisoning. Epsom salt usually acts within from one to two hours, more quickly if taken in hot water and in the morning before breakfast. The ordinary dose as a mild laxative is a heaping teaspoonful; as a cathartic, two to four teaspoonfuls. The taste may be improved, if necessary, by the addition of a little lemon juice and sugar.

Besides its chief use as a saline cathartic, magnesium sulphate is used to a considerable extent externally in saturated solution as an antiphlogistic and antipruritic in erysipelas, ivy poisoning, cellulitis and other local inflammations. Use on compresses saturated with solution.

Dose.—The pure salt to the third potency. Locally 1:4 in water in septic conditions, erysipelas, orchitis, boils, etc.

MAGNOLIA GRANDIFLORA
(Magnolia)

Rheumatism and cardiac lesions are prominent features in the symptomatology of this drug. *Stiffness* and soreness. Alternating pains between spleen and heart. Patient tired and stiff. Soreness when quiet. Erratic shifting of pains.

Heart.—Oppression of chest with inability to expand the lungs. Feeling of a large bolus of food which distressed the stomach. Suffocated feeling when walking fast or lying on left side. Dyspnœa. Crampy pain in heart. Angina pectoris. Endocarditis and pericarditis. Tendency to faint. *Sensation as if heart had stopped beating.* Pain around heart accompanied by itching of the feet.

Extremities.—Stiffness and sharp erratic pains; worse in joints. *Feet itch.* Numbness in left arm. Rheumatic pain in clavicles. Shooting in all limbs.

Modalities.—*Worse*, damp air, lying on left side; in morning on first rising. *Better*, dry weather, motion; intermenstrual flow. [*Ham.; Bovista; Bell.; Elaps.*]

Relationship.—Compare: *Rhus.; Dulcam.; Aurum.*

Dose.—Third potency.

MALANDRINUM
(Grease in Horses)

A very effectual protection against small-pox. Ill effects of vaccination. [*Thuja; Silica.*] Efficacious in clearing of the remnants of cancerous deposits (Cooper).

Skin.—Scab on upper lip, with stinging pain when torn off. Aching in forehead. *Dry, scaly; itching; rhagades of hands and feet in cold weather and from washing.* Toes feel scalded and itch terribly. Bone-like protuberances.

Dose.—Thirtieth potency and highest.

MANCINELLA
(Hippomane—Manganeel Apple)

Skin symptoms most marked. Dermatitis, with excessive vesiculation, oozing of sticky serum and formation of crusts. To be remembered in mental depressed states at puberty and at climacteric, with exalted sexuality. [*Hering.*] *Loss of vision.* Pain in the *thumb*.

Mind.—Silent mood, sadness. Wandering thoughts. *Sudden vanishing of thought.* Bashful. *Fear of becoming insane.*

Head.—Vertigo; head feels light, empty. Scalp itches. Hair falls out after acute sickness.

Nose.—Illusions of smell; of gunpowder, dung, etc. Pressure at root of nose.

Mouth.—Feels peppery. Copious, offensive saliva. Taste of blood. Burning of fauces. Dysphagia from constriction of throat and œsophagus.

Stomach.—Continual choking sensation rising from stomach. Vomiting of ingesta, followed by griping and copious stools. Burning pains and black vomit.

Extremities.—Icy coldness of hands and feet. Pain in thumb.

Skin.—Intense erythema. *Vesicles.* Fungoid growths. Erysipelas. *Large blisters, as from scalds.* Heavy, brown crusts and scabs. *Pemphigus.*

Relationship.—Compare: *Croton; Jatropha; Canth.; Anacard.*

Dose.—Sixth, to thirtieth potency.

MANGANUM ACETICUM

(Manganese Acetate)

Manganum causes anæmia with destruction of the red corpuscles. Jaundice, nephritis with albuminuria. Fatty degeneration of liver. Paralysis agitans. *Cellulitis*, subacute stage, promotes suppuration and hastens regeneration.

Symptoms of chronic poisoning, according to Professor von Jaksch, were involuntary laughter and involuntary weeping and walking backwards. Strongly exaggerated reflexes and physical disturbances, evidenced by men making fun of each other's gait. Paraplegia progressive; wasting, feeble and staggering gait.

Inflammation of bones or joints, with nightly digging pains. Asthmatic persons who cannot lie on a feather pillow. Syphilitic and chlorotic patients with general anæmia and paralytic symptoms often are benefitted by this drug. Gout. Chronic arthritis. For speakers and singers. Great accumulation of mucus. Growing pains and weak ankles. General soreness and aching; every part of the body feels sore when touched; early tuberculosis.

Head.—Anxiety and fear; *better lying down*. Feels large and heavy, with rush of blood; pain from above downward. Field of vision contracted. Stolidy mask-like face.

Mouth.—Nodes on palate. Toothache; *worse*, anything cold. [*Coff.* opposite.] Hemming all the time. Low, monotonous voice.

Nose.—Dry, obstructed. Chronic catarrh, with bleeding, dryness; *worse in cold damp weather*.

Ears.—Feel stopped; cracking on blowing nose. *Pain from other parts extends to ears*. Deafness *in damp weather*. Whistling tinnitus.

Alimentary Canal.—Tongue sore and irritable with ulcers or warts. Flatulence; chronic enlargement of liver.

Respiratory.—*Chronic hoarseness*. Larynx dry, rough, constricted. Tuberculosis of larynx. Cough; worse evening, and *better lying down* and worse in damp weather. Mucus difficult to loosen. Stitches in larynx extending to ear. Heat in chest. Hæmoptysis. *Every cold rouses up a bronchitis*. [*Dulc.*]

MANGANUM ACETICUM

Female.—Derangements of menstruation, amenorrhœa; menses too early and scanty, in anæmic subjects. *Flushes of heat at climacteric.*

Extremities.—Muscular twitching. Cramps in calves. Stiffness in muscles of legs. Inflammation of bones and joints with insupportable nightly digging pains. *Every part of body feels sore when touched.* Cannot walk backwards without falling. *Tending to fall forward. Walks stooping forward.* Legs feel numb. Wilson's disease. Paralysis agitans. Peculiar slapping gait, walks on metacarpo-phalangeal joint; walks backwards. Ankles painful. Bones very sensitive. Shiny red swelling of joints. *Knees pain* and itch. Rheumatism of feet. Intolerable pain in skin of lower limbs. Burning spots about joints. Periosteal inflammation. Suppuration of skin around joints.

Sleep.—Languor and sleepiness. Vivid dreams. Sleepy very early in evening.

Skin.—Suppuration of skin around joints. Red, elevated spots. *Itching;* better, scratching. Deep cracks in bends of elbows, etc. Psoriasis and pityriasis. Burning around ulcers. *Chronic eczema* associated with amenorrhœa, worse at menstrual period or at menopause.

Modalities.—*Worse,* cold wet weather, change of weather. *Better,* lying down (cough).

Relationship.—Compare: *Colloidal Manganese* (Boils and other staphylococcal infections); *Mangan, mur.* (painful ankles, bone-pains); *Mangan. oxydat.* (pain in tibia, dysmenorrhœa, colic, and diarrhœa. Easily fatigued and heated; sleepy. Stolid, mask-like facies; low monotonous voice "Economical Speech." Muscular twitching, cramps in calves; stiff leg muscles; occasional uncontrallable laughter. Peculiar slapping gait. Similar symptoms to paraylsis agitans, progressive lenticular degenerations and pseudo sclerosis. Workers in Mangan. binoxide are frequently affected with bulbar paralysis. Use 3x homœopathically.) *Mangan. sulph.* (liver affections, excess of bile; a powerful intestinal stimulant); *Argent.; Rhus.; Sulph.*

Antidotes: *Coff.; Merc.*

Dose.—Third to thirtieth potency.

MANGIFERA INDICA
(Mango Tree)

One of the best general remedies for passive hæmorrhages, uterine, renal, gastric, pulmonary and intestinal. Rhinitis, sneezing, pharyngitis, and other acute throat troubles, suffocative sensation as if throat would close. Relaxation of mucous membrane of alimentary canal. Catarrhal and serous discharges, chronic intestinal irritation. Varicose veins. Drowsiness. Atonic conditions, poor circulation, relaxed muscles.

Skin.—Itching of palms. Skin as if sunburnt, swollen. White spots, intense itching. Lobes of ears and lips swollen.

Relationship.—Compare: *Erigeron; Epilobium.*

Dose.—Tincture.

MEDORRHINUM
(The Gonorrhœal Virus)

A powerful and deep-acting medicine, often indicated for chronic ailments due to suppressed gonorrhœa. For women with chronic pelvic disorders. Chronic *rheumatism*. Great disturbance and irritability of nervous system. Pains intolerable, tensive; nerves quiver and tingle. Children dwarfed and stunted. Chronic catarrhal conditions in children. Nose dirty, tonsils enlarged, thick yellow mucus from nostrils; lips thickened from mouth breathing. State of collapse and *trembling all over*. History of sycosis. Often restores a gonorrhœal discharge. Intensity of all sensations. Œdema of limbs; dropsy of serous sacs. Disseminated sclerosis.

Mind.—Weak memory. Loses the thread of conversation. Cannot speak without weeping. *Time passes too slowly.* [*Cannab. ind.; Arg. n.*] Is in a great hurry. Hopeless of recovery. Difficult concentration. Fears going insane. [*Mancinella.*] Sensibility exalted. Nervous, restless. Fear in the dark and of some one behind her. Melancholy, with suicidal thoughts.

Head.—Burning pain in brain; worse, occiput. Head heavy and drawn backward. Headache from jarring of cars, exhaustion, or hard work. Weight and pressure in vertex. Hair dry, crispy. Itching of scalp; dandruff.

Eyes.—Feels *as if she stared* at everything. Eyeballs ache. Feels as if sticks in eyes. Lids irritated.

Ears.—Partial deafness, pulsation in ears. Quick, darting pains in right ear.

Nose.—Intense itching. Coldness of tip. Posterior nares obstructed. Chronic nasal and pharyngeal catarrhs.

Face.—Pallor, acne, blotches of reddish color. *Small boils* break out during menses.

Mouth.—Tongue coated brown and thick, blistered; canker sores. Blisters on inner surface of lips and cheeks.

Stomach.—Coppery taste and eructations of sulphuretted hydrogen. Ravenous hunger soon after eating. *Very thirsty.* Cravings for liquor, salt, sweets, etc., warm drinks. Pernicious vomiting of pregnancy.

Abdomen.—Violent pain in liver and spleen. Rests more comfortably lying on abdomen.

Stool.—Can pass stool only by leaning very far back. Painful lump sensation on posterior surface of sphincter. Oozing of fetid moisture. *Intense itching of anus.*

Urine.—Painful tenesmus when urinating. *Nocturnal enuresis.* Renal colic. [*Berb.; Ocim.; Pareir.*] Urine flows very slowly.

Female.—Intense pruritus. Menses *offensive*, profuse, dark, clotted; stains difficult to wash out, urinates frequently at that time. *Sensitive spot near os uteri.* Leucorrhœa thin, acrid, excoriating, fishy odor. Sycotic warts on genitals. Ovarian pain, worse left side, or from ovary to ovary. *Sterility.* Metrorrhagia. Intense menstrual colic. Breasts *cold*, sore, and sensitive.

Male.—Nocturnal emissions, followed by great weakness. *Impotence.* Gleet; whole urethra feels sore. Urethritis. Enlarged and painful prostate with frequent urging and painful urination.

Respiratory.—Much oppression of breathing. Hoarse while reading. Pain and soreness through chest and mammæ. Incessant, dry, night cough. Asthma. Incipient consumption. Larynx feels sore. Dyspnœa; cannot exhale. [*Samb.*] Cough: better lying on stomach.

Extremities.—Pain in back, with burning heat. Legs heavy; ache all night; *cannot keep them still.* [*Zinc.*] Ankles easily turn when walking. Burning of hands and feet. Finger-joints enlarged, puffy. Gouty concretions. *Heels and balls of feet tender.* [*Thuja.*] Soreness of soles. Restless; better, clutching hands.

Skin.—Yellow. Intense and incessant *itching;* worse night and when thinking of it. Fiery red rash about anus in babies. Copper-colored spots. Favus. Tumors and abnormal growth.

Fever.—Wants to be fanned all the time. Chills up and down back; coldness of legs, hands, and forearms. Flashes of heat in face and neck. Night-sweat and hectic.

Sleep.—Dreams she is drinking. *[Ars.; Phos.]* Sleeps in knee-chest position.

Modalities.—*Worse,* when thinking of ailment, *from daylight to sunset,* heat, inland. *Better,* at the seashore, lying on stomach, damp weather. [*Caust.*]

Relationship.—Compare:(Lactation: *Galega; Lactuca;) Sulph.; Syphil.; Zinc.*

Dose.—The very highest potencies only of service. Must not be repeated often.

MEDUSA

(Jelly-fish)

Whole face puffed and œdematous—eyes, nose, ears, lips.

Skin.—Numbness; burning, pricking heat. Vesicular eruption, especially on face, arms, shoulders, and breasts. *Nettle rash.* [*Apis; Chloral.; Dulc.*]

Female.—Marked action on *lacteal glands.* The secretion of milk was established after lack of it in all previous confinements.

Relationship.—Compare: *Pyrarara; Physalia* (urticaria); *Urtica; Homar.; Sep.*

MEL CUM SALE
(Honey with Salt)

Prolapsus uteri and chronic metritis, especially when associated with subinvolution and inflammation of the cervix. The special symptom leading to its selection is a *feeling of soreness across the hypogastrium from ileum to ileum*. Uterine displacements, and in the commencement of metritis. Sensation as if bladder were too full. Pain from sacrum towards pubes. Pain as if in ureters.

Dose.—Third to sixth potency. Honey for itching of anus and worms.

MELILOTUS
(Yellow Melilot—Sweet Clover)

Congestions and hæmorrhages seem to be the special manifestations of this drug. Violent congestive and nervous headaches. Infantile spasms. Epilepsy from blow on head. *Pain* and *debility* point to it. Coldness but also increase of temperature; tenderness, and pain. Muscular system depressed. Dreams and emissions.

Mind.—Unable to fix mind. Memory treacherous. Stupor. Wants to run away and hide. Delusions; thinks every one is looking at her, fears to talk loud, and wants to run away, etc.

Head.—Headache with retching, vomiting, sense of pressure over orbits, pallor, cold hands and feet, black spots before eyes. Heavy, oppressed; *frontal, throbbing*, undulating sensation in brain. *Sick headache;* relieved by epistaxis or *menstrual flow*. *Fullness all over head*. Eyes heavy; blurred sight; wants to close them tightly for relief. *Neuralgia* around and over right side of head and neck. Scalp sore and tender to touch.

Nose.—Stopped up, *dry*, must breathe through mouth; dry, hard clinkers in nose; *profuse epistaxis*.

Face.—Intensely red and flushed, with throbbing carotids. [*Bell.*]

Stool.—Difficult, painful, constipated. Anus feels constricted. full, *throbs*. No desire until there is a large accumulation. [*Bry.; Alum.*]

Female.—Menses *scanty, intermit*, with nausea and bearing-down. Sticking pain in external parts. Dysmenorrhœa. Ovarian neuralgia.

Respiratory.—Feels as if smothering, especially from rapid walking. Hæmoptysis. Weight on chest. Tickling in throat with cough.

Extremities.—Pain in knee; wants to stretch leg, but does not relieve. Joints sore. Skin and extremities cold. Numbness and aching in knee-joints.

Modalities.—*Worse*, rainy, changeable weather, approach of storm, motion; 4 p. m.

Relationship.—Compare: *Melilotus alba*—(White Clover)—practically the same action. (Hæmorrhages, congestive headaches, engorged blood vessels, spasms.) *Amyl; Bell.; Glon.*

Dose.—Tincture, for inhaling; lower potencies.

MENISPERMUM
(Moonseed)

A remedy for megrim, associated with restlessness and dreams. Pain in spine. Dryness, itching all over. Dry mouth and throat.

Head.—Pressure *from within outward*, with *stretching and yawning* and pain down back. Sick headache; pain in forehead and temples, moving to occiput. Tongue swollen and much saliva.

Extremities.—Pain in back, thighs, elbows, shoulders. Legs sore, as if bruised.

Relationship.—Compare: *Cocculus; Bryon.*

Dose.—Third potency.

MENTHA PIPERITA
(Peppermint)

Stimulates the cold-perceiving nerves so just after taking it, a current of air at the ordinary temperature seems cold. Marked action on respiratory organs and skin. Useful in gastrodynia, flatulent cold.

Abdomen.—Bloated, disturbing sleep. Infantile colic. Bilious colic with great accumulation of gas.

Respiratory.—Voice husky. Tip of nose sore to touch. Throat dry and sore, as if pin crosswise in it. *Dry cough, worse from air into larynx, tobacco smoke, fog,* talking; *with irritation in suprasternal fossa* [*Rumex.*] *Trachea painful to touch.*

Skin.—Every scratch becomes a sore. Itching of arm and hand when writing. Vaginal pruritus. Herpes zoster. [*Ars.; Ran. bulb.*]

Relationship.—Compare: *Rumex; Laches.; Mentha pulegium*—European pennyroyal—(pain in bones of forehead and extremities). *Mentha viridis*—Spearmint—(scanty urine with frequent desire).

Dose.—Tincture, 1 to 20 drops, to thirtieth potency. Locally, in pruritus vaginæ.

MENTHOL

The stearopten from the essential oil of Mentha. Mucous membrane of naso-pharynx and spinal nerve plexus, producing neuritic pains and paretnesias. Menthol has proved curative in acute nasal catarrh; in acute eustachian catarrh; pharyngitis; laryngitis; neuralgias, etc. (Wm. B. Griggs, M. D.) Itching, especially *pruritus* vulvæ.

Head.—Frontal headache, pain over frontal sinus, descends to eyeballs. Mental confusion. Supra orbital pain over left eye. Pain in face above zygoma with numbness. Pain in eyeballs. Coryza with post-nasal dripping. Cold sensation in nose. Eustachian tubes feel blocked and some deafness.

Respiratory.—Tickling in the fauces. Stabbing pains in the precordia, radiating over entire chest. Short, dry cough, worse smoking. Asthmatic breathing, with congestive headache.

Extremities.—Muscular pain in cervical region. Soreness of lumbar muscles.

Relationship.—Compare: *Kali bich.; Spigel.*

Dose.—Sixth potency. Externally for itching, use 1 per cent. solution or ointment.

MENYANTHES
(Buck-bean)

A remedy for certain headaches, intermittent fever. Coldness of abdomen. Twitchings. Sensation of tension and compression. Fidgets and urinary difficulties in women. Diabetes.

Head.—Pressing in vertex; *better, hard pressure with hand.* Pressing-together pain. Weight pressing on brain with every step on ascending. Pain from nape over whole brain; better, stooping, sitting; worse, going upstairs. Cracking in jaw and twitching of facial muscles.

Stomach.—No thirst at any time. Ravenous hunger; passing away after eating a little. Desire for meat. Sensation of coldness extending up to œsophagus.

Abdomen.—Distended and full; increased by smoking tobacco. Coldness of abdomen.

Extremities.—*Icy coldness of hands and feet.* Cramp-like pain. As soon as patient lies down, *legs jerk and twitch.*

Fever.—Coldness predominates; felt most acutely in abdomen and legs and tip of nose.

Modalities.—*Worse*, during rest, ascending. *Better*, pressure on affected part, stooping, motion.

Relationship.—Compare: *Caps.; Puls.; Calc.; Phos. ac.; Sang.*

Antidote: *Camph.*

Dose.—Third to thirtieth potency.

MEPHITIS
(Skunk)

A great medicine for *whooping-cough*. In order to insure its full success, it should be given in the lower dilutions from 1x to 3x. Suffocative feeling, asthmatic paroxysms, spasmodic cough; cough so violent, seems as if each spell would terminate life. Child must be raised up, gets blue in face, cannot exhale. Mucous rales through upper part of chest. Patient wants to bathe in ice-cold water.

Mind.—Excited, full of fancies. Can neither sleep nor work.

Eyes.—Pain from overexertion; blur; unable to distinglish letters; conjunctiva red; eyes hot and painful.

Mouth.—Painful jerks in root of teeth. Bloated face. Coppery taste, as after eating onions.

Respiratory.—Sudden contraction of glottis, when drinking or talking. *Food goes down wrong way.* False croup; *cannot exhale. Spasmodic and whooping-cough. Few paroxysms in day-time, but many at night;* with vomiting after eating. Asthma, as if inhaling sulphur; cough from talking; hollow, deep, with rawness, hoarseness, and pains through chest. *Violent spasmodic cough; worse at night.*

Sleep.—Awakes at night with rush of blood to lower legs. Vivid dream of water, fire, etc.

Relationship.—Compare: *Dros.; Coral.; Sticta.*

Dose.—First to third potency. Has a very short action.

MERCURIALIS PERENNIS
(Dog's Mercury)

Great exhaustion and drowsiness. Tumor at ensiform appendix, very sensitive. Affections of the muscular fibres of stomach, intestines, bladder.

Head.—Vertigo on going down stairs. Head confused. Pain as from a band tightly across forehead. Nostrils sore, conscious of nose, feels as if she had two noses.

Mouth.—Great dryness of mouth and throat; tongue feels heavy and dry, numb. Burning blisters of tongue, lips and cheeks. Ulcers on palate, tonsils and back of pharynx. Dryness of throat.

Female.—*Amenorrhœa*, scanty menses, accompanied with orgasms. Pains and swelling of breasts. Dysmenorrhœa.

Relationship.—Compare: *Borax; Croton; Euphorb.*

Dose.—Third potency.

MERCURIUS—HYDRARGYRUM
(Quicksilver)

Every organ and tissue of the body is more or less affected by this powerful drug; it transforms healthy cells into decrepid, inflamed and necrotic wrecks, decomposes the blood, producing a profound anemia. This malignant medicinal force is converted into useful life saving and life preserving service if employed homœopathically, guided by its clear cut symptoms. The lymphatic system is especially affected with all the membranes and *glands,* and internal organs, bones, etc. Lesions produced by mercury very similar to those of syphilis. Very often indicated in the *Secondary* stage of syphilis where there is a febrile chloro-anemia, rheumatoid pains behind sternum, around joints, etc.; ulceration of mouth and throat, falling of the hair, the eruptions and ulcerations of mouth and throat, etc. These are the special conditions and stages to which Mercur is homœopathic and where the 2x will do surprising work. Again, hereditary syphilis manifestations, are within its range; bullæ, abscesses, snuffles, marasmus, stomatitis or destructive inflammations. *Tremors* everywhere. Weakness with ebullitions and tremblings from least exertion. All Mercury symptoms are *worse at night,* from warmth of bed, from damp, cold, rainy weather, *worse during perspiration.* Complaints increase with the sweat and rest; all associated with a great deal of weariness, prostration, and trembling. A human "thermometer." Sensitive to heat and cold. Parts are much swollen, with raw, sore feeling; the profuse, oily perspiration does not relieve. *Breath,* excretions and body smell foul. Tendency to formation of pus, which is thin, greenish, putrid; streaked with thin blood.

Mind.—Slow in answering questions. Memory weakened, and loss of will-power. Weary of life. Mistrustful. Thinks he is losing his reason.

Head.—Vertigo, when *lying on back.* Band-feeling about head. One-sided, tearing pains. *Tension about scalp, as if bandaged.* Catarrhal headaches; much heat in head. Stinging, burning, fetid eruptions on scalp. Loss of hair. Exostosis, with feeling of soreness. Scalp tense; oily sweat on head.

Eyes.—Lids red, thick, swollen. *Profuse, burning, acrid discharge.* Floating black spots. *After exposure to glare of fire; foundrymen.* Parenchymatous keratitis of syphilitic origin with burning pain. Iritis, with hypopyon.

Ears.—Thick, *yellow discharge;* fetid and bloody. *Otalgia. worse warmth of bed;* at night. sticking pains. Boils in external canal. [*Calc. pic.*]

Nose.—Much sneezing. Sneezing *in sunshine. Nostrils raw, ulcerated;* nasal bones swollen. Yellow-green, fetid, pus-like discharge. Coryza; acrid discharge, but too thick to run down the lip; worse, warm room. Pain and *swelling of nasal bones, and caries, with greenish fetid ulceration.* Nosebleed at night. Copious discharge of corroding mucus. Coryza, with sneezing; sore, *raw,* smarting sensation; worse, damp weather; *profuse, fluent.*

Face.—Pale, *earthy,* dirty-looking, puffy. Aching in facial bones. Syphilitic pustules on face.

Mouth.—Sweetish metallic taste. *Salivary secretions greatly increased;* bloody and viscid. Saliva fetid, coppery. Speech difficult on account of trembling tongue. *Gums spongy,* recede, bleed easily. Sore pain on touch and from *chewing.* Whole mouth *moist.* Crown of teeth decay. Teeth loose, feel tender and elongated. *Furrow in upper surface of tongue lengthwise.* Tongue heavy, *thick; moist coating; yellow, flabby, teeth-indented;* feels as if burnt, wich ulcers. *Fetid odor* from mouth; can smell it all over room. Alveolar abscess, worse at night. *Great thirst, with moist mouth.*

Throat.—Bluish-red swelling. Constant desire to swallow. Putrid sore throat; worse right side. *Ulcers* and inflammation appearing at every change in weather. Stitches into ear on swallowing; fluids return through nose. Quinsy, with difficult swallowing, *after pus has formed.* Sore, raw, smarting, burning throat. Complete loss of voice. Burning in throat, as from hot vapor ascending.

Stomach.—Putrid eructations. *Intense thirst for cold drinks.* Weak digestion, with *continuous hunger.* Stomach sensitive to touch. Hiccough and regurgitation. Feels replete and constricted.

Abdomen.—Stabbing pain, with chilliness. Boring pain in right groin. Flatulent distention, with pain. Liver enlarged; sore to touch, indurated. Jaundice. Bile secreted deficiently.

Stool.—Greenish, *bloody and slimy, worse at night; with pain and tenesmus. Never-get-done feeling.* Discharge accompanied by chilliness, sick stomach, cutting colic, and tenesmus. Whitish-gray stools.

Urine.—Frequent urging. Greenish discharge from urethra; burning in urethra on beginning to urinate. Urine dark, scanty, bloody, albuminous.

Male.—Vesicles and ulcers; soft chancre. Cold genitals. Prepuce irritated; itches. Nocturnal emissions, stained with blood.

Female.—Menses profuse, with abdominal pains. Leucorrhœa excoriating, greenish and bloody; *sensation of rawness in* parts. *Stinging pain* in ovaries. [*Apis.*] Itching and burning; worse, after urinating; better, washing with cold water. Morning sickness, with profuse salivation. Mammæ painful and full of milk at menses.

Respiratory.—Soreness from fauces to sternum. *Cannot lie on right side.* [Left side, *Lycop.*] Cough, with yellow mucopurulent expectoration. Paroxysms of two; worse, night, and from warmth of bed. Catarrh, with chilliness; dread of air. Stitches from lower lobe of right lung to back. Whooping-cough with nosebleed. [*Arnica.*] Cough worse, tobacco smoke.

Back.—Bruised pain in small of back, especially when sitting. Tearing pain in coccyx; better, pressing on abdomen.

Extremities.—Weakness of limbs. Bone-pains and in limbs; worse, night. Patient very sensitive to cold. Oily perspiration. *Trembling extremities, especially hands; paralysis agitans.* Lacerating pain in joints. Cold, clammy sweat on legs at night. Dropsical swelling of feet and legs.

Skin.—Almost *constantly moist.* Persistent dryness of the skin contraindicates mercurius. Excessive odorous viscid perspiration; worse, night. *General tendency to free perspiration, but patient is not relieved thereby.* Vesicular and pustular eruptions. Ulcers, irregular in shape, edges undefined. Pimples around the main eruption. *Itching;* worse from warmth of bed. Crusta lactea; yellowish-brown crusts, considerable suppuration. Glands swell every time patient takes cold. Buboes. Orchitis. [*Clemat.*; *Hamam.*; *Puls.*]

Fever.—Generally gastric or bilious, with profuse nightly perspiration; debility, slow and lingering. Heat and shuddering alternately. Yellow perspiration. *Profuse perspiration without relief. Creeping chilliness;* worse in the evening and into night. Alternate flashes of heat in single parts.

Modalities.—*Worse*, at night, wet, damp weather, lying on right side, perspiring; warm room and warm bed.

Relationship.—Compare: *Capparis coriaccea* (polyuria, glandular affections, mucous diarrhœa; influenza); *Epilobium*—Willow herb–(chronic diarrhœa with tenesmus and mucous discharges; ptyalism, dysphagia; wasting of body and much debility; cholera infantum); *Kali hyd.* (in hard chancre); *Mercur. acet.* (Congestion with stiffness, dryness and heat of parts affected. Eyes inflamed, burn and itch. Lack of moisture. Throat dry, talking difficult. Pressure in lower sternum; chancre in urethra; tenia capitis favosa margin of ulcers painful): *Mercurius auratus* (psoriasis and syphilitic catarrh; brain tumors; lues of nose and bones; ozæna; swelling of testicles); *Mercurius bromatus* (secondary syphilitic skin affection); *Mercurius nitrosus*—Nitrate of Mercury—(especially in postular conjunctivitis and keratitis; gonorrhœa and mucous patches, with *sticking pains;* syphilides); *Mercurius phosphoricus* (nervous diseases from syphilis; exostoses); *Mercurius præcipitatus ruber* (suffocative attacks at night on lying down *while on the point of falling asleep*, obliged to jump up suddenly which relieves; gonorrhœa; *urethra felt as a hard string;* chancroid; phagedænic ulcer and bubo; pemphigus, mucous patches, eczema with rhagades and fissures, barber's itch; blepharitis, internally and externally; leaden heaviness in occiput, with otorrhœa); *Mercurius tannicus* (syphilides in patients with gastro-intestinal diseases, or, if very sensitive, to ordinary mercurial preparations); *Erythrinus*—South American Red Mullet Fish—(in pityriasis rubra and syphilis; red rash on chest; pityriasis); *Lolium temulentum* (in *trembling* of hands and legs); *Mercur. cum kali* (inveterate colds, acute facial paralysis). *Henchera*—Alum root—(Gastro-enteritis nausea, vomiting of bile and frothy mucous; stools watery, profuse, slimy, tenesmus, never get done feeling. Dose, 2 to 10 drops of tincture).

Compare: *Mez.; Phos.; Syph.; Kali mur.; Æthiops.*
Antidote: *Hep.; Aur.; Mez.*
Complementary: *Badiaga.*

Dose.—Second to thirtieth potency.

MERCURIUS CORROSIVUS
(Corrosive Sublimate)

This salt leads all other remedies in tenesmus of the rectum, which is incessant, and is not relieved by the stool. The tenesmus often involves the bladder as well. Bright's disease. Gonorrhœa; second stage, with continuous tenesmus. Destroys the secreting portions of the kidneys. This process is slow, but sure. Albuminuria in early pregnancy. (*Phosph.* later and at full term.)

Head.—Delirium, stupor. Frontal pain, congestion of head, with burning in cheeks. Drawing pain in periosteum of skull.

Eyes.—Pain behind eyeballs, as if forced out. Phlyctenulæ; deep ulcers on cornea. Excessive photophobia and *acrid lachrymation*. *Iritis*, ordinary or syphilitic. (Give in association with atropin locally for prevention of adhesions.) Pain severe at night; burning, shooting, tearing. Little tendency to pus formation. *Iris muddy in color, thick, and neither contracts nor dilates.* Retinitis albuminuric, ophthalmia neonatorum. *Lids œdematous*, red, excoriated. *Severe burning. Soreness of the eyes.*

Nose.—Excessive coryza. Ozæna, with perforation of septum nasi. [*Kali bich.*] Rawness and smarting in nostrils. Post-nasal swelling, mucous membrane dry, red, and covered with bloody mucus.

Ears.—Violent pulsations. Fetid pus.

Face.—Swollen. Red, puffy. Lips black, swollen. Sordes. Facial neuralgia within the bones.

Mouth.—Teeth loose. Gums purple, swollen, and spongy. Tongue swollen and inflamed. Salivation. Pyorrhœa. Ptyalism. Taste salty and bitter.

Throat.—*Red, swollen, painful, intensely inflamed. Uvula swollen. Swallowing painful.* Most pain is *post-nasal with sharp pains to ears. Burning pain, with great swelling; worse, slight external pressure.* All glands about thorax swollen.

Stomach.—Incessant, green, bilious vomiting. Epigastrium very sensitive.

Abdomen.—Bruised sensation; cæcal region and transverse colon painful. Bloated; very painful to least touch.

Stool.—Dysentery; tenesmus, not relieved by stool; incessant. Stool hot, bloody, slimy, offensive, with cutting pains and shreds of mucous membrane.

Respiratory.—Pain in larynx as cut with knife. Aphonia. Cough, with bloody expectoration. Pulse rapid and intermittent. Stitches through side of chest.

Urine.—Intense burning in urethra. Urine hot, burning, scanty or *suppressed;* bloody, *greenish discharge. Albuminous. Tenesmus of bladder.* Stabbing pain extending up urethra into bladder. Perspiration after urinating.

Male.—Penis and testes enormously swollen. Chancres assume phagedænic appearance. *Gonorrhœa;* urethra orifice red, swollen; glans sore and hot. Discharge greenish, thick.

Fever.—Chilly from slightest exposure. Profuse perspiration; surfaces cold.

Modalities.—*Worse,* evening, night, acids. *Better,* while at rest.

Relationship.—Compare: *Ars.; Lach.; Leonurus—Motherwort* (Influences pelvic organs, allays spasm and nervous irritability, promotes secretion and reduces febrile excitement. Valuable in suppressed menses and *lochia;* dysentery; vomiting, frightful pains in abdomen, violent thirst. Tongue dry and cracked). *Monsonia*—An African plant belonging to the Geraniaceæ—(Used for dysentery in material doses).

Antidote: *Calcium sulphide* is antidotal to Bichloride poisoning. Use intravenous injection of 7½ grains in 7½ ozs. boiled water.

Dose.—Sixth potency. In solution 1 : 1000, hypodermically injected under conjunctiva in chorodcitis with progressive myopia. Stops immediately the severe aching pain behind eyeballs. (Dr. G. D. Hallet.)

MERCURIUS CYANATUS
(Cyanide of Mercury)

Acute infections, pneumonia, nephritis. Its action is similar to that of the toxines of infectious diseases. Great and rapid prostration, tendency toward hæmorrhages, from the different orifices, of dark fluid blood, cyanosis, rapid respiration and heart action, albuminuria and twitching and jerking of muscles. Typhoid pneumonia.

Livid states from great struggling, where suffocation is imminent and paralysis of lung threatening; great sweat.

Affects most prominently the buccal cavity. This, together with marked prostration, gives it a place in the treatment of *diphtheria*, where it has achieved unquestioned great results. Malignant types, with prostration. Coldness and nausea. Syphilitic ulcers when perforation threatens.

Head.—Great excitement, fits of passion; fury; talkativeness. Atrocious headache. Eyes sunken; face pale.

Mouth.—Covered with ulcerations. Tongue pale. Free salivation. Fetor of breath. Pain and swelling of salivary glands. Astringent taste. *Ulcerations* of mouth have a gray membrane.

Throat.—Feels raw and sore. Mucous membranes broken down, ulcerated. Looks raw in spots, especially in public speakers. Hoarseness, and talking is painful. *Necrotic destruction of soft parts of palate and fauces*. Intense redness of fauces. Swallowing very difficult. Dark blood from nose. Diphtheria of the larynx and nose. [*Kali bich.*]

Stomach.—Nausea, vomiting, bilious, bloody; hiccough; abdomen painful, tender to pressure.

Rectum.—Intolerable pain. Redness around anus. Frequent hæmorrhage; stools with tenesmus. Discharge of fetid liquid with gangrenous odor. Black stools.

Urinary.—Amber color, painful, albuminous, scanty. Nephritis with great debility and chilliness. Suppression of urine.

Skin.—Moisture, with icy coldness.

Dose.—Sixth to thirtieth potency. Aggravation is apt to occur from potencies below the sixth.

MERCURIUS DULCIS
(Calomel)

Has marked effect on catarrhal inflammation of ear, and useful in Eustachian catarrh, deafness. Diarrhœa, with soreness of anus. *Prostatitis*. Remittent bilious attacks. *Pallor, flabby bloatedness*, and turgid flaccidity. Inflammation with plastic exudate. Especially indicated in systems disposed to remittent bilious fevers; in peritonitis and meningitis *with plastic exudate*. Dropsies due to combined renal and cardiac diseases, especially with jaundice (Hale). Cirrhosis of the liver, especially in the hypertrophic form. Use 1x (Jousset).

Ears.—Otitis media; closure of Eustachian tube; ear troubles of scrofulous children; membrana tympani retracted, thickened and immovable.

Mouth.—Offensive breath; salivation; sore gums. Ulcers. Tongue black. Constant flow of dark, putrid saliva; very offensive. Ulceration of throat, with dysphagia. Granular pharyngitis.

Stomach.—Nausea and vomiting. Cyclic vomiting of infants. [*Cup. ars.; Iris.*]

Stool.—Scanty, bloody mucus, with bile, and *constant desire*, without tenesmus. Dark-green, watery, with griping. *Anus sore* and burning. Dysentery; small stools of *mucus and blood, covered with bile*.

Skin.—*Flabby and ill nourished*. Swollen glands. Phagedenic ulcers. Copper-colored eruptions.

Relationship.—Compare: *Kali mur.*

Dose.—Third to sixth trituration. For palliative (non-homœopathic) purposes, to secure evacuation of bowels, two or three-grain doses of first decimal trituration, repeated several times every hour.

MERCURIUS IODATUS FLAVUS
(Proto-iodide of Mercury)

Throat affections, with greatly swollen glands and characteristic coating of tongue. Worse, right side. Chancre; induration remains long time. Swollen inguinal glands, large and hard. *Mammary tumors*, with tendency to much warm perspiration and gastric disturbances.

Tongue.—*Coated thickly; yellow at the base.* Tip and edges may be red and take imprint of teeth.

Throat.—Lacunar tonsillitis. When only the superficial part of the tonsil is involved. Cheesy exudates with offensive breath. Swelling begins on right side. Small ulcers on posterior pharynx. Easily detached patches on inflamed pharynx and fauces; *worse on right tonsil;* much tenacious mucus. Sensation of a lump. *Constant inclination to swallow.*

Relationship.—Compare: *Plum. iod.* (in mammary tumors).

Dose.—Second trituration.

MERCURIUS IODATUS RUBER
(Bin-iodide of Mercury)

Diphtheria and ulcerated sore throats, especially on left side, with much glandular swelling. Chronic suppurating buboes. Hard chancres. Old cases of syphilis in scrofulous patients. Early stages of cold, especially in children.

Throat.—*Fauces dark red;* swallowing painful. Phlegm in nose and throat. Disposition to hawk, with sensation of a lump in throat. *Stiffness of muscles of throat and neck.*

Nose.—Coryza and dull hearing; right side of nose hot. Hawks mucus from posterior nares. Turbinated bones swollen. Boggy mucous membrane of nose and throat; closure of Eustachian tube, opening with a pop.

Mouth.—Gums swollen; toothache; glands swollen. Scalded feeling on tongue. Aphthæ. Profuse saliva. Tongue feels stiff at base, and pains on moving.

Throat.—Diphtheria; submaxillary glands painfully engorged, fauces dark red; *worse on left tonsil*. Parenchymatous tonsillitis. Will often abort peritonsillitis if given frequently. Cough from elongated uvula, with sore throat. Laryngeal troubles with aphonia.

Skin.—Small fissures and cracks; hard papules; *Hunterian chancre*; syphilitic ulcers. Bubo. Sarcocele.

Dose.—Third trituration. Mercuric iodide is far more active as a bactericide than the other mercurials, including the chloride.

MERCURIUS SULPHURICUS—
HYDRARG. OXYD. SUB-SULPH.

(Turpethum Minerale—Yellow Sulphate of Mercury)

Watery stools, burning in anus. Sore tip of tongue. Œdema of legs. Sneezing from direct rays of sun. Diarrhœa early in the morning; stool bursts out in a hot stream of yellow matter. Intense evacuations, like rice-water. Scanty, clear, scalding urine. *Intense dyspnœa;* must sit up. Respiration rapid, short; burning in chest. *Hydrothorax.* [*Ars.*] Cardiac pain and weakness.

Relationship.—Compare: *Mercur. acet.* (cutting in urethra when last drop is flowing out).

METHYLENE BLUE
(One of the Aniline Dyes)

A remedy for neuralgia, neurasthenia, malaria; *typhoid*, here it diminishes the tympanites, delirium, and fever; pus infection. Tendency to tremor, chorea and epilepsy. Nephritis (acute parenchymatous), scarlatinal nephritis. Urine acquires a green color. Bladder irritation from its use antidoted by a little nutmeg. Surgical kidney with large amount of pus in urine. Gonorrhœal rheumatism and cystitis. Backache, sciatica. Later states of apoplexy (Gisevius).

Dose.—3x attenuation. A 2 per cent. solution locally, in chronic otitis with foul smelling discharge.

A 1 per cent. aqueous solution for ulcers and abscesses of cornea.

MEZEREUM
(Spurge Olive)

Skin symptoms, affections of bones, and neuralgias most important, especially about teeth and face. Bruised, weary feeling in joints, with drawing and stiffness. *Pains of various kinds, with chilliness* and *sensitiveness to cold air*. Bone pains. Eruptions after vaccination. Burning, darting sensation in the muscles; subsultus tendinum. Pains shoot upward and seem to draw patient up out of bed. Semi-lateral complaints. *Patient is very sensitive to cold air.*

Head.—Hard work to talk. Headache; worse from talking. Stupefying headache in right side. Affections of external head; scaly eruption, white scabs. Head covered with *thick, leathery crusts, under which pus collects*. Violent neuralgia about face and teeth, running towards ear, at night; *worse, eating;* better near hot stove. Roots of teeth decay. Teeth feel elongated.

Nose.—Sneezing, coryza, interior of nose, excoriated. Post-nasal adenoids.

Ears.—Feel too much open, *as if tympanum was exposed to the cold air and it blew into the ear*. Desire to bore fingers in.

Eyes.—*Ciliary neuralgia after operations.* Especially after removal of eyeball. Pains radiate and shoot downward, *with cold feeling and stiffness of bone*.

Face.—Red. Eruption around mouth, with coryza.

Stomach.—Desire for ham-fat. Burning in tongue, extending to stomach. *Mouth waters.* Nausea felt in throat; better, eating. Chronic gastritis; burning, corroding pain; nausea, vomiting, chocolate color. *Gastric ulcer* with much burning.

Abdomen.—Swelling of glands with large abdomen in children. Pressure in inguinal ring. Flatulent colic, with shivering and difficult respiration.

Rectum.—Constipation after confinement. Prolapse of rectum. Diarrhœa, with small, white particles. *Green discharges.* Constipation, with hepatic and uterine inertia. Constriction of anus, stitches and prolapse of rectum.

Urine.—Red flakes float on top of urine. Hot, bloody. Biting, burning in forepart of urethra at the close of micturition.

Hæmaturia preceded by cramp pain in the bladder. After urinating, a few drops of blood are passed.

Female.—Menses too frequent, soon, profuse. Leucorrhœa like albumen; very corroding.

Male.—*Enlargement of testicles.* Violent sexual desire. Gonorrhœa, with hæmaturia.

Respiratory.—Soreness and burning in bones of thorax. Constriction across chest. Cough; worse, eating, irritation lower than can be reached, on taking a warm drink.

Extremities.—Pain in neck and back; worse, motion and at night; intolerant of all touch. *Pain and burning in tibia and long bones.* Legs and feet go to sleep. Pain in hip and knee.

Skin.—Eczema; *intolerable itching;* chilliness with pruritus; worse in bed. Ulcers itch and burn, surrounded by vesicles and shining, fiery-red areola. Zona, with burning pain. *Bones, especially long bones, inflamed and swollen; caries, exostosis; pain worse night, touch, damp weather.* [*Merc.; Syph.*] *Eruptions ulcerate and form thick scabs under which purulent matter exudes.* [*Chrysophanic acid.*]

Modalities.—*Worse,* cold air; night, evening until midnight, warm food, touch, motion. *Better,* open air.

Relationship.—Compare: *Dirca palustris*—Leather wood—(a gastro-intestinal irritant inducing salivation, emesis and purgation; cerebral hyperæmia, neuralgic pains, with depression, palpitation, and dyspnœa); *Merc.; Phyt.; Rhus; Guaiac.; Syph.*

Antidotes: *Kali hyd.; Merc.*

Dose.—Sixth to thirtieth potency.

MICROMERIA
(Yerba Buena)

A California mint-like plant acting on stomach and bowels. Used as a tea to cure colic and relieve flatulence. Is a pleasant beverage and febrifuge, blood purifyer and tonic.

Stomach.—Nausea; pain in stomach and bowels; flatulence.

Dose.—Tincture.

MILLEFOLIUM
(Yarrow)

An invaluable remedy for various types of hæmorrhages; blood bright red. Incarcerated hernia; small-pox, with great pain in pit of stomach. After operations for stone. Bad effects from fall from a height; overlifting. *Continued high temperature.* Hæmoptysis.

Head.—Vertigo when moving slowly. Sensation as if he had forgotten something. The head seems full of blood. Convulsions and epilepsy from suppressed menses. *Piercing thrusts of pain.*

Nose.—*Nosebleed.* [*Erecht.*] Piercing pain from eyes to root of nose.

Stool.—Hæmorrhage from bowels. Bleeding hæmorrhoids. *Urine bloody.* [*Senec. aur.*]

Female.—Menses early, profuse, protracted. Hæmorrhage from uterus; bright red, fluid. *Painful varices during pregnancy.*

Respiratory.—Hæmoptysis in incipient phthisis. Cough, with bloody expectoration, in suppressed menses or hæmorrhoids. Violent palpitation.

Relationship.—Compare: *Ficus venosa (Pakur).* Hæmorrhage from bowels and lungs. *Acalypha* and *Helix tosta*—Snail—(in hæmoptysis, diseases of chest, consumption); also, *Secale; Ipec.; Erecht.; Geran.; Hamam.*

Dose.—Tincture, to third potency.

MITCHELLA
(Partridge-berry)

Bladder symptoms accompany complaints, especially uterine congestion.

Urinary.—Irritation at neck of bladder, with urging to urinate. [*Eup. purp.; Apis.*] Dysuria. Catarrh of bladder.

Female.—Cervix dark red, swollen. Dysmenorrhœa and uterine hæmorrhage; blood bright red.

Relationship.—Compare: *Chimaph.; Senecio; Uva; Geran.; Gossyp.*

Dose.—Tincture.

MOMORDICA BALSAMINA
(Balsam Apple)

Griping, colic, pain in back and hypogastrium with painful and excessive menses. Accumulation of flatus in splenic flexure of colon. Dropsy.

Head.—Dizzy, contents of head feel lighter; mist before eyes.

Abdomen.—Rumbling, griping, colicky pains, starting from back, spreading over abdomen.

Female.—Painful and profuse menses; labor-like pains, followed by gushes of blood; pain at small of back coming towards front of pelvis.

Relationship.—*Momordica charantia*—Indian variety—(more severe symptoms—intestines full of yellow watery fluid, discharged *explosively*—cramps, thirst, prostration. Choleraic symptoms. Similar to Croton, Elaterium. Use 3x.)

Dose.—Tincture. Used also externally as a liniment and poultice for burns, chapped hands, etc.

MORPHINUM
(An Alkaloid of Opium)

Morphine bears the same relation to Opium as Atropine to Belladonna—i. e., represents its nervous side. It is less stimulating, less convulsant, and more decidedly hypnotic. Constipates less and affects contractility of the bladder more. It is less diaphoretic and more pruritic.

Mind.—*Profound depression.* Irritable, fault-finding, hysterical. *Shock induced by terror. Dream-like state.*

Head.—*Vertigo from the least movement of the head.* Headache, with sensation of being "wound-up." Bursting pain; head drawn back.

Eyes.—Bluish, drooping lids. *Itching* of eyes. Delusion of vision on closing eyes. Staring, injected; diverging strabismus. Pupils unequally contracted. *Look unsteady.* Ptosis. *Paresis of recti interni.*

Ears.—Left ear throbs painfully; better, heat. *Seems to hear circulation all over body.*

Face.—*Dusky red or pallid lividity of face, lips, tongue, mouth or throat.*

Nose.—Sneezing in paroxysms. *Itching* and tingling on end of nose.

Mouth.—*Very dry.* Tongue dry, brown violet in middle. Thirst. Loss of appetite, *with aversion to meat.*

Throat.—Dry and constricted. Pharynx paralyzed, swallowing almost impossible; better hot drinks, worse solids.

Stomach.—Nausea *incessant and deathly*, faintness, constant retching. Vomiting of green fluid. *Nausea and vomiting on rising up.*

Abdomen.—Distended. Acute pain in abdomen and along spinal column. *Tympanitis.*

Rectum.—Diarrhœa watery, brown, or black with horrible tenesmus. Constipation; stools large, dry, knotty, with tendency to bruise and fissure.

Urinary.—Paresis of bladder. *Strangury. Slow and difficult urination.* Retention of prostatic hypertrophy. *Uræmia*, acute and chronic.

Male.—Impotency. Pain in right spermatic cord. [*Oxal. ac.*]

Heart.—*Alternation of tachycardia and bradycardia.* Cardiac muscular tissue is intact, even if severely exhausted. Pulse small, weak, dicrotic.

Respiratory.—Faint and struggling for breath; *diaphragmatic paralysis;* hiccough; dyspnœa, paroxysmal, on first falling asleep. [*Lach.; Grindel.*] Cheyne-Stokes respiration. Chest tight. Pain in middle of sternum. Dry, hard, *teasing*, exhausting cough, worse at night. Strangling cough, with viscid mucus sputum; thin, scanty, but sounds loose and abundant.

Back.—Pain along spine. Weakness of loins. Aching across lumbo-sacral region; cannot walk erect. [*Cimicif.*]

Extremities.—Staggering gait. *Numbness.*

Skin.—*Livid;* purple spots; zoster-like herpes. *Itching.* Skin lost its elasticity. Urticaria appearing at climaxis.

Nervous.—Restlessness and hyperæsthesia; trembling, twitching, jerking, convulsions. *Extremely susceptible to pain.* Pain causes twitching and jerking of limbs. Violent and *sudden* neuralgic pains and sudden fainting. *Delirium, melancholic in character.* Neuralgias *intensely painful;* left supraorbital; right intercostal, better from heat; *multiple neuritis.* Sore feeling all over. *Bed feels too hard.* Aggravation after sleep. [*Lach.*] Neuralgia after zoster. [*Mezer.*]

Sleep.—Yawning, *drowsy;* prolonged, deep sleep. Sleepless; restless sleep, with frequent startings. Sleepy, but cannot sleep.

Fever.—Chills. Icy coldness. Burning heat; profuse sweat.

Dose.—Third to sixth trituration.

MOSCHUS
(Musk)

A remedy for hysteria and nervous paroxysms, *fainting fits* and convulsions, catalepsy, etc. The characteristic condition being aggravation by cold; there is great sensitiveness to air. Much nervous trembling and frequent fainting. Great flatulence. Diseases do not follow a normal course. *Coldness.* Tension in muscles, skin and mind.

Mind.—*Uncontrollable laughter.* Scolding. Anxiety, with palpitation; starting as if frightened. Sexual hypochondriasis.

Head.—Compressive pain over root of nose. Pressure on top of head. Vertigo on least motion; sensation as if falling from a great height. Scalp sensitive. Sounds in ears as from the report of a cannon.

Stomach.—Desire for black coffee, stimulants. Aversion to food. Everything tastes flat. With stomach symptoms, anxiety in chest. Distended. Faints when eating. Abdomen greatly distended. *Spasmodic, nervous hiccough.* [*Hydrocy. ac.; Sulph. ac.; Ignat.; Cajap.*]

Male.—*Violent desire;* involuntary emissions. Impotence, associated with diabetes. [*Coca.*] Premature senility. Nausea and vomiting after coition.

Female.—Menses too early, too profuse, with disposition to faint. [*Nux m.; Veratr.*] Sexual desire, with intolerable titillation in parts. Drawing and pushing in the direction of the genitals; sensation as if menses appear.

Urine.—Profuse urination. *Diabetes.*

Respiratory.—Tightness of chest, is obliged to take a deeper breath. Sudden constriction of larynx and trachea. *Difficult respiration; chest oppressed;* hysterical spasm of chest; asthma. Spasm of glottis. Impending paralysis of lungs. Asthma, with intense anxiety, fear, and smothering sensation. *Cough ceases, mucus cannot be expectorated.* Globus hystericus.

Heart.—Hysterical palpitation. Trembling around heart. Weak pulse and fainting.

Modalities.—*Better*, in open air, rubbing. *Worse*, cold. The open air is felt very, very cold.

Relationship.—Compare: *Nux mosch.; Asaf.; Valer.; Sumbul.; Ign.; Castor.*

Compatible: *Ambra.*

Antidotes: *Camph.; Coff.*

Dose.—First to third potency.

MUREX
(Purple Fish)

The symptoms of the female sexual organs are most prominent, and have been clinically verified. Especially adapted to nervous, lively, affectionate women. Patient weak and run down.

Mind.—Great sadness, anxiety, and dread.

Stomach.—Sinking, all-gone sensation in stomach. [*Sep.*] Hungry, must eat.

Female.—Conscious of a womb. Pulsation in neck of womb. *Desire easily excited.* Feeling as if something was pressing on a sore spot in the pelvis; worse sitting. *Pain from right side of womb to right or left breast. Nymphomania.* Least contact of parts causes *violent sexual excitement*. Sore pain in uterus. Menses irregular, profuse, frequent, large clots. Feeling of protrusion. Prolapse; enlargement of uterus, with pelvic tenesmus and sharp pains, extending toward breasts; aggravated lying down. Dysmenorrhœa and chronic endometritis, with displacement. *Must keep legs tightly crossed.* Leucorrhœa green or bloody, alternate with mental symptoms and aching in sacrum. Benign tumors in breasts. Pain in them during menstrual period.

Urinary.—Urine frequent at night; smells like Valerian; constant urging. [*Kros.*]

Modalities.—*Worse*, least touch.

Relationship.—Compare: *Plat.; Lil.; Sep.* (the latter lacks sexual erethism of *Murex.*)

Dose.—Third to thirtieth potency.

MURIATICUM ACIDUM
(Muriatic Acid)

This acid has an elective affinity for the blood, producing a septic condition similar to that found in low fevers with high temperature and great prostration. Patient becomes so weak she slides down the bed. Decomposition of fluids. Involuntary stools while passing urine. Hæmorrhages. Mouth and anus chiefly affected.

Mind.—Irritable and peevish; fretful. *Loud moaning.* Great restlessness. Sad, taciturn; *suffers in silence.*

Head.—Vertigo; *worse lying on right side;* occiput heavy as if filled with lead. Sound of voice is intolerable. Pain as if brain were crushed.

Nose.—*Hæmorrhage;* much sneezing.

Face.—Lower jaw fallen; pimples and freckles; lips raw, dry, cracked.

Mouth.—Tongue, pale, swollen, dry, leathery, paralyzed. Deep ulcers on tongue. Hard lumps in tongue. Epithelioma; edges bluish-red. [*Carbol. ac.*] Aphthous mouth. Gums and glands swollen. Fetid breath. *Sordes on teeth.*

Throat.—Uvula swollen. Ulcers and false membrane. Œdematous, dark, raw. Attempted swallowing produces spasm and choking.

Stomach.—Cannot bear sight or thought of meat. At times, ravenous appetite and constant desire to drink. Achlorhydria and fermentation of food.

Rectum.—Tendency to involuntary evacuations while urinating. *Hæmorrhoids most sensitive to all touch;* even sheet of toilet paper is painful. Anal itching and prolapsus ani while urinating. *Hæmorrhoids during pregnancy; bluish, hot, with violent stitches.*

Heart.—Pulse rapid, *feeble, and small. Intermits every third beat.*

Urine.—Cannot urinate without having bowels move at same time.

Female.—Menses appear too soon. Leucorrhœa. During menses, soreness of anus. Ulcer in genitals.

Extremities.—Heavy, painful, and weak. Tottering gait. Pain in tendo-Achilles.

Skin.—Papular and vesicular eruptions, with great itching. [*Rhus.*] Carbuncles; foul-smelling ulcers on lower extremities. Scarlet fever, livid, with petechiæ; scanty eruption. Eczema on back of hands.

Fever.—Cold extremities. Heat without thirst. Typhoid types, stupid. Hæmorrhages. Restlessness. Involuntary discharges. Bed-sores. Pulse rapid and feeble. Excessive prostration.

Modalities.—*Worse*, in damp weather, before midnight. *Better*, lying on left side.

Relationship.—Compare: *Phos. ac.; Ars.; Bapt.* Follows well after *Bry.* and *Rhus.*

Antidote: *Bryonia.*

Dose.—First to third potency.

MYGALE LASIODORA
(Black Cuban Spider)

Weakness, palpitation, nervousness, fear, like other spider preparations. Chorea is the principal therapeutic field of this Sexual symptoms are important.

Mind.—Delirious, restless, sad; fears death; despondent.

Face.—*Twitching of facial muscles.* Mouth and eyes open in rapid succession. Hot and *flushed.* Tongue dry and parched; put out with difficulty. Head jerked to one side. Grating of teeth at night.

Stomach.—Nausea, with dim sight. Aversion to food. Excessive thirst.

Male.—Violent erections. Chordee. [*Kali brom.; Camph.*]

Extremities.—Unsteady gait. *Constant motion of whole body.* Tremulous. Intense redness in streaks, following course of lymphatics. Twitching of limbs. Restless hands. Convulsive, *uncontrollable movements of arms and legs.* Limbs drag while walking.

Relationship.—Compare: *Agar.; Tarant.; Cupr.; Zizia.*

Modalities.—*Better*, during sleep. *Worse.* in morning.

Dose.—Third to thirtieth potency.

MYOSOTIS
(Forget-me-not)

Chronic bronchitis and phthisis. Night-sweats.

Respiratory.—Cough with profuse muco-purulent expectoration, gagging and vomiting during cough; worse while or after eating. Bronchorrhœa. Pain in left lung (lower); painful while coughing and sensitive to percussion.

Dose.—Tincture to second potency.

MYRICA
(Bayberry)

Marked action on the liver, with jaundice and mucous membranes. Persistent sleeplessness. *Jaundice.*

Mind.—*Despondent, irritable,* indifferent. *Gloomy.*

Head.—Scalp feels tight. Headache, with drowsiness; yellow sclerotica; aching in eyeballs. Pressure in vertex and forehead. *Dull, heavy aching in temples and forehead on waking in the morning.* Pain and stiffness in nape of neck.

Face.—Yellow. Itching and stinging. Creeping sensation.

Mouth.—Tongue furred, with bad taste in mouth, and nausea. *Tenacious, thick, nauseous secretion.* Tender, spongy, and bleeding gums. [*Merc.*]

Throat.—Constricted and rough feeling, with a constant desire to swallow. Stringy mucus; detached with difficulty.

Stomach.—Taste bitter and nauseous, with offensive breath. Complete loss of appetite, but with a feeling of fullness in the stomach after a hearty meal. Strong desire for acids. Weak, sinking feeling in the epigastrium, approaching nausea; increased after eating; relieved by rapid walking.

Abdomen.—Dull pain in the region of the liver. Complete jaundice, with bronze-yellow skin; loss of appetite. Fullness in the stomach and abdomen. Scanty, yellow, frothy urine.

Stool.—Constant discharge of flatus when walking. Urging to stool, with no other results than the expulsion of a great amount of flatus. Loose, light-colored stool; ash-colored and destitute of bile.

Urinary.—Dark, frothy, scanty, high-colored, biliary.

Sleep.—Disturbed, bad dreams and frequent waking; insomnia.

Extremities.—Staggering gait. Pain under shoulder-blades and back of neck, in all muscles, in hollow of right foot.

Skin.—Yellow and itching. *Jaundice.* Creeping sensation, as of insects.

Relationship.—Compare: *Ptel.; Cornus cir.; Chelid.; Lept.; Fagop.*

Antidote: *Digit. (jaundice).*

Dose.—Tincture, to third potency.

MYRISTICA SEBIFERA
(Brazilian Ucuba)

A remedy of great antiseptic powers. Inflammation of skin, cellular tissue and periosteum. Traumatic infections. Parotitis. Fistulas. Carbuncles. *Specific action in panaritium.* Pain in the finger nails with swelling of the phalanges. Hands are stiff, as if from squeezing something a long time. Coppery taste and burning in throat. Tongue white and cracked. Phlegmonous inflammations. Hastens suppuration and shortens its duration. Often does away with use of the knife. Inflammation of middle ear, suppurative stage. Fistula in ano. Acts more powerfully often than Hepar or Silica.

MYRTUS COMMUNIS
(Myrtle)

The leaves contain Myrtol, an active antiseptic. Chest pains, as found often in consumptives, call for this remedy. Incipient phthisis. Nerve sedative and stimulant to mucous membranes, bronchitis, cystitis and pyelitis.

Chest.—Stitching pain *in left breast, running through to shoulder-blade.* [*Illic.; Therid.; Pix.*] Dry, hollow cough, with tickling in chest. Worse in the morning. Sensation of burning in left chest.

Relationship.—Compare: *Myrtus Chekan* (Chronic bronchitis with dense, yellowish sputum, difficult to detach. Copious expectoration keeps patient distressed and coughing).

Dose.—Third potency.

NAJA TRIPUDIANS
(Virus of the Cobra)

Naja produces a typical bulbar paralysis (L. J. Boyd). Causes no hæmorrhage but only œdema, hence the victims of this reptile frequently bear very little sign of external injury, a small scratch or puncture being the only indication where the fangs have worked their havoc. The tissue lying beneath the wound is colored dark purple, and a large quantity of viscid blood-like fluid collects in the vicinity of the wound. An intense burning pain at the spot bitten is the first symptom. In man there follows an interval before fresh symptoms occur. The average is about an hour. Once developed, the symptoms follow a rapid course. A feeling of intoxication is produced, followed by a loss of power over the limbs. The patient is bereft of speech, swallowing, and the control over the movement of the lips. The saliva is ejected in large quantities, the respiration gradually becomes slower and slower, and at length ceases. Conscious all time. Is not a hæmorrhagic or septic, medicine like Lachesis and Crotalus. Its action settles around the heart; valvular troubles. Marked surging of blood upwards, marked dyspnœa, inability to lie on left side. Hypertrophy, and valvular lesions. *Organs seem to be drawn together.* Very susceptible to cold. With heart symptoms, pain in forehead and temples. Diseases primarily depending upon degeneration of motor cells. Control of sphincters lost.

Mind.—Broods constantly over imaginary troubles. Suicidal insanity. [*Aur.*] Depressed. Aversion to talking. Blurred speech. Melancholy. Dreads to be left alone. Fear of rain.

Head.—*Pain in left temple and in left orbital region, extending to occiput, with nausea and vomiting.* Hay-fever, with dry larynx. Suffocative spells after sleeping. [*Lach.*] Eyes staring. Ptosis of both lids.

Ears.—Illusions of hearing; otalgia; chronic otorrhœa, black discharges; smells like herring brine.

Respiratory.—Grasping at throat, with sense of choking. *Irritating, dry cough, dependent on cardiac lesions.* [*Spong.; Lauroc.*] Sticky mucus and saliva. Asthmatic constriction in evening. Asthma beginning with coryza

Heart.—Dragging and anxiety in præcordia. Feeling of weight on heart. Angina pains extending to nape of neck, left shoulder and arm with anxiety and fear of death. With the heart symptoms pain in forehead and temples. Pulse *irregular in force*. Threatened paralysis of heart, body cold, pulse slow, weak, irregular, tremulous. *Acute and chronic endocarditis.* Palpitation. Stitching pain in region of heart. *Damaged heart after infectious diseases.* Marked symptoms of *low* tension. [*Elaps, Vipera.*]

Female.—Neuralgia of left ovary; often serviceable in obscure pain in left groin, especially in post-operative cases; *seems to be drawn to heart.*

Sleep.—Profound, like a log, with stertorous breathing, a typical reptilian state.

Modalities.—*Worse*, from use of stimulants; *better*, from walking or riding in open air.

Relationship.—Compare: Serpent poisons generally. *Bungarus Fasciatus* (Banded Krait). This venom produces a condition like an acute polioencephalitis and myelitis, both symptomatically and histologically. *Lach.; Crotal.; Spig.; Spong.*

Dose.—Sixth to thirtieth potency.

NAPHTHALINE
(A chemical compound from Coal-tar; Tar Camphor)

Coryza, hay-fever, phthisis pulmonalis, also gonorrhœa have been influenced favorably by this drug. Pyelonephritis. Irritation of the periphery of the urinary apparatus. Whooping-cough.

Head.—Lying as if stupefied by a narcotic. Restless. Face pale yellowish hue.

Eyes.—Marked affinity for the eye. It produces detachment of the retina; papillo-retinal infiltration; deposits in patches upon the retina; amblyopia and consecutive amaurosis; sparkling synchisis; soft cataract. Exudation in the retina, choroid and ciliary body. Cataract. *Opacity of the cornea.*

Urine.—Irresistible desire. Meatus red, swollen, and œdema of prepuce. Black urine. Cutting pain down penis. Pain in bladder. Terribly offensive odor of decomposing ammoniacal urine

Respiratory.—Sneezing; eyes inflamed; painful; head hot. *Hay-fever. Spasmodic asthma;* better in open air. Soreness in chest and stomach; must loosen clothing. *Dyspnœa* and sighing inspiration. Emphysema in the aged with asthma. *Whooping-cough,* long and continued paroxysms of coughing, unable to get a respiration. Acute laryngo-tracheitis. Bronchitis when the spasmodic element is associated with tenacious expectoration and oppression. (Cartier.)

Skin.—Dermatitis; itching infiltration. Eruptions at corners of mouth and pigmentation around nails.

Non-homœopathic Uses.—For worms, and especially pinworms, one-gramme dose. Externally in skin diseases, five per cent. ointment.

Relationship.—Compare: *Dros.; Corall.; Coccus. Terpin. hydrat.* (Whooping-cough, hay asthma and bronchial affections. 1-2 grain doses).

Dose.—Third trituration.

NARCISSUS
(Daffodil)

Symptoms of nausea followed by violent vomiting and diarrhœa.

Daffodil bulbs contain an alkaloid the action of which, according to authorities, varies as to whether the alkaloid is extracted from the flowering bulb or from the bulb after flowering. Thus in the former case the alkaloid *produces dryness of the mouth, checks cutaneous secretions, dilates the pupil of the eye, quickens the pulse, and slows and weakens the heart contractions.* On the other hand, the alkaloid from the bulbs after flowering *produces copious salivation, increases cutaneous secretion, contracts the pupil of the eye, produces slight relaxation of the pulse, and slight faintness and nausea.*—*The Lancet.*

A remedy for cough and bronchitis. Continuous cough. Coryza; frontal headache. Convulsive stage of whooping-cough.

Skin.—Erythema of a papular, vesicular and pustular type, aggravation in wet weather.

Dose.—First attenuation.

NATRUM ARSENICUM
(Arseniate of Sodium)

A remedy for nasal catarrh, with headache, pain at root of nose, dry and painful eyes. Psoriasis. [*Ars.; Chrysoph. ac.; Thyroid.*] Bronchitis of children over seven years. Facilitates the termination of the cold and conserves strength and appetite. (Cartier.)

Head.—Floating sensation on turning head quickly; aching in frontal region and root of nose, over orbits. Headache; worse, pressure and tobacco smoke.

Nose.—Watery discharge; drops into throat. *Feels stopped; pain at root.* Dry crusts, on removal, leave mucous membrane raw. Post-nasal dropping of thick, bland, yellowish mucus. *Crusts in nose.*

Eyes.— Catarrhal conjunctivitis and blepharitis marginalis. Eyes feel weak, stiffness of balls and tendency of lids to close. Feel heavy and droop. Lachrymation in wind. Agglutination in morning. Dry, painful, burning; soon tire. Œdema of orbital region. Supraorbital pain.

Throat.—Dark, *purplish, swollen, œdematous;* red and glassy.

Respiratory.—Racking cough, with profuse greenish expectoration. *Oppression of chest and about heart,* and also larynx. Miner's asthma. Lungs feel as though smoke had been inhaled.

Extremities.—Aching in arms; worse in shoulder. Pain in anterior crural nerves. Joints stiff. Feels tired all over. Knee-joints crack.

Relationship.—Compare: *Ars.; Kali carb.; Apis.*

Dose.—Third to thirtieth potency.

NATRUM CARBONICUM
(Carbonate of Sodium)

All the Natrums stimulate cellular activity and increase oxidation and metabolism. Great debility *caused by summer heat;* chronic effects of sunstroke: exhaustion; anæmic; milky, watery skin; very weak ankles, are all peculiar Natrum carbonicum conditions.

NATRUM CARBONICUM

Mind.—Unable to think; difficult, slow comprehension. Mental weakness and depression; worries; very sensitive to noise; colds, change of weather. Anxious and restless during thunder storm; worse from music. [*Ambra.*] Marked gayety. Sensitive to presence of certain individuals.

Head.—Aches from *slightest mental exertion*, worse from *sun or working under gas-light*. [*Glon.*] Feels too large. Oversensitive of hearing. Head aches with return of hot weather. Vertigo from exposure to sun.

Nose.—All troubles of external nose which may attain a morbid size—pimples and puffiness. Constant coryza; obstruction of nose. Catarrh; *bad smell of nasal secretion.* Many troubles of external nose. [*Caust.*] *Posterior nasal catarrh. Hawking much mucus from throat; worse, slightest draught.*

Face.—Freckles, *yellow spots, pimples.* Swelling of upper lip. Pale, with blue rings around eyes and swollen lids.

Stomach.—Feels swollen and sensitive. Ill effects of drinking cold water when overheated. Waterbrash. Hungry at 5 a. m. *Very weak digestion*, caused by slightest error of diet. Averse to milk. Depressed after eating. Bitter taste. Old dyspeptics, always belching, have sour stomach and rheumatism. Dyspepsia relieved by soda biscuits.

Bowels.—Sudden call to stool. Escapes with haste and noise. *Yellow substance like pulp of orange in discharge.* Diarrhœa from milk.

Female.—Induration of cervix. Pudenda sore. Bearing-down sensation. [*Sep.; Murex.*] Heaviness; worse, sitting; better, by moving. Menses late, scanty, like meat-washings. [*Nitric. ac.*] Leucorrhœal discharge, offensive, irritating, preceded by colic.

Respiratory.—Dry cough, when coming into warm room from out of doors. Cough with coldness of left side of breast.

Sleep.—Wakes too early in morning. Amorous dreams. Drowsy during day.

Extremities.—Old sprains. Great weakness of limbs, especially in morning. *Easy dislocation and spraining of ankles.* Foot bends under. [*Caust.*] Soreness between toes and fingers. Heel and tendo-Achilles affected. Chapped hands. The hollow of the knee is painful on motion. Icy cold up to knees.

Skin.—Inclination to perspire easily, or dry, rough, cracked skin. Eruption on finger-tips, knuckles and toes. Vesicular eruption in patches and circles. Veins full. Soles of feet raw and sore.

Modalities.—*Worse*, sitting, from music, summer *heat*, mental exertion, *thunder storm*. Least draught, changes of weather, sun. *Better*, by moving, by boring in ears and nose.

Relationsh p.—Compare: *Sodii bicarbonas* (in vomiting of pregnancy with acetonuria, 30 grains in water spread over twenty-four hours); *Nat. sulph.; Caust.; Natr. cacodyl.* (Foul breath and mouth with bad odor. Dry dermatitis of the skin of abdomen. Malignant growths. (In phthisis, 5 centigrams hypodermically, daily. Increase number of red blood corpuscles to double. Also in *malignant disease*). *Arsynal*—(Disodium methylarsenate). Introduced by M. A. Gautier, for phthisis in the second stage 4 to 6 centigrammes per day for one week followed by a week's intermission. But much smaller doses, i. e., 1x to 3x are followed by improvement, lessened fever, night sweat and hæmoptysis ceasing.

Antidote: *Ars.; Camph.*

Dose.—Sixth potency.

NATRUM CHLORATUM
(Labarraque's Solution)

In congested and atonic states of the uterus and its ligaments, with hepatic disorders. Chronic catarrhal diseases of the middle ear. *Flabby, debilitated constitution*. Both hands swollen in morning. Phlegmatic. Depressed, faint.

Head.—Vertigo, with aching across forehead. Swimming feeling, as if top of head would float off. Bleeding of nose in clots.

Mouth.—Sore irritable spots along sides of tongue and throat, gums sore, tongue swollen; aphthous ulceration. Putrid taste. Furred tongue, large, flabby, indented. Cough with aphonia.

Stomach.—*Drowsy after meals*.

Urine.—Dark, with albumen and casts. Diffuse nephritis. Much pain across small of back.

Female.—Feeling as if uterus were pushed up on sitting down. [*Ferr iod.*] Feels as if it opened and shut. Violent metrorrhagia. Leucorrhœa and backache. Passive, bearing-down from heavy condition of uterus. Womb is heavy, sodden, with tendency to prolapse. Subinvolution.

Extremities.—Hands swollen every morning. Extreme weakness *in ankles* and knees.

Relationship.—Compare: *Aur. mur. nat.; Calc.; Sepia; Heliotropium* (uterine displacement, with active bearing-down sensation and loss of voice; membranous dysmenorrhœa).

Antidotes: *Pulsat.; Guaiacum.*

Dose.—Fifteen to tweny drops of Labarraque's solution in water. Third attenuation made with dilute alcohol, lower with water.

NATRUM MURIATICUM
(Chloride of Sodium)

The prolonged taking of excessive salt causes profound nutritive changes to take place in the system, and there arise not only the symptoms of salt retention as evidenced by dropsies and œdemas, but also an alteration in the blood causing a condition of anæmia and leucocytosis. There seems also to be a retention in the tissues of effete materials giving rise to symptoms loosely described as gouty or rheumatic gout. The provings are full of such symptoms. (Dr. Stonham.) A great remedy for certain forms of intermittent fever, anæmia, chlorosis, many disturbances of the alimentary tract and skin. Great debility; most weakness felt in the morning in bed. *Coldness.* Emaciation most notable in neck. Great liability to take cold. *Dry mucous membranes.* Constrictive sensation throughout the body. *Great weakness and weariness.* Oversensitive to all sorts of influences. Hyperthyroidism. Goitre. Addison's disease. Diabetes.

Mind.—Psychic causes of disease; ill effects of grief, fright, anger, etc. Depressed, particularly in chronic diseases. *Consolation aggravates.* Irritable; gets into a passion about trifles. Awkward, hasty. Wants to be alone to cry. **Tears with laughter.**

NATRUM MURIATICUM

Head.—Throbs. *Blinding* headache. Aches as if a thousand little hammers were knocking on the brain, in the morning on awakening, *after menstruation*, from *sunrise to sunset*. Feels too large; cold. Anæmic headache of school-girls; nervous, discouraged, broken down. Chronic headache, semi-lateral, congestive, from sunrise to sunset, with pale face, nausea, vomiting; periodical; from eyestrain; menstrual, Before attack, numbness and tingling in lips, tongue and nose, relieved by sleep. Frontal sinus inflammation.

Eyes.—Feel bruised, *with headache in school children*. Eyelids heavy. *Muscles weak and stiff*. Letters run together. Sees sparks. Fiery, zigzag appearance around all objects. Burning in eyes. Give out on reading or writing. Stricture of lachrymal duct with suppuration. Escape of muco-pus when pressing upon sac. Lachrymation, burning and acrid. Lids swollen. Eyes appear wet with tears. *Tears stream down face on coughing*. [*Euph.*] *Asthenopia* due to insufficiency of *internal recii muscles*. [*Gels.* and *Cup. acet.*, when due to *external* muscles.] *Pain in eyes when looking down*. Cataract *incipient*. [*Secale.*]

Ears.—Noises; roaring and ringing.

Nose.—*Violent, fluent coryza*, lasting from one to three days, then changing into stoppage of nose, making breathing difficult. Discharge thin and watery, *like raw white of egg*. Viloent sneezing coryza. *Infallible for stopping a cold commencing with sneezing*. Use thirtieth potency. *Loss of smell and taste*. Internal soreness of nose. Dryness.

Face.—Oily, shiny, as if greased. Earthy complexion. *Fever-blisters*.

Mouth.—Frothy coating on tongue, with bubbles on side. Sense of dryness. Scorbutic gums. *Numbness, tingling of tongue*, lips, and nose. Vesicles and burning on tongue, as if there was a hair on it. Eruptions around mouth and *vesicles like pearls on lips*. Lips and corners of mouth dry, ulcerated, and cracked. Deep crack in middle of lower lip. *Tongue mapped*. [*Ars.; Rhus; Tarax.*] Loss of taste. Large vesicle on lower lip, which is swollen and burns. Immoderate thirst.

Stomach.—Hungry, yet loose flesh. [*Iod.*] Heartburn, with palpitation. Unquenchable thirst. *Sweats while eating*. Crav-

NATRUM MURIATICUM

ing for salt. Aversion to bread, to anything slimy, like oysters; fats. Throbbing in pit. Sticking sensation in cardiac orifice.

Abdomen.—Cutting pain in abdomen. Distended. Pain in abdominal ring on coughing.

Rectum.—Burning pains and stitching after stool. Anus contracted, *torn, bleeding*. Constipation; stool dry, crumbling. [*Am. m.; Mag. m.*] Painless and copious diarrhœa, preceded by pinching pain in abdomen.

Urine.—Pain just *after* urinating. [*Sars.*] Increased, involuntary when walking, coughing, etc. Has to wait a long time for it to pass *if others are present*. [*Hep.; Mur. ac.*]

Male.—Emission, even after coitus. Impotence with retarded emission.

Female.—Menses irregular; usually profuse. Vagina dry. Leucorrhœa acrid, watery. Bearing-down pains; worse in morning. [*Sep.*] Prolapsus uteri, with cutting in urethra. Ineffectual labor-pains. Suppressed menses. [Follow with *Kali carb.*] Hot during menses.

Respiratory.—Cough from a tickling in the pit of stomach, accompanied by stitches in liver and spurting of urine. [*Caust.; Squilla.*] Stitches all over chest. Cough, with bursting pain in head. Shortness of breath, especially on going upstairs. [*Calc.*] Whooping-cough with *flow of tears with cough*.

Heart.—Tachycardia. Sensation of coldness of heart. Heart and chest feel constricted. Fluttering, palpitating; intermittent pulse. Heart's pulsations shake body. *Intermits on lying down.*

Extremities.—Pain in back, *with desire for some firm support.* [*Rhus; Sep.*] Every movement accelerates the circulation. *Palms hot and perspiring.* Arms and legs, but especially knees, feel weak. *Hangnails.* Dryness and cracking about finger-nails. *Numbness and tingling* in fingers and lower extremities. Ankles weak and turn easily. Painful contraction of hamstrings. [*Caust.*] Cracking in joints on motion. *Coldness of legs* with congestion to head, chest, and stomach.

Sleep.—Sleepy in forenoon. Nervous jerking during sleep. Dreams of robbers. Sleepless from grief.

Skin.—Greasy, oily, especially on hairy parts. Dry eruptions, especially on margin of hairy scalp and bends of joints. Fever blisters. Urticaria; itch and burn. Crusty eruptions in *bends of limbs, margin of scalp,* behind ears. [*Caust.*] Warts on palms of hands. Eczema; raw, red, and inflamed; worse, eating salt, at seashore. Affects hair follicles. Alopecia. Hives, itching after exertion. *Greasy* skin.

Fever.—Chill between 9 and 11 a. m. Heat; violent thirst, increases with fever. Fever-blisters. *Coldness of the body,* and *continued chilliness* very marked. Hydræmia in chronic malarial states with weakness, constipation, loss of appetite, etc. Sweats on every exertion.

Modalities.—*Worse,* noise, music, warm room, lying down; about 10 a. m., at seashore, mental exertion, consolation, *heat,* talking. *Better,* open air, cold bathing, going without regular meals, lying on right side; pressure against back, tight clothing.

Relationship.—Complementary to *Apis; Sepia; Ign.* Compare: *Aqua marina*—Isotonic plasma. Marine plasma is a sea water taken some miles from shore and some depth below surface, filtered and diluted with twice as much pure fresh water. It acts primarily on the blood, as in intoxications, scrofulous conditions, enteritis. It disintoxicates in cancer (administered subcutaneously in the treatment of diseases of skin, kidneys and intestines, *gastro-enteritis, and tuberculosis*). *Scrofulous affection of children.* Lymphadenitis. Lupus, eczema, varicose ulcers. A great "blood purifier and vitalizer." Potentized sea-water in weakness, lack of reaction; symptoms worse seaside. Goitre.) *Sal marinum* sea salt, (indicated in chronic enlargements of glands, especially cervical. Suppurating glands. It appears likely to become a most useful remedy as an auxiliary, if not as a principal, in the treatment of diseases in patients of a strumous diathesis. Also useful in constipation.) *Natrum selenicum* (laryngeal phthisis with expectoration of small lumps of bloody mucus and slight hoarseness.) *Natrum silicum* (hæmophilia; scrofulous bone affections; given intravenously every 3 days for *senile pruritus*); [*Dolichos. Fagopyr.*] *Ignat.; Sep.; Thuja; Graph.; Alum.*

Antidotes: *Ars.; Phos.; Spir. nit. dulc.*

Dose.—Twelfth to thirtieth and higher. The very highest potencies often yield most brilliant results. And in infrequent dosage.

NATRUM NITRICUM
(Nitrate of Sodium)

A Rademacherian remedy for *inflammations*. Hæmoptysis. Hæmaturia. Purpura hæmorrhagica. Hæmorrhagic Variola. Drowsiness. Pains of tabes. *Influenza*. Hæmorrhages from mucous membranes, particularly nasal. Hæmoglobinuria. Uric acid diathesis. Asthma with urine supersaturated with solids. Anemia and hydræmia. Exhaustion, must rest frequently when walking.

Head.—Dull. Indisposed to mental and bodily exertion. Pressing inwardpain. Otalgia. Inward pressing in malar bones. *Nosebleed.*

Stomach.—Sour risings. Aversions to coffee. Flatulence, with pressure in pit of stomach and pain in chest; worse motion, better eructation.

Abdomen.—Abdominal muscles painfully contracted towards the spine. Distended. Difficult stool; feels as if more remained to pass.

Heart.—Pain in region of heart. Pulse slower and softer.

Dose.—Second trituration, also watery solution; 1 dram of salt to 8 oz. water. Dram doses.

NATRUM PHOSPHORICUM
(Phosphate of Sodium)

Natrum phosphoricum is the remedy for conditions arising from excess of lactic acid, often resulting from too much sugar. Ailments, with *excess of acidity*. Sour eructations and taste. Sour vomiting. *Yellow, creamy coating at the back of the roof of mouth and tongue.* Inflammation of any part of the throat, with sensation of a lump in throat. Flatulence, with sour risings. Colic, with symptoms of worms. Cracking of joints. *Jaundice* (1x trit.). Oxaluria.

Mind.—Imagines, on waking at night, that pieces of furniture are persons; that he hears footsteps in next room. *Fear.*

Head.—Feels dull in the morning, full feeling and throbbing.

Eyes.—Discharge of *golden-yellow, creamy matter* from the eyes. Dilation of one pupil. Whites of eyes dirty yellow.

Ears.—One ear red, hot, frequently itchy, accompanied by gastric derangements and acidity.

NATRUM PHOSPHORICUM

Nose.—Offensive odor. Itching of nose. Naso-pharyngeal catarrh, with thick, yellow, offensive mucus.

Face.—Paleness of bluish, florid appearance of face.

Mouth.—Canker sores of lip and cheeks. *Blisters on tip of tongue*, with stinging in evening. *Thin, moist coating on the tongue. Yellow, creamy coating at the back part of the roof of the mouth. Dysphagia.* Thick, creamy membrane over tonsils and soft palate.

Stomach.—*Sour eructations, sour vomiting, greenish diarrhœa.* Spits mouthful of food.

Male.—Emissions without dreams, with *weakness in back and trembling in limbs*. Desire without erection. Gonorrhœa.

Female.—Menses too early; pale, thin, watery. Sterility, with acid secretions from vagina. Leucorrhœa; discharge creamy or honey-colored, or acid and watery. Sour-smelling discharges from uterus. Morning sickness, with sour vomiting.

Extremities.—Rheumatism of the knee-joint.

Back.—Weariness; aching in wrists and finger-joints. Hamstrings sore. *Synovial crepitation.* Rheumatic arthritis.

Skin.—Yellow. Itching in various parts, *especially of ankles. Hives.* Smooth, red, shining. Erysipelas. Feet icy cold in daytime, burn at night. Swelling of lymphatic glands.

Relationship.—Compare: *Natrum lactic.* (rheumatism and gout; gouty concretions; rheumatism with diabetes); *Natrum nitrosum* (angina pectoris. Cyanosis, fainting, copious liquid stools at night; throbbing and fullness; faintness, nervous pain in head, nausea, eructations, blue lips). *Natrum silicofluoricum —Salufer—*(a cancer remedy; tumors, bone affection, caries, lupus, ethmoidits. Must be used carefully); *Nat. selen.* (chronic laryngitis and laryngeal phthisis; hoarseness of singers, expectorate small lumps of mucus with frequent clearing of throat); *Nat. sulphurosum* (diarrhœa, with *yeasty stools*); *Nat. sulphocarbol.* (pyæmia; purulent pleurisy, 3 to 5 grains every three hours); *Nat. telluricum* (breath has odor of garlic; night-sweats of phthisis) *Calc.; Robin.; Phos.* In oxaluria 1x four times daily prevents formation of calculi; keeps the oxal. of lime in solution (Schwartz).

Dose.—Third to twelfth trituration. In Jaundice 1x. Nor-

homœopathically, Phosphate Soda used hypodermically for Morphine habit, by Dr. M. J. Luys. Phosphate Soda, 75 gr. daily, for constitutional iodism, thyroidism and Grave's disease.

NATRUM SALICYLICUM
(Salicylate of Sodium)

Has an extensive range of action affecting the head, ear, throat, kidneys and liver and on metabolism. Hæmorrhages, especially epistaxis. Produces marked effects upon the internal ear, with vertigo, deafness, noises in ears and loss of bone conduction, hence, its use in Meniere's disease. *One of the best remedies for the prostrating after-effects of influenza.* Lassitude, drowsiness, listlessness, tremor. Incipient dementia. Increases the quantity of bile. Follicular tonsillitis.

Head.—Perfectly rational periods, alternate with manifestations of insanity of a sombre character. *Vertigo; worse*, raising head. All objects seem to move to the right. Dull headache and confusion. Fibrositis of the scalp

Eyes.—Retinal hæmorrhage, albuminuric retinitis with hæmorrhage. Iridocychitis due to traumatism with infection, and in sympathetic disease secondary to it. (Dr. Gradel.)

Ears.—*Tinnitus* of a low tone. Deafness. Auditory vertigo.

Chest.—Dyspnœa; breathing noisy, shallow, panting; pulse irregular. Complete loss of voice.

Skin.—Œdema, urticaria, red in circumscribed patches. Tingling and itching. Pemphigoid eruption.

Relationship.—Compare: *Lobelia purpurascens* (drowsiness; dizzy headache between eyebrows; cannot keep eyes open; tongue white—feels paralyzed as also do the heart and lungs; intense prostration of all vital forces; deadly chill, without shivering; useful for the low, nervous prostration of grippe); *Gaulth.; China. Pyrus malus*—Crab apple tree—(Labyrinthine vertigo. Dr. Cooper).

Dose.—Third potency.

Non-Homœopathic Uses.—In acute articular rheumatism, lumbago, sciatica, etc. Usual doses, ten to twenty grains every three hours. Must be used carefully, as it is often destructive of kidney tissue Ordinary allopathic doses allay the pain of dysmenorrhœa and promote menstrual flow.

NATRUM SULPHURICUM
(Sulphate of Sodium—Glauber's Salt)

A liver remedy, especially indicated for the so-called hydrogenoid constitution, where the complaints are such as are due to living in damp houses, basements, cellars. They are worse in rainy weather, water in any form. *Feels every change from dry to wet;* cannot even eat plants growing near water, nor fish. Always feels best in warm, dry air. Clinically, it has been found a valuable remedy for *spinal meningitis,* head symptoms *from injuries to head,* mental troubles therefrom. Every spring, return of skin affections. Tendency to warts. Fingers and toes affected. Chronic gout. [*Lycop.*]

Mind.—Lively music saddens. Melancholy, with periodical attacks of mania. Suicidal tendency; *must exercise restraint.* Inability to think. Dislikes to speak, or to be spoken to.

Head.—Occipital pain. Piercing stitches in ears. Vertigo; relieved by sweat on head. Bursting feeling on coughing. Hot feeling on top of head. Boring in right temple, preceded by burning in stomach. Ill-effects of falls and injuries to the head, and mental troubles arising therefrom. Dreams of running water.

Ears.—Sticking pain, earache, lightning-like stitches in damp weather.

Nose.—Nasal catarrh, with thick, yellow discharge and salty mucus. Coryza. Epistaxis. Ethmoiditis.

Eyes.—Conjunctiva yellow. Granular lids. *Photophobia.* [*Graphites.*]

Mouth.—Slimy, thick, tenacious, white mucus. *Bitter taste,* blisters on palate.

Throat.—Thick, yellow mucus, drops from posterior nares.

Stomach.—Vomits sour. *Brown, bitter coating on tongue.* Yellow complexion. Thirst for something cold. Bilious vomiting, *acid* dyspepsia, with heartburn and flatulence.

Abdomen.—Duodenal catarrh; hepatitis; icterus and vomiting of bile; liver sore to touch, with sharp, stitching pains; cannot bear tight clothing around waist, worse, lying on left side. *Flatulency;* **wind** colic in ascending colon; worse, before breakfast. Burning in abdomen and anus. Bruised pain and

NATRUM SULPHURICUM 467

urging to stool. Diarrhœa yellow, watery stools. *Loose morning stools;* worse, after spell of wet weather. Stools involuntary, when passing flatus. *Great size of the fæcal mass.*

Urine.—Loaded with bile. Brick-dust sediment. Excessive secretion. Diabetes.

Female.—Nosebleed during menses, which are acrid and profuse. Burning in pharynx during menstruation. Herpetic vulvitis. *Leucorrhœa* yellowish-green, *following gonorrhœa in female.* Leucorrhœa with hoarseness.

Male.—Condylomata; soft, fleshy excrescenses; greenish discharges. Gonorrhœa; discharge thick, greenish; little pain.

Respiratory.—Dyspnœa, during damp weather. *Must hold chest when coughing.* Humid asthma; rattling in chest, at 4 and 5 a. m. *Cough,* with thick ropy, greenish expectoration; chest feels all gone. Constant desire to take deep, long breath. *Asthma in children,* as a constitutional remedy. Delayed resolution in pneumonia. Springs up in bed the cough hurts so; holds painful side. [*Bry.*] Pain through *lower left chest.* Every fresh cold brings on attack of asthma.

Back.—Itching when undressing. Violent pains in back of neck, *and at base of brain.* Piercing pain between scapulæ. Spinal meningitis; opisthotonos.

Extremities.—Swelling of axillary glands. Inflammation around root of nails. Burning in soles; œdema of feet; itching between toes. Gout. Pain in limbs, compels frequent change in position. Run-arounds. Pain in hip-joints, worse left, worse, stooping. Stiffness of knees, cracking of joints. Rheumatism, worse in damp cold weather.

Skin.—Itching while undressing. Jaundiced, watery blisters. Sycotic excrescences; wart-like red lumps all over body.

Modalities.—*Worse,* music (makes her sad); lying on left side; dampness of basement, damp weather. *Better,* dry weather, pressure, changing position.

Relationship.—Compare: *Natrum succinate* (5 gr. every 3 hours. Catarrhal jaundice). *Malaria officinalis*—decomposed vegetable matter—(Has evident power to cause the disappearance of the plasmodium of malaria. Malarial cachexia. General sense of weariness. Spleen affections. Malaria and rheumatism. Functional hepatic diseases. Sixth potency and higher.) *Natrum choleinicum*—Fel Tauri Depuratum—(constipation; chronic gastric and intestinal catarrh; cirrhotic liver; diabetes; *nape of neck pains; tendency to sleep after eating;* much flatus; ascites); *Momordica*—Balsam Apple—(Colic, dysmenorrhœa with gushes of blood.) *Pulmo vulpis*—Wolf's lung (persistent shortness of breath causing a paroxysm of asthma on the slightest motion. Strong, sonorous bubbling rales. 1x trit.). *Peumus Boldus*—Boldo—(atonic states of stomach and intestinal canal; liver states following malaria. Burning weight in region of liver and stomach, bitter taste, languor; abscess of liver; asthma, bronchitis, catarrh, œdema of lungs); *Natrum iodat.* (Incipient rheumatic endocarditis; chronic bronchitis, rheumatism and tertiary syphilis. Chronic catarrhal affections, arteriosclerosis. Here various symptoms, as *angina pectoris*, vertigo, dyspnœa become less marked after continued use of 5-10 grs., 3 times a day.) *Natrum hyposulph.* (liver-spots, locally and internally); *Sulph.; Thuja; Merc.; Stilling.*

Complementary: *Ars.; Thuja.*

Dose.—First to twelfth trituration.

NICCOLUM

(Metallic Nickel)

Periodical nervous sick headaches, with asthenopia, weak digestion, constipation. Catarrh. Suits debilitated, nervous, literary patients, with frequent headaches, dyspepsia and constipation.

Head.—Cracking in cervical vertebræ when moving the head. Pain on top as from a nail. Pressure on vertex, in morning; worse till noon and in warm room. Stitches. Objects appear too large. Migraine; first on left side. Twitching of upper lip.

Nose.—Violent sneezing; stopped up. Nasal catarrh, with redness and swelling at tip of nose. Acute pain at root of nose, extending to vertex and through temples.

Throat.—Sore, right side with great tenderness; *soreness to touch externally*. Strangulated feeling.

Gastric.—Gone, empty feeling in epigastrium, *without desire for food*. Acute gastralgia with pains extending to shoulder.

Thirst and *intense hiccough*. Sour, fetid secretions ooze from molar teeth. Diarrhœa and tenesmus after milk.

Female.—Menses late, scanty, with great debility and burning in eyes. Profuse leucorrhœa; worse, after urinating [*Mag. mur.; Plat.*]; also worse after menses.

Respiratory.—Hoarseness. Dry, hacking cough, with stitches in chest. *Obliged to sit up and hold head. Must put arms on thighs, when coughing.*

Skin.—Itching all over, worse on neck, not relieved by scratching.

Modalities.—*Worse*, periodically, every two weeks; yearly, forenoon. *Better*, in evening.

Dose.—Third trituration.

NICCOLUM SULPHURICUM
(Sulphate of Nickel)

Useful in climacteric disturbances. Periodic neuralgias of malarial origin. Urine and saliva increased. Coppery taste. Weak, asthenopic literary persons with weak digestion and constipation, are worse in morning and suffer from periodic headaches and hoarseness.

Head.—Nervous, uneasy, desire to recline, tired, cannot settle down to any occupation. Periodic headaches, occipital pain, extending down to spine, worse lying on back; sore pain in eyes.

Back.—Stiff, numb sensation, worse in neck. Spine sore. Awakened in morning with burning soles. Spinal pains, legs and arms heavy and weak, cannot lie on back.

Female.—Dull aching in ovaries, with sensation as if menses appear. *Hot flashes*, followed by perspiration on parts touching each other, when separated become dry.

Dose.—Second trituration.

NITRICUM ACIDUM
(Nitric Acid)

Selects for its special seat of action the outlets of the body where the mucous membrane and skin meet: these pain *as from splinters*. *Sticking* pains. Marked improvement of all symptoms while riding in a carriage. Acts best on the dark complexioned and past middle life. Syphilis, after abuse of Mercury. Pains appear and disappear quickly. [*Bell.*] Hydrogenoid constitution. Sycotic remedy.

Blisters and ulcers in mouth, tongue, genitals; bleed easily. Fissures, with pain during stool, as if rectum were torn. All discharges very offensive, especially urine, fæces, and perspiration. Persons who have chronic diseases, and take cold easily and disposed to diarrhœa. Excessive physical irritability. Cachexia, due to syphilis, scrofula, intermittent fever with liver involvement and anemia, etc. Gravel; arthritis. Capillary bleeding after currettage.

Mind.—*Irritable*, hateful, vindictive, headstrong. Hopeless despair. Sensitive to noise, pain, touch, jar. Fear of death.

Head.—Sensation of a *band around head*. Headache from pressure of hat; full feeling; worse from street noises. Hair falls out. Scalp sensitive.

Ears.—Difficult hearing; better by riding in carriage or train. *Very sensitive to noise*, as the rattle of wagons over pavements. [*Coff.; Nux.*] Cracking in ears when chewing.

Eyes.—Double vision; *sharp, sticking pains*. Ulceration of cornea. Gonorrhœal ophthalmia, photophobia, constant lachrymation. Syphilitic iritis.

Nose.—Ozæna. Green casts from nose every morning. Coryza, with sore and bleeding nostrils. Tip red. Stitches, as of a splinter in nose. *Caries of mastoid. Nosebleed*, with chest affections. Chronic nasal catarrh, with yellow, offensive, *corrosive* discharge. Nasal diphtheria, with watery and exceedingly excoriating discharge.

Mouth.—Putrid breath. Salivation. Bleeding of gums. Painful pimples on the sides of the tongue. *Tongue clean, red and wet with center furrow*. Teeth become loose; gums soft and spongy. *Ulcers in soft palate, with sharp, splinter-like pains*. Salivation and fetor oris. *Bloody saliva*.

Throat.—Dry. Pain into ears. Hawks mucus constantly. White patches and *sharp points, as from splinters*, on swallowing.

Stomach.—Great hunger, with sweetish taste. Longing for indigestible things—chalk, earth, etc. Pain in cardiac orifice. Dyspepsia with excess of oxalic acid, uric acid and phosphates in urine and great mental depression. *Loves fat and salt*. [*Sulph.*]

NITRICUM ACIDUM

Abdomen.—Great straining, but little passes. Rectum feels torn. Bowels constipated, with fissures in rectum. Tearing pains during stools. Violent cutting pains *after stools, lasting for hours.* [*Ratanh.*] Hæmorrhages from bowels, profuse, bright. Prolapsus ani. Hæmorrhoids bleed easily. Diarrhœa, slimy and offensive. After stools, irritable and exhausted. Colic relieved from tightening clothes. Jaundice, aching in liver.

Urine.—Scanty, dark, *offensive.* Smells like horse's urine. *Cold on passing.* Burning and stinging. Urine bloody and albuminous. Alternation of cloudy, phosphatic urine with profuse urinary secretion in old prostatic cases.

Male.—Soreness and burning in glans and beneath prepuce. Ulcers; burn and sting; exude, offensive matter.

Female.—External parts sore, with ulcers. [*Hep.; Merc.; Thuja.*] Leucorrhœa brown, flesh-colored, watery, or stringy, offensive. Hair on genitals falls out. [*Natr. m.; Zinc.*] Uterine hæmorrhages. Menses early, profuse, like muddy water, with pain in back, hips and thighs. Stitches through vagina. Metrorrhagia after parturition.

Respiratory.—Hoarseness. Aphonia, with dry hacking cough, from tickling in larynx and pit of stomach. Soreness at lower end of sternum. *Short breath on going upstairs.* [*Ars. Calc.*] Cough during sleep. [*Cham.*]

Extremities.—Fetid foot-sweat, causing soreness of toes, with sticking pain; chilblains on toes. Sweating of palms, hands; cold, blue nails. Offensive sweat in axillæ at night.

Skin.—Warts, large jagged; bleed on washing. Ulcers bleed easily, sensitive; splinter-like pains; zigzag, irregular edges; base looks like raw flesh. Exuberant granulations. Black pores on face, papules worse on forehead.

Modalities.—*Worse,* evening and night, cold climate, and also *hot* weather. *Better,* while riding in carriage. [Reverse: *Cocculus.*]

Relationship.—Complementary: *Ars.; Calad.; Lac can.; Sepia.*

Inimical: *Lach.*

Compare: *Merc.; Kali c.; Thuja; Hepar; Calc.*

Dose.—Sixth potency. As the nitric acid patient begins to improve skin symptoms may appear for a time, a favorable indication.

NITRI SPIRITUS DULCIS
(Sweet Spirits of Nitre)

Sensorial apathy in low fevers when there is stupor, difficulty of arousing patient, is met by this remedy. Dry skin, nausea, flatulence. Salty taste. *Ill-effects of salt* (halophagia). [*Ars.; Phos.*] Catching cold in stormy weather. Acute nephritis following Scarlet fever. Dropsy. Is an excellent diuretic.

Face.—Prosopalgia, with photophobia. Burning in cheeks, *and vomiting, followed by lassitude.* Boring in facial bones; in angles of lower jaw. Very sensitive to cold.

Respiratory.—Very rapid breathing by going only a short walk. Painful constriction beneath sternum.

Modalities.—*Worse,* from mental disturbance, during winter and spring.

Relationship.—Increases the action of Digitalis.

Compare: *Phos. ac.; Lycop.*

Dose.—A few drops of the pure spirits in water every two or three hours.

NITRO-MURIATIC ACID
(Aqua Regia)

Almost a specific in Oxaluria. Removes the distressing skin symptoms resembling psoriasis. Three to five drops three times a day. So-called bilious conditions; torpid liver, hepatitis and early cirrhosis of liver. More adapted to hepatic torpor and gastric catarrh common in hot and damp climates and aggravated by meat eating and alcohol (Hale). Constricted anus. Gravel.

Mouth.—Gums bleed easily. Ptyalism. *Constant drooling at night.* [*Merc.*] Cankers; small, superficial ulceration over inside of mouth and tongue. Metallic taste. [*Cupr. met.*]

Stomach.—Sour eructations, with empty hungry feeling in stomach; not relieved by eating. *Salivation; worse at night.*

Stool.—Constipated, with ineffectual urging. Sphincter constricted. Anus moist and sore.

Urine.—Cloudy. Burning in urethra. Oxaluria.

Dose.—Five to ten drops, well diluted.

NUPHAR LUTEUM
(Yellow Pond-lily)

Produces nervous weakness, with marked symptoms in the sexual sphere.

Male.—Complete absence of sexual desire; parts relaxed; penis retracted. Impotency, with involuntary emissions during stool, when urinating. Spermatorrhœa. Pain in testicles and penis.

Stool.—Entero-colitis. Yellow diarrhœa; worse in the morning. Diarrhœa during typhoid.

Relationship.—Compare, in sexual weakness; *Agnus; Kali brom.; Lycop.; Selen.; Yohimbin.* In diarrhœa: *Chelid.; Gambog.; Sulph.; Nymphæa odorata*—Sweet Water Lily—(early morning diarrhœa, backache); acrid leucorrhœa, offensive ulcers; bronchorrhœa; ulcerative sore throat.)

Dose.—Tincture to sixth potency.

NUX MOSCHATA
(Nutmeg)

Marked tendency to *fainting fits*, with heart failure. Cold extremities, *extreme dryness of mucous membranes* and skin. Strange feeling, with irresistible *drowsiness*. Indicanuria. General inclination to become unconscious during acute attacks. Lypothymia. [*Ignatia.*] Staggers on trying to walk.

Mind.—Changeable; laughing and crying. Confused, impaired memory. Bewildered sense, as in a dream. Thinks she has two heads.

Head.—Vertigo when walking in open air; aches from eating a little too much. Feeling of expansion, *with sleepiness*. Pulsating in head. Cracking sensation in head. Sensitive to slightest touch in a draught of air. Bursting headache; *better hard pressure.*

Eyes.—Objects look larger, very distant, or vanish. Motes before eyes. Mydriasis.

Nose.—Oversensitive to smell; nosebleed, dark blood; dry, stopped up.

Mouth.—Very dry. Tongue adheres to roof of mouth; but

no desire for water. Saliva like cotton. [*Berb.*] Toothache in pregnancy. Tongue numb, paralyzed. *Dryness* of throat.

Stomach.—*Excessively bloated. Flatulent dyspepsia.* Hiccough, and craving for highly-seasoned food. Retrocession of gout to stomach.

Abdomen.—Paralytic weakness of intestines. *Enormously distended.* Stool is soft, and yet is *unable to expel it*, even with long straining. [*Alum.*] *Faintness during or after stool.* Protruding piles.

Female.—Uterine hæmorrhage. Menses too long, dark, thick. Leucorrhœa muddy and bloody. Suppression, with persistent fainting attacks and sleepiness. [*Kali c.*] *Variableness of menstruation, irregularity of time and quantity.*

Respiratory.—Loss of voice from walking against the wind. [*Hep.*] Cough when getting warm in bed.

Heart.—Trembling, fluttering. Sensation as if something grasped heart. Palpitation; pulse intermits.

Extremities.—Pain in right hip to knee; worse, motion, especially going upstairs. Rheumatism from getting feet wet, from exposure to draughts. Rheumatism relieved by dry, warm clothes. Fatigue on slight exertion.

Sleep.—Great drowsiness. (*Indol.*) *Complaints cause sleepiness.* Coma.

Fever.—Chill begins in left hand. (Carbo.) Chilliness and heat without thirst; *want of perspiration. Dry skin* and of inner parts, also of eyes, nose, lips, mouth, tongue, throat, etc.

Modalities.—*Worse*, cold moist wind, cold food, cold washing, lying on painful side, motion, jar. *Better*, warmth, dry weather.

Relationship.—*Oleum myristica*—Oil of Nutmeg—(as a remedy for boils, felons, poisonous ulcers, it has been used in the 2x potency); *Ornithogalum* (flatulence, swollen feeling across lower chest; whenever she turns in bed, *feels as if a bag of water* turned also; gastric ulcer and cancer). *Myristica Sebifera* (phlegmonous inflammations, hastens suppuration; powerful antiseptic. Ulcerative tendency in all tissues. Said to act more powerfully than Hepar and Silica).

Compare: *Nux v.; Puls.; Rhus; Ign.; Asaf.*

Antidotes: *Camph.; Gels.; Valer.*

Dose.—First to sixth potency.

NUX VOMICA
(Poison-nut)

Is the greatest of polychrests, because the bulk of its symptoms correspond in similarity with those of the commonest and most frequent of diseases. It is frequently the first remedy, indicated after much dosing, establishing a sort of equilibrium of forces and counteracting chronic effects.

Nux is pre-eminently the remedy for many of the conditions incident to modern life. The typical Nux patient is rather thin, spare, quick, active, nervous, and irritable. He does a good deal of mental work; has mental strains and leads a sedentary life, found in prolonged office work, overstudy, and close application to business, with its cares and anxieties. This indoor life and mental strain seeks stimulants, coffee, wine, possibly in excess; or, again, he hopes to quiet his excitement, by indulging in the sedative effects of tobacco, if not really a victim, to the seductive drugs, like opium, etc. These things are associated with other indulgences; at table, he takes preferably rich and stimulating food; wine and women play their part to make him forget the close application of the day. Late hours are a consequence; a thick head, dyspepsia, and irritable temper are the next day's inheritance. Now he takes some cathartic, liver pills, or mineral water, and soon gets into the habit of taking these things, which still further complicate matters. Since these frailties are more yielded to by men than women, Nux is pre-eminently a male remedy. These conditions produce an *irritable*, nervous system, hypersensitive and overimpressionable, which Nux will do much to soothe and calm. Especially adapted to digestive disturbances, portal congestion, and hypochondrical states depending thereon. Convulsions, with consciousness; worse, touch, moving. *Zealous fiery temperament.* Nux patients are easily chilled, avoid open air, etc. Nux always seems to be out of tune; inharmonious spasmodic action.

Mind.—Very *irritable;* sensitive to all impressions. Ugly, malicious. *Cannot bear noises, odors, light,* etc. Does not want to be touched. Time passes too slowly. Even the least ailment affects her greatly. Disposed to reproach others. *Sullen, faultfinding.*

Head.—Headache in occiput or over eyes, with *vertigo;* brain feels turning in a circle. Oversensitiveness. *Vertigo, with momentary loss of consciousness.* Intoxicated feeling; worse, morning; mental exertion, tobacco, alcohol, coffee, open air. Pressing pain on vertex, as if a nail driven in. Vertigo in morning and after dinner. Scalp sensitive. Frontal headache, with desire to press the head against something. Congestive headache, associated with hæmorrhoids. *Headache in the sunshine.* [*Glon.; Nat. carb.*] Feels distended and sore within, after a debauch.

Eyes.—Photophobia; much worse in morning. Smarting, dry sensation in inner canthi. Infra-orbital neuralgia, with watering of eyes. Optic nerve atrophy, from habitual use of intoxicants. Paresis of ocular muscles; worse, tobacco and stimulants. Orbital twitching radiating towards the occiput. Optic neuritis.

Ears.—Itching in ear through Eustachian tube. Auditory canal dry and sensitive. Otalgia; worse in bed. Hyperæsthesia of auditory nerves; loud sounds are painful, and anger him.

Nose.—Stuffed up, at night especially. *Stuffy colds, snuffles,* after exposure to dry, cold atmosphere; worse, in warm room. Odors tend to produce fainting. Coryza; fluent in daytime; *stuffed up at night and outdoors;* or alternates between nostrils. Bleeding in morning. [*Bry.*] Arid discharge, but *with stuffed-up feeling.*

Mouth.—Jaws contracted. Small aphthous ulcers, with *bloody saliva.* First half of tongue clean; posterior covered with deep fur; white, yellow, cracked edges. Teeth ache; worse, cold things. Gums swollen, white, and bleeding.

Throat.—*Rough, scraped feeling. Tickling* after waking in morning. Sensation of *roughness,* tightness, and tension. Pharynx constricted. Uvula swollen. *Stitches into ear.*

Stomach.—Sour taste, and *nausea in the morning, after eating. Weight and pain in stomach;* worse, eating, some time after. Flatulence and pyrosis. Sour, bitter eructations. *Nausea and vomiting,* with much retching. Ravenous hunger, especially about a day before an attack of dyspepsia. *Region of stomach very sensitive to pressure.* [*Bry.; Ars.*] Epigastrium bloated, with pressure as of a stone, *several hours after eating.* Desire for stimulants. Loves *fats* and tolerates them well. (*Puls.* opposite.) Dyspepsia from drinking strong coffee. Difficult belching of gas. Wants to vomit, but cannot.

Abdomen.—*Bruised soreness of abdominal walls.* [*Apis.; Sulph.*] Flatulent distention, with spasmodic colic. Colic from uncovering. Liver engorged, with stitches and soreness. Colic, with upward pressure, causing short breath, and desire for stool. *Weakness of abdominal ring region.* Strangulated hernia. [*Op.*] Forcing in lower abdomen towards genitals. Umbilical hernia of infants.

Stool.—Constipation, *with frequent ineffectual urging,* incomplete and unsatisfactory; *feeling as if part remained unexpelled.* Constriction of rectum. Irregular, peristaltic action; hence *frequent ineffectual desire, or passing but small quantities at each attempt. Absence of all desire for defacation is a contra-indication.* Alternate constipation and diarrhœa—after abuse of purgatives. Urging to stool felt throughout abdomen. *Itching, blind hæmorrhoids,* with ineffectual urging to stool; very painful; after drastic drugs. Diarrhœa after a debauch; worse, morning. Frequent small evacuations. Scanty stool, with much urging. Dysentery; stools *relieve pains for a time. Constant uneasiness in rectum.* Diarrhœa, with jaundice. [*Dig.*]

Urine.—Irritable bladder; from spasmodic sphincter. Frequent calls; little and often. Hæmaturia. [*Ipec.; Tereb.*] Ineffectual urging, spasmodic and strangury. Renal colic extending to genitals, with dribbling urine. While urinating, itching in urethra and pain in neck of bladder.

Male.—Easily excited desire. Emissions from high living. Bad effects of sexual excesses. Constrictive pain in testicles. Orchitis. [*Hama.; Puls.*] Spermatorrhœa, with dreams, backache, burning in spine, weakness and irritability.

Female.—Menses *too early,* lasts too long; *always irregular,* blood *black* [*Cycl.; Lach.; Puls.*] with faint spells. *Prolapsus uteri. Dysmenorrhœa,* with pain in sacrum, and constant urging to stool. Inefficient labor-pains; extend to rectum, with desire for stool and frequent urination. [*Lil.*] Desire too strong. Metrorrhagia, with *sensation as if bowels wanted to move.*

Respiratory.—Catarrhal hoarseness, with *scraping in throat.* Spasmodic constriction. *Asthma, with fullness in stomach,* *morning or after eating*. Cough, with sensation as if something were torn loose in chest. *Shallow respiration. Oppressed breathing*. Tight, dry, hacking cough; at times with bloody expectoration. *Cough brings on bursting headache* and bruised pain in epigastric region.

Back.—Backache in lumbar region. Burning in spine; worse, 3 to 4 a. m. Cervico-brachial neuralgia; worse, touch. *Must sit up in order to turn in bed*. Bruised pain below scapulæ. Sitting is painful.

Extremities.—Arms and hands go to sleep. Paresis of arms, with shocks. Legs numb; feel paralyzed; cramps in calves and soles. Partial paralysis, from overexertion or getting soaked. [*Rhus.*] Cracking in knee-joints during motion. Drags his feet when walking. Sensation of sudden loss of power of arms and legs in the morning.

Sleep.—*Cannot sleep after 3 a. m. until towards morning; awakes feeling wretchedly*. Drowsy after meals, and in early evening. Dreams full of bustle and hurry. *Better after a short sleep*, unless aroused.

Skin.—*Body burning hot, especially face; yet cannot move or uncover without feeling chilly*. Urticaria, with gastric derangement. Acne; skin red and blotchy.

Fever.—Cold stage predominates. Paroxysms anticipate in morning. Excessive rigor, with *blueness of finger-nails*. Aching in limbs and back, and gastric symptoms. Chilly; *must be covered* in every stage of fever. Perspiration sour; only one side of body. *Chilliness on being uncovered, yet he does not allow being covered*. Dry heat of the body.

Modalities.—*Worse*, morning, mental exertion, after eating, touch, spices, stimulants, narcotics, dry weather, cold. *Better*, from a nap, if allowed to finish it; in evening, while at rest, in damp, wet weather [*Caust.*], strong pressure.

Relationship.—*Nux* seeds contain copper, notice the cramp-causing proclivities of both. Complementary: *Sulphur; Sepia.*

Inimical: *Zinc.*

Compare: *Strychnia.*

Compare: *Kali carb.; Hydr.; Bry.; Lyc.; Graph.*

Antidotes: *Coff.; Ignat.; Cocc.*

Dose.—First to thirtieth potency and higher. Nux is said to act best given in the evening.

NYCTANTHES ARBOR-TRISTIS
(Paghala-malli—Sad Tree)

Bilious and obstinate remittent fever; sciatica; rheumatism. Constipation of children.

Head.—Anxious and restless; dull headache. Tongue coated.

Stomach.—Burning sensation, better cold application. Thirst, better vomiting.

Abdomen.—Tenderness of liver. Profuse, bilious stool, with nausea. Constipation.

Fever.—Thirst, before and during chill and heat; better vomiting at close of chill; sweat not marked.

Dose.—Tincture, drop doses.

OCIMUM CANUM
(Brazilian Alfavaca)

Is to be remembered in diseases of the kidneys, bladder and urethra. Uric acid diathesis. Red sand in the urine is its chief characteristic, and frequently verified. Swelling of glands, inguinal and mammary. Renal colic, especially right side. Symptoms of renal calculus are pronounced.

Urine.—High acidity, formation of spike crystals of uric acid. Turbid, thick, purulent, bloody; *brick-dust red* or yellow *sediment. Odor of musk. Pain in ureters.* Cramps in kidneys.

Male.—Heat and swelling of left testicle.

Female.—Vulva swollen; darting pain in labia. Nipples painful to least contact. Breasts feel full and tense; itching. Prolapsus vaginæ.

Relationship.—Compare: *Berb.; Hedeoma; Lycop.; Pareir.; Urtica.*

Dose.—Sixth to thirtieth potency.

OENANTHE CROCATA
(Water Dropwart)

Epileptiform convulsions; worse, during menstruation and pregnancy. Puerperal eclampsia; uræmic convulsions. Burning in throat and stomach, nausea and vomiting. Red spots in face. Convulsive facial twitching. Skin affections, especially lepra and ichthyosis.

Head.—Pains all over head, dizzy. Sudden and complete unconsciousness. Furious delirium, giddiness. Countenance livid, eyes fixed, pupils dilated, *convulsive twitching of facial muscles*, trismus, foaming at mouth, locked jaws. Much yawning. Tendency to cry over little things.

Respiratory.—Tickling cough, with rattling in the lower part of the chest, and thick, frothy expectoration. Heavy, spasmodic, stertorous breathing.

Extremities.—Convulsions; opisthotonos. Pain along crural and sciatic nerves, commencing in back. Cold hands and feet. Numbness of hand and foot.

Relationship.—Compare: *Cicuta; Kali brom.*

Dose.—First to sixth potency.

OLEANDER—NERIUM ODORUM
(Rose-laurel)

Has a marked action on the skin, heart and nervous system, producing and curing paralytic conditions with cramp-like contractions of upper extremities. Hemiplegia. Difficult articulation.

Mind.—Memory weak; slow perception. Melancholy, with obstinate constipation.

Head.—Vertigo and diplopia, when looking down. Vertigo, when looking fixedly at an object, and on rising in bed. Pain in brain, as if head would burst. Numb feeling. Dull, unable to think. Indolence. *Eruption on scalp.* Humid, fetid spots *behind ears* [*Graph.; Petrol.*] and occiput, with red, rough, herpetic spots in front. *Corrosive itching on forehead and edge of hair;* worse, heat.

Eyes.—Can see objects only when looking at them sideways. Eyes water on reading. Double vision. *Sensation as if eyes were drawn back into the head.*

Face.—Pale, sunken, with blue rings around eyes. [*Phos. ac.*]

Stomach.—Canine hunger, *with hurried eating,* without appetite. Thirst. Empty belching. Vomiting of food; greenish water. Throbbing in pit.

Abdomen.—Borborygmus, with profuse, fetid flatus. Gnawing around navel. Ineffectual urging. *Undigested fæces. Stool passes when emitting flatus.* Burning pain in anus.

Chest.—Oppression as from a weight; asthmatic when lying down. *Palpitation,* with weakness and empty feeling in chest. Dyspnœa. Obtuse stitches in chest.

Extremities.—*Weakness of lower limbs.* Paralysis of legs and feet. Want of animal heat in limbs. Cold feet. Painless paralysis. Constant cold feet. Swelling, burning stiffness of fingers. Veins on hands swollen. Œdema. Stiffness of joints.

Skin.—Itching, scurfy pimples; herpes; sensitive and numb. Nocturnal burning. *Very sensitive skin;* slightest friction causes soreness and chapping. *Violent itching eruption, bleeding, oozing;* want of perspiration. Pruritus, especially of scalp, which is sensitive.

Modalities.—*Worse,* undressing, rest, friction of clothes.

Relationship.—Compare: *Con.; Nat. m.; Rhus; Caust.; Lathyr.* Oleander contains Oleandrin and also Nerein which latter is said to be closely related if not identical with Digitalin. The pulse becomes slower, more regular, more powerful. *Diuresis;* palpitation, œdema and dyspnœa of valvular disease, disappear.

Antidotes: *Camph.; Sulph.*

Dose.—Third to thirtieth potency.

OLEUM ANIMALE

(Dippel's Animal Oil)

Acts on the nervous system, especially on pneumo-gastric region. Useful in migraine and neuralgia of spermatic cord. Burning pains and stitches. *"Pulled upward"* and *"from behind forward"* pains.

Head.—Tearing pain, with sadness and irritability; worse after dinner; relieved by rubbing. Itching, burning vesicles; better, friction. Malar bones feel pulled forcibly upward. Migrain with polyuria.

Eyes.—Smarting in eyes; misty vision. Glistening bodies before eyes. Lachrymation when eating. Short-sighted. Twitching of lids. [*Agar.*]

Nose.—Watery, excoriating discharge; worse in open air.

Face.—Feels drawn. Cramp-like pains. *Twitching of lips.* Malar bone feels pulled upward. Toothache, *better pressing teeth together.*

Mouth.—Bites cheek while eating. [*Caust.*] Tongue feels sore. Greasy feeling in mouth.

Throat.—Sore, dry, constricted. Air feels cold.

Stomach.—Sensation *as if water were in stomach;* of coldness, of constriction, and of burning; better, eructations.

Abdomen.—Flatulence and rumbling. Ineffectual urging to stool, with burning in anus. After stool, bruised pain in abdomen.

Urine.—*Polyuria.* Greenish urine, frequent and urgent want to urinate, with tenesmus and scanty emission. Itching in urethra.

Male.—Desire increased; ejaculation too soon. Pain along spermatic cord to testicles. *Testicles feel seized and pulled forcibly upward;* worse, right. *Pressure in the perineum.* Prostatic hypertrophy.

Female.—*Early and scant menstruation;* flow black.

Respiratory.—Chest feels constricted. Asthma from suppressed foot-sweat. Oppression. *Stitches in breast from behind forward.*

Extremities.—Sprained feeling in small of back. Cracking of vertebræ on raising head. [*Aloe; Nat. c.; Thuj.*] Restlessness. Rheumatic pain in shoulders. Fish-brine odor of sweat of heels.

Modalities.—*Worse*, after eating, from 2 to 9 p. m. *Better*, by rubbing, eructation, open air.

Relationship.—Compare: *Puls.; Ars.; Silic.; Sepia.*
Antidotes: *Camph.; Op.*

Dose.—Third to thirtieth potency and higher.

OLEUM JECORIS ASELLI
(Cod-liver Oil)

Internally, a nutrient and a hepatic and pancreatic remedy. (Burnett.) Emaciation, lassitude, scrofulous diseases, rheumatic affections. *Atrophy of infants;* emaciation with hot hands and head; restless and feverish at night. *Pains in liver region* Tuberculosis in the beginning.

Chest.—Hoarseness. Sharp stitching pains. Burning spots. *Dry, hacking, tickling cough,* especially at night. Whooping-cough in miserable, scrofulous children. Here give drop doses, increasing daily one drop up to twelve, then descend in the same way (Dahlke). *Soreness through chest.* Hæmoptysis. [*Acalypha; Millef.*] *Palpitation,* accompanies other symptoms. *Yellowness.* Children who cannot take milk.

Extremities.—Aching in elbows and knees, in *sacrum.* Chronic rheumatism, with rigid muscles and tendons. *Burning in palms.*

Fever.—Constantly chilly towards evening. *Hectic fever.* Night-sweats.

Relationship.—Compare: *Cholesterine; Tubercul.; Phosph.; Iod.* One litre of Ol. Jecoris contains 0.4 gram Iod. *Gadus morrhua*—Cod—(frequent breathing, with flapping of alæ nasi; rush of blood to chest; pain in lungs and cough; dry heat in palms).

Dose.—First to third trituration. Locally in *ring-worm,* and nightly rubbing, for dwarfish, emaciated babies.

OLEUM SANTALI
(Oil of Sandalwood)

The action in the urinary and sexual spheres is most utilizable, especially in gonorrhœa. It is also a stimulating, disinfectant expectorant. Two or three drops on sugar will frequently relieve the hacking cough, when but little sputum is expectorated.

Male.—Painful erections; swelling of the prepuce. Thick, yellowish, muco-purulent discharge. Deep pain in perinuem.

Urine.—Frequent, burning, smarting, swelling, and redness of meatus. Stream small and slow. *Acute aching in kidney region.* Sensation of a ball pressing against the urethra; worse, standing. Gleet, with profuse, thick discharge; chronic cystitis.

Dose.—Two to ten m. in capsules.

ONISCUS ASELLUS—MILLEPEDES
(Wood-louse)

Has distinct diuretic properties; hence its use in dropsies. Asthmatic conditions, with bronchial catarrh.

Head.—Boring pain behind right ear in mastoid process. [*Caps.*] Violent pulsation of arteries. [*Pothos; Glonoine.*] Painful pressure above the root of nose.

Stomach.—Persistent pressure in cardiac orifice. Vomiting.

Abdomen.—Distended; *meteorism; very severe colic.*

Urine.—Cutting, burning in urethra. *Tenesmus of bladder and rectum*, with absence of stool and urine.

Relationship.—Compare: *Pothos. fœt.; Canth.*

Dose.—Sixth potency.

ONOSMODIUM
(False Gromwell)

Want of power of concentration and co-ordination. Vertigo, numbness and muscular prostration. Marked association of head and eye symptoms, with muscular tiredness and weariness. A remedy for *migraine*. Headaches from eyestrain and sexual weakness. It produces diminution of sexual desire in both sexes; hence its homœopathicity, in *sexual neurasthenia*. Depressed or lost sexual life in women. Neuralgic pains. General prostration. Acts as if born tired.

Head.—Loss of memory. Nose feels dry. Confused. Dull, heavy, dizzy, pressing upward in occiput. Occipito-frontal pain in morning on waking, *chiefly left side*. Pain in temples and mastoid. [*Capsic.*]

Eyes.—Vision blurred; optic disc hyperæmic, and retinal vessels enlarged. Strained feeling in eyes; worse, using eyes. Eyes heavy and dull, muscular asthenopia; *ocular muscles tense*. Internal eye muscles paretic. *Pain in eyeballs* between orbit and ball, extending to left temple.

Throat.—Severe dryness. Discharge from posterior nares. Raw, scraping. Stuffed feeling in posterior nares. Symptoms worse by cold drinks.

Abdomen.—Craving for ice-water and cold drinks; wants to drink often. Abdomen feels bloated.

Back.—Pain in dorsal and lumbar regions. Numbness and tingling in feet and legs.

Chest.—Sore, aching in breasts; feels swollen and sore. Pain in heart; pulse, rapid, irregular, weak.

Male.—Constant sexual excitement. *Psychical impotence.* Loss of desire. Speedy emissions. Deficient erections.

Female.—Severe uterine pains; bearing-down pains; old pains return. *Sexual desire completely destroyed.* Feels as if menses would appear. Aching in breasts. Nipples itch. Menses too early and too prolonged. Soreness in uterine region. Leucorrhœa, yellow, acrid, profuse.

Extremities.—Pain in back. *Tired and numb* feeling in legs, popliteal spaces, and below knees. *Staggering gait.* Sidewalk seems too high. Pain in left scapular region. Great muscular weakness and weariness.

Modalities.—*Worse*, from motion, jar, and tight clothing. *Better*, when undressed, when lying down on back, from cold drinks, and eating.

Relationship.—Compare: *Nat. mur.; Lilium; Gels.; Ruta.*

Dose.—Thirtieth attenuation.

OOPHORINUM
(Ovarian Extract)

Suffering following excision of the ovaries. *Climacteric disturbances* generally. Ovarian cysts. Cutaneous disorders and acne rosacea. Prurigo.

Relationship.—Compare: *Orchitinum*—Testicular Extract—(after ovariotomy, sexual weakness, senile decay).

Dose.—Low triturations.

OPERCULINA TURPETHUM
(Nishope)

A remedy for plague, fevers, diarrhœa.

Mind.—Delirium associated with restlessness, loquacity. Tendency to escape from bed; ravings, pains cause fainting.

Abdomen.—Watery diarrhœa, profuse with sinking sensation. Cholera morbus. Hæmorrhoids.

Skin.—Lymphatic glands enlarged and indurated. Boils and slowly suppurating abscesses.

OPIUM.—PAPAVER SOMNIFERUM
(Dried Latex of the Poppy)

Hahnemann says that it is much more difficult to estimate the action of Opium than of almost any other drug. The effects of Opium as shown in the insensibility of the nervous system, the depression drowsy stupor, painlessness, and torpor, the general sluggishness and lack of vital reaction, constitute the main indications for the drug when used homœopathically. All complaints are characterized by *sopor*. They are *painless*, and are accompanied by *heavy, stupid sleep, stertorous breathing. Sweaty skin.* Dark, mahogany-brown face. Serous apoplexy—venous, passive congestion. Want of sensitiveness to the action of medicines. Reappearance and aggravation from becoming heated. Opium lessens voluntary movements, contracts pupils, depresses higher intellectual powers, lessens self-control and power of concentration, judgment; stimulates the imagination, checks all secretions except that of the skin. Want of susceptibility to remedies even though indicated. Diseases that originate from fright.

Mind.—Patient wants nothing. *Complete loss of consciousness; apoplectic state.* Frightful fancies, daring, gay, bright. Unable to understand or appreciate his sufferings. Thinks he is not at home. Delirious talking, with wide open eyes.

Head.—Vertigo; *lightness of head in old people.* Dull, heavy, stupid. Delirium. Vertigo after fright. Pain in back of head; great weight there. [*Gels.*] Bursting feeling. Complete insensibility; no mental grasp for anything. Paralysis of brain.

Eyes.—Half-closed, dilated; pupils insensible, *contracted.* Ptosis. [*Gels.; Caust.*] Staring, glassy.

Face.—Red, bloated, *swollen, dark suffused, hot.* Looks intoxicated, besotted. [*Bapt.; Lach.*] Spasmodic facial twitching, especially corners of mouth. Veins of face distended. *Hanging down of lower jaw.* Distorted.

Mouth.—Dry. Tongue black, *paralyzed.* Bloody froth. Intense thirst. Blubbering of lips. Difficult articulation and swallowing.

Stomach.—Vomiting, with colic and convulsions. Fæcal vomiting. Incarcerated hernia. Hungry; no desire to eat.

OPIUM

Abdomen.—Hard, bloated, tympanitic. Lead colic. During colic, urging to stool and discharge of hard fæces.

Stool.—Obstinate constipation; no desire to go to stool. *Round, hard, black balls.* Fæces protrude and recede. [*Thuj.*; *Sil.*] Spasmodic retention of fæces in small intestines. Stools involuntary, black, offensive, frothy. Violent pain in rectum, as if pressed asunder.

Urine.—Slow to start; feeble stream. *Retained* or involuntary, after fright. Loss of power or sensibility of bladder.

Female.—Suppressed menses from fright. Cessation of labor-pains with coma and twitchings. Puerperal convulsions; drowsiness or coma between paroxysms. Threatened abortion and suppression of lochia, from fright, with sopor. Horrible labor-like pains in uterus, with urging to stool.

Respiratory.—Breathing stops on going to sleep; must be shaken to start it again. [*Grindelia.*] Hoarse. *Deep snoring rattling, stertorous breathing.* Difficult, intermittent, de ; unequal respiration. Heat in chest; burning about he .. Cough, with dyspnœa and blue face; with bloody expectoration.

Sleep.—Great drowsiness. [*Gels.*; *Nux mosch.*] Falls into a heavy stupid sleep. Profound coma. Loss of breath on falling asleep. [*Grind.*] Coma vigil. Picking at bedclothes. Very sleepy, but cannot go to sleep. Distant noises, cocks crowing, etc., keep him awake. Child dreams of cats, dogs, black forms. Bed feels so hot cannot lie on it. Pleasant, fantastic, amorous dreams. Shaking chill; then heat, with sleep and sweat. Thirst only during heat.

Fever.—Pulse *full* and *slow*. Heat extending over body. *Hot* perspiration. Fever characterized by stupor, snoring respiration, twitching of limbs, intense thirst and sleepiness. General low temperature with inclination to stupor.

Back and Extremities.—Opisthotonos. Swollen veins of neck. Painless paralysis. [*Oleand.*] *Twitching of limbs.* Numbness. Jerks as if flexors were overacting. Convulsions; worse from glare of light; coldness of limbs.

Skin.—Hot, damp, sweating. Constant desire to uncover. *Hot perspiration over whole body except lower limbs.*

Modalities.—*Worse*, heat, during and after sleep. [*Apis*; *Lach.*] *Better*, cold things, constant walking.

Relationship.—Compare: *Apis; Bell.; Gels.; Nux mosch.; Morphinum* (extreme susceptibility to pain; twitching; tympanites; much itching); *Codein* (dry, teasing, incessant cough; twitching of muscles, especially those of eyelids); *Eschscholtzia* —California Poppy—(a harmless soporific).

Antidote: Acute Opium poisoning. *Atropin* and Black Coffee. Chronic Opium poisoning. *Ipecac; Nux; Passiflora. Berberis* is useful to counteract opium habit.

Dose.—Third to thirtieth and 200th potency.

Non-Homœopathic Preparations and Uses.—*Palliative only* in great pain, sleeplessness, peritonitis, and to check excessive secretion in diarrhœa, diabetes, etc.

Opium (crude).—Official dose, 1 grain.

Laudanum (tincture)—Dose, 5 to 20 drops. Extract of Opium 1/4 to 1 grain.

Paregoric—Tinctura Camphora Composita. Contains in each dram 1/4 grain of Opium equal to 1/30 grain of Morphine. Dose 1/2 to 1 fluid dram for adults. For an infant 3 to 5 drops,

Dover's Powder consists of Opium, Ipecac and Sulphate of Potash. It contains 10% each of Opium and Ipecac. Dose 5 to 15 grains.

Morphine—1/8 to 1/4 grain.

Magendie's solution—16 grains to 1 oz. or 5 drops equal to 1/6 grain.

Codein—1/2 to 1 grain.

Apomorphia—1/20 to 1/10 grain hypodermically.

OPUNTIA—FICUS INDICA
(Prickly Pear)

Diarrhœa, with nausea. *Feels as if bowels were settled down in lower abdomen.* Sick feeling in lower third of abdomen. Enteroptosis with loose and frequent evacuations.

Relationship.—Compare: *Chaparra amargosa* (which Mexican physicians laud as a specific in chronic diarrhœa). *Ricinus communis* (diarrhœa, dysentery, obstinate chronic diarrhœa).

Dose.—Second attenuation.

OREODAPHNE
(California Laurel)

Neuralgic headache, cervico-occipital pain, cerebro-spinal meningitis, atonic diarrhœa, and intestinal colic.

Head.—Dizziness; worse on stooping or moving. Head heavy, eyelids heavy, twitching. Intense aching, *with pressure at inner angle of either orbit*, generally left, extending through brain and across scalp to the base of the occiput; worse, light, noise; better, closing eyes and perfect quiet. Constant, dull ache in *cervical and occipital region*, extending to scapula down spine, into the head; pain into the ears. Great heaviness of head, with constant desire to move the head, which does not relieve. Drooping eyelids. Twitching. Atonic diarrhœa.

Stomach.—Eructations, with nausea and shuddering.

Dose.—First to third potency. Olfaction of the tincture.

ORIGANUM
(Sweet Marjoram)

Acts on nervous system generally, and is effective in masturbation and excessively aroused sexual impulses. Affections of the breasts. [*Bufo.*] Desire for active exercise *impelling her to run*.

Female.—*Erotomania;* powerful lascivious impulses; leucorrhœa; hysteria. Lascivious ideas and dreams.

Relationship.—Compare: *Ferula glauca* (in violent sexual excitement in women; icy coldness in occiput); *Plat.; Valer.; Canth.; Hyos.*

Dose.—Third potency.

ORNITHOGALUM UMBELLATUM
(Star of Bethlehem)

To be considered in chronic gastric and other abdominal indurations, possibly cancer of intestinal tract, especially of stomach and cæcum. Center of action is the pylorus, causing painful contraction with duodenal distention.

Depression of spirits. Complete prostration. Feeling of sickness keeps patient awake at night.

Stomach.—Tongue coated. Agonizing feeling in chest and stomach, starting from pylorus with flatus that rolls in balls from one side to the other, loss of appetite, phlegmy retchings and loss of flesh. Gastric ulceration even with hæmorrhage. *Pains increased when food passes pyloric outlet.* Vomiting of *coffee-ground*-looking matter. Distention of stomach. Frequent belching of offensive flatus. Painful sinking across epigastrium.

Dose.—Single doses of mother tincture and await action.

OSMIUM
(The Element)

Irritation and catarrh of respiratory organs. Eczema. Albuminuria. *Pain in trachea.* Increases and gives odor to local perspiration. Causes *adhesion of the nail fold.*

Head.—Feels as if a band around head. Falling off of hair. [*Kali carb.; Fluor. ac.*]

Nose.—Coryza, with full feeling in nose. Nose and larynx sensitive to air. Small lumps of phlegm from posterior nares.

Eyes.—*Glaucoma;* with iridescent vision. Violent supra- and infra-orbital neuralgia; violent pains and lachrymation. *Green colors surround candle-light.* Conjunctivitis. Increase in intraocular tension, dim sight, photophobia.

Respiratory.—Acute laryngitis; cough and expectoration of tough, stringy mucus. Convulsive cough; feels as though membrane were torn from larynx. Noisy, *dry, hard, cough,* in violent short bursts, coming from low down, shaking the whole body. Talking causes pain in larynx. Hoarse; *pain in larynx;* sore sternum. Twitching of fingers, with spasmodic cough.

Skin.—Eczema, with pruritus. Irritated skin. Itching pimples. Bromidrosis, sweat in axilla smelling of garlic, worse evening and night. Fold remains attached to growing nail.

Relationship.—Compare: *Argent.; Iridium; Selen.; Mangan.*

Dose.—Sixth potency.

OSTRYA VIRGINICA
(Ironwood)

Of great value in anæmia from malaria. Bilious conditions and intermittent fever.

Gastric.—*Tongue yellow; coated at the root.* Loss of appetite. *Frequent nausea*, with dull, frontal headache. Sickening pains.

Dose.—First to third potency.

OVI GALLINAE PELLICULA
(Membrane of Egg-shell)

Sudden pains. Bearing-down sensation. Intolerance of bands on wrists, arms, waist, etc. Backache and pain in left hip. Debility. Pain in heart and left ovary.

Relationship.—Compare: *Calc.; Naja; Ova tosta—Tosta præparata*—Roasted egg-shells—Calcarea ovorum—(leucorrhœa and backache. A feeling as if the spine were broken and wired, or tied together with a string. Pain of cancer. Warts). Also *Egg Vaccine for Asthma*. Much interest is shown in Dr. Fritz Talbot's method to cure one form of asthma in children by the use of egg vaccine. Asthma due to susceptibility of the proteid substance in eggs can be cured by immunizing against egg poisons by repeated doses of egg white. After the skin has been cleansed with soap and alcohol the egg-white is rubbed into a slight scratch.

OXALICUM ACIDUM
(Sorrel Acid)

Although certain oxalates are constant constituents of vegetable food and of the human body, the acid itself is a violent poison when taken internally, producing gastro-enteritis, motor paralysis, collapse, stupor and death.

Influences the spinal cord, and produces motor paralysis. Pains very violent, *in spots* (*Kali bich.*) *worse*, motion, and *thinking of them. Periodical remissions.* Spasmodic symptoms of throat and chest. *Rheumatism of left side. Neurasthenia.* Tuberculosis.

OXALICUM ACIDUM

Head.—Sense of heat. Confusion and vertigo. Headache, before and during stool.

Eyes.—Severe pain in eyes; feel expanded. *Hyperæsthesia of retina.*

Stomach.—Violent pain in epigastrium discharge of flatus relieves. Gastralgia, oyrosis, sensation of coldness below epigastrium. Burning pain, extending upwards; slightest touch causes excruciating pain. Bitter and sour eructation, worse at night. Cannot eat strawberries.

Abdomen.—Pain in upper part and region of navel two hours after eating, with much flatulence. Stitches in liver. Colic. Burning in small spots in abdomen. Diarrhœa from coffee.

Male.—*Terrible neuralgic pains in spermatic cord.* Testicles feel contused and heavy. Seminal vesiculitis.

Urinary.—Frequent and copious. Burning in urethra and pain in glans when urinating. Must urinate when thinking of it. Urine contains oxalates.

Respiratory.—Nervous aphonia with cardiac derangement. [*Coca; Hydrocy. ac.*] Burning sensation from throat down. Breathing spasmodic, with constriction of larynx and chest. Hoarseness. *Left lung painful. Aphonia.* Paralysis of the tensors of vocal cord. *Dyspnœa; short, jerking inspirations.* Sharp pain through lower region of left lung, extending down to epigastrium.

Heart.—Palpitation and dyspnœa in organic heart disease; *worse*, when thinking of it. Pulse feeble. Heart symptoms alternate with aphonia, *angina pectoris; sharp, lancinating pain in left lung coming on suddenly, depriving of breath.* Præcordial pains which dart to the left shoulder. Aortic insufficiency.

Extremities.—Numb, weak, tingling. Pains start from spine and extend through extremities. Drawing and *lancinating pains* shooting down extremities. *Backache;* numb, weak. Myelitis. Muscular prostration. Wrist painful, as if sprained. [*Ulmus.*] Lower extremities blue, cold, insensible. Sensation of numbness. Multiple cerebral and posterior spinal sclerosis. Lancinating pains in various parts; jerking pains.

Skin.—Sensitive, smarting and soreness, worse shaving; mottled, marbled in circular patches. Perspires easily.

Modalities.—*Worse, left* side; slightest touch; light; shaving. Aroused about 3 a. m. with gastric and abdominal pain. *All conditions made worse by thinking about self.*

Relationship.—Compare: *Ars.; Colch.; Arg.; Pic. ac.; Cicer arietinum*—Chick-pea—(Lithiasis, jaundice, liver affections; diuretic). *Scolopendra*—Centipede—(terrible pains in back and loins, extending down limbs; return periodically, commencing in head, to toes. Angina pectoris. Inflammation, pain and gangrene. Pustules and abscesses). *Cæsium*—(Pain in lumbar region and testicle. Headache, darting through temples. Diarrhœa and colic. Languor.)

Lime Water—Antidote to poisoning of Oxal. acid.

Dose.—Sixth to thirtieth potency.

OXYDENDRON—ANDROMEDA ARBOREA
(Sorrel-tree)

A remedy for dropsy—ascites and anasarca. Urine suppressed. Deranged portal circulation. Prostatic enlargement. Vesical calculi. Irritation of neck of bladder. Great difficulty of breathing. Tincture. Compare: *Cerefolius* (dropsy, Bright's disease, cystitis).

OXYTROPIS
(Loco-weed)

Marked action on nervous system. Trembling, sensation of emptiness. Walks backwards. Congestion of spine and paralysis. Pains come and go quickly. Sphincters relaxed. Staggering gait. Reflexes lost.

Mind.—Desires to be alone. Disinclined to work or talk. Worse, thinking of symptoms. [*Oxalic. ac.*] *Mental depression*. Vertigo. [*Granatum.*]

Head.—Vertigo. Full, warm feeling about head. Feeling of intoxication, with loss of vision. Pain in maxillary bones and masseter muscles. Mouth and nose dry.

Eyes.—Sight obscured; pupils contracted; do not respond to light. Paralysis of nerves and muscles of eyes.

Stomach.—Eructations with colicky pains. Epigastrium tender.

Rectum.—Sphincter seems relaxed. Stools slip from anus, like *lumps of jelly*, mushy.

Urine.—Urging to urinate when thinking of it. *Profuse flow.* Pain in kidneys. [*Berberis.*]

Male.—No desire or ability. Pain in testicles and along spermatic cord and down thighs.

Extremities.—Pain along ulnar nerve. Numb feeling about spine. *Staggering gait.* Loss of co-ordination. Patellar tendon reflex lost. Pains come and go quickly, but muscles remain sore and stiff.

Sleep.—Restless, dreams of quarrel.

Modalities.—*Worse*, thinking of symptoms (mono-maniac tendency). *Worse*, every other day. *Better*, after sleep.

Relationship.—Compare: *Astrag.; Lathyr.; Oxal. ac.; Baryta* (Loco plant is rich in Baryta). *Lolium.*

Dose.—Third potency and higher.

PAEONIA
(Peony)

The rectal and anal symptoms are most important. Chronic ulcers on lower parts of body, leg, foot, toe, also breast, rectum.

Head.—Rush of blood to head and face. Nervous. Vertigo when moving. Burning in eyes and ringing in ears.

Rectum.—Biting, *itching in anus;* orifice swollen. Burning in anus after stool; then internal chilliness. Fistula ani, diarrhœa, with anal burning and internal chilliness. Painful ulcer, oozing offensive moisture on perineum. *Hæmorrhoids, fissures, ulceration of anus and perineum, purple, covered with crusts.* Atrocious pains with and after each stool. Sudden, pasty diarrhœa, with faintness in abdomen.

Chest.—Sticking pain in left chest. Heat in chest. Dull shooting from front to back through heart.

Extremities.—Pain in wrist and fingers; knees and toes. Weakness of legs, inhibiting walking.

Sleep.—Terrifying dreams, nightmare.

Skin.—Sensitive, painful. Ulcers below coccyx, around sacrum; varicose veins. Ulcers in general, from pressure, bed-sores, etc. Itching, burning, as from nettles.

Relationship.—Compare: *Glechoma*—Ground Ivy—(rectal symptom). *Haman.; Sil.; Aesc.; Ratanh. (great constriction of anus; stools forced with great effort).*

Antidotes: *Ratanh.; Aloe.*

Dose.—Third potency.

PALLADIUM
(The Metal)

An ovarian remedy; produces the symptom-complex of chronic Oophoritis. Useful where the parenchyma of the gland is not totally destroyed. Acts also on mind and skin. Motor weakness, averse to exercise.

Mind.—Weeping mood. *Love of approbation.* Pride; *easily offended.* Inclined to use violent language. *Keeps up brightly when in company,* much exhausted afterwards, and pains aggravated.

Head.—Feels as if swung backward and forwards. Temporo-parietal neuralgia with pain in shoulder. *Pain across top of head from ear to ear;* worse after an evening's entertainment, with irritability and sour eructations. Sallow complexion.

Abdomen.—Shooting pain from navel to pelvis. Sensation as if intestines were bitten off. Intestines feel strangulated. Soreness of abdomen, swelling in right groin. Flatulency.

Female.—Uterine prolapse and retroversion. Subacute pelvic peritonitis, with right-sided pain and backache; menorrhagia. Cutting pain in uterus; relieved after stool. *Pain and swelling in region of right ovary.* Shooting or burning pain in pelvis and bearing-down; relieved by rubbing. Soreness and shooting pain from navel to breast. Glairy leucorrhœa. Menstrual discharge while nursing. Stitches in right breast near nipple. It is indicated in that gyæcological condition where the disease had its inception in the right ovary, the uterine prolapse and retroversion, the subacute pelvic peritonitis and concomitant symptoms being secondary. (F. Aguilar, M. D.)

Extremities.—Pruritus. Tired feeling in small of back Fleeting, neuralgic pains in extremities. Heavy and tired in limbs. Darting pains from toes to hips. Rheumatic pain in right shoulder; in right hip. Sciatica.

Relationship.—Complementary: *Plat.*
Compare: *Arg.; Helon.; Lil.; Apis.*

Dose.—Sixth to thirtieth potency.

PARAFFINE
(Purified Paraffin)

Valuable in uterine affections. Particularly serviceable, in constipation. Knife-like pains. Pains extend from one part to another, and alternate. Pain in stomach alternates with pain in throat and spine.

Head.—Left side of head and face suffer most; pains stinging and twisting. Pain as if a nail were driven in left side of vertex. Twisting in left ear.

Eyes.—Vision dim; black specks before. Lids red. Sensation as if there were fat on the eyes.

Mouth.—Tearing, twisting pain in teeth down to lower jaw. Full of saliva; feels sticky; bitter taste.

Stomach.—Hungry all the time. Pain across stomach. Pain in stomach alternates with pain in throat and spine, extends to chest with belching. Fixed pain in left hypochondrium, as if parts were being twisted. Palpitation with stomach pains.

Abdomen.—Pain in lower abdomen, extending to genitals, rectum and coccyx; better, sitting.

Rectum.—Frequent desire for stool. *Obstinate constipation in children.* [*Alumina; Nyctanthes.*] Chronic constipation, with hæmorrhoids and continual urging to stool, without result.

Female.—Menses too late, black, abundant. Milky leucorrhœa. Nipples pain when touched, as if sore inside. Stabbing pain in mons veneris. Very hot urine with burning pains in vulva.

Extremities.—Pain in spine extending to inguinal region and in both loins, when ascending the stairs. Feeling of electric shocks in all joints. Wrenching pain in calves, extending into toes, in joints. Feet swollen with tearing in ankles and soles.

Skin.—Burns, even of third degree, with sloughing and sepsis. Wash with sterile water and dry and spray with paraffine, and cover with thin layer of cotton. Useful also in frost bites.

Relationship.—Compare: *Naphthalin; Petrol.; Kreos.; Eupion.*

Dose.—Lower triturations and thirieth potency.

PAREIRA BRAVA—CHONDRODENDRON TOMENTOSUM
(Virgin-vine)

The urinary symptoms are most important. Useful in renal colic, prostatic affections, and catarrh of bladder. Sensation as if bladder were distended, with pain. *Pain going down thigh.*

Urinary.—Black, bloody, thick mucous urine. *Constant urging; great straining; pain down thighs during efforts to urinate.* Can emit urine only when he goes on his knees, pressing head firmly against the floor. Feeling of the bladder being distended and neuralgic pain in the anterior crural region. [Staph.] Dribbling after micturition. [Selen.] *Violent pain in glans penis.* Itching along urethra; urethritis, with prostatic trouble. Inflammation of urethra; becomes almost cartilaginous.

Relationship.—Compare: *Parietaria* (renal calculi; nightmare, patient dreaming of being buried alive); *Chimaphila* (chronic catarrhal congestion following cystitis; acute prostatitis; feeling of a ball in perineum when sitting); *Fabiana*, see *Pichi* (dysuria; post-gonorrhœal complications; gravel; vesical catarrh); *Uva.; Hydrang.; Berber.; Ocim.; Hedeom.*

Dose.—Tincture, to third potency.

PARIS QUADRIFOLIA
(One-berry)

Head symptoms marked and verified. Sensation of expansion and consequent tension. Coldness of right side of body, left hot. Catarrhal complaints, stuffed feeling at root of nose. Disorder of sense of touch.

Mind.—Imaginary foul smells. Feels too large. *Garrulous,* prattling, vivacious.

Head.—Sensation as if scalp were contracted and bones scraped. Soreness of top of head; cannot brush hair. Aches, as from *pulling a string from eyes to occiput.* Occipital headache, with a feeling of weight. Head feels very large, expanded. Scalp sensitive. Numb feeling on left side of head.

Eyes.—Affections of the eyebrows. Eyes feel heavy, as if they were projected; *sensation of a string through eyeballs.* Expanded, as though lids did not cover.

Face.—Neuralgia; hot stitches in left malar bone, which is very sore. Has relieved in inflammation of the antrum, where eye symptoms co-existed.

Mouth.—*Tongue dry when awaking*—Coated white, *without thirst*, with bitter or diminished taste.

Respiratory.—Stuffed condition and fullness at root of nose. Periodical, painless *hoarseness*. Cough as from vapor of sulphur in trachea. Constant hawking, on account of viscid, green mucus in larynx and trachea.

Extremities.—Sense of *weight and weariness in nape of neck* and across shoulders. Neuralgia, beginning in left intercostal region, and extending into left arm. Arm becomes stiff, fingers clenched. Neuralgia of coccyx; pulsating, sticking, when sitting. *Fingers often feel numb.* Numbness of upper limbs. Everything feels rough.

Relationship.—Compare: *Pastinaca—Parsnip*—(Loquacity; delirium tremens; illusions of vision; intolerance of milk; Roots used dietetically, cooked in water or as broth or as salad for consumptives and "kidney stones.") *Sil.; Calc.; Nux; Rhus.*

Incompatible: *Ferr. phos.*

Antidote: *Coff.*

Dose.—Third potency.

PARTHENIUM—ESCOBA AMARGO
(Bitter-broom)

A Cuban remedy for fevers, especially malarial. Increased flow of milk. Amenorrhœa and general debility. Cheyne-Stokes breathing. After Quinine.

Head.—Aches, extending to nose; feels swelled; pain in frontal eminence. Eyes heavy; eyeballs ache. Ringing in ears. Pain at root of nose; feels swollen. Aching in teeth. *Teeth feel on edge;* too long. Disordered vision. Tinnitus and pain in ears.

Abdomen.—Pain in left hypochondrium. Spleen affections.

Modalities.—*Worse*, after sleep, sudden motion. *Better*, after rising, and walking about.

Relationship.—Compare: *China; Ceanoth.; Helianth.*

PASSIFLORA INCARNATA
(Passion-flower)

An efficient anti-spasmodic. Whooping-cough. **Morphine habit.** Delirium tremens. Convulsions in children; neuralgia. Has a quieting effect on the nervous system. Insomnia, produces normal sleep, no disturbance of cerebral functions, neuroses of children, worm-fever, teething, spasms. *Tetanus.* Hysteria; puerperal convulsions. Painful diarrhœa. Acute mania. *Atonic condition* generally present. *Asthma*, 10-30 gtt. every ten minutes for a few doses. Locally, in erysipelas.

Head.—Violent ache as if top of head would come off—eyes felt as if pushed out.

Stomach.—Leaden, dead feeling after or between meals; flatulence and sour eructations.

Sleep.—Restless and wakeful, resulting from exhaustion. Especially in the feeble, infants and the aged. Insomnia of infants and the aged, and the mentally worried, and overworked, with tendency to convulsions. Nocturnal cough.

Dose.—Large doses of mother tincture are required—thirty to sixty drops, repeated several times.

PAULLINIA SORBILIS
(Guarana)

Contains a large percentage of Caffein, which may explain its use as a remedy for certain forms of sick headache.

Head.—Intellectual excitement. Sick headache in persons who have used tea and coffee in excess. Throbbing headache after use of liquor.

Bowels.—Stools profuse, bloody, bright green; flakes intermixed; odorless. Cholera infantum.

Skin.—Chloasmata on temples and arms. Urticaria. [*Dulc.; Apis; Chloral.*]

Sleep.—Uncontrollable sleepiness and heaviness of head, with flushed face after eating.

Dose.—Must be given in material doses—fifteen to sixty grains of the powder.

PENTHORUM
(Virginia Stonecrop)

A remedy for coryza, with rawness and wet feeling in nose. Throat feels raw. Chronic disorders of mucous membranes, with irritability. Chronic post-nasal catarrh; chronic pharyngitis, mucous membrane purple and relaxed. Posterior nares feel moist and raw; nose and ears feel full. Aphonia, hoarseness, relaxed vocal cords. Hypersecretion of mucous membranes. Itching of anus and burning in rectum. Trouble in pharyngeal vault and Eustachian tube.

Nose.—*Constant wet feeling in nose*, which no amount of blowing will relieve. Discharge thick, pus-like, streaked with blood. *Post-nasal catarrh of puberty.*

Dose.—Not very active, and better adapted to chronic affections; its use should be persisted in for some time. Lower potencies.

Relationship.—Compare: *Penthorun* often follows *Pulsat. Sang.; Hydr.*

PERTUSSIN
(Coqueluchin)

Taken from the glairy and stringy mucus containing the virus of whooping-cough. Introduced by John H. Clarke for the treatment of whooping-cough and other spasmodic coughs.

Relationship.—Compare: *Drosera; Corallium; Cuprum; Naphthal; Mephitis; Passiflor.; Coccus Cacti; Magnes. phos.*

Dose.—The thirtieth potency.

PETROLEUM
(Crude Rock-oil)

Strumous diathesis, especially the dark type, who suffer from catarrhal conditions of the mucous membranes, gastric acidity and cutaneous eruptions.

Very marked skin symptoms, acting on sweat and oil glands. Ailments are worse during the winter season. Ailments from riding in cars, carriages, or ships; lingering gastric and lung

PETROLEUM

troubles; chronic diarrhœa. *Long-lasting complaints* follow mental states—fright, vexation, etc. Chlorosis in young girls with or without ulceration of the stomach.

Mind.—Marked aggravation from mental emotions. Loses his way in streets. Thinks he is double, or some one else lying alongside. *Feels that death is near, and must hurry to settle affairs.* Irritable, easily offended, vexed at everything. *Low-spirited, with dimness of sight.*

Head.—Sensitive, *as of a cold breeze blowing on it.* Feels numb, as if made of wood; *occiput heavy, as of lead.* [*Opium.*] *Vertigo on rising*, felt in occiput, as if intoxicated, or like sea-sickness. *Moist eruption on scalp;* worse, back and ears. Scalp sore to touch, followed by numbness. Headache, must hold temples to relieve; provoked by shaking while coughing. Use thirtieth.

Eyes.—Loss of eyelashes. Dim sight; far-sighted; cannot read fine print without glasses; blenorrhœa of lachrymal sac; *marginal blepharitis.* Canthi fissured. Skin around eyes dry and scurfy.

Ears.—Noise unbearable, especially from several people talking together. Eczema, intertrigo, etc., in and behind ears, with intense itching. Parts sore to touch. Fissures in meatus. Dry catarrh, with deafness and noises. Ringing and cracking in ears. Chronic Eustachian catarrh. Diminished hearing.

Nose.—*Nostrils ulcerated, cracked, burn;* tip of nose itches. Epistaxis. Ozæna, with scabs and muco-purulent discharge.

Face.—Dry; feels constricted, as if covered with albumin.

Stomach.—Heartburn; hot, sharp, sour eructation. Distension. Feeling of great emptiness. Strong aversion to fat food, meat; worse, eating cabbage. *Hunger,* immediately after stool. *Nausea,* with accumulation of water in mouth. Gastralgia when stomach is empty; relieved by constant eating. [*Anac.; Sep.*] Ravenous hunger. Must rise at night and eat. [*Psorin.*] Odor of garlic.

Abdomen.—*Diarrhœa only in the daytime;* watery, gushing and *itching of anus.* After cabbage; with empty feeling of stomach.

Male.—Herpetic eruption on perineum. Prostate inflamed and swollen. Itching in urethra.

Female.—Before menses, throbbing in head. [*Kreos.*] Leucorrhœa, profuse, albuminous. [*Alum.; Bor.; Bov.; Calc. p.*] Genitals sore and moist. Sensation of moisture. [*Eup. purp.*] Itching and mealy coating of nipple.

Respiratory.—Hoarseness. [*Carbo; Caust.; Phos.*] Dry cough and oppression of chest at night. Cough produces headache. Oppression of chest; worse, cold air. Dry cough at night, coming deep from chest. Croup and laryngeal diphtheria.

Heart.—Sensation of coldness. [*Carb. an.; Nat. mur.*] Fainting, with ebullitions, heat, and palpitation.

Back.—Pain in nape of neck, stiff and painful. Weakness in small of back. Coccyx painful.

Extremities.—Chronic sprains. Fetid sweat in axillæ. Knees stiff. *Tips of fingers rough, cracked, fissured every winter.* Scalding sensation in knee. Cracking in joints.

Skin.—Itching at night. Chilblains, moist, itch and burn. Bed-sores. *Skin dry, constricted, very sensitive, rough and cracked, leathery.* Herpes. Slightest scratch makes skin suppurate. [*Hepar.*] Intertrigo; psoriasis of hands. *Thick, greenish crusts, burning and itching; redness, raw; cracks bleed easily.* Eczema. Rhagades *worse in winter.*

Fever.—Chilliness, followed by sweat. Flushes of heat, particularly of the face and head; worse at night. Perspiration on feet and axillæ.

Modalities.—*Worse, dampness,* before and during a thunderstorm, from riding in cars, *passive motion; in winter,* eating, from mental states. *Better,* warm air; lying with head high; dry weather.

Relationship.—Compare: *Carbo; Graph.; Sulph.; Phos.* Complementary: *Sepia.*
Antidotes: *Nux; Coccul.*

Dose.—Third to thirtieth and higher potencies. Material doses often better.

PETROSELINUM
(Parsley)

The urinary symptoms give the keynots for this remedy. *Piles with much itching.*

Urinary.—Burning, tingling, from perineum throughout whole urethra; *sudden urging to urinate;* frequent, voluptuous tickling in fossa navicularis. Gonorrhœa; *sudden, irresistible desire to urinate; intense biting, itching, deep in urethra;* milky discharge.

Stomach.—Thirsty and hungry, but desire fails on beginning to eat or drink.

Relationship.—Compare: *Apiol*—the active principle of Parsley—(in dysmenorrhœa); *Canth.; Sars.: Cannab.; Merc.*

Dose.—First to third potency.

PHASEOLUS
(Dwarf-bean)

Heart symptoms quite pronounced. Diabetes.

Head.—Aches chiefly in forehead or orbits from fullness of brain; worse any movement or mental exertion.

Eyes.—Pupils dilated, insensible to light. Eyeballs painful to touch.

Chest.—Breathing slow and sighing. Pulse rapid. *Palpitation.* Sick feeling about heart, with weak pulse. Right ribs sore. Dropsical effusion into pleura or pericardium.

Urinary.—Diabetic urine.

Heart.—Fearful palpitation and feeling that death ia approaching.

Relationship.—Compare: *Cratæg.; Lach.*

Dose.—Sixth and higher. A decoction of the shells as a drink for diabetes, but look out for severe headache.

PHELLANDRIUM
(Water Dropwort)

The respiratory symptoms are most important, and have been frequently verified clinically. A very good remedy for the *offensive expectoration and cough in phthisis*, bronchitis, and emphysema. Tuberculosis, affecting generally the middle lobes. *Everything tastes sweet.* Hæmoptysis, hectic and colliquative diarrhœa.

Head.—*Weight on vertex; aching and burning in temples and above eyes.* Crushing feeling in vertex. Vertigo, dizzy when lying down.

Eyes.—Ciliary neuralgia; worse any attempt to use eyes: burning in eyes. Lachrymation. Cannot bear light. Headache; involving nerves going to eye.

Female.—*Pain in milk ducts;* intolerable between nursing. Pain in nipples.

Chest.—*Sticking pain through right breast near sternum, extending to back near shoulders.* Dyspnœa, and continuous cough, early in morning. Cough, with profuse and fetid expectoration; compells him to sit up. Hoarseness.

Fever.—Hectic; profuse and debilitating perspiration; intermittent, with pain in arms. Desire for acids.

Extremities.—Tired feeling when walking.

Relationship.—Compare: *Con.; Phyt.; Sil.; Ant. iod.; Myosotis arvensis.*

Dose.—Tincture, to sixth potency. In phthisis not below the sixth.

PHOSPHORICUM ACIDUM
(Phosphoric Acid)

The common acid "debility" is very marked in this remedy, producing a nervous exhaustion. *Mental debility* first; later physical. A congenial soil for the action of Phos. acid is found in young people who grow rapidly, and who are overtaxed, mentally or physically. Whenever the system has been exposed to the ravages of acute disease, excesses, grief, loss of vital fluids, we obtain conditions calling for it. Pyrosis, flatulence, diarrhœa, diabetes, rhachitis and periosteal inflammation. Neurosis in stump, after amputation. Hæmorrhages in typhoid. Useful in relieving pain of cancer.

Mind.—Listless. Impaired membory. [*Anac.*] *Apathetic, indifferent.* Cannot collect his thoughts or find the right word. Difficult comprehension. Effects of grief and mental shock. Delirium, with great stupefaction. Settled despair.

Head.—Heavy; *confused.* Pain as if temples were crushed together. Worse, *shaking* or *noise. Crushing headache. Pressure on top.* Hair gray early in life; falls out. Dull headache after coition; from eye-strain. [*Nat. m.*] *Vertigo toward evening, when standing or walking.* Hair thins out, turns gray early.

Eyes.—*Blue rings around.* Lids inflamed and cold. Pupils dilated. Glassy appearance. Averse to sunlight; sees colors as if a rainbow. Feel too large. Ambylopia in masturbators. Optic nerves seem torpid. *Pain as if eyeballs were frocibly pressed together and into head.*

Ears.—Roaring, with difficult hearing. Intolerant of noise.

Nose.—Bleeding. Bores fingers into nose. *Itching.*

Mouth.—Lips dry, cracked. Bleeding gums; retract from teeth. Tongue swollen, dry, with viscid, frothy mucus. Teeth feel cold. At night, bites tongue involuntarily.

Face.—Pale, earthy; feeling of tension as from dried albumen. Sensation of coldness of one side of face.

Stomach.—Craves juicy things. Sour risings. Nausea. *Symptoms following sour food and drink.* Pressure as from a weight, with sleepiness after eating. [*Fel tauri.*] *Thirst for cold milk.*

Abdomen.—Distention and fermentation in bowels. Enlarged spleen. [*Ceanoth.*] *Aching in umbilical region.* Loud rumbling.

Stool.—Diarrhœa, *white,* watery, involuntary, *painless,* with much flatus; not specially exhausting. Diarrhœa in weakly, delicate rachitic children.

Urine.—Frequent, profuse, watery, *milky. Diabetes.* Micturition, preceded by anxiety and followed by burning. *Frequent urination at night.* Phosphaturia.

Male.—Emissions at night and at stool. Seminal vesiculitis. [*Oxal. acid.*] Sexual power deficient; testicles tender and swollen. Parts relax during embrace. [*Nux.*] Prostatorrhœa, even when passing a soft stool. Eczema of scrotum. Œdema of prepuce, and swollen glans-penis. Herpes preputialis. Sycotic excrescences. [*Thuja.*]

Female.—Menses too early and profuse, with pain in liver. Itching; yellow leucorrhœa after menses. Milk scanty; health deteriorated from nursing.

Respiratory.—Chest troubles develop after brain-fag. Hoarseness. Dry cough from tickling in chest. Salty expectoration. Difficult respiration. *Weak feeling in chest from talking.* [*Stann.*] *Pressure behind the sternum*, rendering breathing difficult.

Heart.—Palpitation in children who grow too fast; after grief, self-abuse. Pulse irregular, intermittent.

Back.—Boring pain between scapulæ. Pain in back and limbs, as if beaten.

Extremities.—Weak. Tearing pains in joints, bones, and periosteum. Cramps in upper arms and wrists. *Great debility*. Pains at night, *as if bones were scraped*. Stumbles easily and makes missteps. Itching, between fingers or in folds of joints.

Skin.—Pimples, acne, blood-boils. Ulcers, with very offensive pus. Burning red rash. Formication in various parts. *Falling out of the hair.* [*Nat. mur.; Selen.*] Tendency to abscess after fevers.

Sleep.—*Somnolency.* Lascivious dreams with emissions.

Fever.—Chilliness. *Profuse sweat during night and morning.* Low types of fever, with dull comprehension and stupor.

Modalities.—*Better*, from keeping warm. *Worse*, exertion, from being talked to; loss of vital fluids; sexual excesses. Everything impeding circulation causes aggravation of symptoms.

Relationship.—Compare: *Oenothera biennis*—Evening primrose—(Effortless diarrhœa with nervous exhaustion. Incipient hydrocephaloid. Whooping-cough and spasmodic asthma). *Nectranda amare.* (Watery diarrhœa, dry tongue, colic, bluish ring around sunken eyes, restless sleep.) *China; Nux; Pic. ac.; Lactic ac.; Phos.*

Antidotes: *Coffea.*

Dose.—First potency.

PHOSPHORUS
(Phosphorus)

Phosphorus irritates, inflames and degenerates mucous membranes, irritates and inflames serous membranes, inflames spinal cord and nerves, causing paralysis, destroys bone, especially the lower jaw and tibia; disorganizes the blood, causing fatty degeneration of blood vessels and every tissue and organ of the body and thus gives rise to hæmorrhages, and hæmatogenous jaundice.

Produces a picture of destructive metabolism. Causes yellow atrophy of the liver and sub-acute hepatitis. Tall, slender persons, narrow chested, with thin, transparent skin, weakened by loss of animal fluids, with great nervous debility, emaciation, amative tendencies, seem to be under the special influence of Phosphorus. Great susceptibility to external impressions, to light, sound, odors, touch, electrical changes, thunder-storms. *Suddenness* of symptoms, sudden prostration, faints, sweats, shooting pains, etc. Polycythæmia. Blood extravasations; *fatty degenerations*, cirrhosis, caries, are pathological states often calling for Phosphorus. Muscular pseudo-hypertrophy, neuritis. Inflammation of the respiratory tract. Paralytic symptoms. Ill effects of Iodine and excessive use of salt; worse, *lying on left side*. Tertiary syphilis, skin lesions, and nervous debility. *Scurvy. Pseudo-hypertrophic paralysis.* Ataxia and adynamia. Osteo myelitis. Bone fragility.

Mind.—Great lowness of spirits. Easily vexed. Fearfulness, as if something were creeping out of every corner. Clairvoyant state. Great tendency to start. Over-sensitive to external impressions. Loss of memory. Paralysis of the insane. Ecstasy. Dread of death when alone. Brain feels tired. Insanity, with an exaggerated idea of one's own importance. Excitable, produces heat all over. Restless, fidgety. *Hypo*-sensitive, indifferent.

Head.—Vertigo of the aged, *after rising*. [*Bry.*] *Heat comes from spine.* Neuralgia; parts must be kept warm. Burning pains. Chronic congestion of head. Brain-fag, with *coldness of occiput*. Vertigo, with faintness. Skin of forehead feels too tight. Itching of scalp, dandruff, falling out of hair in large bunches.

Eyes.—Cataract. Sensation as if everything were covered with a mist or veil, or dust, or something pulled tightly over eyes. Black points seem to float before the eyes. Patient sees better by shading eyes with hand. Fatigue of eyes and head even without much use of eyes. *Green halo about the candlelight.* [*Osmium.*] *Letters appear red.* Atrophy of optic nerve. Œdema of lids and about eyes. Pearly white conjunctiva and long curved lashes. Partial loss of vision from abuse of tobacco. [*Nux.*] Pain in orbital bones. Paresis of extrinsic muscles. Diplopia, due to deviation of the visual axis. Amaurosis from sexual excess. Glaucoma. Thrombosis of retinal vessels and degenerative changes in retinal cells. Degenerative changes where soreness and curved lines are seen in old people. Retinal trouble with lights and hallucination of vision.

Ears.—*Hearing difficult*, especially to human voice. Re-echoing of sounds. [*Caust.*] Dullness of hearing after typhoid.

Nose.—Fan-like motion of nostrils. [*Lyc.*] Bleeding; *epistaxis instead of menses.* Over-sensitive smell. [*Carbol. ac.; Nux.*] Periostitis of nasal bones. Foul imaginary odors. [*Aur.*] Chronic catarrh, *with small hæmorrhages;* handkerchief is always bloody. *Polypi; bleeding easily.* [*Calc.; Sang.*]

Face.—Pale, sickly complexion; blue rings under eyes. Hippocratic countenance. Tearing pain in facial bones; circumscribed redness in one or both cheeks. *Swelling and necrosis of lower jaw.* [*Amphisbæna; Hecla lava.*]

Mouth.—Swelled and easily *bleeding gums*, ulcerated. Toothache after washing clothes. Tongue *dry, smooth, red* or white, not thickly coated. Persistent bleeding after tooth extraction. Nursing sore mouth. Burning in œsophagus. Dryness in pharynx and fauces. *Thirst for very cold water.* Stricture of œsophagus.

Stomach.—Hunger soon after eating. Sour taste and sour eructations after every meal. Belching large quantities of wind, after eating. *Throws up ingesta by the mouthfuls.* Vomiting; *water is thrown up as soon as it gets warm in the stomach. Post-operative vomiting.* Cardiac opening seems contracted, too narrow; the food scarcely swallowed, comes up again. [*Bry.; Alum.*] Pain in stomach; relieved by cold food, ices. Region of stomach painful to touch, or on walking. Inflammation of stomach, with burning extending to throat and bowels. *Bad effects of eating too much salt.*

Abdomen.—Feels cold. [*Caps.*] Sharp, cutting pains. *A very weak, empty, gone sensation* felt in whole abdominal cavity. Liver congested. Acute hepatitis. Fatty degeneration. [*Carbon. tetrachlorid.; Ars. Chlorof.*] Jaundice. Pancreatic disease. Large, yellow spots on abdomen.

Stool.—*Very fetid stools and flatus.* Long, narrow, hard, like a dog's. Difficult to expel. *Painless,* copious *debilitating* diarrhœa. Green mucus, with grains like sago. Involuntary; seems as if anus remained open. *Great weakness after stool.* Discharge of blood from rectum, during stool. *White,* hard stools. Bleeding hæmorrhoids.

Urine.—Hæmaturia, especially in acute Bright's disease. [*Canth.*] Turbid, brown, with red sediment.

Male.—Lack of power. *Irresistible desire;* involuntary emissions, with lascivious dreams.

Female.—Metritis. Chlorosis. Phlebitis. Fistulous tracks after mammary abscess. Slight hæmorrhage from uterus between periods. Menses too early and scanty—not profuse, *but last too long.* Weeps before menses. Stitching pain in mammæ. Leucorrhœa profuse, smarting, corrosive, instead of menses. Amenorrhœa, with vicarious menstruation. [*Bry.*] *Suppuration of mammæ,* burning, watery, offensive discharge. Nymphomania. Uterine polyps.

Respiratory.—Hoarseness; worse evenings. *Larynx very painful.* Clergyman's sore throat; violent tickling in larynx while speaking. Aphonia, worse evenings, with rawness. *Cannot talk on account of pain in larynx.* Cough from tickling in throat; *worse, cold air,* reading, laughing, *talking,* from going from warm room into cold air. Sweetish taste while coughing. Hard, dry, tight, racking cough. Congestion of lungs. Burning pains, heat and oppression of chest. *Tightness across chest; great weight on chest.* Sharp stitches in chest; *respiration quickened, oppressed. Much heat in chest.* Pneumonia, with oppression; *worse, lying on left side.* Whole body *trembles,* with cough. Sputa rusty, blood-colored, or purulent. Tuberculosis in tall, rapidly-growing young people. Do not give it too low or too frequently here, it may but hasten the destructive degeneration of tubercular masses. Repeated hæmoptysis. [*Acal.*] Pain in throat on coughing. Nervous coughs provoked by strong odors, entrance of a stranger; worse in the presence of strangers; worse lying upon left side; in cold room.

Heart.—Violent palpitation with anxiety, while lying on left side. Pulse rapid, small, and *soft*. Heart dilated, especially right. Feeling of warmth in heart.

Back.—Burning in back; pain as if broken. *Heat between the shoulder-blades.* Weak spine.

Extremities.—Ascending sensory and motor paralysis from ends of fingers and toes. Stitches in elbow and shoulder joints. Burning of feet. Weakness and trembling, from every exertion. Can scarcely hold anything with his hands. Tibia inflamed and becomes necrosed. *Arms and hands become numb.* Can lie only on right side. Post-diphtheritic paralysis, with formication of hands and feet. *Joints suddenly give way.*

Sleep.—Great drowsiness, especially after meals. Coma vigil. Sleeplessness in old people. Vivid dreams of fire; of hæmorrhage. Lascivious dreams. Goes to sleep late and awakens weak. *Short naps and frequent wakings.*

Fever.—Chilly every evening. Cold knees at night. *Adynamic with lack of thirst*, but unnatural hunger. Hectic, with small, quick pulse; viscid night-sweats. Stupid delirium. Profuse perspiration.

Skin.—*Wounds bleed very much, even if small;* they heal and break out again. Jaundice. Little ulcer outside of large ones. Petechiæ. Ecchymosis. *Purpura hæmorrhagia. Scurvy.* Fungous hematodes and excrescences.

Modalities.—*Worse*, touch; physical or mental exertion; twilight; warm food or drink; change of weather, from getting wet in hot weather; evening; lying on left or painful side; during a thunder-storm; ascending stairs. *Better*, in dark, lying on right side, cold food; cold; open air; washing with cold water; sleep.

Relationship.—Complementary: *Ars.; Cepa; Lyc.; Silica. Sanguisuga* 30—Leech—(*Persistent hæmorrhages;* effects of use of leeches.) *Phosph. pentachloride* (great soreness of mucous membrane of *eyes* and nose, throat and chest sore).

Incompatible: *Caust.*

Compare: *Tuberculinum* follows *Phosphor* well and complements its action. *Phosphorus hydrogenatus* (crumbling teeth; hyperæsthesia; locomotor ataxia); *Amphisbæna* (right jaw swollen and painful). *Thymol* (Typical sexual neurasthenia; irritable stomach; aching throughout lumbar region; worse, mental and physical exertion); *Calc.*; *Chin.*; *Antim.*; *Sep.*; *Lyc.*; *Sulph.* In Pneumonia, Pneumococin 200 and Pneumotoxin (Cahis) taken from the Diplococcus lanceolatus of Fraenkel. Pneumonia and paralytic phenomena; pleuritic pain and pain in ilio-cœcal region (Cartier).

Antidote: Antidote to Phosph. Poisoning: *Turpentine* with which it forms an insoluble mass. Also *Potass permang. Nux. Phos.* antidotes the nausea and vomiting of *chloroform* and ether.

Dose.—Third to thirtieth potency. Should not be given too low or in too continuous doses. Especially in tuberculous cases. It may act as Euthanasia here.

PHYSALIS—SOLANUM VESICARIUM
(Alkekengi—Winter Cherry)

Marked urinary symptoms confirming its ancient uses in gravel, etc. Lithiasis; marked diuretic action. Languor and muscular weakness.

Head.—Vertigo, hazy feeling; memory weakened; desire to talk constantly. Throbbing pain, heavy over eyes in forehead. Facial paralysis. Dryness of mouth.

Extremities.—Stiff limbs; tonic cramps. Paralysis. When walking, every jar seems repeated in the head.

Fever.—Chilly in open air. Feverish in evening. Sweat during stool, with creeping sensation, with abundant urine. Pain in liver during fever.

Respiratory.—Cough. Hoarse voice; throat irritated; chest oppressed, causing insomnia. Stabbing in chest.

Urinary.—Acrid, foul, retained, abundant. Polyuria. Sudden inability to hold it in women. Nocturnal incontinence. *Enuresis.*

Skin.—Excoriation between fingers and toes; pustules on thighs; nodes on forehead.

Modalities.—*Worse*, cold camp evening. After geing heated.

Dose.—Tincture to third attenuation. The juice of the berries is used in dropsical conditions and irritable bladder.

PHYSOSTIGMA
(Calabar Bean)

This remedy and its active principle, *Eserine*, form a valuable addition to Materia Medica. Stimulates heart, raises blood pressure, and increases peristalsis. Causes contraction of the pupil and of the ciliary muscles. Induces a condition of snort-sightedness. *Spinal irritation*, loss of motility, prostration, with very sensitive vertebræ. Fibrillary tremors. Rigidity of muscles; paralysis. Depresses the motor and reflex activity of the cord and causes loss of sensibility to pain, muscular weakness, followed by complete paralysis, although muscular contractility is not impaired. Paralysis and tremors, chorea. Meningeal irritation, with rigidity of muscles. *Tetanus* and trismus. Polymyelitis anterior. Eserine is used locally to produce contraction of pupil.

Head.—Constant pain on top; vertigo, with constrictive feeling of head. Pain over orbits; *cannot bear to raise eyelids*. Cerebro-spinal meningitis; general tetanic rigidity. Spastic conditions of the face-muscles.

Eyes.—Night-blindness [Opposite: *Bothrops*]; photophobia; *contraction of pupils; twitching of ocular muscles*. Lagophthalmus. Muscæ volitantes; flashes of light; partial blindness. *Glaucoma;* paresis of accommodation; astigmatism. Profuse lachrymation. *Spasm of ciliary muscle, with irritability after using eyes. Increasing myopia.* Post-diphtheritic paralysis of eye and accommodation muscles.

Nose.—Fluent coryza; burning and tingling of nostrils; nose stuffed and hot. Fever-blisters around nostrils.

Mouth.—*Tongue feels sore on tip.* Feeling as if a ball came up throat.

Throat.—Strong heart-pulsation felt in throat.

PHYSOSTIGMA

Stomach.—Great pain immediately after eating. Sensitive to pressure in epigastric region. Pain extends into chest and down arms. Gastralgia; chronic constipation.

Female.—Irregular menstruation, with palpitation. Congestion of eyes. Rigid muscles.

Heart.—Feeble pulse; palpitation; spasmodic action, with feeling of pulsation through the whole body. Beats of heart distinctly perceptible in chest and head. *Fluttering of heart felt in throat.* Fatty degeneration. [*Cup. ac.*]

Extremities.—*Pain in right popliteal space.* Burning and tingling in spine. Hands and feet numb. Sudden jerking of limbs on going to sleep. Tetanic convulsions. Locomotor ataxia. Numbness in paralyzed parts, crampy pains in limbs.

Relationship.—Compare: *Eserine*—the alkaloid of Physostigma—(slows action of heart and increases arterial tension; in ciliary spasm and spasmodic *astigmatism* due to irregular action of ciliary muscles; blepharo-spasms; *pupils contracted.* Twitching of lids, soreness of eyeballs, blurring of vision *after using eyes*, pains around eyes and head). Used locally to contract the pupil. *Eserine* contracts the pupils dilated by *Atropin*, but not those dilated by *Gelsemium*. Internally 6x.)

Eserin Salicylate (post-operative intestinal paralysis; meteorism. Hypodermically 1/60-1/40 gr.).

Compare also: *Muscarin; Conium; Curare; Gels.; Thebainum* (tetanus); *Piperazinum*—(Uric acid conditions. Pruritus. Gout and urinary calculi. *Constant backache.* Skin dry, urine scanty. Rheumatic urthritis. Give one grain daily in carbonated water. First and second decimal trituration three times a day.)

Antidote: *Atropia*. In full medicinal doses will relieve most of the effects of *physostigmine*.

Dose.—Third potency. The neutral sulphate of Eserine is instilled into the eye, from one-half to four grains to one ounce distilled water, to induce *contraction of pupil*, in mydriasis, injuries to the eye, iritis, corneal ulcers, etc.

PHYTOLACCA
(Poke-root)

Aching, soreness, restlessness, prostration, are general symptoms guiding to Phytolacca. Pre-eminently a glandular remedy. Glandular swellings with heat and inflammation. Has a powerful effect on fibrous and osseous tissues; fasciæ and muscle sheaths; acts on scar tissue. Syphilitic bone pains; chronic rheumatism. Sore throat, quinsy, and diphtheria. Tetanus and opisthotonos. Decrease of weight. Retarded dentition.

Mind.—Loss of personal delicacy, disregard of surrounding objects. Indifferent to life.

Head.—Vertigo on rising. Brain feels sore. Pain from frontal region backward. Pressure in temples and over eyes. Rheumatism of scalp; pains come on every time it rains. Scaly eruption on scalp.

Eyes.—*Smarting.* Feeling of sand under lids. Tarsal edges feel hot. Fistula lachrymalis. [*Fluor. ac.*] *Abundant lachrymation, hot.*

Nose.—Coryza; flow of mucus from *one nostril and from posterior nares.*

Mouth.—Teething children with irresistible desire *to bite the teeth together*. Teeth clenched; lower lip drawn down; lips everted; jaws firmly set; chin drawn down on sternum. Tongue *red tip*, feels rough and scalded; bleeding from mouth; blisters on side. Mapped, indented, fissured, with yellow patch down center. Much stringy saliva.

Throat.—*Dark red or bluish red.* Much pain at root of tongue; soft palate and tonsils swollen. Sensation of a lump in throat. [*Bell.; Lach.*] *Throat feels rough, narrow, hot. Tonsils swollen,* especially right; dark-red appearance. *Shooting pain into ears on swallowing.* Pseudo-membranous exudation, grayish white; thick, tenacious yellowish mucus, difficult to dislodge. *Cannot swallow anything hot.* [*Lach.*] Tension and pressure in parotid gland. Ulcerated sore throat and diphtheria; *throat feels very hot; pain at root of tongue extending to ear.* Uvula large, dropsical. *Quinsy; tonsils and fauces swollen,* with burning pain; cannot swallow even water. *Mumps. Follicular pharyngitis.*

Abdomen.—Sore spot in right hypochondrium. Rheumatism of abdominal muscles. Colic at navel. Burning griping pains. Bruised feeling through epigastrium and abdomen. Constipation of the aged and those with weak heart. Bleeding from rectum.

Urine.—Scanty, suppressed, *with pain in kidney region*. Nephritis.

Female.—Mastitis; *mammæ hard and very sensitive*. Tumors of the breasts with enlarged axillary glands. Cancer of breast. Breast is hard, painful and of purple hue. Mammary abscess. When child nurses, *pain goes from nipple all over body*. Cracks and small ulcers about nipples. Irritable breasts, before and during menses. Galactorrhœa. [*Calc.*] Menses too copious and frequent. Ovarian neuralgia of right side.

Male.—Painful induration of testicles. *Shooting along perineum to penis*.

Heart.—Feeling as if heart leaped into throat. [*Pod.*] Shock of pain in cardiac region alternating with pain in right arm.

Respiratory.—Aphonia. Difficult breathing; dry hacking, tickling cough; worse at night. [*Mentha; Bellad.*] Aching pains in chest, through mid-sternum; with cough. Rheumatism of lower intercostals.

Back.—Aching pains in lumbar region; pains streaking up and down spine into sacrum. Weakness and dull pain in region of kidneys. Back stiff, especially in morning on rising and during damp weather.

Extremities.—Shooting pain in right shoulder, with stiffness and inability to raise arm. (see *Heart.*) Rheumatic pains; worse in morning. *Pains fly like electric shocks*, shooting, lancinating, shifting rapidly. [*Puls.; Kali bich.*] Pain in under side of thighs. Syphilitic sciatica. *Aching of heels;* relieved by elevating feet. Pains like shocks. Pain in legs, patient dreads to get up. Feet puffed; pain in ankles and feet. Neuralgia in toes.

Fever.—High fever, alternating with chilliness and great prostration.

Skin.—Itches, becomes dry, shrunken, pale. Papular and pustular lesions. Most useful in early stages of cutaneous diseases. *Disposition to boils*, and when sloughing occurs. Squamous eruptions. Syphilitic eruptions. Swelling and induration of glands. *Venereal buboes*. Scarlatina-like rash. Warts and moles.

Modalities.—*Worse*, sensitive to electric changes. Effects of a wetting, when it *rains*, exposure to *damp*, cold weather, night, exposure, motion, right side. *Better*, warmth, dry weather, rest.

Relationship.—Compare: Tincture of *Phytolacca Berry* (sore throats and in the treatment of obesity); *Bry.; Rhus; Kali hyd.; Merc.; Sang.; Arum triph.*

Inimical: *Mercur.*

Antidotes: Milk and salt; *Bellad.; Mezer.*

Dose.—Tincture, to third potency. Externally for mastitis.

PICRICUM ACIDUM
(Picric Acid) (Trinitrophenol)

Causes degeneration of the spinal cord, with paralysis. Brain-fag and sexual excitement. Acts upon the generative organs probably through the lumbar centers of the spinal cord; prostration, weakness and pain of back, pins and needle sensation in extremities. *Neurasthenia.* [*Oxal. ac.*] Muscular debility. Heavy tired feeling. Myelitis with spasms and prostration. Writer's palsy. Progressive, pernicious anæmia. *Uræmia* with complete anuria. A one per cent. solution applied on lint, is the best application for burns until granulations begin to form. Sallow complexion.

Mind.—Lack of will-power; disinclined to work. Cerebral softening. Dementia with prostration, sits still and listless.

Head.—Head pains; *relieved by bandaging tightly. Occipital pain;* worse, slightest mental exertion. Vertigo and noises in ear. Boils *within* ears and back of neck. After prolonged mental strain, with anxiety and dread of failure at examination. Brain fag.

Eyes.—Chronic catarrhal conjunctivitis with copious, thick yellow discharge.

Stomach.—Bitter taste. Aversion to food.

Urinary.—*Scanty;* complete anuria. Dribbling micturition. Urine contains much indican, granular cylinders and fatty degenerated epithelium. Inflammation of kidneys with profound weakness, dark, bloody, scanty urine. Nightly urging.

Male.—Emissions profuse, followed by great exhaustion, without sensual dreams. *Priapism;* satyriasis. Hard erections, with pain in testicles and up cord. Prostatic hypertrophy, especially in cases not too far advanced.

Female.—Pain in left ovary and leucorrhœa before menstruation. Pruritus vulvæ.

Extremities.—Burning along spine. *Great weakness. Tired, heavy feeling all over body, especially limbs; worse, exertion.* Feet cold. Cannot get warm. Acute ascending paralysis.

Modalities.—*Worse*, least exertion, especially mental, after sleep, wet weather. A summer or hot weather remedy; patient is worse then. *Better*, from cold air, cold water, tight pressure.

Relationship.—Compare: *Oxal. ac.; Gels.; Phos.; Sil.; Arg. nit.* Compare: *Zinc. pic.* (facial palsy and paralysis agitans); *Ferr. pic.* (buzzing in ears, deafness; chronic gout; epistaxis; prostatic troubles); *Calc. pic.* (boils in and around ears).

Dose.—Sixth potency.

PILOCARPUS MICROPHYLLUS
(Jaborandi)

Pilocarpus is a powerful glandular stimulant and the most efficient diaphoretic. Its most important effects are diaphoresis, salivation and myosis. Hot flushes, nausea, salivation and profuse perspiration. The face, ears and neck become in a few minutes after a dose of Jaborandi deeply flu)hed, and drops of perspiration break out all over the body whilst at the same time the mouth waters and saliva pours out in an almost continuous stream. Other secretions, lachrymal, nasal, bronchial and intestinal also but in less degree. The sweat and saliva produced by a single dose is often enormous in quantity, not infrequently half a pint.

Is homœopathic to *abnormal sweats*, and has achieved great success in *night-sweats* of consumptives. Acts upon the thyroid and its sudorific action may possibly be due to it. *Exophthalmic goitre*, with increased heart's action and pulsation of arteries; tremors and nervousness; heat and sweating; bronchial irritation. A valuable remedy in limiting the duration of mumps.

Eyes.—*Eye strain* from whatever cause. Irritability of the ciliary muscle. Eyes easily tire from slightest use. Heat and burning in eyes on use. Headache; smarting and pain in globe on use. Everything at a distance appears hazy; vision becomes indistinct every few moments. Retinal images retained long after using eyes. Irritation from electric or other artificial light. *Pupils contracted;* do not react to light. Staring eyes. *Near-sighted.* Vertigo and nausea after using eyes. *White spots before eyes. Smarting* pain in eyes. Lids twitch. Atrophic choroiditis. Spasm of the accommodation while reading.

Ears.—Serous exudation into the tympanitic cavities. Tinnitus. [*Pilocarpin* 2x.]

Mouth.—Saliva viscid, like white of egg. Dryness. Free salivation, *with profuse sweating.*

Stomach.—Nausea on looking at objects moving; vomiting; pressure and pain in stomach.

Abdomen.—Diarrhœa, painless; during day with flushed face and profuse sweat.

Urinary.—Scanty; pain over pubes with much urging.

Heart.—Pulse irregular, dicrotic. Oppression of chest. Cyanosis; collapse. Nervous cardiac affections.

Respiratory.—Bronchial mucous membrane inflamed. Much inclination to cough and difficult breathing. Œdema of lungs. Foamy sputa. Profuse, thin, serous expectoration. Slow, sighing respiration.

Skin.—*Excessive perspiration from all parts of the body.* Persistent dryness of skin. Dry eczema. Semi-lateral sweats. Chilliness with sweat.

Relationship.—Compare: *Amyl. nit.; Atrop.; Physos.; Lycop; Ruta. Pilocarpin mur.,* (Meniere's disease, rapidly progressive phthisis, with free hæmorrhages, profuse sweating, 2x trit.) Atropine is the antagonist to Pilocarpin, in dose of one one-hundredth grain for one-sixth of Pilocarpin.

Dose.—Third potency.

Non-Homœopathic Uses.—Chiefly as a powerful and rapid diaphoretic. It is of most service in renal disease, especially with uræmia, eliminating both water, and urea. Scarlatinal dropsy. Contra-indicated *in heart failure, and in post-puerperal uræmia,* and in senile cases.

Dose.—One-eighth to one-fourth grain hypodermically.

PINUS SYLVESTRIS
(Scotch Pine)

Has been found of real use in the treatment of *weak ankles* and tardiness in walking, in scrofulous and rachitic children. Emaciation of lower extremities. Pinus sylvestris combines rheumatic, bronchial and urticarious symptoms; the chest seems thin and to give way.

Extremities.—Stiffness; gouty pain in all joints, especially finger-joints. Cramps in calves.

Skin.—Nettle-rash. Itching all over, especially about joints and on abdomen. Nose itches.

Relationship.—Compare: *Pinus Lambertina*—Sugar Pine—(constipation, amenorrhœa, abortion). *Pinus Lambertina* sap is a decided carthartic. Delayed and painful menstruation.)

Also, *Abies can.; Abies nig.*

Dose.—Tincture, to third potency.

PIPER METHYSTICUM
(Kava-kava)

The intoxication produced by *Kava* is of a silent and drowsy character with incoherent dreams, loss of muscular power.

Urinary and skin symptoms have been verified. Marked modality. *Arthritis deformans*. Colic with flatulence.

Mind.—Very sensitive. Exaltation of mind. *Amelioration of pains for a time by diverting attention*. Restless desire to change position.

Urine.—Increased. Burning during micturition, gonorrhœa, and gleet. Cystitis. *Chordee*.

Skin.—Scaly. Fall of scales leaves *white spots*, which often ulcerate. *Leprosy*. Ichthyosis.

Extremities.—Pain in right arm. Hands feel paralyzed. Pain in thumb-joint.

Relationship.—Compare: *Chaulmoogra*—Taraktogenos—(The oil and its derivatives are to a certain extent effective in the treatment of *leprosy*, especially in early cases.)

Bixa orellana, a South American plant related to Chaulmoogra, recommended for leprosy, eczema and elephantiasis.

Modalities.—*Better*, by turning mind to another topic; changing position.

Dose.—Tincture, and lower potencies.

PIPER NIGRUM
(Black Pepper)

Sensation of burning and pressure everywhere.

Mind.—Sad, apprehensive. Unable to concentrate; starts at any noise.

Head.—Heavy headache, as if temples were pressed in; pressure in nasal and facial bones. Eyes inflamed and burning. Red burning face. Bursting aching in eyeballs. Nose itches; sneezing; nosebleed. Lips dry and cracked.

Throat.—Sore, feels raw, burns. Burning pain in tonsils.

Stomach.—Gastric discomfort. Full feeling. Great thirst. Flatulence. Tympanites. Colic and cramps.

Chest.—Dyspnœa, cough with pain in chest in spots, feels as if spitting blood. Palpitation, cardiac pain, slow intermittent pulse. Great flow of milk.

Urinary.—Burning in bladder and urethra. Difficult micturition. Bladder feels full, swollen; frequent inclination without success. Priapism.

Dose.—Low attenuations.

PITUITARY GLAND

Pituitary exercises a superior control over the growth and development of the sexual organs, stimulates muscular activity and overcomes uterine inertia. Its influence over unstriped muscular fibre is marked. Cerebral hæmorrhage. Will check hæmorrhage and add absorption of clot. Uterine inertia in second stage of labor where os is fully dilated. High blood pressure, chronic nephritis, prostatitis. Ten drops after meals. (Dr. Geo. Fuller.) Vertigo, difficult mental concentration, confusion and fullness deep in frontal region. Use 30th potency.

Relationship.—*Pituitrin*—(Is a vaso-constrictor and parturient. Used chiefly for its action on the uterus either to aid in childbirth or to check bleeding after delivery. In doses of 1 c.c.m. intravenously to stimulate labor pains, expulsive period only. Contra indicated in myocarditis, nephritis and arteriosclerosis. A watery solution made from the posterior protion of the gland is put up in ampules containing about 15 minims each and is considered the hypodermic dose. No effect per os.)

PIX LIQUIDA
(Pine-tar)

Tar and its constituents act on various mucous membranes.

Its skin symptoms most important. A great cough medicine. Bronchial irritation after influenza. [*Kreosot.; Kali bich.*] Scaly eruptions. Much itching. *Constant vomiting of blackish fluid, with pain in stomach.* Alopecia. [*Fluor. ac.*]

Chest.—*Pain at a spot about the third left costal cartilage where it joins the rib.* Rales through the lungs, and *muco-purulent sputum;* offensive odor and taste. Chronic bronchitis.

Skin.—Cracked; *itches intolerably;* bleeds on scratching. Eruptions on *back of hands.*

Relationship.—Compare its constituents: *Kreosot.; Petrol.; Pinus; Eupion; Terebinth.; Carbolic acid.*

Dose.—First to sixth potency.

PLANTAGO MAJOR
(Plantain)

Has considerable clinical reputation in the treatment of earache, toothache, and enuresis. Sharp pain in eyes, reflex from decayed teeth or inflammation of middle ear. Eyeball very tender to touch. Pain plays between teeth and ears. Pyorrhœa alveolaris. Depression and insomnia of chronic Nicotinism. Causes an aversion to tobacco.

Head.—Periodical prosopalgia, worse 7 a. m. to 2 p. m., accompanied with flow of tears, photophobia; pains radiate to temples and lower face.

Ears.—Hearing acute; noise painful. Sticking pain in ears. Neuralgic earache; *pain goes from one ear to the other through the head.* Otalgia, with toothache. Loud noises go through one.

Nose.—Sudden, yellowish, watery discharge.

Mouth.—Teeth ache and are sensitive and sore to touch. Swelling of cheeks. Salivation; teeth feel too long; worse, cold air and contact. Toothache, better while eating. Profuse flow of saliva. Toothache, with reflex neuralgia of eyelids.

Stool.—Wants to defecate; goes often, but cannot. Piles so bad, can hardly stand. Diarrhœa, with brown watery stools.

Urine.—Profuse flow; *nocturnal enuresis.* [*Rhus arom.; Caust.; Bellad.*]

Skin.—Itching and burning; papulæ. Urticaria, chilblains. [*Agar.; Tamus.*]

Relationship.—Compare: *Kalm.; Cham.; Puls.*

Dose.—Tincture, and lower potencies. Local use in toothache in hollow teeth, otorrhœa, pruritus, and Poison-oak. Incised wounds.

PLATANUS OCCIDENTALIS
(Sycamore-Buttonwood)

Tarsal tumors. Apply the tincture. Both acute and old neglected cases, where destruction of tissue occurred and cicatricial contraction caused marked deformity of lid, restored to practically normal conditions. Acts best in children. Must be used for some time. Ichtyosis.

PLATINA
(The Metal)

Is pre-eminently a woman's remedy. Strong tendency to paralysis, anæsthesia, localized *numbness and coldness* are shown. Hysterical spasms; pains increase and decrease gradually. [*Stannum.*] Tremulousness.

Mind.—Irresistible impulse to kill. Self-exaltation; *contempt for others.* Arrogant, proud. Weary of everything. Everything seems changed. Mental troubles, associated with suppressed menses. Physical symptoms disappear as mental symptoms develop.

Head.—Tense, pressing pain, confined to a small spot. *Cramp-like, squeezing pain.* Constriction about forehead and right temples. *Numbness, with headache.*

Eyes.—*Objects look smaller than they are.* Twitching of lids. [*Agar.*] Eyes feel cold. Cramp-like pain in orbits.

Ears.—Feels numb. Cramp-like twinges. Roaring and rumbling.

Face.—Prosopalgia, with numb feeling in malar bones, as if the parts were between screws. Pain at root of nose, as if squeezed in a vise. *Coldness, creeping, and numbness*, in whole right side of face. Pains increase and decrease gradually. [*Stann.*]

Stomach.—Fermentation, much flatulence; *constriction;* ravenous hunger; persistent nausea, with anxiety and weakness.

Abdomen.—Painter's colic. Pain in umbilical region; extending through to back. Pressing and bearing down in abdomen, extending into pelvis.

Stool.—Retarded; fæces scanty; evacuated with difficulty. Adheres to rectum, like soft clay. *Sticky stool.* Constipation of travelers, who are constantly changing food and water. Stool as if burnt.

Female.—Parts hypersensitive. Tingling internally and externally. [*Kali brom.; Orig.*] Ovaries sensitive and burn. Menses too early, too profuse, *dark-clotted*, with spasms and painful bearing-down, chilliness, and sensitiveness of parts. Vaginismus. Nymphomania. Excessive sexual development; vaginismus. Pruritus vulvæ. Ovaritis with sterility. Abnormal sexual appetite and melancholia.

Extremities.—Tightness of thighs, as if too tightly wrapped. Numb and weary sensation. Feel paralyzed.

Sleep.—Sleeps with legs far apart. [*Chamom.*]

Modalities.—*Worse*, sitting and standing; evening. *Better*, walking.

Relationship.—Compare: *Rhodium; Stann.; Valer.; Sep.* Compare, also: *Platinum muriaticum* (this remedy has achieved beneficial results after Iodide of Potash failed to cure in syphilitic affection; violent occipital headaches, dysphagia, and syphilitic throat and bone affections; caries of bones of feet); *Plat. mur. nat.* (polyuria and salivation); *Sedum acre* (sexual irritability, relieves irritation of nerve centers and gives rest).

Antidote: *Puls.* Platina antidotes the bad effects of lead.

Dose.—Sixth trituration to thirtieth potency.

PLUMBUM METALLICUM
(Lead)

The great drug for general sclerotic conditions. Lead paralysis is chiefly of extensors, forearm or upper limb, from center to periphery with partial anasthesia or excessive hyperasthesia, preceded by pain. Localized neuralgic pains, neuritis. The blood, alimentary and nervous systems are the special seats of action of Plumbum. Hæmatosis is interfered with, rapid reduction in number of red corpuscles; hence pallor, icterus, anæmia. Constrictive sensation in internal organs.

Delirium, coma and convulsions. Hypertension and arteriosclerosis. *Progressive muscular atrophy.* Infantile paralysis. Locomotor ataxia. Excessive and rapid emaciation. Bulbar paralysis. Important in peripheral affections. The points of attack for Plumbum are the neuraxons and the anterior horns. Symptoms of multiple sclerosis, posterior spinal sclerosis. Contractions and boring pain. All the symptoms of acute Nephritis with amaurosis and cerebral symptoms. *Gout.* (Chronic).

Mind.—*Mental depression. Fear of being assassinated.* Quiet melancholy. Slow perception; loss of memory; amnesic aphasia. Hallucinations and delusions. Intellectual apathy. Memory impaired. [*Anac.; Baryta.*] Paretic dementia.

Head.—Delirium alternating with colic. Pain as if a ball rose from throat to brain. Hair very dry. *Tinnitus.* [*Chin.; Nat. salic.; Carbon. sulph.*]

Eyes.—Pupils contracted. Yellow. Optic nerve inflamed. Intraocular, suppurative inflammation. *Glaucoma,* especially if secondary to spinal lesion. Optic neuritis, central scotoma. Sudden loss of sight after fainting.

Face.—*Pale and cachetic.* Yellow, corpse-like; cheeks sunken. Skin of face greasy, shiny. Tremor of naso-labial muscles.

Mouth.—Gums swollen, pale; *distinct blue lines along margins of gums.* Tongue tremulous, red on margin. Cannot put it out, seems paralyzed.

Stomach.—Contraction in œsophagus and stomach; pressure and tightness. *Gastralgia* Constant vomiting. Solids cannot be swallowed.

PLUMBUM METALLICUM

Abdomen.—Excessive colic, *radiating to all parts of body. Abdominal wall feels drawn by a string to spine.* Pain causes desire to stretch. Intussusception; strangulated hernia. *Abdomen retracted.* Obstructed flatus, with intense colic. Colic alternates with delirium and pain in atrophied limbs.

Rectum.—Constipation; *stools hard, lumpy, black, with urging and spasm of anus.* Obstructed evacuation from impaction of fæces. [*Plat.*] Neuralgia of rectum. *Anus drawn up with constriction.*

Urinary.—Frequent, ineffectual tenesmus. Albuminous; low specific gravity. *Chronic interstitial nephritis*, with great pain in abdomen. Urine scanty. Tenesmus of bladder. Emission drop by drop.

Male.—*Loss of sexual power.* Testicles drawn up, feel constricted.

Female.—*Vaginismus*, with emaciation and constipation. *Induration of mammary glands.* Vulva and vagina hypersensitive. Stitches and burning pains in breasts. [*Apis; Con.; Carb. an.; Sil.*] Tendency to abortion. Menorrhagia with sensation of string pulling from abdomen to back. Disposition to yawn and stretch.

Heart.—Cardiac weakness. Pulse soft and small, dichrotic. Wiry pulse, cramp-like constriction of peripheral arteries.

Back.—Spinal cord sclerosed. Lightning-like pains; temporarily better by pressure. Paralysis of lower extremities.

Skin.—Yellow, dark-brown liver spots. Jaundice. Dry. Dilated veins of forearms and legs.

Extremities.—Paralysis of single muscles. Cannot raise or lift anything with the hand. Extension is difficult. Paralysis from overexertion of the extensor muscles in piano, players. [*Curare.*] Pains in muscles of thighs; *come in paroxysms. Wrist-drop.* Cramps in calves. Stinging and tearing in limbs, also twitching and tingling, numbness, pain or tremor. Paralysis. Feet swollen. Pain in atrophied limbs alternates with colic. Loss of patellar reflex. Hands and feet cold. Pain in *right big toe* at night, very sensitive to touch.

Modalities.—*Worse*, at night, motion. *Better*, rubbing, hard pressure, physical exertion. [*Alumen.*]

Relationship.—Compare: *Plumb. acet.* (painful cramps in paralyzed limbs; severe pain and muscular cramps in gastric ulcer; locally, as an application (non-homœopathic) in moist eczema, and to dry up secretions from mucous surfaces. Care must be used, as sufficient lead can be absorbed to produce lead poison, one to two drams of the *liquor plumbi subacetatis* to the ounce of water; also in pruritus pudendi, equal parts of the *liquor plumbi* and *glycerin*). *Plumb. iodat.* (Has been used empirically in various forms of paralysis, sclerotic degenerations, especially of spinal cord, atrophies, arterio-sclerosis, pellagra. *Indurations of mammary glands, especially when a tendency to become inflamed appears; sore and painful.* Indurations of great hardness and associated with a very dry skin. Lancinating pains of *Tabes.*) Compare: *Alumina; Plat.; Opium; Podoph.; Merc.; Thall. Plectranthus* (paralysis, spastic, spinal form); *Plumb. chromicum* (convulsions, with terrible pains; pupils greatly dilated; retracted abdomen); *Plumb. phosph.* (loss of sexual power; *locomotor ataxia*).

Antidotes: *Plat.; Alum.; Petrol.*

Dose.—Third to thirtieth potency.

PODOPHYLLUM
(May-apple)

Is especially adapted to persons of bilious temperament. It affects chiefly the *duodenum*, small intestines, liver, and *rectum*. The Podophyllum disease is a gastro-enteritis with colicky pain and bilious vomiting. Stool is watery with jelly-like mucus, painless, *profuse*. Gushing and offensive. Many troubles during pregnancy; pendulous abdomen after confinement; prolapsus uteri; painless cholera morbus. Torpidity of the liver; portal engorgement with a tendency to hæmorrhoids, hypogastric pain, fullness of superficial veins, jaundice.

Mind.—Loquacity and delirium from eating acid fruits. Depression of spirits.

Head.—Vertigo, with tendency to fall forward. Headache, dull pressure, worse morning, with heated face and bitter taste; *alternating with diarrhœa. Rolling of head from side to side*, with moaning and vomiting and eyelids half closed. Child perspires on head during sleep.

Mouth.—Grinding the teeth at night; *intense desire to press the gums together.* [*Phytol.*] Difficult dentition. *Tongue broad, large, moist.* Foul, putrid taste. *Burning sensation of tongue.*

Stomach.—Hot, sour belching; nausea and vomiting. Thirst for large quantities of cold water. [*Bry.*] Vomiting of hot, frothy mucus. Heartburn; gagging or empty retching. Vomiting of milk.

Abdomen.—Distended; heat and emptiness. *Sensation of weakness or sinking.* Can lie comfortably only on stomach. Liver region painful, *better rubbing part.* Rumbling and shifting of flatus in ascending colon.

Rectum.—Cholera infantum and morbus. Diarrhœa of long standing; *early in morning; during teething, with hot, glowing cheeks* while being bathed or washed; in hot weather after acid fruits. Morning, painless diarrhœa when not due to venous stasis or intestinal ulceration. Green, watery, *fetid, profuse,* gushing. *Prolapse of rectum* before or with stool. Constipation; clay-colored, hard, dry, difficult. Constipation alternating with diarrhœa. [*Ant. crud.*] Internal and external piles.

Female.—Pain in uterus and *right ovary, with shifting noises along ascending colon.* Suppressed menses, with pelvic tenesmus. *Prolapsed uteri,* especially after parturition. Hæmorrhoids, with prolapsus ani during pregnancy. Prolapsus from overlifting or straining; during pregnancy.

Extremities.—Pain between shoulders, under right scapula, in loins and lumbar region. Pain in right inguinal region; shoots down inner thigh to knees. Paralytic weakness on left side.

Fever.—Chill at 7 a. m., with pain in hypochondria, and knees, ankles, wrists. *Great loquacity* during fever. Profuse sweat.

Modalities.—Worse, in early morning, in hot weather, during dentition.

Relationship.—Compare: *Mandragora*—also called mandrake—(must not be confounded with *Podoph.* Great desire for sleep; exaggeration of sounds and enlarged vision. Bowels inactive; stools large, white and hard). *Aloe; Chelid.; Merc.; Nux; Sulph. Prunella*—Self-heal—(Colitis).

Dose.—Tincture to sixth potency. The 200th and 1000th seem to do good work in cholera infantum, when indicated.

POLYGONUM PUNCTATUM (Hydropiper)
(Smartweed)

Metrorrhagia, also Amenorrhœa in young girls. *Varicosis;* hæmorrhoids and rectal pockets. Burning in stomach followed by feeling of coldness in the pit of the stomach.

Abdomen.—Griping pain, with great rumbling, nausea, and liquid fæces. *Flatulent colic.*

Rectum.—Interior of anus studded with itching eminence. *Hæmorrhoids.* Liquid fæces.

Urinary.—Painful constriction at neck of bladder.

Female.—Aching pains in hips and loins. *Sensation as if hips were being drawn together.* Sensation of weight and tension within pelvis. Shooting pains through breasts. Amenorrhœa.

Skin.—*Superficial ulcers and sores on lower extremities*, especially in females at climacteric.

Relationship.—Compare: *Carduus mar.* (ulcers); *Hamam.; Senecio; Polygonum persicaria* (renal colic and calculi; *gangrene); Polygonum sagittatum*—arrow-leaved. Tear-thumb—(2x for *pains of nephritic colic;* suppurative nephritis; lancinating pains along spine; itching of hard palate; burning inner side of right foot and ankle. C. M. Boger); *Polygonum aviculare*—knot-grass—(in material doses of tincture, found useful in phthisis pulmonalis and intermittent fever, and especially in *arterio-sclerosis.* Erythema).

Dose.—Tincture.

POLYPORUS PINICOLA
(Pine Agaric)

Useful in intermittent, remittent and bilious fevers, with headache, yellow tongue, constant nausea, faintness at episgastrium, and constipation. Similar to its botanical relative, *Polyp. officinalis*, or *Boletus laricis, q. v.* Deep dull, severe pain in shin bones, preventing sleep.

Fever.—Great lassitude, congestion of head, with vertigo, face hot and flushed, prickling sensation all over; restless at night from pain in wrists and knee; rheumatic pains; profuse perspiration. Headache about 10 a. m., with pain in back, ankles and legs increasing until 3 p. m., then gradually better.

POPULUS CANDICANS
(Balm of Gilead)

Seems to have a remarkable power over acute colds, especially when accompanied by a deep, hoarse voice, or even aphonia. General insensibility of surface (worse, back and abdomen); rubbing and pounding borne without pain, and is grateful on account of warmth produced. Finger-ends thickened, horny; insensible to pinching and pricking. Instantaneous voice-producer. [*Coca.*]

Head.—Discusses her symptoms with every one. Hot head with cold extremities. Cold-sores on lips. [*Nat. mur.*] Tongue feels thick and numb. Burning irritation of eyes, nose, mouth, throat, and air passages.

Respiratory.—*Acute hoarseness.* Throat and nostrils burn. Sits bent forward with dry cough. Pharynx and larynx feel dry, and the voice weak and toneless. Rawness and soreness of chest and throat. Cough of children caused by naso-pharyngeal catarrh; mucus drops from posterior nares.

Dose.—Tincture.

POPULUS TREMULOIDES
(American Aspen)

The gastric and urinary symptoms point to its usefulness in dyspepsia and catarrh of the bladder, especially in old people. Good remedy in vesical troubles after operations and in pregnancy. Cystitis. Fullness of head, and sensation of heat of the surfaces of the body. *Night-sweats. Ague.*

Stomach.—*Indigestion, with flatulence and acidity.* Nausea and vomiting.

Urine.—Severe tenesmus; painful scalding. Urine contains mucus and pus. Prostate enlarged. Pain behind pubis, at end of urination.

Relationship.—Compare: *Nux; China; Cornus flor.; Cannabis; Cantharis.*

Dose.—Tincture or *Populin* trit. 1x.

POTHOS FOETIDUS
(Skunk-cabbage—Ictodes)

For asthmatic complaints; worse from inhaling any dust. *Hysteria.* Erratic spasmodic pains. "Will-o'-the-wisp" like character of its subjective symptoms and its physometric property are special features. (Samuel Jones.) *Inflation and tension in the abdomen.* Millar's asthma.

Head.—Absent-minded, irritable. Headache in *single spots,* with *violent pulsation of temporal arteries.* Outward drawing from glabella. Better in open air. [*Puls.*] Red swelling across the bridge of the nose.

Abdomen.—*Inflation and tension* in abdomen.

Respiratory.—Spasmodic croup. Troublesome respiration, with sudden feeling of anguish and sweat.

Sneezing, with pain in throat. Pain in chest, with difficult breathing. Tongue feels numb. *Asthma; relieved by stool.*

Dose.—Tincture and lower potencies.

PRIMULA VERIS
(Cowslip)

Cerebral congestion, with neuralgia; migraine; rheumatic and gouty pains.

Head. -Sensation of a band around head; cannot keep hat on. [*Carbol. ac.*] Skin of forehead tense. Fear of falling when standing up. Violent vertigo, as if everything turned around. Buzzing in ears; better in open air.

Respiratory.—Cough, with burning and pricking in respiratory tracts. Weak voice.

Urinary.—Urine smells strongly of violets. [*Terebinth.*]

Extremities.—Right axillary muscles painful. Weight and lassitude in limbs, especially the *shoulders.* Burning in hollow of right hand. Drawing pain in thumb and big toe.

Relationship.—Compare: *Cyclamen; Ranunc.; Œnothera*—Evening Primrose—(exhausting, watery diarrhœa; cholera infantum; hydrocephaloid); *Primula farinosa*—the wild Primrose—(dermatitis, especially on index fingers and thumbs).

Dose.—Third potency.

PRIMULA OBCONICA
(Primrose)

The poison of the Primrose occurs in its *glandular hairs*, which break easily and discharge an irritating fluid which is absorbed into the skin.

But skin symptoms of poisoning appear in sensitive patients even without coming in direct contact with the plant, mere nearness being sufficient, just like Poison ivy. Intermittency of symptoms; worse right side. Pain in liver and spleen. Deep infiltration and tension of tissues; blisters. *Paralyzed sensation. Weakness.* Pharyngeal soreness alternates with diminished facial irritation.

Face.—Moist eczema. Papular eruption on chin. Burns at night. Urticaria-like eruption. Eyelids swollen.

Extremities.—Eczema on arms, wrists, forearms, hands. papular and excoriated. Rheumatic pain around shoulder. Palms dry and hot. Cracking over joints and fingers. Eruption between fingers. Purple blotches on back of hands, palmar surface stiff. Blisters on fingers.

Skin.—*Great itching*, worse at night, red and swollen like erysipelas. Tumefied. *Small papules on a raised base.* Skin symptoms accompanied by febrile symptoms.

Relationship.—Compare: *Rhus; Fagopyrum* (Antidotal). *Humea Elegans*, similar skin symptoms.

PROPYLAMIN—TRIMETHYLAMINUM
(Distilled Herring-brine)

In acute rheumatism, dissipates fever and pain in a day or two. Rheumatic prosopalgia, and rheumatic metastases, especially heart lesions.

Extremities.—*Pain in wrists and ankles;* worse, slightest motion. [*Bry.*] Great restlessness and thirst. Rheumatism, needle held in fingers gets too heavy. *Tingling and numbness of fingers.* Pain in wrist and ankle, unable to stand.

Relationship.—(*Chenopodium vulvaria.* The plant has an odor of decaying fish and contains a large amount of Propylamine. Weakness in lumbar and lower dorsal region.)

Dose.—Ten to fifteen drops, in about six ounces of water; teaspoonful doses every two hours.

PRUNUS SPINOSA
(Black-thorn)

Special action on the urinary organs and head. Very valuable in certain neuralgias, anasarca, and especially œdema pedum. Ankle and foot feel sprained. *Ciliary neuralgia.* [*Spig.*]

Head.—Pressing-asunder pain beneath skull. *Shooting from right frontal bone through brain to occiput. Pain in right eyeball, as if it would burst.* Piercing toothache, as if teeth were pulled out; worse, taking anything warm.

Eyes.—*Ciliary neuralgia.* Bursting pain in right eyeball, shooting like lightning through the brain to occiput. *Sudden pain in left eye as if it would burst, better by lachrymation.* Irido-choroiditis. Opacity of vitreous humor. Eyes feel as if bursting.

Abdomen.—Ascites. Cramp-like pain in bladder region; worse, walking.

Rectum.—Hard, nodular stool, with rectal pain, as if angular body were pressed inward. Burning in anus after slimy diarrhœa.

Urine.—Tenesmus of bladder. Ineffectual effort to urinate. *Hurriedly impelled to urinate; the urine seems to pass as far as glans, and then returns and causes pain in urethra.* Neuralgic dysuria. *Must press a long time before urine appears.*

Respiratory.—Wheezing when walking. Oppression of chest; anxious, short respiration. Angina pectoris. Furious beating of heart; worse, slightest motion.

Skin.—Herpes zoster. *Dropsy.* Itching on tips of fingers, as if frozen.

Relationship.—Compare: *Lauroc.; Prunus padus*—Birdcherry—(sore throat, pressure behind sternum and sticking pain in rectum); *Prunus Virginiana*—Wild Cherry—(*heart tonic;* relieves the flagging and distended ventricle; irritable heart; dilatation of right heart; *cough, worse at night on lying down;* weak digestion, especially in elderly people; chronic bronchitis; increases muscular tone); *Pyrus*—Mountain Ash—(irritation of eyes; constriction around waist; spasmodic pains in uterus, bladder, heart, cold-water sensation in stomach, coldness extends up œsophagus; neuralgic and gouty pains).

Dose.—Third to sixth potency.

PSORINUM
(Scabies Vesicle)

The therapeutic field of this remedy is found in so-called psoric manifestations. Psorinum is a cold medicine; wants the head kept warm, *wants warm clothing* even in summer. *Extreme sensitiveness to cold.* Debility, independent of any organic disease, especially the weakness remaining after acute disease. *Lack of reaction*, i. e., phagocytes defective; when well-chosen remedies fail to act. Scrofulous patients. Secretions *have a filthy smell*. Profuse sweating. Cardiac weakness. Skin symptoms very prominent. Often gives immunity from cold-catching. Easy perspiration when walking. Syphilis, inherited and tertiary. *Offensive discharges.*

Mind.—Hopeless; despairs of recovery. *Melancholy*, deep and persistent; religious. Suicidal tendency.

Head.—Awakens at night with pain as from blow on head. Chronic headaches; hungry during attacks; with vertigo. Hammering pain; brain feels too large; worse, change of weather. Dull, pressive pain in occiput. Humid eruption on scalp; hair matted. Hair dry.

Eyes.—Agglutinated. Blepharitis. *Chronic ophthalmia, that constantly recurs.* Edges of lids red. Secretion acrid.

Mouth.—Obstinate rhagades at corners. Tongue, gums ulcerated; tough mucus of foul taste adheres to soft palate.

Nose.—Dry, coryza, with stoppage of nose. Chronic catarrh; dropping from posterior nares. Acne rosacea.

Ears.—Raw, red, *oozing scabs around ears.* Sore pain behind ears. Herpes from temples over ears to cheeks. *Offensive discharge from eczema around ears. Intolerable itching.* Chronic otorrhœa. *Most fetid pus from ears*, brownish, offensive.

Face.—Swelling of upper lip. Pale, delicate. *Humid eruption on face.* Sickly.

Throat.—Tonsils greatly swollen; painful swallowing, with pain in ears. Profuse, offensive saliva; tough mucus in throat. Recurring quinsy. *Eradicates tendency to quinsy.* Hawking up of cheesy, pea-like balls of disgusting smell and taste. [*Agar.*]

Stomach.—Eructations like bad eggs. *Very hungry always; must have something to eat in the middle of the night.* Nausea: vomiting of pregnancy. Pain in abdomen after eating.

Stool.—Mucous, *bloody, excessively fetid, dark fluid.* Hard, difficult stool, with blood from rectum and burning piles. *Constipation of infants,* in pale, sickly scrofulous children.

Female.—*Leucorrhœa* fetid, lumpy, with much backache and *debility.* Mammæ swollen and painful. Pimples oozing an acrid fluid that burns and excoriates the glands.

Respiratory.—Asthma, with dyspnœa; worse, sitting up; better, lying down and keeping arms spread wide apart. Dry, hard cough, with great weakness in chest. *Feeling of ulceration under sternum.* Pain in chest; better, lying down. Cough returns every winter, from suppressed eruption. *Hay-fever* returning irregularly every year.

Extremities.—Weakness of joints, as if they would not hold together. *Eruption around finger-nails.* Fetid foot-sweats.

Skin.—Dirty, dingy look. Dry, lustreless, rough hair. *Intolerable itching.* Herpetic eruptions, especially on scalp and bends of joints with itching; worse, from warmth of bed. Enlarged glands. Sebaceous glands secrete excessively; oily skin. Indolent ulcers, slow to heal. Eczema behind ears. Crusty eruptions all over. Urticaria after every exertion. Pustules near finger-nails.

Fever.—Profuse, offensive perspiration; night-sweats.

Sleep.—Sleepless from intolerable itching. Easily startled.

Modalities.—*Worse,* coffee; Psorinum patient does not improve while using coffee. *Worse,* changes of weather, in hot sunshine, from cold. *Dread of least cold air or draft. Better,* heat, warm clothing, even in summer.

Relationship.—Complementary: *Sulphur.*

Compare: *Pediculus*—Head-louse—(psoric manifestations in children. Eruption on dorsum of hands, feet, neck. Prurigo; pellagra. Unusual aptitude for study and work). *Pediculus* (Cooties) transmit typhus and trench fever.) In lack of reaction compare *Calcarea* and *Natrum ars. Gaertner.* (Pessimistic, lack of confidence, subjective troublesome eye symptoms, fear of heights. Urticaria. Use 30th and 200th. (Wheeler.)

Dose.—Two hundredth and higher potencies. Should not be repeated too often. *Psorinum* requires something like 9 days before it manifests its action, and even a single dose may elicit other symptoms lasting for weeks. (Aegedi.)

PTELEA
(Wafer-ash)

Is a remarkable remedy in stomach and liver affections. The aching and heaviness in the region of the liver is *greatly aggravated by lying* on the left side. *Atonic states of stomach.* Asthma.

Head.—Feels dull and stupid. *Pain from forehead to root of nose; pressing-outward pain. Frontal headache;* worse, noise, motion, night, rubbing eyes, with acidity. Temples as if pressed together.

Mouth.—*Excess of saliva,* with dry *bitter taste.* Tongue coated white or yellow; feels rough, swollen. *Papillæ red and prominent.* [*Arg. n.*] Coating may be brownish-yellow.

Stomach.—Weight and fullness. Griping in epigastric region, with dryness of mouth. Eructations, nausea, vomiting. Constant sensation of corrosion, heat and burning in stomach. Stomach feels empty after eating. *Stomach and liver symptoms associated with pain in limbs.*

Abdomen.—Much weight and pain in right side; heavy, aching feeling, relieved by lying on right side. Liver sore, swollen, sensitive to pressure. Retraction of abdomen.

Respiratory.—Feeling of pressure on lungs and of suffocation, when lying on back. *Asthma;* dyspnœa; cramp-like pain in cardiac region.

Sleep.—Restless, with frightful dreams; nightmare, awakes languid and unrefreshed.

Modalities.—*Worse,* lying on left side; early morning. *Better,* eating sour things.

Relationship.—Compare: *Mercur.; Magn. mur.; Nux; Chelid.*

Dose.—First to thirtieth potency.

PULEX IRRITANS
(Common Flea)

Marked urinary and female symptoms.

Head.—Very impatient, cross, and irritable. Frontal headache, with *enlarged feeling of eyes. Face wrinkled and old-looking.*

Mouth.—Metallic taste. Sensation of a thread in throat. Thirsty, especially during headache.

Stomach.—Breath and taste foul. Intense nausea, with vomiting, purging, and faintness. Stool very offensive. Abdomen bloated.

Urine.—Scanty with frequent urging, with pressure on bladder and burning in urethra. Flow stops suddenly followed by pain. Urine foul. Cannot retain urine; must attend to the call without delay. Irritable bladder before menses.

Female.—Menses delayed. Increased flow of saliva during. Intense burning in vagina. Leucorrhœa, profuse, foul, staining a greenish yellow; stains of menses and leucorrhœa very hard to wash out. Backache. [*Oxal. ac.*]

Back.—Aches, weak; drawing of muscles below scapulæ.

Fever.—Feels a glow all over, like being over steam; *chilly*, while sitting beside the fire.

Skin.—Prickly itching. Sore spots all over. Skin emits foul odor.

Modalities.—*Better*, sitting or lying down. *Worse*, left side: moving about.

Dose.—The higher potencies.

PULSATILLA
(Wind Flower)

The weather-cock among remedies.

The disposition and mental state are the chief guiding symptoms to the selection of Pulsatilla. It is pre-eminently a female remedy, especially for mild, gentle, yielding disposition. Sad, crying readily; weeps when talking; *changeable*, contradictory. *The patient seeks the open air; always feels better there*, even though he is chilly. Mucous membranes are all affected. *Discharges thick, bland, and yellowish-green.* Often indicated after abuse of Iron tonics, and after badly-managed measles. *Symptoms ever changing. Thirstless, peevish, and chilly.* When first serious impairment of health is referred to age of puberty. Great sensitiveness. Wants the head high. Feels uncomfortable with only one pillow. Lies with hands above head.

PULSATILLA

Mind.—Weeps easily. Timid, irresolute. Fears in evening to be alone, dark, ghosts. Likes sympathy. Children like fuss and caresses. Easily discouraged. Morbid dread of the opposite sex. Religious melancholy. Given to extremes of pleasure and pain. Highly emotional. Mentally, an April day.

Head.—Wandering stitches about head; pains extend to face and teeth; vertigo; better in open air. Frontal and supraorbital pains. Neuralgic pains, commencing in *right temporal region, with scalding lachrymation of affected side. Headache from overwork.* Pressure on vertex.

Ears.—Sensation as if something were being forced outward. Hearing difficult, as if the ear were stuffed. Otorrhœa. Thick, bland discharge; offensive odor. External ear swollen and red. Catarrhal otitis. Otalgia, worse at night. Diminishes acuteness of hearing.

Eyes.—*Thick, profuse, yellow, bland discharges.* Itching and burning in eyes. Profuse lachrymation and secretion of mucus. *Lids inflamed, agglutinated. Styes.* Veins of fundus oculi greatly enlarged. Ophthalmia neonatorum. Subacute conjunctivitis, with dyspepsia; worse, in warm room.

Nose.—Coryza; stoppage of right nostril, pressing pain at root of nose. Loss of smell. Large green fetid scales in nose. Stoppage in evening. Yellow mucus; abundant in morning. Bad smells, as of old catarrh. Nasal bones sore.

Face.—Right-sided neuralgia, with profuse lachrymation. Swelling of lower lip, which is cracked in middle. Prosopalgia towards evening till midnight; chilly, with pain.

Mouth.—Greasy taste. *Dry mouth, without thirst;* wants it washed frequently. Frequently licks the dry lips. *Crack in middle of lower lip. Yellow or white tongue, covered with a tenacious mucus.* Toothache; relieved by holding cold water in mouth. [*Coff.*] Offensive odor from mouth. [*Merc.; Aur.*] Food, especially bread, tastes bitter. Much *sweet* saliva. *Alterations of taste,* bitter, bilious, greasy, salty, *foul.* Loss of taste. Desire for tonics.

Stomach.—*Averse to fat food, warm food, and drink.* Eructations; *taste of food remains a long time;* after ices, fruits, pasty. *Bitter taste,* diminished taste of all food. Pain as from subcutaneous ulceration. *Flatulence.* Dislikes butter. [*Sang.*]

Heartburn. Dyspepsia, with great tightness after a meal; must loosen clothing. *Thirstlessness*, with nearly all complaints. Vomiting of food eaten long before. Pain in stomach an hour after eating. [*Nux.*] Weight as from a stone, especially in morning on awakening. Gnawing, hungry feeling. [*Abies c.*] Perceptible pulsation in pit of stomach. [*Asaf.*] All-gone sensation, especially in tea drinkers. Waterbrash, with foul taste in the morning.

Abdomen.—Painful, distended; loud rumbling. Pressure as from a stone. Colic, with chilliness in evening.

Stool.—Rumbling, watery; worse, night. *No two stools alike.* After fruit. [*Ars.; Chin.*] Blind hæmorrhoids, with itching and sticking pains. Dysentery; mucus and blood, with chilliness. [*Merc.; Rheum.*] *Two or three normal stools daily.*

Urine.—Increased desire; *worse when lying down.* Burning in orifice of urethra during and after micturition. Involuntary micturition at night, while coughing or passing flatus. After urinating, spasmodic pain in bladder.

Female.—Amenorrhœa. [*Cimicif.; Senec.; Polygon.*] Suppressed menses from wet feet, nervous debility, or chlorosis. Tardy menses. Too late, scanty, thick, dark, *clotted, changeable, intermittent.* Chilliness, nausea, downward pressure, painful, flow intermits. Leucorrhœa acrid, burning, creamy. Pain in back; tired feeling. Diarrhœa during or after menses.

Male.—Orchitis; pain from abdomen to testicles. Thick, yellow discharge from urethra; late stage of gonorrhœa. Stricture; urine passed only in drops, and stream interrupted. [*Clemat.*] *Acute prostatitis.* Pain and tenesmus in urinating, *worse lying on back.*

Respiratory.—Capricious hoarseness; comes and goes. *Dry cough in evening and at night; must sit up in bed to get relief; and loose cough in the morning,* with copious mucous expectoration. *Pressure upon the chest and soreness.* Great soreness of episgastrium. Urine emitted with cough. [*Caust.*] Pain as from ulcer in middle of chest. Expectoration bland, thick, bitter, greenish. Short breath, anxiety, and palpitation when lying on left side. [*Phos.*] Smothering sensation on lying down.

Sleep.—*Wide awake in the evening;* first sleep restless.

Wakes languid, unrefreshed. Irresistible sleepiness in afternoon. Sleeps with hands over head.

Back.—Shooting pain in the nape and back, between shoulders; in sacrum after sitting.

Extremities.—Drawing, tensive pain in thighs and legs, with restlessness, sleeplessness and *chilliness*. *Pain in limbs, shifting rapidly;* tensive pain, *letting up with a snap.* Numbness around elbow. Hip-joint painful. Knees swollen, with tearing, drawing pains. Boring pain in heels toward evening; *suffering worse from letting the affected limb hang down.* [*Vipera.*] Veins in forearms and hands swollen. Feet red, inflamed, swollen. Legs feel heavy and weary.

Skin.—Urticaria, after rich food, with diarrhœa, from delayed menses, worse undressing. *Measles.* Acne at puberty. Varicose veins.

Fever.—*Chilliness*, even in warm room, *without thirst.* Chilly with pains, in spots, worse evening. Chill about 4 p. m. Intolerable burning heat at night, with distended veins; heat in parts of body, coldness in other. One-sided sweat; pains during sweat. *External heat is intolerable, veins are distended.* During apyrexia, headache, diarrhœa, loss of appetite, nausea.

Modalities.—*Worse*, from heat, rich fat food, after eating, towards evening, warm room, lying on left or on painless side, when allowing feet to hang down. *Better*, open air, motion, cold applications, cold food and drinks. though not thirsty.

Relationship.—*Penthorum*, often indicated after Pulsatilla in later colds. *Ionesia Asoca*—Saraca indica—(*Amenorrhœa*, Menorrhagia—acts powerfully on female organs. Abdominal pain). *Atriplex* (Uterine symptoms, amenorrhœa; hysteria, coldness between shoulders, dislike of warm food, craves strange foods, palpitation, sleeplessness). *Pulsatilla Nuttaliana*, identical effects.

Compare: *Cyclamen; Kaii bich.; Kali sulph.; Sulphur.*

Pimenta—Allspice—(one-sided neuralgias, parts of body hot and cold).

Anagyris (headache, amenorrhœa).

Complementary: *Coffea; Chamom.; Nux.*

Dose.—Third to thirtieth attenuation.

PYROGENIUM
(Artificial Sepsin)

This remedy was introduced by English Homœopathists, prepared from decomposed lean beef allowed to stand in the sun for two weeks and then potentized. The provings and most of the clinical experience have been obtained from this preparation. But, subsequently, Dr. Swan potentized some septic pus, which preparation has also been proved and clinically applied. There does not seem to be any marked difference in their effects.

Pyrogen is the great remedy for *septic states*, with intense restlessness. "In septic fevers, especially puerperal, Pyrogen has demonstrated its great value as a homœopathic dynamic antiseptic." (H. C. Allen.) Hectic, typhoid, typhus, ptomaine poisoning, diphtheria, dissecting wounds, sewer-gas poisoning, chronic malaria, after-effects of miscarriage, all these conditions at times may present symptoms calling for this unique medicine. *All discharges are horribly offensive*—menstrual, lochial, diarrhœa, vomit, sweat, breath, etc. Great pain and violent burning in abscesses. Chronic complaints that date back to septic conditions. Threatening heart failure in zymotic and septic fevers. Influenza, typhoid symptoms.

Mind.—Full of anxiety and insane notions. Loquacious. Thinks he is very wealthy. *Restless*. Feels if crowded with arms and legs. Cannot tell whether dreaming while awake or asleep.

Head.—Painless throbbing. Fan-like motion of alæ nasi. [*Lyc.; Phos.*] Bursting headache with restlessness.

Mouth.—Tongue red and *dry*, clean, cracked, smooth, as though varnished. Throat dry, articulation difficult. Nausea and vomiting. Taste terribly fetid. Breath horrible.

Stomach.—Coffee-grounds vomiting. Vomits water, when it becomes warm in stomach.

Abdomen.—Intolerable tenesmus of both bladder and rectum. Bloated, sore, cutting pain.

Stool.—Diarrhœa; horribly offensive, brown-black, painless, involuntary. Constipation, with complete inertia [*Opium*]; obstinate from impaction. Stools large, black, carrion-like, or small black balls.

Heart.—Tired feeling about heart. *Palpitation.* Sensation as if heart were too full. Always can hear her heart beat. Pulse abnormally rapid, *out of proportion to the temperature.* Pain in region of left nipple. Conscious of heart.

Female.—Puerperal peritonitis, with extreme fetor. Septicæmia following abortion. Menses horribly offensive. Uterine hæmorrhages. Fever at each menstrual period, consequent upon latent pelvic inflammation. *Septic puerperal infection.* Pelvic calculitis. Inflammatory exudate. Post-operative cases, with overwhelming sepsis.

Fever.—Coldness and chilliness. *Septic fevers.* Latent pyogenic condition. Chill begins in back. Temperature rises rapidly. Great heat with profuse hot sweat, but *sweating does not cause a fall in temperature.*

Extremities.—Throbbing in vessels of neck. Numbness of hands, arms, feet. Aching in all limbs and bones. *Bed feels too hard.* [*Arn.*] Great debility in the morning. Soreness; better by motion. [*Rhus.*] Rapid decubitus of septic origin.

Skin.—Small cut or injury becomes much swollen and inflamed—discolored. Dry.

Sleep.—Seems to be in semi-sleep. Dreams all night.

Modalities.—Relief from motion.

Relationship.—Compare: *Streptoccin* (anti-febrile action; septic symptoms in infectious diseases). Rapid in its action, especially in its effect on temperature;) *Staphyloccin* in diseases where the staphylococcus is the chief bacterial factor, as acne, abscess, furuncle; empyema, endocarditis, etc.); *Sepin* —A toxin of Proteus vulgaris, prepared by Dr. Shedd, same symptoms as Pyrogen, of which it is the main constituent; *Echinacea; Carbo; Ars.; Lach.; Rhus; Bapt.*

Complementary: *Bryon.*

Dose.—Sixth to thirtieth and higher potencies. Should not be repeated too frequently.

QUASSIA—PICRAENA EXCELSA
(Quassia-wood)

Acts on gastric organs as a tonic. [*Gentian; Hydr.*] Seems to possess marked action on eyes, producing amblyopia and cataract. Pain in right intercostal muscles above the liver. Pressure and stitches in liver, and sympathetically in spleen.

Stomach.—Atonic dyspepsia, with gas and acidity. Heartburn and gastralgia. Regurgitation of food. Abdomen feels empty and retracted. Dyspepsia after infectious diseases; especially grip, dysentery. Tongue dry or with brown sticky coating. Cirrhosis of liver with ascites.

Urinary.—Excessive desire—impossible to retain urine; copious micturition day and night. As soon as the child wakes up the bed is drenched.

Extremities.—Inclination to yawn and stretch. [*Rhus.*] Sensation of coldness over back. Prostration, with hunger. Cold extremities, with sensation of internal coldness. [*Heloderma.*]

Dose.—First to third potency, or spoonful doses of Aqua Quassiæ

QUERCUS GLANDIUM SPIRITUS
(Spirit distilled from Tincture of Acorn Kernels)

Used first by Rademacher for chronic spleen affections; *spleen-dropsy*. Antidotes effects of Alcohol. Vertigo; deafness, with noises in head. *Takes away craving for alcoholics;* give dose as below for several months. Dropsy and liver affections. Useful in gout, old malarial cases with flatulence.

Relationship.—Compare: *Angelica* (in tincture, five drops, three times daily, produces disgust for liquor; also for atony of different organs, dyspepsia, nervous headache, etc.; chronic bronchitis to increase expectoration.) *Ceanoth.; Lach.; Nat. mur.; Helianthus* (spleen enlarged and painful.)

Dose.—Ten drops to a teaspoonful of the distilled spirit three to four times a day. A passing diarrhœa often appears for a time when using it. Curative effect. Quercus acts well in trituration of the acorn 3x in splenic cases, flatulence, old malaria and alcoholic history. (Clark.)

QUILLAYA SAPONARIA
(Chile Soap-bark)

Produces and cures symptoms of acute catarrh, sneezing and sore throat. *Most effective in the beginning of coryza,* frequently checking its further development. Colds with sore throat; heat and dryness of throat. Cough with difficult expectoration. Squamous skin.

Relationship.—Compare: *Kali hyd.; Gels.; Cepa.; Squilla. Saponaria* (sore throat, involuntary urination). Senega.

Dose.—Tincture and first potency.

RADIUM
(Radium Bromide)

An important addition to the Materia Medica, especially since the provings by Diffenbach have precisionized its use. Radium brom. of 1,800,000 radio-activity was employed. Found effective in the treatment of rheumatism and gout, in skin affections generally, acne rosacea, nævi, moles, ulcers and cancers. Lowered blood pressure. *Severe aching pains all over,* with restlessness, better moving about. Chronic rheumatic arthritis. Lateness in appearance of symptoms. Ulcers due to Radium burns, take a long time to heal. Marked increase in the polymorphonuclear neutrophiles. Great weakness.

Mind.—Apprehensive, depressed; fear of being alone in the dark; great desire to be with people. Tired and irritable.

Head.—Vertigo, with pain in back of head, left when in bed. Occipital and vertex pain, accompanying severe lumbar aching. Severe pain over right eye, spreading back to occiput and to vertex, better in open air. Head feels heavy. Frontal headache. Both eyes ache. Itching and dryness of nasal cavities, better in open air. Aching pain in angle of right lower jaw. Violent trifacial neuralgia.

Mouth.—Dryness of mouth. Metallic taste. Prickling sensation on end of tongue.

Stomach.—Empty feeling in stomach. Warm sensation in stomach. Aversion to sweets, ice-cream. Nausea and sinking sensation, belching of gas.

Abdomen.—Pain, violent cramps, rumbling, full of gas; pain over McBurney's point, and at location of sigmoid flexure. Much flatulence. Alternating constipation and loose movements. Pruritus ani and piles.

Urinary.—Increased elimination of solids, particularly of chlorides. Renal irritation, albuminuria, granular and hyaline casts. Nephritis with rheumatic symptoms. Enuresis.

Female.—Pruritus vulvæ. Delayed and irregular menstruation and backache. Aching pains in abdomen over pubes when flow comes on. Right breast sore, relieved by hard rubbing.

Respiratory.—Persistent cough with tickling in suprasternal fossa. Dry, spasmodic cough. Throat dry, sore, chest constricted.

Back.—Aching in back of neck. Pain and lameness in cervical vertebræ, worse dropping head forward, better standing, or sitting erect. *Lumbar and sacral* backache, pain appears to be in *bone*, continued motion relieves. Backache between shoulders and lumbar-sacral region, better after walking.

Extremities.—Severe pain in all the limbs, *joints*, especially in knee and ankles, sharp pains in shoulders, arms, hands and fingers. Legs, arms and neck feel hard and brittle, as though they would break on moving. Arms feel heavy. Cracking in shoulder. *Pain in toes*, calves, hip-joint, popliteal spaces. Muscles of legs and hips sore. *Arthritis*, aching pains, *worse* at night. Dermatitis of the fingers. Trophic changes in the finger nails.

Skin.—Small pimples. Erythema and dermatitis, with itching, burning, swelling and redness. Necrosis and ulceration. *Itching all over body*, burning of skin, as if afire. Epithelioma.

Sleep.—Restless. Sleepiness with lethargy. Dreams vivid, busy. Dreams of fire.

Fever.—Cold sensation internally, with chattering of teeth until noon. Internal chilliness followed by heat of the skin, associated with bowel movements and flatulence.

Modalities.—*Better*, open air, continued motion, hot bath, lying down, pressure. *Worse*, getting up.

Relationship.—Compare: *Anacardium* (the ulceration produced by it is like *Radium*. It may appear elsewhere than on place of contact and appear late). Compare: *X-Ray; Rhus; Sepia; Uranium; Ars.; Pulsat.; Caustic.*

Antidotes: *Rhus ven.; Tellur.*

Dose.—Thirtieth and twelfth trituration.

RANUNCULUS BULBOSUS
(Buttercup)

Acts especially upon the muscular tissue and skin, and its most characteristic effects are upon the chest walls, like pleurodynia. *Bad effects of Alcohol; delirium tremens.* Spasmodic hiccough. Hydrothorax. Shocks throughout the whole body. Sensitive to air and touch. Chronic sciatica.

Head.—Irritable, pains in forehead and eyeballs. Creeping sensation in scalp. Pressing pain in forehead from within outward.

Eyes.—Day-blindness; mist before eyes; pressure and smarting in eyes, as from smoke. Pain over right eye; better, standing and walking. Herpes on cornea. Vesicles on cornea, with intense pain, photophobia, and lachrymation.

Chest.—Various kinds of pains and *soreness, as if bruised in sternum*, ribs, intercostal spaces, and both hypochondria. *Intercostal rheumatism. Chilliness in chest when walking in open air.* Stitches in chest, between shoulder-blades; worse, inspiring, moving. Rheumatic pain in chest, as from subcutaneous ulceration. *Tenderness of abdomen to pressure. Muscular pain along lower margin of the shoulder-blade;* burning in small spots from sedentary employment.

Skin.—*Burning and intense itching; worse, contact.* Hard excrescences. *Herpetic eruptions*, with great itching. *Shingles; bluish vesicles.* Itching in palms. Blister-like eruption in palms. Corns sensitive. Horny skin. Finger-tips and palms chapped. Vesicular and pustular eruptions.

Modalities.—*Worse*, open air, motion, contact, atmospheric changes, wet, stormy weather, evening. Cold air brings on all sorts of ailments.

Relationship.—Incompatible: *Sulph.; Staph.*

Compare: *Ranunc. acris* (pain in lumbar muscles and joints

by bending and turning body); *Ranunc. glacialis*—Reindeer flower Carlina—(Pulmonary affections; broncho-pneumonical Influenza—enormous weight in head with vertigo and sensation as of impending apoplexy; night-sweats—more on thighs); *Ranunc. repens* (crawling sensation in forehead and scalp in evening in bed); *Ranunc. flammula* (ulceration; gangrene of arm). Compare, also: *Bry.; Croton; Mez.; Euphorb.*

Antidotes: *Bry.; Camph.; Rhus.*

Dose.—Mother tincture, in ten to thirty drop doses in delirium tremens; third to thirtieth potency generally. Chronic sciatica, apply tincture to heel of affected leg (M. Jousset).

RANUNCULUS SCELERATUS
(Marsh Buttercup)

Is more irritating than others of this botanical family, as seen in the skin symptoms. *Boring, gnawing pain very marked. Pemphigus.* Periodical complaints. Fainting with pain in stomach.

Head.—Gnawing in one spot left of vertex. Frightful dreams about corpses, serpents, battles, etc. Fluent coryza, with sneezing and burning micturition.

Mouth.—Teeth and gums sensitive. *Tongue mapped.* Denuded patches. Mouth sore and raw. *Burning and rawness of tongue.*

Abdomen.—Sensation of a plug behind umbilicus. *Pain over region of liver, with sensation as if diarrhœa would set it.* Pressure as of a plug behind right false ribs; worse, deep inspiration.

Chest.—Integument sensitive. Bruised pain and weakness in the chest every evening. *Sore burning behind xiphoid cartilage.*

Skin.—*Vesicular eruption, with tendency to form large blisters. Acrid exudation, which makes surrounding parts sore.*

Extremities.—*Boring pain.* Sudden burning sticking *in right toe.* Corns, with burning and soreness, especially when feet hang down. Gout in fingers and toes.

Dose.—First to third potency.

RAPHANUS
(Black Garden Radish)

Produces pain and stitches in liver and spleen. Increases of bile and salivary secretion. Symptoms will not appear if salt is used with the Radish. Great accumulation and incarceration of flatulence. "Globus" symptoms. Seborrhœa, with greasy skin. Pemphigus. Hysteria; chilliness in back and arms. Sexual insomnia. [*Kali brom.*] Nymphomania. *Post-operative gas pains.*

Head.—Sadness, aversion to children, especially girls. Headache, brain feels tender and sore. Œdema of lower eyelids. Mucus in posterior nares.

Throat.—Hot-ball feeling from uterus to throat, stopping there. Heat and burning in throat.

Stomach.—Putrid eructations. Burning in epigastrium, followed by hot eructation.

Abdomen.—Retching and vomiting, loss of appetite. Distended, *tympanitic, hard. No flatus emitted upward or downward.* Griping about navel. Stool liquid, frothy, profuse, brown, with colic, and pad-like swelling of intestines. Vomiting of faecal matter.

Female.—Nervous irritation of genitals. Menses very profuse and long-lasting. *Nymphomania*, with aversion to her own sex and to children, and sexual insomnia.

Urine.—Turbid, with yeast-like sediment. Urine more copious, thick like milk.

Chest.—Pain in chest extends to back and to throat. Heavy lump and coldness in center of chest.

Relationship.—Compare: *Momordica* (worse, near splenic flexure); *Carbo; Anarc.; Arg. nit.; Brassica.*

Dose.—Third to thirtieth potency.

RATANHIA
(Krameria—Mapato)

The rectal symptoms are most important, and have received much clinical confirmation. It has cured pterygium. *Violent hiccough.* Cracked nipples. [*Graph.; Eup. ar.*] *Pin worms.*

Head.—Bursting in head after stool, and when sitting with head bent forward. Sensation as if scalp from nose to vertex were stretched.

Stomach.—Pain like knives cutting the stomach.

Rectum.—Aches, as if full of broken glass. Anus aches and burns for hours after stool. Feels constricted. Dry heat at anus, with sudden knife-like stitches. Stools must be forced with great effort; protrusion of hæmorrhoids. *Fissures of anus, with great constriction, burning like fire*, as do the hæmorrhoids; temporarily relieved by cold water. Fetid, thin diarrhœa; stools burn; burning pains before and after stools. Oozing at anus. *Pin-worms.* [*Sant.; Teuc.; Spig.*] Itching of anus.

Relationship.—Compare: *Pæon.; Croton* (rectal neuralgia); *Sanguin. nit.* (diseases of rectum); *Macuna prurens—Dolichos—piles, with* burning; hæmorrhoidal diathesis); *Silico-sulpho-calcite of Aluminà; Slag*—blast iron furnace cinder—(anal itching, piles, and constipation; housemaid's knee); abdominal flatulent distension and lumbago. Analogue to Lycopod.

Dose.—Third to sixth potency. Locally, the Cerate has proved invaluable in many rectal complaints.

RHAMNUS CALIFORNICA
(California Coffee-tree)

One of the most positive remedies for rheumatism and *muscular pains*. Pleurodynia, lumbago, gastralgia. Vesical tenesmus; *dysmenorrhœa* of myalgic origin; pain in head, neck, and face. *Inflammatory rheumatism*, joints swollen, painful; tendency to metastasis; profuse sweat. Rheumatic heart (Webster).

Provings of students. 2x potency.

Mind.—Nervous, restless, irritable. Lassitude; mentally dull and dazed; unable to concentrate mind on studies.

Head.—*Dizzy* full feeling. Heavy bruised sensation; better, from pressure. *Bursting* feeling with every step. Soreness, especially in occiput and vertex, worse, bending over. Dull pain in left temple. Dull aching in frontal region (left), extending backwards and over forehead. Deep, right-sided frontal headache. Twitching eyelids.

Ears.—*Dullness of hearing.* Soreness, deep under right tragus on swallowing.

Face.—Flushed, hot and glowing. Outward pressure from malar processes.

Mouth.—Canker sore between gums and lips. Tongue coated, with clean, pink central patch.

Throat.—Dry, rough. Soreness on right side and tonsil.

Bowels.—*Constipation* with some flatus. Tenesmus and dry stool. Flatulent diarrhœa.

Genito-urinary.—Increased urination. Tickling in anterior urethra, small morning drop (no previous gonorrhœa). Sexual desire increased.

Respiratory.—Substernal oppression. Tenderness on pressure of right intercostal muscles.

Heart.—Variation of pulse. Slow pulse.

Extremities.—Unable to control muscular action. Legs sore. Walked like a drunken man.

Modality.—Symptoms worse in evening.

Relationship.—*Rhamnus cathartica* or *Rhamnus Frangula*—European Buckthorn—a rheumatic remedy—(abdominal symptoms, colic, diarrhœa; hæmorrhoids, especially chronic). *Rhamnus Purshiana—Cascara Sagrada*—(palliative in constipation, as an intestinal tonic, and dyspepsia dependent thereon. 10-15 drops of tincture).

Dose.—Tincture in 15-drop doses every four hours.

RHEUM
(Rhubarb)

Of frequent use in children with sour diarrhœa; difficult dentition. *Whole child smells sour.*

Mind.—Impatient and vehement; desires many things and cries. [*Cina.*]

Head.—Sweat on hairy scalp; constant and profuse. *Cool sweat on the face, especially about mouth and nose.*

Mouth.—Much saliva. Sensation of coolness in teeth. Difficult teething; restless and irritable. Breath smells sour. [*Cham.*]

Stomach.—Desire for various kinds of food, but soon tires of all. Throbbing in pit. Feels full.

Abdomen.—Colicky pain about navel. Colic when uncovering. Wind seems to rise up to chest.

Rectum.—Before stool, unsuccessful urging to urinate. *Stools smell sour*, pasty, with shivering and tenesmus, and burning in anus. Sour diarrhœa during dentition. Colicky, even ineffectual urging to evacuate altered fæcal stools.

Modalities.—*Worse*, uncovering, after eating, moving about.

Relationship.—Compare: *Mag. phos.; Hep.; Pod.; Cham.; Ipec.*

Antidotes: *Camph.; Cham.*

Complementary: *Mag. carb.*

Dose.—Third to sixth potency.

RHODIUM
(Metal Chemical Element)

(Proved by MacFarlan with the 200th potency.)

Nervous and tearful. Frontal headache; shocks through head. Fleeting neuralgic pains in head, over eyes, in ear, both sides of nose, teeth. Loose cold in head. Lips dry. Nausea especially from sweets. Dull headache. Stiff neck and rheumatic pain down left shoulder and arm. Itching in arms, palms and face. Loose stools with gripings in abdomen. Hyper-active peristalsis, tenesmus after stool. More urine passed. Cough scratchy, wheezy. Thick, yellow mucus from chest. Feels weak, dizzy and a tired feeling.

RHODODENDRON
(Snow-rose)

Rheumatic and gouty symptoms well marked. Rheumatism in the hot season. The modality (worse before a storm) is a true guiding symptom.

Mind.—Dread of a storm; particularly afraid of thunder. Forgetful.

Head.—Aching in temples. Tearing pain in bones. Headache; worse, wine, wind, cold and wet weather. Pain in eyes before a storm. *Ciliary neuralgia*, involving eyeball, orbit, and head. Heat in eyes when using them.

Eyes.—Muscular asthenopia; darting pains through eyes from head, worse before a storm.

Ears.—Difficult hearing, with whizzing and ringing in ears. Hearing better in the morning; noises come on after patient has been up a few hours.

Face.—Prosopalgia; violent jerking pain involving dental nerves, from temple to lower jaw and chin; *better, warmth and eating*. Toothache in damp weather and before a storm. Swollen gums. Stumps of teeth are loosened.

Chest.—Violent pleuritic pains running downward in left anterior chest. Breathless and speechless from violent pleuritic pains running down the anterior chest. Stitches in spleen from fast walking. Crampy pain under short ribs.

Male.—Testicles, worse left, swollen, painful, drawn up. Orchitis; glands feel crushed. Induration and swelling of testes after gonorrhœa. *Hydrocele*. [*Sil.*]

Extremities.—Joints swollen. Gouty inflammation of great toe-joint. *Rheumatic tearing in all limbs*, especially right side; worse, at rest and in stormy weather. Stiffness of neck. Pain in shoulders, arms, wrists; worse when at rest. Pains in bones in spots, and reappear by change of weather. *Cannot sleep unless legs are crossed.*

Modalities.—*Worse*, before a storm. *All symptoms reappear in rough weather*, night, towards morning. *Better*, after the storm breaks, warmth, and eating.

Relationship.—Compare: *Ampelopsis* (hydrocele and renal dropsy); *Dulc.; Rhus; Nat. sulph.*

Dose.—First to sixth potency.

RHUS AROMATICA
(Fragrant Sumach)

Renal and urinary affections, especially *diabetes*. Enuresis due to vesical atony; senile incontinence. Hæmaturia and cystitis come within the range of this remedy.

Urine.—*Pale*, albuminous. *Incontinence. Severe pain at beginning or before urination*, causing great agony in children. Constant dribbling. *Diabetes*, large quantities of urine of low specific gravity. [*Phos. ac.; Acet. ac.*]

Dose.—Tincture, in rather material doses.

RHUS GLABRA
(Smooth Sumach)

Epistaxis and *occipital headache*. *Fetid flatus*. Ulceration of mouth. *Dreams of flying through the air*. [*Sticta.*] *Profuse perspiration arising from debility*. [*China.*] It is claimed that this remedy will so disinfect the bowels that the flatus and stools will be free from odor. It acts well in putrescent conditions with tendency to ulceration.

Mouth.—Scurvy; nursing sore mouth. [*Veronica.*] Aphthous stomatitis.

Relationship.—Said to be antidotal to the action of Mercury, and has been employed in the treatment of secondary syphilis after mercurialization.

Dose.—Tincture. Usually locally to soft, spongy gums, aphthæ, pharyngitis, etc. Internally, first potency.

RHUS TOXICODENDRON
(Poison-ivy)

The effects on the skin, rheumatic pains, mucous membrane affections, and a typhoid type of fever, make this remedy frequently indicated. Rhus affects fibrous tissue markedly—joints, tendons, sheaths—aponeurosis, etc., producing pains and stiffness. Post-operative complications. *Tearing asunder pains*. Motion always "limbers up" the Rhus patient, and hence he feels better for a time from a change of position. Ailments from strains, overlifting, getting wet while perspiring. Septic conditions. Cellulitis and infections, carbuncles in early stages. [*Echinac.*] Rheumatism in the cold season. *Septicæmia*.

Mind.—Listless, sad. Thoughts of suicide. *Extreme restlessness, with continued change of position*. Delirium, with fear of being poisoned. [*Hyos.*] *Sensorium becomes cloudy. Great apprehension at night, cannot remain in bed.*

Head.—Feels as if a board were strapped on the forehead. Vertigo when rising. *Heavy* head. Brain feels loose and as if struck against skull on walking or rising. Scalp sensitive; worse on side lain on. Headache in occiput [*Rhus rad.*]; painful to touch. Pain in forehead and proceeds thence backward. Humid eruptions on scalp; itching greatly.

Eyes.—Swollen, red, œdematous; *orbital cellulitis. Pustular inflammations.* Photophobia; profuse flow of yellow pus. Œdema of lids, suppurative iritis. Lids inflamed, agglutinated, swollen. Old injured eyes. Circumscribed corneal injection. Intensive ulceration of the cornea. Iritis, after exposure to cold and dampness, and of rheumatic origin. Eye painful on turning it or pressing, can hardly move it, as in acute retrobulbar neuritis. Profuse gush of hot, scalding tears upon opening lids.

Ears.—Pain in ears, with sensation as if something were in them. Lobules swollen. Discharge of bloody pus.

Nose.—Sneezing; coryza from getting wet. Tip of nose red, sore, ulcerated. Swelling of nose. Nosebleed on stooping.

Face.—*Jaws crack when chewing.* Easy dislocation of jaw. [*Ign.; Petrol.*] *Swollen face,* erysipelas. Cheek bones sensitive to touch. Parotitis. Facial neuralgia, with chilliness; worse, evening. *Crusta lactea.* [*Calc.; Viol. tric.*]

Mouth.—Teeth feel loose and long; gums sore. Tongue red and cracked; *coated, except red triangular space at the tip;* dry and red at edges. Corners of mouth ulcerated; fever-blisters around mouth and chin. [*Nat. mur.*] *Pain in maxillary joint.*

Throat.—Sore, with *swollen glands.* Sticking pain on swallowing. Parotitis, left side.

Stomach.—Want of appetite for any kind of food, with unquenchable thirst. *Bitter taste.* [*Cupr.*] Nausea, vertigo, and bloated abdomen after eating. *Desire for milk.* Great thirst with dry mouth and throat. Pressure as from a stone. [*Bry., Ars.*] *Drowsy after eating.*

Abdomen.—Violent pains, relieved by lying on abdomen. Swelling of inguinal glands. Pain in region of ascending colon. Colic, compelling to walk bent. Excessive distention after eating. Rumbling of flatus on first rising, but disappears with continued motion.

Rectum.—Diarrhœa of blood, slime, and reddish mucus. Dysentery, with tearing pains down thighs. Stools of cadaverous odor. Frothy, painless stools. Will often abort a beginning suppurative process near the rectum. Dysentery.

Urinary.—Dark, turbid, high-colored, scanty urine, with white sediment. Dysuria, with loss of blood.

Male.—Swelling of glands and prepuce—dark-red erysipelatous; scrotum thick, swollen, œdematous. *Itching intense.*

Female.—Swelling, with intense itching of vulva. Pelvic articulations stiff when beginning to move. Menses early, profuse, and prolonged, acrid. *Lochia thin, protracted, offensive diminished [Puls.; Secale], with shooting upwards in vagina.* [Sep.]

Respiratory.—Tickling behind upper sternum. *Dry, teasing cough from midnight until morning, during a chill, or when putting hands out of bed.* Hæmoptysis from overexertion; blood bright red. Influenza, with aching in all bones. [*Eup. perf.*] Hoarseness from overstraining voice. [*Arn.*] Oppression of the chest, cannot get breath with sticking pains. Bronchial coughs in old people, worse on awaking and with expectoration of small plugs of mucus.

Heart.—Hypertrophy from overexertion. Pulse quick, weak, irregular, intermittent, with numbness of left arm. *Trembling and palpitation when sitting still.*

Back.—Pain between shoulders on swallowing. *Pain and stiffness in small of back; better, motion, or lying on something hard;* worse, while sitting. Stiffness of the nape of the neck.

Extremities.—Hot, painful swelling of joints. *Pains tearing in tendons, ligaments, and fasciæ.* Rheumatic pains spread over a large surface at nape of neck, loins, and extremities; better motion. [*Agaric.*] Soreness of condyles of bones. *Limbs stiff, paralyzed. The cold fresh air is not tolerated; it makes the skin painful.* Pain along ulnar nerve. Tearing down thighs. *Sciatica;* worse, cold, damp weather, at night. Numbness and formication, after overwork and exposure. Paralysis; trembling after exertion. Tenderness about knee-joint. Loss of power in forearm and fingers; crawling sensation in the tips of fingers. Tingling in feet.

Fever.—Adynamic; restless, trembling. Typhoid; tongue dry and brown; sordes; bowels loose; great restlessness. Intermittent; chill, with dry cough and restlessness. During heat, uticaria. Hydroa. Chilly, as if cold water were poured over him, followed by heat and inclination to stretch the limbs.

Skin.—Red, swollen; *itching intense.* Vesicles, herpes; *urticaria;* pemphigus; erysipelas; vesicular suppurative forms. Glands swollen. *Cellulitis.* Burning eczematous eruptions with tendency to scale formation.

Sleep.—*Dreams of great exertion.* Heavy sleep, as from stupor. Sleepless before midnight.

Modalities.—*Worse,* during sleep, cold, wet rainy weather and after rain; at night, *during rest,* drenching, when lying on back or right side. *Better,* warm, dry weather, motion; walking, change of position, rubbing, warm applications, from stretching out limbs.

Relationship.—Complementary: *Bry.; Calc. fluor. Phytol.* (Rheumatism). In urticaria follow with *Bovista.*

Inimical: *Apis.*

Antidotes: Bathing with milk and Grindelia lotion very effective. *Ampelopsis Trifolia*—Three-leaf Woodbine—(Toxic dermatitis due to vegetable poisons—30 and 200. Very similar to Rhus poisoning. Desensitizing against Ivy poisoning by the use of ascending doses of the tincture by mouth or by hypodermic injections is recommended by old school authorities, but is not as effective as the homœopathic remedies especially *Rhus* 30 and 200 and *Anacard.,* etc. *Anacard.; Croton.; Grindelia; Mezer.; Cyprip.; Plumbago* (eczema of vulva); *Graph.*

Compare: *Rhus radicans* (almost identical action); characteristics are, burning in tongue, tip feels sore, pains are often semilateral and in various parts, often remote and successive. Many symptoms are better after a storm has thoroughly set in, especially after an electric storm. Has pronounced *yearly* aggravation. [*Laches.*] *Rhus radicans* has headache in *occiput* even pain in nape of neck and from there pains draw over the head *forwards.*) *Rhus diversiloba*—California Poison-oak— (antidote to Rhus; violent skin symptoms, with frightful itching; much swelling of face, hands and genitals; skin very sensitive; eczema and erysipelas, great nervous weakness, tired from least effort; goes to sleep from sheer exhaustion); *Xerophyllum* (dysmenorrhœa and skin symptoms). Compare, also: *Arn.; Bapt.; Lach.; Ars.; Hyosc.; Op.* (stupefaction more profound). *Mimosa*—Sensitive Plant—(rheumatism, knee stiff, lancinating pains in back and limbs. Swelling of ankles Legs tremble).

Dose.—Sixth to thirtieth potency. The 200th and higher are antidotal to poisoning with the plant and tincture.

RHUS VENENATA
(Poison-elder)

The skin symptoms of this species of Rhus are most severe.

Mind.—Great melancholy; no desire to live, gloomy.

Head.—Heavy, frontal headache; worse, walking or stooping. Eyes nearly closed with great swelling. Vesicular inflammation of ears. Nose red and shiny. Face swollen.

Tongue.—Red at tip. Fissured in middle. Vesicles on under side.

Abdomen.—Profuse, watery, white stools in morning, 4 a. m., with colicky pains; expelled with force. Pain in hypogastrium before every stool.

Extremities.—Paralytic drawing in right arm, especially wrist, and extending to fingers.

Skin.—Itching; relieved by hot water. *Vesicles. Erysipelas; skin dark red.* Erythema nodosum, with nightly itching and pains in long bones.

Relationship.—Antidote: *Clematis*. The California Poison-oak (Rhus diversiloba) is identical with it. It antidotes *Radium* and follows it well. Compare: *Anacard*.

Dose.—Sixth to thirtieth potency.

RICINUS COMMUNIS—BOFAREIRA
(Castor-oil)

Has marked action on gastro-intestinal tract. *Increases the quantity of milk* in nursing women. Vomiting and purging. Languor and weakness.

Head.—Vertigo, occipital pain, congestive symptoms, buzzing in ears. Face pale, twitching of mouth.

Stomach.—Anorexia with great thirst, burning in stomach, pyrosis, nausea, *profuse vomiting*, pit of stomach sensitive. Mouth dry.

Abdomen.—Rumbling with contraction of recti muscles, colic, incessant diarrhœa with purging. Rice water stools with cramps and chilliness.

Stool.—Loose, incessant, painless, with painful cramps in muscles of extremities. Anus inflamed. Stools green, slimy, and bloody. Fever, emaciation, somnolence.

Relationship.—Compare: *Resorcin* (summer complaint with vomiting); destroys organic germs of putrifaction; *Cholos terrapina* (cramps of muscles). *Ars.; Verat.*

Dose.—Third potency. Five drops every four hours for increasing flow of milk; also locally a poultice of the leaves.

ROBINIA
(Yellow Locust)

The remedy for hperchlorhydria. In cases where albuminoid digestion is too rapid and starch digestion is perverted. The gastric symptoms with the most *pronounced acidity* are well authenticated, and are the guiding symptoms. The acidity of Robinia is accompanied by frontal headache. *Intensely acrid eructations.* Acrid and greenish vomiting, colic and flatulence, nightly burning pains in stomach and constipation with urgent desire.—*Acidity of children.* Stools and perspiration sour. Incarcerated flatus.

Head.—Dull, throbbing, frontal pain; worse, motion and reading. Gastric headache with acid vomiting.

Stomach.—Dull, heavy aching. Nausea; *sour* eructations; profuse vomiting of an *intensely sour* fluid. [*Sulph. ac.*] Great distention of stomach and bowels. Flatulent colic. [*Cham.; Diosc.*] Sour stools; child smells sour.

Female.—Nymphomania. Acrid, fetid leucorrhœa. Discharge of blood between menstrual periods. Herpes on vagina and vulva.

Relationship.—*Magnes. phos.; Arg. nit.; Orexine tannate.* (Hyperchlorhydria; deficient acid and slow digestion; 14 hourly doses).

Dose.—Third potency. Must be continued a long time.

ROSA DAMASCENA
(Damask Rose)

Useful in the beginning of hay-fever, with involvement of Eustachian tube.

Ear.—Hardness of hearing; tinnitus. *Eustachian catarrh.* [*Hydr.; Merc. dulc.*]

Relationship.—Compare: in hay-fever: *Phleum pratense*—Timothy grass—(Hay-fever with asthma; watery coryza, itching of nose and eyes; frequent sneezing, dyspnœa. Use 6-30 potency. Rabe.) *Succin. acid; Sabad.; Euph.; Psor.; Kali hyd.; Naphth.*

Dose.—Lower potencies.

RUMEX CRISPUS
(Yellow Dock)

Is characterized by pains, numerous and varied, neither fixed nor constant anywhere. Cough caused by an incessant tickling in the throat-pit, which tickling runs down to the bifurcation of the bronchial tubes. Touching the throat-pit brings on the cough. Worse from the least cold air; so that all cough ceases by covering up all the body and head with the bedclothes. Rumex diminishes the secretions of mucous membranes, and at the same time exalts sensibility of the mucous membranes of the larynx and trachea. Its action upon the skin is marked, producing an intense itching. *Lymphatics enlarged* and secretions perverted.

Stomach.—Tongue sore at edges; coated; sensation of hard substance in pit of stomach; hiccough, pyrosis, nausea; *cannot eat meat; it causes eructations, pruritus.* Jaundice after excessive use of alcoholics. Chronic gastritis; aching pain in pit of stomach and shooting in the chest; extends towards the throat-pit, worse any motion or talking. Pain in left breast after meals; *flatulence.*

Respiratory.—Nose dry. *Tickling in throat-pit causes cough. Copious mucous discharge* from nose and trachea. *Dry, teasing cough, preventing sleep. Aggravated by pressure, talking, and especially by inspiring cool air and at night.* Thin, watery, frothy expectoration by the mouthful; later, stringy and tough. Rawness of larynx and trachea. Soreness behind sternum, especially left side, in region of left shoulder. *Raw pain under clavicle.* Lump in throat.

Stool.—Brown, watery, diarrhœa *early in morning,* with cough, driving him out of bed. Valuable in advanced phthisis. [*Seneg.; Puls.; Lycop.; Ars.*] Itching of anus, with sensation as of a stick in rectum. Piles.

Skin.—Intense itching of skin, especially of *lower extremities; worse, exposure to cold air when undressing.* Urticaria; contagious prurigo.

Modalities.—Worse, in evening, from inhaling cold air; left chest; uncovering.

Relationship.—Compare: *Caust.; Sulph.; Bell.;* Rumex contains chrysophanic acid to which the skin symptoms correspond. *Rumex acetosa*—Sheep sorrel—(Gathered in June and dried, used locally for Epithelioma of face. (Cowperthwaite.) Dry, unremitting short cough, and violent pains in the bowels; uvula elongated; inflammation of œsophagus; also cancer); *Rumex obtusifolius—Lapathum—*Broad-leaf dock—(nosebleed and headache following; pain in kidneys; leucorrhœa).

Dose.—Third to sixth potency.

RUTA GRAVEOLENS
(Rue-bitterwort)

Acts upon the periosteum and cartilages, eyes and uterus. Complaints from straining *flexor tendons* especially. Tendency to the formation of deposits in the periosteum, tendons, and about joints, especially wrist. Overstrain of ocular muscles. All parts of the body are painful, *as if bruised.* Sprains (after *Arnica*). Lameness after sprains. Jaundice. *Feeling of intense lassitude, weakness and despair.* Injured "bruised" bones.

Head.—Pain as from a nail; after excessive intoxicating drinks. Periosteum sore. Epistaxis.

Eyes.—*Eye-strain followed by headache. Eyes red, hot, and painful from sewing or reading fine print.* [*Nat. mur.; Arg. nit.*] *Disturbances of accommodation.* Weary pain while reading. Pressure deep in orbits. Tarsal cartilage feels bruised. Pressure over eyebrow. Asthenopia.

Stomach.—Gastralgia of aching, gnawing character.

Urinary.—Pressure in neck of bladder after urinating; painful closure. [*Apis.*] Constant urging to urinate, feels bladder full.

Rectum.—*Difficult fæces*, evacuated only with straining. Constipation, alternating with mucous, frothy stools; discharge of blood with stool. When sitting, tearing stitches in rectum. *Carcinoma affecting lower bowel. Prolapsus ani* every time the bowels move, after confinement. Frequent, unsuccessful urging to stool. Protrusion of rectum when stooping.

Respiratory.—Cough with copious, thick, yellow expectoration; chest feels weak. Painful spot on sternum; short breath with tightness of chest.

Back.—Pain in nape, back and loins. Backache better pressure and lying on back. Lumbago worse morning before rising.

Extremities.—Spine and limbs feel bruised. Small of back and loins pain. Legs give out on rising from a chair, hips and thighs so weak. [*Phos.; Con.*] Contraction of fingers. Pain and stiffness in wrists and hands. Ganglia. [*Benzoic ac.*] Sciatica; worse, lying down at night; pain from back down hips and thighs. Hamstrings feel shortened. [*Graph.*] *Tendons sore.* Aching pain in tendo-Achilles. *Thighs pain when stretching the limbs.* Pain in bones of feet and ankles. Great restlessness.

Modalities.—*Worse*, lying down, from cold, wet weather.

Relationship.—Compare: *Ratanhia; Carduus.* Rectal (irritation); *Jaborandi; Phyt.; Rhus; Sil.; Arn.*

Antidote: *Camph.*

Complementary: *Calc. phos.*

Dose.—First to sixth potency. Locally, the tincture for ganglia and as a lotion for the eyes.

SABADILLA

(Cevadilla Seed. Asagræa Officialis)

Action on mucous membrane of the nose and the lachrymal glands, producing coryza and symptoms like *hay-fever*, which have been utilized homœopathically. *Chilliness;* sensitive to cold. Ascarides, with reflex symptoms (nymphomania; convulsive symptoms). Children's diarrhœa with constant cutting pains.

Mind.—Nervous, timid, easily startled. Has erroneous notions about himself. Imagines that he is very sick; that parts are shrunken; that she is pregnant; that she has cancer; delirium during intermittents.

Head.—Vertigo with sensation as though all things were turning around each other, accompanied by blackness before eyes and sensation of fainting. Dullness and oppression. Oversensitiveness to odors. *Thinking produces headache and sleeplessness.* *Eyelids red, burning.* *Lachrymation.* Difficult hearing.

Nose.—*Spasmodic sneezing, with running nose.* Coryza, with severe frontal pains and redness of eyes and lachrymation. Copious, watery, nasal discharge.

Throat.—Sore; *begins on left side.* [*Lach.*] Much tough phlegm. Sensation of a skin hanging loosely; must swallow it. *Warm food and drink relieve.* Empty swallowing most painful. Dry fauces and throat. Sensation of a lump in throat with *constant* necessity to swallow. Chronic sore throat; worse, from cold air. Tongue as if burnt.

Stomach.—Spasmodic pain in stomach with dry cough and difficult breathing. *No thirst.* Loathing for strong food. Canine appetite for sweets and farinaceous food. Pyrosis; copious salivation. Cold, empty feeling in stomach. *Desire for hot things.* Sweetish taste.

Female.—Menses too late; come by fits and starts. *Intermit* [*Kreos.*; *Puls.*] (due to transient and localized congestion of womb alternating with chronic anæmic state).

Fever.—*Chill predominates;* from below upwards. Heat in head and face; hands and feet icy cold, with chill. Lachrymation during paroxysm. Thirstless.

Extremities.—Cracking of skin under and beneath toes; inflammation under toe-nails.

Skin.—Dry, like parchment. Horny, deformed, *thickened nails.* Hot, burning, creeping, crawling sensation. Itching in anus.

Modalities.—*Worse,* cold and cold drinks, full moon. *Better,* warm food and drink, wrapped up.

Relationship.—Complementary: *Sepia.* Compare: *Vera-*

trina (is alkaloid of Sabadilla, *not* of Veratrum, locally in neuralgias, and for removal of dropsy. Five grains to two drams Lanolin, rubbed on inside of thighs, causes diuresis). *Colch.; Nux; Arundo* and *Pollatin. Phleum pratense*—Timothy—Hay-fever—Potentized—12—specific to many cases and evidently acts in a desensitizing manner. (Rabe.) *Cumarinum* (hay-fever).

Antidotes: *Puls.; Lycop.; Conium; Lach.*

Dose.—Third to thirtieth potency.

SABAL SERRULATA
(Saw Palmetto)

Sabal is homœopathic to irritability of the genito-urinary organs.

General and sexual debility. Promotes nutrition and tissue building. Head, stomach, and ovarian symptoms marked. Of unquestioned value in prostatic enlargement, *epididymitis*, and urinary difficulties. Acts on membrano-prostatic portion of urethra. Iritis, with prostatic trouble. *Valuable for undeveloped mammary glands. Fear of going to sleep.* Languor, apathy and indifference.

Head.—Confused, full; dislikes sympathy; makes her angry. Vertigo, with headache. Neuralgia in feeble patients. Pain runs up from nose and centers in forehead.

Stomach.—Belching and acidity. Desire for milk. [*Rhus; Apis.*]

Urinary.—Constant desire to pass water at night. *Enuresis;* paresis of sphincter vesicæ. Chronic gonorrhœa. Difficult urination. Cystitis with prostatic hypertrophy.

Male.—*Prostatic troubles;* enlargement; discharge of prostatic fluid. Wasting of testes and *loss of sexual power.* Coitus painful at the time of emission. *Sexual neurotics.* Organs feel cold.

Female.—Ovaries tender and enlarged; *breasts shrivel.* [*Iod.; Kali iod.*] Young female neurotics; suppressed or perverted sexual inclination.

Respiratory.—Copious expectoration, with catarrh of nose. Chronic bronchitis. [*Stann.; Hep.*]

Relationship.—Compare: *Phosph. ac.; Stigmata maydis; Santal.; Apis.* In prostatic symptoms: *Ferr. pic.; Thuja; Picric acid* (more sexual erethism). *Populus tremul.;* (prostatic enlargement with cystitis).

Dose.—Mother tincture, ten to thirty drops. Third potency often better. The tincture must be prepared from the *fresh berries* to be effective.

SABINA
(Savine)

Has a special action on the uterus; also upon serous and fibrous membranes; hence its use in gout. *Pain from sacrum to the pubis. Hæmorrhages, where blood is fluid and clots together.* Tendency to miscarriage, especially at third month. *Violent pulsations;* wants windows open.

Mind.—*Music is intolerable,* produces nervousness.

Head.—Vertigo with suppressed menses. Bursting headache, suddenly coming and going slowly. Rush of blood to head and face. Drawing pains in masseter muscles. Teeth ache when chewing.

Stomach.—Heartburn. Desire for lemonade. Bitter taste. [*Rhus.*] Lancinating pain from pit of stomach across back.

Abdomen.—Bearing-down, constrictive pain. Colic, mostly in hypogastric region. Tympanitic distention.

Rectum.—Sense of fullness. Constipation. *Pain from back to pubis.* Hæmorrhoids, with bright red blood; bleed copiously.

Urine.—Burning and throbbing in region of kidneys. Bloody urine; much urging. Bladder inflamed with throbbing all over. Inflammation of urethra.

Male.—Inflammatory gonorrhœa, with pus-like discharge. Sycotic excrescences. Burning, sore pain in glans. Prepuce painful with difficulty in retracting it. Increased desire.

Female.—*Menses profuse, bright.* Uterine pains extend into thighs. Threatened miscarriage. Sexual desire increased. Leucorrhœa after menses, corrosive, offensive. Discharge of blood between periods, with sexual excitement. [*Ambr.*] Retained placenta; intense after-pains. Menorrhagia in women who aborted readily. Inflammation of ovaries and uterus after abortion. Promotes expulsion of moles from uterus. [*Canth.*] *Pain from sacrum to pubis, and from below upwards shooting up the vagina.* Hæmorrhage; partly clotted; worse *from least motion.* Atony of uterus.

Back.—*Pain between sacrum and pubis from one bone to another.* Paralytic pain in small of back.

Extremities.—Bruised pains in anterior portion of thighs. Shooting in heels and metatarsal bones. *Arthritic pain in joints.* Gout; worse, in heated room. Red, shining swelling. Gouty nodosities. [*Ammon. phos.*]

Skin.—Fig-warts, with intolerable itching and burning. Exuberant granulations. [*Thuj.; Nit. ac.*] *Warts.* Black pores in skin.

Modalities.—*Worse*, from least motion, heat, warm air. *Better*, in cool fresh air.

Relationship.—Complementary: *Thuja.*

Compare: *Sanguisorba* (Venous congestion and passive hæmorrhages; varices of lower extremities; dysentery. *Long lasting, profuse menses* with congestion to head and limbs in sensitive, irritable patients. *Climacteric* hæmorrhages. Use 2x attenuation.) *Sanguisuga*—The leech—(Hæmorrhages, especially bleeding from anus. Use 6x). *Rosmarinus* (menses too early; violent pains followed by uterine hæmorrhage. Head heavy, *drowsy*. Chilly with icy coldness of lower extremities without thirst, followed by heat. Memory deficient). *Croc.; Calc.; Trill.; Ipec.; Millef.; Erig.*

Antidote: *Puls.*

Dose.—Locally, for warts, tincture. Internally, third to thirtieth potency.

SACCHARUM OFFICINALE—SUCROSE
(Cane-sugar)

According to the great Dr. Hering, a large proportion of chronic diseases of women and children are developed by using too much sugar.

Sugar is an antiseptic. Combats infection and putrefaction; has a solvent action on fibrin and stimulates secretion by the intense osmotic changes induced, thus rinsing out the wound with serum from within outward, favoring healing. Leg ulcers.

Sugar must be considered a sustainer and developer of the musculature of the heart and hence useful in failure of compensation and a variety of cardio-vascular troubles. Acts as a nutrient and tonic, in wasting disorders, anæmia, neurasthenia, etc., increasing weight and power.

Opacity of cornea. Dim sight. *Acidity and anal itching.* Cold expectoration. Myocardial degeneration.

Fat, bloated, large-limbed children, who are *cross, peevish,* whining; capricious; want dainty things, tidbits, and refuse substantial food. Œdema of feet. Headache every seven days

Relationship.—Compare: *Saccharum lactis*—Sugar of milk—lactose—(diuresis; amblyopia; *cold pains*, as if produced by fine, icy cold needle with tingling, as if frost bitten; great physical exhaustion. *Sugar of milk* in large doses to develop the Bacillus acidophilus to correct putrefactive intestinal conditions and also constipation.)

Dose.—Thirtieth potency and higher. Locally in gangrene. One ounce of lump sugar morning and evening valuable adjunct in the treatment of obstinate cases of heart failure due to deficient heart muscle without valvular lesion. Epilepsy; blood with reduced sugar content irritates the nervous system with tending to convulsions.

Sugar as an oxytocic has its most suitable application towards the end of labor when there is no mechanical obstruction and delay is due to uterine inertia. 25 grammes dissolved in water, several times every half hour.

Compare: *Saccharin* (hinders both the salivary and peptic ferment actions with consequent dyspepsia. Prof. Lewin believes its action to be on the secretory cells themselves and it has caused pain (right hypogastrium), loss of appetite, diarrhœa and wasting).

SALICYLICUM ACIDUM
(Salicylic Acid)

The symptoms point to its use in rheumatism, dyspepsia, and *Meniere's disease*. Prostration after influenza; also tinnitus aurium and deafness. Hæmaturia.

Head.—Vertigo; tendency to fall to left side. Headache; confusion in head on rising suddenly. Incipient coryza. Piercing pain in temples.

Eyes.—Retinal hæmorrhage. Retinitis after influenza, also albuminuric.

Ears.—*Roaring and ringing in ears.* Deafness, with vertigo.

Throat.—Sore, red and swollen. Pharyngitis; swallowing difficult.

Stomach.—*Canker sores,* with burning soreness and fetid breath. *Flatulence; hot, sour belching.* Putrid fermentation. *Fermentative dyspepsia.* Tongue purplish, leaden-colored; foul breath.

Stools.—Putrid diarrhœa; gastro-intestinal derangements, especially in children; stools like green frog's spawn. [*Magn. carb.*] Pruritus ani.

Extremities.—Knees swollen and painful. Acute articular rheumatism; worse, touch and motion, profuse sweat. Pain shifts. Sciatica, burning pain; worse at night. Copious foot-sweat and ill affects where suppressed.

Skin.—Itching vesicles and pustules; better by scratching. Sweat without sleep. Urticaria. Hot and burning skin. Purpura. Herpes zoster. Necrosis and softening of bones.

Relationship.—Compare: *Salol* (rheumatic pain in joints, with soreness and stiffness, headache over eyes; urine violet-smelling); *Colch.; China; Lact. ac.* Spiræa and Gaultheria contain salicyl. acid.

Dose.—Third decimal trituration. In acute articular rheumatism, 5 grains every 3 hours. (Old school dose.)

SALIX NIGRA
(Black-willow)

Has a positive action on the generative organs of both sexes Hysteria and nervousness. Libidinous thoughts and lascivious dreams. Controls genital irritability. Moderates sexual passion. Satyriasis and erotomania. In acute gonorrhœa, with much erotic trouble; chordee. After masturbation; spermatorrhœa.

Face.—Red, swollen, especially the end of nose—eyes bloodshot and sore to touch and on motion. Roots of hair hurt. Epistaxis.

Female.—Before and during menses much nervous disturbance, pain in ovaries; difficult menstruation. Ovarian congestion and neuralgia. Menorrhagia. Bleeding with uterine fibroid. Nymphomania.

Male.—Painful movement of the testicles.

Back.—Pain across sacral and lumbar region. Unable to step out quickly.

Relationship.—Compare: *Yohimbin.; Canth.*

Dose.—Material doses of the tincture, thirty drops.

SALVIA OFFICINALIS
(Sage)

Controls excessive sweating when circulation is enfeebled; of less use in phthisis *with night-sweats* and suffocating tickling cough. Galactorrhœa. Exerts a tonic influence on the skin.

Respiratory.—Tickling cough, especially in consumption.

Skin.—Soft, relaxed, with enfeebled circulation and cold extremities. *Colliquative perspiration.*

Relationship.—Compare: *Chrysanthemum Leucanthemum*—Ox-eye Daisy. Has specific action on sudoriparous glands. Quiets nervous system like *Cypripedium*. Right sided tearing pain in bones of jaw and temple. Pain in teeth and gums, worse touch, better warmth. Irritable and tearful. Here use 12x. *Insomnia and night-sweats.* For colliquative sweating and hyperæsthesia of nervous system. Material doses of tincture.) *Phelland.; Tuberc.; Salvia sclerata* (tonic influence on nervous system; dose, teaspoonful to one pint hot water, as inhalent for sponging). *Rubia tinctorum*—Madder—A remedy for the spleen. [*Ceanothus.*] Chlorosis and amenorrhœa; tuberculosis. Anæmia; undernourished conditions; splenic anæmia. Dose, 10 drops of tincture).

Dose.—Tincture, in twenty-drop doses, in a little water. The effects manifest themselves quickly two hours after taking a dose, and they persist for from two to six days.

SAMBUCUS NIGRA
(Elder)

Acts especially on the respiratory organs. Dry coryza of infants, snuffles, œdematous swellings. *Profuse sweat* accompanies many affections.

Mind.—Sees images when shutting eyes. *Constant fretfulness.* Very easily frightened. Fright followed by suffocative attacks.

Face.—Turns blue with cough. Red, burning spots on cheeks. Heat and perspiration of face.

Abdomen.—Colic, with nausea and flatulence; frequent watery, slimy stools.

Urine.—Profuse urine with dry heat of skin. Frequent micturition, with scanty urine. Acute nephritis; dropsical symptoms, with vomiting.

Respiratory.—Chest oppressed with pressure in stomach, and nausea. Hoarseness with tenacious mucus in larynx. Paroxysmal, *suffocative cough, coming on about midnight*, with crying and dyspnœa. Spasmodic croup. Dry coryza. *Sniffles of infants;* nose dry and obstructed. Loose choking cough. When nursing child must let go of nipple, nose blocked up, cannot breathe. *Child awakes suddenly, nearly suffocating, sits up, turns blue. Cannot expire.* [*Meph.*] Millar's asthma.

Extremities.—Hands turn blue. Œdematous swelling in legs, insteps, and feet. Feet icy cold. Debilitating night-sweats. [*Salvia; Acet. ac.*]

Fever.—Dry heat while sleeping. *Dreads uncovering. Profuse sweat over entire body during waking hours.* Dry, deep cough precedes the fever paroxysm.

Skin.—Dry heat of skin during sleep. Bloated and swollen; general dropsy; *profuse sweat on waking.*

Modalities.—*Worse*, sleep, during rest, after eating fruit. *Better*, sitting up in bed, motion.

Relationship.—Compare: *Ipec.; Meph.; Opium; Sambucus Canadensis* (great vlaue in dropsies; large doses required—fluid extract, ¼ to 1 teaspoonful three times daily).

Antidotes: *Ars.; Camph.*

Dose.—Tincture, to sixth potency.

SANGUINARIA
(Blood Root)

Is a right-sided remedy pre-eminently, and affects chiefly the mucous membranes, especially of the respiratory tract. It has marked vaso-motor disturbances, as seen in the circumscribed redness of the cheeks, flashes of heat, determination of blood to head and chest, distention of temporal veins, burning in palms and soles, and has been found very applicable to climacteric disorders. *Burning* sensations, like from hot water. Influenzal coughs. Phthisis. *Sudden stopping of catarrh of respiratory tract followed by diarrhœa. Burning* in various parts is characteristic.

Head.—Worse *right* side, sun headache. Periodical sick headache; pain begins in occiput, spreads upwards, and *settles over eyes, especially right. Veins and temples are distended*. Pain better lying down and sleep. Headaches return at climacteric; every seventh day. [*Sulph.; Sabad.*] Pain in small spot over upper left parietal bone. Burning in eyes. Pain in the back of head "like a flash of lightning."

Face.—Flushed. Neuralgia; pain extends in all directions from upper jaw. *Redness and burning of cheeks. Hectic flush.* Fullness and tenderness behind angle of jaws.

Nose.—Hay-fever. Ozæna, with profuse, offensive yellowish discharges. *Nasal polypi.* Coryza, followed by diarrhœa. Chronic rhinitis; membrane *dry* and congested.

Ears.—Burning in ears. Earache with headache. Humming and roaring. Aural polypus.

Throat.—Swollen; worse, right side. Dry and constricted. Ulceration of mouth and fauces, with dry, burning sensation. Tongue white; feels scalded. Tonsillitis.

Stomach.—Aversion to butter. Craving for piquant things. Unquenchable thirst. Burning, vomiting. Nausea, with salivation. Sinking, faint all-gone feeling. [*Phos.; Sep.*] Spitting up of bile; gastro-duodenal catarrh.

Abdomen.—Diarrhœa as coryza improves. Pain over region of liver. Diarrhœa; bilious, liquid, gushing stool. [*Nat. sulph.; Lycop.*] Cancer of rectum.

SANGUINARIA

Female.—Leucorrhœa fetid, corrosive. Menses offensive, profuse. Soreness of breasts. Uterine polypi. Before, menses, itching of axillæ. Climacteric disorders.

Respiratory.—Œdema of larynx. Trachea sore. Heat and tension behind the sternum. Aphonia. *Cough of gastric origin;* relieved by eructation. Cough, with burning pain in chest; worse, right side. Sputum tough, *rust-colored*, offensive, almost impossible to raise. Spasmodic cough after influenza and *after whooping-cough.* Cough returns with every fresh cold. Tickling behind sternum, causes a constant hacking cough; worse at night on lying down. Must sit up in bed. Burning soreness in right chest, through to right shoulder. Severe soreness under right nipple. Hæmoptysis from suppressed menses. *Severe dyspnœa* and constriction of chest. Offensive breath and purulent expectoration. Burning in chest as of hot steam from chest to abdomen. Fibroid phthisis. Pneumonia; better, lying on back. Asthma with stomach disorders. [*Nux.*] Valvular disease with lung development, phosphates in urine and loss of flesh. Sudden stoppage of catarrh of air passages brings on diarrhœa.

Extremities.—Rheumatism of right shoulder, left hip-joint and nape of neck. *Burning in soles and palms.* Rheumatic pains in places least covered by flesh; not in joints. Toes and soles of feet burn. Right-sided neuritis; better touching the part.

Skin.—Antidotes: *Rhus poisoning.* Red, blotchy eruptions; worse in spring. Burning and itching; worse by heat. Acne, with scanty menses. Circumscribed red spots over malar bones.

Modalities.—*Worse,* sweets, right side, motion, touch. Better, acids, sleep, darkness.

Relationship.—Complementary: *Tart. em.*

Compare: *Justicia* (bronchial catarrh, coryza, hoarseness; oversensitive). *Digitalis* (Migraine). *Bell.; Iris; Melil.; Lach.; Ferr.; Op.*

Dose.—Tincture in headaches; sixth potency in rheumatism.

SANGUINARINA NITRICA
(Nitrate of Sanguinarine)

Is of use in polypus of the nose. Acute and chronic catarrh. Acute pharyngitis. (*Wyethia*) Smarting and burning in throat and chest especially under sternum. *Influenza*. Lachrymation, pains in eyes and head, sore scalp; *sense of obstruction*. Chronic follicular pharyngitis.

Nose.—*Feels obstructed. Profuse, watery mucus, with burning pain.* Enlarged turbinates at beginning of hypertrophic process. Secretion scant, tendency to dryness. Small crusts which bleed when removed. Post-nasal secretions adherent to nasopharynx, dislodged with difficulty. Dry and burning nostrils; watery mucus, with pressure over root of nose. Nostrils plugged with thick, yellow, bloody mucus. *Sneezing*. Rawness and soreness in posterior nares.

Throat.—Rough, dry, *constricted, burning*. Right tonsil sore, swallowing difficult.

Mouth.—Ulceration on the *side* of the tongue.

Respiratory.—Short, hacking cough, with expectoration of thick, yellow, sweetish mucus. *Pressure behind center of sternum*. Dryness and burning in throat and bronchi. *Tickling cough*. Chronic nasal, laryngeal, and bronchial catarrh. Voice altered, deep, hoarse.

Relationship.—Compare: *Sanguin. tartaricum* (exophthalmos; *mydriasis;* dim vision); *Arum triph.; Psorin.; Kal. bich.*

Dose.—Third trituration.

SANICULA (AQUA)
(The Water of Sanicula Springs, Ottawa, Ill.)

Has been found a useful remedy in enuresis, seasickness, constipation, etc. Rickets.

Head.—Dread of downward motion. [*Borax.*] *Profuse sweat on occiput* and in nape of neck, during sleep. [*Calc.; Sil.*] Photophobia. Lachrymation in cold air or from cold application. Profuse scaly dandruff. Soreness behind ears.

Throat.—Thick, ropy, tenacious mucus.

Mouth.—Tongue large, flabby, burning; must protrude it to keep cool. Ringworm on tongue.

Stomach.—Nausea and vomiting from car-riding. Thirst; drink little and often. [*Ars.; Chin.*] Is vomited as soon as it reaches the stomach.

Rectum.—Stools large, heavy and painful. *Pain in whole perineum.* No desire until a large accumulation. After great straining only partially expelled; recedes, crumbles at verge of anus. [*Mag. mur.*] Very offensive odor. Excoriation of skin about anus, perineum, and genitals. Diarrhœa; changeable in character and color; after eating.

Female.—Bearing-down, as if contents of pelvis would escape; better, rest. Desire to support parts. Soreness of uterus. Leucorrhœa with *odor of fish-brine or old cheese.* [*Hepar.*] Vagina feels large.

Back.—Dislocated feeling in sacrum and better lying on right side.

Extremities.—Burning of soles of feet. [*Sulph.; Lach.*] *Offensive foot-sweat.* [*Sil.; Psor.*] Cold, clammy sweat of extremities.

Skin.—Dirty, greasy, brownish, wrinkled. Eczema, fissured hands and fingers. [*Petrol.; Graph.*]

Modalities.—*Worse, moving arms backward.*

Relationship.—Compare: *Abrot.; Alum.; Calc.; Sil.; Sulph.* Sanicula Aqua must not be confounded with the Sanicle (poolroot or wood marsh), also called *Sanicula.* This is used in various nervous affections, resembling Valeriana. It is used as a vulnerary, resolvent for sanguineous extravasations, and as an astringent. Has not been proved.)

Dose.—Thirtieth potency.

SANTONINUM

(Santonin)

Is the active principle of Santonica, the unexpanded flower heads of *Artemisia Maritima*—Cina., which see.

The eye stymptoms and those of the urinary tract are most prominent. It is of unquestioned value in the treatment of worm diseases, as gastro-intestinal irritation, *itching of nose*, restless sleep, twitching of muscles. Ascaris lumbricoides, and thread worms, but not tapeworms. *Night cough* of children. *Chronic cystitis*. Laryngeal crises and lightning pains of tabes.

Head.—Occipital headache, with *chromatic hallucinations*. *Itching of nose*. Bores into nostrils.

Eyes.—Sudden dimness of sight. *Color blindness;* Xanthopsia. Strabismus due to worms. Dark rings about eyes.

Mouth.—Fetid breath, depraved appetite; thirsty. Tongue deep-red. *Grinding of teeth*. Nausea; better after eating. Choking feeling.

Urinary.—Urine greenish if acid and reddish purple if alkaline. *Incontinence and dysuria*. *Enuresis*. Feeling of fullness of bladder. Nephritis.

Relationship.—Compare: *Cina; Teucr.; Napth.; Nat. phos.; Spigel.*

Dose.—Second to third trituration. Lower preparations are often toxic. Do not give to a child with fever or constipation.

SAPONARIA
(Soap Root)

Of great use in the treatment of acute colds, coryza, sore throat, etc. Will often "break up" a cold.

Mind.—Utter indifference to pain or possible death. Apathetic, *depressed, with sleepiness*.

Head.—Stitching pain, *supraorbital;* worse, left side, evening, motion. Throbbing over orbits. Congestions to head; tired feeling in nape. *Coryza*. Sensation of drunkenness with constant endeavor to go left-wards. Left-sided trigeminal neuralgia, especially supraorbital. Stopped up feeling in nose, also itching and sneezing.

Eyes.—Violent eye pains. Hot stitches deep in eyeball. Ciliary neuralgia; worse, left side. Photophobia. Exophthalmos, worse reading and writing. Increased intraocular pressure. Glaucoma.

Stomach.—Difficult swallowing. Nausea, heartburn; full feeling not relieved by eructation.

Heart.—Impulse weak; pulse less frequent. Palpitation with anxiety.

Modalities.—*Worse*, at night, mental exertion, left side.

Relationship.—Compare: *Saponin*—a glucosidal principle found in Quillayá, Yucca, Senega, Dioscorea and other plants. (Tired, indifferent. *Pain in left temple, eye*, photophobia, hot stitches deep in eye. Fifth nerve affections. Migraine. Much pain *before* the mentsrual flow; severe sore throat, worse right side; tonsils swollen, worse in warm room. Sharp burning taste and violent sneezing.)

Compare, also: *Verbasc.; Coccul.* (both containing Saponin). *Quillaya;* (Anagallis, *Agrostema,* Helonias, Sarsaparilla, Paris, Cyclamen and others contain Saponin).

SARCOLACTIC ACID

Is apparently formed in muscle tissue during the stage of muscle exhaustion. Differs from ordinary Lactic acid in its relation to polarized light.

It represents a much broader and more profoundly acting drug and its pathogenesis is quite dissimilar from the normal acid. Proved by Wm. B. Griggs, M. D., who found it of great value in the most violent form of *Epidemic influenza, especially with violent and retching and greatest prostration*, when Arsenic had failed. Spinal neurasthenia, muscular weakness, dyspnœa with myocardial weakness.

General Symptoms.—Tired feeling with *muscular prostration*, worse any exertion. Sore feeling all over, worse in afternoon. Restless at night. Difficulty in getting to sleep. Tired feeling in morning on getting up.

Throat.—Constriction in pharynx. Sore throat with tightness in naso-pharynx. Tickling in throat.

Stomach.—Nausea. Uncontrollable vomiting even of water followed by extreme weakness.

Back and Extremities.—Tired feeling in back and neck and shoulders. Paralytic weakness. Wrist tires easily from writing. Extreme weakness from climbing stairs. Stiffness of thigh and calves. Arms feel as if no strength in them. Cramp in the calves.

Dose.—Sixth to 30th potency. The 15x most marked action (Griggs).

SARRACENIA PURPUREA
(Pitcher-plant)

A remedy for variola. Visual disorders. Congestion to head, with irregular heart action. Chlorosis. Contains a very active proteolytic enzyme. Sick headache; throbbing in various parts, especially in neck, shoulders and head, which feels full to bursting.

Eyes.—Photophobia. Eyes feel swollen and sore. Pain in orbits. Black objects move with the eye.

Stomach.—Hungry all the time, even after a meal. Sleepy during meals. Copious, painful vomiting.

Back.—Pains shooting in *zig-zag* course from lumbar region to middle of scapula.

Extremities.—Limbs weak; bruised pain in knees and hip-joints. Bones in arm pain. *Weak between shoulders.*

Skin.—Variola, aborts the disease, arrests pustulation.

Relationship.—Compare: *Tartar. em.; Variol.; Maland.*

Dose.—Third to sixth potency.

SARSAPARILLA
(Smilax)

Renal colic; marasmus and periosteal pains due to venereal disease. Eruptions following hot weather and vaccinations; boils, and eczema. Urinary symptoms well marked.

Mind.—Despondent, sensitive, easily offended, ill humored and taciturn.

Head.—*Pains cause depression.* Shooting pain from above right temporal region. Pains *from occiput to eyes*. Words reverberate in ear to the root of nose. Periosteal pains due to venereal disease. Influenza. Scalp sensitive. *Eruptions on face and upper lip*. Moist eruption on scalp. Crusta lactea beginning in face.

Mouth.—Tongue white; *aphthæ; salivation;* metallic taste; no thirst. Fetid breath.

Abdomen.—Rumbling and fermentation. *Colic and backache at same time.* Much flatus; cholera infantum.

SARSAPARILLA

Urinary.—Urine scanty, slimy, flaky, sandy, *bloody*. Gravel. Renal colic. *Severe pain at conclusion of urination. Urine dribbles while sitting.* Bladder distended and tender. *Child screams before and while passing urine.* Sand on diaper. Renal colic and dysuria in infants. *Pain from right kidney downward.* Tenesmus of bladder; urine passes in thin, feeble stream. Pain at meatus.

Male.—Bloody, seminal emissions. Intolerable stench on genitals. Herpetic eruption on genitals. Itching on scrotum and perineum. Syphilis; squamous eruption and bone pains.

Female.—Nipples small, withered, *retracted. Before menstruation, itching and humid eruption of forehead.* Menses late and scanty. Moist eruption in right groin before menses.

Skin.—*Emaciated, shriveled, lies in folds* [*Abrot.*; *Sanic.*], dry, flabby. Herpetic eruptions; ulcers. Rash from exposure to open air; dry, itching; *comes on in spring;* becomes crusty. Rhagades; skin cracked on hands and feet. Skin hard, indurated. Summer cutaneous affections.

Extremities.—Paralytic, tearing pains. Trembling of hands and feet. Burning on sides of fingers and toes. Onychia, ulceration around ends of fingers, cutting sensation under nails. Rheumatism, bone pains; worse at night. Deep rhagades on fingers and toes; burn under nails. Tetter on hands; ulceration around ends of fingers. [*Psorin.*] Cutting sensation under nails. [*Petrol.*] Rheumatic pains after gonorrhœa.

Modalities.—*Worse,* dampness at night, after urinating, when yawning, in spring, before menses.

Relationship.—Complementary: *Merc.; Sep.*

Compare: *Berb.; Lycop.; Nat. m.; Petrol.; Sassafras; Saururus*—Lizard's tail—(Irritation of kidneys, bladder, prostate and urinary passages. Painful and difficult micturition; cystitis with strangury). *Cucurbita citrellus*—Watermellon. (Infusion of the seed acts promptly in painful urination with constriction and backache, relieves pain and stimulates flow.)

Antidote: *Bell.*

Dose.—First to sixth potency.

SCROPHULARIA NODOSA
(Knotted Figwort)

A powerful medicine whenever *enlarged glands* are present. Hodgkin's disease.

A valuable skin remedy. Has a specific affinity for the breast; very useful in the dissipation of breast tumors. *Eczema of the ear*. Pruritus vaginæ. Lupoid ulceration. *Scrofulous swellings*. [*Cistus.*] *Painful hæmorrhoids*. Tubercular testis. Ephithelioma. Nodosities in the breasts. [*Scirrhinum.*] Pain in all flexor muscles.

Head.—Vertigo felt in vertex, greater when standing; drowsiness; pain from forehead to back of head. Eczema behind ear. Crusta lactea.

Eyes.—Distressing photophobia. [*Conium.*] Spots before eyes. Stitches in eyebrow. Sore eyeballs.

Ears.—Inflammation about auricle. Deep ulcerated auricle. Eczema around ear.

Abdomen.—*Pain in liver* on pressure. Colic below navel. Pain in sigmoid flexure and *rectum*. *Painful*. bleeding, protruding *piles*.

Respiratory.—Violent dyspnœa, oppression of chest with trembling. Pain about bifurcation of trachea. Asthma in scrofulous patients.

Skin.—Prickling itching, worse back of hand.

Sleep.—*Great drowsiness;* in morning and before and after meals with weariness.

Modalities.—Worse lying on right side.

Compare: *Lobel. erinus; Ruta; Carcinosin; Conium; Asterias*.

Dose.—Tincture and first potency. Apply locally to cancerous glands also *Semper. viv*.

SCUTELLARIA LATERIFLORA
(Skullcap)

This is a nervous sedative, where *nervous fear* predominates. *Cardiac irritability*. Chorea. Nervous irritation and spasms of children, during dentition. *Twitching of muscles*. Nervous weakness after influenza.

Mental.—*Fear of some calamity.* Inability to fix attention. [*Æthus.*] Confusion.

Head.—*Dull, frontal headache.* Eyes feel pressed outwards. Flushed face. Restless sleep and frightful dreams. *Must move about.* Night terrors. Migraine; worse, over right eye; *aching in eyeballs.* Explosive headaches of school teachers with frequent urination; headaches in front and base of brain. Nervous sick headaches, worse noise, odor light, better night; rest, 5 drops of tincture.

Stomach.—Nausea; sour eructations; hiccough; pain and distress.

Abdomen.—Gas, fullness and distention, colicky pain and uneasiness. Light colored diarrhœa

Male.—Seminal emissions and impotency, with fear of never being better.

Sleep.—Night-terrors; sleeplessness; sudden wakefulness; frightful dreams.

Extremities.—Twitchings of muscles; must be moving. Chorea. Tremors. Sharp stinging pains in upper extremities. Nightly restlessness. Weakness and aching.

Relationship.—Compare: *Cyprip.; Lycopus.*

Dose.—Tincture and lower potencies.

SECALE CORNUTUM—CLAVICEPS PURPUREA
(Ergot)

Produces contraction of the unstriped muscular fibers; hence a constringent feeling throughout the whole body. This produces an anæmic condition, coldness, numbness, petechiæ, mortification, gangrene. A useful remedy for old people with shriveled skin—thin, scrawny old women. All the Secale conditions are *better from cold;* the whole body is pervaded by a sense of great heat. Hæmorrhages; continued oozing; *thin,* fetid, watery black blood. *Debility, anxiety, emaciation, though appetite and thirst may be excessive.* Facial and abdominal muscles twitch. Secale decreases the flow of pancreatic juice by raising the blood pressure. (Hinsdale.)

Head.—Passive, congestive pain (rises from back of head), with pale face. Head drawn back. Falling of hair; dry and gray. *Nosebleed,* dark, oozing.

SECALE CORNUTUM

Eyes.—Pupils dilated. Incipient cataract, senile especially in women. *Eyes sunken and surrounded by a blue margin.*

Face.—*Pale, pinched, sunken.* Cramps commence in face and spread over whole body. Livid spots on face. *Spasmodic distortion.*

Mouth.—Tongue dry, *cracked; blood like ink exudes,* coated thick; viscid, yellowish, cold livid. *Tingling of tip of tongue, which is stiff.* Tongue swollen, paralyzed.

Stomach.—*Unnatural ravenous appetite; craves* acids. *Thirst* unquenchable. Singultus, nausea; vomiting of blood and coffee-grounds fluid. Burning in stomach and abdomen; tympanites. Eructations of bad odor.

Stool.—Cholera-like stools, with coldness and cramps. *Olive-green, thin, putrid, bloody, with icy coldness and intolerance of being covered, with great exhaustion. Involuntary stools;* no sensation of passing fæces, anus wide open.

Urine.—Paralysis of bladder. Retention, with unsuccessful urging. Discharge of black blood from bladder. Enuresis in old people.

Female.—Menstrual colic, with coldness and intolerance of heat. Passive hæmorrhages in feeble, cachectic women. Burning pains in uterus. *Brownish, offensive leucorrhœa.* Menses irregular, copious, dark; *continuous oozing of watery blood* until next period. Threatened abortion about the *third* month. [Sab.] During labor no expulsive action, though everything is relaxed. After-pains. Suppression of milk; breasts do not fill properly. Dark, offensive lochia. Puerperal fever, putrid discharges, tympanitis, coldness, suppressed urine.

Chest.—Angina pectoris. Dyspnœa and oppression, with cramp in diaphragm. Boring pain in chest. Præcordial tenderness. Palpitation, with contracted and intermittent pulse.

Sleep.—Profound and long. Insomnia with restlessness, fever, anxious dreams. *Insomnia of drug and liquor habitues.*

Back.—Spinal irritation, tingling of lower extremities; can bear only slightest covering. *Locomotor ataxia.* Formication and numbness. Myelitis.

Extremities.—Cold, dry hands and feet of excessive smokers with feeling of fuzziness in fingers. Trembling, staggering gait.

Formication, pain and spasmodic movements. Numbness. Fingers and feet bluish, shriveled, *spread apart or bent backwards*, numb. *Violent cramps. Icy coldness of extremities.* Violent pain in finger-tips, tingling in toes.

Skin.—Shriveled, numb; mottled dusky-blue tinge. Scleræma and œdema neonatorum. Raynaud's disease. Blue color. *Dry gangrene*, developing slowly. *Varicose ulcers. Burning sensation;* better by cold; *wants parts uncovered*, though cold to touch. Formication; petechiæ. Slight wounds continue to bleed. Livid spots. Boils, small, painful, with green contents; mature slowly. *Skin feels cold to touch*, yet covering is not tolerated. *Great aversion to heat. Formication under skin.*

Fever.—*Coldness;* cold, dry skin; cold, clammy sweat; excessive thirst. Sense of internal heat.

Modalities.—*Worse*, heat, *warm covering*. *Better*, cold, *uncovering*, rubbing, stretching out limbs.

Relationship.—Compare: *Ergotin.* (Beginning arteriosclerosis progressing rather rapidly. Increased blood pressure: 2x trit. Edema, gangrene and purpura hæmorrhagia; when Secale, though indicated, fails); *Pedicularis Canadensis* (symptoms of locomotor ataxia; spinal irritation); *Brassica napus*—Rape-seed—(dropsical swellings, scorbutic mouth, voracious appetite, tympanitis, dropping of nails, gangrene); *Cinnamon.; Colch.; Ars.; Aurum mur.* 2x (locomotor ataxia); *Agrostema*—Corn-cockle—active constituent is *Saponin*, which causes violent sneezing and sharp burning taste; burning in stomach, extends to œsophagus, neck and breast; (vertigo, headache, difficult locomotion, burning sensation); *Ustilago; Carbo; Pituitrin* (dilated os, little pain, no progress. Dose, ½ c.c., repeat in half hour, if necessary. Hypodermically contraindicated in first stage of labor, valvular lesions or deformed pelvis).

Antidotes: *Camph.; Opium.*

Dose.—First to thirtieth potency. *Non-homœopathic use.*—In hæmorrhages of the puerperium, after the uterus is entirely emptied, when it fails to contract satisfactorily and in secondary puerperal hæmorrhage the result of incomplete involution of the uterus, give one-half to one dram of the fluid extract. Re_ member Pagot's law. "As long as the uterus contains anything, be it child, placenta, membranes, clots, never administer Ergot."

SEDUM ACRE
(Small Houseleek)

Hæmorrhoidal pains, like those of anal fissures; constricting pains, worse few hours after stool. *Fissures*.

Relationship.—Compare: *Mucuna urens* (hæmorrhoidal diathesis and diseases depending thereon); *Sedum telephium* (uterine hæmorrhages, also of bowels and rectum; *menorrhagia, especially at climacteric*); *Sedum repens—S. alpestre—(cancer;* specific action on abdominal organs; pain, loss of strength).

Dose.—Tincture to sixth potency.

SELENIUM
(The Element Selenium)

Selenium is a constant constituent of bones and teeth.

Marked effects on the genito-urinary organs, and often indicated in elderly men, especially for prostatitis and sexual atony. *Great debility;* worse, heat. Easy exhaustion, mental and physical, in old age. Debility after exhausting diseases.

Mind.—Lascivious thoughts, with impotency. Mental labor fatigues. *Extreme sadness*. Abject despair, uncompromising melancholy.

Head.—Hair falls out. *Pain over left eye; worse, walking in sun, strong odors and tea*. Scalp feels tense. Headache from tea drinking.

Throat.—Incipient tubercular laryngitis. Hawking and raising transparent lumps of mucus every morning. *Hoarseness*. Cough in morning, with expectoration of bloody mucus. Hoarseness of singers. Much clear, starchy mucus. [*Stann.*]

Stomach.—Desire for brandy and other strong drink. Sweetish taste. Hiccough and eructations after smoking. After eating, pulsation all over, especially abdomen.

Abdomen.—Chronic liver affections; liver painful, *enlarged, with fine rash over liver region*. Stool constipated, hard and accumulated in rectum.

Urinary.—Sensation in the tip of urethra as if a biting drop were forcing its way out. Involuntary dribbling.

Male.—Dribbling of semen during sleep. Dribbling of prostatic fluid. Irritability after coitus. *Loss of sexual power*, with lascivious fancies. *Increases desire, decreases ability.* Semen thin, odorless. Sexual neurasthenia. On attempting coition, penis relaxes. *Hydrocele.*

Skin.—Dry, scaly eruption in palms, with itching. *Itching about the ankles* and folds of skin, between fingers. Hair falls out from brows, beard, and genitals. Itching about finger-joints and between fingers; in palms. Vesicular eruption between fingers. [*Rhus; Anac.*] Seborrhœa oleosa; comedones *with an oily surface of the skin;* alopecia. *Acne.*

Extremities.—Paralytic pains in small of back in the morning. Tearing pain in hands, at night.

Sleep.—*Sleep prevented by pulsation in all vessels,* worse abdomen. Sleepless until midnight, awakens early and always same hour.

Modalities.—*Worse,* after sleep, in hot weather, from Cinchona, draught of air, coition.

Relationship.—Incompatible: *China; Wine.*

Compare: *Agnus; Calad.; Sulphur; Tellur.; Phosph. acid.* Antidotes: *Ign.; Puls.*

Dose.—Sixth to thirtieth potency. Colloidal Selenium injection for inoperable cancer. Pain, sleeplessness, ulceration and discharge are markedly diminished.

SEMPERVIVUM TECTORUM
(Houseleek)

Is recommended for herpes, zoster and *cancerous tumors*. Scirrhous induration of tongue. Mammary carcinoma. Ringworm. Hæmorrhoids.

Mouth.—Malignant ulcers of mouth. Cancer of tongue. [*Galium.*] Tongue has ulcers; *bleed easily,* especially at night; much soreness of tongue with *stabbing* pains. Whole mouth very tender.

Skin.—Erysipelatous affections. *Warts* and corns. Aphthæ. Flushed surface and stinging pains.

Relationship.—Compare: *Sedum acre*—small Houseleek—(scorbutic conditions; ulcers, intermittent fever). [*Galium;*

Kali cyanat.] *Oxalis acetosella*—Wood sorrel—(The inspissated juice used as a cautery to remove cancerous growths of the lips). *Cotyledon. Ficus Carica*—(Fig)—The milky juice of the freshly broken stalk applied to warts; causes their disappearance.

Dose.—Tincture and 2 decimal, also fresh juice of plant. Locally for bites of insects, stings of bees, and poisoned wounds, warts.

SENECIO AUREUS
(Golden Ragwort)

Its action on the female organism has been clinically verified. Urinary organs also affected in a marked degree. Backaches of congested kidneys. Early cirrhosis of liver.

Mind.—Inability to fix mind upon any one subject. Despondent. Nervous and irritable.

Head.—Dull, stupefying headache. *Wavelike dizziness* from occiput to sinciput. *Sharp pains over left eye, and through left temple.* Fullness of nasal passages; burning; *sneezing;* profuse flow.

Face.—Teeth very sensitive. *Sharp, cutting pain* left side. *Dryness* of fauces, throat, and mouth.

Stomach.—Sour eructations; nausea.

Throat.—Dry mouth, throat, and fauces. Burning in pharynx, raw feeling in naso-pharynx, must swallow, though painful.

Abdomen.—Pain around umbilicus; spreads all over abdomen; better, stool. Thin, watery stool, intermingled with hard lumps of fæces. [*Ant. crud.*] *Straining at stool; thin, dark, bloody, with tenesmus.*

Urinary.—Scanty, high-colored, *bloody*, with much mucus and *tenesmus. Great heat and constant urging.* Nephritis. Irritable bladder of children, with headache. Renal colic [*Pareira; Ocim.; Berb.*]

Male.—Lascivious dreams, with involuntary emissions. *Prostate enlarged.* Dull, heavy pain in spermatic cord, extending to testicles.

Female.—*Menses retarded*, suppressed. *Functional amenorrhœa of young girls* with backache. Before menses, inflammatory conditions of throat, chest, and bladder. After menstruation commences. these improve. Anæmic dysmenorrhœa with urinary disturbances. Premature and too profuse menses. [*Calc.; Erig.*]

Respiratory.—Acute inflammatory conditions of upper respiratory tract. Hoarseness. *Cough loose*, with labored inspiration. Chest sore and raw. Dyspnœa on ascending. [*Calc.*] Dry teasing cough, stitching chest pains.

Sleep.—Great drowsiness, with unpleasant dreams. Nervousness and sleeplessness.

Relationship.—Compare: *Senecio Jacobæa* (cerebro-spinal irritation, rigid muscles, chiefly of neck and shoulders; also, in cancer); *Aletris; Caulop.; Sep.*

Dose.—Tincture, to third potency. *Senecin*, first trituration.

SENEGA
(Snakewort)

Catarrhal symptoms, especially of the respiratory tract, and distinct eye symptoms of a paralytic type, are most characteristic. Circumscribed spots in chest left after inflammations.

Mind.—Suddenly remembers unimportant regions which he saw long ago. Inclined to quarrel.

Head.—Dullness, with pressure and weakness of eyes. Pain in temples. *Bursting* pain in forehead.

Eyes.—Hyperphoria, better by bending head backwards. Acts on the rectus superior. Blepharitis; lids dry and crusty. [*Graph.*] Dryness, with sensation *as if too large for orbits.* Staring. Lachrymation. Flickering; must wipe eyes frequently. Objects look shaded. Muscular asthenopia. [*Caust.*] Double vision; better only by bending head backward. Opacities of the vitreous humor. Promotes absorption of fragments of lens, after operation.

Nose.—Dry. Coryza; much watery mucus and sneezing. Nostrils feel peppery.

Face.—Paralysis of left side of face. Heat in face. Burning vesicles in corners of mouth and lips.

Throat.—Catarrhal inflammation of throat and fauces, with scraping hoarseness. Burning and rawness. Sensation as if membrane had been abraded.

Respiratory.—Hoarseness. Hurts to talk. Bursting pain in back on coughing. Catarrh of larynx. Loss of voice. Hacking cough. Thorax feels too narrow. *Cough often ends in a sneeze. Rattling in chest.* [*Tart. emet.*] Chest oppressed on ascending. Bronchial catarrh, *with sore chest walls;* much mucus; sensation of oppression and weight of chest. *Difficult raising of tough, profuse mucus,* in the aged. Asthenic bronchitis of old people with chronic interstitial nephritis or chronic emphysema. Old asthmatics with congestive attacks. *Exudations in Pleura.* Hydrothorax. [*Merc. sulph.*] Pressure on chest as though lungs were forced back to spine. Voice unsteady, vocal cords partially paralyzed.

Urinary.—Greatly diminished; loaded with shreds and mucus; scalding before and after urinating. *Back,* bursting distending pain in kidney region.

Modalities.—*Worse,* walking in open air, during rest. *Better,* from sweat; *bending head backwards.*

Relationship.—Compare: *Caust.; Phos.; Saponin; Ammon.; Calc.; Nepeta cataria*—Catnip (to break up a cold; infantile colic: hysteria).

Dose.—Tincture, to thirtieth potency.

SENNA
(Cassia Acutifolia)

Is of much use in infantile colics when the child seems to be *full of wind.* Oxaluria, with excess of urea; increased specific gravity. Where the system is broken down, bowels constipated, muscular weakness, and waste of nitrogenous materials, Senna will act as a tonic. Ebullitions of blood at night. *Acetonæmia,* prostration, fainting, constipation with colic and flatulence. Liver enlarged and tender.

Stool.—Fluid yellowish, with pinching pains before. Greenish mucus; never-get-done sensation. [*Merc.*] Burning in rectum, with strangury of bladder. *Constipation,* with colic and flatulence. Liver enlarged and tender, stools hard and dark, with loss of appetite, coated tongue, bad taste, and *weakness.*

Urine.—Specific gravity and density increased; hyperazoturia, oxaluria, phosphaturia, and acetonuria.

Relationship.—Compare: *Kali carb.; Jalapa.*

Antidotes: *Nux; Cham.*

Dose.—Third to sixth potency.

SEPIA
(Inky Juice of Cuttlefish)

Acts specially on the portal syster , with venous congestion. Stasis and thereby ptosis of viscera and weariness and misery Weakness, yellow complexion, bearing-down sensation, especially in women, upon whose organism it has most pronounced effect. Pains extend down to back, chills easily. Tendency to abortion. Hot flashes at menopause with weakness and perspiration. Upward tendency of its symptoms. Easy fainting. "Ball" sensation in inner parts. Sepia acts best on brunettes. All pains are from below up. One of the most important uterine remedies. Tubercular patients with chronic hepatic troubles and uterine reflexes. *Feels cold* even in warm room. Pulsating headache in cerebellum.

Mind.—*Indifferent* to those loved best. Averse to occupation, to *family*. Irritable; easily offended. Dreads to be alone. *Very sad.* Weeps when telling symptoms. Miserly. Anxious toward evening; indolent.

Head.—Vertigo, with sensation of something rolling round in head. Prodromal symptoms of apoplexy. Stinging pain from within outward and upward mostly left, or in forehead, with nausea, vomiting; worse indoors and when lying on painful side. Jerking of head backwards and forwards. Coldness of vertex. Headache in *terrible shocks* at menstrual nisus, with scanty flow. Hair falls out. Open fontanelles. Roots of hair sensitive. Pimples on forehead near hair.

Nose.—*Thick, greenish discharge;* thick plugs and crusts. *Yellowish saddle across nose.* Atrophic catarrh with greenish crusts from anterior nose and pain at root of nose. Chronic nasal catarrh, especially post-nasal, dropping of heavy, lumpy discharges; must be hawked through the mouth.

Eyes.—Muscular asthenopia; black spots in the field of vision; asthenic inflammations, and in connection with uterine trouble. Aggravation of eye troubles morning and evening. Tarsal tumors. Ptosis, ciliary irritation. Venous congestion of the fundus.

Ears.—*Herpes behind ears on nape of neck.* Pain as if from sub-cutaneous ulceration. Swelling and eruption of external ear.

Face.—Yellow blotches; pale or sallow; yellow about mouth. Rosacea; saddle-like brownish distribution on nose and cheeks.

Mouth.—Tongue white. Taste salty, putrid. Tongue foul, but clears during menses. Swelling and cracking of lower lip. Pain in teeth from 6 p. m. till midnight; worse on lying.

Stomach.—*Feeling of goneness; not relieved by eating.* [*Carb. an.*] Nausea at smell or sight of food. Nausea worse lying on side. *Tobacco dyspepsia.* Everything tastes too salty. [*Carbo veg.; Chin.*] Band of pain about four inches wide encircling hypochondria. *Nausea in morning before eating.* Disposition to vomit after eating. Burning in pit of stomach. Longing for *vinegar*, acids, and pickles. Worse, after milk, especially when boiled. Acid dyspepsia with bloated abdomen, sour eructations. Loathes fat.

Abdomen.—*Flatulent*, with headache. *Liver sore and painful; relieved by lying on right side.* Many brown spots on abdomen. Feeling of relaxation and bearing-down in abdomen.

Rectum.—Bleeding at stool and fullness of rectum. Constipation; large, hard stools; *feeling of a ball in rectum;* cannot strain; with great tenesmus and pains shooting *upward.* Dark-brown, round balls glued together with mucus. Soft stool, difficult. Prolapsus ani. [*Pod.*] *Almost constant oozing from anus.* Infantile diarrhœa, *worse from boiled milk*, and rapid exhaustion. *Pains shoot up* in rectum and vagina.

Urinary.—Red, *adhesive*, sand in urine. Involuntary urination, *during first sleep.* Chronic cystitis, slow micturition, with bearing-down sensation above pubis.

Male.—Organs cold. Offensive perspiration. Gleet; discharge from urethra only during night; no pain. Condylomata surround head of penis. Complaints from coition.

Female.—Pelvic organs relaxed. *Bearing-down sensation as if everything would escape through vulva* [*Bell.; Kreoso; Lac c.; Lil. t.; Nat. c.; Pod.*]; must cross limbs to prevent protrusion.

or press against vulva. Leucorrhœa yellow, greenish; with much itching. Menses *too late and scanty*, irregular; *early and profuse;* sharp clutching pains. Violent stitches upward in the vagina, from uterus to umbilicus. *Prolapse* of uterus and vagina. Morning sickness. Vagina painful, especially on coition.

Respiratory.—Dry, fatiguing cough, apparently coming from stomach. Rotten-egg taste with coughing. Oppression of chest morning and evening. Dyspnœa; worse, after sleep; better, rapid motion. Cough in morning, with profuse expectoration, tasting salty. [*Phos.; Ambr.*] Hypostatic pleuritis. Whooping-cough that drags on. Cough excited by tickling in larynx or chest.

Heart.—Violent, intermittent palpitation. Beating in all arteries. Tremulous feeling with flushes.

Back.—*Weakness in small of back. Pains extend into back.* Coldness between shoulders.

Extremities.—Lower extremities lame and stiff, tension as if too short. Heaviness and bruised feeling. *Restlessness in all limbs*, twitching and jerkings night and day. Pain in heel. Coldness of legs and feet.

Fever.—Frequent flushes of heat; sweat from least motion. General lack of warmth of body. Feet cold and wet. Shivering, with thirst; worse, towards evening.

Skin.—Herpes circinatus in isolated spots. Itching; not relieved by scratching; worse in bends of elbows and knees. Chloasma; herpetic eruption on lips, about mouth and nose. Ringworm-like eruption every spring. Urticaria on going in open air; better in warm room. Hyperidrosis and bromidrosis. Sweat on feet, worse on toes; intolerable odor. Lentigo in young women. Ichthyosis with offensive odor of skin.

Modalities.—*Worse*, forenoons and evenings; washing, laundry-work, dampness, left side, after sweat; cold air, before thunder-storm. *Better*, by *exercise*, pressure, warmth of bed, hot applications, drawing limbs up, cold bathing, after sleep.

Relationship.—Complementary: *Nat. mur.; Phosph.* Nux intensifies action. *Guaiacum* often beneficial after *Sepia*.

Inimical: *Lach.; Puls.*

Compare: *Lil.; Murex· Silica; Sulph.; Asperula*—Nacent

oxygen—Distilled water charged with the gas—(leucorrhœa of young girls and uterine catarrh); *Ozonum (sacral* pain; tired feeling through pelvic viscera and perineum); *Dictamnus*—Burning Bush—(Soothes labor pains); (metrorrhagia, leucorrhœa, and constipation; also somnambulism). *Lapathum.* (Leucorrhœa with constriction and expulsive effort through womb and pain in kidneys).

Dose.—Twelfth, 30th and 200th potency. Should not be used too low or be repeated too frequently. On the other hand Dr. Jousset's unique experience is that it should be continued for some time in strong doses. 1x twice a day.

SERUM ANGUILLAR ICHTHYOTOXIN
(Eel Serum)

The *serum of the eel* has a toxic action on the blood, rapidly destroying its globules. The presence of albumin and renal elements in the urine, the hemoglobinuria, the prolonged anuria (24 and 26 hours), together with the results of the autopsy, plainly demonstrate its elective action on the kidneys. Secondarily, the liver and the heart are affected, and the alterations observed are those usually present in infectious diseases.

From all these facts it is easy to infer, *a priori*, the therapeutical indications of the *serum of the eel*. Whenever the kidney becomes acutely affected, either from cold or infection or intoxication, and the attack is characterized by *oliguria, anuria* and *albuminuria*, we will find the *eel's serum* eminently efficacious to re-establish diuresis, and in rapidly arresting albuminuria. When during the course of *heart-disease*, the kidney, previously working well, should suddenly become affected and its function inhibited; and when besides we observe cardiac irregularities and a marked state of asystolia, we may yet expect good results from this serum. But to determine here the choice of this remedy is not an easy matter. While *digitalis* presents in its indications, the well-known symptomatic trilogy: *arterial hypertension, oliguria and œdema;* the *serum of the eel* seems better adapted to cases of *hypertension and oliguria, without œdema.* We should bear in mind that the elective action of the eel's serum is on the kidney, and I believe we can well assert that if *digitalis* is a cardiac, the *eel's serum* is a renal remedy. So far, at least, the clinical observations published seem to confirm this distinction. The serum of the eel has given very small results in attacks of asystolia; but it has been very efficacious in *cardiac uremia*. There, where *digitalis* is powerless, the *serum of the eel* has put an end to the renal obstruction and produced an abundant diuresis. But its really specific indication seems to be for *acute nephritis a frigori*. (Jousset.)

Subacute nephritis. Heart diseases, in cases of failure of compensation and impending asytole. The experiments of Dr. Jousset have amply demonstrated the rapid hæmaturia, albuminuria and oliguria caused by it. In the presence of acute nephritis with threatening uræmia we should always think of this serum. Very efficacious in functional heart diseases. Mitral insufficiency, asystolia with or without œdema, dyspnœa and difficult urinary secretion.

Relationship.—Great analogy exists between eel serum and the venom of the *Vipera*.

Compare, also: *Pelias; Lachesis*.

Dose.—Attenuations are made with glycerine or distilled water, the lower 1x to 3 in heart disease, the higher in sudden renal attacks.

SILICEA
(Silica. Pure Flint)

Imperfect assimilation and consequent defective nutrition. It goes further and produces neurasthenic states in consequence, and increased susceptibility to nervous stimuli and exaggerated reflexes. Diseases of bones, caries and necrosis. Silica can stimulate the organism to re-absorb fibrotic conditions and scar-tissue. In phthisis must be used with care, for here it may cause the absorption of scar-tissue, liberate the disease, walled in, to new activities. (J. Weir.) Organic changes; it is deep and slow in action. Periodical states; abscesses, quinsy, headaches, spasms, epilepsy, feeling of coldness before an attack. Keloid growth. Scrofulous, rachitic children, with large head, open fontanelles and sutures, distended abdomen, slow in walking. *Ill effects of vaccination. Suppurative processes.* It

SILICEA

is related to all fistulous burrowings. Ripens abscesses since it promotes suppuration. Silica patient is cold, chilly, hugs the fire, wants plenty warm clothing, hates drafts, hands and feet cold, worse in winter. Lack of vital heat. Prostration of mind and body. Great sensitiveness to taking cold. *Intolerance of alcoholic stimulants.* Ailments attended with *pus formation.* Epilepsy. *Want of grit,* moral or physical.

Mind.—Yielding, *faint-hearted, anxious.* Nervous and excitable. *Sensitive* to all impressions. Brain-fag. Obstinate, headstrong children. Abstracted. Fixed ideas; thinks only of *pins,* fears them, searches and counts them.

Head.—Aches from fasting. Vertigo from looking up; *better, wrapping up warmly; when lying on left side.* [*Magnes. mur.; Strontia.*] *Profuse sweat of head,* offensive, and extends to neck. Pain begins at occiput, and spreads over head and settles over eyes. Swelling in the glabella.

Eyes.—Angles of eyes affected. *Swelling of lachrymal duct.* Aversion to light, especially daylight; it produces dazzling, sharp pain through eyes; eyes tender to touch; worse when closed. Vision confused; letters run together on reading. *Styes.* Iritis and irido-choroiditis, with pus in anterior chamber. *Perforating* or sloughing ulcer of cornea. Abscess in cornea after traumatic injury. Cataract in office workers. After-effects of keratitis and ulcus cornæ, clearing the opacity. Use 30th potency for months.

Ears.—Fetid discharge. Caries of mastoid. Loud pistol-like report. Sensitive to noise. *Roaring in ears.*

Nose.—Itching at point of nose. Dry, hard crusts form, *bleeding when loosened.* Nasal bones sensitive. Sneezing in morning. Obstructed and loss of smell. Perforation of septum.

Face.—Skin cracked on margin of lips. Eruption on chin. Facial neuralgia, throbbing, tearing, face red; worse, cold damp.

Mouth.—*Sensation of a hair on tongue.* Gums sensitive to cold air. Boils on gums. Abscess at root of teeth. Pyorrhœa. [*Merc. cor.*] Sensitive to cold water.

Throat.—Periodical quinsy. *Pricking as of a pin in tonsil.* Colds settle in throat. *Parotid glands swollen.* [*Bell.;. Rhus; Calc.*] Stinging pain on swallowing. Hard, cold swelling of cervical glands.

Stomach.—Disgust for meat and *warm food*. On swallowing food, it easily gets into posterior nares. Want of appetite; thirst excessive. Sour eructations after eating. [*Sepia; Calc.*] Pit of stomach painful to pressure. Vomiting after drinking. [*Ars.; Verat.*]

Abdomen.—Pain or painful cold feeling in abdomen, better external heat. Hard, bloated. Colic; cutting pain, with constipation; yellow hands and blue nails. Much rumbling in bowels. Inguinal glands swollen and painful. Hepatic abscess.

Rectum.—Feels paralyzed. *Fistula in ano.* [*Berb.; Lach.*] Fissures and hæmorrhoids, *painful, with spasm of sphincter. Stool comes down with diffculty; when partly expelled, recedes again.* Great straining; rectum stings; closes upon stool. Fæces remain a long time in rectum. *Constipation always before and during menses;* with irritable sphincter ani. Diarrhœa of cadaverous odor.

Urinary.—Bloody, involuntary, with red or yellow sediment. Prostatic fluid discharged when straining at stool. Nocturnal enuresis in children with worms.

Male.—Burning and soreness of genitals, with eruption on inner surface of thighs. Chronic gonorrhœa, with thick, fetid discharge. Elephantiasis of scrotum. Sexual erethism; nocturnal emissions. Hydrocele.

Female.—A milky [*Calc.; Puls.; Sep.*], acrid leucorrhœa, during urination. Itching of vulva and vagina; very sensitive. Discharge of blood between menstrual periods. Increased menses, with paroxysms of *icy coldness over whole body.* Nipples very sore; ulcerated easily; drawn in. Fistulous ulcers of breast. [*Phos.*] Abscess of labia. Discharge of blood from vagina every time child is nursed. Vaginal cysts. [*Lyc.; Puls.; Rhod.*] Hard lumps in breast. [*Conium.*]

Respiratory.—Colds fail to yield; sputum persistently mucopurulent and profuse. Slow recovery after pneumonia. Cough and sore throat, with expectoration of little granules like shot, which, when broken, smell very offensive. Cough with expectoration in day, bloody or purulent. Stitches in chest through to back. *Violent cough when lying down, with thick, yellow lumpy expectoration;* suppurative stage of expectoration. [*Bals. Peru.*]

Back.—Weak spine; very susceptible to draughts on back. Pain in coccyx. Spinal irritation after injuries to spine; diseases of bones of spine. Potts' disease.

Sleep.—*Night-walking;* gets up while asleep. Sleeplessness, with great orgasm of blood and heat in head. Frequent starts in sleep. Anxious dreams. Excessive gaping.

Extremities.—Sciatica, pains through hips, legs and feet. Cramp in calves and soles. Loss of power in legs. Tremulous hands when using them. Paralytic weakness of forearm. *Affections of finger nails*, especially if white spots on nails. Ingrowing toe-nails. *Icy cold and sweaty feet. The parts lain on go to sleep.* Offensive sweat on feet, hands, and axillæ. Sensation in tips of fingers, as if suppurating. Panaritium. Pain in knee, as if tightly bound. Calves tense and contracted. Pain beneath toes. Soles sore. [*Ruta.*] *Soreness in feet from instep through to the sole. Suppurates.*

Skin.—*Felons, abscesses, boils, old fistulous ulcers.* Delicate, pale, waxy. Cracks at end of fingers. Painless swelling of glands. Rose-colored blotches. Scars suddenly become painful. Pus offensive. *Promotes expulsion of foreign bodies from tissues.* Every little injury suppurates. Long lasting suppuration and fistulous tracts. Dry finger tips. Eruptions itch only in daytime and evening. *Crippled nails.* Indurated tumors. Abscesses of joints. After impure vaccination. Bursa. Lepra, nodes, and coppery spots. *Keloid growths.*

Fever.—Chilliness; very sensitive to cold air. Creeping, shivering over the whole body. Cold extremities, even in a warm room. Sweat at night; worse towards morning. *Suffering parts feel cold.*

Modalities.—*Worse*, new moon, in morning, from washing, during menses, uncovering, lying down, damp, lying on left side, cold. *Better*, warmth, wrapping up head, summer; in wet or humid weather.

Relationship.—Complementary: *Thuja; Sanic.; Puls.; Fluor. ac.* Mercurius and Silica do not follow each other well.

Compare: *Black Gunpowder* 3x. (Abscesses, boils, carbuncles, limb purple. Wounds that refuse to heal; accident from bad food or water.—Clarke.) *Hep.; Kali phos.; Pic. ac.; Calc.; Phos.; Tabasheer; Natrum silicum* (tumors, hæmophilia, arthritis; dose, three drops three times daily, in milk); *Ferrum cyanatum* (epilepsy; neuroses, with irritable weakness and hyper-sensitiveness, especially of a periodical character). *Silica marina*—Sea-sand—(Silica and Natrum mur. symptoms. *Inflamed glands* and commencing suppuration. Constipation. Use for some time 3x trit.) *Vitrum—Crown glass*—(Potts' disease, after Silica, necrosis, discharge thin, watery, fetid. Much pain, fine *grinding* and *grating* like grit.) *Arundo donax* (acts on excretory and generative organs; suppuration, especially chronic, and where the ulceration is fistulous, especially in long bones. Itching eruption on chest, upper extremities and behind eard).

Dose.—Sixth to thirtieth potency. The 200th and higher of unquestioned activity. In malignant affections, the lowest potencies needed at times.

SILPHIUM
(Rosin-weed)

Is used in various forms of asthma and chronic bronchitis Catarrh of bladder. Catarrhal influenza. Dysentery; attack preceded by constipated stools covered with white mucus.

Respiratory.—Cough with expectoration *profuse*, stringy, forthy, light-colored. Excited by sense of mucus rattling in chest and worse by drafts of air. Constriction of lungs. Catarrh, with copious, stringy, mucous discharges. Desire to hawk and scrape throat. Irritation of posterior nares, involving mucous membranes of nasal passages with constriction of supra-orbital region.

Relationship.—Compare: *Aral.; Copaiv.; Tereb.; Cubeb.; Samb.; Silphion cyrenaicum* (phthisis pulmonum, with incessant cough, profuse night-sweats, emaciation, etc.); *Polygonum aviculare* (has been found useful in phthisis, when given in material doses of the mother tincture); *Salvia* (tickling cough). *Arum dracontium* (loose cough at night on lying down). *Justicia adhatoda* (bronchial catarrh, hoarseness, oversensitive).

Dose.—Third **potency.** Lower *triturations* preferred by some.

SINAPIS NIGRA—BRASSICA NIGRA
(Black Mustard)

Is of use in hay-fever, coryza, and pharyngitis. Dry nares and pharynx, with thick, lumpy secretion. Small-pox.

Head.—Scalp hot and itches. *Sweat on upper lip and forehead.* Tongue feels blistered.

Nose.—Mucus from posterior nares feels *cold*. Scanty, *acrid* discharge. *Stoppage of left nostril all day*, or in afternoon and evening. Dry, hot, with lachrymation, sneezing; hacking cough; better lying down. *Nostrils alternately stopped.* Dryness of anterior nares.

Respiratory.—Cough is relieved by lying down.

Throat.—Feels scalded, hot, inflamed. Asthmatic breathing. Loud coughing-spells with barking expiration.

Stomach.—*Offensive breath*, smelling like onions. [*Asaf.; Armorac.*] Burning in stomach, extending up œsophagus, throat, and mouth, which is full of canker sores. Hot sour eructations. *Colic; pains come on while bent forward; better, sitting up straight.* Sweat better when nausea comes on.

Urinary.—Pain in bladder, frequent *copious* flow day and night.

Back.—Rheumatic pain in intercostal and lumbar muscles; sleeplessness from pain in back and hips.

Relationship.—Compare: *Sulph.; Capsic.; Colocy.; Sinapis alba*—White Mustard—(throat symptoms marked, especially *pressure and burning, with obstruction in œsophagus;* sensation of a lump in œsophagus behind the Manubrium Sterni and with much eructation; similar symptoms in rectum). *Mustard oil* by inhalation (acts on the sensory nerve endings of the trigeminal. Relieves pain in middle ear disease and in painful conditions of nose, nasal cavities, and tonsils.)

Dose.—Third potency.

SKATOL

Represents the ultimate end of proteid decomposition and is a constituent of human fæces.

Acne with auto-intoxication dependent upon intestinal decomposition.

Stomach and abdominal symptoms and frontal headache. Sluggishness with no ambition. Desire to curse and swear.

Mind.—Lack of concentration; impossible to study; *despondent;* desire to be with people. Irritable. Felt mean towards everyone.

Head.—Frontal headache, worse over left eye, in the evening, *better by short sleep.*

Gastric.—Tongue coated, *foul taste.* Salty taste to all cereals. *Belching.* Appetite increased. Light, yellow, narrow, *very offensive* stool. Intestinal dyspepsia.

Urinary.—Frequent, scanty, burning, difficult.

Sleep.—Increased desire to sleep; wakes unrefreshed, half doped feeling.

Relationship.—Compare: *Indol.; Baptis.; Sulph.*

Dose.—Sixth potency.

SKOOKUM-CHUCK

Chuck—Water and Skookum—Strong
(Salts from Water from Medical Lake near Spokane, Wash.)

Has strong affinity for skin and mucous membranes—An anti-psoric medicine.

Otitis media. Profuse, ichorous, cadaverously smelling discharge. Lithæmia. *Catarrh.* Urticaria. *Skin affections. Eczema. Dry skin. Hay-fever.* Profuse coryza and constant sheezing.

Relationship.—*Saxonite*—(appears to have remarkable cleansing, deodorizing and soothing properties for the skin. (Cowperthwaite.) Eczema, scalds, burns, sores and hæmorrhoids).

Dose.—Third trituration.

SOLANUM LYCOPERSICUM— LYCOPERSICUM ESCULENTUM
(Tomato)

Marked symptoms of rheumatism and influenza. Severe aching pains all over body. *Pains left after influenza.* Head always shows signs of acute congestion. Hay-fever, with marked aggravation from breathing the least dust. Frequent urination and profuse watery diarrhœa.

Head.—Bursting pain, beginning in occiput and spreading all over. Whole head and scalp feels sore, bruised, after pain has ceased.

Eyes.—Dull, heavy; pupils contracted; eyeballs feel contracted; aching in and around eyes. Eyes suffused.

Nose.—Profuse, watery coryza; drops down throat. Itching in anterior chamber; worse, breathing any dust; better, indoors.

Heart.—Decided decrease in pulse rate with anxiety and apprehensiveness.

Respiratory.—Voice husky. Pain in chest, extending to head. Hoarseness; constant desire to clear throat. Expulsive cough, deep and harsh. Chest oppressed; dry, hacking cough coming on at night and keeping one awake.

Urine.—Constant dribbling *in open air*. Must rise at night to urinate.

Extremities.—Aching through back. Dull pain in lumbar region. *Sharp pain in right deltoid and pectoralis muscles*. Pain deep in middle of right arm. Rheumatic pain in right elbow and wrist, and hands of both sides. Intense aching in lower limbs. Right crural neuralgia. Tingling along right ulnar nerve.

Modalities.—*Worse*, right side, open air, continued motion, jars, noises. *Better*, warm room, tobacco.

Relationship.—Compare: *Bellad.* (follows well); *Eup. perf.*; *Rhus*; *Sanguin.*; *Caps.*

Dose.—Third to thirtieth potency.

SOLANUM NIGRUM
(Black Nightshade)

Used with success in ergotism, with tetanic spasms and stiffness of whole body, with mania. Marked action on head and eyes. *Meningitis.* Chronic intestinal toxæmia. Brain irritation during dentition. Restlessness of a violent and convulsive nature. Formication with contraction of extremities.

Head.—Furious delirium. Vertigo; terrible headache and complete cessation of the mental faculties. Night terrors. *Congestive* headache.

Nose.—Acute coryza; *profuse, watery discharge from right nostril;* left stopped up, with chilly sensation, alternating with heat.

Eyes.—Pain over both eyes. Alternate dilatation and contraction of pupils; weak sight; floating spots.

Respiratory.—Constrictive feeling in chest, with difficult breathing; cough with tickling in throat. Expectoration *thick, yellow.* Pain in *left* chest, sore to touch.

Fever.—Alternation of coldness and heat. Scarlet fever; eruption in spots, large and vivid.

Relationship.—Compare: *Bellad.; Solanum Carolinense*—Horse-nettle—(convulsions and epilepsy, twenty to forty-drop doses; is of great value in grand mal of idiopathic type, where the disease has begun beyond age of childhood; hystero-epilepsy, also in whooping-cough); *Solan. mammosum*—Apple of Sodom—(pain in left hip-joint); *Solan. oleraceum* (swelling of mammary gland, with profuse secretion of milk); *Solan. tuberosum* (cramps in calves and contraction of fingers; spitting through closed teeth); *Solan. vesicarium* (recommended in facial paralysis); *Solaninum aceticum* (threatening paralysis of the lungs in the course of bronchitis in the aged and children must cough a long time before able to raise expectoration; *Solan. pseudocaps.* (acute pains, in lower abdomen); *Solan. tuberos. ægrotans*—Diseased potato—(prolapse of the rectum, patulous anus; offensive breath and odor of body; tumors of rectum look like decayed potato; dreams of pools of blood); *Solanum tuberosum*—Potato berries—(cramps in the calves of the legs and fingers).

Dose.—Second to thirtieth potency.

SOLIDAGO VIRGA
(Golden-rod)

Inhalation of the pollen has caused hæmorrhage from the lungs in phthisis. *Repeated colds of tuberculosis* (2x). *Feeling of weakness,* chilliness alternating with heat; naso-pharyngeal catarrh, burning in throat, pains in limbs and thoracic oppression. Pain in region of kidneys, with dysuria. *Kidneys sensi-*

tive to pressure. Bright's disease. Hay-fever when Solidago is the exciting cause. Here give 30th potency or higher.

Eyes.—Injected, watery, burning, stinging.

Nose.—Nares irritated with abundant mucus secretion; paroxysms of sneezing.

Stomach.—Bitter taste, especially at night; coated tongue with very scanty brown and sour urine.

Respiratory.—Bronchitis, cough with much purulent expectoration, blood-streaked; oppressed breathing. Continuous dyspnœa. Asthma, with nightly dysuria.

Female.—Uterine enlargement, organ pressed down upon the bladder. *Fibroid tumors.*

Urine.—Scanty, reddish brown, thick sediment, dysuria, gravel. *Difficult and scanty.* Albumen, blood, and slime in urine. Pain in kidneys extend forward to abdomen and bladder. [*Berb.*] *Clear and offensive urine.* Sometimes makes the use of the catheter unnecessary.

Back.—Backache of congested kidneys. [*Senec. aur.*]

Skin.—Blotches, especially on lower extremities; *itch.* Exanthema of lower extremities, with urinary disturbances, dropsy and threatened gangrene.

Relationship.—*Iodoform* 2x antidotes poison of Golden-rod. *Arsenic. Agrimonia.* (Pain in region of kindeys.)

Dose.—Tincture, to third potency. Oil of Solidago, 1 oz. to 8 oz. Alcohol. 15 drops doses to promote expectoration in bronchitis and bronchial asthma in old people. (Eli G. Jones.)

SPARTIUM SCOPARIUM—CYSTISUS SCOPARIUS

(Broom)

Spartein sulphate increases the strength of the heart, slows it and reduces the blood pressure. It continues the good effects of Veratrum and Digitalis without any of the undesirable effects of either. (Hinsdale.)

The effect of spartein sulphate (the alkaloid of Broom) is to cause a *lowering* of the systolic and diastolic pressures of the provers. Sphygmograms also show a condition of lowered blood-pressure. It depresses the heart by poisonous action exerted on the myocardium and this, with the stimulating action of the drug upon the vagus, accounts for the lowered blood pressure and reduced pulse rate. It weakens the cardiac contraction. The total amount of urine is increased. The drug has, therfore, diuretic properties and is useful in dropsy.

Albuminuria. Cheyne-Stokes respiration. Irregular heart following grip and various infections. Hypotension. Used palliatively in physiological dosage to combat arterial hypertension, arterio-sclerosis. Very useful hypodermically 1/10 to 1/4 grain in sustaining heart after stopping habit of Morphia. Spartium is indicated when primarily the muscles of the heart and especially the nervous apparatus is affected. Acts rapidly and lasts three to four days. Does not disturb digestion. Nephritis.

Heart—Tobacco heart. Angina pectoris. Irregular action, disturbed rhythm due to gas, etc., feeble in nervous hysterical patients. Myocardial degeneration, failing compensation. Hypotension. Spartein in 2 gr. doses for water-logged cases, cannot lie down. Here it produces much comfort. Has specific action upon the kidneys, enabling them to eliminate and relieve the distress upon the heart.

Stomach.—Great accumulation of gas in gastro-intestinal canal, with mental depression.

Urinary.—Burning along urinary tract or in pudendum. *Profuse flow of urine.*

Dose.—For non-homœopathic use (palliative as above), one to two grains t. i. d. by mouth, exerts a definite action upon the kidneys that will enable them to relieve the distress upon the heart. It is a safe drug and prompt in its action. Hypodermically, not less than 1/4 of a grain. Doses as high as 2 grains by mouth three times a day are safe (Hinsdale).

Homœopathically. First to third trituration.

SPIGELIA

(Pinkroot)

Spigelia is an important remedy in pericarditis and other diseases of the heart, because the provings were conducted with the greatest regard for objective symptoms and the subjective symptoms are by innumerable confirmations proved to be correct (C. Hering).

Has marked elective affinity for the eye, heart, and nervous system. Neuralgia of the fifth nerve is very prominent in its effects. Is especially adapted to anæmic, debilitated, rheumatic, and scrofulous subjects. Stabbing pains. Heart affections and neuralgia. *Very sensitive to touch. Parts feel chilly; send shudder through frame.* A remedy for symptoms due to the presence of worms. *Child refers to the navel as the most painful part.* [*Granat.; Nux mosch.*]

Mind.—Afraid of sharp, pointed things, pins, needles, etc.

Head.—*Pain beneath frontal eminence and temples, extending to eyes.* [*Onos.*] Semi-lateral, involving left eye; pain violent, throbbing; worse, making a false step. Pain as if a band around head. [*Carbol. ac.; Cact.; Gels.*] Vertigo, hearing exalted.

Eyes.—Feel too large; *pressive pain on turning them.* Pupils dilated; photophobia; rheumatic ophthalmia. *Severe pain in and around eyes, extending deep into socket.* Ciliary neuralgia, a true neuritis.

Nose.—Forepart of nose always dry; *discharge through posterior nares.* Chronic catarrh, with post-nasal dropping of bland mucus.

Mouth.—Tongue fissured, painful. Tearing toothache; worse, after eating and cold. *Foul odor from mouth.* Offensive taste.

Face.—*Prosopalgia, involving eye, zygoma, cheek, teeth, temple,* worse, stooping, touch, from morning until sunset.

Heart.—Violent palpitation. Præcordial pain and great aggravation from movement. Frequent attacks of palpitation, especially with foul odor from mouth. Pulse weak and irregular. Pericarditis, with sticking pains, palpitation, dyspnœa. Neuralgia extending to arm or both arms. Angina pectoris. Craving for hot water which relieves. Rheumatic carditis, trembling pulse; whole left side sore. *Dyspnœa; must lie on right side with head high.*

Rectum.—Itching and crawling. Frequent ineffectual urging to stool. Ascarides.

Fever.—Chilliness on the slightest motion.

Modalities.—*Worse*, from touch, motion, noise, turning, washing, concussion. *Better*, lying on right side with head high; inspiring.

Relationship.—Compare: *Spigelia Marylandica* (maniacal excitement, paroxysmal laughing and crying, loud, disconnected talking, vertigo, dilated pupils, congestions); *Acon.; Cact.; Cimicif.; Arnica* (Spigela is a chronic Arnica); *Cinnab.* (supra-orbital pain); *Naja; Spong.* (*heart*); *Sabad.; Teucr.; Cina* (worm symptoms).

Antidote: *Pulsat.*

Dose.—Sixth to thirtieth potency for neuralgic symptoms; second to third potency for inflammatory symptoms.

SPIRAEA ULMARIA
(Hardhack)

Burning and pressure in œsophagus, feels contracted but not made worse by swallowing. *Morbidly conscientious.* Relieves irritation of the urinary passages; influences the prostate gland; checks gleet and prostatorrhœa; has been used for eclampsia, epilepsy, and hydrophobia. Bites of mad animals. Heat in various parts. (Salicylic acid is found in Spiræa.)

SPIRANTHES
(Lady's Tresses)

Has been used for milk-flow in nursing women, lumbago and rheumatism, colic, with drowsiness and spasmodic yawning. Is an anti-phlogistic remedy akin to Acon. its symptoms showing congestion and inflammation. Acidity and burning in œsophagus with eructation.

Female.—Pruritus; vulva red; dryness and burning in vagina. Burning pain in vagina during coition. Leucorrhœa, bloody.

Extremities.—Sciatic pain, especially right side. Pain in shoulders. Swelling of veins of hands. Pain in all articulations of hands. Coldness of feet and toes.

Fever.—Flushes of heat. Sweat on palms. Hands alternately hot and cold.

Dose.—Third potency

SPONGIA TOSTA

(Roasted Sponge)

A remedy especially marked in the symptoms of the respiratory organs, cough, croup, etc. Heart affections and often indicated for the tubercular diathesis. Children with fair complexion, lax fiber; swollen glands. *Exhaustion and heaviness of the body after slight exertion, with orgasm of blood to chest, face. Anxiety and difficult breathing.*

Mind.—Anxiety and fear. Every excitement increases the cough.

Head.—Rush of blood; bursting headache; worse, forehead.

Eyes.—Watering; gummy or mucus discharge.

Nose.—Fluent coryza, alternating with stoppage. Dryness; chronic, dry, nasal catarrh.

Mouth.—Tongue dry and brown; full of vesicles.

Throat.—Thyroid gland swollen. Stitches and dryness. Burning and stinging. Sore throat; worse after eating sweet things. Tickling causes cough. Clears throat constantly.

Stomach.—Excessive thirst, *great hunger*. Cannot bear tight clothing around trunk. Hiccough.

Male.—*Swelling of spermatic cord and testicles, with pain and tenderness.* Orchitis. Epididymitis. Heat in parts.

Female.—Before menses, pain in sacrum, hunger, *palpitation. During menses,* wakes with suffocative spells. [*Cupr.; Iod.; Lach.*] Amenorrhœa, with asthma. [*Puls.*]

Respiratory.—Great dryness of all air-passages. *Hoarseness; larynx dry, burns, constricted.* Cough, dry, barking, croupy; larynx sensitive to touch. *Croup; worse, during inspiration and before midnight.* Respiration short, panting, *difficult; feeling of a plug in larynx. Cough abates after eating or drinking,* especially warm drinks. The dry, chronic sympathetic cough or organic heart disease is relieved by Spongia. [*Naja.*] Irrepressible cough from a spot deep in chest, as if raw and sore. Chest weak; can scarcely talk. Laryngeal phthisis. Goitre, with suffocative spells. Bronchial catarrh, with wheezing, asthmatic cough, worse cold air, with profuse expectoration and suffocation; worse, lying with head low and in hot room. Oppression and heat of chest, with sudden weakness.

Heart.—Rapid and violent palpitation, with dyspnœa; cannot lie down; also feels best resting in horizontal position. *Awakened suddenly after midnight with pain and suffocation;* is flushed, hot, and frightened to death. [*Acon.*] Valvular insufficiency. Angina pectoris; faintness, and anxious sweat. Ebullition of blood, veins distended. *Surging of heart into chest, as if it would force out upward.* Hypertrophy of heart, especially right, with asthmatic symptoms.

Skin.—*Swelling and induration of glands;* also exophthalmic; cervical glands swollen with tensive pain on turning head, painful on pressure; goitre. Itching; measles.

Sleep.—*Awakes in a fright, and feels as if suffocating.* Generally worse after sleep, or sleeps into an aggravation. [*Lach.*]

Fever.—*Attacks of heat with anxiety;* heat and redness of face and perspiration.

Modalities.—*Worse,* ascending, wind, before midnight. *Better,* descending, lying with head low.

Relationship.—Compare: *Acon.; Hep.; Brom.; Lach.; Merc. prot.; Iod.* (Goitre.)

Dose.—Second trituration, or tincture to third potency.

SQUILLA MARITIMA
(Sea-onion)

A slow acting remedy. Corresponds to ailments requiring several days to reach their maximum. Persistent, dull, rheumatic pains permeate the body. A spleen medicine; stitches under left free ribs. Important heart and kidney medicine. *Broncho-pneumonia.*

Acts especially on mucous membranes of the respiratory and digestive tracts, and also upon the kidneys. Valuable in chronic bronchitis of old people with mucous rales, dyspnœa, and scanty bronchitis of old people with mucous rales, dyspnœa, and scanty urine.

Eyes.—Feel irritable; child bores into them with fists. Sensation as if swimming in cold water.

Stomach.—Pressure like a stone

Respiratory.—Fluent coryza; margins of nostrils feel sore. Sneezing; throat irritated; short, dry cough; must take a deep breath. *Dyspnœa and stitches in chest,* and painful contraction of abdominal muscles. *Violent,* furious, exhausting cough, with much mucus; profuse, salty, slimy expectoration, and with *involuntary spurting of urine and sneezing. Child rubs face with fist during cough.* [*Caust.; Puls.*] Cough provoked by taking a deep breath or cold drinks, from exertion, change from warm to cold air. Cough of measles. Frequent calls to urinate at night, passing large quantities. [*Phos. ac.*] *Sneezing with coughing.*

Heart.—A cardiac stimulant affecting the peripheral vessels and coronary arteries.

Urinary.—Great urging: *much watery urine. Involuntary spurting of urine when coughing.* [*Caustic; Puls.*]

Skin.—Small, red spots over body, with prickling pain.

Extremities.—Icy cold hands and feet, with warmth of the rest of the body. [*Menyanthes.*] Feet get sore from standing. Tender feet with shop girls.

Modalities.—*Better,* rest; *worse,* motion.

Relationship.—Compare: *Digit.; Strophant.; Apocyn. can.; Bry.; Kali carb.* Squilla follows *Digitalis,* if this fails to relieve water-logged cases.

Dose.—First to third potency.

STANNUM
(Tin)

Chief action is centered upon the nervous system and respiratory organs. Debility is very marked when Stannum is the remedy, especially the debility of chronic bronchial and pulmonary conditions, characterized by profuse muco-purulent discharges upon tuberculosis basis. *Talking causes a very weak feeling in the throat and chest. Pains that come and go gradually,* call unmistakably for Stannum. Paralytic weakness; spasms; paralysis.

Mind.—Sad, anxious. *Discouraged.* Dread of seeing people.

Head.—Aching in temples and forehead. Obstinate acute coryza and influenza with cough. Pain worse motion; *gradually increasing and decreasing* as if constricted by a band; forehead feels pressed inwards. Jarring of walking resounds painfully in head. Drawing pains in malar bones and orbits. Ulceration of ringhole in lobe of ear.

Throat.—Much adhesive mucus, difficult to detach; efforts to detach cause nausea. Throat dry and stings.

Stomach.—Hunger. *Smell of cooking causes vomiting.* Bitter taste. Pain better pressure, but sore to touch. Sensation of *emptiness in stomach.*

Abdomen.—Cramp-like colic around navel, with a feeling of emptiness. *Colic relieved by hard pressure.*

Female.—*Bearing-down sensation.* Prolapsus, with *weak, sinking feeling in stomach.* [Sep.] *Menses early and profuse.* Pain in vagina, upward and back to spine. Leucorrhœa, with great debility.

Respiratory.—Hoarse; mucus expelled by forcible cough. Violent, dry cough in evening until midnight. Cough excited by *laughing*, singing, talking; worse lying on right side. During day, with *copious green, sweetish*, expectoration. Chest feels sore. *Chest feels weak;* can hardly talk. Influenzal cough from noon to midnight with scanty expectoration. Respiration short, oppressive; stitches in left side when breathing and lying on same side. *Phthisis mucosa. Hectic fever.*

Sleep.—Sleeps with one leg drawn up, the other stretched out.

Extremities.—Paralytic weakness; drops things. Ankles swollen. Limbs suddenly *give out when attempting to sit down.* Dizziness and weakness *when descending.* Spasmodic twitching of muscles of forearm and hand. Fingers jerk when holding pen. Neuritis. Typewriters' paralysis.

Fever.—Heat in evening; *exhausting night-sweats*, especially towards morning. Hectic. Perspiration, principally on forehead and nape of neck; debilitating; smelling musty, or offensive.

Modalities.—*Worse*, using voice (*i. e.*, laughing, talking, singing), lying on right side, warm drinks. *Better*, coughing or expectorating, hard pressure.

Relationship.—Complementary: *Puls.*

Compare: *Stann. iod.* 3x. (Valuable in chronic chest diseases characterized by plastic tissue changes. Persistent inclination to cough, excited by tickling dry spot in the throat, apparently at root of tongue. Dryness of throat. Trachial and bronchial irritation of smokers. Pulmonary symptoms; cough, loud, hollow, ending with expectoration. [Phellandrium.] State of purulent infiltration. *Advanced* phthisis sometimes when Stann. jod has not taken effect, an additional dose of Iodine in milk caused the drug to have its usual beneficial effect. (Stonham.) Compare: *Caust.; Calc.; Sil.; Tuberc.; Bacil.; Helon. Myrtus chekan* (chronic bronchitis, cough of phthisis, emphysema, with gastric catarrhal complications and thick, yellow difficult sputum. Old persons with weakened power of expectoration.)

Dose.—Third to thirtieth potency.

STAPHYSAGRIA
(Stavesacre)

Nervous affections with marked irritability, diseases of the genito-urinary tract and skin, most frequently give symptoms calling for this drug. Acts on teeth and alveolar periosteum. Ill effects of anger and insults. *Sexual sins and excesses. Very sensitive.* Lacerated tissues. Pain and nervousness after extraction of teeth. Sphincters lacerated or stretched.

Mind.—Impetuous, *violent outbursts of passion*, hypochondriacal, sad. *Very sensitive* as to what others say about her. Dwells on sexual matters; prefers solitude. Peevish. Child cries for many things, and refuses them when offered.

Head.—Stupefying headache; passes off with yawning. Brain feels squeezed. Sensation of a ball of lead in forehead. Itching eruption above and behind ears. [*Oleand.*]

Eyes.—Heat in eyeballs, dims spectacles. *Recurrent styes. Chalazæ.* [*Platanus.*] Eyes sunken, with blue rings. Margin of lids itch. Affections of angles of eye, particularly the inner. Lacerated or incised wounds of cornea. Bursting pain in eyeballs of syphilitic iritis.

Throat.—*Stitches flying to the ear on swallowing, especially left.*

Mouth.—Toothache during menses. *Teeth black and crumbling.* Salivation, spongy gums, bleed easily. [*Merc.; Kreos.*] Submaxillary glands swollen. After eating feels sleepy. Pyorrhœa. [*Plantago.*]

Stomach.—Flabby and weak. Desire for stimulants. Stomach feels relaxed. *Craving for tobacco.* Canine hunger, even when stomach is full. Nausea after abdominal operations.

Abdomen.—Colic after anger. Hot flatus. Swollen abdomen in children, with much flatus. Colic, with pelvic tenesmus. *Severe pain following an abdominal operation.* Incarcerated flatus. Diarrhœa after drinking cold water, with tenesmus. *Constipation* (2 drops tincture night and morning), hæmorrhoids, with enlarged prostate.

Male.—Especially after self-abuse; persistent dwelling on sexual subjects. Spermatorrhœa, with sunken features; guilty look; emissions, with backache and weakness and sexual neurasthenia. Dyspnœa after coition.

Female.—*Parts very sensitive*, worse sitting down. [*Berb.; Kreos.*] *Irritable bladder in young married women.* Leucorrhœa. Prolapsus, with sinking in the abdomen; aching around the hips.

Urinary.—*Cystocele* (locally and internally). Cystitis in lying-in patients. Ineffectual urging to urinate in *newly married* women. Pressure upon bladder; feels as if it did not empty. *Sensation as if a drop of urine were rolling continuously along the channel.* Burning in urethra during micturition. Prostatic troubles; frequent urination, burning in urethra *when not urinating.* [*Thuja; Sabal; Ferr. pic.*] Urging and pain *after* urinating. Pain after lithotomy.

Skin.—Eczema of head, ears, face, and body; thick scabs, dry, and itch violently; *scratching changes location of itching.* Fig-warts pedunculated. [*Thuja.*] Arthritic nodes. Inflammation of phalanges. Night-sweats.

Extremities.—Muscles, especially of calves, feel bruised. *Backache; worse in morning before rising.* Extremities feel beaten and painful. Joints stiff. *Crural neuralgia.* Dull aching of nates extending to hip-joint and small of back.

Modalities.—Worse, anger, indignation, grief, mortification, loss of fluids, onanism, sexual excesses, tobacco; least touch on affected parts. *Better*, after breakfast, warmth, rest at night.

Relationship.—Inimical: *Ranunc. bulb.*

Complementary: *Caust.; Colocy.*

Compare: *Ferrum pyrophos.* (tarsal cysts); *Colocy.; Caust.; Ign.; Phos. ac.; Calad.*

Antidote: *Camph.*

Dose.—Third to thirtieth potency.

STELLARIA MEDIA
(Chickweed)

Induces a condition of stasis, congestion, and sluggishness of all functions. Morning aggravation.

Sharp, *shifting*, rheumatic pains in all parts very pronounced. *Rheumatism;* darting pains in almost every part; stiffness of joints; parts sore to touch; worse, motion. *Chronic rheumatism. Shifting pains.* [*Puls.; Kali sulph.*] Psoriasis. Enlarged and inflamed gouty finger joints.

Head.—General irritability. Lassitude, indisposition to work. Smarting and burning in eyes, feel protruded. Dull, frontal headache; worse in morning and left side with sleepiness. Neck muscles stiff and sore. Eyes feel protruded.

Abdomen.—*Liver engorged, swollen, with stitching pain and sensitive to pressure.* Clay-colored stools. Hepatic torpor. Constipation or alternating constipation and diarrhœa.

Extremities.—Rheumatoid pains in different parts of the body. Sharp pain in small of back, over kidneys, in gluteal region, extending down thigh. Pain in shoulders and arms. *Synovitis.* Bruised feeling. Rheumatic pains in calves of legs.

Modalities.—*Worse*, mornings, warmth, tobacco. *Better*, evenings, cold air, motion.

Relationship.—Compare: *Pulsat.* (similar in rheumatism, pains shifting, worse rest, warmth; better cold air).

Dose.—Tincture, externally. Internally, 2x potency.

STERCULIA
(Kola-nut)

Neurasthenia. Regulates the circulation, is tonic and antidiarrhœic, regulates cardiac rhythm and acts diuretically. Weak heart.

The remedy for the drinking habit. It promotes the appetite and digestion, and lessens the craving for liquor. *Asthma.* Gives power to endure prolonged physical exertion without taking food and without feeling fatigued.

Relationship.—*Coca.*

Dose.—Three to ten drops, even one dram doses, three times a day.

STICTA
(Lungwort)

Offers a set of symptoms like coryza, bronchial catarrh and influenza, together with nervous and *rheumatic* disturbances. There is a general feeling of dullness and malaise, as when a cold is coming on; dull, heavy pressure in forehead, catarrhal conjunctivitis, etc. *Rheumatic stiffness of neck.*

Mind.—*Feels as if floating in air.* [*Datura arborea.; Lac. Can.*] Confusion of ideas; *patient must talk.*

Head.—Dull headache, with dull heavy pressure in forehead and *root of nose. Catarrhal headache before discharge appears.* Burning in eyes and soreness of balls. Sensation as if scalp were too small. Burning in eyelids.

Nose.—*Feeling of fullness at the root of the nose.* [*Nux.*] Atrophic rhinitis. [*Calc. fluor.*] *Dryness of nasal membrane. Constant need to blow the nose, but no discharge.* Dry scabs, especially in evening and night. *Hay-fever;* incessant sneezing. [*Sabad.*]

Female.—Scanty flow of milk.

Abdomen.—Diarrhœa; stools profuse, frothy; worse, morning. Urine increased, with soreness and aching in bladder.

Respiratory.—Throat raw; dropping of mucus posteriorly. *Dry, hacking cough during night; worse, inspiration.* Tracheitis, facilitates expectoration. Loose cough in morning. Pain through chest from sternum to spinal column. Cough after measles [*Sang.*]; *worse towards evening and when tired. Pulsation from right side of sternum down to abdomen.*

Extremities.—Rheumatic pain in right shoulder joint, deltoid, and biceps. Swelling, heat, redness of joints. *Spot of inflammation and redness over affected joint.* Pain severe and drawing. Chorea-like spasms; legs feel floating in air. *Housemaid's knee.* [*Rhus; Kali hyd.; Slag.*] Shooting pains in knees. Joints and neighboring muscles red, swollen, painful. Rheumatic pains precede catarrhal symptoms.

Modalities.—*Worse*, sudden changes of temperature.

Relationship.—Compare: *Datura arborea—Bougmancia candida* (cannot concentrate thoughts; brain floats in thousands of problems and grand ideas. Floating sensation as if ideas were floating outside of brain. Headache, heartburn. Burning sensation around cardiac end of stomach, extending to œsophagus with sense of constriction. Heat and fullness over liver region.) *Cetraria*—Iceland Moss (chronic diarrhœa, phthisis, bloody expectoration. Is used as a decoction and boiled with milk as an expectorant and nutrient in bronchorrhœa, catarrh, etc.) Also compare: *Eryng.; Dros.; Stilling.; Rumex; Sambuc.*

Dose.—Tincture, to sixth potency.

STIGMATA MAYDIS—ZEA
(Corn-silk)

Has marked urinary symptoms, and has been used with success in organic heart disease, with much œdema of lower extremities and scanty urination. Enlarged prostate and retention of urine. Uric and phosphatic Gonorrhœa. Cystitis.

Urinary.—Suppression and *retention*. Dysuria. Renal lithiasis; nephritic colic; blood and red sand in urine. Tenesmus after urinating. Vesical catarrh. Gonorrhœa. Cystitis.

Shucks (as a decoction used for chronic malaria, teaspoonful doses freely. Dr. E. C. Lowe, England).

Dose.—Tincture in ten-to fifty-drop doses.

STILLINGIA
(Queen's Root)

Chronic periosteal rheumatism, syphilitic and scrofulous affections. Respiratory symptoms well marked. Torpor of lymphatics; torpid liver, with jaundice and constipation.

Mind.—*Gloomy forebodings;* depressed.

Respiratory.—Dry, spasmodic cough. Larynx constricted, with stinging in fauces. Trachea feels sore when pressed. *Hoarseness* and chronic laryngeal affections of public speakers.

Urinary.—Urine colorless. *Deposits white sediment;* urine milky and thick.

Extremities.—Aching pains in *bones* of extremities and back.

Skin.—Ulcers; chronic eruptions on hands and fingers. *Enlarged cervical glands.* Burning, itching of legs; worse, exposure to air. Exostosis. Scrofuloderma; syphilis, secondary eruption and later symptoms. Valuable for intercurrent use.

Modalities.—*Worse*, in afternoons, damp air, motion. *Better*, in morning, dry air.

Relationship.—Compare: *Staphis.; Mercur.; Syphil.; Aur.; Corydalis* (syphilitic nodes).

Dose.—Tincture and first potency.

STRAMONIUM
(Thorn-apple)

The entire force of this drug seems to be expended on the brain, though the skin and throat show some disturbance. Suppressed secretions and excretions. Sensation as if limbs were separated from body. Delirium tremens. Absence of pain and muscular mobility especially of muscles of expression and of locomotion. Gyratory and graceful motions. Parkinsonism.

Mind.—*Devout, earnest, beseeching and ceaseless talking.* Loquacious, garrulous, laughing, singing, swearing, praying, rhyming. Sees ghosts, hears voices, talks with spirits. Rapid changes from joy to sadness. Violent and lewd. Delusions about his identity; thinks himself tall, double, a part missing. Religious mania. Cannot bear solitude or darkness; *must have light and company.* Sight of water or anything glittering brings on spasms. Delirium, with desire to escape. [*Bell.; Bry.; Rhus.*]

Head.—*Raises head frequently from the pillow.* Pain in forehead and over eyebrows, beginning at 9 a. m.; worse until noon. Boring pain, preceded by obscure vision. Rush of blood to head; staggers, with tendency to fall forward and to the left. Auditory hallucinations.

Eyes.—Seem prominent, *staring wide open;* pupils dilated. Loss of vision; complains that it is dark, *and calls for light. Small objects look large.* Parts of the body seem enormously swollen. Strabismus. All objects look black.

Face.—Hot, red; circumscribed redness of cheeks. Blood rushes to face; distorted. *Expression of terror.* Pale face

Mouth.—Dry; dribbling of viscid saliva. Aversion to water. *Stammering.* Risus sardonicus. Cannot swallow on account of spasm. Chewing motion.

Stomach.—Food tastes like straw. Violent thirst. Vomiting of mucus and *green* bile.

Urine.—*Suppression*, bladder empty.

Male.—*Sexual erethism*, with indecent speech and action. Hands constantly kept on genitals.

Female.—*Metrorrhagia*, with *loquacity, singing,* praying. Puerperal mania, with characteristic mental symptoms and profuse sweatings. Convulsions after labor.

Sleep.—Awakens terrified; screams with fright. Deep snoring sleep. Sleepy, but cannot sleep. [*Bell.*]

Extremities.—*Graceful, rhythmic motions.* Convulsions of upper extremities and of isolated groups of muscles. *Chorea;* spasms partial, constantly changing. *Violent pain in left hip.* Trembling, twitching of tendons, staggering gait.

Skin.—Shining red flash. *Effects of suppressed eruption in scarlatina*, with delirium, etc.

Fever.—Profuse sweat, which does not relieve. Violent fever.

Modalities.—*Worse,* in dark room, when alone, looking at bright or shining objects, after sleep, on swallowing. *Better,* from bright light, company, warmth.

Relationship.—Compare especially: *Hyoscy.* and *Bellad.* It has less fever than *Bellad.*, but more than *Hyos*. It causes more functional excitement of the brain, but never approaches the true inflammatory condition of *Bellad.*

Antidotes: *Bellad.; Tabac.; Nux.*

Dose.—Thirtieth potency and lower.

STRONTIA

(Carbonate of Strontia)

Rheumatic pains, chronic sprains, stenosis of œsophagus. Pains make patient faint or sick all over. Chronic *sequelæ of hæmorrhages*, after operations with much oozing of blood and coldness and prostration. Arterio-sclerosis. High blood pressure with flushed face pulsating arteries, threatened apoplexy. Violent involuntary starts. Affections of bones, especially femur. Restlessness at night, smothering feeling. *For shock after surgical operations. Neuritis*, great sensitiveness to cold.

Head.—*Vertigo with headache and nausea.* Distensive pressure. Aches from nape of neck, spreading upwards; better wrapping head up warmly. [*Sil.*] Flushes in face; violent pulsating. Supraorbital neuralgia; pains increase and decrease slowly. [*Stann.*] Bloody crusts in nose. Face red; burns, itches. Itching, redness and burning of nose.

Eyes.—Burning and redness of eyes. Pain and lachrymation on using eyes, with dancing and chromatic alterations of objects looked at.

Stomach.—Loss of appetite, aversion to meat, craves bread and beer. Food tasteless. Eructations after eating. Hiccough causes chest pains; cardialgia.

Abdomen.—Sticking in abdominal ring. Diarrhœa; *worse at night; continuous urging;* better towards morning. Burning in anus lasts a long time after stool. [*Ratanh.*] Uncomfortable fullness and swelling of abdomen.

Extremities.—Sciatica with œdema of ankle. Rheumatic pain in right shoulder. Rheumatism with diarrhœa. Gnawing as if in marrow of bones. Cramps in calves and soles. *Chronic spasms, particularly of ankle-joint.* Œdematous swelling. Icy-cold feet. Rheumatic pains, especially in joints. Veins of hands engorged.

Fever.—Heat, with aversion to uncover or undress.

Skin.—Moist, itching, burning eruption; better in open air, especially warm sunshine. *Sprains of ankle-joint, with œdema.* Violent perspiration at night.

Modalities.—*Better* immersing in *hot water; worse*, change of weather; from being quiet; when beginning to move; great sensitiveness to cold.

Relationship.—Compare: *Arnica; Ruta; Sil.; Baryta c.; Carbo.; Stront. jodat.* (arterio-sclerosis.) *Strontium brom.* (often gives excellent results where a bromide is indicated. Vomiting of pregnancy. Nervous dyspepsia. It is anti-fermentative and neutralizes excessive acidity.) *Stront. nit.* (Morbid cravings; headache and eczema behind ears.)

Dose.—Sixth trituration and thirtieth potency.

STROPHANTHUS HISPIDUS
(Kombe-seed)

Strophanthus is a muscle poison; it increases the contractile power of all striped muscles. Acts on the heart, *increasing the systole and diminishes the rapidity*. May be used with advantage to tone the heart, and run off dropsical accumulations. In small doses for weak heart; it feels enlarged. In mitral regurgitation, where œdema and dropsy have supervened. [*Digit.*] Strophantus occasions no gastric distress, has no cumulative effects, is a greater diuretic, and is safer for the aged, as it does not affect the vaso-motors. In pneumonia and in severe prostration from hæmorrhage after operations and acute diseases After the long use of stimulants; *irritable heart* of tabacco-smokers. Arterio-sclerosis; rigid arteries of aged. Restores tone to a *brittle* tissue, especially of the heart muscle and valves. Especially useful in failing compensation dependent upon fatty heart. Hives. Anæmia with palpitation and breathlessness. Exophthalmia goitre. Corpulent persons.

Head.—Temporal pains with double vision, impaired sight; brilliant eyes, flushed face. Senile vertigo.

Stomach.—Nausea with special disgust for alcohol and so aids in treatment of dipsomania. Seven drops of tincture.

Urinary.—Increased secretion; scanty and albuminous.

Female.—Menorrhagia; uterine hæmorrhage; uterus heavily congested. Aching pain through hips and thighs during climacteric.

Respiratory.—*Dyspnœa*, especially on ascending. Lungs congested. Œdema of lungs. Bronchial and cardiac asthma.

Heart.—Pulse quickened. Heart's action weak, rapid, irregular, due to muscular *debility;* and *insufficiency*. Cardiac pain.

Skin.—Urticaria, especially more chronic forms.

Extremities.—Swollen, dropsical. Anasarca.

Relationship.—Compare: *Digit.* (but is slower than *Strophant.* in its action); *Phos. ac.* (weak heart, irregular pulse, fluttering sensation in cardiac region, palpitation during sleep, fainting).

Dose.—Tincture and 6x potency. In more acute cases, five to ten drops of the tincture three times a day.

STRYCHNINUM

(Alkaloid of Nux Vomica)

Its primary function is to stimulate the motor centers and the reflex action of the spinal cord. Homœopathic to spasms of muscles, cramps from an undue reflex excitability of the cord, spasms of the bladder, etc. Strychnin stimulates the central nervous system, mental activities, special senses rendered more acute. Respiration increased. All reflexes are made more active. Stiffness in muscles and face and neck. Opisthotonos. Tetanic convulsions with opisthotonos. The muscles relax between paroxysms; worse slightest touch, sound, odor. Influences more directly the spinal cord and is less appropriate in visceral derangements than Nux. *Tetanus*. Explosive nervousness. The pains and sensations come *suddenly* and return at *intervals*.

Head.—Restless. *Over-irritability*. Full and bursting headache, with heat in eyes. Vertigo, with roaring in ears. Jerking of head forwards. Scalp sore. Itching of scalp and nape.

Eyes.—Hot, painful, protruding, staring. Pupils dilated. Sparks before eyes. Spasmodic contraction of ocular muscles; twitching and trembling of lids.

Ears.—Hearing very acute; burning, itching, and roaring in ears.

Face.—Pale, anxious, livid. Jaws stiffened; lower jaw spasmodically closed.

Throat.—Dry, contracted; feeling of a lump. Deglutition impossible. Burning along and spasms of œsophagus. Violent itching in roof of mouth.

Stomach.—Constant retching. Violent vomiting. Nausea of pregnancy.

Abdomen.—Sharp pain in abdominal muscles, griping pain in bowels.

Rectum.—Fæces discharged involuntarily during spasms. Very obstinate constipation.

Female.—Desire for coitus. [*Canth.; Camph.; Fl. ac.; Lach.; Phos.; Plat.*] Any touch on body excites a voluptuous sensation.

Respiratory.—*Spasm of muscles* about larynx. Excessive

dyspnœa. Sharp, contractive pains in muscles of chest. Persistent cough, recurring after influenza.

Back.—*Rigidity of cervical muscles.* Sharp pain in nape and down spine. Back stiff; violent jerks in spinal column. *Icy sensation down spine.*

Extremities.—Limbs stiff. Rheumatism with stiff joints. *Violent jerking, twitching, and trembling.* Tetanic convulsions and opisthotonos; spasms provoked by slightest touch and attempt to move. Shocks in the muscles. *Cramp-like pains.*

Fever.—Cold chills down spine. Perspiration in a stream down head and chest. Lower extremities cold.

Skin.—Itching of whole body, especially nose. Icy sensation down the spine.

Modalities.—*Worse*, morning; touch; noise; motion; after meals. *Better*, lying on back.

Relationship.—Compare: *Eucalyptus* (neutralizes ill effects of *Strychnin*). *Strych. ars.* (Paresis in the aged, relaxed musculature. Prostration. Psoriasis; chronic diarrhœa with paralytic symptoms: compensatory hypertrophy of heart with beginning fatty degeneration; marked dyspnœa when lying down; œdema of lower extremities, urine scanty, high specific gravity, heavily loaded with glucose. Diabetes. 6x trit.). *Strych. et Ferr. cit.* (chlorotic and paralytic conditions; dyspepsia, with vomiting of ingesta; 2x and 3x trit.); *Strychnin. nit.* (2x and 3x. Said to remove craving for alcohol. Use for two weeks); *Strychnin. sulph.* (Gastric atony); *Strych. valerin.* (exhaustion of brain-power; women of high nervous erethism; 2x trit.). Compare: *Cicuta; Arnica* (tetanus).

Dose.—Third to thirtieth potency. For non-homœopathic use, to produce its direct physiological effects in paralysis the dose will range from one-fiftieth to one-twentieth of a grain, repeated three times a day. Under twelve years of age, one-fiftieth to one two-hundredth of a grain. *Strych.*, hypodermically, is capable of arresting progressive muscular atrophy, and is a certain stimulant to the respiratory centers, and is useful in embarrassed breathing, in the course of pneumonia especially. Is an antidote to Chloral, used in asphyxia from gas and chloroform and early stages of Opium poisoning. Dose, one one-hundredth to one-sixtieth grain every three hours.

STRYCHNIA PHOSPHORICA
(Phosphate of Strychnin)

This drug acts through the cerebro-spinal system upon muscles, causing twitching, stiffness, weakness and loss of power; upon circulation, producing irregularity of pulse, and upon the mind, producing lack of control, *uncontrollable desire to laugh* and disinclination to use the brain. Very irregular pulse. Tachycardia. Rapid and weak pulse. Useful in chorea, hysteria, acute asthenia after acute fevers. Symptoms *worse* motion, *better* rest and in open air. An excellent remedy in anæmia of spinal cord; paralysis; burning, aching, and weakness of spine; pain extends to front of chest; tenderness on pressure in mid-dorsal region; cold, clammy feet; *hands and axillæ covered with clammy perspiration*. Atelectasis and break in the compensation of a hypertrophied heart; the beginning of fatty degeneration of the heart muscle. (Royal.)

Dose.—Third trituration.

SUCCINUM
(Electron. Amber)—(A Fossil Resin)

Nervous and hysterical symptoms. Asthma. Affections of spleen.

Head.—Fear of trains and close places. Headache, lachrymation, sneezing.

Respiratory.—Asthma, incipient phthisis, chronic bronchitis, pains in chest. Whooping-cough.

Relationship.—Compare: Do not confound with Ambergris (Ambra). *Succinic acid.* (Hay-fever. Paroxysmal sneezing, dropping of watery mucus from nostrils; asthma. Inflammation through respiratory tract; causing asthma, chest pains, etc.; itching of eyelids and canthi and nose worse drafts. Use 6 to 30th potency). Compare: *Arundo, Wyethia, Sabadilla, Sinapis.*

Dose.—Third trituration. Five drop doses of the oil.

SULFONAL
(A Coal-tar Product)

Vertigo of cerebral origin, cerebellar disease, ataxic symptoms and chorea, present a field for the homœopathic employment of this drug. *Profound weakness*, gone, faint feeling, and despondency. Loss of control of sphincter. Muscular incoordination.

Mind.—Mental confusion, incoherency, illusions; apathetic. *Alternation of happy, hopeful states with depression and weakness.* Extreme irritability.

Head.—Dropsy, stupid; pain on attempting to raise head. Double vision; heavy look about eyes; tinnitus, aphasia; *tongue as if paralyzed. Eyes bloodshot and restless.* Vertigo, unable to rise. Double vision; ptosis; tinnitus; dysphagia, difficult speech.

Urinary.—Albuminuria, with casts. Scanty. Pink color. Constant desire to urinate; scanty, brownish red. Hæmatoporphyrinuria.

Respiratory.—Congestion of lungs; stertorous breathing. Sighing dyspnœa.

Extremities.—Ataxic movements, *staggering gait;* cold, weak, trembling; legs seem too heavy. Extreme restlessness; muscular twitchings. Knee-jerks disappear. Stiffness and paralysis of both legs. Anæsthesia of legs.

Sleep.—Fidgety, wakeful, drowsy. Insomnia.

Skin.—Itching, bluish purpura. Erythema.

Relationship.—*Trional;* insomnia associated with physical excitement; (vertigo, loss of equilibrium, ataxia, nausea, vomiting, diarrhœa, stertorous breathing, cyanosis, tinnitus, hallucinations).

Dose.—Third trituration.

Non-Homœopathic Uses.—As a hypnotic. Dose, ten to thirty grains in hot water. Takes about two hours to act.

SULPHUR
(Sublimated Sulphur)

This is the great Hahnemannian anti-psoric. Its action is centrifugal—from within outward—having an elective affinity for the skin, where it produces heat and *burning*, with itching; made worse by heat of bed. Inertia and relaxation of fiber; hence feebleness of tone characterizes its symptoms. *Ebullitions of heat, dislike of water, dry and hard hair and skin, red orifices, sinking feeling at stomach about* 11 a. m., *and cat-nap sleep;* always indicate Sulphur homœopathically. *Standing* is the worst position for sulphur patients, it is always uncomfortable. Dirty, filthy people, prone to skin affections. Aversion to being washed. *When carefully-selected remedies fail to act, especially in acute diseases*, it frequently arouses the reactionary powers of the organism. *Complaints that relapse. General offensive character of discharge and exhalations*. Very red lips and face, flushing easily. Often great use in beginning the treatment of chronic cases and in finishing acute ones.

Mind.—Very forgetful. Difficult thinking. Delusions; thinks rags beautiful things—that he is immensely wealthy. Busy all the time. Childish peevishness in grown people. Irritable. Affections vitiated; *very selfish*, no regard for others. Religious melancholy. Averse to business; loafs—too lazy to arouse himself. Imagining giving wrong things to people, causing their death. Sulphur subjects are nearly always irritable, depressed, thin and weak, even with good appetite.

Head.- -Constant *heat on top of head*. [*Cup. sulph.; Graph.*? Heaviness and fullness, pressure in temples. Beating headache; worse, stooping, and with vertigo. Sick headache recurring periodically. Tinea capitis, dry form. *Scalp dry*, falling of hair; worse, washing. *Itching; scratching causes burning*.

Eyes.—*Burning* ulceration of margin of lids. Halo around lamp-light. Heat and *burning in eyes*. [*Ars.; Bell.*] Black motes before eyes. First stage of ulceration of cornea. Chronic ophthalmia, with much burning and itching. Parenchymatous keratitis. Cornea like ground glass.

Ears.—Whizzing in ears. Bad effects from the suppression of an otorrhœa. Oversensitive to odors. Deafness, preceded by exceedingly sensitive hearing; catarrhal deafness.

Nose.—Herpes across the nose. Nose stuffed indoors. Imaginary foul smells. *Alæ red and scabby.* *Chronic dry catarrh; dry scabs and readily bleeding.* Polypus and adenoids.

Mouth.—Lips dry, *bright red,* burning. *Bitter taste* in morning. Jerks through teeth. Swelling of gums; throbbing pain. Tongue white, with red tip and borders.

Throat.—Pressure as from a lump, as from a splinter, as of a hair. Burning, redness and dryness. Ball seems to rise and close pharynx.

Stomach.—Complete loss of, or excessive appetite. Putrid eructation. Food tastes too salty. Drinks much, eats little. *Milk disagrees.* Great desire for sweets. [*Arg. nit.*] *Great acidity,* sour eructation. Burning, painful, weight-like pressure. *Very weak and faint about* 11 a. m.; must have something to eat. Nausea during gestation. Water fills the patient up.

Abdomen.—Very sensitive to pressure; internal feeling of rawness and soreness. Movements as of something alive. [*Croc.; Thuj.*] Pain and soreness over liver. Colic after drinking.

Rectum.—Itching and burning of anus; piles dependent upon abdominal plethora. Frequent, unsuccessful desire; hard, knotty, insufficient. Child afraid on account of pain. *Redness around the anus,* with itching. *Morning diarrhœa, painless, drives out of bed,* with prolapsus recti. Hæmorrhoids, oozing and belching.

Urine.—Frequent micturition, especially at night. *Enuresis,* especially in scrofulous, untidy children. Burning in urethra during micturition, lasts long after. Mucus and pus in urine; *parts sore over which it passes.* *Must hurry,* sudden call to urinate. *Great quantities of colorless urine.*

Male.—Stitches in penis. Involuntary emissions. Itching of genitals when going to bed. Organs cold, relaxed and powerless.

Female.—Pudenda *itches.* *Vagina burns.* Much offensive perspiration. Menses too late, short, scanty, and difficult; thick, black, *acrid, making parts sore.* Menses preceded by headache or suddenly stopped. Leucorrhœa, burning, excoriating. Nipples cracked; smart and burn.

Respiratory.—Oppression and burning sensation in chest. *Difficult respiration; wants windows open.* Aphonia. Heat, throughout chest. Red, brown spots all over chest. Loose cough; worse talking, morning, greenish, purulent, sweetish expectoration. *Much rattling of mucus.* Chest feels heavy; stitches, with heart feeling too large and palpitating. *Pleuritic exudations.* Use Tinctura sulphuris. Stitching pains shooting through to the back, worse lying on back or breathing deeply. Flushes of heat in chest rising to head. *Oppression, as of a load on chest.* Dyspnœa in middle of night, relieved by sitting up. *Pulse more rapid in morning* than in evening.

Back.—Drawing pain between shoulders. Stiffness of nape. Sensation as if vertebræ glided over each other

Extremities.—Trembling of hands. *Hot, sweaty hands.* Rheumatic pain in left shoulder. Heaviness; paretic feeling. Rheumatic gout, with itching. *Burning in soles and hands at night.* Sweat in armpits, smelling like garlic. Drawing and tearing in arms and hands. Stiffness of knees and ankles. Cannot walk erect; *stoop-shouldered.* Ganglion.

Sleep.—Talks, jerks, and twitches during sleep. Vivid dreams. Wakes up singing. Wakes frequently, and becomes wide awake suddenly. *Catnaps;* slightest noise awakens. Cannot sleep between 2 and 5 a. m.

Fever.—*Frequent flashes of heat. Violent ebullitions of heat throughout entire body.* Dry skin and great thirst. Night sweat, on nape and occiput. Perspiration of single parts. Disgusting sweats. Remittent type.

Skin.—*Dry, scaly, unhealthy; every little injury suppurates.* Freckles. *Itching, burning; worse scratching and washing.* Pimply eruption, pustules, rhagades, hang-nails. Excoriation, especially in folds. [*Lyc.*] Feeling of a band around bones. Skin affections after local medication. *Pruritus,* especially from warmth, in evening, often recurs in spring-time, in damp weather.

Modalities.—*Worse,* at rest, when standing, *warmth in bed,* washing, bathing, in morning, 11 a. m., night, from alcoholic stimulants, periodically. *Better, dry, warm weather,* lying on right side, from drawing up affected limbs.

Relationship.—Complementary: *Aloe; Psorin.; Acon.; Pyrarara* (a fish caught in the Amazon, clinically used for various skin affections). Lepra, tuberculides, syphilides, varicosities, etc.

Compare: *Acon.* (Sulph. often follows in acute diseases); *Mercur.* and *Calcarea* are frequently useful *after* Sulphur, not before. Lyc.; Sep.; Sars.; Puls.; *Sulphur hydrogenisatum* (delirium, mania, asphyxia); *Sulphur terebinthinatum* (chronic rheumatic arthritis; chorea); *Tannic acid* (Nasal hæmorrhage; elongated uvula; gargle; constipation). *Magnes. artiflcialis* (great hunger in evening, profuse sweat on face, bruised pain in joints, rectal constriction after stool).

Magnetis polus Articus (anxious, *coldness of eyes as if a piece of ice lay in orbit*, increased flow of saliva, constipation, sopor, trembling, abdominal flatulence).

Magnetis polus Australis (dryness of lids, easy dislocation of ankle, *ingrowing toe-nails*, aching in patella, shooting in soles).

Compare in adenoids: *Agraphis*.

Dose.—Acts in all potencies from the lowest to the highest. Some of the best results are obtained from the higher, and not too frequent doses. The twelfth potency is a good one to begin treatment with, going higher or lower according to the susceptibility of the patient. In chronic diseases, 200th and upward. In *torpid* eruptions the *lowest* potencies.

SULPHUR IODATUM
(Iodide of Sulphur)

Obstinate skin affections, notably in *barber's itch* and *acne*. Weeping eczema.

Throat.—Uvula and tonsils enlarged and reddened. Swollen. Tongue thick. Parotid hypertrophied.

Skin.—Itching on ears, nose, and in urethra. Papular eruption on face. Cold-sores on lips. Boils on neck. Barber's itch. *Acne*. Lichen planus. Arms covered with itching rash. **Hair** feels as if erect.

Dose.—Third trituration.

SULPHURICUM ACIDUM
(Sulphuric Acid)

The "debility" common to acids shows itself here, especially in the digestive tract, giving a very relaxed feeling in the stomach, with craving for stimulants. *Tremor and weakness;* everything must be done in a hurry. *Hot flushes,* followed by perspiration, with trembling. Tendency to gangrene following mechanical injuries. Writer's cramp. Lead poisoning. Gastralgia and hypochlorrhydria. Purpura hæmorrhagia.

Mind.—Fretful, impatient. Unwilling to answer questions; hurried.

Head.—Right-sided neuralgia; painful shocks; skin feels pinched. Sensation as if brain was loose in forehead and falling from side to side. [*Bell.; Rhus.*] Concussion of brain where skin is cold, body bathed in cold sweat. Compressive pain in side of occiput; *relieved by holding the hands near the head.* Pain of outer parts, as if there were subcutaneous ulceration; painful to touch. *Thrust in right temple as if plug were pressed in.*

Eyes.—Intra-ocular hæmorrhage following traumatism. Great chemosis of conjunctiva, with aching and sharp pain.

Mouth.—Aphthæ; gums bleed readily. Offensive breath. Pyorrhœa.

Stomach.—Heartburn; *sour eructations; sets teeth on edge.* [*Robin.*] *Craving for alcohol. Water causes coldness of stomach;* must be mixed with liquors. *Relaxed feeling in stomach.* Averse to smell of coffee. Sour vomiting. Desire for fresh food. *Hiccough.* Coldness of stomach relieved by applied heat. Nausea with chilliness.

Abdomen.—Weak feeling, with dragging into the hips and small of back. *Feeling as if hernia would protrude,* especially left side.

Rectum.—Piles; oozing dampness. Rectum feels as if it had a big ball. Diarrhœa, fetid, black, with sour odor of body, and empty faint feeling in abdomen.

Female.—Menstruation early and profuse. Erosion of cervix in the aged; easily bleeding. Acrid, burning leucorrhœa, often of bloody mucus.

Respiratory.—Respiration rapid with shooting in cervical muscles and movement of wings of nose; *larynx moves up and down violently.* Bronchitis in children with short, teasing cough.

Extremities.—Cramp-like paralytic contraction in arms, hands; jerking of fingers while writing.

Skin.—Bad effects from mechanical injuries, with bruises and livid skin. Ecchymosis. Petechiæ. *Purpura hæmorrhagica.* Livid, red, itching blotches. Hæmorrhage of black blood from all outlets. Cicatrices turn red and blue and become painful. Chilblains with gangrenous tendency. Carbuncles, boils and other staphylococcic and streptococcic infections.

Modalities.—*Worse,* from excess of heat or cold in forenoon and evening. *Better,* from warmth, and lying on affected side.

Relationship.—Complementary: *Puls.*

Compare: *Arn.; Calend.; Led.; Sep.; Calc.*

Dose.—Sulphuric acid mixed with three parts of alcohol, ten to fifteen drops three times daily for several weeks, has been successfully used to subdue the craving for liquor. For homœopathic purposes second to thirtieth potency.

SULPHUROSUM ACIDUM

(Sulphurous Acid. H_2SO_3)

Sulphurous acid, (tonsillitis (as a spray), acne rosacea, *ulcerative stomatitis,* pityriasis versicolor).

Head.—Anxious, furious, disposed to fight. Headache better by vomiting. Ringing in ears.

Mouth.—Ulcerative inflammation of mouth. Tongue red or bluish-red. Coated.

Stomach.—Loss of appetite. Obstinate constipation.

Respiratory.—Persistent choking cough with copious expectoration. Hoarseness, constriction of chest. Difficult breathing.

Female.—Fluor albus. Debility.

Dose.—As a spray in tonsillitis. According to Ringer, ten to fifteen minims taken ten minutes before each meal will remedy pyrosis and prevent fermentation and flatulence. It also removes thrush. Homœopathically, third attenuation.

SUMBUL—FERULA SUMBUL
(Musk-root)

Has many hysterical and nervous symptoms, and is of use in neuralgic affections and anomalous, functional, cardiac disorders. *Numbness on becoming cold.* Numbness on left side. *Insomnia* of delirium tremens (fifteen drops of tincture). Sensation as if water dropped down spine. Asthma. A tissue remedy for sclerosed arteries.

Head.—Emotional and fidgety. Dull in morning, clear in evening. Mistakes in writing and adding. Comedones. Tenacious, yellow, mucus in nose.

Throat.—Choking constriction; constant swallowing. Belching of gas from stomach. Spasm of pharyngeal muscles. Tenacious mucus in throat.

Heart.—*Nervous palpitation.* Neuralgia around left breast and left hypochondriac region. *Cardiac asthma.* Aching in left arm, heavy, numb and weary. Loses breath on any exertion. Pulse irregular.

Female.—Ovarian neuralgia. *Abdomen full, distended, and painful.* Climacteric flushes.

Urinary.—*Oily pellicle on surface of urine.*

Modalities.—*Worse,* active exercise; left side.

Relationship.—Compare: *Asaf.; Mosch.*

Dose.—Tincture, to third potency. Dr. W. McGeorge advises the 2x every 3 hours for arterio-sclerosis.

SYMPHORICARPUS RACEMOSA
(Snowberry)

This drug is highly recommended for the persistent *vomiting of pregnancy*. Gastric disturbances, fickle appetite, nausea, waterbrash, bitter taste. *Constipation.* Nausea during menstruation. Nausea, *worse any motion. Averse to all food. Better,* lying on back.

Dose.—Second and third potency.
200th has proved curative.

SYMPHYTUM
(Comfrey—Knitbone)

The root contains a crystalline solid, that stimulates the growth of epithelium on ulcerated surfaces. It may be administered internally in the treatment of gastric and duodenal ulcers. Also in gastralgia, and externally in pruritus ani. Injuries to sinews, tendons and the periosteum. Acts on joints generally. Neuralgia of knee.

Of great use in wounds penetrating to perineum and bones, *and in non-union of fractures;* irritable stump after amputation, irritable bone at point of fracture. Psoas abscess. *Pricking pain* and soreness of periosteum.

Head.—Pain in occiput, top and forehead; changing places. Pain comes down bone of nose. Inflammation of inferior maxillary bone, hard, red, swelling.

Eye.—*Pain in eye after a blow of an obtuse body.* For traumatic injuries of the eyes no remedy equals this.

Relationship.—Compare: *Arn.; Calc phos.*

Dose.—Tincture.

Externally as a dressing for sores and ulcers and pruritus ani.

SYPHILINUM
(The Syphilitic Virus—A Nosode)

Utter prostration and debility in the morning.

Shifting rheumatic pains. Chronic eruptions and rheumatism.

Ichthyosis. Syphilitic affections. Pains from darkness to daylight; decrease and increase gradually. Hereditary tendency to alcoholism. *Ulceration of* mouth, nose, genitals, skin. *Succession of abscesses.*

Mind.—Loss of memory; remembers everything previous to his illness. Apathetic; *feels as if going insane or being paralyzed. Fears the night,* and the suffering from exhaustion on awakening. Hopeless; *despairs of recovery.*

Head.—Linear pains from temple across, or from eyes backward; cause sleeplessness and delirium at night. *Falling of the hair.* Pain in bones of head. Top of head feels as if coming off. Stupefying cephalalgia.

Eyes.—*Chronic, recurrent, phlyctenular inflammation of cornea;* successive crops of phyctenules and abrasions of epithelial layer of cornea; photophobia intense, lachrymation profuse. Lids swollen; *pain intense at night;* ptosis. Tubercular iritis. Diplopia; one image seen below the other. Feeling of cold air blowing on eye. [*Fluor. ac.*]

Ears.—Caries of ossicles in ear of syphilitic origin.

Nose.—Caries of nasal bones, hard palate and septum, with perforation; ozæna.

Mouth.—Teeth decay at gum; edges serrated, dwarfed. Tongue coated, teeth-indented; deep longitudinal cracks. Ulcers smart and burn. *Excessive flow of saliva; it runs out of mouth when sleeping.*

Stomach.—*Craves alcohol.*

Rectum.—Feels tied up with strictures. Enemas very painful. Fissures, prolapse.

Extremities.—Sciatica; worse at night; better about daybreak. Rheumatism of shoulder-joint, at insertion of deltoid. Run-around. Severe pain in long bones. Redness and rawness between toes. [*Sil.*] Rheumatism, muscles are caked in hard knot or lumps. *Always washing the hands.* Indolent ulcers. Muscles contracted in hard knots.

Female.—Ulcers on labia. Leucorrhœa *profuse, thin, watery, acrid,* with sharp, knife-pain in ovaries.

Respiratory.—Aphonia; chronic asthma in summer, wheezing and rattling. [*Tart. emet.*] Cough dry, hard; worse at night; windpipe sensitive to touch. [*Lach.*] Lancinating pains from base of heart to apex at night.

Skin.—Reddish-brown eruption, with a disagreeable odor. Extreme emaciation.

Relationship.—Compare: *Merc.; Kal. hyd.; Nit. ac.; Aur.; Alum.*

Modalities.—*Worse,* at night, sundown to sunrise, seashore, in summer. *Better,* inland and mountains, during day, moving about slowly.

Dose.—The highest potencies only, and in infrequent doses.

SYZYGIUM JAMBOLANUM
(Jambol Seeds—Enlexing, active principle)

Has an immediate effect of increasing the blood sugar, glycosuria results.

A most useful remedy in diabetes mellitus. *No other remedy causes in so marked degree the diminution and disappearance of sugar in the urine. Prickly heat in upper part of the body;* small red pimples itch violently. Great thirst, weakness, emaciation. Very large amount of urine, specific gravity high. Old ulcers of skin. Diabetic ulceration. The seeds powdered, ten grains three times a day; also, the tincture.

Relationship.—Compare: *Insulin*—An aqueous solution of an active principle from pancreas which affects sugar metabolism. If administered at suitable intervals in diabetes mellitus, the blood sugar is maintained at a normal level and the urine remains free of sugar. Overdosage is followed by weakness and fatigue and tremulousness and profuse sweating.

TABACUM
(Tobacco)

The symptomatology of Tabacum is exceedingly well marked. The nausea, giddiness, death-like pallor, vomiting, icy coldness, and sweat, with the intermittent pulse, are all most characteristic. Has marked antiseptic qualities, antidotal to cholera germs. Complete prostration of the entire muscular system. Collapse. Gastralgia, enteralgia, *seasickness*, cholera infantum; cold, but *wants abdomen uncovered*. Vigorous peristaltic activity. diarrhœa. Produces high tension and arteriosclerosis of the coronary arteries. Should prove the most homœopathic drug for angina pectoris, with coronaritis and high tension (Cartier). Constriction of throat, chest, bladder, rectum. Pallor, breathlessness, hard-cordlike pulse.

Mind.—Sensation of excessive wretchedness. *Very despondent.* Forgetful. Discontented.

Head.—Vertigo *on opening eyes;* sick headache, with deathly nausea; periodical. Tight feeling as from a band. Sudden pain, as if struck by a hammer. Nervous deafness. Secretion from eyes, nose and mouth increased.

Eyes.—Dim sight; sees as through a veil; strabismus. *Amaurosis;* muscæ volitantes. Central scotoma. Rapid blindness without lesion, followed by venous hyperæmia and atrophy of optic nerve.

Face.—Pale, blue, pinched, sunken, collapsed, covered with cold sweat. [*Ars.; Verat.*] Freckles.

Throat.—Nasopharyngitis and tracheitis, *hemming,* morning cough, sometimes with vomiting. Hoarseness of public speakers.

Stomach.—Incessant nausea; worse, smell of tobacco smoke [*Phos.*]; vomiting on least motion, sometimes of fecal matter. *during pregnancy with much spitting. Seasickness; terrible faint, sinking feeling at pit of stomach.* Sense of relaxation of stomach, with nausea. [*Ipec.*] Gastralgia; pain from cardiac end extending to left arm.

Abdomen.—Cold. *Wants abdomen uncovered.* It lessens the nausea and vomiting. Painful distension. Incarcerated hernia.

Rectum.—Constipation; rectum paralyzed, prolapsed. Diarrhœa, sudden, watery, with nausea and vomiting, prostration, and cold sweat; discharges look like sour milk, thick, curdled, watery. Rectal tenesmus.

Urinary.—Renal colic; violent pain along ureter, left side.

Heart.—Palpitation when lying on left side. Pulse intermits, feeble, imperceptible. Angina pectoris, pain in præcordial region. Pain radiates from center of sternum. Tachycardia. Bradycardia. *Acute dilatation* caused by shock or violent physical exertion (Royal).

Respiratory.—Difficult, violent constriction of chest. Præcordial oppression, with palpitation and pain between shoulders. Cough followed by hiccough. Cough dry, teasing, must take a swallow of cold water [*Caust.; Phos.*]. Dyspœna, with tingling down left arm when lying on left side.

Extremities.—Legs and hands icy cold; limbs tremble. Paralysis following apoplexy. [*Plumb.*] Gait shuffling, unsteady. Feebleness of arms.

Sleep.—Insomnia with dilated heart, with cold, clammy skin and anxiety.

Fever.—Chills, with *cold sweat.*

Modalities.—*Worse,* opening eyes; evening; extremes of heat and cold. *Better,* uncovering, open fresh air.

Relationship.—Compare: *Hydrobromic acid; Camph.; Verat.; Ars.* Compare: *Nicotinum* (Alternate tonic and clonic spasms, followed by general relaxation and trembling; nausea, cold sweat, and speedy collapse; head drawn back, contraction of eyelids and masseter muscles; muscles of neck and back rigid; hissing respiration from spasm of laryngeal and bronchial muscles).

Antidote: Vinegar; sour apples. *Camphor* in the physiological antagonist. *Ars.* (chewing tobacco); *Ign.;* (smoking); *Sep.* (neuralgia and dyspepsia); *Lycop.* (impotency); *Nux* (bad taste due to tobacco); *Calad.* and *Plantag.* (cause aversion to tobacco); *Phosph.* (tobacco heart, sexual weakness).

Dose.—Third to thirtieth and higher potencies.

TANACETUM VULGARE
(Tansy)

Abnormal lassitude. Nervous and tired feeling. "Half dead, half alive feeling" all over. Of use in chorea and reflex spasms (worms). Said to be a specific against effects of poison ivy.

Head.—Heavy, dull, confused. Headache with least exertion.

Mental.—Irritable, sensitive to noise. Mental fatigue nausea and vertigo, worse in a closed room.

Ears.—Roaring and ringing; voice sounds strange; *ears seem to close up suddenly.*

Abdomen.—Pain in bowels; relieved by stool. Desire for stool immediately after eating. *Dysentery.*

Female.—Dysmenorrhœa, with bearing-down pains, tenderness, drawing in groins. Menses suppressed; later, profuse.

Respiratory.—Hurried, labored, stertorous respiration. Frothy mucus obstructs the air-passages.

Relationship.—Compare: *Cimicif.; Cina; Absinth. Nux* follows well.

Dose.—Tincture, to third potency.

TANNIC ACID
Tannin—(Digallic Acid)

Mostly used locally against excessive secretion of mucous membranes, to contract tissue and check hæmorrhage. In Osmidrosis, corrects fetor of the perspiration. Obstinate nervous coughs. Hæmaturia. Obstinate constipation. Pain in abdomen, sensitive to pressure. Intestines can be felt like cylindrical enlargements. One-half per cent solution.

Relationship.—Gallic acid q. v.

TARENTULA CUBENSIS
(Cuban Spider)

A toxæmic medicine, septic conditions. *Diphtheria.* Adapted to the most severe types of inflammation and pain, early and persistent prostration. Various forms of malignant suppuration. Purplish hue and burning, stinging pains. Bubo. It is the remedy for *pain of death; soothes the last struggles. Pruritus, especially about genitals.* Restless feet. Intermittent septic chills. Bubonic plague. As a curative and preventive remedy especially during the period of invasion.

Head.—Dizziness after heat and hot perspiration. Dull ache on top of head. Shooting pain through left eye across frontal region.

Gastric.—Stomach feels hard, sore. Loss of appetite, except for breakfast.

Back.—Itches across kidney region.

Extremities.—Hands tremble, turgid with blood.

Urinary.—Retention. Cannot hold urine on coughing.

Skin.—Red spots and pimples. Feels puffed all over. *Carbuncles*, burning, stinging pains. Purplish hue. Gangrene. Abscesses, where pain and inflammation predominate. Scirrhus of breasts. "Senile" ulcers.

Sleep.—Drowsiness. Sleep restless. Sleep prevented by harsh cough.

Relationship.—Compare: *Ars.; Pyrog.; Crotal.; Echin.; Anthrac.; Bellad.; Apis*.

Modalities.—*Better*, smoking. *Worse*, night.

Dose.—Sixth to thirtieth potency.

TARENTULA HISPANIA
(Spanish Spider)

Remarkable nervous phenomena; hysteria with chlorosis; *chorea*, dysmenorrhœa, spinal irritability. Bladder tenesmus. *Constriction* sensations. Formication. *Extreme restlessness;* must keep in constant motion even though walking aggravates. Hysterical epilepsy. Intense sexual excitement.

Mind.—Sudden alteration of mood. Foxy. Destructive impulses; *moral relaxation*. Must constantly busy herself or walk. *Sensitive to music*. Averse to company, but wants some one present. Ungrateful, discontented. Guided by whims.

Head.—Intense pain, as if thousands of needles were pricking into brain. *Vertigo*. Wants hair brushed or head rubbed.

Male.—Sexual excitement; lasciviousness reaching almost to insanity; seminal emissions.

Heart.—Palpitation; præcordial anguish, sensation as if heart twisted and turned around.

Female.—Vulva dry and hot, with much itching. Profuse menstruation, with frequent erotic spasms. *Pruritus vulvæ; nymphomania*. Dysmenorrhœa, with very sensitive ovaries.

Extremities.—Weakness of legs; choreic movements. Numbness of legs. Multiple sclerosis, with trembling. *Twitching and jerking*. Yawning with uneasiness of legs, must move them constantly. Extraordinary contractions and movements.

Modalities.—*Worse*, motion, contact, noise. *Better*, in open air, *music*, bright colors, rubbing affected parts. *Worse*, seeing others in trouble.

Relationship.—Compare: *Agar.; Ars.; Cupr.; Mag. phos.*
Antidotes: *Lach*.

Dose.—Sixth to thirtieth potency.

TARACUM
(Dandelion)

For gastric headaches, bilious attacks, with characteristically mapped tongue and jaundiced skin. Cancer of bladder. Flatulence. *Hysterical tympanites*.

Head.—Sensation of great heat on top of head. *Sterno-mastoid* muscle very painful to touch.

Mouth.—Mapped tongue. Tongue covered with a white film; feels raw; comes off in patches, leaving *red, sensitive spots*. Loss of appetite. Bitter taste and eructations. Salivation.

Abdomen.—Liver enlarged and indurated. Sharp stitches in left side. Sensation of bubbles bursting in bowels. Tympanites. Evacuation difficult.

Extremities.—Very restless limbs. *Neuralgia of knee; better, pressure.* Limbs painful to touch.

Fever.—Chilliness after eating, worse drinking; *finger tips cold. Bitter taste.* Heat without thirst, in face, *in toes.* Sweat on falling asleep.

Skin.—*Profuse night-sweats.*

Modalities.—*Worse,* resting, lying down, sitting. *Better.* touch.

Relationship.—Compare: *Choline,* a constituent of Taraxacum root, has given encouraging results in the treatment of cancer. Choline is closely related to *Neurin,* it is the "Cancronie" of Prof. Adamkiewicz (E. Schlegel.) *Bry.; Hydrast.; Nux. Tela aranea* (nervous asthma and sleeplessness).

Dose.—Tincture, to third potency. In cancer 1-2 drams fluid extract.

TARTARICUM ACIDUM
(Tartaric Acid)

Found in grapes, pineapple, sorrel and other fruits. It is an antiscorbutic antiseptic, stimulating the mucous and salivary secretions.

Dullness and lassitude. Great weakness, with diarrhœa, with dry and brown tongue. Pain in heels. [*Phytol.*]

Stomach.—Excessive thirst, continued vomiting burning in throat and stomach. Dyspepsia with copious secretion of mucus.

Abdomen.—Pain around umbilicus and region of loins. Stool color of coffee-grounds (worse at night), with brown and dry tongue, and dark-green vomiting.

Dose.—Third trituration. The pure acid 10-30 grains dissolved in water.

TAXUS BACCATA
(Yew)

In pustular diseases of skin and night-sweats. Also in gout and chronic rheumatism.

Head.—Supra-orbital and temporal pain on right side, with lachrymation. Pupils dilated. Face puffy and pale.

Stomach.—*Saliva hot*, acrid. Nausea. Pain in pit of stomach and region of navel. After eating, cough. Feeling of pins and needles at pit of stomach; of *emptiness*, must eat frequently (compare the coniferæ).

Skin.—Large, flat, itching pustules. Badly smelling night-sweats. Podagra. Erysipelas.

Dose.—Tincture, to third potency.

TELLURIUM
(The Metal Tellurium)

Marked skin (herpes circinatus), spinal, eye and ear symptoms. Very *sensitive back*. Pains all over body. Offensive discharges. Slow development of symptoms. [*Radium.*] Sacral and sciatic pains.

Head.—Neglectful and forgetful. Pain in left side of head and in forehead above left eye. Distortion and twitching of left facial muscles; when speaking left angle of mouth drawn upwards and to left. Fear of being touched in sensitive places. Congestion to head and nape of neck, followed by weakness and faintness in stomach. Itching of scalp; red spots.

Eyes.—Lids *thickened, inflamed*, itching. Pterygium; pustular conjunctivitis. Cataract, following ocular lesions; aids the absorption of infiltrations in iris and choroid.

Ears.—*Eczema behind ear. Catarrh of middle ear, discharge acrid, smells like fish-pickle. Itching, swelling, throbbing in meatus.* Deafness.

Nose.—Coryza, lachrymation and hoarseness; better in open air. [*Cepa.*] Obstructed; hawks salty phlegm from posterior nares.

Stomach.—Craving for apples. Empty and weak feeling. Heartburn.

Rectum.—Prutitus ani et perinei after every stool.

Back.—Pain in sacrum. *Pain from last cervical to fifth dorsal vertebra*, very sensitive; worse touch. [*Chin. s.; Phosph.*] *Sciatica;* worse right side, *coughing, straining*, and at night, with sensitive vertebral column. *Contraction of tendons in bends of knees.*

Skin.—Itching of hands and feet. Herpetic spots; *ringworm.* [*Tuberc.*] *Ring-shape lesions*, offensive odors from affected parts. Barber's itch. Stinging in skin. *Fetid exhalations.* [*Sulph.*] Offensive foot-sweat. Eczema, back of ears and occiput. Circular patches of eczema.

Modalities.—*Worse*, while at rest at night, cold weather, from friction, coughing, laughing, lying on painful side, touch.

Relationship.—Compare: *Radium; Selenium; Tetradymite* —crystals from Georgia and North Carolina containing *Bismuth, Tellurium* and *Sulphur*—(coccygodynia, ulceration of nails; pains in hands, in small spots, ankles, heels, and tendo-Achilles); *Sep.; Ars.; Rhus.*

Dose.—Sixth potency and higher. Takes long time to develop its action, which is very prolonged.

TEREBINTHINA
(Turpentine)

Has a selective affinity for *bleeding mucous surfaces*. Tympanites and urinary symptoms very marked. Inflammation of kidneys, with hæmorrhages—dark, passive, fetid. Bright's disease preceded by dropsy (Goullon). Drowsiness and strangury. Coma. *Unbroken chilblains*.

Head.—Dull pain like from a band around the head. [*Carb. ac.*] Vertigo, with vanishing of vision. Disturbed sense of equilibrium. Tired and difficult concentration of thoughts. Cold in head with sore nostrils with disposition to bleed.

Eyes.—Ciliary neuralgia over right eye. Intense pain in eye and side of head. Amblyopia from alcohol.

Ears.—Own voice sounds unnatural; humming as of a seashell, talking loudly is painful. Otalgia.

TEREBINTHINA

Mouth.—Tongue *dry, red sore, shining;* burning in tip, with prominent papillæ. [*Arg. n.; Bell.; Kali b.; Nux m.*] Breath cold, foul. Choking sensation in throat. Stomatitis. Dentition.

Stomach.—Nausea and vomiting; heat in epigastric region.

Abdomen.—*Enormous distention.* Diarrhœa; stools watery, greenish, fetid, bloody. Pain before flatus with and relief after stool. Hæmorrhage from bowels. Worms; lumbrici. Abdominal dropsy; pelvic peritonitis. Fainting after every stool. Entero-colitis, with hæmorrhage and ulceration of bowels.

Urinary.—*Strangury, with bloody urine.* Scanty, suppressed, *odor of violets.* Urethritis, with painful erections. [*Canthar.*] Inflamed kidneys following any acute disease. Constant tenesmus.

Female.—Intense *burning in uterine region.* Metritis; puerperal peritonitis. Metrorrhagia with burning in uterus.

Respiratory.—Difficult breathing; lungs feel distended; hæmoptysis. Bloody expectoration.

Heart.—Pulse rapid, small, thready, intermittent.

Back.—*Burning pain in region of kidneys.* Drawing in right kidney extending to hip.

Skin.—Acne. Erythema; itching pustular, vesicular eruption; urticaria. Purpura, ecchymosis, dropsies. Scarlatina. Chilblains; with excessive itching and pulsative pains. Aching soreness of the muscles.

Fever.—Heat, with violent thirst, dry tongue, profuse cold, clammy sweat. Typhoid with tympanites, hæmorrhages, stupor, delirium. Prostration.

Relationship.—Compare: *Alumen; Secale; Canth.; Nit. ac. Terebene* 1x; (chronic bronchitis and winter coughs; subacute stages of inflammation of respiratory tract. Loosens secretion, relieves tightened feeling, makes expectoration easy). *Neurotic coughs.* Huskiness of public speakers, and singers. Cystitis when urine is alkaline and offensive.)

Ononis - spinosa—Rest Harrow—(Diuretic, Lithontriptic. Chronic nephritis; diuretic effects like *Juniper;* calculus nosebleed, worse washing face).

Antidote: *Phos.*

Dose.—First to sixth potency.

TEUCRIUM MARUM
(Cat-thyme)

Nasal and rectal symptoms marked. *Polypi*. Affections of children. Suitable after too much medicine has been taken. Oversensitiveness. *Desire to stretch*. A remedy of first importance in chronic nasal catarrh with atrophy; large, offensive crusts and clinkers. *Ozæna. Loss of sense of smell.*

Head.—Excited, tremulous feeling. Frontal pain; worse, stooping. Strengthens brain after delirium tremens.

Eyes.—Smarting in canthi; lids red and puffy; tarsal tumor. [*Staph.*]

Ears.—Hissing and ringing otalgia.

Nose.—Catarrhal condition of both anterior and posterior nostrils. *Mucous polypus*. Chronic catarrh; *discharge of large, irregular clinkers*. Foul breath. *Crawling in nostrils*, with lachrymation and sneezing. Coryza, with stoppage of nostrils.

Stomach.—Vomiting of large quantities of dark-green masses. Constant hiccough, attended with pain in back. Unnatural appetite. Hiccough on eating, after nursing.

Respiratory.—Dry cough, tickling in trachea; *mouldy taste in throat* when hawking up mucus, expectoration profuse.

Extremities.—Affection of finger-tips and joints of toes. Tearing pains in arms and legs. *Pain in toe-nails*, as if they had grown into flesh.

Rectum.—*Itching of anus, and constant irritation in the evening in bed. Ascarides, with nightly restlessness*. Crawling in rectum after stool.

Sleep.—Restless, with twitching, choking, and starting up frightened.

Skin.—Itching causes tossing about all night. Very dry skin. Suppurating grooves in the nails.

Relationship.—Compare: *Teucrium scorodonia*—Wood-sage (in tuberculosis with muco-purulent expectoration; dropsy; orchitis and *tuberculous epidymitis; especially* in young, thin individuals with tuberculosis of lungs, glands; bones and urogenitals, 3x). *Cina; Ignat.; Sang.; Sil.*

Dose.—First to sixth potency. Locally for polypi, dry powder.

THALLIUM
(The Metal Thallium)

Thallium seems to influence the endocrines, especially the thyroid and adrenalin. Most horrible neuralgic, spasmodic, shooting pains. Muscular atrophy. Tremors. Relieves the violent pains in locomotor ataxia. *Paralysis of lower limbs.* Pain in stomach and bowels, like electric shocks. Paraplegia. *Alopecia* following acute, exhausting diseases. Night sweats. Polyneuritis. Dermal trophic lesions.

Extremities.—*Trembling. Paralytic feeling.* Lancinating pains, like electric shocks. Very tired. Chronic myelitis. Numbness in fingers and toes, with extension up lower extremities, involving lower abdomen and perineum. *Paralysis of lower limbs.* Cyanosis of extremities. Formication, beginning in fingers and extending through pelvis, perineum and inner thighs to feet.

Relationship.—Compare: *Lathyr.; Caust.; Arg. nit.; Plumbum.*

Dose.—Lower trituration to thirtieth potency.

THASPIUM AUREUM—ZIZIA
(Meadow Parsnip)

Hysteria, epilepsy, chorea, hypochondirasis, come within the sphere of this remedy.

Mind.—Suicidal; depressed; laughing and weeping moods alternate.

Head.—Pressure on top, in right temple, associated with backache.

Male.—Great lassitude following coitus. Sexual power increased.

Female.—Intermittent neuralgia of left ovary. Acrid, profuse leucorrhœa, with retarded menses.

Respiratory.—Dry cough, with stitches in chest. Dyspnœa.

Extremities.—Unusual tired feeling. *Chorea, especially during sleep. Fidgety legs.* [*Tarant.*] Lameness in arms and spasmodic twitching.

Modalities.—Worse, *during sleep*.

Relationship.—Compare: *Agar.; Stram.; Tarant.; Cicuta; Æthusa*.

Dose.—Tincture, to third potency.

THEA
(Tea)

Nervous sleeplessness, heart troubles, palpitation, and dyspepsia of old tea-drinkers. Produces most of the sick headaches Tabacum antidotal (Allen).

Head.—Temporary mental exaltation. Ill-humored. Sick headache radiating from one point. Sleepless and restless. Hallucinations of hearing. Cold damp feeling at back of head.

Stomach.—Sinking sensation at epigastrium. *Faint, gone feeling*. [*Sep.; Hyd.; Oleand.*] Craves acids. Sudden production of wind in large quantities.

Abdomen.—Borborygmi. Liability to hernia.

Female.—Soreness and tenderness in ovaries.

Heart.—Anxious oppression. Præcordial distress. Palpitation; unable to lie on left side. Fluttering. Pulse rapid, irregular, intermittent.

Sleep.—Sleepy in daytime; sleepiness at night, with vascular excitement and restlessness, and dry skin. Horrible dreams cause no horror.

Modalities.—*Worse*, night, on walking in open air, after meals. *Better* warmth; warm bath.

Relationship.—Antidote: *Kali hypophos.; Thuja; Ferr.; Kali hyd*. (Material doses for tea-taster's cough.)

Dose.—Third to thirtieth potency.

Theine ¼-½ grain hypodermically for sciatica and supra-orbital neuralgia.

THERIDION
(Orange-spider)

Nervous hyperæsthesia. Has affinity for the tubercular diathesis. Vertigo, sick headache, peculiar pain around heart region, phthisis florida, scrofula have all been treated successfully with this remedy. *Sensitive to noise; it penetrates the* body, *especially teeth*. Noises seem to strike on painful spots over the body. Rachitis, caries, necrosis. Phthisis, stitch high up in left apex. [*Anthrax.*] Where the indicated remedy does not hold long.

Mind.—Restless; finds pleasure in nothing. Time passes too quickly.

Head.—Pain worse anyone walking over floor. *Vertigo, with nausea and vomiting on least motion*, particularly when closing eyes.

Eyes.—Luminous vibrations before eyes; sensitive to light. Pressure behind eyeballs. Throbbing over left eye.

Nose.—Discharge yellowish, thick, offensive; ozæna. [*Puls.; Thuja.*]

Stomach.—Seasickness. Nausea and vomiting when closing eyes and on motion. [*Tabac.*] Stinging pain on left side over anterior aspect of spleen. Burning in liver region.

Respiratory.—Pain in upper left chest. [*Myrt.; Pix.; Anis.*] *Pain in left floating ribs. Cardiac anxiety and pain.* Pinching in left pectoral muscle.

Back.—Sensitiveness between vertebræ; avoids pressure on spine. Stinging pains.

Skin.—*Stinging thrusts everywhere.* Sensitive skin in thighs. Itching sensations.

Modalities.—*Worse*, touch; pressure; on shipboard; riding in carriage; closing eyes; jar; noise; coitus; left side.

Dose.—Thirtieth potency.

THIOSINAMINUM—RHODALLIN

(A Chemical Derived from Oil of Mustard-seed)

A resolvent, externally and internally, for *dissolving scar tissue*, tumors, enlarged glands; lupus, strictures, adhesions. Ectropion, opacities of cornea, cataract, ankylosis, fibroids, scleroderma. Noises in ear. Suggested by Dr. A. S. Hard for retarding old age. A remedy for Tabes dorsalis, improving the lightning pains. Gastric, vesicle and rectal crises. Stricture of rectum, 2 grains twice daily.

Ear.—Arterio-sclerotic *vertigo*. *Tinnitus*. Catarrhal deafness with cicatricial thickening. Subacute suppurative otitis media, formation of fibrous bands impeding free movement of the ossicles. Thickened drum. Deafness due to some fibrous change in the nerve.

Dose.—Inject under skin, or, into the lesion a 10 per cent. solution in glycerine and water, 15-30 drops twice a week. Internally in capsules ½ grain daily. Obstinate arterio-sclerotic ailments in doses of ½ grain, never more, 3 times a day. Vertigo and arthritis (Bartlett). 2x attenuation.

THLASPI BURSA PASTORIS—CAPSELLA
(Shepherd's Purse)

Is an anti-hæmorrhagic and anti-uric-acid remedy. Albuminuria during gestation. Chronic neuralgia. Renal and vesical irritation. Hæmorrhage from uterine fibroid with aching in back or general bruised soreness. Aching between scapulæ. Uterine hæmorrhage, with cramps and expulsion of clots. Craves buttermilk. Effects of suppressed uterine disease. (Burnett.)

Head.—Eyes and face puffy. Frequent epistaxis. Vertigo; worse, rising. Frontal pain; worse toward evening. Scaly eruption behind ears. Tongue white, coated. Mouth and lips cracked. Sharp pain over right eye drawing eye upwards.

Nose.—Bleeding in nasal operations. Especially passive hæmorrhage.

Male.—Spermatic cord sensitive to concussion of walking or riding.

Female.—Metrorrhagia; too frequent and copious menses. Hæmorrhage, with violent uterine colic. Every alternate period very profuse. Leucorrhœa before and after menses; bloody, dark, offensive; *stains indelibly*. *Sore pain in womb on rising*. Scarcely recovers from one period before another begins.

Urinary.—Frequent desire; urine *heavy*, phosphatic. Chronic cystitis. Dysuria and spasmodic retention. Hæmaturia. Accumulation of gravel. Renal colic. *Brick-dust sediment*. Urethritis; urine runs away in little jets. Often replaces the use of the catheter.

Relationship.—Compare: *Urtica; Croc.; Trill.; Millefol.*

Dose.—Tincture, to sixth potency.

THUJA OCCIDENTALIS
(Arbor vitæ)

Acts on skin, blood, gastro-intestinal tract, kidneys, and brain. Its relation to the production of pathological vegetations condylomate, warty excrescences, spongy tumors is very important. Moist mucous tubercles. Bleeding fungus growths. Nævus. Excess of venosity.

The main action of Thuja is on the skin and genito-urinary organs, producing conditions that correspond with Hahnemann's sycotic dyscrasia, whose chief manifestation is the formation of wart-like excrescences upon mucous and cutaneous surfaces—fig-warts and condylomata. Has a specific antibacterial action, as in gonorrhœa and vaccination. Suppressed gonorrhœa, salpingitis. *Ill-effects of vaccination.* Sycotic pains, i. e., tearing in muscles and joints, worse at rest, better in dry weather, worse damp humid atmosphere; lameness. *Hydrogenoid constitutions*, whose blood is morbidly hydroscopic, so that damp air and water are inimical. Complaints from moonlight. *Rapid exhaustion and emaciation.* Left-sided and chilly medicine. Variola, aborts the pustule and prevents the suppurating fever. *Vaccinosis*, viz., inveterable skin troubles, neuralgia, etc.

Mind.—*Fixed ideas*, as if a strange person were at his side; as if soul and body were separated; as if something alive in abdomen. [*Croc.*] Emotional sensitiveness; music causes weeping and trembling.

Head.—Pain as if pierced by a nail. [*Coff.*; *Ign.*] Neuralgia from tea. [*Selen.*] Left-sided headache. White, scaly dandruff; hair dry and falling out. Greasy skin of face.

Eyes.—Ciliary neuralgia; iritis. Eyelids agglutinated at night; dry, scaly. Styes and tarsal tumors. [*Staph.*] Acute and subacute inflammation of sclera. Sclera raised in patches, and looks bluish-red. Large, flat phlyctenules; *indolent*. Recurring episcleritis. Chronic scleritis.

Ears.—Chronic otitis; discharge purulent. Creaking when swallowing. Polypi.

Nose.—Chronic catarrh; thick, green mucus; blood and pus. On blowing nose, pain in teeth. Ulceration within the nostrils. Dryness of nasal cavities. Painful pressure at root.

Mouth.—Tip of tongue very painful. *White blisters on side close to root, painfully sore.* Teeth decay next to gums; very sensitive; gums retract. Drinks fall audibly into stomach. Ranula; varicose veins on tongue and mouth. Pyorrhœa alveolaris.

Stomach.—Complete loss of appetite. Dislike for fresh meat and potatoes. Rancid eructations after fat food. Cutting pain in epigastrium. Cannot eat onions. Flatulence; pain after food; sinking sensation in epigastrium before food; thirst. Tea-drinking dyspepsia.

Abdomen.—Distended; indurations in abdomen. Chronic diarrhœa, worse after breakfast. Discharges forcibly expelled; gurgling sound. Brown spots. *Flatulence and distention; protruding here and there.* Rumbling and colic. Constipation, with violent rectal pain, causing stool to recede. [*Sil.; Sanic.*] Piles swollen; pain worse sitting, with stitching, burning pains at the anus. Anus fissured; painful to touch, with warts. *Movements as of something living* [*Crocus*], without pain.

Urinary.—Urethra swollen, inflamed. Urinary stream split and small. Sensation of trickling after urinating. Severe cutting *after*. [*Sars.*] Frequent micturition accompanying pains. Desire sudden and urgent, but cannot be controlled. Paralysis sphincter vesicæ.

Male.—Inflammation of prepuce and glans; pain in penis. Balanitis. *Gonorrhœal rheumatism. Gonorrhœa.* Chronic induration of testicles. Pain and burning felt near neck of bladder, with frequent and urgent desire to urinate. Prostatic enlargement. [*Ferr. pic.; Thiosinaminum; Iod.; Sabal.*]

Female.—Vagina *very sensitive.* [*Berb.; Kreos.; Lyssin.*] Warty excrescences on vulva and perineum. Profuse leucorrhœa; thick, greenish. Severe pain in left ovary and left inguinal region. Menses scanty, retarded. *Polypi;* fleshy excrescences. Ovaritis; worse left side, at every menstrual period. [*Lach.*] Profuse perspiration before menses.

Respiratory.—Dry, hacking cough in afternoon, with pain in pit of stomach. Stitches in chest; worse, cold drinks. *Asthma in children.* [*Nat. sulph.*] Papilloma of larynx. Chronic laryngitis.

Extremities.—When walking, limbs feel as if made of wood or glass, and would break easily. Tips of fingers swollen, red, feel dead. Muscular twitchings, weakness and trembling. Cracking in joints. Pain in heels and tendo-Achilles. Nails brittle. Ingrowing toe nail.

Skin.—Polypi, tubercles, *warts* epithelioma, næva, carbuncles; ulcers, especially in ano-genital region. Freckles and blotches. Perspiration sweetish, and strong. Dry skin, with brown spots. Zona; herpetic eruptions. Tearing pains in glands. Glandular enlargement. Nails crippled; brittle and soft. *Eruptions only on covered parts;* worse after scratching. Very sensitive to touch. Coldness of one side. Sarcoma; polypi. *Brown spots on hands and arms.*

Sleep.—Persistent insomnia.

Fever.—Chill, beginning in thighs. Sweat *only on uncovered parts*, or all over except head, when sleeping; profuse, sour, smelling like honey. Orgasm of blood in the evening, with throbbing in the blood-vessels.

Modalities.—*Worse*, at night, from heat of bed; at 3 a. m. and 3 p. m., from cold, damp air; after breakfast; fat, coffee; vaccination. *Better*, left side; while drawing up a limb.

Relationship.—Compare: (Hydrogenoid constitution: *Calcar.; Silica; Nat. sulph.; Aranea; Apis; Pulsat.*) *Cupressus australis* (sharp, prickling pain; general feeling of warmth; rheumatism and gonorrhœa). *Cupressus Lawsoniana* (acts like Thuja; *terrible pains in the stomach*). *Sphingurus* (falling out of hair from beard; pain in jaw-joint and zygoma); *Sil.; Maland.* (vaccination); *Medorrh.* (suppressed gonorrhœa); *Merc.; Cinnab.; Terebinth.; Juniperus; Sabin.; Sil.; Canth.; Cannab.; Nit. ac.; Puls.; Ant. tart.; Arborin* is a non-alcoholic preparation of *Thuja*.

Antidotes: *Merc.; Camph.: Sabin.* (warts).

Complementary: *Sabina; Ars.; Nat. sulph.; Silica.*

Dose.—Locally, for warts and excrescences, tincture, or cerate. Internally, tincture to thirtieth potency.

THYMOL
(Thyme Camphor)

A remedy having a wide field in genito-urinary diseases. It is indicated in pathological emissions, priapism and prostatorrhœa. The provings show an action limited to the sexual organs, producing a typical sexual neurasthenia. Specific for hookworm disease. [*Chenopodium.*]

Mental.—Irritable, arbitrary, must have his own way. Craves company. Energy gone.

Back.—Tired, aching throughout lumbar region. Worse, mental and physical labor.

Male.—Profuse, nightly, seminal emissions with lascivious dreams of a perverted character. Priapism. Urinary burning and subsequent dribbling of urine. Polyuria. Urates increased. Phosphates decreased.

Sleep.—Awakes tired and unrefreshed. Lascivious and fantastic dreams.

Relationship.—Compare: *Carbon Tetrachloride* as a remedy for Hookworms, according to Dr. Lambert, Suva, Fiji who employed it in 50,000 cases.

"1. Carbon tetrachloride is a vermifuge and vermicide of great potency, and has shown itself to be the best vermifuge for the treatment of hookworm in a country where the disease predominates.

"2. It gives little discomfort to the patient, is palatable, required no preparation of the patient, and when pure is apparently not toxic—all of which features are of advantage in a popular campaign.

"W. G. Smillie, and S. B. Pessoa, of Sao Paulo, Brazil, also have found carbon tetrachloride to be extremely efficient in removing hookworms. A single dose of 3 Cc. given to adults has been proved to remove 95 per cent. of all the hookworms harbored."

Modalities.—Thymol. *Worse*, mental and physical labor.

Dose.—Sixth attenuation.

THYMUS SERPYLLUM
(Wild Thyme)

Respiratory infections of children; dry nervous asthma, whooping-cough, severe spasms but little sputum.

Ringing in ears with feeling of pressure in head. Burning in pharynx, sore throat worse empty swallowing; blood vessels distended, dark.

Dose.—Tincture.

THYROIDINUM
(Dried Thyroid Gland of the Sheep)

Thyroid produces anæmia, emaciation, muscular weakness, sweating, headache, nervous tremor of face and limbs, tingling sensations, paralysis. Heart rate increased, exophthalmus and dilatation of pupils. *In myxœdema and cretinism* its effects are striking. Rheumatoid arthritis. Infantile wasting. Rickets. Delayed union of fractures. In half grain doses twice a day over a considerable period said to be *effective in undescended testicle* in boys. Thyroid exercises a general regulating influence over the mechanism of the organs of nutrition, growth and development. Thyroid weakness causes decided craving for large amount of sweets.

Of use in psoriasis; and *tachycardia*. Arrested development in children. Improves the memory. *Goitre.* Excessive obesity. Acts better with pale patients, rather than those of high color. Amblyopia. *Mammary tumor. Uterine fibroid.* Great weakness and hunger, yet loses flesh. *Nocturnal enuresis. Agalactea.* Begin treatment early in pregnancy. Dose 1½ gr. 2 to 3 times daily. *Vomiting of pregnancy* (give early in morning before patient gets up). *Fibroid tumors of the breast,* 2x trit. Dilates arterioles. [*Adrenalin contracts them.*] Sensation of faintness and nausea. Marked sensitiveness to cold Hypothyroidism after acute diseases, i. e., weakness. Easy fatigue, weak pulse, tendency to fainting, palpitation, cold hands and feet, low blood pressure, chilliness and sensitive to cold. (Thyroid 1x 3 times daily.) Has a powerful diuretic action in myxodema and various types of œdema.

Mind.—Stupor, alternating with restless melancholy. Irritable, worse least opposition; goes into a rage over trifles.

Head.—Feeling of lightness in brain. *Persistent frontal* headache. Eyeballs prominent. Face flushed; lips burn. Tongue thickly coated. Fullness and heat. Face flushed. Bad taste in mouth.

Heart.—Weak, frequent pulse, with inability to lie down. *Tachycardia.* [*Naja.*] Anxiety about chest, *as if constricted. Palpitation from least exertion.* Severe heart pain. Ready excitability of heart. Heart's action weak, with numbness of fingers.

Eyes.—Progressive diminution of sight with central scotoma. [*Carbon. sulf.*]

Throat.—Dry, congested, raw, burning; worse left side.

Stomach.—Desire for sweets and thirst for cold water. Nausea worse riding in car. Flatulence, much flatus in abdomen.

Urinary.—Increased flow; polyuria; some albumen and sugar. *Enuresis* in weakly children who are nervous and irritable (½ gr. night and morning). Urine smells of violets, burning along urethra, increase of uric acid.

Extremities.—Rheumative arthritis with tendency to obesity, coldness and cramps of extremities. Peeling of skin of lower limbs. Cold extremities. Aching pains. Œdema of legs. Trembling of limbs and entire body.

Respiratory.—Dry, painful cough with scanty, difficult expectoration and burning in pharynx.

Skin.—*Psoriasis* associated with adiposity (*not* in developing stage). Skin *dry*, impoverished. Cold hands and feet. *Eczema.* Uterine fibroids. *Browny swelling.* Swelling of glands of stony hardness. Sluggish cases. Jaundice with prutitus. Ichthyosis, lupus. Itching without eruption, worse night.

Relationship.—Compare: *Spongia; Calc.; Fucus; Lycopus; Iodothyrine,* (the active principle isolated from thyroid gland, a substance rich in Iodine and nitrogen, affects metabolism, reducing weight, may produce glycosuria. Use cautiously in obesity, for a fatty heart may not be able to maintain the accelerated rhythm. Milk contains the internal secretion of the thyroid.) *Thymus gland extract* (arthritis deformans; metabolic osteoarthritis, 5-grain tablets 3 times daily). High potencies very efficient in exophthalmic goitre.

Dose.—Crude Thyroid at times; better sixth to thirtieth potency. If the crude Thyroid is taken (two to three grains or more daily); the pulse should be watched. Must not be given in physiological doses where with feeble heart there is high blood pressure and not in tubercular patients.

TILIA EUROPA
(Linden)

Of value in muscular weakness of the eye; hæmorrhage o thin, pale blood. Puerperal metritis. Diseases of the antrum. [*Kali hyd.; Chelid.*]

Head.—*Neuralgia* (first right, then left side), *with veil before eyes*. Confusion, with dimness of vision. Much sneezing, with fluent coryza. Bleeding from nose.

Eyes.—Sensation as of gauze before eyes. [*Calc.; Caust.; Nat. m.*] Binocular vision imperfect.

Female.—*Intense sore feeling about uterus;* bearing-down, with hot sweat, but without relief. Much slimy leucorrhœa when walking. [*Bov.; Carb. an.; Graph.*] Soreness and redness of external genitals. [*Thuj.; Sulph.*] Pelvic inflammation, tympanites, abdominal tenderness and hot sweat which does not relieve.

Skin.—Urticaria. Violent itching, and burning like fire after scratching. Eruption of small, red itching pimples. *Sweat warm and profuse* soon after falling asleep. Sweat increases as rheumatic pains increase.

Modalities.—*Worse*, in afternoon and evening; in warm room, heat of bed. *Better*, cool room, motion.

Relationship.—Compare: *Lilium; Bellad.*

Dose.—Tincture, to sixth potency.

TITANIUM
(The Metal)

Is found in the bones and muscles. Has been used in lupus and tuberculosis processes, externally, also in skin disease, nasal catarrh, etc. Apples contain 0.11 per cent. of Titan. Imperfect vision, the peculiarity being that *half an object* only could be seen at once. Giddiness with *vertical hemiopia*. Also, sexual weakness, with *too early ejaculation* of semen in coitus. Bright's disease. Eczema, lupus, rhinitis.

Dose.—Lower and middle potencies.

TONGO—DIPTRIX ODORATA
(Seeds of Coumarouna—a tree in Guiana)

Useful in neuralgia; pertussis.

Head.—Tearing pain in supra-orbital nerve, with heat and throbbing pain in head and epiphora. Confused, especially the occiput, with somnolence and a sort of intoxication. Trembling in right upper lid. Coryza; nose stopped, must breathe through mouth.

Extremities.—Tearing pains in hip-joints, femur, and knee, especially left side.

Relationship.—*Melilotus. Anthoxanthum, Asperula,* and *Tonga* contain *Coumarin,* the active principle. Compare them in hay-fever; also, *Trifol.; Napth.; Sabad.*

Dose.—Tincture and lower potencies.

TORULA CEREVISIAE
(Saccharomyces) (Yeast Plant)

Introduced by Drs. Lehman and Yingling. Not proved, hence clinical symptoms only but many have been verified. Sycotic remedy Anaphylactic states produced by proteins and enzymes (Yingling).

Head.—Aching back of head and neck. Headache and sharp pains all over. Worse from constipation. Sneezing and wheezing. Catarrhal discharge from posterior nares. Irritable and nervous.

Stomach.—Bad taste. Nausea. Poor digestion. Belching of gas in stomach and abdomen. Soreness all over abdomen. Sense of fulness. Rumbling, pains shift, flatulence. *Constipation.* Sour, yeasty, mouldy odor from discharges.

Extremities.—Backache, tired and weak from elbows and knees down. Hands cold like ice and go to sleep easily.

Sleep.—Disturbed with much restlessness.

Skin.—Boils, recurrent. Itching eczema around ankles. Tinea versicolor.

Dose.—Pure yeast cake or potencies from 3rd to high. Yeast poultices are much used in skin diseases, boils and swelling.

TRIBULUS TERRESTRIS
(Ikshugandha)

An East Indian drug useful in urinary affections, expecially dysuria, and in debilitated states of the sexual organs, as expressed in seminal weakness, ready emissions and impoverished semen. Prostatitis, calculous affections and sexual neurasthenia. It meets the auto-traumatism of masturbation, correcting the emissions and spermatorrhœa. Partial impotence caused by overindulgence of advancing age, or when accompanied by urinary symptoms, incontinence, painful micturition, etc.

Dose.—Ten to twenty drops of the tincture three times daily.

TRIFOLIUM PRATENSE
(Red Clover)

Produces most marked ptyalism. Feeling of fullness with congestion of salivary glands, followed by increased copious flow of saliva. Feeling as if mumps were coming on. *Crusta lactea;* dry, scaly crusts. Stiff neck. *Cancerous diathesis.*

Head.—Confusion and headache on awaking. Dullness in anterior brain. Mental failure, loss of memory.

Mouth.—*Increased flow of saliva.* [*Merc.; Syphil.*] Sore throat, with hoarseness.

Respiratory.—Coryza like that which precedes hay-fever; thin mucus, with much irritation. *Hoarse and choking; chills with cough at night.* Cough on coming into the open air. Hay-fever. Spasmodic cough; *whooping cough,* paroxysms; worse at night.

Back.—Neck stiff; cramp in sterno-cleido muscles; relieved by heat and irritation.

Extremities.—Tingling in palms. Hands and feet cold. Tibial ulcers.

Relationship.—Compare: *Trifolium repens*—White clover—. (Prophylactic against mumps, feeling of congestion in salivary glands, pain and hardening, especially submaxillary; worse, lying down. Mouth filled with watery saliva, *worse lying down*. Taste of blood in mouth and throat. Sensation as if heart would stop, with great fear, better sitting up or moving about; worse, when alone, with cold sweat on face.)

Dose.—Tincture.

TRILLIUM PENDULUM
(White Beth-root)

A general hæmorrhagic medicine, *with great faintness* and *dizziness*. Chronic diarrhœa of bloody mucus. Uterine hæmorrhage. Threatened abortion. *Relaxation of pelvic region*. Cramp-like pains. Phthisis with purulent and copious expectoration and spitting of blood.

Head.—Pain in forehead; worse, noise. Confused; eyeballs feel too large. Vision blurred; everything looks bluish. *Nosebleed*. [*Millef.; Melilot.*]

Mouth.—Hæmorrhage from gums. *Bleeding after tooth extraction*.

Stomach.—Heat and burning stomach rising up in œsophagus. Hæmatemesis.

Rectum.—Chronic diarrhœa; discharge bloody. Dysentery; passage almost pure blood.

Female.—Uterine hæmorrhages, *with sensation as though hips and back were falling to pieces; better tight bandages*. Gushing of bright blood on least movement. Hæmorrhage from fibroids. [*Calc.; Nitr. ac.; Phos.; Sulph. ac.*] Prolapse, with great bearing-down. Leucorrhœa copious, yellow, stringy. [*Hydras.; Kali b.; Sabin.*] Metrorrhagia at climacteric. *Lochia suddenly becomes sanguinous*. Dribbling of urine after labor.

Respiratory.—Cough, with spitting of blood. Copious, purulent expectoration. Hæmoptysis. Aching at end of sternum. Suffocative attack of irregular breathing with sneezing. Shooting pains through chest.

Relationship.—Compare: *Trillium cernum* (eye symptoms) everything looks bluish; greasy feeling in mouth); *Ficus* (hæmorrhages; menorrhagia, hæmaturia, epistaxis, hæmatemesis, bleeding piles); *Sanguisuga*—Leech—(hæmorrhages; bleeding from anus). *Ipec.; Sab.; Lach.; Hamam.*

Dose.—Tincture and lower potencies.

TRIOSTEUM PERFOLIATUM
(Fever-root)

Triosteum is a very valuable remedy in diarrhœa attended with colicky pains and nausea, *numbness of lower limbs after stool*, and increased flow of urine; also in influenza. Quiets nervous symptoms. [*Coffea.; Hyos.*] Biliousness. Bilious colic.

Head.—Occipital pain, with nausea on rising, followed by vomiting. Influenza, with aching pains all over, and heat in the limbs. *Ozæna;* frontal pain.

Stomach.—Loathing of food; nausea on rising, followed by vomiting and cramps. Stools watery, frothy.

Extremities.—Stiffness of all joints; calves numb; aching in bones. Rheumatic pain in back. Pains in limbs.

Skin.—Itching welts. *Urticaria* from gastric derangement.

Dose.—Sixth potency.

TRINITROTOLUENE
(T.N.T.)

Symptoms found in munition workers handling T.N.T. who inhale and ingest it and also absorb some through the skin. They were compiled by Dr. Conrad Wesselhoeft and published in the December, 1926 number of the Journal of the American Institute of Homœopathy.

The destructive action of T.N.T. on the red blood corpuscles is responsible for the anemia and the jaundice with their secondary symptoms. The hemoglobin is changed so it cannot act satisfactorily as an oxygen carrier and as a result we have breathlessness, dizziness, headache, faintness, palpitation, undue fatigue, muscle cramps and cyanosis; also drowsiness, depression and insomnia. Later stages of the poisoning produce toxic jaundice and aplastic anemia. The jaundice is the result of cellular destruction in contrast to obstructive jaundice.

Head.—Depression and headache (frontal). Aversion to company, apathetic and weeps easily. Faintness, dizziness, mental sluggishness; delirium, convulsions, coma. Face very dark.

Respiratory.—Nose dry with stuffed sensation. Sneezing, coryza, burning of trachea, choking weight on chest; dry, convulsive cough, raising mucous plugs.

Gastro-Intestinal.—Bitter taste, much thirst, sour regurgitation; dull burning behind the ensiform; nausea, vomiting, constipation followed by diarrhœa with cramps.

Cardio Vascular.—Palpitation, tachycardia, bradycardia, intermittent pulse.

Urinary.—High colored urine, burning on urination, sudden desire, incontinence and retention.

Skin.—Hands stained yellow. Dermatitis, nodular erythema, vesicles, itching and burning; puffiness. *Tendency to hæmorrhage* under the skin and from the nose. *Tired pain in back of knees.*

Modalities.—*Worse*, alcohol (falls after one or two drinks of whisky). *Tea* (marked aversion).

Relationship.—Compare: *Zinc.; Phosph.; Cina; Ars.; Plumbum.*

Dose.—Thirtieth potency has been used with success.

TRITICUM—AGROPYRON REPENS
(Couch-Grass)

An excellent remedy in excessive irritability of the bladder, dysuria, cystitis, gonorrhœa.

Nose.—Always blowing nose.

Urinary.—Frequent, *difficult*, and painful urination. [*Pop.*] Gravelly deposits. Catarrhal and purulent discharges. [*Pareira.*] Strangury, pyelitis; enlarged prostate. Chronic cystic irritability. Incontinence; constant desire. Urine is dense and causes irritation of the mucous surfaces.

Relationship.—Compare: *Tradescantia;* (Hæmorrhage from ear and upper air passages; painful urination, urethral discharge; scrotum inflamed). *Chimaph.; Senecio; Populus trem.; Buchu; Uva.*

Polytrichum Juniperinum—Ground Moss—(Painful urination of old people; dropsy, urinary obstruction and suppression).

Dose.—Tincture or infusion by boiling two ounces in a quart of water until it is reduced to a pint. To be taken in four doses in 24 hours.

TROMBIDIUM
(Red acarus of the fly)

Has a specific place in the treatment of dysentery. Symptoms *are worse by food and drink*.

Abdomen.—Much pain before and after stool; stool only after eating. Griping in hypochondrium in morning. Congestion of the liver, with urgent, loose, stools on rising. Brown, thin, bloody stools, with tenesmus. During stool, sharp pain in left side, shooting downward. Burning in anus.

Dose.—Sixth to thirtieth potency.

TUBERCULINUM
(A Nucleo-protein, a Nosode from Tubercular Abscess)

Tuberculinum is indicated in renal affections, but caution is necessary, for where skin and intestines do not perform normally even high potencies are dangerous. In chronic cystitis, brilliant and permanent results. (Dr. Nebel Montreux.)

Of undoubted value in the treatment of *incipient tuberculosis*. Especially adapted to the light-complexioned, narrow-chested subjects. Lax fiber, low recuperative powers, and very susceptible to changes in the weather. Patient always tired; motion causes intense fatigue; aversion to work; wants constant changes. When *symptoms are constantly changing and well-selected remedies fail to improve, and cold is taken from the slightest exposure*. Rapid emaciation. Of great value in epilepsy, neurasthenia and in nervous children. Diarrhœa in children running for weeks, extreme wasting, bluish pallor, exhaustion. Mentally deficient children. Enlarged tonsils. Skin affections, *acute articular rheumatism*. Very sensitive, mentally and physically. General exhaustion. Nervous weakness. Trembling. Epilepsy. Arthritis.

Mind.—Contradictory characteristics of Tuberculinum are mania and melancholia; insomnia and sopor. Irritable, especially when awakening. *Depressed*, melancholy. *Fear of dogs. Animals especially.* Desire to use foul language, curse and swear.

Head.—Subject to deep brain headaches and intense neuralgias. Everything seems strange. Intense pain, as of an iron band around head. Meningitis. When critical discharges appear, sweat, polyuria, diarrhœa, exanthema, repeating the dose only when crises come on. Nocturnal hallucinations, awakes frightened. Plica polonica. [*Vinca.*] Crops of small boils, intensely painful, successively appear in the nose; *green, fetid pus.*

Ears.—Persistent, offensive otorrhœa. *Perforation in membrana tympani, with ragged edges.*

Stomach.—Averse to meat. All-gone, hungry sensation. [*Sulph.*] Desire for cold milk.

Abdomen.—Early-morning, sudden diarrhœa. [*Sulph.*] Stools dark-brown, offensive, discharged with much force. Tabes mesenterica.

Female.—*Benign mammary tumors.* Menses too early, too profuse, long-lasting. *Dysmenorrhœa. Pains increase with the establishment of the flow.*

Respiratory.—*Enlarged tonsils.* Hard, dry cough during sleep. Expectoration thick, easy; profuse bronchorrhœa. Shortness of breath. Sensation of suffocation, even with plenty of fresh air. Longs for cold air. Broncho-pneumonia in children. Hard, hacking cough, profuse sweating and loss of weight, rales all over chest. Deposits begin in apex of lung. (Repeated doses.)

Back.—Tension in nape of neck and down spine. Chilliness between shoulders or up the back.

Skin.—Chronic eczema; itching intense; worse at night. *Acne* in tuberculous children. Measles; psoriasis [*Thyroid.*]

Sleep.—Poor; wakes early. Overpowering sleepiness in daytime. Dreams vivid and distressing.

Fever.—Post-critical temperature of a remittent type. Here repeat dose every two hours. (MacFarlan.) Profuse sweat. General chilliness.

Modalities.—*Worse*, motion, music; before a storm; standing; dampness; from draught; early morning, and after sleep. *Better*, open air.

Relationship.—Compare: *Koch's lymph* (*acute and chronic parenchymatous nephritis;* produces pneumonia, broncho-pneumonia, and congestion of the lungs in tuberculous patients, and is a remarkably efficacious remedy in lobular pneumonia—*broncho-pneumonia*); *Aviare*—Tuberculin from birds—(acts on the apices of the lungs; has proved an excellent remedy in influenzal bronchitis; symptoms similar to tuberculosis; relieves the debility, diminishes the cough, improves the appetite, and braces up the whole organism; acute broncho-pulmonary diseases of children; itching of palms and ears; cough, acute, inflammatory, irritating, incessant, and tickling; loss of strength and appetite); *Hydrast.* (to fatten patients after Tuberc.): *Formic acid* (tuberculosis, chronic nephritis, malignant tumors; pulmonary tuberculosis, not in third stage, however; lupus; carcinoma of breast and stomach; Dr. Krull uses injections of solutions corresponding to the third centesimal potency; these must not be repeated before six months). Compare: *Bacil.; Psorin.; Lach. Kalagua* (tuberculosis; garlicky odor of all secretions and breath). *Teucrium scoradonia.* Compare: *Thuja.* (Vaccinosis may block the way of action of *Tuberculin* until Thuja has been given and then acts brilliantly. (Burnett.)

Complementary: *Calcarea; China; Bryon.*

Dose.—*Tuberculin* needs more frequent repetition in children's complaints than nearly every other chronic remedy. (H. Fergie Woods.) Thirtieth and much higher, in infrequent doses. When Tuberculinum fails *Syphilinum* often follows advantageously, producing a reaction.

"The use of Tuberculinum in phthisis pulmonalis demands attention to the following points: In apyretic purely tubercular phthisis results are marked, provided the eliminative organs are in good order, but nothing below the 1000th should be used, unless absolutely necessary. With patients where strepto-staphylo-pneumococci are in the bronchi; where also after washing the sputum, a pure "t. b." bacilli-mass remains, the same treatment is indicated. With mixed infection—found in the majority of cases—where the sputum swarms with virulent micro-organisms in addition to the "t. b.," other procedure is necessary. If the heart is in good shape, a single dose of Tuberculinum 1000-2000 is given, provided there are no marked indications for other remedies. With due attention to temperature and possible excretions, the dose is allowed to work until effects are no longer observed, eight days to eight weeks. Usually a syndrome then presents, permitting the accurate choice of an antipsoric Silica, Lycopodium, Phosphorus, etc. After a while the picture again darkens and now a high potency of the isopathic remedy corresponding to the most virulent and prominent micro-organism found in the sputum is given: Staphylo-, Strepto-, or Pneumococcin. The accurate bacteriological analysis of the sputum is absolutely essential; the choice of the ison again clears the picture, and so, proceeding on the one side etiologically (where these isopathica have not yet been proved); on the other side symptomatically with antipsoric remedies, the disease is dominated.

My own experience warns, in the case of mixed infection, against the use of Strepto-, Staphylo-, or Pneumococcin below the 500th. I use them only from 2000 to 1000, having seen terrible aggravations from the 30, 100, 200, with a lowering temperature from 104 to 96. Hence the admonition, which need not concern scoffers, but those alone who wish to avail themselves of a potent weapon. The toxins used as remedies are, like Tuberculinum, prepared from pure and virulent cultures.

And cases, seemingly condemned to speedy death, are brought in a year or two back to normal temperature, though, of course, sacrificing a large portion of lung tissue. This result is sure when the patient can and will take care of himself, where the heart has withstood the toxin and the stomach and liver are in good function. Further, climatic variations must be avoided. With the great mineral metabolism of the phthisic, diet regulation is imperative, and should be preponderately vegetable, together with the addition of psysiological salts in low potency, Calcarea carb., 3x, 5x, Calcarea phos., 2x, 6x, and intercurrently according to indications organ-remedies as Cactus Tr. 30, Chelidonium Tr. 30, Taraxacum Tr., Nasturtium Tr., Urtica urens Tr., Tussilago farfara Tr., Lysimachia numularia Tr., for short periods.

The first dose of Tuberculinum in any difficult case is, however, the most weighty prescription. The remedy should not be given without a most careful cardiac examination. As the surgeon before the anæsthetic, so must the physician know the heart before administering this drug, especially to children, and seniles—and to young seniles. He who observes this rule will have fewer clinical reproaches on his conscience. When Tuberculinum is contraindicated, recourse must be had to the nearest antipsoric.

The above caution applies also to asthma, pleuritis, peritonitis in scrofulous (tuberculous) subjects." [Dr. Nebel Montreux

TURNERA
(Damiana)

Said to be of use in sexual neurasthenia; impotency. Sexual debility from nervous prostration. Incontinence of old people. Chronic prostatic discharge. Renal and cystic catarrh; *frigidity of females*. Aids the establishment of normal menstrual flow in young girls.

Dose.—Tincture and fluid extract—ten- to forty-drop doses.

TUSSILAGO PETASITES
(Butter-burr)

Has some action on the urinary organs, and found useful in gonorrhœa. Affections of pylorus.

Urinary.—Crawling in urethra.

Male.—Gonorrhœa; yellowish, thick discharge. Erections, with urethral crawling. Pain in spermatic cord.

Relationship.—Compare: *Tussilago fragrans* (pylorus pain, plethora and corpulency); *Tussilago farfara* (coughs); as an intercurrent medicine in phthisis pulmonalis. (See Tuberculinum.)

Dose.—Tincture.

UPAS TIENTE
(Upas-tree—Strychnos Tiente)

Produces *tonic spasms, tetanus, and asphyxia*.

Head.—Disinclined for mental work. Irritable. Dull headache deep in brain.

Eyes.—*Pain in eyes and orbits, with conjunctivitis.* Dull sunken eyes. Styes.

Mouth.—Herpes on lips. Burning on the tongue. Pain in mouth, as from a splinter. [*Nit. ac.*]

Male.—Desire increased, with loss of power. *Dull backache,* as after excessive coitus.

Chest.—Lancinating pain throughout right lung toward the liver, stopping breathing. Violent palpitation; sensation of heaviness in stomach.

Skin.—Numb hands and feet. Hangnails inflamed; itching and redness of roots of nails.

Relationship.—Compare: *Upas antiaris*—resinous exudation of *Antiarus toxicaria,* (a deadly poison to the muscular system. It suspends both voluntary muscular action and that of the heart without causing convulsions. Used in Java as an arrow poison (Merrell). Differs in producing *clonic spasms,* violent vomiting, diarrhœa, great prostration). *Oxal. ac. Upas* when Bryonia fails (typhoid).

Antidote: *Curare.*

Dose.—Third to sixth potency.

URANIUM NITRICUM
(Nitrate of Uranium)

Causes glycosuria and increased urine. Is known to produce nephritis, diabetes, degeneration of the liver, high blood pressure and dropsy. Its therapeutic keynote is *great emaciation, debility and tendency to ascites and general dropsy.* Backache and delayed menses. Dry mucous membranes and skin.

Head.—Ill-tempered; dull, heavy pain. Nostrils sore, with purulent, acrid discharge. Mental depression.

Eyes.—Lids inflamed and agglutinated; *styes.*

Stomach.—Excessive thirst; nausea; *vomiting. Ravenous appetite;* eating followed by flatulence. *Boring pain in pyloric region. Gastric and duodenal ulcers.* Burning pain. *Abdomen bloated.* Gas, second only to Lycop.

Urinary.—Copious urination. *Diuresis.* Incontinence of urine. *Diabetes.* Emaciation and tympanites. *Burning in* *urethra*, with very acid urine. *Unable to* retain urine without pain. *Enuresis.* [*Mullein oil.*]

Male.—Complete impotency, with nocturnal emissions. Organs cold, relaxed, sweaty.

Relationship.—Compare: *Syzygium; Phos. ac.; Lact. ac.; Arg. nit.; Kali bich.; Ars.; Phloridzin* (a glucosidal principle obtained from the bark of the root of the apple and other fruit trees. Produces diabetes and fatty degeneraion of the liver; intermittent fever. Daily doses, 15 grains. Phlorizin causes glycosuria. No hyperglycemia results. It compels the secretory epithelium of the kidney to break down serum albumin into sugar. There is no increase in blood sugar.)

Dose —Second trituration.

UREA
(Carbamide)

Tuberculosis. Lumps. Enlarged glands. Renal dropsy, with symptoms of general intoxication. Gouty eczema. Albuminuria, diabetes; uræmia. Urine thin and of low specific gravity. A hydrogogue diuretic in the treatment of dropsies. 10 grains every 6 hours.

Relationship.—Compare: *Uric acid* (gout, gouty eczema, rheumatism, lipoma); *Urinum* (acne, boils, scurvy, dropsy); *Urtica; Tubercul.; Thyroid*.

URTICA URENS
(Stinging-nettle)

A remedy for agalactia and *lithiasis*. Profuse discharge from mucous surfaces. Enuresis and urticaria. Spleen affections. *Antidotes ill-effects of eating shellfish.* Symptoms return at the same time every year. Gout and uric acid diathesis. Favors elimination.

Rheumatism associated with urticaria-like eruptions. Neuritis.

Head.—Vertigo, headache with spleen pains.

Abdomen.—Diarrhœa chronic disease of large intestine characterized by large secretion of mucus.

Male.—Itching of scrotum, keeps him awake; scrotum swollen.

Female.—*Diminished secretion of milk.* Uterine hæmorrhage. Acid and excoriating leucorrhœa. *Pruritus vulvæ, with stinging, itching,* and œdema. Arrests flow of milk after weaning. Excessive swelling of breasts.

Extremities.—Pain in acute gout deltoid; pain in ankles, wrists.

Skin.—*Itching blotches. Urticaria,* burning heat, with formication; violent itching. Consequences of suppressed nettle-rash. Rheumatism alternates with nettle-rash. Burn confined to skin. Urticaria nodosa. [*Bov.*] Erythema, with burning and stinging. *Burns and scalds. Chicken-pox.* [*Dulc.*] Angioneurotic œdema. Herpes labialis with sensation of heat and itching. Itching and stinging of scrotum.

Fever.—General heat in bed with soreness over abdomen. Fever of gout. Tropical fever.

Modalities.—*Worse,* from snow-air; water, cool moist-air, touch.

Relationship.—Compare: *Medusa; Nat. mur.; Lac. can.; Ricin* (diminished mammary secretion); *Bombyx; Rhus; Apis; Chloral.; Astac.; Puls.* (urticaria); *Boletus luridus* and *Anacard.* (urticaria tuberosa); *Lycop.* and *Hedeoma* (uric acid conditions); *Formica.*

Dose.—Tincture and lower potencies.

USNEA BARBATA
(Tree-moss)

Is a remedy in some forms of congestive headache; sunstroke.

Head.—Bursting feeling, *as if temples would burst, or the eyes burst out of the sockets.* Throbbing carotids.

Relationship.—Compare: *Glonoine; Bellad.*

Dose.—Tincture, drop doses.

USTILAGO MAYDIS
(Corn-smut)

Flabby condition of uterus. Hæmorrhage. Congestion to various parts, especially at climacteric. **Crusta lactea.** [*Viola tric.*]

Head.—Very depressed. Full feeling. Nervous headache from menstrual irregularities. Aching in eyeballs, with much lachrymation.

Male.—Uncontrollable masturbation. Spermatorrhœa, with erotic fancies and amorous dreams. Emissions, with irresistible tendency to masturbation. Dull pain in lumbar region, with great despondency and mental irritability.

Female.—Vicarious menstruation. Ovaries burn, pain, swell. Profuse menses after miscarriage; discharge of blood from slightest provocation; bright red; partly clotted. Menorrhagia at climaxis. [*Calc. c.; Lach.*] Oozing of dark blood, clotted, forming long black strings. Uterus hypertrophied. *Cervix bleed easily.* Postpartum hæmorrhage. Profuse lochia.

Fever.—Abundant sweat. Pulse at first accelerated then enfeebled. Palpitations.

Extremities.—Muscular debility, *sensation of boiling water along the back*. Clonic and tetanic movements. Muscular contractions, especially of lower limbs.

Skin.—Alopecia. Tendency to small boils. Skin dry; eczema; copper-colored spots Pruritus; sunburn. Psoriasis. (Internally and externally.)

Relationship.—Compare: *Secale; Sabin.; Zea Italica.* (Possess curative properties in skin diseases, particularly in psoriasis and eczema rubrum. Mania for bathing. Impulse to suicide, particularly by drowning. Easily angered. Appetite increased, voracious, alternating with disgust for food. Pyrosis, nausea, vomiting, better drinking wine.)

Dose.—Tincture, to third potency.

UVA URSI
(Bearberry)

Urinary symptoms most important. Cystitis, with bloody urine. Uterine hæmorrhage. Chronic vesical irritation, with pain, tenesmus, and catarrhal discharges. *Burning after the discharge of slimy urine.* Pyelitis. Calculous inflammation. Dyspnœa, nausea, vomiting, pulse small and irregular. Cyanosis. Urticaria without itching.

Urinary.—Frequent urging, with severe spasms of bladder;

burning and tearing pain. Urine contains blood, pus, and much tenacious mucus, with clots in large masses. Involuntary; green urine. Painful dysuria.

Relationship.—Compare: *Arbutin* (a crystallized glucoside of Uva; found also in Kalmia, Gaultheria and other genera of the family of *Eriaceæ;* given in doses of 3 to 8 grains with sugar three times a day. Used as an urinary antiseptic and diuretic. *Arctosphylos manzanita* (acts on renal and reproductive organs. Gonorrhœa, vesical catarrh, diabetes, menorrhagia. Tincture of leaves). *Vaccinum myrtillus*—Huckleberries—(dysentery; typhoid, keeps intestines aseptic and prevents absorption and reinfection).

Dose.—Tincture, five to thirty drops. In pyelitis a trituration of the leaves.

VACCININUM
(Nosode—From vaccine matter)

Vaccine poison is capable of setting up a morbid state of extreme chronicity, named by Burnett Vaccinosis, symptoms like those of Hahnemann's Sycosis. Neuralgias, inveterate skin eruptions, chilliness, indigestion with great flatulent distension (Clark). Whooping-cough.

Mind.—Irritable, impatient ill-humored, nervous.

Head.—Frontal headache. Forehead and eyes feel as if split. Inflamed and red lids.

Skin.—Hot and dry. Pimples and blotches. Eruption like variola.

Relationship.—Compare: anti-vaccinal remedies; *Variolin; Malandrinum;* Thuja, powerful adjuvants in treatment of malignant disease.

Dose.—Sixth to 200th potency.

VALERIANA
(Valerian)

Hysteria, over-sensitiveness, nervous affections, when apparently well-chosen remedies fail. Hysterical spasms and affections generally. *Hysterical flatulency.*

Mind.—Changeable disposition. Feels light, as if floating in air. Over-sensitiveness. [*Staph.*] Hallucinations at night. *Irritable.* Tremulous.

Head.—Sensation of great coldness. Pressure in forehead. Feeling of intoxication.

Ears.—*Earache from exposure to draughts and cold.* Nervous noises. Hyperæsthesia.

Throat.—*Sensation as if a thread were hanging down throat.* Nausea felt in throat. Pharynx feels constricted.

Stomach.—Hunger, with nausea. Erucatations foul. Heartburn with gulping of rancid fluid. Nausea, with faintness. *Child vomits curdled milk in large lumps after nursing.*

Abdomen.—Bloated. Hysterical cramps. Thin, watery diarrhœa, *with lumps of coagulated milk, with violent screaming in children.* Greenish, papescent, bloody stool. Spasms in bowels after food and at night in bed.

Respiratory.—Choking on falling asleep. Spasmodic asthma; convulsive movements of the diaphragm.

Female.—Menses late and scanty. [*Puls.*]

Extremities.—Rheumatic pains in limbs. *Constant jerking.* Heaviness. Sciatica; *pain worse standing and resting on floor* [*Bell.*]; better walking. Pain in heels *when sitting*.

Sleep.—Sleepless, with nightly itching and muscular spasms. Worse on waking.

Fever.—Long lasting heat, often with sweat on face. *Heat predominates.* Sensation of icy coldness. [*Heloderma; Camp.; Abies c.*]

Relationship.—Compare: *Asaf.; Ign.; Croc.; Castor.; Amm. valer.* (in neuralgia, gastric disturbance, and great nervous agitation). Insomnia especially during pregnancy and menopause. Feeble, hysterical nervous patients.

Dose.—Tincture.

VANADIUM
(The Metal)

Its action is that of an oxygen carrier and a catalyzer, hence its use in wasting diseases. Increases amount of hæmoglobin, also combines its oxygen with toxines and destroys their virulence. Also increases and stimulates phagocytes.

A remedy in degenerative conditions of the liver and arteries. Anorexia and symptoms of gastro intestinal irritation; albumen, casts and blood in urine. Tremors; vertigo; hysteria and melancholia; neuro-retinitis and blindness. Anæmia, emaciation. Cough dry, irritating and paroxysmal, sometimes with hæmorrhages. Irritation of nose, eyes and throat. Tuberculosis, chronic rheumatism, diabetes. *Acts as a tonic to digestive function* and in early tuberculosis. Arterio-sclerosis, sensation as if heart was compressed, as if blood had no room in the aorta. Anxious pressure on whole chest. Fatty heart. Degenerative states, has brain softening. Atheroma of arteries of brain and liver. Compare: *Ars.; Phos. Ammon. vanad.* (fatty degeneration of liver.)

Dose.—6-12 potency. The best form is Vanadiate of Soda, 2 mg. daily, by mouth.

VANILLA—PLANIFOLIA
(Vanilla)

Marked skin irritation resembling milk Poison-oak; is sometimes produced by handling the beans, also by local use of vanilla essence in a hair wash. Vanilla is supposed to stimulate the brain and sexual propensities. Do not use the synthetic Vanilla extract. Various disorders of the nervous system and circulation are produced in workers with Vanilla. Is an emmagogue and aphrodisiac. Menses prolonged.

Dose.—Vanilla, 6th to 30th, has been found effective in curing the skin affection.

VARIOLINUM
(Lymph from Small-pox Pustule)

Used for "internal vaccination." Seems to be efficacious in protecting against, modifying and aiding in the cure of small-pox.

Head.—Morbid fear of small-pox. Deafness. Pain in occiput. Inflamed eyelids.

Respiratory.—Oppressed breathing. Throat feels closed. Cough with thick viscid, bloody mucus. Feeling of a lump in right side of throat.

Extremities.— *Excruciating backache. Aching in legs.* Tired all over with restlessness. Wrists pain. Pains shift from back to abdomen.

Fever.—Hot fever, with intense radiating heat. Profuse, bad-smelling sweat.

Skin.—Hot, dry. Eruption of pustules. *Shingles.*

Relationship.—Compare: *Vaccin.* (same action); *Malandrinum*—the morbid product of the grease of the horse (a prophylactic of small-pox and a remedy for the ill-effects of vaccination; chronic eczema following vaccination).

Dose.—Sixth to thirtieth potency.

VERATRUM ALBUM
(White Hellebore)

A perfect picture of *collapse,* with *extreme coldness, blueness, and weakness,* is offered by this drug. Post-operative shock with cold sweat on forehead, pale face, rapid, feeble pulse. *Cold perspiration on the forehead,* with nearly all complaints. *Vomiting, purging, and cramps in extremities.* The *profuse,* violent retching and vomiting is most characteristic. Surgical shock. Excessive dryness of all mucous surfaces. *"Coprophagia"* violent mania alternates with silence and refusal to talk.

Mind.—Melancholy, with stupor and mania. Sits in a stupid manner; notices nothing; *Sullen indifference.* Frenzy of excitement; shrieks, curses. Puerperal mania. Aimless wandering from home. *Delusions of impending misfortunes.* Mania, with desire to cut and tear things. [*Tarant.*] Attacks of pain, with delirium driving to madness. Cursing, howling all night.

Head.—Contracted features. *Cold sweat on forehead. Sensation of a lump of ice on vertex.* Headache, with nausea, vomiting, diarrhœa, pale face. Neck too weak to hold head up.

Eyes.—Surrounded by dark rings. Staring; turned upwards. without lustre. Lachrymation with redness. Lids dry heavy.

Face.—Features sunken. *Icy coldness of tip of nose and face.* Nose grows more pointed. Tearing in cheeks, temples, and eyes. *Face very pale, blue, collapsed, cold.*

Mouth.—Tongue pale, cold; cool sensation, as from peppermint. Dry in center not relieved by water. Salty saliva. Toothache, teeth feel heavy as if filled with lead.

Stomach.—*Voracious* appetite. *Thirst for cold water, but is vomited as soon as swallowed.* Averse to warm food. Hiccough. *Copious vomiting and nausea; aggravated by drinking and least motion.* Craves fruit, juicy and cold things, ice, salt. Anguish in pit of stomach. Great weakness after vomiting. Gastric irritability with *chronic* vomiting of food.

Abdomen.—Sinking and empty feeling. *Cold feeling* in stomach and abdomen. Pain in abdomen preceding stool. Cramps, knotting abdomen and legs. Sensation as if hernia would protrude. [*Nux.*] Abdomen sensitive to pressure, swollen with terrible colic.

Rectum.—Constipation from inactivity of rectum, with heat and headache. Constipation of babies, and when produced by very cold weather. *Stools large, with much straining until exhausted, with cold sweat.* Diarrhœa, very painful, watery, *copious, and forcibly evacuated*, followed by great prostration. Evacuations of cholera morbus and true cholera when vomiting accompanies the purging.

Respiratory.—Hoarse, weak voice. Rattling in chest. Much mucus in bronchial tubes, that cannot be coughed up. Coarse rales. Chronic bronchitis in the aged. [*Hippozanin.*] Loud, barking, stomach cough, followed by eructation of gas; worse, warm room. Hollow cough, tickling low down, with blue face. Cough comes on from drinking, especially cold water; urine escapes when coughing. Cough on entering warm room from cold air. [*Bryonia.*]

Heart.—Palpitation with anxiety and rapid audible respiration. Pulse irregular, feeble. Tobacco heart from chewing. Intermittent action of heart in feeble persons with some hepatic obstruction. One of the best heart stimulants in homœop. doses. (J. S. Mitchell.)

Female.—Menses too early; profuse and exhausting. *Dysmenorrhœa, with coldness,* purging, *cold sweat. Faints from least exertion.* Sexual mania precedes menses.

Extremities.—Soreness and tenderness of joints. Sciatica;

pains like electric flashes. *Cramps in calves.* Neuralgia in brachial plexus; arms feel swollen, cold, paralytic.

Skin.—Blue, cold, clammy, inelastic; *cold as death.* Cold sweat. Wrinkling of skin of hands and feet.

Fever.—Chill, *with extreme coldness* and thirst.

Modalities.—*Worse,* at night; wet, cold weather. *Better,* walking and warmth.

Relationship.—Compare: *Veratrinum*—alkaloid from seeds of Sabadilla.—(electric pains, electric shocks in muscles, fibrillary twitchings); *Cholos terrepina* (cramps in calves); *Camph.; Cupr.; Ars.; Cuprum ars. (intermittent, cold, clammy sweat); Narcissus poeticus* (gastro-enteritis with much griping and cutting pain in bowels. Fainting, trembling, cold limbs, small and irregular pulse); *Trychosanthes*—(diarrhœa, pain in liver, dizziness after every stool); *Agaric. emetic.* (vertigo; longing for ice-cold water; burning pains in stomach); *Agaric. phalloides* (cholera, cramps in stomach, cold extremities, urine suppressed). *Veratrine* (Increased vascular tension. It relaxes it and stimulates the elimination of toxins by skin, kidneys, and liver).

Dose.—First to thirtieth potency. In diarrhœa, not below the sixth.

VERATRUM VIRIDE
(White American Hellebore)

Paroxysms of auricular fibrillation. Induces fall of both systolic and diastolic blood pressure. Congestions, especially to lungs, base of brain, with nausea and vomiting. Twitchings and convulsions. Especially adapted to full-blooded, plethoric persons. Great prostration. Rheumatism of heart. *Bloated, livid face.* Furious delirium. Effects of sunstroke. *Œsophagitis.* (Farrington.) *Verat. vir,* will raise the opsonic index against the *diploccus pneumonia,* 70 to 109 per cent. Congestive stage and early manifestations of hepatization in pneumonia. Zigzag temperature. Clinically, it is known that such diseases as Tiegel's contracture, Thompson's Disease, athetosis and pseudo-hypertrophic muscular paralysis present a symptomatology quite like that produced by Veratrum vir. upon muscular tissue. (A. E. Hinsdale, M.D.)

Mind.—Quarrelsome and delirious.

Head.—Congestion intense, almost apoplectic. Hot head,

bloodshot eyes. Bloated, livid face. Hippocratic face. Head retracted, *pupils dilated*, double vision. Meningitis. *Pain from nape of neck;* cannot hold head up. Sunstroke; head full, throbbing arteries. [*Bell.; Glon.; Usnea.*] *Face flushed.* Convulsive twitching of facial muscles. [*Agaricus.*] Vertigo with nausea.

Tongue.—White or yellow, *with red streak down the middle.* Feels scalded. Increased saliva.

Stomach.—Thirsty. Nausea and vomiting. Smallest quantity of food or drink immediately rejected. Constrictive pain; increased by warm drinks. *Hiccough;* excessive and painful, with *spasms of œsophagus.* Burning in stomach and œsophagus.

Abdomen.—Pain above pelvis, with soreness.

Respiratory.—Congestion of lungs. Difficult breathing. Sensation of a heavy load on chest. Pneumonia, with faint feeling in stomach and violent congestion. *Croup.* Menstrual colic before the appearance of the discharge with strangury.

Urine.—Scanty with cloudy sediment.

Female.—Rigid os. [*Bell.; Gels.*] Puerperal fever. Suppressed menstruation, with congestion to head. [*Bell.*] Menstrual colic before the appearance of the discharge with strangury

Heart.—Pulse *slow, soft, weak*, irregular, intermittent. Rapid pulse, low tension. [*Tabac.; Dig.*] Constant, dull, burning pain in region of heart. Valvular diseases. *Beating of pulses throughout body.* especially in right thigh.

Extremities.—Aching pain in back of neck and shoulders. Severe pain in joints and muscles. Violent electric-like shocks in limbs. Convulsive twitchings. *Acute rheumatism. Fever.*

Skin.—Erysipelas, with cerebral symptoms. Erythema. Itching in various parts. *Hot sweating.*

Fever.—Hyperthermy in the evening and hypothermy in the morning. Suppurative fevers with great variation of temperature.

Relationship.—Compare: *Gels.; Bapt.; Bell.; Acon.; Ferr. phos.* Antidotes Strychnin—fluid extract, 20-40 drops.

Dose.—First to sixth potency.

VERBASCUM
(Mullein)

Has a pronounced action on the inferior maxillary branch of the fifth pair of the cranial nerves; on the ear; and respiratory tract and bladder. *Catarrhs, and colds, with periodical prosopalgia.* Quiets nervous, and bronchial, and urinary irritation, and cough.

Face.—Neuralgia affecting zygoma, temporo maxillary joint, and ear [*Menyanth.*], particularly of left side, with lachrymation, coryza, and sensation *as if parts were crushed with tongs.* Talking, sneezing, and change of temperature aggravate the pains; also, pressing teeth together. Pains seem to come in flashes, excited by least movement, occurring periodically at same hour in morning and afternoon each day.

Ears.—Otalgia, with a sense of obstruction. Deafness. Dry, scaly condition of meatus (use locally).

Abdomen.—Pain extends deep down, causing contraction of sphincter ani.

Rectum.—Many movements a day, with twisting about navel. Hæmorrhoids, with obstructed, hardened stool. Inflamed and painful piles.

Respiratory.—*Hoarse;* voice deep, harsh; sounds like a trumpet; "basso profundo." Cough; worse at night. Asthma. Soreness in pharynx, cough during sleep.

Urinary.—Constant dribbling. *Enuresis.* Burning urination. Increase with pressure in bladder.

Extremities.—Cramp-like pain in soles, right foot, and knee. Lower extremities feel heavy. Thumb feels numb. Neuralgic pain in left ankle. Stiffness *and soreness of joints of lower extremities.*

Modalities.—*Worse,* change of temperature, talking, sneezing, biting hard (inferior dental nerve): from 9 a. m. to 4 p. m.

Relationship.—Compare: *Rhus arom.; Caust.; Platin.; Sphingurus* (pain in zygoma).

Dose.—*Mullein oil,* (locally, for earache and dry, scaly condition of meatus. Also for teasing cough at night or lying down. Internally, tincture and lower potencies. *Enuresis,* five-drop doses night and morning.

VERBENA
(Blue Vervain)

Affects the skin and *nervous system*. Nervous depression, weakness and irritation and spasms. Promotes the absorption of blood and allays pain in bruises. Vesicular erysipelas. Passive congestion and intermittent fever. One of the remedies for Poison-oak. *Epilepsy*, insomnia, mental exhaustion. In epilepsy, it *brightens up the patient's mental powers* and helps the constipation.

Dose.—Single dose of the tincture. In epilepsy must be continued for a long time. Verbena in the form of a tea as a diuretic drink is used by Vannier (Paris) to aid elimination in tubercular therapy.

VESPA CRABRO
(Live Wasp)

Skin and female symptoms marked. Indurated feeling. Vasomotor symptoms of skin and mucous membranes.

Dizzy, better lying on back. Fainting. Numbness and blindness. Nausea and vomiting, followed by creeping chills from feet upward. Cramping pain in bowels. Axillary glands swollen with soreness of upper arms. Perspiration on parts laid on with itching.

Face.—Painful and swollen. Erysipelatous inflammation of lids. *Chemosis of conjunctiva.* Swelling of mouth and throat, with violent burning pains.

Urinary.—*Burning* with micturition; also itching.

Female.—Menstruation, preceded by depression, pain, pressure, and constipation. *Left ovary markedly affected*, with *frequent burning, micturition;* sacral pains extending up back. *Erosion around external os.*

Skin.—Erythema; *intense itching;* burning. *Boils;* stinging and soreness, relieved by bathing with vinegar. Wheals, macules and swellings with burning, stinging and soreness. Erythema multiforme, *relieved* by bathing with vinegar.

Relationship.—Compare: *Scorpio* (salivation; strabismus; tetanus); *Apis.*

Antidote: *Sempervivum tector.*, locally.

Dose.—Third to thirtieth potency.

VIBURNUM OPULUS
(High Cranberry)

A general remedy for cramps. Colicky pains in pelvic organs. Superconscious of internal sexual organs. Female symptoms most important. *Often prevents miscarriage.* False labor-pains. Spasmodic and congestive affections, dependent upon ovarian or uterine origin.

Head.—Irritable. Vertigo; feels as if falling forward. Severe pain in temporal region. Sore feeling in eyeballs.

Stomach.—Constant nausea; relieved by eating. No appetite.

Abdomen.—*Sudden cramps and colic pains.* Tender to pressure about umbilicus.

Female.—Menses *too late, scanty, lasting a few hours,* offensive in odor, with crampy pains, cramps extend down thighs. [*Bell.*] Bearing-down pains before. Ovarian region feels heavy and congested. Aching in sacrum and pubes, with pain in anterior muscles of thighs [*Xanthox.*]; *spasmodic and membranous dysmenorrhœa.* [*Borax.*] Leucorrhœa, excoriating. Smarting and itching of genitals. Faint on attempting to sit up. *Frequent and very early miscarriage,* causing seeming sterility. Pains from back to loins and womb worse early morning.

Urinary.—Frequent urging. Copious, pale, light-colored urine. Cannot hold water on coughing or walking.

Rectum.—Stools large and hard, with cutting in rectum and soreness of anus.

Extremities.—Stiff, sore feeling in nape of neck. Feels as if back would break. Sacral backache. Lower extremities weak and heavy.

Modalities.—*Worse,* lying on affected side, in warm room, evening and night. *Better,* in open air and resting.

Relationship.—Compare: *Viburnum prunifolium*—Black Haw—(habitual miscarriage; *after-pains;* cancer of the tongue; obstinate hiccough; supposed to be a uterine tonic. Morning sickness; menstrual irregularities of sterile females with uterine displacements.) *Cimicif.; Cauloph.; Sep.; Xanthox.*

Dose.—Tincture, and lower potencies.

VINCA MINOR
(Lesser Periwinkle)

A remedy for skin affections, eczema, and especially plica polonica; also for hæmorrhages and diphtheria.

Head.—Tearing pain in vertex, ringing and whistling in ears. Whirling vertigo, with flickering before eyes. *Spots on scalp, oozing moisture, matting hair together. Corrosive itching of scalp.* Bald spots. *Plica polonica.* Irresistible desire to scratch.

Nose.—Tip gets red easily. Moist eruption on septum. Stoppage of one nostril. *Sores in nose.* Seborrhœa upper lip and base of nose.

Throat.—Difficult swallowing. Ulcers. Frequent hawking. *Diphtheria.*

Female.—Excessive menstruation with great weakness. *Passive uterine hæmorrhages.* [*Ust.; Trill.; Secale.*] Menorrhagia; continuous flow, particulary at climacteric. [*Lach.*] Hæmorrhages from fibroids.

Skin.—Corrosive itching. *Great sensitiveness of skin, with redness and soreness* from slight rubbing. Eczema of head and face; pustules, itching, burning, and offensive odor. Hair matted together.

Relationship.—Compare: *Oleand.; Staph.*

Dose.—First to third potency.

VIOLA ODORATA
(Violet)

Has a specific action on the ear. Affects especially dark-haired patients; supra-orbital and orbital regions; rheumatism in upper parts of the body when on the *right* side. *Worm affections* in children. [*Teuc.*] Locally, for pain due to uterine fibroids. Also against snake-bites, bee-stings. *Tension* extends to upper half of face and ears.

Head.—*Burning of the forehead.* Vertigo; everything in head seems to whirl around. Heaviness of head, with sensation of weakness in muscles of nape of neck. *Scalp tense; must knit the brows. Tendency to pain immediately above eyebrows.* Throbbing under eye and temple. *Headache across the fore-*

head. Acts upon frontal sinuses. Hysterical attacks in tuberculous patients.

Eyes.—Heaviness of lids. Eyeball feels compressed. Flames before eyes. Myopia. Choroiditis. Illusions of vision; fiery, serpentine circles.

Ears.—Shooting in ears. Aversion to music. Roaring and tickling. Deep stitches beneath ears. Deafness; *otorrhœa*. Ear affections with pain in eyeballs.

Respiratory.—Torpor in the end of nose, as from a blow. Dry, short, spasmodic cough and dyspnœa; worse in daytime. Oppression of chest. Pertussis, with hoarseness. *Dyspnœa during pregnancy*. Difficult breathing, anxiety and palpitation, with hysteria.

Extremities.—Rheumatism of the deltoid muscle. Trembling of limbs. *Pressing pain in right carpal and metacarpal joints*. [*Ulmus.*]

Urinary.—*Milky urine;* smells strong. Enuresis in nervous children.

Modalities.—*Worse,* cool air.

Relationship.—Compare: *Ulmus* (formication in feet, numb, creeping pain in legs and feet; rheumatic pains above wrists; numbness, tingling, and full soreness where gastrocnemius gives off its tendon); *Chenopodium (ears; serous or bloody effusion in the labyrinth;* chronic otitis media; *progressive deafness to the voice, but sensitive to sounds* of passing vehicles and other sounds; buzzing; absent or deficient bone conduction; a consciousness of the ear; hearing better for shrill, high-pitched sounds than for low ones); *Aur.; Puls.; Sep.; Ign.; Cina; Cauloph.* (in rheumatism of small joints.)

Dose.—First to sixth potency.

VIOLA TRICOLOR
(Pansy)

The principal uses of this remedy are for eczema in childhood and nocturnal emission accompanied by very vivid dreams.

Head.—Heavy, pressing-outward pain. Eczema of scalp, with swollen glands. Face hot and sweating after eating.

Throat.—Much phlegm, causing hawking; worse in the air. Swallowing difficult.

Urinary.—Copious; disagreeable, cat-like odor.

Male.—Swelling of prepuce, burning in glans. Itching. Involuntary, seminal emissions at stool.

Skin.—*Impetigo.* Intolerable itching. Eruptions, particularly over face and head, with burning, itching; worse at night. Thick scabs, which crack and exude a tenacious yellow pus. Eczema impetigonoides of the face. Sycosis.

Modalities.—*Worse,* winter; 11 a. m. Compare: *Lycop.*

Relationship.—Compare: *Rhus; Calc.; Sepia.*

Dose.—Lower potencies.

VIPERA
(The German Viper)

Viper poisoning causes a temporary increase in reflexes, paresis supervenes, a paraplegia of the lower extremities extending upwards. Resembles acute ascending paralysis of Landry. (Wells.) Has special action on kidneys and induces hæmaturia. Cardiac dropsy.

Indicated in inflammation of veins with great swelling; *bursting sensation. Enlargement of liver.* Ailments of menopause. Œdema of glottis. Poly-neuritis, polio-myelitis.

Face.—Excessively swollen. Lips and tongue swollen, livid, protruding. Tongue dry, brown, black. Speech difficult.

Liver.—Violent pain in enlarged liver, with jaundice and fever; extends to shoulder and hip.

Extremities.—Patient is obliged to keep the extremities elevated. *When they are allowed to hang down, it seems as if they would burst, and the pain is unbearable.* [*Diad.*] *Varicose veins* and acute phlebitis. Veins swollen, sensitive; bursting pain. Severe cramps in lower extremities.

Skin.—Livid. Skin peels in large plates. Lymphangioma, boils, carbuncles, with *bursting* sensation, relieved by elevating parts.

Relationship.—*Pelius berus*—Adder. (Prostration and fainting, faltering pulse, skin yellow, *pain about navel.* Swelling of arm, tongue, right eye; giddiness, nervousness, faintness, sickness, compression of chest, could not breathe properly or take a deep breath; aching and stiffness of limbs, joints stiff, collapsed feeling, great thirst.) *Eel serum* (heart and kidney diseases. Failure of compensation and impending asystole).

Dose.—Twelfth potency.

VISCUM ALBUM
(Mistletoe)

Lowered blood pressure. Dilated blood vessels but does not act on the centers in the medulla. Pulse is slow due to central irritation of the vagus.

The symptoms point especially to rheumatic and gouty complaints; neuralgia, especially sciatica. Epilepsy, *chorea*, and metrorrhagia. *Rheumatic deafness. Asthma.* Spinal pains, due to uterine causes. Rheumatism with *tearing pains.* Hypertensive albuminuria. Valvular disease, with disturbances in sexual sphere. Symptoms like epileptic aura and petit mal.

Head.—Feeling as if whole vault of skull were lifted up. Blue rings around eyes. Double vision. Buzzing and stopped-up feeling in ear. Deafness from cold. Facial muscles in constant agitation. Persistent vertigo.

Respiratory.—Dyspnœa; *feeling of suffocation when lying on left side.* Spasmodic cough. *Asthma,* if connected with gout or rheumatism. Stertorous breathing.

Female.—Hæmorrhage, with pain; blood partly clots and bright red. Climacteric complaints. [*Lach.; Sulph.*] Pain from sacrum into pelvis, with tearing, shooting pains from above downwards. Retained placenta. [*Secale.*] Chronic endometritis. Metrorrhagia. Ovaralgia, especially left.

Heart.—Hypertrophy with valvular insufficiency; pulse small and weak; unable to rest in a reclining position. Palpitation during coitus. Low tension. Failing compensation, dyspnœa worse lying on left side. Weight and oppression of heart; as if a hand were squeezing it; tickling sensation about heart.

Extremities.—Pains alternate in the knee and ankle with shoulder and elbow. *Sciatica. Tearing,* shooting pains in both thighs and upper extremities. A *glow* rises from the feet to the head; seems to be on fire. Periodic pains from sacrum into pelvis, *worse in bed*, with pains into thighs and upper extremities. General tremor, as if all muscles were in state of fibrillary contraction. Dropsy of extremities. Sensation of a spider crawling over back of hand and foot. Itching all over. Compressing pain in feet.

Modalities.—*Worse,* winter, cold, stormy weather; in bed. Movement; lying on left side.

Relationship.—Compare: *Secale; Convallar.; Bry.; Puls.; Rhodod. Guipsine*—active principle—(exalts the hypotensive properties of Viscum). *Hedera Helix*—Ivy—(Intercranial pressure).

Dose.—Tincture and lower potencies.

WYETHIA
(Poison-weed)

Has marked effects on the throat, and has proven an excellent remedy in *pharyngitis,* especially the follicular form. Irritable throats of singers and public speakers. Useful also in hæmorrhoids. Hay-fever symptoms; *itching in posterior nares.*

Head.—Nervous, uneasy, depressed. Dizzy. Rush of blood to head. Sharp pain in forehead.

Mouth.—Feels as if scalded; sensation of heat down œsophagus. Itching of the palate.

Throat.—Constant clearing and hemming. *Dry,* posterior nares; no relief from clearing. *Throat feels swollen;* epiglottis dry and burning. Difficult swallowing. Constant desire to swallow saliva. Uvula feels elongated.

Stomach.—Sense of weight. Belching of wind alternating with hiccough. Nausea and vomiting.

Abdomen.—Pain below ribs of right side.

Stool.—Loose, dark, at night. Itching of anus. Constipation, *with hæmorrhoids;* not bleeding.

Respiratory.—*Dry, hacking cough,* caused by tickling of the epiglottis. Burning sensation in the bronchial tubes. Tendency to get hoarse talking or singing; throat hot, dry. Dry asthma.

Female.—Pain in left ovary, shooting down to knee. Pain in uterus; could outline its contour.

Extremities.—Pain in back; extends to end of spine. Pain right arm, stiffness of wrist and hand. Aching pains all over.

Fever.—Chill at 11 a. m. Thirst for ice-water during chill. No thirst with heat. Profuse sweat all night. Terrific headache during sweat.

Relationship.—Compare: *Arum; Sang.; Lach.*

Dose.—First to sixth potency.

XANTHOXYLUM
(Prickly Ash)

Its specific action is on the nervous system and mucous membranes. Paralysis, especially *hemiplegia*. Painful hæmorrhages, after-pains, *neuralgic dysmenorrhœa*, and rheumatic affections, offer a therapeutic field for this remedy, especially in patients of spare habit and nervous, delicate organization. Indigestion from over-eating or from too much fluid. Sluggish capillary circulation. Neurasthenia, poor assimilation, insomnia, occipital headache. Increases mucous secretion of mouth and stimulates the secretion from all glands with ducts opening in the mouth.

Mind.—Nervous, frightened. Mental depression.

Head.—Feels full. Weight and pain on vertex. Pain over eyes, throbbing pressure over nose, pressure in forehead; head seems divided; ringing in ears. Occipital headache. Sick headache with dizziness and flatulence.

Face.—Neuralgia of lower jaw. Dryness of mouth and fauces. Pharyngitis. [*Wyethia*.]

Abdomen.—Griping and diarrhœa. Dysentery, with *tympanites*, tenesmus; inodorous discharges.

Female.—Menses too early and painful. Ovarian neuralgia, with pain in loins and lower abdomen; worse, *left side*, extending down the thigh, along genito-crural nerves. *Neuralgic dysmenorrhœa*, with neuralgic headaches; pain in *back and down legs*. Menses thick, almost black. *After-pains*. [*Arnica; Cup.; Cham.*] Leucorrhœa at time of menses. Neurasthænic patients who are thin, emaciated; poor assimilation with insomnia and occipital headache.

Respiratory.—Aphonia. Constant desire to take a long breath; oppression of chest. Dry cough, day and night.

Extremities.—Paralysis of left side following spinal disorders. Numbness of left side; impairment of nerves of motion. Hemiplegia. Pain in nape, extending down back. Sciatica; worse, hot weather. Anterior, crural neuralgia. [*Staph.*] Left arm numb. Neuralgic shooting pain, as from electricity, all over limbs.

Sleep.—Hard and unrefreshing; dreams of flying. Sleeplessness in neurasthenics.

Relationship.—Compare: *Gnaph.; Cimicif.; Staph.; Mezer.; Piscidia*—White dogwood—(a nerve sedative. *Insomnia due to worry, nervous excitement, spasmodic coughs; pains of irregular menstruation; regulates the flow. Neuralgic and spasmodic affections. Use tincture in rather material doses.*)

Dose.—First to sixth potency.

XEROPHYLLUM

(Tamalpais Lily. Basket Grass Flower)

Should prove curative in eczematous conditions, poison-oak, early typhoid states, etc.

Mind.—Dull, cannot concentrate mind for study; forgets names; *writes last letters of words first;* misspells common words.

Head.—Feels full, stuffed up, pain across forehead and above eyes. Great pressure at root of nose. Bewildered. Loss of consciousness. Pulsating headache.

Eyes.—Painful, as of sand, smarting; difficult to focus for close work. Eyes feel sore, burn.

Nose.—Stuffed; tightness at bridge of nose; acute nasal catarrh.

Face.—Bloated in morning. Puffy under eyes.

Throat.—Stitching pain upon swallowing.

Stomach.—Feels full and heavy. Eructations sour; offensive, an hour after luncheon and dinner. Vomiting at 2 p. m.

Abdomen.—Intestinal flatulence. In morning rumbling in bowels, with desire for stool.

Rectum.—Constipation, stools hard, small lumps. Difficult, soft stools, with much straining. Much flatus. Bearing-down pain in rectum.

Urine.—Difficulty of retaining; dribbling when walking. Frequent urination at night.

Female.—Bearing-down sensation. Vulva inflamed, with furious itching. Increased sexual desire, with ovarian and uterine pains and leucorrhœa.

Respiratory.—Posterior nares raw; discharge thick, yellow mucus. Sneezing. Trachea sore; lumps feel constricted.

Back.—Feels hot from sacrum to scapulæ. Backache, extending down legs. Pain over kidneys. Heat deep in spine.

Extremities.—Muscular lameness, trembling. Pain in knees. Limbs feel stiff. [*Rhus.*]

Skin.—Erythema, with vesication and intense itching, stinging, and burning. Blisters, little lumps. Skin rough and cracked; feels like leather. Dermatitis, especially around knees. Inflammation resembling poison-oak. Inguinal glands and behind knee swollen.

Modalities.—*Worse*, application of cold water, in afternoon and evening. *Better*, application of hot water, in morning, moving affected part.

Relationship.—Compare: *Rhus; Anacard.: Grindelia.*

Dose.—Sixth potency or higher.

X-RAY

(Vial containing alcohol exposed to X-Ray)

Repeated exposure to Roentgen (X-ray) has produced skin lesions often followed by cancer. Distressing pain. Sexual glands are particularly affected. Atrophy of ovaries and testicles. Sterility. Changes take place in the blood lymphatics and bone marrow. Anæmia and leukæmia. Corresponds to stubbornness as in burns, they refuse to heal. Psoriasis.

Has the property of stimulating cellular metabolism. Arouses the reactive vitality, mentally and physically. Brings to the surface suppressed symptoms, especially sycotic and those due to mixed infections. Its homœopathic action is thus centrifugal, towards the periphery.

Head.—Sticking pains in different parts of head and face. Dull pain in right upper jaw. Stiff neck. Sudden cricks in neck, pains more severe behind ears. Pain in muscles of neck when lifting head from pillow. Fullness in ears, ringing in head.

Mouth.—Tongue dry, rough, sore. Throat painful on swallowing. Nausea.

Male.—Lewd dreams. Sexual desire lost. Re-establishes suppressed gonorrhœa.

Extremities.—Rheumatic pains. General tired and sick feeling. Palms rough and scaly.

Skin.—Dry, itching eczema. Erythema around roots of nails. Skin dry, wrinkled. Painful cracks. Warty growths. Nails thicken. Psoriasis.

Modalities.—*Worse*, in bed, afternoon, evening and night; open air.

Dose.—Twelfth potency and higher.

Compare: *Electricitas.*—Sugar of milk saturated with the current. (Anxiety, nervous tremors, restlessness, palpitation, headaches. Dreads approach of thunder-storms; heaviness of limbs.)

Magnetis Poli Ambo.—The Magnet.—Sugar of milk or distilled water exposed to influence of entire mass. (Burning lancinations throughout the body; pains as if broken in joints, when cartilages of two bones touch; shooting and jerkings; headache as if a nail were driven in; tendency of old wounds to bleed afresh.)

Magnetis Polus Arcticus.—North pole of the magnet.— (Disturbed sleep, somnambulism, cracking in cervical vertebræ, sensation of coldness; toothache.)

Magnetis Polus Australis.—South pole of the magnet.— (Severe pain in inner side of nail of the big toe, *ingrowing toenail;* easy dislocation of joints of foot; feet are painful when letting them hang down.)

YOHIMBINUM
(Coryanthe Yohimbe)

Excites sexual organs and acts on central nervous system and respiratory centre. An aphrodisiac, used in physiological doses. but contraindicated in all acute and chronic inflammations of abdominal organs. Homœopathically, should be of service in congestive conditions of the sexual organs. Causes hyperæmia of the milk glands and stimulates the function of lactation. Menorrhagia.

Head.—Agitation, with flying sensations of heat in face. Disagreeable, metallic taste. Copious salivation. Nausea and eructation.

Sexual.—*Strong and lasting erections*. Neurasthenic impotence. Bleeding piles. Intestinal hæmorrhage. Urethritis.

Fever.—Rigor; intense heat, waves of heat and chilliness, tendency to sweat.

Sleep.—*Sleepless.* Thoughts of events of whole past life keep him awake.

Dose.—As a sexual stimulant, ten drops of a one per cent. solution, or hypodermic tablets of 0.005 gm. Homœopathic dose, third potency.

YUCCA FILAMENTOSA
(Bear-grass)

So-called bilious symptoms, with headache. Despondent and irritable.

Head.—Aches as if top of head would fly off. Arteries of forehead throb. Nose red.

Face.—Yellow; tongue yellow, coated, taking imprint of teeth. [*Merc.; Pod.; Rhus.*]

Mouth.—Taste as of rotten eggs. [*Arnica.*]

Throat.—Sensation as if something hung down from posterior nares; cannot get it up or down.

Abdomen.—Deep pain in right side over liver, going through back. Stool yellowish brown, with bile.

Male.—Burning and swelling of the prepuce, with redness of meatus. Gonorrhœa. [*Cann.; Tussil.*]

Skin.—Erythematous redness.

Dose.—Tincture, to third potency.

ZINCUM METALLICUM
(Zinc)

The provings picture cerebral depression. The word "fag" covers a large part of zinc action. Tissues are worn out faster than they are repaired. Poisoning from suppressed eruptions or discharges. The nervous symptoms of most importance. Defective vitality. Impending brain paralysis. *Period of depression in disease.* Spinal affections. Twitchings. Pain, as if between skin and flesh. Great relief from discharges. Chorea, from fright or suppressed eruption. *Convulsions, with pale face and no heat.* Marked anæmia with profound prostration. It causes a decrease in the number, and destruction of red blood corpuscles. Repercussed eruptive diseases. In chronic diseases with brain and spinal symptoms, trembling, convulsive twitching and fidgety feet are guiding symptoms.

Mind.—Weak memory. *Very sensitive to noise.* Averse to work, to talk. *Child repeats everything said to it.* Fears arrest on account of a supposed crime. Melancholia. *Lethargic, stupid.* Paresis.

Head.—Feels as if he would fall to left side. Headache from the smallest quantity of wine. Hydrocephalus. Rolls head from side to side. Bores head into pillow. *Occipital* pain, with weight on vertex. Automatic motion of head and hands. Brain-fag; headaches of overtaxed school children. *Forehead cool; base of brain hot.* Roaring in head. Starting in fright.

Eyes.—Pterygium; smarting, lachrymation, itching. Pressure as if pressed into head. Itching and soreness of lids and *inner angles.* Ptosis. *Rolling of eyes.* Blurring of one-half of vision; worse, stimulants. *Squinting.* Amaurosis, with severe headache. Red and inflamed conjunctiva; *worse, inner canthus.*

Ears.—Tearing, stitches, and external swelling. Discharge of fetid pus.

Nose.—Sore feeling high up; pressure upon root.

Face.—*Pale* lips, and corners of mouth cracked. Redness and itching eruption on chin. Tearing in facial bones.

Mouth.—Teeth loose. Gums bleed. Gnashing of teeth. Bloody taste. Blisters on tongue. Difficult dentition; child weak; cold and restless feet.

Throat.—Dry; constant inclination to hawk up tenacious mucus. Rawness and dryness in throat and larynx. Pain in muscles of throat when swallowing.

Stomach.—Hiccough, nausea, vomiting of bitter mucus. Burning in stomach, heartburn from sweet things. *Cannot stand smallest quantity of wine. Ravenous hunger* about 11 a. m. [*Sulph.*] Great greediness when eating; cannot eat fast enough. Atonic dyspepsia, feeling as if stomach were collapsed.

Abdomen.—Pain after a light meal, with tympanitis. Pain in spot beneath navel. Gurgling and griping; distended. Faltuent colic, with retraction of abdomen. [*Plumb.*] Enlarged,

ZINCUM METALLICUM

indurated sore liver. Reflex symptoms from floating kidney. *Griping after eating.*

Urine.—Can only void urine when sitting bent backwards. Hysterical retention. Involuntary urination when walking, coughing or sneezing.

Rectum.—Hard, small, constipated stool. *Cholera infantum*, with tenesmus; green mucous discharges. Sudden cessation of diarrhœa, followed by cerebral symptoms.

Male.—Testicles swelled, drawn up. Erections violent. Emissions with hypochondriasis. Falling off of hair (pubic). Drawing in testicles up to spermatic cord.

Female.—Ovarian pain, *especially left; can't keep still.* [*Viburn.*] Nymphomania of lying-in women. Menses too late, suppressed; lochia suppressed. [*Puls.*] Breasts painful. Nipples sore. Menses flow more at night. [*Bov.*] Complaints all *better during menstrual flow.* [*Eupion; Lach.*] *All the female symptoms are associated with restlessness, depression, coldness, spinal tenderness and restless feet.* Dry cough before and during menses.

Respiratory.—Burning pressure beneath sternum. Constriction and cutting in chest. Hoarseness. Debilitating, spasmodic cough; worse, eating sweet things. Child grasps genitals during cough. Asthmatic bronchitis, with constriction of chest. *Dyspnœa better as soon as expectoration appears.*

Back.—Pain in small of back. Cannot bear back *touched.* [*Sul.; Therid.; Cinch.*] Tension and stinging between shoulders. Spinal irritation. *Dull aching about the last dorsal or first lumbar vertebræ; worse sitting.* Burning along spine. Nape of neck weary from writing or any exertion. Tearing in shoulder-blades.

Extremities.—Lameness, *weakness, trembling and twitching* of various muscles. Chilblains. [*Agar.*] *Feet in continued motion; cannot keep still.* Large varicose veins on legs. Sweaty. Convulsions, *with pale face. Transverse pains,* especially in upper extremity. *Soles of feet sensitive.* Steps with entire sole of foot on floor.

Sleep.—Cries out during sleep; body jerks; wakes frightened, stared. Nervous motion of feet when asleep. Loud screaming out at night in sleep without being aware of it. Somnambulism. [*Kali phos.*]

Skin.—*Varicose veins*, especially of lower extremities. [*Puls.*] Formication of feet and legs as from bugs crawling over the skin, preventing sleep. Eczema, especially in the anæmic and neurotic. Itching of thighs and *hollow of knees*. *Retrocession of eruptions.*

Fever.—Frequent, febrile shiverings down back. Cold extremities. Night-sweat. Profuse sweat on feet.

Modalities.—*Worse*, at menstrual period, from touch, between 5 to 7 p. m.; after dinner, from wine. *Better*, while eating, discharges, and appearance of eruptions.

Relationship.—Compare: *Agaric.; Ign.; Plumb.; Argent.; Puls.; Helleb.; Tuberc.* Inimical: *Nux; Cham.* Compare in amelioration by secretions: *Lach.; Stan.; Mosch.*

Compare: *Zincum aceticum* (effects of night-watching and erysipelas; brain feels sore; *Rademacher's solution*, five-drop doses three times a day in water, *for those who are compelled to work, on an insufficient amount of sleep*); *Zinc. bromatum* (dentition, chorea, hydrocephalus; *Zinc. oxydatum*. (Nausea and sour taste. Sudden vomiting in children. Vomiting of bile and diarrhœa. Flatulent abdomen. Watery stools with tenesmus. Debility after grip. Fiery red face, *great drowsiness* with dreamlike unrefreshing sleep. Similar to effect of night watching. Mental and physical exertion (Rademacher). *Zinc. Sulph.*, not repeated frequently (high potency) will clear up opacities of the cornea (McFarland). Corneitis; granular lids; tongue paralyzed; cramps in arms and legs; trembling and convulsions. Hypochrondriasis due to masturbation; nervous headaches); *Zinc. cyanatum* (as a remedy for meningitis and cerebro-spinal meningitis, paralysis agitans, chorea, and hysteria, it has received some attention); *Zinc. ars.* (chorea, anæmia, *profound exhaustion* on slight exertion. Depression and marked involvement of lower extremities); *Zinc. carb.* (post-gonorrhœal throat affections, tonsils swollen, bluish superficial spots); *Zinc. phos.* (herpes zoster 1x); *Zinc. muriat.* (disposition to pick the bedclothes; sense of smell and taste perverted; bluish-green tint of skin; cold and sweaty); *Zinc. phos.* (neuralgia of head and face; lightning-like pains in locomotor ataxia, brain-fag, nervousness, and vertigo; sexual excitement and sleeplessness); *Ammon. valerian* (violent neuralgia, with great nervous agitation); *Zinc. picricum* (facial paralysis; brain-fag, headache in Bright's disease; seminal emissions; loss of memory and energy). Oxide of zinc is used locally as an astringent and stimulant application to unhealthy ulcers, fissures, intertrigo, burns, etc.

Dose.—Second to sixth potency.

ZINCUM VALERIANUM
(Valerinate of Zinc)

A remedy for *neuralgia*, hysteria, angina pectoris, and other *painful* affections, notably in *ovarian affections*. Epilepsy without aura. Hysterical heart-pain. *Facial* neuralgia, violent in left temple and inferior maxillary. Sleeplessness in children. Obstinate *hiccough*.

Head.—Violent, neuralgic, *intermittent headaches*. Becomes almost insane with pain, which is piercing and stabbing. Uncontrollable sleeplessness from pain in head with melancholy.

Female.—*Ovaralgia; pain shoots down limbs*, even to foot.

Extremities.—Severe pain in neck and spine. Cannot sit still; must keep legs in constant motion. Sciatic neuralgia.

Dose.—First and second trituration. Must be continued for some time in treatment of neuralgia.

ZINGIBER
(Ginger)

States of debility in the digestive tract, and sexual system and respiratory troubles, call for this remedy. Complete cessation of function of kidneys.

Head.—Hemicrania; sudden glimmering before eyes; feels confused and empty. Pain over eyebrows.

Nose.—Feels obstructed and dry. Intolerable itching; red pimples.

Stomach.—Taste of food remains long, especially of bread and toast. Feels heavy, like from a stone. *Complaints from eating melons and drinking impure water. Acidity.* [*Calc.;*

Robinia.] Heaviness in stomach on awakening with wind and rumbling, great thirst and emptiness. Pain from pit to under sternum, worse eating.

Abdomen.—Colic, diarrhœa, extremely loose bowels. Diarrhœa from drinking bad water, with much flatulence, cutting pain, relaxation of sphincter. Hot, sore, painful anus during pregnancy. Chronic intestinal catarrh. Anus red and inflamed. Hæmorrhoids hot, painful, sore. [*Aloe.*]

Urinary.—Frequent desire to urinate. Stinging, burning in orifice. Yellow discharge from urethra. Urine thick, turbid, of strong odor, suppressed. Complete suppression after typhoid. After urinating, continues to ooze in drops.

Male.—Itching of prepuce. Sexual desire excited; painful erections. Emissions.

Respiratory.—Hoarseness. *Smarting below larynx;* breathing difficult. *Asthma*, without anxiety, *worse* toward morning. Scratching sensation in throat; stitches in chest. Cough dry, hacking; copious morning sputa.

Extremities.—Very weak in all joints. Back lame. Cramps in soles and palms.

Relationship.—Compare: *Calad.*

Antidote: *Nux.*

Dose.—First to sixth potency.

REPERTORY

MIND

AWKWARD—Lets things fall from hand: Æth.; *Apis;* Bov.; Helleb.; Ign.; Lach.; *Nat. m.;* Nux v.; Tar. h.

BRAIN-FAG—*Æth.;* Ail.; Alfal.; *Anac.;* Anhal.; *Arg. n.;* Avena; Bapt.; *Calc. c.; Calc. p.;* Coca; *Cocc.;* Cupr. m.; *Gels.;* Kali p.; Lecith.; Nat. m.; Nux v.; *Phos. ac.; Phos.;* Picr. ac.; Sil.; *Strych. p.;* Zinc. m.; *Zinc. p.; Zinc. picr.* See Neurasthenia (Nervous System).

CATALEPSY—Trance: Acon.; Art. v.; Camph. monobr.; *Can. ind.;* Cham.; Cic.; *Crot. casc.;* Cur.; Gels.; Graph.; Hydroc. ac.; Hyos.; Lach.; Merc.; *Morph.; Mosch.;* Nux m.; *Op.;* Sabad.; Stram.

CLAIRVOYANCE—*Acon.; Anac.;* Anhal.; *Can. ind.;* Nabulus; Nux m.; *Phos.* See Hallucinations.

COMPREHENSION—Difficult: Agn.; *Ail.; Anac.;* Bapt.; Cocc.; *Gels.; Helleb.;* Lyc.; Nat. c.; *Nux m.;* Oleand.; *Op.; Phos. ac.;* Phos.; Plumb. m.; Xerophyl.; *Zinc. m.* See Memory.

COMPREHENSION—Easy: Bell.; *Coff.;* Lach.

CONSCIOUSNESS—Loss: Absinth.; *Ail.;* Arn.; Atrop.; *Bell.; Can. ind.;* Carb. ac.; *Cic.;* Cupr. ac.; Gels.; Glon.; *Helleb.; Hydroc. ac.; Hyoc.;* Mur. ac.; Nux m.; Œnanthe; *Op.;* Stram.; Xerophyl.; *Zinc. m.*

CRETINISM—Imbecility, Idiocy: Absinth.; *Æth.; Anac.;* Arn.; Bac.; Bar. c.; Bar. m.; *Bufo;* Calc. p.; Helleb.; Ign.; Iod.; Lol.; Nat. c.; Oxytrop.; Phos. ac.; Plumb. m.; Sul.; *Thyr.*

DELIRIUM—Alcoholic (delirium tremens): Acon.; Agar.; Ant. t.; *Atrop.; Bell.; Can. ind.; Caps.;* Chin. s.; Cim.; Dig.; Hyos.; *Hyosc. hydrobr.;* Kali br.; Kali p.; Lach.; Lupul.; *Nux v.;* Op.; Passifl.; Pastin.; *Ran. b.;* Stram.; Strych. n.; Sumb.; Teucr.

Carphologia (picking at bed clothes, flocks)—Agar.; Atrop.; *Bell.;* Helleb.; *Hyos.;* Mur. ac.; Op.; Stram.; Zinc. mur.

Coma Vigil—Cur.; Hyos.; Mur. ac.; Op.; Phos.

Destructive (desire to bark, bite, strike, tear things)—*Bell.; Canth.;* Cupr. m.; Hyos.; Sec.; *Stram.; Ver. a.;* Ver. v.

Effort to escape from bed, or hide—Acon.; *Agar.; Bell.; Bry.;* Cupr. m.; Helleb.; *Hyos.;* Operc.; Op.; Rhus t.; *Stram.; Ver. a.*

Furor, frenzy, ravings—Acon.; Agar.; *Bell.; Canth.;* Cic.; Cupr. m.; *Hyos.;* Merc. cy.; Œnanthe; Solan. n.; *Stram.; Ver. a.*

Lascivious furor—*Canth.; Hyos.;* Phos.; Stram.; Ver. a.

Loquacity, talks incessantly—*Agar.;* Bell.; Can. ind.; *Cim.; Hyos.; Lach.;* Merc. cy.; Oper.; Op.; Stram.; Ver. a.

Merry, dancing, singing—Agar.; *Bell.;* Hyos.; Stram.; Ver. a.

Muttering, low, incoherently—Agar.; *Ail.;* Apis; Arn.; Bapt.; Bell.; Crot.; Helleb.; *Hyos.;* Lach.; *Mur. ac.; Phos. ac.;* Phos.; *Rhus t.;* Stram.; Ver. a.

Rapid answering—Cim.; *Lach.*; Stram.; Ver. **a.**

Slow answering, relapses—Arn.; Bapt.; Diph.; *Helleb.*; Hyos.; Phos. ac.; Phos.; Sul.

Sopor, stupor, coma—Æth.; Agar.; *Ail.*; Am. c.; *Ant. t.*; *Apis*; Arn.; Bapt.; Bell.; Benz. nit.; Camph.; Carb. ac.; Diph.; Gels.; *Helleb.*; Hyos.; Lach.; Laur.; Lob. purp.; Mur. ac.; Nitr. sp. d.; Nux m.; Op.; Phos. ac.; Phos.; Piloc.; *Rhus t.*; Stram.; Tereb.; Thyr.; Ver. a.; Zinc. m.

DEMENTIA—*Agar.*; *Anac.*; Apium v.; *Bell.*; Calc. c.; Calc. p.; Can. ind.; Con.; Helleb.; *Hyos.*; Ign.; *Lil t.*; Merc.; *Nat. sal.*; Op.; Phos. ac.; Phos.; Picr. ac.; Sul.; Ver. a.

Epileptic—Acon.; *Bell.*; Cim.; *Cupr. ac.*; Cupr. m.; Laur.; *Œnanthe*; *Sil.*; Solan. n.; Stram.; Ver. v.

Masturbatic—*Agn.*; Calc. p.; Canth.; Caust.; Damiana; Nux v.; Op.; Phos. ac.; Phos.; Picr. ac.; *Staph.*

Paretic—*Acon.*; Æsc. gl.; Agar.; Ars.; *Bad.*; Bell.; Can. ind.; Cim.; Cupr. m.; Hyos.; Ign.; Iodof.; Merc.; Phos.; Plumb. m.; Stram.; Ver. v.; Zinc. m.

Senile—Anac.; *Aur. iod.*; Bar. ac.; *Bar. c.*; Calc. p.; Con.; Nat. iod.; Phos.; Sec.

Syphilitic—Aur. iod.; *Kali iod.*; Mercuries; Nit. ac.; Sul.

EMOTIONS—**Effects: Anger, bad news, disappointment, vexation:** Acon.; Apis; Ars.; Aur.; Bry.; Caust.; Cham.; Cocc.; Colch.; Col.; Gels.; Grat.; Hyos.; Ign.; Lach.; Nat. m.; *Nux v.*; Phos. ac.; Puls.; Sep.; Staph.

Fright, fear—*Acon.*; Apis; Aur.; Bell.; *Gels.*; Hyos.; Hyper.; Ign.; Nat. m., Morph.; *Op.*; Puls.; Samb.; Ver. a.

Grief, sorrow—Am. m.; Ant. c.; Apis; Aur. m.; Calc. p.; Caust.; Cocc.; Cycl.; Hyos.; *Ign.*; Lach.; Nat. m.; *Phos. ac.*; Plat.; Samb.

Jealousy—Apis; Hyos.; *Lach.*; Staph.

Joy, excessive—Caust.; *Coff.*; Croc.

Nostalgia (homesickness)—*Caps.*; Eup. purp.; Helleb.; *Ign.*; Mag. m.; Phos. ac.; Senec.

Shame, mortification, reserved displeasure—Aur.; Ign.; Nat. m.; *Staph.*

FEARS—**Dread: Being carried or raised:** Bor.; Bry.; Sanic. ac.

Crossing streets, crowds, excitement—*Acon.*; Hydroc. ac.; Plat.

Dark, ghosts—*Acon.*; Ars.; Bell.; Carb. v.; Caust.; Hyos.; Lyc.; Med.; Op.; Phos.; Puls.; Radium; Rhus t.; *Stram.*

Death, fatal diseases, impending evil—*Acon.*; *Agn.*; Anac.; *Apis*; Arg. n.; Ars.; *Aur.*; *Cact.*; Calc. c.; Can. ind.; *Cim.*; *Dig.*; Gels.; Graph.; Hydr.; Ign.; Kali c.; Lac c.; *Lil. t.*; Med.; Naja; Nat. m.; *Nit. ac.*; *Nux v.*; Phaseol.; Phos.; *Plat.*; Pod.; Psor.; Puls.; Rhus t.; Sabad.; Sec.; Sep.; Stann.; Staph.; Still.; Syph.; Ver. a.

Downward motion, falling—*Bor.*; Gels.; Hyper.; *Sanic.*

Heart ceases beating, must move—Gels. (reverse Dig.).

Lectophobia—Can. s.

Loss of reason—*Acon.*; Alum.; *Arg. n.*; *Calc. c.*; Can. ind.; Chlorum; Cim.; Iod.; Kali br.; Lac c.; *Lil. t.*; Lyssin; *Mancin.*; Med.; Plat.; Sep.; Syph.; Ver. **a.**

Motion—*Bry.;* Calad.; Gels.; Mag. p.

Music—Acon.; *Ambra;* Bufo; *Nat. c.;* Nux v.; *Sab.;* Tar. h.; Thuya.

Noises—Acon.; *Asar.;* Bell.; *Bor.;* Calad.; *Cham.;* Cocc.; Ferr.; Ign.; Kali c.; Mag. m.; Med.; Nat. c.; Nit. ac.; *Nux v.;* Phos.; Sil.; Tanac.; Tar. h.; *Ther.;* Zinc. m.

People (anthropophobia)—*Acon.;* Ambra.; Anac.; Aur.; Bar. c.; Con.; Gels.; Ign.; Iod.; Kali p.; Lyc.; Meli.; Nat. c.; Nat. m.; Sep.; Stann.; *Staph.*

Places closed—Succin.

Pointed objects—Sil.; Spig.

Poison—*Hyos.;* Kali br.; Lach.; Rhus t.; Ver. v.

Rain—Naja.

Solitude, aversion to—Ant. t.; Ars.; *Bism.;* Con.; *Hyos.; Kali. c.;* Lac c.; Lil. t.; *Lyc.;* Naja; Phos.; Puls.; Radium; Sep.; *Stram.;* Thymol; Ver. a.

Solitude, desire for—Ambra; Aragal.; *Ars. m.;* Aur.; *Bar. c.;* Bry.; *Bufo;* Cact.; Caps.; *Carbo an.;* Cim.; *Coca;* Cycl.; *Gels.; Ign.;* Iod.; Nat. c.; Nat. m.; *Nux v.;* Oxytr.; Phos. ac.; *Staph.;* Thuya.

Space (agoraphobia)—*Acon.;* Arg. n.; Arn.; *Calc. c.;* Hydroc. ac.; Nux v.

Stage-fright—Anac.; Arg. n.; Gels.

Syphilis—Hyos.

Thunderstorms—Bor.; Electricitas; *Nat. c.;* Phos.; Psor.; Rhod.; Sil.

Touch, contact—*Acon.;* Angust. sp.; *Ant. c.;* Ant. t.; Apis; *Arn.;* Bell.; *Cham.;* Cina; *Cinch.;* Colch.; *Hep.;* Iod.; *Kali c.;* Lach ; Mag. p.; Nit. ac.; Nux m.; *Nux v.;* Phos.; *Plumb.;* Sanic.; Sep.; *Spig.;* Stram.; Sul.; *Tar. h.;* Thuya.

Water (hydrophobia)—Agave; Anag.; Ant. c.; *Bell.; Canth.;* Coccinel.; Fagus; *Hyos.; Lach.;* Laur.; *Lyssin;* Spirea; *Stram.;* Sul.; Tanac.; Ver. a.; Xanth. sp.

HYPOCHONDRIASIS—Alfal.; Aloe; Alum.; *Anac.; Arg. n.;* Ars.; *Aur. m.;* Aur. mur.; Avena; Cact.; *Calc. c.;* Cim.; *Con.;* Ferr. m.; Helon.; Hydroc. ac.; Hyos.; *Ign.;* Kali br.; *Kali p.; Lyc.;* Merc.; Nat. c.; *Nat. m.; Nux v.; Phos. ac.;* Plumb.; Pod.; Puls.; Stann.; *Staph.; Sul.;* Sumb.; Tar. h.; Thasp. a.; Thuya; Val.; *Ver. a.;* Zinc. m.; Zinc. oxy.

HYSTERIA—Acon.; Agn.; *Ambra;* Am. val.; Apis; *Aquil.; Asaf.;* Aster.; Bell.; Cact.; Cajup.; Camph. monobr.; Can. ind.; Castor.; Caul.; Cham.; *Cim.;* Cocc.; Con.; Croc.; *Eup. ar.; Gels.;* Hyos.; *Ign.; Kali p.;* Lil. t.; Mag. m.; *Mosch.;* Myg.; *Nux m.;* Orig.; Phos. ac.; *Phos.; Plat.;* Poth.; *Puls.;* Scutel.; Senec.; *Sep.;* Stram.; Strych. p.; Sumb.; Tar. h.; Ther.; Val.; Zinc. v.

IMAGINATION—**Fancies, hallucinations, illusions: Acute vivid:** *Absinth.;* Acon.; Agar.; Ambra; *Bell.; Can. ind.;* Dub.; *Hyos.;* Kali c.; *Lach.;* Op.; Rhus t.; Scopal.; *Stram.;* Sul.; Ver. a. See Hallucinations.

Away from home, must get there—*Bry.;* Calc. p.; Cim.; Hyos.; Op.

Bed occupied by another person—Petrol.

Bed sinking—Bapt.; Bell.; *Benz.;* Kali c.

Bed too hard—*Arn.; Bapt.;* Bry.; *Morph.; Pyr.;* Ruta.

Being abused or criticized—*Bar. c.;* Cocaine; Hyos.; Ign.; Pallad.; Staph.

Being assassinated—Absinth.; Kali br.; Plumb. m.
Being broken in fragments, scattered about—Bapt.; Daph.; *Petrol.*; Phos.; Stram.
Being crushed by houses—Arg. n.
Being dead—Apis; *Lach.*; Mosch.; Op.
Being demon, curses, swears—Anac.
Being doomed, lost to salvation—Acon.; Ars.; Aur.; Cycl.; Lach.; *Lil. t.*; Lyc.; Meli.; Op.; *Plat.*; Psor.; Puls.; Stram.; Sul.; *Ver. a.*
Being double, (dual personality)—*Anac.*; Bapt.; Can. ind.; Petrol.; *Stram.*; Thuya; Val.
Being enveloped in dark cloud, world black and sinister—Arg. n.; *Cim.*; Lac c.; Puls.
Being frightened by a mouse running from under a chair—*Æth.*; *Cim.*; Lac c.
Being guilty of some committed crime—Ars.; Cina; *Cycl.*; *Ign.*; Nux v.; Ruta; Staph.; *Ver. a.*; Zinc. m.
Being hollow in organs—*Cocc.*; Oxytr.
Being in strange surroundings—*Cic.*; Hyos.; Plat.; Tub.
Being light, spirit-like, hovering in the air—*Asar.*; *Dat. arb.*; *Hyper.*; *Lac c.*; Latrod. has.; Nat. ars.; Op.; Rhus gl.; *Sticta*; *Val.*
Being made of glass, wood, etc.—Eupion; Rhus t.; *Thuya*.
Being occupied about business—*Bry.*; Op.
Being persecuted by his enemies—*Anac.*; Cinch.; *Cocaine*; *Hyos.*; Kali br.; *Lach.*; Nux v.; Plumb. m.; Rhus t.; Stram.
Being poisoned—*Hyos.*; Lach.; Rhus t.; Ver. v.
Being possessed of two wills—*Anac.*; Lach.
Being possessed of brain in stomach—Acon.
Being possessed of two noses—Merc. per.
Being pregnant, or something alive in the abdomen—Croc.; Cycl.; Op.; Sabad.; Sul.; *Thuya*; Ver. a.
Being pursued—*Anac.*; Hyos.; Stram.
Being separated body and soul—*Anac.*; Nit. ac.; Thuya.
Being swollen—Acon.; Aran.; Arg. n.; Asaf.; Bapt.; Bov.; *Can. ind.*; Glon.; Op.; Plat.
Being under superhuman control—*Anac.*; Lach.; Op.; Plat.; Thuya.
Being very sick.—Ars.; Pod.; Sabad.
Being very wealthy—Phos.; *Plat.*; Pyr.; *Sul.*; Ver. a.
Dimensions of things larger—Acon.; Agar.; Arg. n.; Atrop.; Bov.; *Can. ind.*; *Gels.*; Glon.; *Hyos.*; Op.; Paris.
Dimensions of things reversed—Camph. monobr.
Dimensions of things smaller.—Plat.
Duration of time and space lost or confused—Anhal.; *Can. ind.*; Cic.; Glon.; Lach.
Duration of time changed, it passes too rapidly—*Cocc.*; Ther.
Duration of time changed, it passes too slowly—*Alum.*; Ambra; Anhal.; *Arg. n.*; Can. ind.; Med.; Nux m.; Nux v.
Hallucinations—Remedies in general: *Absinth.*; *Agar.*; Ambra; *Anac.*; Anhal.; *Antipyr.*; Ars.; Atrop.; *Bell.*; *Can. ind.*; Cantn.; Cham.;

MIND

Chloral; Cim.; Cocaine; *Crot. casc.*; *Hyos.*; Kali br.; Lach.; Nat. sal.; Nux v.; *Op.*; Phos.; *Stram.*; Sul.; Thea; Trion.; Zinc. mur.

Hallucinations, auditory (bells, music, voices)—Agar.; *Anac.*; *Antipyr.*; Ars.; Bell.; *Can. ind.*; Carbon. s.; *Cham.*; Cocaine; Elaps; Merc.; Naja; Nat. p.; Puls.; *Stram.*; Thea.

Hallucinations, olfactory—*Agn.*; *Anac.*; Ars.; Euph. amy.; *Op.*; Parie; Puls.; Zinc. mur.

Hallucinations, tactile—Anac.; Canth.; *Op.*; Stram.

Hallucinations, visual (animals, bugs, faces)—*Absinth.*; Agar.; Ambra; Anhal.; *Antipyr.*; Ars.; *Atrop.*; *Bell.*; Calc. c.; *Can. ind.*; Cim.; Cocaine; *Hyos.*; Kali br.; Lach.; *Morph.*; Nat. sal.; *Op.*; Pastin.; Phos.; Plat.; Puls.; Sant.; *Stram.*; Sul.; Val.; Ver. a.

INSANITY—See Mania, Melancholia, Dementia.

LOQUACITY—*Agar.*; Ambra; Bell.; Can. ind.; *Cim.*; Cocaine; Eug. j.; *Hyos.*; *Lach.*; Op.; Pastin.; Physal.; *Stram.*; Tar. h.; Val.; Ver. a.

MANIA—Remedies in general: Absinth.; *Acon.*; Agar.; *Anac.*; Arn.; Ars.; Atrop.; Bapt.; *Bell.*; Bry.; *Can. ind.*; *Canth.*; Chloral; *Cim.*; Cinch.; Croc.; *Crot. casc.*; Cupr. ac.; Cupr. m.; Glon.; *Hyos.*; Kali br.; *Lach.*; Laur.; Lil. t.; Lyc.; Merc.; Nat. m.; Nux v.; *Op.*; Orig.; Passifl.; Phos.; Picr. ac.; Piscidia; *Plat.*; Puls.; Rhus t.; Sec.; *Solan. n.*; Spig. mar.; Spong.; Sul. hydr.; Sul.; *Stram.*; Tar. h.; Ust.; *Ver. a.*; Ver. v.

Erotomania (nymphomania, satyriasis)—Ambra; Apis; Bar. m.; Calc. p.; *Can. ind.*; *Canth.*; Ferrula gl.; Ginseng; Grat.; *Hyos.*; Lil. t.; Mancin.; *Murex*; Orig.; Phos.; Picr. ac.; Plat.; Robin.; Salix n.; *Stram.*; Tar. h.; Ver. a.

Lypemania—Ars.; *Aur.*; Caust.; Cic.; *Ign.*; Nux v.; *Puls*.

Monomania (kleptomania, etc.)—*Absinth.*; Cic.; Hyos.; Oxytr.; Plat.; Tar. h.

Puerperal—Agn.; Bell.; *Cim.*; Hyos.; Plat.; Sec.; Senec.; *Stram.*; Ver. a.; Ver. v.

MELANCHOLIA—Remedies in general: Acon.; *Agn.*; Alum.; *Anac.*; Arg. n.; *Ars.*; *Aur.*; Bapt.; Bell.; Cact.; Calc. c.; Camph.; Caust.; *Cim.*; Cinch.; Coca; Coff.; *Con.*; *Cycl.*; Dig.; Ferr. m.; Gels.; Helleb.; Helon.; *Ign.*; Iod.; Kali br.; Lac c.; Lach.; *Lil. t.*; Lyc.; Merc.; *Nat. m.*; Nux m.; *Nux v.*; Op.; Phos. ac.; Phos.; Picr. ac.; *Plat.*; Plumb. ac.; Plumb. m.; Pod.; *Puls.*; *Sep.*; Sil.; Solan. c.; Stram.; Sul.; Tar. h.; Thuya; *Ver. a.*; Ver. v.; Zinc. m.

Pubertic—Ant. c.; *Helleb.*; Mancin.; Nat. m.

Puerperal—Agn.; Bell.; *Cim.*; Nat. m.; Plat.; *Ver. v.*

Religious—Ars.; *Aur. m.*; *Aur. mur.*; Kali br.; Lil. t.; Meli.; Plumb.; Psor.; Puls.; *Stram.*; Sul.; *Ver. a.*

Sexual—Agn.; Aur.; *Cim.*; Con.; *Lil. t.*; Nux v.; Picr. ac.; Plat.; Sep.

MEMORY—Forgetful, weak or lost: Absinth.; Acon.; Æth.; *Agn.*; *Alum.*; Ambra; *Anac.*; Anhal.; *Arg. n.*; Arn.; *Aur.*; Azar.; *Bar. c.*; Calad.; *Calc. c.*; Calc. p.; Camph.; *Can ind.*; Carbo v.; Cocc.; *Con.*; Glycerin; Ichthy.; *Kali br.*; Kali c.; *Kali p.*; *Lac c.*; Lach.; Lecith.; *Lyc.*; Med.; Merc.; *Nat. c.*; *Nat. m.*; Nit. ac.; *Nux m.*; *Nux v.*; Oleand.

MIND

Op.; *Phos. ac.*; *Phos.*; *Picr. ac.*; Plumb. m.; Rhod.; Rhus t.; *Selen.*; Sep.; Sil.; *Sul.*; Syph.; Tellur.; Thyr.; Zinc. m.; Zinc. p.; Zinc. picr.

Cannot remember familiar streets—Can. ind.; *Glon.*; Lach.; Nux m.

Cannot remember names—*Anac.*; Bar. ac.; *Chlorum*; *Euonym.*; Guaiac.; Hep.; Lyc.; Med.; *Sul.*; Syph.; Xerophyl.

Cannot remember right words (amnesic aphasia, paraphasia)—Agar.; Alum.; *Anac.*; Arag.; Arg. n.; Arn.; Calc. c.; Calc. p.; Can. ind.; Cham.; Cinch.; Diosc.; Dulc.; *Kali br.*; Lac c.; Lil. t.; *Lyc.*; *Nux m.*; Phos. ac.; *Plumb. m.*; Sumb.; Xerophyl.

Difficulty or inability of fixing attention—*Æth.*; Agar.; *Agn.*; Aloe; Alum.; *Anac.*; Apis; Arag.; Arg. n.; Bapt.; Bar. c.; Can. ind.; Caust.; *Con.*; Fagop.; *Gels.*; Glon.; Glycerin; Helleb.; Ichthy.; Indol; Irid.; Lac c.; Lyc.; Op.; Nat. c.; *Nux m.*; *Nux v.*; *Phos. ac.*; *Phos.*; *Picr. ac.*; Pituit.; Sep.; Sil.; Staph.; Sul.; Syph.; Xerophyl.; Zinc. m.

Omits letters, words—Benz. ac.; Cereus serp.; Cham.; *Kali br.*; Lac c.; Lach.; *Lyc.*; Meli.; *Nux m.*; Nux v.

Thoughts, rapid—Anac.; Bell.; *Can. ind.*; Cim.; Cinch.; *Coff.*; *Ign.*; Lac c.; Lach.; *Physost.*

Thoughts, slow—Agn.; Caps.; *Carbo v.*; Lyc.; Med.; *Nux m.*; Op.; *Phos. ac.*; *Phos.*; Plumb.; Sec.; Thuya.

Thoughts vanish while reading, talking, writing—*Anac.*; Asar.; Camph.; *Can. ind.*; Lach.; Lyc.; *Nux m.*; Picr. ac.; Staph.

Unable to think—Abies n.; *Æth.*; Alum.; *Anac.*; Arg. n.; Aur. m.; Bapt.; Calc. c.; Can. ind.; Caps.; *Con.*; Dig.; *Gels.*; Glycerin; *Kali p.*; Lyc.; Nat. c.; Nat. m.; *Nux m.*; *Nux v.*; Oleand.; Petrol.; *Phos. ac.*; *Phos.*; *Picr. ac.*; Rhus t.; Sep.; Sil.; Zinc. m.

Weak from sexual abuse—*Agn.*; *Anac.*; Arg. n.; Aur.; Cinch.; Nat. m.; Nux v.; *Phos. ac.*; *Staph.*

MIND—Absence: Acon.; *Agn.*; *Anac.*; Apis; Arag.; Arn.; Bar. c.; *Can. ind.*; *Kali br.*; Kreos.; *Lac c.*; Lach.; Merc.; Nat. m.; *Nux m.*; Phos. ac.; Poth.; Rhus t.; Tellur.; Zinc.

Absence of moral and will power—Abrot.; Acetan.; *Anac.*; Cereus serp.; *Coca*; *Cocaine*; Kali br.; *Morph.*; Op.; Picr. ac.; Strych. p.; *Tar. h.*

Cloudiness, confusion, depression, dullness—*Abies n.*; Acon.; Æsc.; Agar.; *Ail.*; Alfal.; Alum.; *Anac.*; Apis; Aragal.; Arg. n.; Arn.; *Bapt.*; Bar. c.; Bell.; Calc. c.; Can. ind.; Cann. s.; Carbon. s.; Cic.; Cocc.; Colch.; Euonym.; Ferr. m.; *Gels.*; *Glon.*; Glycerin; *Helleb.*; Hyos.; Hyper.; Indol; Irid.; Kali b.; Kali p.; Lac c.; Lecith.; Lyc.; Mancin.; Nat. c.; *Nux m.*; *Nux v.*; *Op.*; *Phos. ac.*; Phos.; Picr. ac.; Piscidia; *Rhus t.*; *Selen.*; Staph.; Stram.; Sulphon.; Xerophyl.; Zinc. m.; Zinc. v.

Excitement, exhilaration—Acon.; Agar.; *Bell.*; *Can. ind.*; *Canth.*; Coca; Cocaine; *Coff.*; Croc.; Eucal.; *Hyos.*; *Lach.*; Merc. cy.; Nux v.; Op.; Paul.; Physost.; Piscidia; *Stram.*; Thea; Ver. a.

MOOD—DISPOSITION—Anxiety felt during thunderstorm: Nat. c.; *Phos.*

Anxiety felt in stomach—Ars.; *Dig.*; Ipec.; Kali c.; *Puls.*; Ver. a.

Anxious—Acon.; Æth.; *Agn.*; Amyl; Anac.; Ant. c.; Arg. n.; *Ars.*; Asaf.; *Aur.*; Bell.; *Bism.*; Bor.; Cact.; *Calc. c.*; Camph.; Can. ind.; Cham.; Cim.; Cinch.; Coff.; Con.; Cupr. m.; *Dig.*; Hep.; *Ign.*; *Kali*

MIND

c.; *Lach.*; *Lil. t.*; Med.; Nat. c.; Nat. m.; Nit. ac.; *Nux v.*; Op.,
Phos.; *Plat.*; Psor.; *Puls.*; Rhus t.; Sec.; *Sep.*; Sil.; Staph.; Stram.;
Sul.; Tab.; Ver. a.

Apathetic, indifferent to everything—Agar.; Agn.; *Apis*; Arg. n.; Arn.;
Ars.; *Bapt.*; Bry.; *Cim.*; *Cinch.*; Con.; Fluor. ac.; *Gels.*; Glycerin;
Helleb.; Hydroc. ac.; *Ign.*; Indol; Laburn.; Lach.; Lil. t.; Merc.; Nat.
m.; Nux m.; Nux v.; *Op.*; *Phos. ac.*; Phos.; Phyt.; *Picr. ac.*; Plat.;
Puls.; Sec.; *Sep.*; *Staph.*; Thuya; Ver. a.

Aversion to mental and physical work—Agar.; Alfal.; *Aloe*; *Anac.*; Aragal.;
Aur. mur.; Bapt.; *Bar. c.*; *Calc. c.*; *Caps.*; *Carb. ac.*; Caust.; *Cinch.*;
Coca; Con.; Cycl.; *Gels.*; Glon.; Helleb.; Indol; *Kali p.*; Lecith.;
Mag. p.; Nat. c.; Niccol. s.; Nit. ac.; *Nux v.*; Oxytr.; Phos. ac.; Phos.;
Picr. ac.; Puls.; Rhamnus cal.; Selen.; Sep.; Sil.; Strych. p.; *Sul.*;
Tanac.; Thymol; Zinc m.

Bashful, timid—*Ambra*; Aur.; *Bar. c.*; Calc. c.; Calc. sil.; Caust.; Coca;
Con.; Graph.; *Ign.*; Kali p.; Lil. t.; Mancin.; Meli.; Phos.; *Puls.*;
Sil.; *Staph.*

Complaining, discontented, dissatisfied—Aloe; Ant. c.; Ars.; Bism.; Bor.;
Bry.; Caps.; *Cham.*; *Cina*; Colch.; Indol; Kali c.; Mag. p.; Nit. ac.
Nux v.; Plat.; Psor.; *Puls.*; Staph.; Sul.; Tab.

Despairing, hopeless, discouraged easily, lack of confidence—*Acon.*; *Agn.*;
Alum.; *Anac.*; Ant. c.; Arg. n.; Arn.; *Ars.*; *Aur.*; Bar. c.; Calc. c.;
Calc. sil.; Caust.; Con.; Gels.; Helleb.; *Ign.*; Iod.; Lil. t.; Nat. m.;
Nit. ac.; Nux v.; Op.; *Phos. ac.*; Phos.; Picr. ac.; Psor.; *Puls.*; Ruta;
Selen.; *Sep.*; Sil.; Staph.; Syph.; Thymol; Ver. a.

Fault-finding, finicky, cautious—Apis; *Ars.*; *Cham.*; Graph.; Helon.;
Morph.; *Nux v.*; *Plat.*; Sep.; Staph.; Sul.; Tar. h.; Ver. a.

Fearlessness, daring—*Agar.*; Bell.; Cocaine; *Op.*; Sil.

Fretful, cross, irritable, peevish, quarrelsome, whining—Abrot.; Acon.;
Æsc.; Æth.; Agar.; Alfal.; Anac.; *Ant. c.*; *Ant. t.*; Apis; Ars.; Aur.;
Bry.; Bufo; Calc. br.; Calc. c.; *Caps.*; Caust.; *Cham.*; *Cina*; Cinch.;
Colch.; *Col.*; Con.; Croc.; Ferr.; Helon.; Hep.; Iberis; *Ign.*; Indol;
Ipec.; Kali c.; *Kali p.*; *Kreos.*; Lac c.; Lil. t.; Lyc.; *Nat. m.*; *Nit. ac.*;
Nux v.; Plat.; Puls.; Radium; Rheum; Sars.; *Sep.*; Sil.; *Staph.*;
Sulphon.; Sul.; Syph.; Thuya; Thymol; Tub.; *Val.*; Ver. a.; Ver. v.;
Zinc. m.

Fretful day and night—*Cham.*; Ign.; Ipec.; Lac c.; *Psor.*; *Stram.*

Fretful day only—Lyc.

Fretful night only—Ant. t.; Jal.; Nux v.; Rheum.

Fretful, so that child cannot bear to be touched, looked at, or spoken to—
Ant. c.; Ant. t.; *Cham.*; *Cina*; Gels.; *Nux v.*; Sanic.; *Sil.*; Thuya.

Fretful, so that child wants different things, but petulantly rejects them—
Ant. t.; Bry.; *Cham.*; *Cina*; Ipec.; Kreos.; Rheum; *Staph.*

Gay, frolicsome, hilarious—Anag.; Bell.; *Can. ind.*; *Coff.*; *Croc.*; Cyprip.;
Eucal.; *Formica*; *Hyos.*; Lach.; Nux m.; Plat.; Spong.; Stram.;
Thea; Val.

Grieving, introspective, sighing—Ail.; Calc. p.; *Cim.*; Dig.; *Iberis*; *Ign.*;
Lyc.; *Mur. ac.*; Nat. m.; Phos. ac.; *Puls.*

Haughty, arrogant, prideful—Bell.; Con.; **Cupr. m.**; **Lach.**; **Lyc.**; *Pall.*; Phos.; *Plat.*; Staph.; *Stram.*; Ver. a.

Haughty, contempt of others—Ipec.; *Plat.*

Haughty, contempt of self—*Agn.*; *Aur.*; Lac c.; Thuya.

Hypersensitive, cannot bear contradiction, vexed at trifles—Acon.; *Anac.*; *Ant. c.*; Arn.; Ars.; Asaf.; Asar.; Aster.; *Aur.*; Bell.; *Bry.*; Canth.; Caps.; *Cham.*; *Cina*; Cinch.; Cocc.; *Colch.*; Col.; Con.; Ferr. m.; Glon.; Helleb.; Helon.; Hep.; *Ign.*; Lach.; Lyc.; Mez.; Morph.; Mur. ac.; *Nat. m.*; Nit. ac.; *Nux v.*; Pall.; Petrol.; Phos.; *Plat.*; Puls.; Sars.; *Sep.*; Sil.; Staph.; Thuya; Thyr.

Hysterical (changeable, vacillatory)—*Acon.*; *Alum.*; *Ambra*; *Asaf.*; Camph. monobr.; *Cast.*; Caust.; *Cim.*; Cob.; Cocc.; Coff.; *Croc.*; Gels.; *Ign.*; Kali p.; Lil. t.; Mang. ac.; *Mosch.*; Nat. m.; *Nux m.*; Phos.; *Plat.*; *Puls.*; Sep.; *Sumb.*; Tar. h.; Thasp.; *Val.*; *Zinc. v.*

Impatient, impulsive—Acon.; *Anac.*; Ant. c.; Arg. n.; *Cham.*; *Col.*; Hep.; Ign.; Ipec.; Med.; *Nat. m.*; Nux v.; Puls.; Rheum; Sep.; *Staph.*; Sul.

Impudent, insulting, malicious, revengeful, spiteful—*Anac.*; Ars.; Bufo; *Cham.*; Cinch.; Cupr.; Lac c.; *Lyc.*; *Nit. ac.*; Nux v.; *Staph.*; Tar. h.

Impudent, teasing, laugh at reproof—Graph.

Indecisive, irresolute—Arg. n.; *Aur.*; *Bar. c.*; *Calc. sil.*; Caust.; *Graph.*; *Ign.*; Nux m.; Nux v.; *Puls.*

Indolent, listless, lethargic, ambitionless—Alet.; Aloe; Anac.; *Apis*; Aur. m.; *Bapt.*; Bar. c.; Berb. aq.; *Bry.*; Calc. c.; *Caps.*; Carb. ac.; Carbo v.; Con.; Cycl.; Dig.; Euphras.; Ferr.; *Gels.*; Glon.; Helon.; Indol; Kali p.; Lecith.; Lil. t.; Merc.; Nat. m.; Nux v.; *Phos. ac.*; Phos.; *Picr. ac.*; Puls.; Ruta; Sarcol. ac.; *Sep.*; Stann.; Sul.; Thymol; Zinc.

Jealous—*Apis*; Hyos.; Ign.; *Lach.*; Nux v.

Melancholic, despondent, depressed, low-spirited, gloomy, apprehensive, "blues"—Abies n.; *Acon.*; *Æsc.*; *Agn.*; Alfal.; *Alum.*; Am. c.; Am. m.; *Anac.*; Ant. c.; Apis; Arg. m.; Arg. n.; *Ars.*; Ars. m.; *Aur.*; Bry.; But. ac.; Cact.; Calc. ars.; Calc. c.; Caust.; *Cim.*; *Cinch.*; Cocc.; Con.; Cupr. m.; *Cycl.*; Dig.; Euonym.; Euphras.; *Graph.*; Helleb.; *Helon.*; Hep.; *Hydr.*; Iberis; *Ign.*; *Indigo*; Indol; Iod.; Kali br.; Kali p.; Lac c.; Lac d.; Lach.; *Lit. t.*; *Lyc.*; Med.; Merc.; Myg.; Myr.; Naja; Nat. c.; *Nat. m.*; Nat. s.; Nit. ac.; Nux m.; *Nux v.*; *Phos. ac.*; Phos.; Plat.; Plumb.; Pod.; Psor.; *Puls.*; Radium; Rhus t.; Sarcol. ac.; Sars.; Senec.; *Sep.*; Sil.; Spig.; *Stann.*; Staph.; Still.; Sul.; Tab.; Thuya; *Tub.*; Ver. a.; Zinc. m.; Zinc. p.

Mild, gentle, yielding—Alum.; *Ign.*; Murex; Phos. ac.; *Puls.*; Sep.; Sil.

Misanthropic, miserly, selfish—Ars.; *Lyc.*; Pall.; Plat.; Sep.; *Sul.*

Nervous, excited, fidgety, worried—Absinth.; *Acon.*; *Ambra*; *Anac.*; Apis; Apium gr.; *Arg. n.*; *Ars.*; Asaf.; *Asar.*; Aur. m.; *Bell.*; *Bor.*; Bov.; But. ac.; Calc. br.; *Camph. monobr.*; Caust.; Ced.; *Cham.*; *Cim.*; Cina; *Coff.*; Con.; Ferr.; *Gels.*; Helon.; Hyos.; *Hyos. hydrobr.*; Iberis; *Ign.*; Kali br.; Kali p.; Lac c.; Lach.; Lil. t.; Mag. c.; Med.; Morph.; Nat. c.; Nux m.; *Nux v.*; *Phos.*; Psor.; Puls.; Sec.; *Sep.*; *Sil.*; Staph.; Stram.; *Sumb.*; Tar. h.; Thea; *Val.*; Zinc. m.; Zinc. p.; Zinc. v.

Obscene, amative—*Canth.*; Hyos.; Lil. t.; Murex; *Phos.*; Puls.; Staph.; Stram.; *Ver. a.*

Restless (mentally and physically)—Absinth.; *Acon.*; Agar.; Ambra; Arag.; *Ars.*; Aur. m.; Bell.; *Bism.*; Camph.; Can. ind.; Canth.; Caust.; Cenchris; *Cham.*; *Cim.*; *Coff.*; *Hyos.*; *Ign.*; Iod.; *Kali br.*; Lac c.; Lach.; Laur.; Lil. t.; Med.; *Morph.*; Mur. ac.; Myg.; Nat. c.; Nat. m.; Nux v.; Op.; Phos.; Phyt.; Plat.; Psor.; *Pyr.*; Radium; *Rhus t.*; Ruta; Sil.; *Stram.*; *Tar. h.*; Urt.; Val.; Ver. a.; Ver. v.; Zinc. m.; Zinc. v.

Sad, sentimental, sighing—*Agn.*; Am. c.; Am. m.; *Ant. c.*; *Aur.*; Cact.; Calc. p.; Carbo an.; Cim.; Cocc.; Con.; *Cycl.*; Dig.; *Graph.*; Iberis; *Ign.*; *Indigo*; Kali p.; Lach.; Lil. t.; Mur. ac.; Naja; Nat c.; *Nat. m.*; Nat. s.; Nit. ac.; Nux v.; Phos. ac.; Phos.; Plat.; Psor.; *Puls.*; Rhus t.; Sec.; *Selen.*; *Sep.*; *Stann.*; Staph.; Sul.; Thuya; Zinc. m.

Sad, weeping from music—Acon.; Ambra; *Graph.*; Nat. c.; Nat. s.; Sab.; Tar. h.; *Thuya.*

Slovenly, filthy—Am. c.; *Caps.*; Merc.; *Psor.*; *Sul.*; Ver. a.

Stubborn, obstinate, self-willed—Agar.; Ant. c.; *Bry.*; Caps.; *Cham.*; Cinch.; Kali c.; *Nit. ac.*; *Nux v.*; Sanic.; Sil.; Staph.

Stupid—Æsc. gl.; *Anac.*; *Apis*; Arn.; *Bapt.*; Bell.; Bry.; Cocc.; *Gels.*; *Helleb.*; Hyos.; Indol; Lach.; *Nux m.*; *Op.*; *Phos. ac.*; Phos.; Rhus t.; Sec.; Stram.; Ver. a.

Suicidal—Alum.; Anac.; *Ant. c.*; *Ars.*; *Aur.*; Cinch.; Fuligo; Ign.; Iod.; Kali br.; *Naja*; Nat. s.; Nit. ac.; *Nux v.*; Psor; Puls.; Rhus t.; Sec.; Sep.; Sil.; Ustil.; Ver. a.

Suspicious, mistrustful—*Anac.*; Anhal.; Caust.; *Cim.*; Hyos.; Lach.; Merc.; Nux v.; Puls.; Staph.; Ver. a.; Ver. v.

Sympathetic—*Caust.*; Cocc.; Puls.

Taciturn, disinclined to be disturbed, or answer questions—Agar.; *Ant. c.*; Ant. t.; Arn.; Bell.; *Bry.*; Cact.; Carbo an.; *Cham.*; *Col.*; *Gels.*; Helleb.; Ign.; Iod.; Mur. ac.; Naja; *Nat. m.*; Nat. s.; Nux v.; Oxytr.; *Phos. ac.*; Phos.; Sars.; Sil.; Sul.

Taciturn, morose, sulky, sullen, unsociable—*Ant. c.*; Ant. t.; Arn.; Aur.; Bry.; *Cham.*; Cim.; *Cinch.*; Col.; Con.; Cupr.; Ign.; Lyc.; Nat. m.; Nux v.; *Plat.*; Puls.; Sanic.; Sil.; Sul.; Tub.; *Ver. a.*; Ver. v.

Tearful, weeping—*Am. m.*; Ant. c.; *Apis*; Ars.; Aur.; Cact.; Calc. c.; Caust.; *Cim.*; Cocc.; Croc.; *Cycl.*; Dig.; *Graph.*; *Ign.*; Lac c.; Lach.; Lil. t.; Lyc.; Mag. m.; *Nat. m.*; Nit. ac.; Nux m.; Phos. ac.; Plat.; *Puls.*; Rhus t.; *Sep.*; Sil.; *Stann.*; Sul.

NIGHT-TERRORS—Acon.; *Aur. br.*; Calc. c.; Cham.; Cic.; *Cina*; Chloral.; Cyprip.; *Kali br.*; Kali p.; Scutel.; Solan. n.; *Stram.*; Tub.; Zinc. m.

PROPENSITY—To be abusive, curse, swear—*Anac.*; Bell.; Canth.; Cereus serp.; *Lac c.*; Lil. t.; *Nit. ac.*; Pall.; *Stram.*; *Tub.*; Ver. a.

To be aimlessly busy—Absinth.; *Arg. n.*; Ars.; Canth.; *Lil. t.*; Sul.; Tar. h.

To be carried—Ant. t.; Ars.; Benz. ac.; *Cham.*; Cina; Ipec.

To be cruel, violent, inhuman—Abrot.; *Absinth.*; *Anac.*; Bell.; Bry.; Canth.; Croc.; *Nit. ac.*; *Nux v.*; Plat.; Staph.; *Stram.*; Tar. h.; Ver. a.

To be destructive, bite, strike, tear clothes—*Bell.*; Bufo; *Canth.*; Cupr. m.; *Hyos.*; Lil. t.; Sec.; *Stram.*; Tar. h.; *Ver. a.*

To be dirty, untidy, filthy—Caps.; *Psor.*; Sil.
To be magnetized—Calc. c.; *Phos.*; Sil.
To be obscene—Anac.; *Canth.*; *Hyos.*; Lach.; Lil. t.; *Phos.*; Plat.; Stram.; Ver. a.
To commit suicide—Alum.; *Ant. c.*; *Ars.*; *Aur.*; Caps.; Cim.; *Ign.*; Kali br.; Merc.; *Naja*; Nat. s.; *Nux v.*; Psor.; Puls.; Rhus t.; Thasp.; Ustil.; Ver. a.
To dance—*Agar.*; Bell.; Cic.; *Croc.*; Hyos.; Sticta; Stram.; *Tar. h.*
To do absurd things—Bell.; Can. ind.; Cic.; *Hyos.*; Lach.; Stram.; Tar. h.
To eat greedily—Lyc.; Zinc. m.
To handle organs—Bufo; Canth.; Hyos.; Ustil.; Zinc.
To hurry—Acon.; Alum.; Apis; *Arg. n.*; *Aur.*; Bell.; Coff.; Ign.; *Lil. t.*; Med.; Nat. m.; *Sul. ac.*; Thuya; Zinc v.
To hurry others—Arg. n.; Can. ind.; *Nux m.*
To kill beloved ones—Ars.; Cinch.; Merc.; *Nux v.*; *Plat.*
To laugh immoderately at trifles—Anac.; *Can. ind.*; *Croc.*; *Hyos.*; Ign.; *Mosch.*; Nux m.; *Plat.*; *Stram.*; *Strych. p.*; Tar. h.; Zinc. oxy.
To lie—*Morph.*; Op.; Ver. a.
To mutilate body—Agar.; *Ars.*; Bell.; Hyos.; Stram.
To perform great things—Cocaine.
To pray, beseech, entreat—Aur. m.; Puls.; *Stram.*; Ver. a.
To repeat everything—Zinc. m.
To scold—Con.; Dulc.; Lyc.; *Mosch.*; Nux v.; Pall.; *Petrol.*; Ver. a.
To sing—*Agar.*; Bell.; Can. ind.; Cic.; *Croc.*; *Hyos.*; Spong.; *Stram.*; Tar. h.; Ver. a.
To slide down in bed—Mur. ac.
To stretch and yawn incessantly—Amyl; Plumb. m.
To talk in rhymes, repeat verses, prophecy—Agar.; Ant. c.; Lach.; Stram.
To tear things—Agar.; *Bell.*; *Cimex*; Cupr. m.; *Stram.*; Tar. h.; *Ver. a.*
To tease, laugh at reproofs—Graph.
To theorize or meditate—*Can. ind.*; Cocc.; Coff.; Sul.
To touch different things—Bell.; Sul.; *Thuya.*
To wander from home—Arag.; *Bry.*; Elat.; Lach.; Ver. a.
To work—Æth.; Aur.; Cereus; *Cocaine*; Coff.; *Eucal.*; Fluor. ac.; *Helon.*; *Lacertus*; Pedic.; Piscidia.

SCREAMS—**Shrill, sudden, piercing**—Apis; *Bell.*; Bor.; Bry.; Calc. c.; Cham.; Cic.; Cina; Cinch.; Cyprip.; Gels.; *Helleb.*; Iodof.; Kali br.; Stram.; Tub.; Ver. a.; *Zinc. m.*

SENSES—**Dulled**—Ail.; Anac.; Bapt.; Caps.; Dig.; Gels.; Helleb.; Phos. ac.; Rhus t.
Hyperacute—*Acon.*; Asaf.; Asar.; Atrop.; Aur.; *Bell.*; Bor.; *Cham.*; Cinch.; *Coff.*; *Colch.*; Ferr. m.; *Ign.*; Lyssin; Morph.; *Nux v.*; Op.; Phos.; Sil.; *Strych.*; Sul.; Tar. h.; Val.; Zinc. m.

SPEECH—**Hurried**—Anac.; Aur.; *Bell.*; *Bry.*; Cocc.; Hep.; Hyos.; Lil. t.; Merc.; Ver. a.
Lost or paralysis (aphasia)—Bar. ac.; *Bar. c.*; *Bothrops*; *Caust.*; Cham.; Chenop.; *Colch.*; Con.; Glon.; *Kali br.*; Kali cy.; Lach.; *Lyc.*; Mez.; Phos.; Plumb. m.; *Stram.*; Sulphon. See Nervous System.

Nasal—Bar. m.; Bell.; Lach.; Phos. ac.

Slow, difficult enunciation, inarticulate, stammering—*Æsc. gl.*; Agar.; Anac.; Anhal.; Atrop.; Bar. c.; Bell.; *Bothrops; Bov.*; Bufo; Can. ind.; *Can. s.; Caust.*; Cereus serp.; Cic.; *Cupr. m.*; Gels.; Hyos.; *Ign.*; Kali br.; Kali cy.; Lach.; Laur.; Merc.; Myg.; Naja; Nat. m.; Nux m.; Oleand.; *Op.; Phos.; Stram.*; Sulphon.; Thuya; Vip.

Slow, monotonous, economical—Mang. ac.; Mang. oxy.

SOMNAMBULISM—Acon.; *Art. v.; Can. ind.*; Cur.; Ign.; *Kali br.*; Kali p.; Phos.; *Sil.; Zinc. m.*

STARTLES—Easily frightened—*Acon.*; Agar.; Apis; *Asar.; Bell.; Bor.*; Calad.; Calc. c.; Carbo v.; *Cham.*; Cim.; Cyprip.; *Ign.*; *Kali br.*: Kali c.; Kali p.; Nat. c.; *Nux v.*; Op.; *Phos.*; Psor.; Samb.; *Seutel.*; Sep.; *Sil.; Stram.*; Sul.; *Tar. h.*; Ther.; Tub.; Zinc. m.

TAEDIUM VITAE (disgust of life)—*Ant. c.*; Ars.; *Aur.; Cinch.*; Hydr.; Lac c.; Lac d.; Kali br.; Naja; Nat. s.; Nit. ac.; *Phos.*; Plat.; Pod.; Rhus t.; Sul.; Tab.; *Thuya;* Ver. a.

HEAD

BRAIN—Abscess—Arn.; Bell.; Crot.; Iod.; Lach.; Op.; Vipera.

Anaemia—Alum.; *Ars.*; Calc. p.; Camph.; *Cinch.*; Ferr. m.; **Ferr. p.**; Kali c.; *Kali p.*; *Nux v.*; Phos.; Sec.; Tab.; Ver. a.; Zinc. m.

Atrophy—*Aur.*; Bar. c.; Fluor. ac.; Iod.; Phos.; Plumb. m.; Zinc. m.

Concussion—*Acon.*; *Arn.*; *Bell.*; Cic.; Ham.; *Hyper.*; Kali iod.; Nat. s.; *Op.*; Sul. ac.

Congestion—(rush of blood to head)—Absinth.; *Acon.*; Act. spic.; Agar.; Ambra; *Amyl*; Arn.; Aster.; Aur.; *Bell.*; *Bry.*; Cact.; Calc. ars.; Carbo v.; Cham.; *Chin. s.*; Cinnab.; *Cinch.*; Coff.; Croc.; Cupr. ac.; Cupr. m.; Ferr. p.; *Ferr. pyroph.*; Gels.; *Glon.*; Hyos.; Ign.; Iod.; Lach.; Lyc.; *Meli.*; Nat. s.; *Nux v.*; Op.; Sang.; Sep.; Sil.; Solan. lyc.; Stram.; *Sul.*; Ver. v.

Congestion, passive—Æsc.; Chloral.; *Cinch.*; Dig.; *Ferr. pyroph.*; Gels.; Helleb.; *Op.*; Phos.

Inflammation (meningitis)—Cerebral (acute and chronic)—Acon.; Æth.; Apis; Apoc. c.; Arn.; Ars.; Bapt.; *Bell.*; *Bry.*; Calc. br.; Calc. c.; Calc. p.; Camph.; Carb. ac.; Chin. s.; Chrom. oxy.; *Cic.*; Cim.; Cinch.; Crot.; Cupr. ac.; *Cupr. m.*; Dig.; Gels.; Glon.; *Helleb.*; Hydroc. ac.; Hyper.; Iod.; Iodof.; Kali iod.; Kreos.; Lach.; Merc. c.; Merc. d.; Mosch.; *Op.*; Ox. ac.; Physost.; Plumb. m.; Phos.; Rhus t.; *Sil.*; Solan. n.; *Sul.*; *Stram.*; *Tub.*; Ver. v.; Vipera; *Zinc. m.* See Hydrocephalus.

Inflammation, basilar—Cupr. cy.; Dig.; Helleb.; Iod.; Sec.; Tub.; *Ver. v.*

Inflammation, cerebro-spinal—*Agar.*; Ail.; *Apis*; Arg. n.; Atrop.; *Bell.*; Bry.; *Cic.*; *Cim.*; Cocc.; *Cupr. ac.*; Echin.; *Gels.*; Glon.; *Helleb.*; Hyos.; Ipec.; Kali iod.; Laburn.; Nat. s.; Op.; Oreodaph.; Physost.; Sil.; Stram.; Sul.; Ver. v.; *Zinc. cy.*; Zinc. m.

Inflammation, traumatic—Acon.; *Arn.*; Bell.; *Hyper.*; Nat. s.; Sil.

Inflammation, tubercular—*Apis*; Bac.; Bell.; Bry.; Calc. c.; Calc. p.; Cocc.; *Cupr. cy.*; Dig.; Glon.; *Helleb.*; Hyos.; Iod.; *Iodof.*; Kali iod.; Op.; Stram.; *Sul.*; Tub.; *Ver. v.*; Zinc. m.; Zinc. oxy.

Paralysis—Alumen; Con.; Cupr. m.; Gels.; Helleb.; Lyc.; Op.; *Plumb.*; Sec.; *Zinc. m.* See Apoplexy (Circulatory System).

Sclerosis (softening, degeneration)—Agar.; Arg. n.; *Aur.*; Bar. c.; Can. ind.; Con.; Kali br.; Kali iod.; Kali p.; Lach.; Lyc.; Nux m.; Nux v.; *Phos.*; Picr. ac.; *Plumb. m.*; Salam.; Vanad.; *Zinc. m.* See Arteriosclerosis (Circulatory System).

Tumors—Apomorph.; Arn.; *Bar. c.*; Bell.; Calc. c.; Con.; Glon.; Graph.; Hydr.; *Kali iod.*; *Plumb. m.*; Sep.

CEREBELLAR DISEASE—Helod.; Sulphon.

FONTANELLES—Tardy closure—Apis; Apoc.; *Calc. c.*; *Calc. p.*; Merc.; Sep.; *Sil.*; *Sul.*; Zinc. m.

HEADACHE (cephalalgia)—Cause: Altitude high: Coca.
Bathing—Ant. c.

HEAD

Beer—Rhus t.
Bright's disease—Am. v.; Zinc. picr.
Candy, sweets—Ant. c.
Catarrh—*Cepa;* Hydr.; Merc.; Puls.; *Sticta.*
Catarrh suppressed—Bell.; *Kali bich.;* Lach.
Coffee—Arum; Ign.; *Nux v.;* Paul.
Constipation—*Aloe;* Alum.; *Bry.;* Collins.; Hydr.; Nit. ac.; *Nux v.;* Op.; Ratanh.
Dancing—Arg. n.
Diarrhoea alternating—*Aloe;* Pod.
Effete matter in system—Asclep. s.
Emotional disturbances—Acetan.; Arg. n.; Cham.; Cim.; Coff.; *Epiph.; Gels.; Ign.;* Mez.; Phos. ac.; *Picr. ac.;* Plat.; Rhus t.; Sil.
Eruptions suppressed—Ant. c.; Psor.; Sul.
Eye-strain—Acetan.; *Cim.; Epiph.; Gels.; Nat. m.; Onosm.;* Phos. ac.; *Ruta;* Tub.
Fasting—Ars.; Cact.; Lach.; *Lyc.;* Sil.
Gastralgia alternating or attending—Bism.
Gastro-intestinal derangements—*Ant. c.;* Bry.; Carbo v.; *Cinch.;* Ipec.; *Iris;* Nux m.; *Nux v.; Puls.;* Rham. c.; Robin.
Hair-cut—Bell.; Bry.
Hat, pressure—Calc. p.; Carbo v.; *Hep.;* Net. m.; Nit. ac.
Hæmorrhage, excesses or vital losses—Carbo v.; *Cinch.;* Ferr.; Ferr. pyroph.; Phos. ac.; Sil.
Hæmorrhoids—Collins.; Nux v.
Ice-water—Dig.
Influenza—Camph.; Lob. purp.
Ironing—*Bry.;* Sep.
Lemonade, tea, wine—Selen.
Liver derangements—Lept.; Nux v.; Ptelea.
Lumbago, alternating with it—Aloe.
Malaria—*Ars.;* Caps., Ced.; *Chin. s.;* Cinch.; Cupr. ac.; *Eup. perf.;* Gels.; *Nat. m.*
Mental exertion or nervous exhaustion—Acetan.; Agar.; Anac.; Arg. n.; Aur. br.; Chionanth.; Cim.; Coff.; *Epiph.; Gels.;* Ign.; *Kali p.;* Mag. p.; *Nat. c.;* Niccol.; *Nux v.;* Phaseol.; Phos. ac.; *Picr. ac.;* Sabad.; Scutel.; Sil.; Zinc. m.
Mercury—Still.
Narcotics, abuse—Acet. ac.
Over-lifting—Calc. c.
Perspiration, suppressed—Asclep. s.; Bry.
Riding against wind—Calc. iod.; *Kali c.*
Riding in cars—*Cocc.;* Graph.; Med.; *Nit. ac.*
Sexual excitement, weakness—Cinch.; Nux v.; Onosm.; *Phos. ac.;* Sil.
Sleep, damp room—Bry.
Sleep, loss—Cim.; Cocc.; *Nux v.*
Spinal disease, chorea—Agar.
Spirituous liquors—Agar.; Ant. c.; Lob. infl.; *Nux v.;* Paul.; Rhod.; *Ruta; Zinc. m.*

702 HEAD

Sunlight or heat—*Bell.;* Cact.; Ferr. p.; *Gels.; Glon.;* Kal.; Lach.; *Nat. c.;* Nux v.; Sang.; Stram.

Syphilis—Ars.; Aur. ars.; *Aur.;* Sars.; Still.; Syph.

Tea—Nux v.; Paul.; *Selen.;* Thuya.

Tobacco—Ant. c.; Calad.; Carb. ac.; *Gels.; Ign.;* Lob. infl.; Nux v.

Traumatism—*Arn.;* Hyper.; Nat. s.

Uraemia—Arn.; Bapt.; Can. ind.; *Glon.;* Hyper.; *Sang.*

Uterine disease, reflex—Aloe; Bell.; *Cim.;* Gels.; Ign.; Puls.; *Sep.;* Zinc. p.

Vaccination—Thuya.

Weather changes—*Calc. p.;* Phyt.

TYPE—Anaemic: Ars.; Calc. p.; *Cinch.;* Cycl.; Ferr. m.; *Ferr. p.;* Ferr. r.; Kal.; Nat. m.; *Phos. ac.;* Zinc. m.

Catarrhal—Ars.; *Bell.;* Bry.; Camph.; *Cepa;* Eup. perf.; Euphras.; *Gels.; Kali bich.;* Lyc.; Menthol; *Merc.;* Nux v.; *Puls.;* Sabad.; Sang.; *Sticta;* Sul.

Chronic—*Arg. n.;* Chin. s.; Cocc.; Lach.; *Nat. m.;* Phos.; Plumb.; Psor.; Sep.; *Sil.;* Thuya; Tub.; *Zinc. m.*

Chronic, old people—Bar. c.; Calc. p.; Iod.; Phos.

Chronic, school girls—*Calc. p.;* Kali p.; *Nat. m.; Phos. ac.; Picr. ac.;* Psor.; Tub.; Zinc. m.

Chronic, sedentary persons—Anac.; *Arg. n.;* Bry.; *Nux v.*

Climacteric—Amyl; Cact.; *Cim.;* Croc.; *Cycl.; Glon.;* Lach.; *Sang.;* Sul.

Congestive—*Acon.;* Amyl; Arg. n.; *Bell.;* Bry.; *Cact.;* Chin. s.; *Ferr. p.; Gels.; Glon.;* Glycerin; Jonosia; Lach.; *Meli.;* Nat. m.; Nux v.; Op.; Phaseol.; *Sang.;* Sil.; Solan. n.; Sul.; Usnea; *Ver. v.*

Congestive, passive—*Chin. s.;* Ferr. p.; *Ferr. pyroph.;* Gels.; Op.; Sil.

Gastric, bilious—Am. picr.; Anac.; *Arg. n.;* Bapt.; *Bry.;* Cham.; Chel.; *Chionanth.;* Cycl.; Eup. perf.; *Ipec.; Iris;* Lob. infl.; Merc. s.; *Nux v.;* Pod.; *Puls.;* Robin.; *Sang.;* Strych.; Tarax.

Hysterical (clavus)—Agar.; Aquil.; *Coff.;* Euonym.; Hep.; *Ign.;* Kali c.; Mag. m.; Nat. m.; Nux v.; *Plat.;* Puls.; Thuya.

Menstrual—Æth.; Avena; Bell.; Cact.; Can. ind.; Can. s.; Chionanth.; *Cim.;* Cinch.; Cocc.; Croc.; *Cycl.;* Ferr. m.; *Glon.;* Glycerin; Kali p.; Lac d.; Lach.; Lil. t.; *Nat. m.; Plat. mur.; Puls.; Sang.; Sep.;* Ustil.; Vib. op.; Xanth.

Migraine, megrim, nervous—Am. c.; Am. val.; *Anac.;* Anhal.; *Arg. n.;* Aspar.; Avena; *Bell.;* Bry.; Caff. citr.; *Calc. ac.;* Calc. c.; *Can. ind.;* Carb. ac.; Ced.; Chionanth.; *Cim.;* Cocc.; *Coff.;* Crot. casc.; *Cycl.; Epiph.; Gels.;* Guar.; *Ign.;* Indigo; *Iris;* Kali bich.; *Kali c.; Lac d.; Lach.; Meli.;* Menisp.; Nat. m.; Niccol.; *Nux v.; Onosm.;* Paul.; *Plat. mur.; Puls.; Sang.;* Saponin; *Scutel.; Sep.;* Sil.; Spig.; Stann.; Sul.; Tab.; Thea; Ther.; Verbasc.; Xanth.; *Zinc. sul.; Zinc. v.;* Zizia.

Neuralgic—*Aconitine;* Æsc.; Arg. n.; *Ars.; Bell.;* Bism.; *Ced.;* Cepa; Chel.; *Chin. s.;* Cim.; Col.; Derris; *Gels.; Mag. p.;* Meli.; Menthol; Oreodaph.; Pall.; Phos.; *Spig.;* Tar. h.; Zinc. v.

Rheumatic, gouty—Act. spic.; Bell.; Bry.; Calc. c.; Colch.; Col.; Derris;

HEAD

Guaiac.; Hep.; Ipec.; Kali s.; Kal.; Lyc.; Nux v.; *Phyt.; Rhus t.;* Sep.; Sil.; Sul.

Uraemic—Arn.; *Glon.;* Hyper.; Sang.

Utero-ovarian—Bell.; *Cim.; Gels.;* Helon.; Ign.; Jonosia; Lil. t.; Plat.; *Puls.;* Sep.; Zinc.

LOCATION—Frontal: *Acon.;* Æsc.; Alfal.; Agar.; Ail.; *Aloe;* Am. c.; *Anac.;* Antipyr.; Arg. n.; Ars.; Aur.; *Bell.; Bry.;* Calc. c.; Carb. ac.; Ced.; *Cepa; Chin. s.;* Chionanth.; Eup. perf.; Euphras.; Gels.; *Glon.; Hydr.;* Ign.; Indol; Iris; *Kali bich.; Lept.;* Meli.; Menisp.; Nat. m.; *Nux v.;* Phos.; Picr. ac.; Prun. sp.; *Ptel.;* Puls.; Robin.; Rhus t.; *Scutel.;* Sil.; Stellar.; Sticta; *Viola od.*

Frontal, extending to eyes, root of nose, face, etc.—Acon.; *Agar.; Aloe;* Ars. m.; Bad.; *Bry.;* Caps.; Ced.; Cepa; Cereus; *Cim.;* Hep.; Ign.; Kali iod.; *Lach.;* Mag. m.; Menthol; Onosm.; *Plat.;* Prun. sp.; *Ptel.; Spig.;* Sticta.

Frontal, extending to occiput, nape of neck and spine—*Bry.;* Euonym.; Gels.; Lac d.; Menisp.; Nux v.; *Oreodaph.;* Prun. sp.; Sep.; Tub.

Occipital—Æth.; Alfal.; Anac.; Avena; *Bry.;* Camph.; Can. ind.; Carbo v.; *Cim.; Cocc.;* Euonym.; Eup. perf.; Ferr. m.; *Gels.;* Gins.; Jugl. c.; Lac c.; Lach.; Lecith.; Niccol. s.; *Nux v.;* Onosm.; Oreodaph.; *Petrol.;* Phos. ac.; *Picr. ac.;* Plat. mur.; Radium; *Rhus gl.; Sang.;* Sep.; *Sil.;* Sul.; Xanth.; Zinc. m.

Occipital extending to eyes and forehead—Arundo; Bell.; Carbo v.; Cim.; Cinch.; *Gels.;* Glycerin; Indol; Lac c.; Mag. m.; Onosm.; Phos. ac.; Picr. ac.; *Rhus r.; Sang.; Sars.; Sil.;* Spig.

Semilateral (hemicrania)—Arg. n.; Ars.; *Bell.; Bry.;* Ced.; Cham.; *Coff.;* Col.; *Cycl.;* Gins.; Glon.; *Ign.;* Jonosia; Kali bich.; Lach.; Nat. m.; Ol. an.; *Onosm.;* Phos.; Prun. sp.; *Puls.; Sang.;* Sep.; *Sil.; Spig.; Stann.;* Thuya.

Semilateral, left side—Nat. m.; Nux v.; *Onosm.;* Saponin; *Spig.*

Semilateral, right side—*Ced.;* Chel.; Iris; Kali bich.; Radium; *Sang.;* Sil.; Tab.

Spinal and cervical—Bell.; *Cim.; Cocc.;* Dulc.; *Gels.; Gossyp.; Helleb.;* Nat. m.; Nat. s.; Niccol. s.; *Oreodaph.;* Phos. ac.; *Picr. ac.;* Scutel.; *Sil.;* Ver. v.

Supraorbital—Acon.; Aconit.; Aloe; *Ars.;* Carb. ac.; *Ced.;* Cereus; *Chin. s.;* Cim.; Cinnab.; Col.; Glon.; Ign.; Indol; Iris; *Kali bich.;* Lyc.; Meli.; Menthol; *Nux v.;* Phell.; Puls.; Viola od.

Supraorbital, left—Act. spic.; Arg. n.; Astrag.; Bry.; Carbo v.; *Ced.;* Cocc.; Euonym.; Menthol; Nux v.; Oreodaph.; Sapon.; Selen.; Senec.; *Spig.;* Tellur.; Xanth.

Supraorbital, right—Arundo; *Bell.;* Bism.; *Chel.; Iris;* Kali bich.; Meli.; Plat.; Sang.; Sil.

Sutures, along—Calc. p.

Temples—*Acon.; Anac.;* Arn.; *Bell.; Bry.;* Caps.; Ced.; *Carb. ac.;* Chin. s.; *Cinch.;* Epiph.; Gels.; *Glon.;* Ign.; Lach.; Naja; *Onosm.,* Oreodaph.; *Phell.;* Phos. ac.; Plat.; Rhus t.; *Sang.; Senec.;* Sep.; Spig.; *Stann.;* Sul. ac.; Usnea.

HEAD

Temples, ear to ear—Antipyr.; Calc. ars.; Menthol; Pall.; Syph.

Vertex (crown of head)—Alumen; Anac.; Act. spic.; Ars.; *Cact.*; Calc. p.; *Cim.*; Cinch.; Gels.; Glon.; Hyper.; *Lach.*; Menyanth.; Naja; Nux v.; Pall.; *Phell.*; *Phos. ac.*; Plat.; Puls.; Radium; Sep.; *Sul.*; Ver. a.

CHARACTER OF PAIN

Aching, dull: Acon.; *Æsc.*; Alfal.; *Aloe*; Ant. c.; *Arg. n.*; Ars.; Azar.; Bapt.; Bell.; But. ac.; Caps.; Carb. ac.; Carbo v.; Card. m.; Cepa; *Cham.*; *Cinch.*; Cocc.; Eyonym.; *Gels.*; *Helleb.*; *Hydr.*; Ichthy.; *Ign.*; Indol; Iris; Kali bich.; *Lept.*; Lil. t.; Menthol; Myr.; Naja; Nat. ars.; *Nux v.*; *Nyctanth.*; Onosm.; Oreodaph.; *Phell.*; Picr. ac.; *Plumb. m.*; Scutel.; *Sil.*; Stann.; *Stellar.*

Boring, digging—*Arg. n.*; *Asaf.*; Aur.; Bell.; *Clem.*; *Col.*; *Hep.*; Nat. s.; Sep.; Stram.

Bruised, battered, sore—Arn.; *Bapt.*; Bellis; Cinch.; Coff.; Euonym.; *Eup. perf.*; *Gel.*; Guarea; *Ign.*; Ipec.; Lyc.; Menthol; *Nux v.*; Phell.; Phos. ac.; *Rhus t.*; Sil.; Tab.

Burning, heat—*Acon.*; Alumen; *Apis*; Arn.; *Ars.*; Aster.; Bell.; Calc. p.; Glon.; Helon.; *Lach.*; Lil. t.; Merc.; Ox. ac.; Phell.; *Phos.*; Sil.; Tongo; Ver. v.; Viola od.

Bursting, splitting—*Acon.*; Bell.; *Bry.*; Cact.; *Caps.*; Cinch.; Daphne; Gels.; *Glon.*; Mag. m.; Meli.; *Nat. m.*; Nux m.; Nux v.; Oleand.; Puls.; Sang.; Sep.; Solan. lyc.; Strych.; *Usnea*; Ver. a.

Constrictive, band-like, squeezing—Acon.; *Anac.*; *Ant. t.*; Antipyr.; *Cact.*; *Carb. ac.*; Carbo v.; Card. m.; Coca; Cocc.; Eup. perf.; *Gels.*; Glon.; Guano; Iod.; Lept.; Merc. per.; *Merc.*; *Nit. ac.*; Osm.; *Plat.*; Spig.; Stann.; *Sul.*; Tar. h.; Tub.

Distensive, full—*Acon.*; Amyl; Arg. n.; Bapt.; *Bell.*; Bov.; *Bry.*; Cact.; *Caps.*; Chin. ars.; Cim.; Cinch.; *Gels.*; *Glon.*; Glyderin; Kali bich.; Menthol; Nux v.; Strych.; *Sul.*; Ver. v.

Drawing—Bism.; *Bry.*; *Caps.*; Carbo v.; Caul.; *Caust.*; *Cham.*; Kali c.; Nux v.

Excruciating, violent—Agar.; Amyl; *Anac.*; Arg. n.; Aur.; *Bell.*; Bry.; *Cim.*; *Cinch.*; *Glon.*; Kali iod.; Meli.; Oreodaph.; Plat. mur.; *Sang.*; Scutel.; Sil.; *Spig.*; Strych.; Zinc. v.

Heaviness—*Acon.*; *Aloe*; Arg. n.; *Bapt.*; Bar. m.; Bell.; *Bry.*; Cact.; Calc. c.; Carbo v.; *Cocc.*; *Gels.*; *Glon.*; Glycerin; Hydr.; Hyper.; *Ign.*; Iris; *Lach.*; Lil. t.; Meli.; *Menyanth.*; Merc.; *Nux v.*; Onosm.; *Op.*; Oreodaph.; Petrol.; *Phell.*; *Phos. ac.*; Phos.; Picr. ac.; *Plat.*; Puls.; Rhus t.; *Sep.*; *Sul.*; Ther.

Periodical, intermittent—Acon.; Am. picr.; Arg. n.; *Ars.*; *Bell.*; Cact.; Ced.; Chel.; *Cinch.*; Eup. perf.; Gels.; Ign.; Kali cy.; Mag. m.; Niccol.; Niccol. s.; *Sang.*; Sep.; *Spig.*; Tab.; Tela ar.; Zinc. v.

Periodical, intermittent, alternate days—*Anhal.*; *Cinch.*

Periodical, intermittent, every third day—seventh day—Eup. perf.

Periodical, intermittent, every seventh day—Calc. ars.; Sabad.; *Sang.*; Sil.; Sul.

Periodical, intermittent, every eighth day—Iris.

Periodical, intermittent, every week or two—Sul.

Periodical, intermittent, every two-three weeks—Ferr. m.

HEAD 705

Periodical, intermittent, every six weeks—Mag. m.
Periodical, intermittent, lasting several days—Tab.
Periodical, with increase and decrease of sun—Glon.; Kal.; Nat. c.; *Nat. m.*; *Sang.*; *Spig.*; Tab.
Piercing, as from nail—*Agar.*; Ananth.; Aquil.; *Coff.*; *Hep.*; *Ign.*; Mag. pol. am.; *Nux v.*; Paraf.; Ruta; Sil.; *Thuya*; Zinc v.
Pressing—*Acon.*; Aloe; *Anac.*; *Bell.*; *Bry.*; Cact.; *Caps.*; Carb. ac.; *Cham.*; *Chel.*; Chionanth.; Cim.; Epiph; *Eup. perf.*; Ferr.; *Glon.*; Hydroc. ac.; *Ign.*; Kali c.; Lach.; Meli.; *Menyanth.*; *Nux v.*; Onosm.; Op.; Oreodaph.; Petrol.; *Phos. ac.*; *P!at.*; Pod.; Puls.; Rhus t.; Sang.; Sep.; Stann.; Sticta; *Sul.*; Sul. ac.; Thasp.; Ver. a.; *Zinc. m.*
Pressing, as from pincers, or vise—Act. spic.; Bism.; *Cact.*; Cham.; Lyc.; Menisp.; *Menyanth.*; Phos. ac.; *Plat.*; Puls.; *Verbasc.*; Viola tr.
Pressing asunder—Arg. n.; *Asaf.*; Aur.; *Bry.*; Carbo an.; *Cim.*; Cinch.; Coral.; Eriod.; *Fagop.*; *Menisp.*; Prun. sp.; *Ptel.*; Stront.
Pressing, dull as from weight—Aloe; Alumen; *Anac.*; *Cact.*; Carbo v.; *Cim.*; Eup. perf.; Hyper.; *Lach.*; Menyanth.; *Naja*; *Nux v.*; Op.; Petrol.; *Phell.*; *Phos. ac.*; Puls.; *Sep.*; *Sul.*; Ther.
Pressing, in small spots—Arg. n.; *Ign.*; *Kali bich.*; Plat.; Poth.; Thuya.
Shifting, shooting, stinging, tearing—Acon.; Æsc.; Apis; Arn.; Ars.; *Bell.*; *Caps.*; *Ced.*; Cim.; *Cinch.*; Col; Ign.; *Iris*; Kali bich.; Kali c.; Lac c.; *Prun. sp.*; Puls.; Sang.; Sil.; Spig.; Vinca.
Shock (electric) like stabbing—Apis; *Aster.*; *Bell.*; Can. ind.; Cic.; Cocc.; *Glon.*; Rhodium; Sang.; *Sep.*; Tab.; Zinc. v.
Stitching, sticking—Acon.; *Æsc.*; Arn.; Ars.; Bell.; *Bry.*; Can. ind.; *Caps.*; Cycl.; *Kali c.*; Niccol.; Puls.; Tar. h.
Stupefying—Arg. n.; *Bell.*; Bry.; Gels.; *Glon.*; Senec.; Staph.; Syph.
Throbbing, beating, hammering, pulsating—*Acon.*; Act. spic.; Amyl; Arg. n.; Ars.; *Bell.*; Bry.; *Cact.*; Can. ind.; *Caps.*; Chin. ars.; Chin. s.; Cim.; *Cinch.*; Croc.; Eup. perf.; *Ferr. m.*; Ferr. p.; Gels.; *Glon.*; Glycerin; Hyper.; *Iris*; *Lac d.*; Lach.; Lyc.; *Meli.*; *Nat. m.*; Nux v.; Paul.; Psor.; Puls.; Sang.; Sep.; Sil.; *Spig.*; *Sul.*; Tongo; Ver. v.

CONCOMITANTS—Anguish, anxiety—Acon.; Ars.; Plat.
Arterial excitement, tension—Acon.; *Bell.*; *Glon.*; Glycerin; Meli.; Poth.; Usnea; *Ver. v.*
Burning along spine—Picr. ac.
Chilliness—*Arg. n.*; Camph.; Lact. v.; Mang. m.; *Puls.*; Sang.; Sil.
Coldness in back and occiput—Berb. v.
Coldness in head—Calc. ac.; Calc. c.; Sep.; Ver. a.
Coldness of hands and feet—Bell.; *Calc. c.*; Ferr. m.; Lach.; Meli.; *Menyanth.*; Naja; Sep.; Sul.; Ver. a.
Colic—Aloe; Cocc.
Constipation—Aloe; Alum.; *Bry.*; Euonym.; *Hydr.*; Lac d.; Niccol.; *Nux v.*; Op.; Plumb. m.
Coryza—Agar.; Camph.; Cepa.
Cough—Arn.; Caps.; Lyc.
Delirium—Agar.; Bell.; Syph.; Ver. a.
Diarrhoea—Aloe; Cham.; Pod.; Ver. a.

Drowsiness—*Ail.;* Ant. t.; Branca; Chel.; Dub.; *Gels.; Indium;* Lept.; Myr.; Stellar.

Ears, burning—Rhus t.

Ears, deafness—Chin. s.; Verbasc.

Ears, roaring—Aur.; *Chin. s.; Cinch.;* Ferr. m.; Sang.; Sulphon.

Ears, stitching—Caps.

Empty feeling in stomach—*Ign.;* Kali p.; *Sep.*

Excitement, emotional—Can. ind.; Pall.

Excitement, sexual—Apis; Plat. mur.

Exhaustion, asthenia—*Ars.;* Aur. br.; *Cinch.; Gels.;* Ign.; Indium; Lac d.; Lob. infl.; *Picr. ac.;* Sang.; Sul.

Eyes: blindness, or visual disturbances, precede or attend—Anhal.; Bell.; *Cycl.;* Epiph.; *Gels.;* Ign.; *Iris; Kali bich.;* Kali c.; Lac c.; *Lac d.; Nat. m.;* Niccol.; Nux v.; Picr. ac.; Pod.; Psor.; *Sang.;* Sil.; Spig.; *Ther.;* Zinc. s.

Eyes, enlarged feeling—Arg. n.

Eyes, heaviness—Aloe.

Eyes, heaviness of, and lids—Bell.; Gels.

Eyes, injection—*Bell.;* Meli.; Nux v.

Eyes, lachrymation—Chel.; Phell.; Rhus t.; Spig.; Taxus.

Eyes, soreness, pain—Aloe; Ced.; *Cim.; Eup. perf.; Gels.;* Homarus; Menthol; Myr.; Nat. m.; Phell.; *Scutel.;* Sil.; *Spig.*

Eyes, vision returns as headache comes on—*Iris;* Lac d.; Nat. m.

Face, flushed, hot—*Acon.;* Amyl; *Bell.;* Cham.; Ferr. p.; Gels.; *Glon.;* Mag. p.; *Meli.;* Naja; Nat. m.; Nux v.; Pod.; *Sang.;* Sep.

Face, pale—Acon.; *Calc. c.;* Cinch.; Ign.; *Lach.;* Lob. infl.; Meli.; Nat. m.; Sil.; Spig.; Tab.; *Ver. a.*

Faintness—Nux v.; Ver. a.

Fever—Acon.; Ars.; *Bell.;* Ferr. p.

Flatulence—Asclep. t.; Calc. ac.; Calc. p.; Can. ind.; *Carbo v.;* Xanth.

Gastralgia, attending or following—Bism.

Gastro-intestinal derangements—Agar.; Aloe; Arg n.; Ars.; *Bry.;* Can. ind.; *Carbo v.; Cinch.;* Iris; Nux v.; Pod.; *Puls.*

Hair, falling out—Ant. c.; Nit. ac.; Sil.

Head nodding—Lamium; Sep.

Head retracted—Bell.; Cocc.; *Gossyp.*

Heart's action labored—Lycopus.

Haemorrhoids—Nux v.

Hunger—Anac.; Cact.; *Epiph.;* Ign.; *Lyc.; Psor.*

Hypochondrium, right, stitches—Æsc.

Irritability—Anac.; *Bry.;* Cham.; Ign.; *Nux v.*

Liver disturbance—Chel.; Jugl. c.; *Lept.;* Nux v.

Loquacity—Can. ind.

Lumbago, alternating—Aloe.

Mental depression, despondency—Aloe; *Arg. n.;* Aur.; *Ign.;* Indol; Iris; Lac d.; Naja; Picr. ac.; Plumb. m.; *Puls.;* Sars.; Sep.; Zinc. m.

Mental weakness—Arg. n.; Nux v.; Sil.

Muscular soreness—Gels.; Rhus t.

HEAD 707

Nausea—Aloe; *Ant. c.*; Ars.; *Bry.*; *Cocc.*; Ferr. m.; Gels.; Indol; *Ipec.*; *Iris*; Lac c.; Lac d.; Lob. infl.; Lob. purp.; Naja; Nat. m.; *Nux v.*; Paul.; Petrol.; *Puls.*; *Sang.*; *Sep.*; Sil.; *Tab.*

Nodules, gouty of scalp—Sil.

Nosebleed—Agar.; Amyl; Ant. c.; Ham.; *Meli.*

Nose, dry, neuralgia—Dulc.

Numbness, tingling, of lips, tongue, nose—Nat. m.

Numbness—Chel.; Indol; Plat.

Occipital soreness—Cim.; Sil.

Oversensitiveness—Ars.; *Bell.*; *Cham.*; Cinch.; Coff.; *Ign.*; *Nux v.*; Sil.; Spig.; Tela ar.

Pains in abdomen—Cina; Col.; Ver. a.

Pains in limbs—Sang.

Pains in lumbar region—Radium.

Palpitation—Cact.; Spig.

Polyuria—Asclep. s.; *Gels.*; *Ign.*; Lac d.; *Sang.*; Scutel.; Sil.

Ptyalism—Fagus; Iris.

Respiratory affections—Lact. v.

Restlessness—*Ars.*; Helleb.; Ign.; Pyr.; Spig.

Scalp, bruised feeling—Æsc.; *Cinch.*; Col.; Sil.

Scotoma—Aspar.

Sleeplessness—*Coff.*; Indium; Syph.; Zinc. v.

Spasmodic symptoms—Ign.

Sweat profuse—Lob. infl.; Tab.

Temporal veins engorged—Carls.; Gels.

Thirst—Pulex.

Tongue coated, fetor oris, etc.—Calc. ac.; Card. m.; Euonym.; Gymnocl.; *Puls.*

Toothache—Sang.

Trembling all over—*Arg. n.*; Bor.; *Gels.*

Vertigo—Acon.; Agrost.; Bry.; Chin. s.; *Cinch.*; *Cocc.*; *Eup. purp.*; *Gels.*; Glon.; Ign.; Lept.; Lob. purp.; *Nux v.*; Pod.; Sep.; Xanth.

Vomiting—Arg. n.; *Ars.*; *Bry.*; Calc. ac.; Cham.; Cinch.; Cocc.; Glon.; *Ipec.*; *Iris*; Lac c.; Lac d.; Lob. infl.; Meli.; Nat. m.; *Nux v.*; Puls.; Robin.; *Sang.*; Sep.; Sil.; Tab.; Ver. a.; Zinc. s.

Yawning—Kali c.; Staph.

MODALITIES—**Aggravation**: **After drugging**: Nux v.

After midnight—Ferr. m.

Afternoon—Ananth.; Bad.; *Bell.*; Cycl.; Eup. purp.; Indol; Lob. infl.; Meli.; Selen.

Air, open—*Ars.*; Bov.; Branca; *Cinch.*; Cocc.; Coff.; Mag. m.; *Nux v.*; Sep.

Anger—Nux v.

Ascending—Ant. c.; Bell.; But. ac.; *Calc. c.*; Conv.; *Menyanth.*

Attention, close—Ign.

Awaking from sleep—Lach.

Beating time—Anhal.

Bending head backward—Glon.

HEAD

Bending head forward—Bell.; Cob.

Closing teeth—Am. c.

Cold, draft of air—*Ars.;* Bell.; *Cinch.;* Eup. purp.; Ferr. p.; Ichth.; Ign.; Iris; Nux v.; Rhod.; Rhus t.; Sil.

Contact, touch—*Bell.; Cinch.,* Ferr. p.; Rhus t.; *Tar. h.*

Coughing—Acon.; Arn.; *Bell.; Bry.; Caps.;* Carbo v.; Iris; Kali c.; *Nat. m.; Nux v.;* Petrol.; Phos.; Sep.; Sul.

Dinking coffee—Act. spic.; Ign.; Nux v.

Drinking milk—Brom.

Eating—Am. c.; Arn.; *Ars.;* Atrop.; *Bry.;* Cact.; Cocc.; Coff.; Gels.; Ign.; Lach.; *Lyc.; Nux v.*

Evening—Aur.; Caust.; *Cepa;* Cycl.; Eup. purp.; Indol; Kali s.; *Puls.;* Thlaspi.

Exertion, mental or physical—Aloe; *Anac.; Arg. n.;* Cocc.; *Epiph.;* Gels.; Nat. c.; *Nux v.;* Phos. ac.; Phos.; *Picr. ac.;* Sep.; Sil.; Tub.

Gradually: crescendo, decrescendo—Plat.; Stann.

Hawking—Conv.

Jar, misstep, etc.—Aloe; *Bell.;* Bry.; Cinch.; Crot.; Ferr. p.; *Glon.;* Lach.; Lyc.; Menyanth.; Rhus t.; Sil.; *Spig.; Ther.*

Left side—Anac.; Ars. m.; *Brom.;* Chin. s.; *Cycl.;* Epiph.; Eup. purp.; *Lach.;* Niccol.; Oreodaph.; Paraf.; Sapon.; *Senec.;* Sep.; *Spig.;* Thuya.

Light—*Bell.;* Ferr.; Lac d.; Lyssin; *Ign.;* Kali bich.; Kali c.; *Nux v.;* Oreodaph.; Phell.; Sang.; Scutel.; Sil.; Tar. h.

Lying down—Ars. m.; *Bell.;* Bov.; Cinch.; Col.; Eup. perf.; Gels.; *Glon.;* Lach.; Lyc.; Rhus t.; Sang.; Ther.

Lying on back of head—Cocc.; Col.

Lying on painful side—Sep.

Menses—Croc.; Lac d.; *Nat. m.;* Sep.

Morning—Æsc.; Alum.; Am. m.; Aspar.; Cycl.; Hep.; Lac d.; Myr.; *Nat. m.;* Niccol.; Nux v.; Phos. ac.; Pod.; Sang.; Spig.; Stellar.; Sul.

Morning on awaking, opening eyes—Bov.; *Bry.;* Graph.; *Nat. m.; Nux v.;* Onosm.; Strych.; Tab.

Motion—Acon.; Anac.; *Apis;* Bell.; Bry.; But. ac.; Cinch.; Cocc.; Gels.; *Glon.;* Glycerin; Ign.; Iris; Lach.; Mag. m.; Menthol; Nat. m.; *Nux v.; Phos. ac.;* Ptel.; Rhus t.; Sep.; *Sil.; Spig.;* Stann.; Ther.

Motion of eyes—Bell.; *Bry.;* Cim.; Col.; Cupr. m.; Gels.; Ichth.; Ign.; Nux v.; Physost.; Puls.; Rhus t.; Spig.

Muscular strain—Calc. c.

Narcotics—Coff.

Night—Ars.; *Aur.;* Bov.; Merc. d.; Ptel.; *Puls.;* Strych.; Sul.; Syph.; Tar. h.

Noises—Acon.; Ars.; Bell.; Coff.; Ferr. p.; *Ign.;* Lac d.; Lachnanth.; Nit. ac.; *Nux v.;* Phell.; *Phos. ac.;* Ptel.; Sang.; Scutel.; *Sil.;* Spig.; Tab.; Tar. h.

Noon—Chin. s.; Sang.; Tab.

Nosebleed—Amyl; Ant. c.

Objects, bright—*Bell.;* Oreodaph.; Phos. ac.; *Sil.;* Spig.

Odors—Coff.; Ign.; Scutel.; *Selen.*

Overheating—Carbo v.; Sil.; Thuya.

HEAD

Pressure—Diosc.; Hep.; Lach.; Nat. ars.; Ptel.; Sil.
Riding in cars—Cocc.; Kali c.; Petrol.
Right side—*Bell.*; Bry.; *Cact.*; Carb. ac.; *Chel.*; Crot.; Hep.; Iris; *Lyc.*; Mez.; *Sang.*; Taxus.
Rising in bed—*Bry.*; Cocc.
Sitting—Cinch.; Rhus t.
Sleep after—Crot. casc.; Ign.; *Lach.*
Stimulants, abuse—Ign.; *Nux v.*
Stool.—Aloe; Ign.; Ox. ac.
Stooping—Acon.; Ars. m.; *Bell.*; Bry.; Glon.; *Ign.*; Lach.; *Nux v.*; Puls.; Rhus v.; Sep.; Sil.; *Spig.*; Sul.
Sun—*Bell.*; *Gels.*; *Glon.*; Kali bich.; Lach.; *Nat. c.*; Nux v.; *Sang.*; *Selen.*; Spig.
Talking—*Cact.*; Coff.; Ign.; Mez.
Tobacco—Carb. ac.; Gels.; Hep.; *Ign.*; Lob. infl.; Nat. ars.
Warmth in general—Aloe; Bry.; Cepa; Euphras.; *Glon.*; Hyper.; Led.; Niccol.; Phos.; *Puls.*; Sep.
Water, sight of—Lyssin.
Weather changes—*Calc. p.*; Dulc.; Guaiac.; *Phyt.*; Psor.; Rhod.; Spig.
Wine—Nux v.; Rhod.; Zinc.
Winter—Aloe; Bism.; Carbo v.; Nux v.; Sabad.; Sul.
Working in black—Ced.

AMELIORATION—After rising: Kali p.
Bending head backward—*Bell.*; Murex.
Bending head forward—Cim.; Hyos.; Ign.
Closing eyes—Ant. t.; Bell.
Cold in general—Aloe; Alumen; Ars.; Bism.; Cepa; Cycl.; Ferr p.; Lyc.; Phos.; Poth.; *Puls.*; Spig.; *Tab.*
Conversation—Dulc.
Dark room—Sang.; Sil.
Eating—Alum.; *Anac.*; Apium gr.; Carls.; *Chel.*; Coca; Kali p.; *Lith. c.*; *Psor.*
Holding hands near head—Carbo an.; Glon.; Petrol.; Sul. ac.
Lying—Anac.; *Bry.*; *Cinch.*; Ferr.; Gels.; Ign.; Lach.; Mag. m.; Nux v.; Phos. ac.; *Sang.*; *Sil.*; Ther.
Lying on painful side—Calc. ars.; Ign.
Lying on painful side with head high—*Bell.*; Gels.
Lying on painful side with head low—Absinth.; Æth.
Menses, during—Bell.; Cepa; Glycerin; Jonosia; Lach.; *Meli.*; Zinc. m.
Mental exertion—*Helon.*; Picr. ac.
Motion, gentle—Cinch.; Glon.; Helon.; Iris; Kali p.; *Puls.*
Motion, hard, continued—Indigo; Rhus t.; Sep.
Nosebleed—Bry.; Bufo; Ferr. p.; Mag. s.; *Meli.*; Psor.; Rhus t.
Open air—Acon.; Act. spic.; *Cepa*; *Coca*; Indol; Jonosia; *Puls.*; Radium; Sep.; Thuya.
Partially closing eyes—*Aloe*; Coccinel.; Oreodaph.
Polyuria—Acon.; Gels.; *Ign.*; *Phos. ac.*; Sang.; Sil.; Ver. a.
Pressure—*Apis*; Arg. n.; *Bell.*; Bry.; Carbo an.; *Cinch.*; Col.; Gels.;

HEAD

Glon.; Ign.; Indigo; Lac c.; Lac d.; Mag. m.; Mag. p.; Menyanth.; Nux m.; Nux v.; Paris; Puls.; Sang.; Sep.; Sil.; Spig.; Thuya; Ver. a.
Raising head—Sulphon.
Rest, quiet—Bell.; Bry.; Cocc.; Gels.; Lith. c.; Menyanth.; Nux v.; Oreodaph.; Puls.; Sang.; Sil.; Spig.
Rubbing—Indigo; Tar. h.
Semierect posture—Bell.
Sleep—Coccinel.; Gels.; Nat. m.; Sang.; Scutel.; Sil.
Smoking—Aran.
Stimulants—Gels.
Stool and expelling flatus—Æth.; Sang.
Stooping—Cina; Ign.; Menyanth.
Sweating—Nat. m.
Tea—Carb. ac.
Thinking of pain—Camph.; Helon.; Ox. ac.
Turning head forward—Ign.
Uncovering head—Glon.; Lyc.
Warmth in general—Am. c.; Cinch.; Col.; Ichthy.; Mag. p.; Nux v.; Phos.; Rhus t.; Sil.
Wrapping or bandaging tightly—Agar.; Apis; Arg. n.; Bell.; Glon.; Ign.; Lac d.; Mag. m.; Picr. ac.; Puls.; Sil.; Stront.

HYDROCEPHALUS—(**acute and chronic**): **hydrocephaloid**: Acon.; Apis; Apoc.; Arg. n.; Arn.; Ars.; Bac.; Bar. c.; Bell.; Bry.; Calc. c.; Calc. p.; Canth.; Carb. ac.; Chin. s.; Cinch.; Cupr. ac.; Cyprip.; Dig.; Gels.; Helleb.; Iod.; Iodof.; Ipec.; Kali br.; Kali iod.; Laburn.; Merc. s.; Œnothera; Op.; Phos.; Pod.; Sil.; Solan. n.; Sul.; Tub.; Ver. a.; Zinc. br.; Zinc. m.; Zinc. mur.

MOTION—**POSITION OF HEAD**—**Boring back into pillow or rolling sideways**:—Apis; Arum; Bell.; Helleb.; Pod.; Zinc. m.
Cannot hold head up, neck so weak—Abrot.; Æth.; Cocc.; Nat. m.; Ver. a.
Drawn back, retracted—Agar.; Art. v.; Bell.; Camph. monobr.; Cic.; Cur.; Hydroc. ac.; Iodof.; Morph.; Nat. s.; Sec.; Stram.; Sul.; Ver. v.
Motion constant, jerking trembling—Agar.; Ant. t.; Ars.; Bell.; Can. ind.; Cham.; Hyos.; Lamium; Myg.; Nux m.; Op.; Stram.; Strych.; Ver. v.; Zinc. m.

SCALP—**Dandruff (seborrhoea)**:—Am. m.; Ars.; Bar. c.; Branca; Bry.; Fluor. ac.; Graph.; Hep.; Heracl.; Iod.; Kali s.; Lyc.; Nat. m.; Phos.; Sanic.; Sep.; Sul.; Sul. iod.; Thuya.

ERUPTIONS—**Boils**: Anac.; Ant. t.; Aur.; Calc. mur.; Calc. s.; Dulc.; Hep.; Jugl. r.; Scrophul.; Sil.
Crusta lactea—Arct. l.; Asatacus; Bar. c.; Calc. c.; Calc. iod.; Calc. s.; Cic.; Clem.; Dulc.; Graph.; Hep.; Kali m.; Lyc.; Merc.; Mez.; Oleand.; Petrol.; Psor.; Rhus t.; Sars.; Scrophul.; Sep.; Sil.; Sul.; Trifol.; Vinca m.; Viola tr.
Eczema—Arct. l.; Astac.; Calc. c.; Clem.; Graph.; Hydr.; Lyc.; Mez.; Oleand.; Petrol.; Psor.; Selen.; Sul.; Tellur.; Viola od.
Erysipelas—Bell.; Euphorb.; Rhus t.
Favus (porrigo, scald head)—Æthiops; Ars.; Ars. iod.; Calc. c.; Calc. iod.;

HEAD

Calc. mur.; Calc. s.; *Dulc.;* Ferr. iod.; Graph.; Hep.; Jugl. r.; Kali s.; Nit. ac.; Sep.; *Sil.;* Sul.; Viola tr.

Growths, tumors, exostoses—Ananth.; Aur. m.; *Calc. fl.;* Cupr. m.; Fluor. ac.; *Hekla; Kali iod.;* Merc. phos.; Merc.; Sil.; Still.

Herpes—Ananth.; Chrys.; Nat. m.; Oleand.; *Rhus t.*

Itching eruptions—Clem.; *Oleand.;* Sil.; Staph.; *Sul.*

Moist, humid eruptions—*Calc. s.;* Clem.; Graph.; Hep.; Lyc.; Merc.; *Mez.; Oleand.; Petrol.;* Psor.; *Rhus t.;* Sep.; Sil.; Staph.; *Vinca.*

Moist, humid eruptions, behind ears—*Graph.;* Lyc.; Oleand.; *Petrol.;* Staph.; Thlaspi; Tub.

Moist, humid eruptions, of margin of hair, nape of neck—*Clem.;* Hydr.; Nat. m.; *Oleand.;* Sul.

Plica polonica—Ant. t.; Bar. c.; Bor.; Graph.; *Lyc.;* Nat. m.; Psor.; Sars.; Tub.; *Vinca;* Viola tr.

Pustules—Arundo; Cic.; *Clem.;* Graph.; Iris; Jugl. c. ; Mez.

Ringworm (tinea capitis)—Ars.; *Bac.;* Bar. m.; Calc. c.; Chrys.; Dulc.; *Graph.;* Kali s.; *Mez.;* Petrol.; *Psor.;* Sep.; Sil.; Sul.; *Tellur.;* Tub.; Viola tr. See Skin.

Scabs, crusts—Ant. c.; Ars.; Calc. s.; Cic.; *Dulc.; Graph.;* Hep.; Lyc.; *Mez.;* Sul.; Trifol.

Scales, dry—*Ars.;* Kali s.; Mez.; *Nat. m.;* Phos.; Phyt.; Psor.; Sanic.; Thlaspi.

Spots, red—Tellur.

Wens—*Bar. c.; Benz. ac.;* Graph.; Hep.; *Kali iod.;* Nit. ac.; Phyt.

HAIR—Brittle, harsh, dry: Bad.; Bell.; Bor.; Graph.; *Kali c.;* Plumb. m.; *Psor.;* Sec.; Staph.; Thuya.

Falling out (alopecia)—*Alum.;* Ant. c.; *Ars.;* Arundo; Aur.; Bac.; Bar. c.; Calc. c.; Calc. iod.; Carbo v.; Chrysar.; *Fluor. ac.; Graph.;* Hyper.; Kali c.; Lyc.; Mancin.; Mez.; *Nat. m.;* Nit. ac.; Petrol.; *Phos. ac.; Phos.;* Pix liq.; *Selen.; Sep.;* Sil.; Strych. ars.; *Syph.; Thallium;* Thuya; Thyr.; Sphingur.; *Vinca;* Zinc. m.

Greasy—Benz. nit.; Bry.; Merc.

Gray, premature—Lyc.; *Phos. ac.;* Sec.; Sul. ac.

Tangled, in bunches—*Bor.;* Fluor. ac.; Lyc.; *Psor.;* Tub.; Vinca.

ITCHING of scalp—Alum.; Ant. c.; *Ars.;* Arundo; Bov.; *Calc. c.;* Carbo v.; Clem.; Graph.; Heracl.; Iodof.; Jugl., r.; Mag. c.; Mancin.; Menisp.; Nit. ac.; *Oleand.;* Phos.; Sep.; Sil.; Strych.; *Sul.;* Tellur.; *Vinca.*

Neuralgia—*Acon.; Cim.;* Hydr.; Phyt.

Numbness—*Acon.;* Alum.; Ferr. br.; *Graph.;* Petrol.

Sensitive to touch, combing—*Acon.;* Apis; Arn.; Ars.; Azar.; *Bell.;* Bov.; Bry.; Carbo v.; Caust.; *Cinch.;* Euonym.; *Eup. perf.; Gels.;* Hep.; Kali bich.; Lachnanth.; Meli.; Merc.; Nat. m.; Nit. ac.; Nux m.; *Nux v.;* Oleand.; *Paris;* Rhus t.; Sep.; *Sil.;* Strych.; Sul.

Sweat—*Calc. c.;* Calc. p.; *Cham.;* Graph.; Helleb.; Hep.; Heracl.; Hyper.; Mag. m.; Merc.; Pod.; *Rheum.;* Sanic.; Sil.

Tension—*Acon.;* Arn.; Asar.; *Bapt.;* Canchal.; Caust.; Iris; *Merc.; Paris;* Ratanh.; Selen.; Sticta; *Viola.*

SENSATIONS—As if a ball, firmly lodged in forehead: Staph.

As if brain were frozen—Indigo.

As if brain were loose, in forehead, falling laterally—Bell.; Bry.; Rhus t.; Sul. ac.

As if hair were pulled, on vertex—Acon.; *Arg. n.*; Kali n.; Lachnanth.; Mag. c.; *Phos.*

As if top would fly off—Acon.; *Can. ind.*; *Cim.* Passif.; Syph.; Visc. a.; Yucca.

Bewildered, confused, stupid, intoxicated feeling—*Absinth.*; Acon.; Ail.; Aloe; Anac.; *Apis*; Aran.; Bapt.; Bell.; *Bry.*; Can. ind.; Carbo v.; Cinch.; Cocc.; Gels.; Glon.; Helleb.; Menthol; Nat. c.; Nux m.; Nux v.; Op.; Phos. ac.; *Phos.*; *Quercus*; Rhus t.; Sep.; *Sul.*; Tanac.; Xerophyl.; Zinc. m.

Bruised, sore feeling, of brain—Arg. m.; *Arn.*; *Bapt.*; Bell.; *Bellis*; Bov.; Cinch.; Eupion; Led.; *Nux v.*; Petrol.; Rhus t.; Ver. a. See Headache.

Burning, head—*Acon.*; Alumen; Apis; Arn.; Ars.; *Aster.*; Bell.; Canth.; Nux v.; *Phos.*; Zinc.

Burning on vertex—Avena; Cupr. s.; Daphne; *Frax. am.*; *Graph.*; Helon.; *Lach.*; Rhus t.; *Sul.*; Tarax.

Bursting—*Acon.*; Arg. n.; *Bell.*; *Bry.*; Caps.; Cinch.; Cocaine; Formica; Gels.; *Glon.*; Nat. c.; Nat. m.; Nux m.

Coldness—*Agar.*; Ars.; Bar. c.; *Calc. c.*; Calc. p.; Calc. sil.; Carbo v.; Con.; Helod.; Laur.; Nat. m.; *Sep.*; Sil.; Val.; Ver. a.

Coldness in occiput—Berb. v.; Calc. p.; Dulc.; Ferrula; *Helod.*; Phos.

Compressed in vise—*Anac.*; Antipyr.; Arg. n.; *Berb. v.*; *Cact.*; Can. ind.; Carb. ac.; Cim.; Coca; *Eup. perf.*; Franciscea; Gels.; Hyper.; Mag. p.; Nit. ac.; *Plat.*; Stann.; Sul.; Tub. See Headache.

Crawling, formication—*Acon.*; Calc. c.; Petrol.; Ran. b.; Ran. rep.; Sul.

Emptiness, hollowness—*Arg. m.*; Caust.; Cocc.; Cupr. ac.; Cupr. m.; Granat.; *Ign.*; Mancin.; *Phos.*; Puls.; Zinc.

Enlarged, full, expanded feeling—Acetan.; *Acon.*; *Arg. n.*; Ars. m.; Bapt.; Bell.; Bov.; Bry.; Cim.; Cocc.; Gels.; Glon.; Jugl. c.; Justicia; Lachnanth.; *Meli.*; Menthol; Nat. c.; *Nux v.*; Oxytr.; Paris; Rhus t.; Usnea; Ver. v.

Gnawing in spot—Nat. s.; Ran. s.

Heaviness—*Acon.*; Agar.; *Aloe*; Arn.; Apis; *Bapt.*; Calc. c.; Chel.; Cim.; Cinch.; *Gels.*; Mur. ac.; Op.; Oreodaph.; *Petrol.*; Phos. ac.; Plat.; Rhus t.; Sep. See Headache.

Lightness—Abies c.; Hyos.; *Jugl. c.*; Mancin.; Nat. ars.; Nat. chlor.

Looseness of brain—Am. c.; Ars.; Bell.; Bry.; Cinch.; Hyos.; Kali c.; *Rhus t.*; Spig.; Sul. ac.; Sul.

Numbness—Alum.; Bapt.; Bufo; Calc. ars.; Cocc.; Con.; Graph.; Kali br.; Oleand.; Paris; Petrol.; *Plat.*

Opening and shutting—Can. ind.; *Cim.*; Cocc.; Lac c.

Tired feeling—*Apis*; Arn.; Chin. ars.; Con.; Ferr. p.; *Phos.*; Zinc. v.

Undulating, surging, wavelike—*Acon.*; Aur.; *Bell.*; Canth.; Chin. s.;

HEAD 713

Cim.; *Cinch.;* *Glon.;* Hep.; Hyos.; Ind.; Lach.; Mag. p.; *Meli.;* Nux v.; Pall.; Rhus t.; Senec.; Sul.
Wild, crazy feeling on vertex—Lil. t.

VERTIGO—Dizziness: Remedies in general: *Absinth.;* Acon.; Adren.; Æsc. gl.; *Æth.;* *Agar.;* *Alum.;* Ambra; Ant. c.; *Apis;* Apomorph.; *Arg. n.;* Arn.; Ars. iod.; Aur. mur.; Bapt.; *Bell.;* Bism.; Bor.; *Bry.;* *Calc. c.;* Can. ind.; *Carb. ac.;* *Carbo v.;* Chenop.; *Chin. s.;* Cim.; *Cinch.;* Coca; Cocc.; Con.; Cycl.; Dig.; Eup. perf.; Ferr. m.; Formal.; *Gels.;* Gins.; *Glon.;* *Granat.;* *Hydroc. ac.;* Iod.; Kali c.; Laburn.; Lach.; *Lith chlor.;* Lol.; Lupul.; Merc. v.; *Morph.;* Mosch.; Nat. sal.; Nicot.; Nux v.; *Op.;* Ox. ac.; Petrol.; *Phos.;* *Picr. ac.;* Pod.; *Puls.;* Quercus; Radium; Sal. ac.; Senec.; Sep.; *Sil.;* Spig.; Stront.; Strych.; Sul.; Tab.; Tar. h.; *Ther.;* Wyeth.

CAUSE AND TYPE—Anæmia of brain: Arn.; Bar. m.; Calc. c.; Chin s..; *Cinch.;* Con.; Dig.; Ferr. carb.; *Ferr.;* Hydroc. ac.; Nat. m.; Sil.
Cerebral origin—Bell.; *Cocc.;* Geis.; Sulphon.; Tab.
Congestion of brain—Acon.; Arn.; *Bell.;* Cinch.; *Cupr. m.;* *Glon.;* Hydroc. ac.; *Iod.;* Nux v.; Op.; Stram.; Sul.
Epileptic—Arg. n.; Calc. c.; *Cupr. m.;* Kal.; Nux v.; *Sil.*
Gastro-enteric derangement—Aloe; *Bry.;* Cinch.; *Cocc.;* Ipec.; Kali c.; Nux v.; *Puls.;* Rham. cal.; *Tab.*
Hysterical—*Asaf.; Ign.;* Val.
Labyrinthic origin (Meniere's disease)—Arn.; Bar. m.; Bry.; Carbon. s.; Caust.; *Chenop.;* *Chin. sal.;* *Chin. s.;* Cinch.; Con.; Ferr. p.; Gels.; Hydrobr. ac.; Kali iod.; *Nat. sal.;* Onosm.; Petrol.; Piloc.; Pyrus; *Sal. ac.;* Sil.; Tab.; *Ther.*
Mal-de-mer—Apomorph.; *Cocc.;* Petrol.; Staph.; Tab.
Mental exertion—*Arg. n.;* Nat. c.; Nux v.
Nervous origin—Ambra; Arg. n.; Cocc.; Nux v.; *Phos.;* Rhus t.; Ther.
Noises—Nux v.; *Ther.*
Odor of flowers—Nux v.; Phos.
Old age (senile changes)—*Ambra;* Ars. iod.; Bar. m.; Bellis; *Con.;* Dig.; *Iod.;* Op.; *Phos.;* Rhus t.; Sul.
Open air—Arn.; Calc. ac.; Canth.; Cycl.; Nux v.
Optical disturbances—Con.; *Gels.;* Piloc.
Pelvic troubles—Aloe; Con.
Sunlight—Agar.; Nat. c.
Worms—Cina; Spig.

OCCURRENCE—Alternates with colic: Col.; Mag. c.; Spig.
Beginning in nape of neck, or occiput—*Gels.;* Iberis; Petrol.; *Sil.*
When ascending stairs—Ars. hydr.; Calc. c.
When closing eyes—Apis; Arn.; Lach.; Mag. p.; *Ther.;* Thuya.
When coughing—Ant. t.
When descending stairs—*Bor.;* Con.; Ferr.; Meph.; *Sanic.*
When eating—Am. c.; Cocc.; Mag. m.; Nux v.; Puls.
When entering warm room—Ars.; *Iod.;* Plat.; Tab.
When frightened—Op.
When in high-ceilinged room—Cupr. ac.

When looking at colored light—Art. v.

When looking at running water—Arg. m.; Brom.; *Ferr. m.;* *Ver. a.*

When looking down—*Bor.;* Oleand.; Kal.; *Spig.*

When looking fixedly—Caust.; Con.; Lach.; Oleand.

When looking up—Calc. c.; Chin. ars.; *Granat.;* Kali p.; Petrol.; *Puls.;* *Sil.;* Tab.

When lying down—Adon. v.; Apis; Calad.; *Con.;* Lach.; Nat. m.; Nux v.; Rhod.; Rhus t.; Sil.; Staph.; *Ther.;* Thuya.

When onening eyes—Lach.; *Tab.*

When reading—Am. c.; Arn.; Cupr. m.; Nat. m.

When riding in carriage—*Cocc.;* Hep.; Lac d.; Petrol.

When rising from bed or chair—*Acon.;* Adon. v.; Bell.; *Bry.;* Can. ind.; *Cocc.;* Con.; Ferr. m.; *Nat. sal.;* *Nux v.;* Oleand.; Op.; Petrol.; Phos.; Rhus t.; Sul.

When rising in morning—*Alum.;* Bry.; Jacar.; *Lach.;* Lyc.; *Nux v.;* Op.; Phos.; Pod.; Puls.

When shaking or turning head—*Acon.;* Calc. c.; *Con.;* Hep.; Kali c.; *Morph.;* Nat. ars.

When standing with eyes closed—Arg. n.; Lathyr.

When stooping—*Acon.;* Bar. c.; Bell.; Bry.; Glon.; Iod.; *Kal.;* Nux v.; Oreodaph.; *Puls.;* *Sul.;* Ther.

When turning eyes—Con.

When turning head—Bry.; Calc. c.; Col.; *Con.;* Kali c.; Menthol; *Morph.;* Nat. ars.

When turning head to left—*Col.;* Con.

When turning in bed—Bell.; *Con.*

When walking—Acon.; Agar.; *Bell.;* *Caust.;* Cinch.; Dig.; *Gels.;* Kali c.; Lach.; Mag. p.; Nit. ac.; Nux m.; *Oreodaph.;* Petrol.; *Phos. ac.;* Rhus t.; *Ther.*

When walking in dark—Stram.

When walking in open air—Agar.; Arn.; *Cycl.;* Dros.; *Nux v.;* Sep.; *Sul.*

When walking over bridge or water—Ferr.; Lyssin.

CONCOMITANTS—**Buzzing, tinnitus:** Arg. n.; Bell.; Carbo v.; Chenop.; *Chin. s.;* Gels.; Picr. ac.; *Strych.;* Val.

Deathly pallor—*Dub.;* Puls.; *Tab.*

Debility, prostration—Ambra; *Arg. n.;* Bapt.; Cinch.; Con.; Echin.; Gels.; *Tab.;* Ver. a.

Dim vision, diplopia, etc.—Arg. n.; Bell.; *Gels.;* Glon.; Nux v.; Val.; Vinca.

Drowsiness, hot head—Æth.

Fainting, unconscious—Acon.; Alet.; Berb. v.; Bry.; Camph.; *Carbo v.;* Glon.; *Nux v.;* Phos.; Sabad.; Tab.

Gastralgia, spasms—Cic.

Head feels elongated, urging to urinate—Hyper.

Headache—Acon.; Agrost.; Apis; Cocc.; *Nux v.*

Intoxicated feeling—Abies c.; Arg. m.; Bell.; Cinch.; Cocc.; Con.; *Gels.;* *Nux v.;* Op.; Oxytr.; Petrol.

Liver disturbances—Bry.; Card. m.; Chel.

HEAD

Nausea, vomiting—Acon.; *Bry.;* *Cocc.;* Euonym.; *Kali bich.;* *Nux v.;* *Petrol.;* Piloc.; *Pod.;* Puls.; Stront.; *Tab.;* Ther.
Nervous phenomena—Ambra; Cocc.; *Gels.; Ign.;* Phos.
Nosebleed—Bell.; Bry.; Carbo an.
Opisthotonos—Cic.
Palpitation, heart symptoms—Æth.; Bell.; *Cact.;* Dig.; Spig.
Pressure at root of nose—Bapt.
Relief from closing eyes—Aloe; Lol.
Relief from food—Alum.
Relief from holding head perfectly still—Con.
Relief from lying down—Apis; Antham.; Aur.; Bry.; Cinch.; *Cocc.;* Nit. ac.; Puls.
Relief from nosebleed—Brom.
Relief from rest—Arn.; Colch.; Cycl.; Spig.
Relief from vomiting—Tab.
Relief from walking in open air—Am. m.; Kali c.; Mag. p.; *Puls.; Rhus t.;* Tab.
Relief from warmth—Mang. m.; Sil.; Stront.
With balancing sensation—Ferr. m.
With staggering, trembling, weakness—*Arg. n.;* Crot.; *Gels.;* Nux v.; Phos. ac.; Stram.
With tendency to fall backward—*Absinth.;* Bell.; Bry.; Kali n.; Nux v.
With tendency to fall forward—Alum.; *Bry.;* Card. m.; Caust.; Chel.; Elaps.; Guarea; Mag. p.; Petrol.; *Pod.;* Spig.; Stram.; Urt.; Vib. op.
With tendency to fall to left—Aur.; Bell.; *Con.;* Dros.; Eup. perf.; Iod.; Sal. ac.; Sil.; Stram.; Zinc.
With tendency to fall to right—Helod.; Kali n.

EYES

BROWS—Hair falls out: *Alum.*; Bor.; Merc.; *Nit. ac.*; Plumb. ac.; Sanic.; Selen.; Sil.

Pimples on—Fluor. ac.; Sil.; Thuya.

Warty growths on—Ananth.

CANTHI (angles)—Itching, smarting: Alum.; Apium gr.; Ars.; Carbo v.; Fluor. ac.; *Gamb.*; Hep.; Lyc.; Nat. m.; Nux v.; Phos.; Succin. ac.; Sul.; Zinc. m.

Sore, raw, fissured—*Ant. c.*; Bor.; Graph.; Petrol.; *Sil.*; Staph.; Zinc. m.

Swollen, red—Agar.; Arg. n.; Cinnab; Graph.; Zinc. m.

CATARACT—Am. c.; Arg. iod.; Calc. c.; *Calc. fl.*; Can. s.; *Caust.*; Chimaph.; Ciner.; Cochlear; Colch.; Con.; Euphras.; Iod.; Kali m.; Led.; Mag. c.; Naph.; Nat. m.; *Phos.*; Platan.; Puls.; Quass.; Santon.; Sec.; Senega; Sep.; *Sil.*; *Sul.*; Tellur.; *Thiosin.*; Zinc.

CHAMBER, anterior, pus in—Hep.; Sil.

Chamber, hemorrhage after iridectomy—Led.

CHOROID—Congestion: Agar.; Phos.; Rhod.; Ruta; *Santon.*

Choroid, Detachment—Acon.; Arn.; Nux v.

Choroid, Extravasation—Ham.

Choroid, Inflammation (choroiditis), Atrophic—Nux v.; Phos.; Piloc.

Choroiditis, disseminated and simple—Ars.; *Bell.*; Bry.; Ced.; Gels.; Ipec.; *Kali iod.*; *Merc.*; Merc. i. r.; Naph.; Phos.; *Prun. sp.*; Santon.; Tab.; Tellur.; Thuya.

Choroiditis, suppurative—Hep.; Rhus t.

Choroiditis, suppurative, with iris involvement—Kali iod.; *Prun. s.*; Sil.

Choroiditis, suppurative, with retinal involvement (syphilitic)—Aur.; *Kali iod.*; Kali m.; Merc. c.; *Merc. i. r.*

CILIARY MUSCLE—Accommodation disturbed: Ipec.; Ruta.

Ciliary muscle, paretic condition—*Arg. n.*; Atrop.; Caust.; Dub.; Gels.; Paris; Physost.

Ciliary muscle, spasm—*Agar.*; Eser.; Ipec.; Jabor.; Lil. t.; *Physost.*; Piloc.

CILIARY NEURALGIA—Ars.; *Ced.*; Chel.; Chenop.; *Cim.*; Cinch.; Cinnab.; Col.; Commocl.; Croc.; Crot. t.; *Gels.*; Lach.; Mez.; Nat. m.; Paris; Phos.; Plant.; *Prun. sp.*; *Rhod.*; Sapon.; Spig. See Pain.

CONJUNCTIVA—Chemosis: *Apis*; Guarea; Hep.; Kali iod.; Rhus t.; Sul. ac.; *Vespa.*

Discharge, acrid—Ars.; Arum; *Euphras.*; Merc. c.; *Merc.*; Psor.; Rhus t.

Discharge, clear mucus—Ipec.; Kali m.

Discharge, creamy, profuse—*Arg. n.*; Calc. s.; Dulc.; Hep.; *Nat. p.*; Nat. s.; Picr. ac.; *Puls.*; Rhus t.; Syph.

Discharge, ropy—Kali bich.

Ecchymoses and injuries—Acon.; *Arn.*; *Ham.*; Lach.; Led.; Nux v.

Foreign bodies, irritation—*Acon.*; Sul.

Granulations, blisters or wart like—Thuya.

EYES

Hyperemia—*Acon.;* Ars.; *Bell.;* Cepa; Ipec.; *Nux v.;* Rhus t.; Sul.; *Thuya.*

Inflammation (conjunctivitis)—Acute and sub-acute catarrhal:—*Acon.;* Apis; *Arg. n.;* Ars.; *Bell.;* Canth.; *Chloral.;* Dub.; Dulc.; *Euphras.;* Ferr. p.; Guarea; *Hep.;* Kali m.; Merc. c.; Merc. per.; *Merc.;* Nat. ars.; Op.; Picr. ac.; *Puls.;* Rhus t.; Sep.; Sticta; Sul.; Upas.

Inflammation, chronic—*Alum.;* Ant. t.; Arg. n.; *Ars.;* Aur. mur.; Bell.; Euphras.; *Kali bich.;* Merc. s.; Picr. ac.; Psor.; *Puls.; Sul.;* Thuya; Zinc. m.

Inflammation, croupous, diphtheritic—Acet. ac.; Apis; Guarea; Iod.; *Kali bich.; Merc. cy.*

Inflammation, follicular (granular)—Apis; Arg. n.; *Ars.;* Aur. m.; *Aur. mur.;* Calc. iod.; Crot. t.; Jequir.; *Kali bich.;* Nat. m.: Phyt.; Puls.; *Thuya;* Zinc. s.

Inflammation, gonorrhoeal—*Acon.;* Ant. t.; Apis; *Arg. n.;* Calc. hypoph.; Hep.; Kali bich.; Merc. c.; *Merc.; Puls.;* Rhus t.; Ver. v.

Inflammation, gonorrhoeal, sympathetic form—*Arg. n.;* Euphras.; Merc.; Puls. See Purulent.

Inflammation, phlyctenular—Ant. t.; *Calc. c.; Calc. picr.;* Con.; Euphras.; Graph.; Ign.; Merc. c.; Puls.; *Rhus t.;* Sil.; Sul.

Inflammation, purulent—*Arg. n.;* Calc. hypoph.; Hep.; *Merc. c.;* Merc.; Puls.; *Rhus t.;* Sil.

Inflammation, pustular—*Ant. t.;* Arg. n.; Ars.; Calc. c.; Graph.; *Hep.;* Jequir.; Kali bich.; *Merc. c.;* Merc. nit.; Puls.; Rhus t.

Inflammation, traumatic—*Acon.;* Arn.; Bell.; *Calend.;* Canth.; Euphras.; Ham.; Led.; Symphyt.

ORNEA—Abscess of: Calc. s.; *Hep.;* Kali s.; Merc. c.; Sil.; Sul.

Ectasia—Calc. p.

Exudation, serous—Apis.

Foreign bodies—*Acon.;* Calc. hypoph.; Hep.; Rhus t.; Sul.

Inflammation, (keratitis)—Acon.; Apis; Ars.; Ars. iod.; *Aur. mur.;* Bell.; Can. s.; Con.; Euphras.; Hep.; Ilex; *Kali bich.;* Kali m.; Merc. c.; Nux v.; Phos.; Sang.; Sul.; Thuya.

Inflammation, arthritic—Clem.; Colch.; Col.

Inflammation, herpetic, vesicular—*Apis;* Ars.; Calc. p.; Euphras.; Ran. b.; Tellur.

Inflammation, interstitial, in persons of hereditary syphilis—Aur. m.; *Aur. mur.;* Can. s.; Merc. c.; Merc. cy.

Inflammation, parenchymatous, syphilitic origin—*Aur. mur.;* Calc. hypoph.; Kali iod.; Kali m.; Merc. s.; Sul.

Inflammation, phlyctenular—*Apis;* Bell.; Calc. c.; *Calc. fl.;* Calc. p.; Con.; *Graph.;* Hep.; Ipec.; *Merc. c.;* Puls.; Rhus t.; Syph.; Thuya.

Onyx—Hep.

Opacities—Arg. n.; Aur.; Aur. mur.; Bar. c.; Cadm. s.; Calc. c.; *Calc. fl.;* Calc. hypoph.; Calc. iod.; *Caust.; Can. s.;* Ciner.; Con.; *Euphras.;* Hep.; Kali bich.; Kali m.; Merc. c.; Merc. s.; *Naph.;* Nit .ac.; Phos.; Puls.; Sacchar. of.; Senega; *Sil.;* Sul.; Thiosinam.; Zinc. m.; Zinc. s.

EYES

Pustules—Ant. c.; Calc. c.; Con.; Crot. t.; Euphras.; *Hep.*; Kali bich.; Kali iod.; Merc. nit.; Nit. ac.

Staphyloma, after suppurative inflammation—*Apis*; Euphras.; Ilex; Physost.

Ulcers—Æthiops antim.; Apis; Arg. n.; Ars.; Aur. mur.; *Calc. c.*; Calc. hypoph.; Calc. iod.; Calc. sil.; *Euphras.*; Graph.; *Hep.*; *Kali bich.*; Kali m.; *Merc. c.*; Merc. i. fl.; Nat. m.; Nit. ac.; Rhus t.; *Sil.*; Sul.; Thuya; Zinc. m.

Ulcers, deep—Ars.; Euphras.; *Kali bich.*; *Merc. c.*: Merc. i. fl.; Merc. i. r.; Sil.

Ulcers, indolent—Calc. c.; *Kali bich.*; *Sil.*; Sul.

Ulcers, superficial, flat—Ars.; Asaf.; Euphras.; Kali m.; Merc.; Nit. ac.

Ulcers, vascular—Aur. m.

Wounds, incised, lacerated—Staph.

EYE-BALLS—**Bad effects from exposure to snow:** Acon.; Cic.

Bad effects from electric or artificial light—Glon.; Jabor.

Bad effects from glare of fire—Acon.; Canth.; Glon.; Merc.

Bad effects from operations—Acon.; Arn.; Asar.; Bry.; Croc.; Ign.; *Led.*; Rhus t.; Senega; Stront.; Thuya.

Bad effects from sight seeing, moving pictures—Arn.

Burning, smarting—*Acon.*; *Ars.*; Ars. m.; Aur. mur.; *Bell.*; Calc. c.; Canth.; *Cepa*; Croc.; *Euphras.*; Fagop.; Ferr. p.; Lept.; Lyc.; Mag. p.; *Merc. c.*; *Nat. ars.*; *Nat. m.*; Op.; Phyt.; Piloc.; Puls.; Ran. b.; Sang.; *Sul.*; *Thuya*; Zinc. m.

Coldness—Alum.; Asar.; Con.; Mez.; Nat. m.; Plat.

Coldness, as if wind blowing under lids—*Croc.*; Fluor. ac.; Syph.; Thuya.

Dryness, heat—*Acon.*; Alum.; Ars.; *Bell.*; Berb. v.; Clem.; Croc.; Grat.; Lyc.; *Merc. c.*; Nat. ars.; Nat. c.; Nat. m.; Nat. s.; Nux m.; Op.; Senega; Sep.; Sticta; *Sul.*; Zinc. m.

Edema of ocular conjunctiva, translucent—Apis.

Enlarged, swollen feeling—Acon.; *Bell.*; Ox. ac.; Paris; Phos. ac.; *Rhus t.*; Sarrac.; *Senega*; *Spig.*; Trill.

Eruptions about—Ant. t.; Crot. t.; Guaiac.

Heat, and flickering, worse in damp weather—Aran.

Heat, and sensitive to air—Clem.; Coral.

Heat—Æsc.; Carbo v.; Indol; Lil. t.; Meph.; Op.; Phos.; *Ruta*; Sapon.; Strych.; *Sul.*

Heaviness—Bapt.; *Gels.*; Meli.; *Onosm.*; Op.; Paris; Parth.; Sep.; Solan. lyc.; Sulphon.

Hemorrhage (inter-ocular)—Arn.; *Ham.*; Lach.; Led.; *Sul. ac.*: Supraren. ext.

Injuries—Acon.; *Arn.*; Calend.; Canth.; Cochlear.; Ham.; Led.; Physost.; *Rhus t.*; Sul. ac.; *Symphyt.*

Itching—Agar.; *Agn.*; Ant. c.; Ars. m.; *Aur. mur.*; Calc. c.; Caust.; Cepa; Croc.; *Fagop.*; Gamb.; *Merc.*; Nux v.; Puls.; *Rhus t.*; Scilla; *Sul.*; Zinc. m.

LOOK—CONDITION—Dull: Ant. c.; *Ant. t.*; Bapt.; Diph.; Merc.; Onosm.; Solan. lyc.

EYES

Fixed, staring, distorted—*Bell.*; Can. ind.; *Cic.*; Cupr m.; Glon.; *Helleb.*; Hyos.; *Morph.*; Œnanthe; Op.; Phos. ac.; Piscidia; *Stram.*; Strych.

Glazed, death-like—*Op.*; Phos. ac.; Zinc. m. See Face.

Glistening, dazzling, brilliant—*Bell.*; Bry.; *Canth.*; Cupr. m.; Hyos.; Merc. c.; *Stram.*; Ver. v.

Looking downwards—*Æth.*; *Hyos*.

Protruding, bulging (exophthalmus)—Amyl; *Bell.*; Clem.; Com. cl.; Ferr. p.; Glon.; Helod.; Lycop.; Paris; Sang. tart.; Sapon.; Spong.; Stellar.; *Stram.*; Strych.; *Thyr*.

Red, blood-shot, suffused—*Acon.*; Æsc.; Ail.; *Bell.*; Cepa; Cinnab.; Dulc.; Gels.; Ham.; Hyos.; Merc. c.; Morph.; Op.; Ruta; Sil.; Sulphon.; Sul.; *Thuya*; Ver. v.

Red, inflamed—*Aeon.*; Ant. c.; Arg. n.; Ars.; Aur. mur.; *Bell.*; Caust.; Clem.; *Euphras.*; Ferr. p.; Hep.; Indol; Ipec.; Jacor.; Lyc.; Merc. s.; Nat. m.; Rhus t.; Sang. n.

Red, raw—Arg. n.; Crot. t.

Red, with yellow vision—Aloe.

Rolling downwards—*Æth.*; Hyos.

Rolling in vertical axis—*Benz. nit.*; Zinc. m.

Rolling on falling asleep—Æth.

Rolling quickly with closed eyes—Cupr. m.

Rolling upwards—Bell.; *Cic.*; Helleb.; Mur. ac.; Œnanthe.

Sensation as if fat on eyes—Paraf.

Sensation as if sand or sticks in—*Acon.*; Alum.; Ars.; *Caust.*; Coccus c.; Euphras.; Ferr. p.; Graph.; *Nat. m.*; Phos.; Phyt.; *Sul*; Xeroph.

Sensation as if wind blowing in eyes—Fluor. ac.

Squinting to relieve pain in forehead—Aloe.

Stiffness—Asar.; Aur.; *Kal.*; Med.; Nat. ars.; Rhus t.

Sunken, surrounded by blue rings—Acet. ac.; Ant. c.; Apium gr.; *Ars.*; *Camph.*; Cinch.; Cupr. m.; Granat.; Helleb.; Ipec.; Nat. c.; *Phos ac.*; Phos.; Sec.; *Staph.*; Upas; *Ver. a.*; Visc. a. See Face.

Syphilitic diseases—Jacar. g.; Kali iod.; Merc. i. fl.; Nit. ac.; Thuya.

Trembling (nystagmus)—*Agar.*; Benz. nit.; Carbon. hydr.; *Cic.*; Gels.; Iod.; Kali iod.; Mag. p.; Physost.

Unable to keep eyes fixed steadily—Arg. n.; Paris.

Whites of, yellow—Brassica; Cham.; *Chel.*; *Cinch.*; Crot.; Dig.; Euonym. tarop.; Iod.; Lach.; Merc.; Myr.; Nat. p.; Nat. s.; *Pod.*; Plumb.; Sep. See Face.

EYELIDS AND MARGINS—**Agglutination:** Agar.; Alum.; *Ant. c.*; Apis; Arg. n.; Bor.; Calc. c.; Caust.; Dig.; *Euphras.*; *Graph.*; Kali bich.; Kali c.; Lyc.; *Merc. s.*; Nat. ars.; Nat. m.; Psor.; *Puls.*; Rhus t.; Sep.; *Sul.*; Thuya; Uran.; Zinc. m.

Blueness—Dig.; Morph.

Drooping (ptosis)—Alum.; Caul.; *Caust.*; *Con.*; Dulc.; *Gels.*; Graph.; Hæmat.; Helod.; Kal.; *Morph.*; Naja; Nat. ars.; Nit. ac.; Nux m.; Nux v.; Op.; Phos.; Plumb.; Rhus t.; *Sep.*; Spig.; Stram.; Sulphon.; Syph.; Upas; Ver. a.; *Zinc. m*.

EYES

Dryness—*Acon.;* Alum.; Ars.; *Bell.; Graph.;* Lith. c.; Nux v.; *Puls.;* Senega; Sep.; Sul.; Zinc. m.

Dryness, scaliness—*Ars.;* Bor.; Sep.; Tellur.; Thuya.

Ectropion—Apis; Graph.; Thiosinam.

Entropion—*Bor.;* Graph.; Nat. m.; Tellur.

ERUPTIONS, growths, blisters, vesicles—Canth.; *Nat. s.;* Pall.; *Rhus t.;* Sep.; *Thuya.*

Chalazae, tarsal tumors—Ant. t.; Calc. c.; Caust.; *Con.;* Ferr. pyropn.; *Kali iod.;* Platanus; Sil.; *Staph.; Thuya;* Zinc. m.

Cysts, sebaceous—*Benz. ac.;* Calc. c.; *Calc. fl.;* Iod.; *Kali iod.;* Merc. s.; Platanus; *Staph.*

Eczema, fissures—Bac.; Chrysarob.; *Graph.; Petrol.;* Staph.; Sul.; Tellur.

Granular lids (trachoma)—*Alum.;* Ars.; Aur. mur.; *Calc. c.;* Cinnab.; Dulc.; *Euphras.;* Graph.; Hep.; Jequir.; *Kali bich.;* Kali m.; Merc. per.; Nat. ars.; Nat. s.; Puls.; Sep.; Sul.; *Thuya;* Zinc. s.

Pustules—Ant. c.; Hep.

Scabs, crusts, scurfs—Arg. n.; *Ars.;* Bor.; Calc. c.; *Graph.;* Kali m.; Lyc.; Senega; Sep.

Styes (hordeolum)—Agar.; Apis; Aur. m. n.; *Calc. picr.;* Con.; *Graph.;* Hep.; Lyc.; Merc.; *Puls.; Sep.; Sil.; Staph.; Sul.;* Thuya; Uran.

Styes, followed by hard nodosities—Con.; Staph.; Thuya.

Ulcers—Arg. n.; *Ars.; Caust.;* Euphras.; *Graph.;* Hep.; Lappa; Lyc.; *Sul.; Tellur.* See Tissues.

Inflammation (blepharitis)—Acute: *Acon.;* Apis; Arg. n.; *Ars.;* Cham.; Dig.; Dulc.; *Euphras.;* Hep.; Kreos.; Merc. i. fl.; *Merc. pr. rub.; Merc. s.;* Nat. ars.; Petrol.; *Puls.;* Rhus t.; Sul.; Upas; Uran.

Inflammation, chronic—*Alum.;* Ant. c.; *Arg. n.;* Aur.; Bar. c.; *Bor.;* Calc. c.; Clem.; Euphras.; *Graph.;* Hep.; Jugl.; Merc. c.; Merc. pr. r.; Petrol.; Psor.; Sep.; *Sil.; Staph.; Sul.; Tellur.*

Inflammation, erysipelatous—*Apis;* Bell.; *Rhus t.;* Vespa.

Redness—Agar.; Am. br.; *Ant. c.;* Apis; Arg. n.; Ars.; *Bell.;* Cinnab.; Clem.; Dig.; Euphras.; Graph.; Hep.; Lyc.; *Merc. c.;* Merc. s.; Rhus t.; Sabad.; *Sul.* See Inflammation.

SENSATIONS—Burning and smarting:—Agar.; Alum.; Apis; *Ars.;* Arundo; Bell., Calc. c.; Cepa; Cham.; Croc.; *Euphras.;* Graph.; Kali bich.; Kali iod.; Lyc.; Merc.; Mez.; Nat. m.; Puls.; Sabad.; *Sul.*

Coldness—Croc.; Phos. ac.

Heaviness—Caul.; *Gels.;* Hæmat.; Helod.; Nat. m.; *Sep.* See Drooping.

Itching—Agar.; Alum.; *Ambros.;* Calc. c.; *Gamb.;* Graph.; Lyc.; Mez.; *Morph.; Puls.;* Rhus t.; Staph.; Succin. ac.; *Sul.;* Tellur.; Zinc.

Pulsation of superciliary muscle—Cina.

Rawness and soreness—*Ant. c.;* Arg. n.; Ars.; Bor.; Euphras.; *Graph.;* Hep.; Merc. c.; Petrol.; Sul.; Zinc. See Belpharitis.

Spasms of eyelids, twitching, (blepharospasm, nictitation)—*Agar.;* Ars.; Atrop.; *Bell.;* Calc. c.; Cham.; Cic.; *Cod.;* Croc.; Eser.; Gels.; Guaiac.; Hyos.; Ign.; Lob. purp.; Mag. p.; Nat. m.; Nicot.; *Nux v.;* Physost.; Puls.; Ruta; Strych.; Sul. ac.

Stiffness—Caust.; Gels.; Kal.; Rhus t.

Swelling (Œdema)—Am. br.; *Apis;* Arg. n.; *Ars.;* Ars. m.; Aur. mur.; Bell.; Calc. c.; Dig.; Euphorb. d.; *Euphras.;* Graph.; Hep.; *Kali c.;* Kali iod.; Merc. c.; Nat. ars.; Nat. c.; Phos.; Puls.; *Rhus t.;* Rhus v.; Sabad.; Sep.

Thickening—*Alum.;* Arg. n.; Calc. c.; *Graph.;* Hep.; Merc.; *Tellur.*

GLAUCOMA—*Acon.;* Atrop.; Aur.; *Bell.;* Bry.; Caust.; Ced.; Cocaine; Col.; Commod.; Croc.; Eser.; *Gels.;* Mag. c.; Nux v.; Op.; *Osm.; Phos.: Physost.;* Prun. sp.; *Spig.;* Supraren. ext.

HYPOPION—Crot. t.; *Hep.;* Merc. c.; Merc.; Plumb.; *Sil.*

IRIDO-CHOROIDITIS—Kali. iod.; Prun. sp.; *Sil.*

Irido-cyclitis, traumatic, with infection and sequelæ—Nat. salic.

IRIS—**Prolapse:** Ant. s. a.; Physost.

IRITIS—**Remedies in general:** *Acon.;* Ars.; Bell.; Ced.; *Cinnab.; Clem.;* Dub.; *Euphras.;* Ferr. p.; Gels.; Grind.; Hep.; Iod.; Kali bich.; Kali iod.; *Merc. c.;* Merc. s.; Puls.; *Rhus t.;* Spig.; Sul.; Syph.; Tellur.; Tereb.; Thuya.

Plastic—*Acon.;* Bry.; Cinnab.; Hep.; *Merc. c.;* Rhus t.; Thuya.

Rheumatic—Arn.; *Bry.;* Clem.; Colch.; *Euphras.;* Formica; Kali bich.; Kal.; Led.; Merc. c.; *Rhus t.;* Spig.; Tereb.; *Thuya.*

Serous—Apis; *Ars.;* Bry.; Ced.; *Gels.;* Merc. c.; Merc.; Spig.

Syphilitic—Asaf.; *Aur.; Cinnab.;* Clem.; Iod.; Kali bich.; *Kali iod.; Merc. c.;* Merc. cy.; Merc. i. fl.; *Nit. ac.;* Sul.; Thuya.

Traumatic—Acon.; *Arn.;* Bell.; *Ham.;* Led.; Rhus t.

Tuberculous—*Ars.;* Kali bich.; Sul.; Syph.; Tub.

LACHRYMAL SAC—**Blemorrhœa:** Ant. t.; Calc. c.; Calend.; *Hep.;* Merc. d.; Nat. m.; Petrol.; *Puls.;* Sil.; Stann.

Dacryo-cystitis—Apis; Fluor. ac.; *Hep.;* Iod.; Merc.; Petrol.; *Puls.; Sil.;* Stann.

Duct closed, from cold, exposure—Calc. c.

Duct, stricture—Nat. m.

Duct, swollen—Graph.; Sil.

Epiphora—Calc. c.; Graph.; Hep.; *Merc. per.;* Merc. s.; *Nat. m.;* Scilla; Sil.; Tongo. See Lachrymation.

Fistula lachrymalis—*Calc. c.;* Caust.; *Fluor. ac.;* Lach.; Merc. c.; Nat. m.; Nit. ac.; Petrol.; Phos.; Phyt.; *Sil.;* Stann.; Sul.

LACHRYMATION—Acon.; *Ambros.;* Antipyr.; Apis; *Ars.;* Ars. m.; Aur.; Calc. c.; Caust.; *Cepa;* Con.; Eugen. j.; *Euphras.;* Guarea; Ipec.; *Kali iod.;* Lyc.; *Merc. c.;* Merc. per.; Merc. s.; Nat. ars.; *Nat. m.;* Phos.; Phyt.; *Puls.;* Rhus t.; *Sabad.;* Sang. n.; Scilla; Sil.; Sticta; Succin.; Sul.; Taxus.

Acrid, burning, hot—Apis; *Ars.;* Ced.; Eugen. j.; *Euphras.;* Graph.; *Kali iod.;* Kreos.; *Merc. c.;* Naph.; *Nat. m.; Rhus t.;* Sul.

Bland—Cepa; *Puls.*

MODALITIES—**Relief in open air:** Cepa.

Worse at night—Apis.

Worse from cold application—Sanic.

Worse from coughing—Euphras.; Nat. m.

Worse from eating—Ol. an.

Worse from foreign bodies in eyes, cold wind, reflection from snow—Acon.

Worse in morning early—Calc. c.

Worse in open air—Calc. c.; Colch.; Lyc.; Phos.; Sanic.; Sil.

LAGOPHTHALMOS—Physost.

MEIBOMIAN GLANDS—Swollen: *Æth.;* Bad.; Clem.; Dig.; Graph.; Hep.; Puls.; Rhus t. See Blepharitis.

OCULAR MUSCLES—Contracted spasmodically: *Agar.;* Cic.; Physost.; Strych.

Ocular muscles, pain—Carbo v.; Cim.; *Onosm.* See Pain.

Ocular muscles, paralysis—Arg. n.; Bell.; *Caust.; Con.;* Euphras.; Gels.; Hyos.; Lach.; Oxytr.; Phos.; Physost.; *Rhus t.; Ruta;* Santon.; Senega; Syph.

Ocular muscles, paralysis, extrinsic—Gels.; Phos.

Ocular muscles, paralysis, intrinsic—Alum.; Con.; Lach.; Nat. m.; Onosm.; Ruta.

Ocular muscles, paralysis superior rectus—Senega.

Ocular muscles, paralysis, weak—*Gels.;* Lach.; Nat. m.; Physost.; *Ruta;* Tilia.

OCULAR TENSION—Decreased:—Apium v.; Ced.; Eser.; Nat. m.; Osm.; Prun. sp.; 'Ran. b.; Rhod.

Increased—See Glaucoma.

OPHTHALMIA—Catarrhal: *Acon.;* Am. m.; Apis; Ars.; Bell.; Cham.; Dulc.; *Euphras.;* Gels.; *Kali bich.;* Merc. c.; Merc.; Nux v.; *Puls.;* Sul.

Chronic—*Alum.;* Arg. n.; Ars.; Con.; Euphras.; *Graph.;* Kali bich.; Lyc.; *Psor.;* Sep.; *Sul.;* Zinc. m.

Follicular, granular—Aur. mur.; Euphras.; Jequir.; *Puls.*

Gonorrhoeal (neonatorum)—Acon.; *Arg. n.;* Bell.; Calc. s.; Can. s.; *Hep.;* Kali s.; *Merc. c.; Merc. pr. rub.; Merc.;* Nit. ac.; *Puls.;* Rhus t.; Syph.; Thuya.

Gonorrhoeal, constitutional—Acon.; *Clem.;* Nit. ac.; Puls.

Purulent—Apis; *Arg. n.;* Calend.; Grind.; *Hep.;* Merc. c.; Merc. pr. rub.; Nat. s.; Plumb.; Puls.; *Rhus t.*

Rheumatic—Acon.; Bell.; Bry.; Calc. c.; Caust.; Clem.; Colch.; Euphras.; Ilex; *Kali bich.;* Led.; Lith. c.; Lyc.; Merc. c.; Merc.; Nux v.; Phyt.; *Rhus t.;* Sil.; Spig.; Sul.

Scrofulous—*Æthiops; Æthiops antim.;* Æth.; Apis; Arg. n.; Ars.; Ars. iod.; Aur.; Aur. mur.; Bar. c.; Bar. iod.; Bell.; *Calc. c.; Calc. iod.;* Can. s.; Cist.; Clem.; *Cochlear.;* Colch.; Con.; *Euphras.; Graph.; Hep.;* Iod.; *Kali bich.;* Merc. c.; Merc. d.; Merc. nit.; Merc. pr. rub.; Nat. m.; *Nit. ac.;* Psor.; Puls.; Rhus t.; Scrophul.; Sil.; *Sul.;* Thuya; Viola tr.; Zinc. s.

Senile—Alum.

Sympathetic—*Bell.;* Bry.; Calend.; Merc.; *Rhus t.;* Sil. See Conjunctivitis.

EYES

Syphilitic—Apis; Asaf.; Gels.; Kali iod.; Merc. c.; Nit. ac.

OPTICAL—Hyperæsthesia:—Chrysar.

OPTIC DESKS—Hyperemic, retinal vessels enlarged:—Bell.; Onosm.

Optic disks, pallor, visual field contracted, retinal vessels shrunken—Acetan.

OPTIC NERVE—Atrophy: Agar.; Arg. n.; Atoxyl; Carbon. s.; Iodof.; Nux v.; *Phos.*; Santon.; *Strych. nit.*; Tab.

Inflammation (neuritis)—*Apis*; Ars.; Bell.; Carbon. s.; Kali iod.; *Merc. c.*; Nux v.; Picr. ac.; Plumb. m.; Puls.; Rhus t.; Santon.; Tab.; Thyr.

Neuritis, choked—Bell.; Bry.; Dub.; Gels.; Helleb.; Nux v.; Puls.; Ver. v.

Neuritis, descending—Ars.; Cupr. m.; Merc. c.

Paralysis—Nux v.; Oxytr.; Phos. ac.

ORBITS—Bony tumors: Kali iod.

Cellulitis—*Apis*; Hep.; Kali iod.; Phyt.; *Rhus t.*; Sil.

Injuries—Acon.; *Arn.*; Ham.; Symphyt.

Pain around—Apis; *Asaf.*; Aur. m.; Bell.; *Cinnab.*; Hep.; Hydrocot.; Ilex; Plat.; Plumb. m.; Spig.

Pain, deep|in—*Aloe;* Gels.; Merc. c.; Phos.: Phyt.; Plat.; Ruta; Sarrac.; *Spig.*; Stann.; Upas. See Pain.

Periostitis—Asaf.; *Aur.*; *Kali iod.*; Merc.; Sil.

PAIN: LOCATION—Ciliary body—Ars.; *Ced.*; Chenop.; Chrom. oxy.; *Cim.*; *Cinnab.*; *Commocl.*; Crot. t.; *Gels.*; Paris; Phos.; Plant.; *Prun. sp.*; Rhod.; *Spig.;* Thuya.

Eyeballs—*Acon.*; Alfal.; Am. br.; Asaf.; Aur.; Azar.; Bapt.; *Bell.*; *Bry.*; *Ced.*; Chel.; Chimap.; *Cim.*; Cinch.; *Clem.*; Cocc.; Col.; *Commocl.*; Con.; Crot. t.; Eser.; *Eup. perf.*; *Euphras.*; Gels.; Grind.; Guarea; Hep.; Indol.; Jabor.; Kali iod.; Kal.; *Lycop.*; Menthol; *Merc. c.*; Nat. m.; Niccol. s.; Nit. ac.; Oleand.; Onosm.; Osm.; Paris; Passif.; Phos.; Phos. ac.; Physost.; Plat.; *Prun. sp.*; *Puls.*; Rhod.; Rhus t.; *Ruta;* Sang.; *Spig.*; Staph,; Symphyt.; Syph.; Tereb.; Ther.; Thuya; Upas; Viola od.

Orbits—*Aloe;* Am. picr.; *Asaf.;* Aur. m.; Chel.; Cim.; Cinnab.; Crot. t.; Gels.; Ilex; *Kali iod.;* Menthol; *Phos.*; Ruta; *Spig.*; Ther.; *Upas.*

Supra-orbital—Asaf.; *Bry.*; Carb. ac.; *Ced.*; *Chin. s.*; Dub.; Gels.; *Kali bich.*; Mag. p.; Meli.; Menthol; Merc. c.; Plat.; Ruta; *Spig.*; Thuya.

TYPE—Aching, sore: Æsc.; Alfal.; Aloe; Arn.; Arg. n.; Bapt.; *Bry.*; Cim.; *Eup. perf.*; Euphras.; Eser.; Gels.; *Ham.*; Led.; Lept.; Menthol; *Nat. m.*; Niccol. s.; Nit. ac.; Onosm.; Radium; Rhus t.; *Ruta*; Sep.; Spig.

Boring—Asaf.; *Aur.*; Col.; Crot. t.; Hep.; Merc. c.

Bruised—*Arn.*; Aur. mur.; Cim.; Cupr. m.; *Gels.*; Hep.; Nat. m.

Burning, smarting—*Acon.*; Am. gummi; *Ars.*; Asaf.; Carbo v.; Cepa; Clem.; Euphras.; Ilex aq.; Indol; Iod.; Jabor.; Lyc.; Merc. c.; *Nat. m.*; *Phos.*; Ran. b.; *Ruta*; Sil.

Enlarged feeling, bursting—Am. br.; Bry.; Cim.; Commocl.; Paris; *Prun. sp.*; Spig.

Neuralgic—*Ars.*; Asaf.; Bell.; Ced.; Chin. s.; Cim.; Cinch.; Cinnab.;

Col.; Commocl.; Crot. t.; *Gels.*, Kali iod.; Kal.; Mag. p.; Meli.; Mez.; Osm.; Phos.; Physost.; *Prun. sp.;* Rhod.; *Spig.*

Periodically, intermittent—Ars.; Asaf.; *Ced.;* Chin. s.; Cinch.; *Spig.*

Piercing, penetrating—Apis; Aur.; Millef.; Rhus t.

Pressing inwards, as if retracted—Aur. mur.; Crot. *t.;* Hep.; Oleand.; *Paris; Phos. ac.*

Pressing outwards—Asar.; *Bry.;* Cim.; *Cocc.;* Col.; Commocl.; Guarea; *Lycop.;* Merc. c.; Passif.; *Spig.;* Ther.

Pressive, crushing—*Acon.;* Asaf.; Aur. mur.; Cinch.; Clem.; Crot. t.; Cupr.; Euphras.; Hep.; Menthol; Nit. ac.; Oleand.; *Paris; Phos. ac.;* Phos.; *Prun. sp.;* Ran. b.; Rhus t.; *Ruta;* Sang.; Sep.; *Spig.*

Sensitive to touch—*Acon.;* Arn.; Ars.; Aur.; *Bell.;* Bry.; Cim.; Clem.; Eup. perf.; *Ham.;* Hep.; Lept.; Rhus t.; Sil.; *Spig.;* Thuya. See Aching.

Shooting, stitching, darting, cutting—Acon.; Asaf.; *Bry.;* Calc. c.; Chimap.; *Cim.; Cinnab.;* Clem.; *Col.;* Euphras.; Graph.; Helleb.; Hep.; *Kali c.;* Kal.; Mag. p.; Merc. c.; *Nit. ac.;* Physost.; Prun. sp.; Rhod.; Rhus t.; Sil.; *Spig.*

Splinter-like—Apis; Aur.; *Hep.;* Med.; Merc.; *Nit. ac.;* Sul.; Thuya.

Stinging—*Apis;* Euphras.; Hep.; Kali c.; Puls.; Thuya.

Strained, stiff feeling—*Guaiac.;* Jabor.; *Kal.;* Med.; *Nat. m.;* Onosm.; Rhus t.; *Ruta.*

Tearing—Ars.; Asaf.; *Aur. mur.;* Bell.; Chel.; Colch.; Crot. t.; Guarea; Merc. c.; *Puls.;* Sil.

Throbbing—Asaf.; *Bell.;* Bry.; Cim.; *Hep.;* Merc.; Ther.

MODALITIES—**Aggravation: At night:** Ars.; Asaf.; Cinnab.; Con.; Euphras.; Hep.; *Kali iod.;* Lyc.; Merc. c.; *Merc. s.;* Puls.; Rhus t.; Sep.; Spig.; *Syph.;* Thuya.

Before a storm—Rhod.

From closing eyes—Sil.

From cold air—*Asar.; Clem.;* Hep.; Mag. p.

From damp, cold, rainy weather—Merc. c.; *Rhus t.;* Spig.

From glare of light—Asar.; Con.; Merc.

From looking down—Nat. m.

From looking up—Chel.

From lying down—Bell.

From motion—Ars.; *Bry.;* Cim.; Crot. t.; Grind.; Indol; Kal.; Rhus t.; *Spig.*

From motion, or use of eyes—*Arg. n.;* Arn.; *Bry.;* Cim.; Euphras.; Kal.; *Nat. m.;* Onosm.; Physost.; Puls.; Rhus t.; *Ruta;* Spig.

From sunlight—Asar.; Merc.

From sunrise to sunset—Kal.; Nat. m.

From touch—*Bry.; Hep.;* Phos.; Plant.

From warmth—Arg. n.; *Commocl.;* Puls.; Sul.; Thuya.

Worse on left side—Menthol; Onosm.; *Spig.;* Ther.

Worse on right side—*Bell.;* Ced.; *Chel.;* Commocl.; Kal.; *Mag. p.;* Prun. sp.; Ran. b.; Ruta.

EYES

AMELIORATION—Cold air, applications: Arg. n.; *Asar.;* Puls.
  Darkness—Con.; Lil. t.
  Lying down on back—Puls.
  Motion—Kali iod.
  Pressure—Arg. n.; Asaf.; Chel.; *Chin. s.; Col.;* Con.; Lil. t.
  Rest—Asaf.; Bry.; Cim.
  Touch, pressure—Asaf.; Chel.
  Warmth—Ars.; *Hep.;* Mag. p.; *Thuya.*

PANNUS—Apis; *Aur. mur.;* Chin. mur.; *Hep.;* Kali bich.; Merc. i. r., Nit. ac. See Cornea.

PAN-OPHTHALMITIS—Hep.; Rhus t.

PERCEPTIVE POWER lost—Kali p.

PHOTOPHOBIA—*Acon.;* Agn.; Ail.; Ant. t.; Apis; *Arg. n.*, *Ars.;* Ars. m.; Asar.; Aur. mur.; *Bell.;* Benzol; Calc. c.; Calc. p.; Cepa; Cim.; Clem.; *Con.;* Croc.; Elaps; *Euphras.; Graph.;* Hep.; *Ign.;* Kali c.; Lil. t.; Lyc.; *Merc. c.; Merc. s.;* Nat. s.; Nux m.; *Nux v.;* Op.; Phos. ac.; Phos.; Psor.; *Puls.; Rhus t.;* Scrophul.; Sil.; Spig.; *Sul.;* Ther.; Zinc.

PTERYGIUM—Am. br.; Apis; Calc. c.; *Can. s.;* Guarea; Lach.; *Ratanh.;* Spig.; *Sul.;* Tellur.; *Zinc. m.*

PUPILS—Contracted (myosis): Acon.; Cina; *Eser.;* Gels.; Helleb.; Ign.; Iodof.; Lonic.; Merc. c.; *Morph.; Op.;* Oxytr.; Phos.; *Physost.;* Piloc.; Solan. n.
  Dilated (mydriasis)—Acetan.; Agar.; *Agn.;* Ail.; Atrop.; *Bell.;* Calc. c.; Camph.; *Cic.;*. Cocaine; Dig.; *Dub.;* Gels.; Glon.; Helleb.; *Hyos.; Iodof.;* Nit. ac.; Nux m.; Œnanthe; Sec.; *Stram.;* Ver. v.; Zinc. m.
  Insensible, poor reaction—Bell.; Benzol; Camph.; *Cic.; Gels.;* Helleb.; Hydroc. ac.; Hyos.; Laur.; Nit. ac.; *Op.;* Phos.; Piloc.; Stram.; *Zinc.*

RETINA—Anemia: Lith. c.
  Apoplexy (hæmorrhage from, traumatism, cough, etc.)—Acon.; *Arn.;* Bell.; Bothrops; Croc.; *Crot.;* Ham.; Lach.; *Led.;* Nat. sal.; Phos.; Symphyt.
  Artery, spasm—Nux v.
  Congestion—Acon.; *Aur.; Bell.;* Carbon. s.; *Dub.;* Ferr. p.; Gels.; Phos.; Puls.; Santon.
  Congestion, from cardiac disease—Cact.
  Congestion, from light, artificial, brilliant—Glon.
  Congestion, from menstrual suppression—Bell.; Puls.
  Congestion, from overuse of eyes—*Ruta;* Santon.
  Detachment—*Aur. mur.;* Dig.; *Gels.;* Naph.; Piloc.
  Edema—*Apis;* Bell.; Canth.; *Kali iod.;* Phos.
  Hyperæsthesia (optical)—*Bell.;* Cim.; Con.; Lil. t.; Macrot.; *Nux v.;* Ox. ac.; Phos.; Strych.
  Inflammation (retinitis), albuminuric and chronic—Crot.; Gels.; Kal.; Merc. c.; Nat. sal.; Phos.; *Plumb. m.;* Sal. ac.
  Inflammation, apoplectic—Glon.; Lach.
  Inflammation, leukemic—Nat. s ; *Thuya.*

EYES

Inflammation, pigmentary—Nux v.; Phos.

Inflammation, proliferating—Kali iod.; Thuya.

Inflammation, punctata albescens—Bell.; Kali iod.; Merc. c.; Merc. i. r.; Naph.; Sul.

Inflammation, simple and serous—*Aur.;* Bell.; *Benz. dinit.;* Bry.; *Dub.;* Gels.; *Merc.;* Picr. ac.; Puls.; Santon.

Inflammation, syphilitic—Iod.; *Kali iod.*

Injuries—Acon.; *Arn.;* Bell.; *Ham ;* Lach.; Led.; Phos.

Thrombosis and degeneration—Ham.; Phos.

SCLEROTICA—Degeneration: Aur.; Bar. mur.; Plumb.

Ecchymosis—*Arn.;* Bell.; Cham.; Ham.; Lach.; *Led.;* Nux v.; Senega.

Inflammation, deep (scleritis)—*Acon.; Ars.;* Aur. mur.; Eryng. aq.; Hep.; Kal.; *Merc. c.;* Sep.; *Spig.;* Thuya.

Inflammation, superficial (episcleritis)—*Acon.;* Bell.; Bry.; Kali iod.; Merc. c.; Rhus t.; Tereb.; *Thuya.*

STRABISMUS (squinting)—Alumen; Alum.; Apis; Apoc.; *Bell.;* Benz. dinit.; Calc. p.; *Cic.;* Cina; Cupr. ac.; Cycl.; *Gels.; Hyos.;* Nux v.; *Santon.;* Sec.; Spig.; *Stram.;* Tab.; Zinc.

Convergent—Cycl.; Jabor.

Dependent on convulsions—Bell.; *Cic.;* Hyos.

Dependent on injuries—Cic.

Dependent on worms—Bell.; *Cina;* Cycl.; Hyos.; Merc.; *Santon.;* Spig.

Divergent—Morph.; Nat. sal.

VISION—AMAUROSIS (blindness): Acon.; Apis; *Aur. m.;* Bell.; Calc. c.; Caust.; Chin. s.; Cinch.; *Con.;* Cycl.; Dulc.; *Gels.;* Hep.; Hyos.; Mancin.; *Merc.;* Mormord.; Naph.; Nat. m.; Nux m.; Nux v.; *Phos.; Plumb. ac.;* Plumb. m.; Santon.; Sep.; Sil.; Stram.; Strych.; Tab.; Vanad.; Zinc. m.

Colors—*Benz. dinit.;* Carbon. s.; Physost.; *Santon.*

Day—Acon.; *Bothrops;* Castor.; Lyc.; Phos.; Ran. b.; Sil.

Hysterical—Phos.; Plat.; Sep.

Night—*Bell.;* Cadm. s.; Cinch.; Helleb.; Hep.; Hyos.; Lyc.; *Nux v.;* Physost.; Puls.; Strych.

Retro-bulbar neuritis—Iodof.

Tobacco—*Nux v.;* Phos.; Piloc.; Plumb. ac.

AMBLYOPIA—(blurred, weak vision): Acon.; *Agar.; Anac.;* Arn.; *Aur.;* Bapt.; *Benz. dinit.; Caust.;* Cinch.; *Con.;* Colch.; *Cycl.;* Dig.; Elaps; Eser.; Euphras.; *Gels.;* Hep.; *Jabor.; Kali c.;* Kali p.; Lil. t.; *Lith. chlor.;* Lyc.; Mag. p.; Naph.; *Nat. m.;* Nux m.; Nux v.; *Onosm.;* Ox. ac.; Osm.; Phos. ac.; *Phos.;* Physost.; Piloc.; *Puls.;* Ran. b.; Rhus t.; *Ruta; Santon.;* Senega; Sep.; Sil.; Stront.; *Tab.;* Thuya; Titan.; Zinc. m.

Objects appear as looking through mist or veil—Agar.; Calc. c.; *Caust.;* Cina; *Croc.;* Cycl.; *Gels.;* Kali c.; Lil. t.; *Mormord.; Nat. m.; Phos.;* Physost.; Plumb.; *Puls.; Ruta; Sep.; Tab.*

Objects appear elongated—Bell.

Objects appear inverted—Bell.; Guarea.

EYES

Objects appear too large—Bov.; Hep.; *Hyos.*; Niccol.; Nux m.; *Ox. ac.*
Objects appear too small—Benz. dinit.; Glon.; Nicot.; *Plat.*; Stram.
Retinal images persist—Jabor.
When reading, eyes easily fatigued—Ammon.; Calc. c.; Cina; *Jabor.*; Nat. ars.; Nat. m.; Phos.; *Ruta*; Sep.; Sul.
When reading, eyes feel pressed asunder or outward, relieved by cold bathing—Asar.
When reading, letters appear red—Phos.
When reading, letters disappear—Cic.; Cocc.
When reading, letters run together—*Agar.*; Bell.; *Calc. c.*; Can. ind.; Cina; Cinch.; Con.; Elaps; Ferr.; Hyos.; Lyc.; *Nat. m.*; Sil.

ASTHENOPIA—(eye-strain, with spasm of accommodation): *Agar.*; Alum.; Am. c.; Am. gutti; Apis; Arg. n.; Arn.; Artem.; Bell.; Carbon. s. *Caust.*; *Cim.*; Cina; Croc.; *Gels.*; Ign.; *Jabor.*; Kali c.; Kal.; *Lac. f.*; *Macrot.*; *Nat. m.*; Niccol. sul.; Nicot.; Nux v.; Onosm.; Paris; *Phos.*; *Physost.*; Rhod.; *Ruta*; Santon.; Senega; Sep.; Stront.
External recti—Cupr. ac.; Gels.
Internal recti—Jabor.; Muscar.; Nat. m.; Physost.; Piloc.
Myopic—Eser.; Lil. t.

ASTIGMATISM—Gels.; *Lil. t.*; Physost.

DIPLOPIA—(double vision): Agar.; Aur.; *Bell.*; Cic.; Con.; *Cycl.*; Dig. *Gels.*; Gins.; *Hyos.*; Nat. m.; *Nit. ac.*; Oleand.; Onosm.; Phos.; Physost.; Plumb.; Sec.; Stram.; Sulphon.; Sul.; Syph.; Ver. v.

HEMIOPIA—Calc. s.; Glon.; Hep.; *Lith. c.*; Lyc.; Mur. ac.; Nat. m.; Titan.; Ver. v.
Left-half—Calc. c.; Lith. c.; Lyc.
Lower-half—Aur.; Digit.
Vertical—Ferr. p.; *Lith. c.*; Morph.; Mur. ac.; *Titan*.

HYPERMETROPIA—Calc. c.; Con.; *Jabor.*; Nat. m.; Petrol.; Ruta; Sep.; Sil.

MYOPIA—Acon.; *Agar.*; Aur. mur.; Bell.; Carbon. s.; Euphras.; Gels.; Lil. t.; Nit. ac.; Phos.; *Physost.*; *Piloc.*; Ruta; Viola od.

OPTICAL ILLUSIONS—(chromopsia, photopsia): Black before eyes: Agar.; *Atrop.*; Bell.; *Carbo v.*; *Carbon. s.*; Cinch.; Cycl.; Dig.; Lach.; Lyc.; Mag. c.; Mag. p.; Merc.; Nat. m.; Phos.; Physost.; Sep.; Stront.; *Tab.*; Zinc.
Blue before eyes—Crot.; Trill. cer.; Trill. p.
Confusion of colors—*Bell.*; Calc. c.; Croc.; Merc.; Puls.; Ruta; Staph.; Stram.
Flashes, flames, flickering—Agar.; Aloe; *Bell.*; Calc. fl.; Caust.; Clem.; *Cycl.*; Glon.; Hep.; Ign.; *Iris*; Lyc.; Phos.; Physost.; Puls.; Senega; Viola od.
Gray—Arg. n.; Conv.; Guarea.
Green—Dig.; Osm.; Phos.
Halo around light—Bell.; Chloral; Hyos.; Sul.
Objects appear white—Chloral.

Objects, brilliant, fantastic, colored, fiery—*Anhal.;* Aur.; Bell.; Cinch.; Cycl.; Nat. m.; Sep.

Red before the eyes—Antipyr.; Apis; Bell.; Dub.; Elaps; Hep.; Phos.; Stront.

Sparks, stars—Aur.; Bell.; Calc. fl.; Caust.; Croc.; Cycl.; Glon.; Lyc.; Naph.; Sil.; Strych.

Spots (muscæ volitantes)—*Agar.;* Anac.; *Atrop.;* Aur.; Carbo v.; Caust.; Cinch.; Colch.; Con.; Cycl.; Cyprip.; Kali c.; Mell.; Merc.; Nit. ac.; Nux v.; Phos.; Physost.; Sep.; Sil.; Sul.; Tab.

Yellow before eyes—*Aloe;* Canth.; Cina; Digitox; *Santon.*

VITREOUS OPACITIES—diffused: Ham.; Hep.; Kali iod.; Merc. c.; Merc i. r.; Thuya.

Turbid—Cholest.; *Kali iod.;* Phos.; Prun. sp.; *Senega;* Solan. n. **Sul.**

EARS

AUDITORY NERVE—Torpor: *Chenop.*

AURICLE—(external ear): Burning, as if frost-bitten—Agar.; Caust.; Sang.

ERUPTIONS—Remedies in general: Ant. c.; Bar. c.; *Calc. c.*; Calc. s.; Graph.; Lyc.; *Mez.*; Petrol.; Rhus t.; Tellur.

Acne—Calc. s.

Eczema around—*Ars.*; Arundo; Bov.; Chrysarob.; *Clem.*; Crot. t.; *Graph.*; Hep.; Kali m.; *Mez.*; Oleand.; Petrol.; Psor.; *Rhus t.*; Sanic.; Scrophul.; Tellur.

Erysipelas—*Apis;* Bell.; Rhus t.; Rhus v.

Fissures—Calc. c.; Graph.

Frost-bites—Agar.; *Apis;* Bell.; Rhus t.

Intertrigo—Petrol.

Herpes—Cistus; Graph.; Psor.; Rhus t.; *Sep.;* Tellur.

Moist, oozing—Ant. c.; Calc. c.; *Graph.;* Hep.; *Mez.;* Petrol.; *Psor.;* Sanic.

Pustules—Ars.; *Hep.;* Psor.

Scabs, scurfs—Chrysar.; Hep.; *Psor.*

Glands, swollen, painful, around—Bar. c.; Bell.; *Calc. c.;* Caps.; Graph.; Iod.; *Merc.*

Itching—*Agar.;* Ars.; Hep.; Nat. p.; *Sul. iod.;* Tub.

Lobe, eruption on—Bar. c.

Lobe, ulceration of ring hole—Stann.

Numbness—Mag. c.; Plat.; Verbasc.

Pain, tearing, with tophi—Berv. v.

Red, raw, sore—Graph.; Petrol.; Sul.

Red, swollen—*Acon.;* Agar.; Anac.; Apis; Bell.; Cinch.; Graph.; Hep.; Kali bich.; Medusa; Merc.; Puls.; *Rhus t.;* Scrophul.; Sul.

Sensitive to touch—Arn.; *Bell.;* Bry.; Caps.; Cinch.; Ferr. p.; *Hep.;* Psor.; Sanic.; Sep.

CERUMEN—Carbo v.; Caust.; Con.; Elaps; Graph.; Lach.; Puls.; Sep.; Spong.

DEAFNESS—HARDNESS OF HEARING—Remedies in general: Agar.; Agraph.; Ambra; Am. c.; Arn.; Ars. iod.; Bar. c.; Bar. mur.; Bell.; Calc. c.; Calc. fl.; Calend.; Carbo an.; Carbon. s.; *Caust.;* Cheiranth.; *Chenop.;* Chin. s.; *Cinch.;* Con.; Dig.; Dulc.; Elaps; Ferr. p.; Ferr. picr.; *Graph.;* Hep.; Hydr.; Hydrobr. ac.; Iod.; Kali ars.; Kali c.; *Kali m.;* Lob. infl.; *Lyc.;* Mang. ac.; *Merc. d.;* Merc. s.; *Mez.;* Nat. c.; *Nat. sal.;* Nit. ac.; *Petrol.;* Phos. ac.; *Phos.;* Psor.; Puls.; Rham. c.; Sal. ac.; Sang. n.; Sep.; *Sil.;* Tellur.; Thiosin.; *Verbasc.;* Viola od.

CAUSE—Abuse of Mercury: Hep.; Nit. ac.

Adenoids and hypertrophied tonsils—*Agraph.;* Aur.; Bar. c.; Calc. p.; Merc.; Nit. ac.; Staph.

Alternate with sensibility of ear—Sil.

Apoplexy—Arn.; Bell.; Caust.; Hyos.; Rhus t.

Bone conduction, deficient, or absent—Chenop.

Catarrh (eustachian, middle ear)—Ars. iod.; Asar.; *Calcareas;* Caust.; Gels.; Graph.; *Hep.;* Hydr.; *Iod.;* Kali bich.; *Kali m.;* Kali s.; Mang. ac.; Menthol; *Merc. d.;* Merc. s.; Petrol.; *Puls* ; Rosa d.; Sang.; Sep.; Sil.; Thiosin.

Cerebral—Chenop.; Mur. ac.

Cold exposure—Acon.; Kali m.; Visc. a.

Concussion—Arn.; Chin. s.

Damp weather—Mang. ac.

Discharge suppressed or eczema—Lob. infl.

Eruption of scalp, suppressed—Mez.

Human voice, difficult to hear—Calc. c.; *Chenop.;* Ign.; Phos.; Sil.; Sul.

Infectious diseases—Arn.; *Bapt.; Gels.;* Hep.; Lyc.; Petrol.; Phos.; Puls.

Nervous exhaustion, and nervous origin—*Ambra;* Anac.; Aur.; *Bell.;* Caust.; Chin. s.; Cinch.; *Gels.; Ign.; Lach.;* Phos. ac.; Phos.; Plat.; Tab.; *Val.*

Nutritional disturbance, in growing children—Calc. c.; Merc. i. r.

Old age—Kali m.; Merc. d.; Phos.

Rheumatico-gouty diathesis—*Ferr. picr.;* Ham.; Kali iod.; Led.; Sil.; Sul.; Visc. a.

Sclerotic condition of conducting media—Ferr. picr.; Thiosin.

Scrofulous diathesis—*Æthiops;* Calc. c.; Merc.; Mez.; Sil.; *Sul.*

Sounds, low toned—Chenop.

Syphilis—Kreos.

Work'ng in water—Calc. c.

Aggravated before menses—Ferr. picr.; Kreos.

Ameliorated from noise, riding in cars—Calend.; *Graph.;* Nit. ac.

EUSTACHIAN TUBES—(catarrh or closure): Alfal.; Alum.; Bar. m.; *Calcareas;* Caps.; *Caust.;* Ferr. iod.; Ferr. p.; Gels.; *Graph.;* Hep.; Hydr.; *Iod.;* Kali bich.; Kali chlor.; *Kali m.;* Lach.; Lob., cer.; Menthol; *Merc. d.;* Merc.; Nit. ac.; Penthor.; Petrol.; Phyt.; *Puls.;* Rosa d.; Sang. n.; *Sil.;* Visc. a.

Eustachian tube inflamed, sub-acute, great pain—Bell.; Caps.

Eustachian tube, tickling inducing swallowing, cough—Gels.; Nux v.; Sil.

EXTERNAL AUDITORY CANAL—Boils, pimples: Bell.; *Calc. picr.;* Hep.; *Merc. s.; Picr. ac.; Sil.;* Sul.

Burning—Ars.; Arundo; *Caps.;* Sang.; Stsych.

Digging and scratching Into—Cina; Psor.

Dryness—Calc. picr.; Carbo v.; Ferr. picr.; *Graph.;* Nux v.; Petrol.; Verbasc.

Exostoses—Calc. fl.; *Hekla;* Kali iod.

Feels, as if distended by air—Mez.; Puls.

Fissures—*Graph.;* Petrol.

Inflammation and pain—*Acon.;* Apis; Ars. iod.; *Bell.;* Bor.; Brachygl.; *Cal. picr.; Cham.; Ferr. p.;* Hep.; Kali bich.; *Kali m.; Merc. s.;* Nit. ac.; Psor.; *Puls.;* Rhus t.; *Tellur.*

EARS

Itching—*Alum.;* Anac.; Calc. c.; Caust.; Elaps; Hep.; Kali bich.; Kali c.; Psor.; *Puls.;* Sabad.; *Sep.;* Sil.; *Sul.; Tellur.;* Viola od.

Polypoid excrescenses, granulations—Alum.; Calc. c.; *Calc. iod.;* Calc. p.; Formica; Kali bich.; Kali iod.; *Kali m.;* Merc. s.; *Nit. ac.;* Phos.; *Sang.;* Sil.; Staph.; Teucr.; *Thuya.*

Scales, epithelial, exfoliated, with scurfy accumulation—Calc. picr.

Sensation, as if drop of water in left ear—Acon.

Sensation, as if heat emanated from—*Æth.;* Caust.

Sensation, as if obstructed—Æth.; *Anac.;* Asar.; Carbon. s.; *Cham.;* Crot.; Glon.; Merc.; Nit. ac.; *Puls.; Verbasc.*

Sensation, as if open too much—Mez.

Sensitive to air, touch—Ars.; Bell.; *Bor.;* Caps.; *Cham.;* Ferr. p.; *Hep.;* Merc.; Mez.; Nux v.; Petrol.; Tellur.

HYPERSENSITIVE—to noises, sounds, voices:—Acon.; Anhal.; *Asar.;* Aur.; *Bell.; Bor.;* Chenop.; Cim.; *Cinch.; Coff.;* Ferr. p.; Ign.; Iod.; Lach.; *Mag. m.; Nat. c.;* Nit. ac.; Nux m.; *Nux v.;* Op.; Petrol.; Phos. ac.; Phos.; Plant.; Puls.; Sang.; Sep.; *Sil.;* Spig.; Tereb.; *Ther.*

LABYRINTH—Bloody, serous effusion, in: Chenop.

Inflamed (otitis interna)—Aur.; Kali iod.; Merc. i. r.

MASTOID PROCESS—Caries: *Aur.;* Caps.; Fluor. ac.; *Nit. ac.;* Sil.

Inflammation (mastoiditis)—*Am. picr.;* Asaf.; *Aur.; Bell.;* Benz. ac.; Canth.; *Caps.;* Hep.; Kali m.; Mag. p.; Menthol; *Onosm.;* Oniscus.; Tellur.

MEMBRANA TYMPANI—Calcareous deposits: Calc. fl.

Inflammation (myringitis)—*Acon.;* Atrop.; Bell.; Bry.; Cinch.; *Hep.* See Otitis.

Perforated—Aur.; Calc. c.; Caps.; Kali bich.; Merc.; *Sil.;* Tellur.; *Tub.*

Thickened—Ars. iod.; Merc. d.; Thiosin.

Thin, white, scaly deposit—Graph.

Ulceration—Kali bich.

OSSICLES—Caries:—Asaf.; *Aur.;* Calc. c.; Caps.; Fluor. ac.; Hep.; Iod.; *Sil.;* Syph.

Petrous bone, tender to touch—*Caps.;* Onosm.

Sclerosis, also petrous portion of temporal bone—Calc. fl.

TYMPANUM (middle ear): Inflammation (otitis):

Catarrhal, acute—*Acon.; Bell.;* Cham.; *Ferr. p.;* Gels.; Hep.; *Kali m.; Merc.;* Puls., Rhus t.; Sil.

Catarrhal, chronic—Agar.; Ars.; *Bar. m.; Calc. c.; Caust.;* Cinch.; Graph.; *Hydr.; Iod.;* Jabor.; Kali bich.; Kali iod.; *Kali m.;* Merc. d.; Nit. ac.; Phos.; Sang.; Teucr. See Eustachian Tubes.

Suppurative, acute (otitis media suppurative, acute)—*Acon.;* Ars.; Ars. iod.; *Bell.;* Bor.; Bov.; Calc. s.; *Caps.; Cham.; Ferr. p.;* Gels.; Guaiac.; *Hep.;* Kali bich.; Kali m.; Merc. s.; *Merc. v.;* Myrist.; *Plant.;* Puls.; Sil.; Thiosin.

Suppurative, chronic—*Æthiops;* Alum.; *Ars. iod.;* Aur.; Bar. m.; *Calc. c.;* Calc. fl.; *Calc. iod.;* Caps.; *Caust.;* Chenop.; Elaps; *Hep.;* Hydr.; Iod.; *Kali bich.;* Kali iod.; Kali m.; Kali p.; *Kali s.;* Kinc; Lapis alb.;

Lyc.; Merc. s.; *Merc. v.*; Naja; Nit. ac.; Psor.; *Puls.*; *Sil.*; *Sul.*; Tellur.; *Thuya*; Viola od.

TYPE OF DISCHARGE—(otorrhœa): **Bloody**—Ars.; Ferr. p.; Hep.; Kali iod.; Merc. s.; *Merc.*; Psor.; Rhus t.; Shook. ch.

Excoriating, thin—*Alum.*; Ars.; Ars. iod.; Calc. iod.; Calc. p.; Cistus; *Iod.*; Merc.; Syph.; *Tellur.*

Muco-purulent, fetid, acrid or bland—Æthiops; Ars. iod.; Asaf.; Aur.; Bor.; *Calc. c.*; *Calc. s.*; Caps.; *Carbo v.*; Elaps; Ferr. p.; Graph.; *Hep.*; Hydr.; Kali bich.; *Kali s.*; Kino; Lyc.; Merc. pr. rub.; Merc. s.; *Merc. v.*; Nat. m.; Psor.; *Puls.*; *Sil.*; Sul.; *Tellur.*; Thuya; Tub.

PAIN (otalgia)—*Acon.*; Antipyr.; Apis; *Bell.*; Bor.; *Caps.*; *Cham.*; Chin. s.; Coff.; Dulc.; *Ferr. p.*; Gels.; *Hep.*; Iod.; Kali bich.; Kali iod.; Mag. p.; Menthol; *Merc. s.*; *Merc. v.*; Naja; *Plant.*; *Puls.*; Sang.; Tereb.; Val.; Viola od.; Visc. a.; *Verbasc.*

TYPE—**Aching, constant**—Caps.; Guaiac.; Merc.

Boring—Am. picr.; *Asaf.*; Aur.; Bell.; *Caps.*; Kali iod.; Sil.; Spig.

Burning—*Ars.*; Caps.; Kreos.; Sang.; Sul.

Cramp-like, pressing, piercing—*Anac.*; Calc. c.; *Cham.*; Kali bich.; Merc.; Puls.

Neuralgic, lancinating, shifting, shooting, paroxysmal—Acon.; *Bell.*; Caps.; Cepa; *Cham.*; Cinch.; Ferr. p.; Kali c.; *Mag. p.*; Nit. ac.; *Puls.*; Sil.; *Spig.*; Viola od.

Pulsating, throbbing—Acon.; *Bell.*; Cact.; Calc. c.; *Ferr. p.*; *Glon.*; Merc. c.; Merc. s.; Puls.; Rhus t.; Tellur.

Stinging—Acon.; Apis; Caps.

Stitching—Bor.; *Cham.*; Ferr. p.; Hep.; Kali bich.; *Kali c.*; Merc.; Nit. ac.; *Plant.*; Puls.; Viola od.

Tearing—*Bell.*; Caps.; *Cham.*; Kali bich.; Kali iod.; Merc. s.; Plant.; Puls.

MODALITIES—**Aggravation: At night**—*Acon.*; Ars.; Bell.; Calc. p.; *Cham.*; Dulc.; Ferr. p.; Hep.; Kali iod.; *Merc.*; *Puls.*; Rhus t.

From cold air—Calc. p.; Caps.; *Cham.*; Hep.; Kali m.; Mag. p.; Sang.

Noise—Bell.; Cham.

Pressure, motion—Menthol.

Warmth—Acon.; Bor.; Calc. p.; *Cham.*; Dulc.; *Merc.*; Nux v.; *Puls.*

Washing face and neck with cold water—Mag. p.

AMELIORATION—**During day**: Acon

From being carried, motion—Cham.

From cold applications—Puls.

From motion, covering—Aur.

From sipping cold water—Bar. m.

From warmth—*Bell.*; Caps.; Cham.; Dulc.; Hep.; *Mag. p.*

In open air—Acon.; Aur.; Ferr. p.; *Puls.*

TINNITUS AURIUM—(noises in ears): **Remedies in general**: Adren.; Am. c.; Antipyr.; Ars.; *Bar. c.*; *Bar. m.*; Bell.; Canchal.; Carbon. s.; *Caust.*; *Chenop.*; Chenop. gl.; *Chin. sal.*; *Chin. s.*; Cim.; *Cinch.*; Cistus dec.; Con.; Dig.; Ferr. p.; Ferr. picr.; *Graph.*; Hep.; Hydr.; Jabor.;

Kali c.; Kali iod.; *Kali m.;* Kali p.; Lach.; Lecith.; Lith. chlor.; Merc.; Merc. d.; Nat. m.; *Nat. sal.;* Parth.; Petrol.; Phos.; Piloc.; Plat.; Plumb. m.; *Puls.;* Sal. ac.; Sang.; *Sang. n.;* Sil.; Sulphon.; Sul.; Viola od.

Buzzing—Am. c.; Anac.; Antipyr.; *Bar. m.;* Calc. c.; Canchal.; Caust.; *Chenop.; Chin. s.;* Cinch.; Dig.; Diosc.; Ferr. p.; Formica; Graph.; Iod.; Iris; Kali p.; Kreos.; Lach.

Cracking, snapping, when blowing nose, chewing, swallowing, sneezing—Ambra; *Bar. c.; Bar. m.;* Calc. c.; Chenop. gl.; Formica; Gels.; *Graph.;* Kali c.; *Kali m.;* Lach.; *Nit. ac.;* Petrol.; Puls.; Sil.; Thuya.

Hissing—Can. ind.; *Chin. s.;* Dig.; Graph.; Teucr.

Humming—Alum.; Anac.; Calc. c.; *Caust.;* Cinch.; Ferr. p.; *Kali p.;* Kreos.; *Lyc.;* Petrol.; Puls.; Sang.; Sep.; Tereb.

Intolerance of music—*Acon.;* Ambra; Bufo; Viola od.

Pulsating, throbbing—Calc. c.; Caust.; *Ferr. p.;* Glon.; Hep.; Hydrobr ac.; Lach.; Merc.; Morph.; Nit. ac.; Puls.

Re-echoing of voice, sounds—Bar. c.; *Bar. m.;* Bell.; *Caust.;* Col.; Lyc.; Phos.; Tereb.

Ringing as of bells—*Bell.;* Calc. fl.; Carbon. s.; Caust.; Cham.; *Chin. s.; Cinch.;* Formica; *Graph.;* Iris; Lach.; Mez.; *Nat. sal.;* Petrol.

Roaring—Aur.; Calc. c.; Caust.; *Chin. s.;* Cinch.; Elaps; Ferr. p.; *Graph.;* Kreos.; *Lyc.;* Merc. d.; Merc.; Nat. m.; Nat. sal.; Nit. ac.; Petrol.; Phos. ac.; *Puls.;* Sal. ac.; Sang.; *Sil.;* Strych.; Viola od.

Roaring, relieved by music—Ign.

Rushing—Ferr. p.; Gels.; Puls.

Singing—*Chin. s.;* Dig.; Graph.; Lach.; Puls.

Whizzing—Bar. m.; Bell.; *Hep.;* Rhod.; Sul.

NOSE

AFFECTIONS, syphilitic—Asaf.; *Aur.;* Aur. mur.; *Cinnab.;* Fluor. ac.; *Kali bich.; Kali iod.;* Merc. c.; Sil.

BONES—Caries: Asaf.; *Aur.;* Aur. mur.; Cadm. s.; Kali bich.; Merc. i. r.; Merc.; *Phos.* See Tissues (Generalities).
Pain—*Asaf.; Aur.;* Cinnab.; *Hep.;* Kali iod.; Lach.; *Merc.;* Puls.; *Sil.*
Periostitis—Asaf.; *Aur.;* Merc.; *Phos.* See Tissues.
Ulceration—Asaf.; *Hekla;* Hep.; Kali bich. See Tissues.

EXTERNAL NOSE—ERUPTIONS, growths—Acne: Ars.; *Ars. br.; Aster.;* Bor.; *Caust.;* Clem.; Elaps; Kali br.; Nat. c.; Sil. ; Zing.
Eczema—Bals. per.; Iris; Sars.
Erysipelas—Bell.; Canth.; Rhus t.
Freckles—Phos.; Sul.
Furuncles—Cadm. s.; Cur.; *Hep.;* Sil.
Herpes—Acon. lyc.; Alum.; Bell.; Mur. ac.; Nat. m.; *Sep.;* Sul.
Lupus—Ars.; Aur. mur.; Kali bich.; Kreos.; Thuya; X-ray.
Pustules—*Hep.;* Petrol.; Psor.; Sil.
Scales—*Caust.*
Warts—Caust.; Thuya. See Skin.
Inflammation—Acon.; Agar.; *Apis; Aur.;* Aur. mur.; *Bell.;* Bor.; Carbo an.; Ferr. iod.; *Ferr. picr.;* Fluor. ac.; Graph.; *Hep.;* Hippoz.; *Kali iod.;* Medusa; Merc. c.; Naph.; Nat. c.; *Nit. ac.;* Sil.; Sul.
Itching—*Agar.; Cina;* Filix m.; *Ign.;* Iod.; Phos. ac.; Pin. syl.; Teucr.; Zing.
Numbness—Nat. m.
Redness—Agar.; Alum.; *Apis;* Ars.; Bell.; *Bor.;* Iod.; *Kali iod.;* Nat. c.; Psor.; Rhus t.; Rhus v.; Yucca; Zinc.
Soreness to touch—Alum.; Aur. m.; Bry.; Calc. c.; *Cinnab.;* Con.; Graph.; *Hep.;* Kali bich.; Lachnanth.; Lith. m.; *Merc.; Nit. ac.;* Rhus t.; Sil.
Varicose veins—Carbo v.
Yellow saddle—Sep.

ALAE—(wings): Burning, hot, biting: Ars.; Chenop. gl.; *Sang. n.;* Senega; Sinap.; Sul.
Dryness—Chlorum; Helleb.; *Sang. n.*
Eczema—Ant. c.; Bals. per.; Bar. c.; *Graph.; Petrol.*
Eruptions, growths, cracks, crusts, ulcerations—Alum.; *Ant. c.; Arum;* Aur.; Aur. m. n.; Bov.; *Calc. c.;* Caust.; Condur.; Coral.; *Graph.;* Ign.; *Kali bich.;* Kali c.; Lyc.; Merc.; *Nit. ac.; Petrol.;* Sul.; Tereb.; *Thuya.*
Fanning—*Ant. t.;* Brom.; *Chel.;* Gadus m.; Kali br.; *Lyc.; Phos.;* Pyr.; Sul. ac.
Herpes—Dulc.; Nat. m.; Physost.; Sil.
Itching—Carbo v.; *Cina;* Nat. p.; *Santon.;* Sil.; Sul.
Red, inner angles—Agar.; Merc. s.; Plumb. ac.; Sul.
Soreness to touch—*Alum; Ant. c.;* Ars.; *Arum;* Aur. mur.; Calc. c.; Cop.;

NOSE

Coral.; Fagop.; *Graph.*; *Hep.*; *Kali bich.*; Merc. c.; Merc.; *Nit. ac.*; Petrol.; Scilla; Uran.

Sooty, dirty nostrils—Helleb.

Throbbing—Acon.; Brom.

TIP—Blueness:—Carbo an.; *Dig.*

Burning—Bell.; Bor.; Ox. ac.; Rhus t.

Cold, pale, pointed—Apis; *Ars.*; Calc. p.; *Camph.*; Carbo v.; *Cinch.*; Helleb.; *Tab.*; *Ver. a.* See Face.

Congestion—Am. c.

ERUPTIONS, growths—Acne: Am. c.; Caust.; Sep.

Cracks—Alum.; *Graph.*; Petrol.

Furuncles—Ananth.; Bor.

Herpes—*Æth.*; Clem.; Conv.; Dulc.; Nat. m.

Knobby—Aur.

Pustules—Kali br.

Scales—Caust.; Nat. c.

Ulcers—Bor.; Rhus t.

Tumors—Ananth.; Carbo an.

Warts—Caust.

Inflammation—Bell.; Bor.; Cistus; Euphorbia; Niccol.; Nit. ac.; **Rhus t.**; Sep.

Itching—Carbo an.; Caust.; *Cina*; *Morph.*; Petrol.; Santon.; Sil.

Redness—Bell.; *Bor.*; Calc. c.; *Caps.*; Kali iod.; Kali n.; Niccol.; **Nit. ac.**; *Rhus t.*; Salix; *Sil.*; Sul.; Vinca m.

Soreness to touch—Bor.; Hep.; *Mentha*; Rhus t.

Tingling—Bell.; *Morph.*

Torpor, as from blow—Viola od.

INTERNAL NOSE—Abscess of septum: Acon.; *Bell.*; Calc. c.; *Hep.*; Sil.

Bleeding (epistaxis): Remedies in general—Abrot.; *Acon.*; Agar.; Ambros.; Am. c.; *Arn.*; Ars.; Bell.; *Bry.*; Cact.; Calc. c.; Carbo v.; *Cinch.*; Croc.; Crot. casc.; Elaps; Ferr. ac.; *Ferr. p.*; Ferr. picr.; Ficus; *Ham.*; *Ipec.*; Kali c.; Kali chlor.; Lach.; *Meli.*; Merc.; *Millef.*; **Mur. ac.**; Nat. nit.; Nat. sal.; *Nit. ac.*; Nux v.; Oniscus; Osm.; *Phos.*; **Puls.**; Sec.; Sep.; Sul.; *Thlaspi*; Tilia; *Trill.*; Vipera.

CAUSE—Blowing nose: Agar.; Aur. m.; Bov.; Carbo v.; Caust.; *Graph.*; Phos.; Sec.; Sep.; Sul.

Cough—Arn.

Eating—Am. c.

Hemophilia—Ars.; Crot.; Ham.; Ipec.; *Lach.*; Phos.

Hæmorrhoids, suppressed—Nux v.

Menses, absent (vicarious)—*Bry.*; *Ham.*; Lach.; Nat. s.; *Phos.*; **Puls.**; Sep.

Motion, noise, light—Bell.

Operations—Thlaspi.

Recurrent cases—Ars.; Ferr. p.; Millef.; Phos.

Stooping—Rhus t.

Straining—Carbo v.

Symptomatic (fevers, purpura)—Arn.; Ham.; Ipec.; Lach.; Phos.; Rhus t.
Traumatism—Acet. ac.; *Arn.*; Ham.; Millef.
Washing—*Am. c.;* *Ant. s. a.;* Arn.; Kali c.; Mag. c.

OCCURRENCE AND CONCOMITANTS—At night during sleep—*Merc. s.;* Nux v.

In children growing rapidly—Abrot.; Arn.; *Calc. c.;* Croc.; Phos.
In daily attacks—Carbo v.
In morning from washing face—Am. c.; Arn.; *Kali c.;* Oniscus.
In morning on awaking, arising, etc.—Aloe; Ambra; Bov.; *Bry.;* Cinch.; Lach.; Nux v.
In old people—Agar.; *Carbo v.*
Persistent, with goose flesh—Camph.
Preceded by heat and pain in head—Nux v.
With biliousness—Chel.
With chest affections—Ham.; Nit. ac.
With chronic vertigo—Sul.
With face congested, red—Bell.; *Meli.;* Nux v.
With face pale—Carbo v.; Ipec.
With prostration—Carbo v.; Cinch.; Diph.
With relief of chest symptoms—Bov.
With relief of headache—Ham.; *Meli.*
With tightness, pressure at root of nose—Ham.

TYPE OF BLOOD—Black, stringy: Croc.; Crot.; Merc. s.

Bright red—*Acon.;* Bell.; Bry.; Carbo v.; Erecht.; *Ferr. p.;* Ipec.; *Millef.;* *Trill.*
Coagulated—Cinch.; Nat. chlor.; Nux v.
Dark, fluid—Arn.; *Ham.;* Lach.; Mur. ac.; Sec.
Non-coagulable, passive, profuse—Bry.; Carbo v.; Crot.; *Ham.;* Phos.; Thlaspi; Trill.

BLOWS NOSE continually—Am. c.; Bor.; Hydr.; Lac c.; Mag. m.; *Sticta;* Tritic.

Boring, digging into—*Arum;* *Cina;* Helleb.; Phos. ac.; *Santon.;* Teucr.; Zinc. m.
Burning, smarting—Acon.; Æsc.; Am. m.; *Ars.;* *Ars. iod.;* Arum; Bar. c.; Brom.; Caps.; Cepa; Cop.; Hep.; *Hydr.;* Kaolin; Merc. c.; *Merc. s.;* Penthor.; Sabad.; *Sang.;* Sang. n.; Sinap.
Coldness—*Æsc.;* *Camph.;* *Cistus;* Coral.; Hydr.; Lith. c.; Ver. a.
Congestion, violent—Bell.; Cupr. m.; *Meli.*
Dryness—Acon.; Æsc.; *Am. c.;* Bell.; Calc. c.; *Camph.;* Con.; Cop.; Glycerin; *Graph.;* Kali bich.; Kali c.; Kali iod.; Lemna; *Lyc.;* Nat. m.; Nit. ac.; Nux m.; *Nux v.;* Onosm.; Petrol.; *Phos.;* Rumex; *Samb.;* *Sang.;* Sang. n.; Senec.; Sep.; Sil.; Sinap.; *Sticta;* Sul. See Stoppage.

ERUPTIONS, growths—Furuncles, pimples: Sil.; Tub.; Vinca.

Lupus—*Ars.;* Calc. c.; Cic.; Hydr.; *Hydrocot.;* Merc.; Rhus t.; Sul.; Tub.
Nodular swelling—Ars.
Papilloma—Caust.; Nit. ac.; *Thuya.*

NOSE

Polypi—Cadm. s.; *Calc. c.;* Calc. iod.; Calc. p.; Caust.; *Cepa;* Con.; Formica; Kali bich.; Kali n.; Lemna m.; Merc. i. r.; Nit. ac.; *Phos.;* Psor.; *Sang.;* Sang. n.; Staph.; *Teucr.; Thuya;* Wyeth.

Scabs, crusts, plugs, clinkers—*Alum.;* Ant. c.; *Arum;* Aur., Bor.; Cadm. s.; Calc. fl.; Cop.; Dulc.; Elaps; *Graph.;* Hep.; *Hydr.; Kali bich.;* Lemna m.; *Lyc.;* Nat. ars.; Nat. m.; Nit. ac.; *Puls.;* Sang. n.; *Sep.;* Sil.; Sticta; Sul.; *Teucr.;* Thuya.

Ulcerations, exocriations—Alum.; Ars.; Ars. iod.; Arum; Aur.; Bor.; Cepa; *Graph.;* Hep.; *Hydr.; Kali bich.;* Kali c.; Kreos.; Merc. c.; Merc.; *Nit. ac.;* Ran. s.; *Sil.;* Thuya; *Vinca.*

HARDNESS (rhino-sclerma)—Aur. m. n.; Calc. fl.; Con.

Inflammation (rhinitis): Acute, catarrhal from pollen irritation, HAY FEVER, rose cold, summer catarrh: *Ambros.; Aral.;* Ars.; *Ars. iod.;* Arum; Arundo; Benz. ac.; Cepa; Chin. ars.; Cocaine; Cupr. ac.; Dulc.; Euphorb. pil.; *Euphras.;* Gels.; Hep.; Ipec.; Kali iod.; Kali s. chrom.; *Lach.;* Linum usit.; Merc. i. fl.; *Naph.;* Nat. iod.; Nat. m.; Nux v.; Pollantin; *Psor.; Ran. b.;* Rosa d.; *Sabad.;* Sang.: *Sang. n.; Sil.; Sinap.;* Skook. ch.; Solid.; *Sticta;* Supraren. ext.; Trifol.; Tub.

Inflammation, acute, catarrhal, ordinary cold in head: *Acon.;* Æsc.; Am. c.; Am. m.; *Ars.; Ars. iod.; Arum;* Avena; Bell.; Brom.; *Bry.;* Camph.; *Cepa;* Cham.; *Dulc.;* Eup.; perf.; *Euphras.;* Ferr. p.; *Gels.;* Glycerin; Hep.; *Hydr.;* Hydroc. ac.; *Iod.; Justicia; Kali bich.; Kali iod.;* Lach.; Menthol; *Merc. s.; Nat. ars.; Nat. m.; Nux v.;* Phos.; Puls.; *Quill.;* Sabad.; Samb.; Sang.; *Sang. n.;* Solid.; *Sticta;* Tereb.; Ther.; Tromb.

CONCOMITANTS—Aching in limbs: Acon.; Bry.; *Eup. perf.; Gels.*

Chilliness (initial stage)—*Acon.;* Bapt.; *Camph.;* Caps.; Ferr. p.; *Gels.;* Merc. i. r.; *Nat. m.;* Nux v.; Phyt.; *Quill.;* Sapon.

Predisposition to colds—Agraph.; Alum.; Ars.; Bac.; Bar. c.; *Calc. c.;* Calc. iod.; Calc. p.; Calend.; Dulc.; Ferr. p.; Gels.; *Hep.;* Hydr.; Kali c.; Merc.; *Nat. m.;* Nux v.; Phos.; *Psor.;* Sep.; Solid.; *Sul.; Tub*

CORYZA—Dry (stuffy colds, snuffles): Acon.; Ambros.; *Am. c.;* Am. m.; Arum; *Calc. c.;* Camph.; Caust.; *Cham.;* Cistus; Con.; Dulc.; Elaps; Glycerin; Graph.; *Hep.;* Iod.; *Kali bich.; Kali c.;* Lach.; *Lyc.;* Menthol; *Nat. m.;* Nit. ac.; *Nux v.;* Osm.; Puls.; *Samb.;* Sep.; Sil.; *Sinap.; Sticta;* Teucr. See Stoppage.

Alternately dry and fluent—Am. c.; *Ars.; Lac c.;* Lach.; Mag. m.; *Nat. ars.; Nux v.;* Puls.; Quill.; *Sinap.;* Solan. n.; Spong.

Coryza, fluent, watery (running cold)—Æsc.; Agraph.; *Ail; Ambros.;* Am. m.; Am. phos.; *Aral.;* Ars.; *Ars. iod.; Arum;* Brom.; *Cepa;* Cycl.; Eucal.; Eup. perf.; *Euphras.; Gels.;* Hydr.; Iod.; Ipec.; *Justicia;* Kali chlor.; *Kali iod.;* Merc. c.; *Merc. s.;* Narcissus; *Nat. ars.; Nat. m.; Quill.; Sabad.; Sang. n.;* Scilla; Sil.; Solan. n.; *Trifol.*

Coryza, periodic—Ars.; Cinch.; Nat. m.; Sang.

Coryza, with chronic tendency—Am. c.; Calc. c.; Calc. iod.; *Con.; Graph.;* Hep.; *Kali bich.;* Kali iod.; *Puls.;* Sars.; *Sil.;* Sul.;

Coryza, with palpitation, especially in aged—Anac.

Coryza, with thick mucus—*Aur.*; Ferr. iod.; *Hep.*; *Kali bich.*; **Kali s.**; *Merc. s.*; Penthor.; *Puls.*; Sang. n.; Sep.; *Sticta.*
Coryza, worse in evening—Cepa; Glycerin; Puls.
Coryza, worse in newborn—Dulc.
Coryza, worse in warm room, better in open air—Ars.; Cepa; Nux v.
Cough—Alum.; *Bell.*; Bry.; *Cepa*; Dros.; Euphras.; *Justicia*; Lyc.; Nux v.; Sang.; Sinap.; *Sticta.*
Fever, low type, in old people—Bapt.
Headache—Acon.; Ars.; Bell.; *Bry.*; Cepa; Camph.; Cinch.; Eup. perf.; *Gels.*; Kali bich.; *Kali iod.*; Nat. ars.; *Nux v.*; Sabad.; Sang.
Hoarseness, aphonia—Ars.; *Caust.*; Cepa; Hep.; Osm.; Phos.; Pop. c.; Tellur.; Verbasc.
Infants, with snuffles—Acon.; *Am. c.*; Bell.; *Cham.*; Dulc.; Elaps; *Hep.*; Merc. i. fl.; *Nux v.*; *Samb.*; Sticta; Sul.
Insomnia—Ars.; Cham.
Lachrymation, sneezing—Acon.; Ambros.; Am. phos.; Aral.; *Ars.*; Ars. iod.; Camph.; *Cepa*; Cham.; *Cycl.*; Eup. perf.; *Euphras.*; *Gels.*; Ipec.; *Justicia*; Kali chlor.; *Kali iod.*; Menthol; Merc. s.; Naph.; *Nat. m.*; Nux v.; Quill.; *Sabad.*; Scilla; Sinap.; Solid.; Sticta. See Lachrymation.
Photophobia—Ars.; Bell.; Cepa; *Euphras.*
Prostration, lassitude—Ars.; Ars. iod.; Bapt.; Gels.; Quill.
Respiration, asthmatic—Ant. t.; *Aral.*; *Ars. iod.*; Bad.; *Ipec.*; Naph.
Inflammation, acute, croupous, fibrinous—*Am. caust.*; Apis; Ars.; Echin.; Hep.; *Kali bich.*; Lach.; Merc. s.; Nit. ac.
Inflammation, chronic atrophic (sicca)—*Alum.*; Am. c.; Aur.; *Calc. fl.*; Cinnab.; Elaps; Fluor. ac.; Graph.; *Hep.*; *Kali bich.*; Kali iod.; Kali s. chrom.; *Lemna m.*; *Lyc.*; Merc.; Sabal; *Sep.*; *Sticta*; *Sul.*; Teucr.; Wyeth.
Inflammation, chronic catarrhal—*Alum.*; Am. br.; *Am. m.*; Ars. iod.; Aur. mur.; Bals. per.; Brom.; *Calc. c.*; Calc. p.; Cub.; Elaps; *Eucal.*; *Hep.*; Hippoz.; *Hydr.*; *Kali bich.*; Kali c.; Kali iod.; Kreos.; Lemna m.; Med.; Merc. i. r.; *Merc. s.*; *Nat. c.*; Nat. m.; Nat. s.; Nit. ac.; Phos.; Psor.; *Puls.*; Sabad.; Sang.; Sang. n.; *Sep.*; Sil.; Spig.; Sticta; Teucr.; Ther.; Thuya.
Inflammation, purulent in children—Alum.; Arg. n.; *Calc. c.*; Cycl.; Hep.; Iod.; *Kali bich.*; *Lyc.*; Nat. c.; Nit. ac.

TYPE OF DISCHARGE IN RHINITIS—**Acrid, watery, fluent, hot, or thin mucus:** Ambros.; Am. caust.; *Am. m.*; *Aral.*; *Ars.*; *Ars. iod.*; Arum; Bell.; Carbo v.; *Cepa*; Cham.; Eucal.; *Gels.*; Glycerin; *Iod.*; *Kali iod.*; Kreos.; Lach.; Merc. c.; Merc.; Mur. ac.; Naph.; *Nat. ars.*; *Nat. m.*; Nit. ac.; Sabad.; Sang.; Sang. n.; Scilla; Sul.; Trifol.
Albuminous, clear mucus—*Æsc.*; Calc. c.; Camph.; Graph.; Hydr.; Kali bich.; Kali iod.; *Kali m.*; Lac c.; Menthol; *Nat. m.*; Phos.
Bland mucus—*Euphras.*; Jugl. c.; Kali iod.; *Puls.*; Sep.
Bloody mucus—Ail.; A.g. n.; Ars.; *Arum*; Aur.; Echin.; *Hep.*; Hydr.; Kali bich.; Merc. c.; *Merc. i. r.*; Penthor.; *Phos.*; Sang. n.; Sil.; Thuya.
Green, yellow, fetid (purulent or muco-purulent)—Alum.; Ars.; Ars. iod.;

Arum; Aur.; *Bals. per.;* *Calc. c.;* Calc. iod.; Calc. s.; *Dulc.;* **Eucal.;** Hep., *Hydr.;* *Kali bich.;* Kali iod.; *Kali s.;* *Lyc.;* Med.; **Merc.;** Nat. c.; *Nat. s.;* Nit. ac.; Penthor.; Phos.; *Puls.;* Sang. n.; *Sep.;* Sil.; Ther.; Thuya; Tub.

Membranous formation—*Am. caust.;* Echin.; Hep.; *Kali bich.* See Croupous Rhinitis.

Offensive, fetid—Ars. iod.; Asaf.; *Aur.;* Bals. per.; *Calc. c.;* Echin.; Elaps; Eucal.; Graph.; *Hep.;* *Hydr.;* *Kali bich.;* Kali iod.; Merc. s.; Nat. c.; Nit. ac.; Psor.; *Puls.;* Sang.; Sep.; *Sil.;* *Sul.;* Ther.; Tub.

Profuse—Ail; Am. m.; Aral.; *Ars.;* *Ars. iod.;* Arum; Bals. per.; Calc. iod.; Cepa; *Euphras.;* Hep.; *Hydr.;* *Kali bich.;* *Kali iod.;* *Merc.;* Nux v.; *Puls.;* Sang.; Sang. n.; Sep.; Thuya.

Salty-tasting—Aral.; Tellur.

Scabs, crusts, plugs—*Alum.;* Ant. c.; Aur.; Aur. mur.; Bor.; Calc. fl.; Calc. sil.; Caust.; Elaps; Fagop.; *Graph.;* Hep.; *Hydr.;* *Kali bich.;* Kaolin; Lemna m.; *Lyc.;* Merc. i. fl.; Nat. ars.; Nit. ac.; Petrol.; Psor.; *Puls.;* Sep.; Sil.; Sticta; *Sul.;* *Teucr.;* Ther.; Thuya.

Thick—Alum.; Am. brom.; *Calc. c.;* Hep.; Hydr.; *Kali bich.;* **Merc. c.;** Merc. s.; Nat. c.; Penthor.; *Puls.;* Sep.; Ther.; Thuya.

Unilateral—Calc. s.; Calend.; Phyt.

Viscid, ropy, stringy—*Bov.;* Gall. ac.; *Hydr.;* *Kali bich.;* Myr.; **Sticta;** Sumb.

ITCHING in nose—*Agn.;* Am. c.; Ars. iod.; *Arundo;* Aur.; Brom.; Cepa; *Cina;* Fagop.; Glycerin; *Hydr.;* Nat. m.; Ran. b.; Rosa d.; **Sabad.;** Sang.; *Santon.;* Sep.; Sil.; *Teucr.;* *Wyeth.*

Nervous disturbance—Agar.

Numbness, tingling—Acon.; Jugl. c.; *Nat. m.;* Plat.; Ran. b.; Sabad.; Sang.; Sil.; *Sticta.*

OZAENA—Odor:—Alum.; Ars. iod.; *Asaf.;* Aur. m.; *Aur. mur.;* *Cadm. s.;* Calc. c.; Calc. fl.; Carb. ac.; Diph.; Elaps; Ferr. iod.; Graph.; *Hep.;* Hippoz.; *Hydr.;* Hydrast. mur.; *Iod.;* *Kali bich.;* Kali c.; Kali chrom.; Kali iod.; Kali p.; Kreos.; Lach.; Lemna m.; Merc. i. fl.; Merc. pr. rub.; *Merc. s.;* Nit. ac.; Phos. ac.; Phos.; *Psor.;* *Puls.;* Sep.; Sil.; Teucr.; Ther.; Thuya; *Triost.*

Syphilitic—Asaf.; *Aur.;* Aur. mur.; Crot.; *Fluor ac.;* **Kali bich.;** **Kali iod.;** *Nit. ac.;* Syph.

PAIN in—Aching in dorsum, better from pressure—Agn.

Boring, gnawing—Asaf.; *Aur.;* Brom.; Kali iod.; Merc. i. r.

Burning—Æsc.; *Ars.;* *Ars. iod.;* Arum; Chrom. ac.; *Kali iod.;* **Lach.;** Merc. c.; *Sang.* See Burning.

Cramp-like—Plat.; Sabad.

Pressing at root of nose—*Acon.;* Alum.; Arum; Caps.; *Cepa;* Cinnab.; Gels.; Hep.; Iod.; *Kali bich.;* Kali iod.; Menyanth.; Nat. ars.; *Nux v.;* Oniscus; *Paris;* Plat.; Puls.; Ran. b.; Ruta; *Sang. n.;* Sep.; **Sticta;** Ther.

Pressing in frontal sinuses—Gels.; Ign.; Iod.; Kali bich.; *Kali iod.;* Merc.; Nux v.; Sang.; *Sticta.*

Sharp to ears—Merc. c.

Splinter-like, sticking—*Aur.*; *Hep.*; Kali bich.; *Nit. ac*

String-like to ear—Lemna m.

Throbbing—Bell.; *Hep.*; Kali iod.

Violent shooting, from occiput to root of nose, from suppressed discharge—Kali bich.

POSTERIOR NARES—(naso-pharynx): Inflammation of: Acute: Acon.; Camph.; Cistus; Gels.; Kali bich.; Menthol; *Merc. c.*: Nat. ars.; Wyeth. See Rhinitis, Pharyngitis.

Chronic—Aur.; Calc. fl.; Elaps; Fagop.; *Hydr.*; *Kali bich.*; Kali c.; Merc. c.; Penthor.; Sep.; *Spig.*; *Sticta*; Sul.; Thuya.

Chronic with dropping of mucus-Remedies in General: Alum.; Am. br.; Ant. c.; Ars. iod.; Aur.; Calc. sil.; *Coral.*; Echin.; Glycerin; *Hydr.*; Irid.; *Kali bich.*; Kali m.; *Lemna m.*; Merc. i. r.; Nat. c.; *Penthor.*; *Phyt.*; *Sang. n.*; Sinap. n.; *Spig.*; Sticta; Teucr.; Ther.; Wyeth.

Clear, acrid, thin mucus—Ars. iod.

Clear mucus—Cepa; *Kali m.*; Nat. m.; Solan. lyc.

Lumpy—Osm.; Teucr.

Thick, tenacious, yellow, or white mucus—Alum.; Am. br.; Ant. c.; Calc. sil.; Coral.; *Hydr.*; *Kali bich.*; Lemna m.; Menthol; Merc. i. fl.; Nat. c.; Sang. n.; Sep.; Spig.

Tumors—Chrom. ac.; Osm.

Wet, raw feeling—Penthor.

SENSE OF SMELL—Diminished: *Alum.*; *Cycl.*; Helleb.; *Hep.*; Kali c.; Menthol; Mez.; Rhod.; Sil.; Tab.

Hypersensitive—*Acon.*; Agar.; Aur.; *Bell.*; *Carb. ac.*; Carbo v.; *Cham.*; Cinch.; Coff.; *Colch.*; Graph.; Ign.; Lyc.; Mag. m.; *Nux v.*; *Phos.*; Sang.; Sabad.; *Sep.*; Sul.

Hypersensitive to flowers—Graph.

Hypersensitive to food—Ars.; Colch.; Sep.

Hypersensitive to tobacco—Bell.

Lost (anosmia) or perverted—*Alum.*; Am. m.; amyg. pers.; *Anac.*; Apoc. andr.; Aur.; Bell.; Calc. c.; *Hep.*; Ign.; Iod.; Justicia; *Kali bich.*; Lemna m.; *Mag. m.*; Nat. m.; Nit. ac.; *Puls.*; Sang.; Sep.; Sil.; Sul.; Teucr.; Zinc. mur.

Parosmia (illusions)—Agn.; *Anac.*; Apoc. andr.; Ars.; Aur.; *Bell.*; Calc. c.; Coral.; Diosc.; Graph.; Ign.; *Kali bich.*; Mag. m.; *Merc.*; Nit. ac.; Nux v.; Phos.; *Puls.*; Sang.; Sul.

SENSITIVENESS of nose to air, touch—*Æsc.*; Alum.; Ant. c.; Aral.; Ars.; Arum; Aur.; Aur. mur.; Bell.; Calc. c.; Camph.; *Hep.*; Kali bich.; Kaolin; *Merc.*; Nat. m.; Osm.; Sil.

SINUSES—(antrum, frontal, sphenoidal): Affections in general: Ars.; *Asaf.*; Aur. m.; Bell.; Calc. c.; Camph.; Eucal.; *Hep.*; *Iod.*; Kali bich.; *Kali iod.*; Kali m.; Lyc.; *Merc. i. fl.*; Merc.; Mez.; Phos. ac.; *Phos.*; Sil.; Spig.; *Sticta*; Teucr.

Catarrh of frontal sinuses—Ammoniacum; Ign.; Iod.; *Kali bich.*; *Kali iod.*; Lyc.; Menthol; Merc. i. fl.; Nat. m.; Nux v.; Sabad.; Sticta; Thuya.

NOSE

Pain and swelling of antrum—Phos.; Spig.

Syphilitic affections—Aur.; *Kali iod.*; Nit. ac.

SNEEZING—(sternutation): Acon.; Ambros.; Am. m.; *Aral.; Ars.;* Ars. iod.; Arum; Arundo; Calc. c.; Camph.; *Cepa; Cycl.;* Eup. perf.; Euphorbia; *Euphras.; Gels.;* Ichthy.; Iod.; *Ipec.;* Kali bich.; *Kali iod.;* Lob. cer.; Menthol; Merc.; Naph.; Nat. m.; Nit. ac.; Nux v.; Rosa d.; Rhus t.; *Sabad.;* Succin. ac.; Sang.; *Sang. n.;* Sapon.; Scilla; Senec.; Senega; Sinap.; *Sticta.*

Sneezing, chronic tendency—Sil.

Sneezing, ineffectual—*Ars.;* Carbo v.; Sil.

Sneezing, worse coming into warm room: rising from bed: handling peaches—Cepa.

Sneezing, worse in cool air—Ars.; Hep.; Sabad.

Sneezing, worse in evening—Glycerin.

Sneezing, worse in morning—Camph.; Caust.; *Nux v.;* Sil.

Sneezing, worse immersing hands in water—Lac. d.; Phos.

STOPPAGE—Stuffiness: *Acon.;* Ambros.; *Am. c.;* Am. m.; Anac.; Apoc.; Ars.; Ars. iod.; *Arum; Aur.;* Aur. m. n.; *Calc. c.;* Camph.; Caust.; *Cham.;* Con.; Cop.; Elaps; Eucal.; Fluor. ac.; *Formica;* Glycerin; Graph.; Helianth.; *Hep.; Kali bich.;* Kali c.; Kali iod.; Lemna m.; *Lyc.;* Menthol; Nat. ars.; Nat. c.; Nat. m.; Nit. ac.; *Nux v.;* Paris; Penthor.; Petrol.; *Puls.;* Radium; Sabad.; *Samb.;* Sang. n.; Sapon.; Sep.; Sil.; *Sinap.;* Spong.; *Sticta.*

Stoppage, alternating nostrils—Acon.; Am. c.; Bor.; *Lac c.;* Mag. m.; *Nux v.*

Swelling—Antipyr.; Ars.; *Ars. iod.; Aur.;* Aur. s. a.; Bar. c.; Bell.; Calc. c.; Hep.; *Kali bich.; Lemna m.; Merc. c.;* Merc. i. r.; *Nit. ac.;* Sabad.; Sang.; Sep. See Inflammation.

ULCERATION OF SEPTUM—Alum.; Aur.; Brom.; Calc. c.; Carb. ac.; Fluor. ac.; Hippoz.; *Hydr.; Kali bich.;* Kali iod.; Merc. c.; Nit. ac.; *Sil.;* Vinca.

Ulceration, syphilitic—*Aur.;* Aur. mur.; Coral.; Kali bich.; *Kali iod.;* Lach.; Merc. aur.; *Nit. ac.*

Wet feeling not relieved by blowing—Penthor.

FACE

APPEARANCE—CONDITION—Anemic, alabaster-like, waxen: *Acet. ac.;* Apis; Ars.; Calc. p.; Ferr. m.; Lach.; Merc. c.; Nat. c.; Sep.; Sil.

Bloated, puffy—Æth.; *Am. benz.;* Apis; Ars.; Bor. ac.; Bothrops; Calc. c.; Ferr. m.; *Kali c.;* Helleb.; Hyos.; Lach.; Medusa; *Merc. c.; Op.; Phos.;* Taxus; Xerophyl.

Bloated about eyes—*Am. benz.;* Ars.; Bor. ac.; Elaps; *Merc. c.;* Nat. c.; *Phos.;* Rhus t.; Thlaspi; Xerophyl.

Bloated about lower eyelids—*Apis;* Xerophyl.

Bloated about upper eyelids—Kali c.

Blue, livid (cyanosis)—Absinth.; Am. c.; *Ant. t.;* Arg. n.; *Ars.;* Aur.; *Camph.;* Carbo an.; *Carbo v.;* Chlorum; *Cic.;* Cina; Cinnab.; Crot.; *Cupr. ac.;* Cupr. m.; *Dig.;* Ferr.; *Hydroc. ac.; Ipec.;* Lach.; *Laur.; Morph.;* Œnanthe; Op.; Phenac.; Rhus t.; *Samb.;* Sec.; Strych.; *Tab.; Ver. a.* See Circulatory System.

Blue rings around, dull looking eyes—*Abrot.;* Acet. ac.; *Ars.;* Berb .v.; Bism.; Calc. c.; *Camph.; Cina; Cinch.;* Cycl.; Ipec.; Nat. c.; *Œnanthe; Phos. ac.; Phos.;* Santon.; Sec.; Sep.; Spig.; Stann.; *Staph.;* Tab.; *Ver. a.;* Zinc. m.

Blushing—Ambra; *Amyl;* Carbo an.; Carls.; *Coca;* Ferr.; Stram.; Sul.

Bronzed—Ant. c.; Nit. ac.; Sec.; Spig.

Brown spots on—Caul.; Sep.

Coppery look—Alum.; Nit. ac.

Distorted—Absinth.; Art. v.; Bell.; Camph.; *Cic.;* Cupr. ac.; *Cupr. m.;* Crot.; Helleb.; Hyos.; Nux v.; *Op.;* Sec.; *Stram.*

Earthy, dirty, sallow, cachectic—*Acet. ac.;* Ars.; Berb. v.; Calc. p.; Camph.; *Carbo v.; Caust.;* Chel.; *Cinch.;* Ferr.; Glycerin; Hydr.; Iod.; *Lyc.;* Merc. c.; Merc.; *Nat. m.;* Nux v.; Phos. ac.; Phos.; Picr. ac.; *Plumb. m.; Psor.; Sanic.;* Sec.; Sep.; Spig.; *Staph.;* Sul.

Expression anxious, suffering—Acon.; *Æth.;* Ars.; Bor.; *Camph.;* Canth.; Cina; Cinch.; Iod.; Kreos.; Merc. c.; Plumb.; *Stram.;* Strych.; Tab.; *Ver. a.*

Expression drowsy, stupid—Ail.; Apis; *Bapt.;* Can. ind.; *Gels.;* Helleb.; *Op.;* Rhus t.

Expression stolid, mask-like—Mang. ac.

Greasy, shiny, oily—*Nat. m.;* Plumb.; Psor.; Sanic.; Selen.; Thuya.

Hippocratic (sickly, sunken, deathly cold)—Acon.; Æth.; Ant. t.; Arn.; Ars.; Berb. v.; *Camph.; Carbo v.;* Cinch.; Cyprip.; Helleb.; Lach.; Merc. cy.; Plumb. m.; Pyr.; *Sec.; Tab.; Ver. a.;* Zinc. m.

Jaundiced, yellow—*Ars.;* Berb. v.; Blatta am.; Bry.; Calc. c.; Carbo v.; Chel.; *Chionanth.; Cinch.;* Crot.; *Dig.;* Hep.; Hydr.; Iod.; Kali c.; Lach.; Lyc.; Merc.; *Merc. d.;* Myr.; Nat. m.; Nat. p.; Nat. s.; *Nux v.;* Ol. j. as.; Petrol.; Picr. ac.; *Plumb. m.;* Pod.; Sep.; *Tarax.;* Yucca. See Jaundice.

Pale—Abrot.; *Acet. ac.;* Ant. t.; Apis; Arg. n.; Ars.; Bell.; Berb. v.; Bor.; Calc. c.; Calc. p.; *Camph.; Carbo v.; Cina;* Cinch.; Cupr. m.;

FACE

Cycl.; Dig.; *Ferr. ac.*; *Ferr. m.*; *Ferr. mur.*; Ferr. red.; Glon.; Helleb.; *Ipec.*; Kali c.; Lach.; Lecith.; Med.; *Merc. c.*; Merc. d.; *Morph.*; Nat. c.; Nat. m.; Nit. ac.; Phos. ac.; Phos.; *Plumb. m.*; *Puls.*; Pyr.; *Santon.*; Sec.; Sep.; Sil.; Spig.; Stann.; Staph.; *Tab.*; *Ver. a.*; Zinc. m.

Parchment-like—Ars.

Red, becomes deathly pale on rising—*Acon.*; Ver. a.

Red, dark, dusky, besotted, bloated—*Ail.*; Apis; Ars. m.; *Bapt.*; Bothrops; Bry.; Carb. ac.; Diph.; *Gels.*; Hyos.; Lach.; *Morph.*; Nux v.; *Op.*; Rhus t.; Stram.

Red, distorted—Bell.; *Cic.*; Cupr. ac.; *Cupr. m.*; Crot.; Hyos.; Op.; *Stram.*

Red, flushed after eating—Alum.; Carbo an.; Carls.; Coral.; Stront.

Red, flushed, from emotion, pain, exertion—Acon.; *Ferr. m.*; Ign.; Meli.

Red, flushed, hot, florid—Acet. ac.; *Acon.*; Agar.; *Amyl*; *Aster.*; Bapt.; *Bell.*; Canth.; Caps.; *Ferr. p.*; Gels.; *Glon.*; Glycerin; Kreos.; *Meli.*; Myg.; Op.; Quercus; Rhamnus c.; *Sang.*; *Stram.*; Sul.; *Ver. v.*

Red, semi-lateral—Acon.; *Cham.*; *Cina*; Dros.; Ipec.; *Nux v.*

Red, though cold—Asaf.; Caps.

Sensitive, after neuralgia—Cod.

Sweating—*Acet. ac.*; Amyl; *Ant. t.*; Ars.; *Cham.*; Glon.; Samb.; Sil.; *Tab.*; *Ver. a.*; Viola tr.

Sweating, cold—*Ant. t.*; *Ars.*; Camph.; *Carbo v.*; Cina; Euphorbia; *Lob. infl.*; *Tab.*; *Ver. a.*; Zinc. mur.

Sweating, in small spots, while eating—Ign.

Sweating on forehead—Cham.; Euphorbia; Op.; *Ver. a.*

Swelling—*Acon.*; Ant. ars.; Antipyr.; *Apis*; Ars.; Ars. m.; *Bell.*; Cepa; Colch.; *Helleb.*; Lach.; *Merc. c.*; Œnanthe; Op.; Phos.; *Rhus t.*; Rhus v.; Ver. a.; Vespa; Vipera.

Swelling from toothache—Bell.; Cham.; Coff.; Mag. c.; *Merc.*

Wrinkled, shrivelled, old-looking—Abrot.; *Arg. n.*; Bar. c.; Bor.; Calc. p.; Con.; *Fluor. ac.*; Iod.; Kreos.; Lyc.; *Nat. m.*; Op.; *Psor.*; *Pulex*; *Sanic.*; Sars.; Sec.; Sil.; Sul.

BONES—(facial): Caries: Aur. m.; Cistus; Fluor. ac.; Hekla.

Exostoses—Fluor. ac.; Hekla.

Inflammation—Aur. m.

Pains—Alum.; Arg. n.; Astrag.; *Aur.*; Carbo an.; Caust.; Dulc.; *Hep.*; Merc.; Nit. sp. d.; *Phos.*; *Sil.*; Zinc.

Sensitive—Aur.; *Hep.*; Kali bich.; Mez. See Jaws.

CHEEKS—Bites when chewing, talking—Caust.; *Ign.*; Ol. an.

Burning—Agar.; Euphorb.; Ferr. p.; Nit. sp. d.; Phos. ac.; Phos.; Sul. See Sensation.

Eruptions—*Ant. c.*; Dulc.; Graph.; *Led.*; *Mez.* See Eruptions on face.

Lumpy—Antipyr.

Pains—Agar.; August.; Ver. a. See Prosopalgia.

Redness—Brom.; *Caps.*; *Cic.*; Coff.; Colch.; Euphorbia; Euphras.; *Meli.* See Red Face.

Redness, unilateral—*Acon.*; *Cham.*; Cina; Dros.; Ipec.; *Nux v.*

Spots, circumscribed, red, burning—Benz. ac.; Bry.; *Cina;* Ferr. mur.; Lachnanth.; *Phos.;* Samb.; *Sang.;* Stram.; Sul.

Swelling—*Acon.;* Bell.; Bov.; *Calc. fl.;* Euphorb.; Kali m.; *Plant.;* Plat. See Swelling of Face.

Tingling, numbness—*Acon.;* Plat.

Ulcers, wart-like—Ars.

Yellow saddle in uterine disease—Sep.

CHIN—Eruptions: *Ant. c.;* Aster.; *Cic.;* Dulc.; *Graph.;* *Hep.;* Nat. m.; Phos. ac.; Rhus t.; Sep.; Sil.; *Sul. iod.;* Zinc.

ERUPTIONS ON FACE—Acne rosacea—*Ars. br.;* Carbo an.; Chrysar.; *Eug. j.; Kreos.;* Ophor.; Psor.; Sul.; Sulphurous ac.

Acne simplex—Ambra; *Ant. c.; Bell.; Berb. aq.;* Calc. p.; Calc. s.; Carbo v.; Cim.; Clem.; Con.: Crot. t.; *Eug. j.;* Graph.; Ind.; *Jugl. r.;* Kali ars.; Kali br.; Kali c.; *Led.;* Med.; Nat. m.; *Nux v.;* Phos. ac.; *Sul.;* Thuya.

Angioma—Abrot.

Blotches—*Berb. aq.;* Kali c.; Nux v.

Cancer, open, bleeding—Cistus.

Chilblains—Agar.

Comedones—*Abrot.;* Eug. j.; Jugl. r.; Nit. ac.; *Sul.*

Crusta-lactea—Calc. c.; Hep.; Merc. pr. rub.; *Rhus t.;* Sil.; Viola tr. See Scalp.

Eczema—Anac.; *Ant. c.; Ars.;* Calc. c.; Carb. ac.; *Crot. t.;* Dulc.; *Graph.;* Hep.; Led.; Merc. pr. rub.; *Mez.;* Nat. m.; Sep.; Sil.; *Sul.;* Sul. iod.; *Vinca;* Viola tr.

Epithelioma—Ars.; Kali s.; Lob. erin.

Erysipelas—Anac. oc.; Ananth.; *Apis; Bell.;* Bor.; *Canth.;* Carbo an.; *Euphorb.;* Ferr. mur.; *Graph.;* Gymnocl.; Hep.; *Rhus t.;* Sep.; Solan. c.; Ver. v.

Erythema—Ars. iod.; *Bell.;* Condur.; Echin.; Euphorbia; *Graph.;* Nux v.

Furuncles—Alum.; *Ant. c.;* Calc. p.; *Hep.; Led.;* Med.

Herpes (tetter)—Anac. oc.; Canth.; Clem.; *Dulc.;* Euphorb.; Limulus; Lyc.; *Nat. m.; Rhus t.;* Sep.

Humid, moist—Ant. c.; Cic.; Dulc.; *Graph.;* Hep.; Mez.; Psor.; Rhus t.; Viola tr.

Itching eruption on forehead during menses—Eug. j.; Psor.; Sang.; Sars.

Lentigo (freckles)—Am. c.; Iris germ.; Graph.; Lyc.; *Mur. ac.;* Nat. c.; *Nit. ac.;* Phos.; Sep.; *Sul.;* Tab.; Thuya.

Lupus—Cistus.

Pustules—*Ant. c.;* Bell.; Calc. c.; *Calc. s.; Cic.;* Graph.; *Hep.;* Indium; Merc.; Psor.

Rough, harsh—*Berb. aq.;* Kali c.; *Petrol.;* Sul.

Scabs, crusts, scurfs—Ars.; Cic.; Cistus; Dulc.; Graph.; Hep.; Mez.; Rhus t.

Scales—Ars.; Euphorbia.

Spots, copper-colored—Benz. ac.; *Carbo an.;* Lyc.; Nit. ac.

Spots, red—*Berb. aq.;* Euphorbia; Kali bich.; *Kali c.;* Œnanthe: Petrol.

Spots, yellow—Nat. c.; *Sep.*

FACE 745

SYPHILIDAE—Areolæ, papules:—Kali iod.
 Copper spots—Carbo an.; Lyc.; *Nit. ac.*
 Crusts, areolæ—Nit. ac.
 Pustules—Kali iod.; Nit. ac.
 Tubercles—Alum.; Carbo an.; Fluor. ac.
 Ulcer, eroding—Con.
 Warts—Calc. s.; Castorea; *Caust.*; Kali c.
 Whiskers, eruptions—Hep.
 Whiskers, falling out—Graph.; Selen. See Scalp.
 Whiskers, itching—Calc. c. See Skin.

FOREHEAD feels contracted, wrinkled—Bapt.; Bellis; Grat.; *Helleb.*; Lyc.; Phos.; Primula.
 Glabella, swelling—Sil.

JAWS—Cracking when chewing: Am. c.; Granat.; Lac c.; *Nit. ac.*; *Rhus t.*
 Dislocated easy—Ign.; Petrol.; *Rhus t.*; Staph.
 Growths, swelling—Amphis.; *Calc. fl.*; Hekla; Plumb.; Thuya.
 Pain—Acon.; Agar.; Alum.; Am. m.; Am. picr.; *Amphis.*; August.; Arum; Astrag.; Aur. m.; Bapt. conf.; Calc. caust.; Carbo an.; *Caust.*; Merc.; Phos.; Rhus t.; Sang.; *Sphingur.*; Spig.; Xanth.
 Stiffness (trismus, lockjaw)—Absinth.; *Acon.*; Arn.; Bell.; Carbon. oxy.; Caust.; Cham.; Cic.; Cupr. ac.; *Cupr. m.*; Cur.; Dulc.; Hydroc. ac.; *Hyper.*; *Ign.*; Merc. c.; *Morph.*; Nerium; Nicot.; Nux v.; Œnanthe; Physost.; Solan. n.; Stram.; *Strych.*; Ver. a.
 Trembling—Alum.; *Ant. t.*; Cadm. s.; *Gels.*

LOWER JAW—Caries, necrosis:—Amphis.; Angust.; *Phos.*; Sil.
 Chewing motion—Acon.; Bell.; Bry.; *Helleb.*; Stram.
 Epulis—Plumb. ac.; Thuya.
 Hanging down, relaxed—Arn.; Ars.; Gels.; *Helleb.*; Hyos.; Lach.; Lyc.; Mur. ac.; Op.
 Nodes, painful—Graph.
 Pain—Caust.; Chin. s.; Cinch.; Sil.; Spig.; Xanth. See Jaws.
 Swelling—Amphis.; Aur. m. n.; Merc.; *Phos.*; Sil.; Symphyt.

UPPER JAW—Affections of Antrum of Highmore: Arn.; Bell.; Chel.; Commocl.; Euphorb. amyg.; Hep.; *Kali iod.*; Kali s.; Mag. c.; Merc. c.; Paris; *Phos.*; Sil.; Tilia.
 Pain—Astrag.; Calc. p.; Euphorbia; *Fluor. ac.*; Merc. i. r.; *Phos.*; Polygon.; *Spig.*
 Tumor—Hekla.

MUSCLES—(facial) Distortion (risus sardonicus): *Cic.*; Cupr. ac.; Hydroc ac.; Op.; *Sec.*; Stram.; Strych.; Tellur.
 Pain—Anac.; Angust.; Cocc.; Colch.; Oxytr.; Sab. See Prosopalgia.
 Paralysis—Bell's palsy: Acon.; Alum.; *Am. phos.*; Bell.; Cadm. s.; *Caust.*; Cocc.; Cur.; *Dulc.*; Formica; Gels.; *Graph.*; Hyper.; *Kali chlor.*; *Kali iod.*; Merc. c. k.; Physal.; Rhus t.; Ruta; *Senega*; Zinc. pier.
 Left side—Cadm. s.; Senega.
 Right side—Bell.; Caust.

FACE

Stiffness—Absinth.; Acon.; *Agar.*; Bapt.; *Caust.*; Gels.; Helod.; Nux v.; Rhus t. See Trismus.

Twitching, spasmodic—Agar.; Arg. n.; *Bell.*; Caust.; Cham.; *Cic.*; *Cina*; Gels.; Hyos.; *Ign.*; Laburn.; Laur.; Menyanth.; *Myg.*; Nux v.; Œnanthe; Op.; Sec.; Stram.; Tellur.; Visc. a.

PROSOPALGIA—Pain (face-ache):

TYPE—Congestive, inflammatory, neuralgic: Acon.; *Agar.*; Aran.; Arg. n.; *Ars.*; *Bell.*; Cact.; *Caps.*; Caust.; *Ced.*; Cepa; *Cham.*; Chin. ars.; *Chin. s.*; Cim.; *Cinch.* Coff.; *Col.*; Ferr.; *Gels.*; Hekla; *Kali iod.*; Kali p.; Kal.; *Mag. p.*; Menthol; Merc. c.; Merc. s.; *Mez.*; Nit. sp. d.; Phos.; *Plant.*; *Plat.*; Puls.; Radium; Rhodium; *Rhus t.*; Sang.; Sil.; *Spig.*; Stann.; Sul.; Thuya; Tilia; *Verbasc.*; Zinc. p.; *Zinc. v.*

Reflex, from decayed teeth—Coff. tosta; Hekla; Merc. s.; *Mez.*; Staph.

Rheumatic—*Acon.*; Act. sp.; *Caust.*; Cham.; Colch.; Col.; *Dulc.*; Puls.; *Rhod.*; Rhus t.; Spig.

Syphilitic (mercurial)—*Kali iod.*; Mez.; Nit. ac.

Toxic (malarial, quinine)—Ars.; Cinch.; Ipec.; Nat. m.

LOCATION—Eyes: Ars.; *Cim.*; Clem.; Nux v.; Paris; *Spig.*; Thuya. See Eyes.

Jaw, lower—*Amphis.*; Calc. c.; Lach.; Nit. sp. d.; Plat.; Radium; *Rhod.*; Xanth.; Zinc. v.

Jaw, upper—*Amphis.*; Bism.; *Calc. caust.*; Cham.; Col.; Dulc.; Euphorb. amyg.; Graph.; Iris; *Kali cy.*; *Kali iod.*; Kal.; *Kreos.*; Mez.; Paris; Sang.; Thuya; *Verbasc.*

Jaw, upper, (infra-orbital)—Colch.; Iris; Mag. p.; *Mez.*; Nux v.; Phos.; Verbasc.

Jaw, upper, to teeth, temples, ears, eyes, malar bones—*Act. sp.*; Arg. n.; Ars.; Bell.; Bism.; *Cham.*; Clem.; *Coff.*; *Col.*; Dulc.; *Kali cy.*; *Mez.*; Phos.; Plant.; Rhod.; Sang.; *Spig.*; Thuya; *Verbasc.*

Malar bones (zygoma)—Angust.; Arg. m.; Aur.; *Calc. caust.*; Caps.; *Cim.*; Col.; Hydrocot.; Lecith.; Menthol; Ol. an.; Mag. c.; Mez.; Paris; *Plat.*; Rhus t.; *Sphingur.*; *Spig.*; Strych.; Thuya; *Verbasc.*; Zinc. m.

Unilateral, left—*Acon.*; Arg. n.; *Col.*; Coral.; Hydrocot.; *Lach.*; Paris; Plat.; Sapon.; Senec.; *Spig.*; *Verbasc.*; Zinc. v.

Unilateral, right—Aran.; *Cact.*; Caps.; Ced.; Clem.; Coff.; Colch.; Hyper.; Kal.; Mag. p.; *Mez.*; Puls.

TYPE OF PAIN—Cramp-like drawing, pressing: Angust.; Bism.; Bry.; *Cact.*; Cocc.; Col.; *Mez.*; *Plat.*; Thuya; Ver. a.; *Verbasc.*

Cutting, tearing, jerking, stitching, rending—Acon.; Amphis.; *Ars.*; Aur.; Caust.; *Cham.*; Cinch.; *Col.*; Dulc.; Hyper.; Mag. p.; Merc.; Mez.; Nux v.; Phos.; *Puls.*; Rhodium; Rhod.; Senec.; Sil.; *Spig.*

Fine line of pain coursing along the nerve—Caps.; Cepa.

Gradual onset and cessation—Plat.; *Stann.*

Gradual onset and sudden cessation—Arg. m.; *Bell.*; Puls.

Hot needles, penetrating—Ars.

Icy needles, penetrating—Agar.

Lancinating, paroxysmal, lightning-like, radiating—Arg. n.; Ars.; *Bell.*;

FACE

Cocc.; *Col.*; Gels.; Graph.; Hep.; *Kali iod.*; Kreos.; Mag. p.; *Nux v.*; Phos.; Plant.; *Rhodium*; Sang.; *Spig.*; *Strych.*; Zinc. m.

Periodical, intermittent—Cact.; Ced.; Chin. s.; *Cinch.*; *Col.*; Graph.; Mag. p.; Plant.; *Spig.*; Ver. a.; Verbasc.

CONCOMITANTS—**Acid, sour eructations**: Arg. n.; Nux v.; Verbasc.

Canine hunger, preceded by coldness—Dulc.

Catarrh (coryza, lachrymation)—Verbasc.

Cheek, dark red—Spig.

Chilliness—Col.; Dulc.; *Mez.*; *Puls.*; Rhus t.

Gastralgia, alternating—Bism.

Lachrymation—Bell.; Ipec.; Nux v.; Plant.; *Puls.*; Verbasc.

Mental irritability—Cham.; Coff.; Kreos.; Nux v.

Numbness—*Acon.*; Menthol; *Mez.*; Plat.; Rhus t.

Photophobia—Nit. sp. d.; Plant.

Ptosis—Gels.

Restlessness, palpitation—Spig.

Salivation, stiff neck—Mez.

Tenderness to touch—Acon.; Bell.; *Cinch.*; Col.; *Hep.*; Mez.; Paris; Spig.; Verbasc.

Twitching about face—Agar.; Bell.; *Colch.*; Kali c.; Nux v.; Thuya; *Zinc. m.*

Vision veiled—Tilia.

MODALITIES—**Aggravation: From acids, motion, emotion**: Kali c.

From chewing, opening mouth—Angust.; Cocc.; Helleb.; Hep.; Mez.

From cold, dry exposure—*Acon.*; Coff.; Kal.; Mag. c.; Mag. p.; Nit. sp. d.

From cold, wet exposure—Col.; *Dulc.*; Mag. m.; Rhus t.; *Sil.*; *Spig.*; Thuya.

From contact, touch—Bell.; Caps.; *Cinch.*; Col.; *Cupr. m.*; Hep.; Mag. p.; *Mez.*; Paris; *Spig.*; Verbasc.

From eating, drinking—Bism.; Iris; *Mez.*

From eating motion—Col.; Phos.; Verbasc.

From eating, motion, stooping, jar, etc.—*Bell.*; Ferr. p.; *Spig.*

From morning until sunset—Spig.

From motion, noise—Ars.; Chin. s.; Cinch.; *Spig.*

From pressure—Caps.

From rest—Mag. c.; Plat.; Rhus t.

From talking, motion, sitting or lying on unaffected side—Kreos.

From talking, sneezing, change of temperature, pressure of teeth—Verbasc.

From tea—Selen.; Spig.; Thuya.

From thinking of pain—Aur.

From tobacco—Sep.

From warmth—Cham.; Glon.; Kali s.; Merc. s.; Mez.; *Puls.*

In afternoon—Cocc.

In daytime—Ced.; Plant.; Spig.

In evening, night—*Ars.*; Caps.; Mag. c.; Merc. s.; Mez.; *Puls.*; Rhus t.

AMELIORATION—**From chewing**—Cupr. ac.

From cold applications, cold—Bism.; *Clem.*; Kali p.; Phos.; *Puls.*

From eating—Rhod.

From kneeling, and pressing head firmly against floor—Sang.
From motion, open air—Thuya.
From pressure—Cinch.; *Col.;* Mag. m.; *Rhod.*
From rest—Col.; Nux v.
From rubbing—Acon.; *Plat.*
From warmth—Ars.; Calc. c.; *Col.;* Cupr. ac.; Mag. m.; *Mag. p.;* Mez.; Thuya. See Modalities.

SENSATIONS—**Burning heat:** *Agar.;* Agrost.; Ant. c.; *Ars.;* Arum; *Canth.;* Caps.; *Cham.;* Euphorbia; Kali c.; Nat. c.; Sang.; Senega; Sil.; Stront.; *Sul.;* Viola tr.

Cobwebs dried on, as if—Alum.; *Bar. c.;* Bor.; Brom.; Euphorbia; *Graph.;* Phos. ac.; *Ran. s.*

Coldness—Abrot.; *Agar.;* Ant. t.; *Camph.;* Carbo v.; Dros.; *Helod.;* Phos. ac.; *Plat.;* Ver. a. See Hippocratic Face.

Contracted, wrinkled feeling, in forehead—*Bapt.;* Bellis; Grat.; *Helleb.;* Phos.; Primula.

Formication (numbness, tingling, crawling)—*Acon.;* Agar.; Colch.; Gymnocl.; Helod.; Myr.; Nux v.; *Plat.*

Itching—*Agar.;* Ant. c.; *Mez.;* Myr.; Nat. m.; Rhus t.; Sep.; Stront.

TIC-DOULOUREUX–*Acon.; Aconit.;* Ananth.; Arg. n.; *Ars.; Bell.;* Caps.; Cim.; *Coccinel.;* Colch.; Cupr. m.; *Gels.;* Glon.; Graph.; Kali c.; Kali chlor.; *Kali iod.; Mag. p.;* Mez.; Nat. s.; Nux v.; *Phos.;* Rhus t.; Sep.; **Stann.;** Staph.; Sul.; *Strych.; Thuya;* Verbasc.; Zinc. m. See **Prosopalgia**, Trifacial Neuralgia.

MOUTH

BREATH, cold—Ant. t.; Ars.; *Camph.*; Carbo v.; Cistus; Cupr. m.; Euphorb. dath.; *Helod.*; Jatropha; *Tab.*; Tereb.; *Ver. a*.

Breath, offensive (fetor oris)—Abies n.; Alum.; Ambra; Anac.; *Ant. c.*; *Arn.*; *Ars.*; *Aur.*; Bapt.; Bor.; Bry.; Calc. c.; Caps.; *Carb. ac.*; Carbo v.; Chel.; Cinch.; Cistus; Daphne; *Diph.*; Graph.; Helleb.; *Hep.*; Indol.; *Iod.*; Kalagua; Kali chlor.; Kali per.; Kali p.; *Kali tell.*; Kreos.; Lach.; Merc. c.; Merc. cy.; Merc. d.; *Merc. s.*; Mur. ac.; *Nat. tell.*; Nit. ac.; Nux v.; *Petrol.*; Phyt.; Psor.; *Puls.*; Quercus; Rheum; *Sep.*; Sinap.; Spig.; Stann.; Sul. ac.; Tereb.

Breath offensive, after meals only—Cham.; Nux v.; Sul.

Breath offensive, in evening or night—Puls.; Sul.

Breath offensive, in girls at puberty—Aur. m.

Breath offensive, in morning only—*Arn.*; Bell.; Nux v.; Sil.; Sul.

EXTERNAL MOUTH—Commissures (corners): Color: pearly white about: Æth.; *Cina*; Santon.

Color, yellow about—Sep.

Cracks, ulcerations—Am. m.; *Ant. c.*; Ars.; *Arum*; Arundo; Bov.; *Condur.*; Echin.; Eup. perf.; *Graph.*; Helleb.; *Hep.*; Nat. m.; *Nit. ac.*; Petrol.; Rhus t.; Sec.

Eruptions around—Ant. c.; *Ars.*; Aster.; Echin.; *Graph.*; *Hep.*; Naph.; Mez.; Mur. ac.; *Nat. m.*; Petrol.; Senega.

LIPS—Black:—*Ars.*; Bry.; *Merc. c.*; Vipera.

Blue, cyanosed—Ars.; *Camph.*; Carbo an.; Carbo v.; Cupr. *m.*; Cupr. *s.*; *Dig.*; Hydroc. ac.; Sec.; *Ver. a.*; Zinc. See Face.

Burning, hot, parched—Acon.; Arn.; *Ars.*; Arum; *Bry.*; Caps.; Illic.; Nat. m.; Phos.; Rhus t.; *Sul.*; Thyr.

Cancer—Acet. ac.; *Ars.*; Ars. iod.; Clem.; Commocl.; Condur.; Con.; Hydr.; Kreos.; Lyc.; Sep.; Tab.; Thuya.

Chewing motion—Acon.; *Bell.*; Bry.; Helleb.; Stram.

Cold sores, herpes, hydroa—Agar.; Ars.; Calc. fl.; *Caps.*; Dulc.; Frax. am.; Hep.; Med.; *Nat. m.*; *Rhus t.*; Rhus v.; Sep.; Sul. iod.; Upas.

Cracks, ulcerations—Ant. c.; *Ars.*; *Arum*; Bry.; Carbo v.; Carbon. s.; *Clem.*; Condur.; Echin.; Glycerin; *Graph.*; Kali bich.; Merc. pr. rub.; Mur. ac.; Nat. m.; *Nit. ac.*; Phos.; *Rhus t.*; Sil.

Cracks, ulcerations in middle of lower lip—Am. c.; Graph.; *Hep.*; Nat. m.; Puls.; Sep.

Distortion—*Art. v.*; Cadm. s.; *Cic.*; Cupr. ac.; Cur.; Stram.

Dryness—Acon.; Ant. c.; *Bry.*; Chionanth.; Cinch.; Euonym.; Glycerin; Helleb.; *Helon.*; Mur. ac.; *Nat. m.*; Nux m.; Phos. ac.; Puls.; Rhus t.; Senec.; Sep.; *Sul.*; Zinc. m. See Burning.

Eczema—*Ant. c.*; Aur. mur.; Bov.; Calc. c.; Graph.; Lyc.; *Mez.*; *Rhus v.*

Eruptions—Acne: Bor.; Psor.; Sars.; Sul. iod.

Exfoliation—Con.; Sep.

Foam at the mouth—Absinth.; Cic.; Cupr. ac.; *Cupr. m.*; Hydroc. ac.; Hyos.; Lyssin; Œnanthe; Op. See Convulsions (Nervous System).

Glued together—Can. ind.; Helon.
Licks them frequently—Puls.
Numbness, tingling—Acon.; Crot.; Echin.; Nat. m.
Pain, soreness—Arum; Bor.; Calc. c.; Illic.; Nat. m.; Rhus t.; Rhus v.; Sep.
Picks them until they bleed—Arum; Helleb.; Zinc. m.
Red, bleeding—Arum; Kreos.
Red, crimson—Aloe; Sul.; Tub.
Swelling—Antipyr.; Apis; Bov.; Bry.; Caps.; Medusa; Merc. c.; Rhus v.; Vipera.
Swelling of lower—Puls.; Sep.
Swelling of upper—Apis; Bell.; Calc. c.; Hep.; Nat. c.; Nat. m.; Psor.; Rhus t.
Twitching, spasmodic—Agar.; Art. v.; Cim.; Gels.; Ign.; Myg.; Niccol.; Op.; Strych.
Ulcer, cancerous—Ars.

INNER MOUTH—(buccal cavity): **Bleeding, after tooth extraction:** Arn.; Bov.; Cinch.; Ham.
Burning, smarting—Acon.; Aesc.; Apis; Ars.; Arum; Bell.; Bor.; Bry.; Caps.; Canth.; Carb. ac.; Carbo v.; Colch.; Ferr. p.; Iris; Merc. c.; Sang.; Sul.; Tarax.; Vespa.
Canker-sores—Agave; Ant. c.; Arg. n.; Ars.; Bor.; Caps.; Carbo v.; Echin.; Hydr.; Kali bich.; Kali chlor.; Lach.; Lyc.; Merc. c.; Merc.; Mur. ac.; Nat. hypochlor.; Nat. m.; Nit. ac.; Phyt.; Sal. ac.; Sul. ac.; Sul. See Aphthous Stomatitis.
Coldness—Camph.; Cistus; Coccinel.; Sinap. n.; Ver. a.
Dryness—Acon.; Aesc.; Alum.; Apis; Ars.; Bell.; Bor.; Bry.; Cupr.; Dub.; Hyos.; Iris ten.; Kali bich.; Kali p.; Lach.; Lyc.; Merc. c.; Merc. per.; Morph.; Mur. ac.; Nat. m.; Nat. s.; Nux m.; Op.; Phos.; Puls.; Radium; Rhus t.; Sang.; Senec.; Sep.; Tereb.
Dryness, with great thirst—Acon.; Ars.; Bry.; Rhus t.; Sul., Ver. a.
Dryness, yet no thirst—Apis; Lach.; Lyc.; Nux m.; Paris; Puls.; Sabad.
Glands, salivary cellular tissue inflamed—Anthrac.; Bry.; Hep.; Merc.; Mur. ac.
Inflammation (stomatitis)—in general: Acon.; Alum.; Arg. n.; Arum; Bapt.; Bell.; Bor.; Caps.; Corn. c.; Hydr.; Kali chlor.; Kali m.; Merc. c.; Merc. s.; Nat. m.; Nit. ac.; Nux v.; Ran. s.; Sep.; Sinap. n.; Sul.; Sul. ac.; Vespa.
Inflammation, aphthous (thrush)—Æth.; Ant. t.; Ars.; Bapt.; Bor.; Bry.; Carbo v.; Eup. arom.; Hydr.; Hydrast. m.; Kali chlor.; Kali m.; Merc. c.; Merc. s.; Mur. ac.; Nat. m.; Nit. ac.; Rhus gl.; Sars.; Semperv. t.; Sul. ac.; Sul.
Inflammation, follicular, vesicular—Anac.; Ananth.; Canth.; Caps.; Kali chlor.; Hydrast. m.; Mag. c.; Nat. m.; Mur. ac.; Rhus t.; Sul.
Inflammation, gangrenous (noma, cancrum oris)—Ars.; Bapt.; Hydr.; Kali chlor.; Kali p.; Kreos.; Lach.; Merc. c.; Merc. s.; Mur. ac.; Sec.; Sul. ac.
Inflammation, mercurial—Bapt.; Carbo v.; Hep.; Hydr.; Mur. ac.; Nit. ac.

MOUTH

Inflammation, ulcerative—Agave; Alnus; *Arg. n.*; *Ars.*; Arum; Bapt.; Bor.; Chlor.; *Cinnab.*; Coryd.; *Hep.*; *Hydrast. m.*; Kali bich.; *Kali chlor.*; Kali cy.; Mag. c.; Menthol; *Merc. c.*; *Merc. s.*; *Mur. ac.*; *Nit. ac.*; Nit. mur. ac.; Phos.; *Rhus gl.*; Sul. ac.; Sulphurous ac.; **Tarax.**

Itching—Arundo; Bor.; Kali bich.

Mucous membrane glossy, as if varnished—*Apis*; Nit. ac.; Tereb.

Mucous membrane inflamed from burns—Apis; Canth.

Mucous membrane pallid—Ferr. m.; Morph.

Mucous membrane red, dusky—*Bapt.*; Lach.; Morph.; *Phyt.*

Mucous membrane red, tumid, with gray-based ulcers—Kali chlor. See Stomatitis.

Pain—Apis; *Arum*; Bell.; Bor.; Hep.; *Merc.*; *Nit. ac.*; Upas. See Stomatitis.

Pain from plate of teeth, worse on touch, eating—Alumen; Bor.

PALATE—Aphthæ: Agave.

Blisters—Nat. s.

Coating, creamy—Nat. p.

Constriction, scratching—Acon.

Dryness—Carbo an.

Edema—Apis.

Elongated—Strych. See Uvula.

Itching, tickling—*Arundo;* Gels.; Wyeth.

Necrosis, caries—*Aur.;* Merc. cy.

Red, swollen—Acon.; *Apis;* Aur.; Bell.; Fluor. ac.; *Kali iod.;* Merc. c.

Ulceration, rawness—Ant. c.; *Arum; Cinnab.;* Hep.; Merc. c.; Merc. per.; *Nit. ac.;* Sul. ac.; Tarax. See Throat.

Wrinkled; pain on chewing, nursing—Bor.

PTYALISM—Saliva, increased: *Acet. ac.;* Allium s.; Anac.; Ant. c.; *Arum;* Bapt.; Bism.; Bry.; Cham.; Chionanth.; Cinch.; Colch.; Cupr. m.; Daphne; Dig.; Dulc.; *Epiph.; Euphorb.;* Granat.; Hep.; *Iod.; Ipec.; Iris; Jabor.;* Kali chlor.; *Kali iod.;* Kali perm.; Lac c.; Lact. ac.; *Lob. infl.;* Merc. c.; Merc. cy.; Merc. d.; Merc. i. r.; *Merc. s.;* Mez.; Muscar.; Nat. m.; *Nit. ac.; Nit. mur. ac.;* Phos.; *Piloc.;* Pod.; Ptel.; *Puls.;* Rhus t.; Sang.; Sars.; Sep.; Sul.; *Syph.;* Tab.; Trifol.

After eating—Allium s.

During pregnancy—Acet. ac.; *Granat.; Iod.; Jabor.;* Lact. ac.; *Merc.;* Muscar.; Nit. ac.; Piloc.; Sep. See Pregnancy (Female Sexual System).

During sleep—*Cham.;* Coccinel.; Lact. ac.; *Merc.;* Rheum; *Syph.*

From mercurialization—*Hep.;* Iod.; *Iris;* Kali chlor.; Nit. ac.

Saliva acrid, hot—Ars.; *Arum;* Bor.; Daphne; *Kali chlor.;* Kreos.; **Merc.;** *Nit. ac.;* Taxus.

Bitter—*Ars.;* Atham.; Bry.; Kali s.; *Puls.;* Sul.

Bloody—Antipyr.; *Ars.;* Mag. c.; *Merc.; Nit. ac.;* Nux v.

FETID, offensive—Ars.; *Iod.;* Kreos.; Mancin.; Merc. d.; *Merc. s.;* **Nit.** *ac.;* Psor.; Rheum.

Frothy, cotton-like—Alet.; Aqua mar.; *Berb. v.;* Bry.; Canth.; Lyssin; *Nux m.;* Nux v.; Phos. ac.; Sul.

Metallic—Bism.; Cham.; Cocc.; *Cupr. m.*; *Merc.*; *Nit. ac.*; Zinc.
Milky—Plumb. oxy.
Mucus—Bell.; Colch.; *Dulc.*; *Nit. ac.*; Phos. ac.; *Phos.*; Puls.
Ropy, tenacious, slimy, soapy—Am. m.; Ant. c.; Arg. n.; Dulc.; *Epiph.; Hydrast. m.*; Hydr.; Iod.; Iris; *Kali bich.*; Kali chlor.; Lyssin; *Merc. s.*; *Merc. v.*; Myr.; Nat. m.; Piloc.; *Puls.*; Tarax.
Salty—Ant. c.; *Euphorb.*; Lact. ac.; *Merc. c.*; *Nat. m.*; Phos.; Sep.; Ver. a.
Sour—*Iris*; *Nit. ac.*; Nux v.; Paris; Pod.
Sweetish—Cupr. m.; Merc.; Plumb. ac.; *Puls.*; Stann.
Watery—Asar.; Bism.; Iod.; Jabor.; Lob. infl.; *Nat. m.*; Phos.; Trifol.
ULCERATIONS—Soreness of mouth: Alum.; *Arg. n.*; *Ars.*; *Arum*; *Bor.*; Caps.; *Hep.*; *Hydrast. mur.*; Hydr.; Kali chlor.; *Merc. c.*; *Merc. s.*; *Mur. ac.*; *Nit. ac.*; Nux m.; Phyt.; *Ran. s.*; *Rhus gl.*; Semperv. t.; Sinap. n.; Sul. ac.; Tarax. See Stomatitis (Ulcerative).
Ulcerations, syphilitic mucous patches—*Cinnab.*: Kali bich.; *Merc. c.*; Merc. nit.; Merc. pr. rub.; Merc. s.; *Nit. ac.*; Still.; *Thuya* See Male Sexual System.
Varicose veins—Ambra; Thuya.

TONGUE

COATING—COLOR—Blackish—*Ars.;* Bapt.; Camph.; Lach.; Lyc.; **Merc. c.;** *Merc. cy.;* Merc. d.; Merc. v.; *Op.;* Phos.; Rhus t.; Vipera.

Bluish, livid, pale—Ars.; *Cupr. s.;* Dig.; *Gymnocl.;* Merc. cy.; *Morph.;* Op.; Mur. ac.; *Sec.;* Ver. a.; Vipera.

Brownish—Am. c.; Ant. t.; *Ars.;* Bapt.; *Bry.;* Cupr. ars.; Echin.; Hyos.; Med.; *Merc. cy.;* Morph.; Mur. ac.; Nat. s.; Phos.; Sec.; Vipera.

Brown center—*Bapt.;* Phos.; Plumb. m.

Brownish, dry—*Ail.;* Ant. t.; *Ars.;* Bapt.; *Bry.;* Kali p.; *Lach.; Rhus t.;* Spong.; Tart. ac.; Vipera.

Clean—Ars.; *Asar.; Cina;* Cinch.; *Coryd.;* Dig.; *Ipec.;* Mag. p.; Nit. ac.; *Pyr.; Rhus t.;* Sep.

Clean anteriorly, coated posteriorly—Nux v.

Clean at menstrual nisus, foul after flow ceases—Sep.

Dark streak in center, typhoid tongue—Arn.; Bapt.; Mur. ac.

Flabby, moist, with imprints of teeth—Ars.; Chel.; *Hydr.;* Kali bich.; Merc. c.; *Merc. d.; Merc. s.;* Nat. p.; *Pod.;* Pyr.; *Rhus t.;* Sanic.; Stram.; Yucca.

Frothy, with bubbles on side—Nat. m.

Furred—Ant. t.; Ars.; *Bapt.;* Canth.; *Card. m.;* Chin. ars.; Coca; Ferr. picr.; Gels.; Guaiac.; Lyc.; Myr.; *Nux v.;* Puls.; Rumex. See White.

Grayish-white base—Kali m.

Greenish—Nat. s.; Plumb. ac.

Mapped—Ant. c.; *Ars.;* Kali bich.; Lach.; Merc. v.; *Nat. m.;* Nit. ac.; Ox. ac.; Phyt.; Ran. s.; Rhus t.; *Tarax.;* Tereb.

Mapped, with red, insular patches—Nat. m.

Red—Acon.; *Apis;* Ars.; *Bell.; Bor. ac.; Canth.;* Crot.; Diph.; Gels.; Hyos.; *Kali bich.;* Lach.; Merc. c.; Mez.; Nux v.; *Pyr.; Rhus t.;* Tereb.

Red, dry, especially center—Ant. t.; Rhus t.

Red edges—Amyg. pers.; Ant. t.; Ars.; Bapt.; *Bell.;* Canth.; Card. m.; *Chel.;* Echin.; Kali bich.; Lac c.; Lach.; Merc. c.; Merc. i. fl.; *Merc.;* Nit. ac.; Pod.; *Rhus t.;* Rhus v.; Sul.; Tarax.

Red edges, white center—*Bell.;* Rhus t.

Red in center, or streaks—Ant. t.; *Ars.;* Caust.; Crot.; Ver. v.

Red, papillæ pale, effaced—Allium s.

Red, papillæ prominent—Ant. t.; *Arg. n.;* Ars.; *Bell.;* Kali bich.; Lyc.; Mez.; Nux m.; *Ptel.;* Tereb.

Red, raw—Ars.; *Arum;* Canth.; Tarax.

Red, shining, glossy, as if varnished—Apis; *Canth.;* Crot.; Jal.; *Kali bich.;* Lach.; *Nit. ac.;* Phos.; *Pyr.;* Rhus t.; *Tereb.*

Red spots, sensitive—Ran. s.; *Tarax;* Tereb.

Red tip—Amyg. pers.; *Arg. n.;* Ars.; Cycl.; Merc. i. fl.; Phyt.; *Rhus t.;* Rhus v.; Sul.

Red, wet, central furrow—Nit. ac.

Strawberry—*Bell.;* Fragar.; Sapon.

Unilateral—*Daphne;* Lob. infl.; Rhus t.

White-furred, slimy, pasty—Acon.; Æsc.; Ant. c.; Ant. t.; Arg. n.; Arn.; Bapt.; Bell.; Bism.; Bry.; Calc. c.; Carbo v.; Card. m.; *Chel.;* Cinch.; Cycl.; Ferr. ; Glon.; Hedeoma; *Hydr.;* Ipec.; Kali c.; Kali chlor.; Kali m.; Lac c.; Lob. infl.; Lyc.; Merc. c.; *Merc.;* Mez.; Nat. m.; Nux v.; Ox. ac.; Paris; Petrol.; Phos.; *Puls.;* Sep.; Sul.; Tarax.; Ver. v.

Yellow, dirty, thick coating—*Æsc.;* Bapt.; Bry.; Carbo v.; Cham.; *Chel.;* Chionanth.; *Cinch.;* Ferr.; *Hydr.;* Indol; *Kali bich.;* Kali s.; Lept.; Lyc.; Merc. d.; Merc. i. fl.; *Merc.;* Myr.; Nat. p.; *Nat. s.;* Nux v.; Ostrya; Pod.; *Puls.;* Sang.; Sul.; *Yucca.*

Yellow patch in center—Bapt.; Phyt.

CONDITIONS—Anæsthesia—Carbon. s.

Atrophy—Mur. ac.

Biting—Absinth.; Hydr.; Hyos.; *Ign.;* Illic.; Phos. ac.; Sec.

Burning, smarting scalded feeling—Acon.; Apis; *Ars.;* Arum; Bapt.; Bell.; Berb. v.; Canth.; Caps.; Carbo an.; Caust.; Col.; *Iris;* Lyc.; Merc. c.; Mez.; *Mur. ac.;* Nat. m.; Phos. ac.; Pod.; Ran. s.; *Sang.;* Sanic.; Sinap.; Sul.

Burning tip—*Ars.;* Bar. c.; Calc. c.; Caps.; *Iris;* Lathyrus; Physost.; *Sang.;* Tereb.

Coldness—Acet. ac.; *Camph.;* Carbo v.; *Cistus;* Helod.; Hydroc. ac.; Sec.; *Ver. a.*

Dryness—Acon.; Ail.; Ant. t.; Apis; *Ars.;* Bapt.; *Bell.;* Bry.; Calc. c.; Colch.; Hyos.; Kali bich.; Kali c.; Lach.; Leonur.; Merc. c.; Merc.; Morph.; *Mur. ac.;* Nat. m.; *Nux m.;* Paris; Phos. ac.; Phos.; Puls.; Pyr.; Rhus t.; Sul.; Tereb.; Ver. v.; Vipera.

ERUPTIONS, growths—Cancer: Alumen; Apis; Ars.; Aur.; Aur. m. n.; Crot.; Galium; Hoang nan; Kali chlor.; *Kali cy.;* Mur. ac.; Semperv. t.; *Thuya;* Vib. pr.

Cracks, excoriations—Ananth.; *Ars.;* Arum; Arundo; Bapt.; Bell.; Bor. ac.; Bor.; Bry.; Cham.; *Kali bich.;* Lach.; Leonur.; Nat. m.; *Nit. ac.;* Phyt.; Plumb. ac.; Pyr.; Ran. s.; *Rhus t.;* Rhus v.; Semperv. t. See Ulcerations.

Epithelioma—Ars.; Carb. ac.; Chrom. ac.; *Hydr.; Kali cy.;* Mur. ac.; *Thuya.*

Furrows lengthwise, in upper part—Merc.

Growths, nodules—Ars. hydr.; *Aur.;* Aur. m. n.; Castor.; *Gall. ap.;* Mur. ac.; Nit. ac.; *Thuya.*

Psoriasis—*Cast. eq.;* Kali bich.; *Mur. ac.*

Ranula—Ambra; *Calc. c.;* Ferr. p.; Fluor. ac.; Merc. s.; Nit. ac.; *Thuya.*

Ring worm—Nat. m.; Sanic. See Red edges.

Ulcerations—Apis; *Arg. n.;* Ars.; Ars. hydr.; Bapt.; Fluor. ac.; Kali bich.; Lyc.; *Merc.;* Mur. ac.; *Nit. ac.; Nit. mur. ac.;* Sang. n.; Semperv. t.; Syph.; Thuya.

Ulcerations, syphilitic—Aur.; *Cinnab.;* Fluor. ac.; *Kali bich.;* Lach.; Merc.; Mez.; *Nit. ac.*

Veins, varicose—Ambra; *Ham.;* Thuya.

Vesicles, blisters—Am. c.; Apis; Berb. v.; Bor.; *Canth.;* Carbo an.; La-

TONGUE

cert.; *Lyc.*; Merc. per.; Mur. ac.; *Nat. p.*; *Nat. m.*; Nit. ac.; Phyt.; *Rhus t.*; Sul. ac.; *Sul.*; Thuya.

Warts—Aur. mur.; Mang. ac.

Hard, induration of—Alumen; Aur. m.; *Calc. fl.*; Mur. ac.; Semperv. t.; *Sil.*

Heaviness—Caust.; Colch.; Gels.; Guaco; Merc. per.; Mur. ac.; Nux v.

Inflammation (glossitis)—*Acon.*; *Apis*; Ars.; Bell.; Canth.; Crot.; *Lach.*; Merc. c.; Merc.; *Mur. ac.*; Ox. ac.; Phyt.; Ran. s.; *Sul. ac.*; *Vipera*. See Swelling.

Numbness, tingling—*Acon.*; Con.; Echin.; *Gels.*; Ign.; Lathyrus; Merc. per.; *Nat. m.*; Nux m.; Nux v.; Plat.; Radium; Rheum; Sec.

Pain—Acon.; *Ars.*; Arum; Bell.; Kali ars.; Kali iod.; Merc. v.; *Nit. ac.*; *Phyt.*; Ruta; Semperv. t.; *Thuya*. See Soreness.

Paralysis—Acon. cam.; Acon.; Anac.; Arn.; Ars.; Bar. c.; *Bell.*; *Bothrops*; Can. ind.; *Caust.*; Cocc.; *Con.*; Cupr.; *Cur.*; *Dulc.*; *Gels.*; Guaco; Hyos.; Lach.; Lob. purp.; *Mur. ac.*; Nux m.; Oleand.; Op.; *Plumb. m.*; Sec.; Stram.; Zinc. s. See Nervous System.

Protrusion, difficult—Anac.; *Apis*; Ars.; Calc. c.; *Caust.*; Crot.; Dulc.; Guaco; Gels.; Hyos.; *Lach.*; Merc.; Mur. ac.; *Myg.*; Nat. m.; Pyr.; Plumb. m.; Stram.; Sulphon; Tereb.

Protrusion, snake-like—Absinth.; Crot.; *Cupr.*; *Lach.*; Lyc.; Merc.; Sanic.; *Vipera*.

Rawness, roughness—Apis; *Ars.*; *Arum*; *Canth.*; Dulc.; *Nit. ac.*; Phyt.; *Ran. s.*; Tarax.

Sensation, as if hair on tongue—Allium s.; Kali bich.; Nat. m.; *Sil.*

Sensation, as if swollen, enlarged—Absinth.; Æth.; *Anac.*; Crot.; Nux v.; Ptel.; Puls.

Soreness—*Apis*; *Arum*; Cistus; Kali c.; Merc. c.; Mur. ac.; *Nit. ac.*; Ox. ac.; Phelland.; Physost.; *Ran. s.*; *Rhus t.*; Semperv. t.; Sep.; Sil.; *Tereb.*; Thuya.

Spasm—Acon.; Bell.; Ruta; Sec. See Trembling.

Stiffness—Con.; *Dulc.*; Hyos.; Lac c.; Merc. i. r.; Nicol.; Sec.; Stram.

Swelling—*Acon.*; *Apis*; Ars.; Arum; Aster.; Bapt.; *Bell.*; Bism.; Cajup.; *Canth.*; *Crot.*; Diph.; Fragar.; Kali tell.; Lach.; Mag. p.; *Merc. c.*; *Mez.*; *Mur. ac.*; Œnanthe; Ox. ac.; Pelias; Ruta; Thuya; *Vespa*; *Vipera*.

Trembling—*Absinth.*; *Agar.*; *Agraricin*; Apis; Ars.; *Bell.*; Camph.; Caust.; Cham.; Gels.; *Lach.*; *Merc.*; Plumb.; **Stram.**

TASTE

LOST—Amyg. per.; Ant. c.; Bry.; Cycl.; Formal.; Gymnema; Justicia; Lyc.; Mag. c.; *Mag. m.*; *Nat. m.*; Pod.; *Puls.*; Sang.; Sil.; Sul.

PERVERTED—ALTERED—In general: Æsc.; *Alum.*; Ant. t.; *Arg. n.*; Arn.; Ars.; Calc. c.; Camph.; Carbo v.; Chel.; *Cinch.*; Cycl.; Fagop.; *Gymnema;* Hydr.; Kali c.; Lyc.; Mag. c.; Mag. m.; Merc. c.; *Merc. s.; Nat. m.*; Nit. ac.; *Nux v.*; Paris; Pod.; *Puls.*; Rheum; Sep.; Sul.; Zinc. mur.

After eating—Ars.; Carbo v.; *Nat. m.*; Nit. ac.; Zinc.

After sleep—Rheum.

Acid, astringent, sour—Aloe; Am. c.; *Calc. c.*; Carbo v.; Cham.; Cinch.; Euphorbia; Hep.; *Hydr.*; Ign.; Iris; Kali c.; Lob. infl.; *Lyc.*; *Mag. c.*; Nat. p.; Nit. ac.; *Nux v.*; Phos. ac.; Phos.; *Puls.*; Sep.; *Sul.*

Bitter, bilious—*Acon.*; Aloe; Ars.; *Atham.*; Bapt.; *Bry.*; Camph.; *Card. m.*; *Cham.*; *Chel.*; *Cinch.*; *Col.*; Cupr.; Dig.; *Hydr.*; Ipec.; Kali c.; *Lyc.*; Merc. c.; *Myr.*; Nat. m.; Nat. s.; *Nux v.*; Paris; Pod.; Ptel.; *Puls.*; Rhus t.; Sabad.; *Sep.*; Stann.; *Sul.*; Tarax.

Bitter from tobacco—*Asar.*; Euphras.; Puls.

Bloody-like—*Alum.*; Chel.; Kali c.; Mancin.; *Nit. ac.*; Sil.; Sul.; Trifol.; Zinc.

Coppery, metallic—Æsc.; Arg. n.; Ars.; Bism.; Cocc.; *Cupr. ars.*; *Cupr. m.*; Lact. ac.; *Lob. infl.*; Merc. c.; Nit. mur. ac.; Nux v.; *Rhus t.*; Sul.

Delicate, changeable—Coff.; *Puls.*

Disgusting, putrid, foul, slimy—*Arn.*; Aur. mur.; Bor.; Calc. c.; *Carbo v.*; Chel.; Ferr. m.; Graph.; Hep.; Indol; Led.; Lemna m.; Lyc.; Merc. c.; *Merc.*; Nat. m.; Nat. s.; Nux v.; Petrol.; Phos.; Pod.; *Puls.*; Pyr.; Sep.; Yucca.

Flat, insipid, straw-like, pappy—Ant. c.; Ant. t.; *Ars.*; Bapt.; Bor.; *Cinch.*; *Cycl.*; Euphor. amyg.; *Ferr. m.*; Glycerin; Ign.; Kali s.; Nux m.; *Puls.*

Greasy, fatty, pasty—Arn.; Carbo v.; Caust.; Euonym.; Ol. an.; Phos.; *Puls.*; Trill. cer.

Peppery—Hydr.

Perverted in morning—Fagop.; Graph.; Hydr.; *Nux v.*; Puls.

Salty—Ant. c.; Ars.; *Bell.*; Cadm. s.; *Carbo v.*; Cinch.; *Cycl.*; Merc. c.; *Merc.*; *Puls.*; Sep.; Sul.; Zinc. m.

Sweet—Agar.; *Apoc. andr.*; Bism.; Chel.; Cupr. m.; Dig.; Glycerin; *Merc.*; *Nit. ac.*; Phelland.; *Plumb.*; Puls.; *Pyr.*; Sabad.; Selen.; Stann.

GUMS

BLEEDING easily—*Agave;* Alum.; Ambra; Ant. c.; *Arg. n.;* Arn.; Ars.; Bapt.; Benz. ac.; Bor.; Calc. c.; *Carbo v.;* Cistus; Crotal.; Echin.; Hep.; *Iod.; Kreos.;* Lach.; Merc. c.; *Merc.;* Nit. c.; Phos.; Plant.; Sep.; Sil.; Staph.; Sul. ac.; Sul.; Zinc.

Bleeding protractedly, after tooth extraction—Ars.; Bov., *Ham.; Kreos.;* Phos.; Trill.

Blue line along margin—Plumb.

Burning—Antypr. See Pain.

Cold feeling—Coccinel.

Desire to press teeth together—Phyt.; Pod.

Epulis—Calc. c.; Plumb.; *Thuya.*

Inflammation (gumboil)—*Acon.;* Bell.; Bor.; *Calc. fl.;* Calc. s.; Cham.; *Hekla;* Hep.; Kreos.; Merc. c.; *Merc.;* Phos.; Rhus t.; *Sil.* See Pain, Swelling.

Painful after tooth extraction—Arn.; Sep.

Painful, sore, sensitive—Alum.; Am. c.; Arg. n.; *Bapt.;* Bell.; Bor.; Calc. c.; *Carbo v.;* Caust.; *Cham.;* Dolichos; *Hep.;* Kreos.; *Merc.;* Nit. ac.; Plant.; Rhus t.; *Sil.;* Sul.; Thuya.

Red seam (strophulus)—*Ant. c.;* Apis; *Cham.;* Kali p.; *Puls.;* Rhus t.

Scorbutic (soft, spongy, receding)—*Agave;* Alum.; Ant. c.; Arn.; Ars.; Bapt.; *Carbo v.;* Cistus; Echin.; Hep.; *Iod.;* Kali c.; Kali chlor.; Kali p.; *Kreos.; Merc.; Mur. ac.;* Nat. m.; *Nit. ac.; Phos.;* Staph.; Sul.; Thuya.

Swelling—*Apis;* Bell.; Bism.; Calc. c.; Caust.; *Cham.;* Cistus; Graph.; Kreos.; Lach.; Mag. m.; Merc. c.; Merc. d.; *Merc. i. r.; Merc. v.;* Mur. ac.; Nit. ac.; *Phos.;* Plumb.; Rhod.; Sep.; Sil.; Staph.; Sul.; Tereb.

Ulceration (pyorrhœa alveolaris)—Aur.; *Bapt.;* Carbo v.; *Caust.; Cistus;* Emetine; Kali c.; Kreos.; *Merc. c.; Merc.; Nit. ac.;* Phos.; *Plant.; Sep.; Sil.; Staph.;* Sul. ac.; Thuya.

TEETH

ALVEOLAR abscess—Hep.; Merc.; Sil.

Black, dark, crumbling—Ant. c.; *Kreos.*; Merc.; Phos. hydr.; *Staph.*; Syph.; Thuya.

Caries, decay, premature—Calc. c.; Calc. fl.; *Calc. p.*; Cocc.; Fluor. ac.; Hekla; *Kreos.*; Merc.; *Mez.*; Phos.; *Plant.*; Sil.; *Staph.*; Tub.

Caries at crown—Merc.; *Staph.*

Caries at root—*Merc.*; Mez.; Sil.; Syph.; *Thuya.*

Cupped, dwarfed, serrated—Staph.; *Syph.*

DENTITION—(teething difficult, delayed): Acon.; *Bell.*; Bor.; Calc. c.; *Calc. p.*; Caust.; *Cham.*; Cheiranth.; *Coff.*; *Cupr.*; Gels.; *Hekla;* Kali br.; *Kreos.*; Mag. p.; Merc.; Nux v.; Passifl.; Phyt.; *Pod.*; Puls.; *Sil.*; Solan. n.; Staph.; Sul.; *Tereb.*; Zinc. br.; Zinc. m.

With cerebral, nervous symptoms—Acon.; Agar.; *Bell.*; *Cham.*; Cim.; Cyprip.; Dolichos; *Helleb.*; Kali br.; *Pod.*; Solan. n.; Tereb.; *Zinc.*

With compression of gums—Cic.; Phyt.; Pod.

With constipation, general irritation, cachexia—*Kreos.*; Nux v.; Op.

With convulsions—*Bell.*; Calc. c.; *Cham.*; Cic.; Cupr.; Glon.; Kali br.; *Mag. p.*; Solan. n.; Stann.; Zinc. br.

With cough—Acon.; Bell.; Ferr. p.; Kreos.

With deafness, otorrhœa, stuffiness of nose—Cheiranth.

With diarrhœa—Æth.; *Calc. c.*; *Calc. p.*; *Cham.*; Ferr. p.; Ipec.; Kreos.; Mag. c.; Merc.; Oleand.; Phos.; *Pod.*; Puls.; Rheum; *Sil.*

With effusion threatened, in brain—*Apis*; Helleb.; Tub.; *Zinc. m.*

With eye symptoms—Bell.; Calc. c.; Puls.

With insomnia—Bell.; Cham.; *Coff.*; *Cyprip.*; Kreos.; Passifl.; Scutel.; Tereb.

With intertrigo—Caust.; Lyc.

With milk indigestion—Æth.; Calc. c.; *Mag. m.*

With salivation—Bor.

With sour smell of body, pale face, irritability—Kreos.

With weakness, pallor, fretfulness, must be carried rapidly—Ars.

With worms—*Cina*; Merc.; Stann.

FEEL cold—*Coccinel.*; Gamb.; Phos. ac.; Rheum.

Feel loose—Alum.; Am. c.; Arn.; Bism.; Calc. fl.; Cardo v.; Hyos.; Lyc.; *Merc. c.*; *Merc.*; Nit. ac.; *Plant.*; Rhus t.; Sil.; Zinc.

Feel numb—Plat.

Feel sensitive to cold, chewing, touch—*Acon.*; Ars.; Bell.; Carbo v.; Cham.; *Coff.*; *Fluor. ac.*; Gymnocl.; Merc.; Parth.; Plant.; Staph. See Pain.

Feel too long—Bry.; Carbo v.; Caust.; *Cham.*; Clem.; Lyc.; Mag. c.; *Merc.*; *Mez.*; Parth.; Plant.; Ratanh.; Rhus t.

Feel warm—Fluor. ac.

FISTULA DENTALIS—Calc. fl.; Caust.; *Fluor. ac.*; Nat. m.; *Sil.*; Staph.; Sul.

GRINDING—Apis; *Bell.*; Can. ind.; *Cic.*; Cina; Helleb.; Myg.; *Phyt.*; Plant.; *Pod.*; Santon.; Spig.; Zinc.

ODONTALGIA—Toothache—Remedies in general: Acon.; Agar.; Ant. c.; Antipyr.; Apis; *Ars.*; Atrop.; *Bell.*; *Bry.*; Calc. c.; Carb. ac.; Carbo v.; *Cham*; *Clem.*; Coccinel.; *Coff.*; Col.; Ferr. m.; Gels.; Glon.; Hekla; Ign.; Kali c.; *Kreos.*; Lach.; *Mag. c.*; *Mag. p.*; *Merc.*; Nux v.; Ox. ac.; Phos.; Phyt.; *Plant.*; Puls.; Sep.; Spig.; *Staph.*; Tab.; Ther.; Thuja.

CAUSE—Coffee: Cham.; Ign.

Cold bathing—Ant. c.

Decayed teeth—Cham.; *Kreos.*; *Merc.*; Mez.; Staph.

Dental pulp, inflamed—Bell.

Drafts, or cold exposure—Acon.; Bell.; Bry.; *Calc. c.*; Cham.; Merc.; Puls.; Rhod.; Sil.

Extraction of teeth—Arn.; Staph.

Menses, during—Bar. c.; Cham.; Sep.; *Staph.*

Nursing baby—Cinch.

Pregnancy—Alum.; *Calc. c.*; Cham.; *Mag. c.*; Nux m.; Puls.; Ratanh.; Sep.; Tab. See Female Sexual System.

Tea—Thuja.

Tobacco-smoking—*Clem.*; Ign.; Plant.; *Spig.*

Washing clothes—Phos.

LOCATION—Decayed teeth: Ant. c.; Cham.; *Kreos.*; Mag. c.; *Merc.*; Mez.; Nux v.; Staph.; Thuya.

Eye-teeth—Ther.

Lower—Antipyr.; Caust.; Merc.; Staph.; Verbasc.

Molars—Antipyr.; Bry.; Caust.

Roots of teeth—Meph.; *Merc.*; Staph.

Sound teeth—Arg. n.; Caust.; Cham.; Plant.; Spig.; Staph.

Upper teeth—Bell.; Fluor. ac.

TYPE—Neuralgic, congestive: Acon.; Aran.; Ars.; *Bell.*; Ced.; *Cham.*; *Coff.*; Dolichos; Ferr. picr.; *Ign.*; Mag. c.; Mag. p.; Merc. v.; Plant.; *Spig.* See Odontalgia.

Rheumatic—Acon.; *Bry.*; Cham.; Chin. s.; Colch.; Guaiac.; Merc.; Puls.; Rhod.

TYPE OF PAIN—Aching: Cham.; Kreos.; Merc.; Mez.; Staph.

Burning—*Ars.*; Bell.; Sil.

Drawing, jerking, tearing—*Bell.*; *Cham.*; Chimap.; Coff.; Cycl.; Kreos.; Meph.; *Merc.*; *Nux v.*; Prun. sp.; *Puls.*; Rhod.; Sep.; Sil.; *Spig.*; Sul.

Gnawing boring—Calc. c.; Carbo v.; Mez.; Nux v.; Plant.; Puls.; Sil.; Staph.

Periodical—Ars.; Chin. s.; Coff.

Shock-like—Am. c.; Aran.; Nux v.

Shooting—Calc. c.; *Cham.*; Kali c.; Mag. c.; *Nux v.*; Phos.; Sep.; Sil.

Stitching—*Bry.*; Cham.; Nit. ac.; Puls.

Throbbing—Acon.; *Bell.*; Coccinel.; Glon.; Kali c.; Mag. c.; *Merc.*; Sil.; See Odontalgia.

CONCOMITANTS—Distraction of the mind: Acon.; Cham.

Heat, thirst, fainting—Cham.

Neuralgia of lids, reflex—Plant.

Rush of blood to head, loose feeling of teeth—Hyos.

Soreness of teeth—Bell.; Merc.; Plant.; Zinc. m.

Swelling about jaws, cheeks—Bell.; Bor.; Cham.; *Hekla;* Hep.; Lyc.; *Merc.;* Sil. See Gumboil.

MODALITIES—AGGRAVATION—After midnight: Ars.

At night—Ant. c.; Aran.; *Bell.;* Caust.; *Cham.; Clem.; Mag. c.;* Mag. p.; *Merc.;* Mez.; *Puls.;* Sep.; Sil.; Sul.

From blowing nose—Culex; Thuya.

From change of weather—Aran.; Merc.; *Rhod.*

From cold foods, drinks—Calc. c.; Lach.; Mag. p.; *Merc.;* Nux v.; Staph.; Sul.

From cold in general—Ant. c.; Calc. c.; Hyos.; Lyc.; Mag. c.; Merc.; Nux v.; Plant.; *Sil.;* Spig.; Sul.

From contact, touch—Bell.; Calc. fl.; Caust.; Cinch.; Kali c.; Mag. m.; Mez.; Plant.; *Staph.*

From eating—Ant. c.; Bell.; Bry.; *Calc. c.;* Cham.; Chimap.; *Kali c.;* Mag. p.; Mez.; Nux v.; *Puls.;* Sil.; *Spig.;* Staph.; Zinc.

From exertion of mind or body—Chimap.; Nux v.

From lying down, rest, quiet—*Aran.;* Mag. c.; Nat. s.; *Ratanh.;* Sep.

From shrill sounds—Ther.

From smoking tobacco—Clem.; Ign.; *Spig.*

From warm food—*Bism.;* Bry.; Calc. c.; *Caust.; Clem.; Coff.;* Merc.; *Puls.;* Sil.

In intervals between meals—Ign.

In morning—Hyos.

Warmth in general—*Cham.; Merc.;* Prun. sp.; *Puls.;* Sep.

Windy weather, thunder storms—Rhod.

AMELIORATION—Cold air: Nat. s.; Puls.

Cold drinks—*Bism.;* Bry.; Chimap.; *Coff.;* Ferr. m.; Ferr. p.; Nat. s.; Puls.

Eating—Ign.; Plant.; *Spig.*

Hot liquids—*Mag. p.*

Lying down—Spig.

Mouth open, sucking in air—Mez.

Pressure external—Bry.; Cinch.

Pressure of teeth—Cinch.; *Ol. an.;* Staph.

Rubbing cheek—Merc.

Sweat in general—Cham.; *Chenop. gl.*

Walking about—Mag. c.; Ratanh.

Warmth—*Ars.;* Cinch.; Lyc.; *Mag. p.;* Merc.; Nux v.

Wet finger—Cham.

RIGG'S DISEASE—Calc. ren.; Merc.; Sil. mar.

SORDES and deposits—*Ail.;* Alum.; Ars.; *Bapt.; Echin.;* Hyos.; Iod.; Kali p.; Merc. c.; *Mur. ac.;* Phos. ac.; Plant.; *Rhus t.*

THROAT

ADENOID VEGETATIONS—*Agraph.*; Bar. c.; Calc. c.; *Calc. fl.*; *Calc. iod.*; *Calc. p.*; Chrom. ac.; Iod.; Kali s.; Lob. syph.; Mez.; **Psor.**; *Sang. n.*; Sul.; Thuya.

DIPHTHERIA—Remedies in general: Ail.; *Apis*; *Ars.*; Ars. iod.; Arum; *Bapt.*; *Bell.*; *Brom.*; Calc. chlor.; *Canth.*; Carb. ac.; *Crot.*; *Diph.*; Echin.; Guaiac.; *Kali bich.*; Kali chlor.; *Kali m.*; *Kali per.*; Lac c.; *Lach.*; Lachnanth.; Led.; Lob. infl.; *Lyc.*; *Merc. c.*; *Merc. cy.*; Merc. i. fl.; Mer. i. r.; *Mur. ac.*; Naja; *Nit. ac.*; *Phyt.*; Rhus t.; Sang.; Sul.; Tar. c.; Vinca.; Zinc. m.

TYPE—Ataxic: Ars.; Bell.; Lach.; Mosch.; Phos.

Laryngeal—Apis; *Brom.*; Canth.; Chlorum; Diph.; *Hep.*; Iod.; *Kali bich.*; Lac c.; *Merc. cy.*; Petrol.; Phos.; Samb.; Spong.

Malignant—*Ail.*; Apis; Ars.; *Carb. ac.*; Chin. ars.; Crot.; Diph.; *Echin.*; Kali p.; Lac c.; *Lach.*; *Merc. cy.*; Mur. ac.; Pyr.

Nasal—*Am. c.*; Am. caust.; *Kali bich.*; Lyc.; Merc. cy.; *Nit. ac.*

CONDITIONS—Extension downwards: Iod.; *Kali bich.*; Lac c.; Merc. cy.

Extension left to right—Lac c.; *Lach.*; Sabad.

Extension right to left—Lyc.

Extension upward—Brom.

With croup—Acet. ac.; *Brom.*; Hep.; *Iod.*; *Kali bich.*; Kali m.; Lach.; Merc. cy.; Phos.; Samb.; Spong.

With drooling—Lac c.; Merc. cy.

With objective symptoms only: painless type; deficient reaction; sopor, stupor, epistaxis—Diph.

With post-diphtheritic paralysis—*Arg. n.*; *Caust.*; Cocc.; Con.; Curare; Diph.; *Gels.*; Kali p.; Lach.; Oleand.; *Phos.*; Plumb.; Rhus t.; Sec.

With prostration from beginning—Ail.; *Apis*; *Ars.*; Bapt.; Canth.; *Carb. ac.*; Crot.; *Diph.*; Kali per.; *Lach.*; *Merc. cy.*; Mur. ac.; Phyt.

With spasm of glottis—Mosch.; Samb.

With urine scanty—Apis; Ars.; Canth.; Lac c.; Merc. cy.; Naja.

OESOPHAGUS—Burning, smarting: Acon.; *Am. caust.*; Asaf.; Ars.; *Canth.*; Caps.; Carb. ac.; *Crot. t.*; Gels.; *Iris*; *Merc. c.*; Mez.; Ox. ac.; *Phos.*; Sang.; Sinap. a.; Strych.

Constriction—Abies n.; *Alum.*; Am. m.; Asaf.; Bapt.; Bell.; Cact.; *Cajup.*; Caps.; *Cic.*; Condur.; Gels.; Hyos.; Ign.; *Lyssin*; Merc. c.; Naja; *Phos.*; Plat.; Plumb.; Rhus t.; Stram.; Ver. v.

Dryness—*Acon.*; *Bell.*; Cocc.; *Mez.*; *Naja.*

Inflammation (esophagitis)—Acon.; Alum.; Ars.; *Bell.*; Merc. c.; *Naja*; Phos.; Sul. ac.; Ver. a.

Pain—*Am. caust.*; Cocc.; Gels.; *Phos.*

Spasm (esophagismus)—Aconitin; Arg. cy.; Asaf.; *Bapt.*; Bar. c.; *Bell.*; Canth.; Cic.; Hyos.; *Ign.*; Lach.; Lyssin; Merc. c.; *Naja*; Stram.; Strych.; *Ver. v.* **See Pharynx.**

THROAT

FAUCES—Anesthesia: Kali br.

Burning heat—Acon.; Æsc.; Bell.; *Canth.*; *Caps.*; Carb. ac.; Gels.; *Phos.*; *Phyt.*; Sinap. n.; Still.

Dryness—Acon.; Æsc.; Bell.; Canth.; Caps.; Gels.; Jugl. c.; *Nux m.*; Phos.; *Phyt.*; Sabad.; Senec.

Inflammation—Ail.; Apis; *Bell.*; Ferr. p.; *Kali bich.*; Menthol; Merc. i. fl.; Merc. s.

Necrosis—Merc. cy.

Redness—*Bell.*; Carb. ac.; Ferr. p.; Gymnocl.; Menthol; *Merc. cy.*; Merc. i. r.; Mez.; Naja; Puls.

Roughness, sensitive—Æsc.; Coccus; Dros.; *Nux v.*; Phos.; *Phyt.*

Tingling—*Acon.*; Echin.; Phyt.

Ulceration—Coryd.; *Kali bich.*; Merc. i. r.; *Nit. ac.*; Sang. See Pharynx

PHARYNX—Abscess (retro-pharyngeal): Antipyr.; Bell.; Bry.; *Hep.*; Lach.; *Merc.*; Nit. ac.; Phos.; *Sil.*

Abscess, predisposition to—Calc. c.; *Calc. iod.*; Ferr. p.; *Kali iod.*; *Sil.*

Adherent crusts—Elaps; Kali bich.; Kali m.

Anesthesia—Gels.; *Kali br.*

Burning, smarting, scalded feeling—Acon.; Æsc.; *Am. caust.*; Apis; *Ars.*; Ars. iod.; *Arum;* Aur.; Bar. c.; Bell.; Camph.; *Canth.*; *Caps.*; Carb. ac.; *Caust.*; Cocaine; Con.; Glycerin; Guaiac.; Hydr.; *Iris;* Kali bich.; *Kali per.*; Kreos.; Lyc.; *Merc. c.*; Merc. i. fl.; Merc.; *Mez.*; Nat. ars.; Nit. ac.; Phos.; *Phyt.*; Pop. c.; Quill.; *Sang.*; Sang. n.; Senec.; *Sul.*; Wyeth.

Coldness—Cistus.

Constriction, spasmodic—*Acon.*; Æsc.; Agar.; Alum.; Apis; *Arg. n.*; Ars.; Arum; Asaf.; Bapt.; *Bell.*; Bothrops; Cact.; Calc. c.; Cajup.; *Canth.*; *Caps.*; Cic.; Cocaine; Cupr. m.; *Hyos.*; *Ign.*; Lach.; *Merc. c.*; Mez.; Morph.; Nux v.; *Phyt.*; Plumb. m.; Puls.; Ratanh.; *Sang.*; *Sang. n.*; Sarcol. ac.; *Stram.*; *Strych.*; Sumb.; Val.

DYSPHAGIA—Deglutition painful, difficult: Remedies in general: Agar.; Ail.; Alum.; Amyg. pers.; Anac.; Apis; Ars.; Atrop.; *Bapt.*; *Bell.*; Bothrops; Bry.; *Cajup.*; *Canth.*; *Caps.*; Carb. ac.; *Cic.*; Cocc.; Con.; Cocaine; Cur.; Dub.; Fluor. ac.; Grat.; Hep.; Hydroc. ac.; *Hyos.*; *Ign.*; Iod.; Kali bich.; Kali br.; Kali c.; Kali chlor.; Kali m.; Kali perm.; *Lac c.*; *Lach.*; Lyc.; Lyssin; *Merc. c.*; Merc. cy.; Merc. i. fl.; Merc. i. r.; *Merc. s.*; *Merc. v.*; Nat. p.; *Nit. ac.*; Phos.; *Phyt.*; Pop. c.; Psor.; Sang.; Sang. n.; Senec.; *Stram.*; Strych.

Can swallow only liquids—*Bapt.*; Bar. c.; Cham., Nat. m.; Plumb.; *Sil.*

Can swallow only solids, liquids descend with difficulty—*Alumen;* Bell.; Bothrops; Bry.; Cact.; *Canth.*; *Crot.*; Gels.; *Hyos.*; Ign.; Lach.; *Lyssin;* Merc. c.; Sil.

Choking when eating, drinking—Abies n.; *Anac.*; Cajup.; *Can. s.*; Glon.; *Kava;* Merc. c.; Mur. ac.; Niccol.; Nit. ac.; *Phyt.*; Santon.; Sumb.

Food descends "wrong way"—*Anac.*; Can. s.; Kali c.; *Meph.*; Nat. m.

Food regurgitates, per nasum—*Bell.*; Diph.; Kali perm.; *Lach.*; Lyc.; *Merc. c.*; Merc. v.

THROAT

Liquids descend with gurgling sound—Ars.; *Cupr. ac.*; Hydroc. ac.; *Laur.*; Thuya.

Swallows food and drink hastily—*Anac.*; *Bell.*; Bry.; Coff.; Helleb.; Hep.; Oleand.; Zinc. m.

DEPOSITS—**Membranous**—*Acet. ac.*; Apis; Brom.; Carb. ac.; *Kali bich.*; Kali m.; Kali perm.; Lach.; Merc. cy.; Mur. ac.; *Nit. ac.*; Phyt. See Diphtheria.

Dryness—*Acon.*; *Æsc.*; Agar.; *Alum.*; *Apis*; *Ars.*; Asaf.; *Atrop.*; *Bell.*; *Bry.*; *Canth.*; *Caps.*; Caust.; Cistus; Cocaine; Cocc.; Dros.; *Dub.*; Ferr. p.; *Guaiac.*; Hep.; Hyos.; Justicia; Kali bich.; Kali c.; Kali chlor.; *Lach.*; Lemna m.; *Lyc.*; Merc. c.; Merc. per.; Merc.; Mez.; Morph.; Nat. m.; Nat. s.; Nit. ac.; *Nux m.*; Onosm.; Phos.; *Phyt.*; Puls.; Quill.; Rhus t.; *Sabad.*; *Sang.*; Sang. n.; Sarcol. ac.; Sep.; *Spong.*; Strych.; Sul.; *Wyeth*.

Edema—Ail.; *Apis*; Ars.; Kali perm.; Lach.; Mag. p.; Mur. ac.; *Nat. ars.*; Phos.; Phyt.; Rhus t.

Erysipelas—*Apis*; Bell.; *Canth.*; Euphorb. of.; Lach.; *Rhus t.*

Globus hystericus—*Ambra*; *Aquil.*; *Asaf.*; Bell.; Gels.; Hyos.; *Ign.*; Kali p.; Lach.; Lob. infl.; Mag. m.; Mancin.; *Mosch.*; *Nux m.*; Plat.; Raph.; *Val.* See Hysteria.

HAWKING—**Hemming (clearing throat)**:—*Æsc.*; *Alum.*; Am. m.; *Arg. m.*; *Arg. n.*; *Arum*; Bry.; Calc. c.; *Canth.*; Carbo v.; *Caust.*; Cistus; Cocc.; *Coccus*; Con.; *Coral.*; Eucal.; Guaiac.; Gymnocl.; *Hep.*; Hepat.; *Hydr.*; Iberis; Justicia; *Kali bich.*; Kali c.; *Kali m.*; Lach.; *Lyc.*; Merc. i. fl.; *Merc. i. r.*; *Nat. c.*; *Nat. m.*; Nit. ac.; *Nux v.*; *Phos.*; *Phyt.*; Psor.; *Selen.*; Sep.; Silph s.; Spong.; *Stann.*; Sul.; *Tab.*; Trifrol. pr.; Vinca m.; Viola tr.; *Wyeth.* See Chronic Pharyngitis.

Hawking with cheesy, fetid, lumps—*Agar.*; Kali bich.; Kali m.; Mag. c.; Merc. i. r.; *Psor.*; Sec.; Sil. See Follicular Pharyngitis.

Hawking, with fetid pus—Antipyr.; *Hep.*; Lyc.; Sil.

Hawking, with gelatinous, viscid, gluey mucus; difficult raising—*Æsc.*; Aloe; *Alum.*; Am. br.; Am. m.; *Arg. n.*; *Arum*; *Canth.*; Carbo v.; *Caust.*; Cistus; Coca; *Coccus*; Euphras.; *Hydr.*; Iberis; *Kali bich.*; Kali c.; Lach.; *Merc. i. fl.*; *Merc. i. r.*; Myr.; Nat. c.; Nat. m.; Nat. s.; Nux v.; Petrol.; Phos. ac.; Phos.; *Phyt.*; Psor.; *Rumex*; Sang.; *Selen.*; Sep.; Silph. s.; *Stann*.

Hollow feeling, as if pharynx had disappeared—Lach.; Phyt.

Inclination to swallow constantly—*Æsc.*; Asaf.; *Bell.*; Caust.; Lac c.; *Lach.*; Lact. ac.; Lyssin; *Merc. i. fl.*; *Merc.*; Myr.; Phyt.; Sumb.; Wyeth.

INFLAMMATION-**(Pharyngitis)**: **Atrophic (sicca)**: Æsc.; *Alum.*; Dub.; Arg. n.; Ars. iod.; Kali bich.; Nux v.; Sabal.

Inflammation, catarrhal, acute—*Acon.*; *Æsc.*; Apis; Arg. n.; *Bell.*; Bry.; Canth.; *Caps.*; Caust.; Cistus; Eucal.; Ferr. p.; *Gels.*; Glycerin; Guaiac.; Gymnocl.; *Hep.*; Iod.; *Justicia*; *Kali bich.*; Kali c.; Kali m.; Lach.; Lachnanth.; Led.; Menthol; Merc. c.; Mer. i. fl.; Merc. i. r.; *Merc.*; Naja; Nat. ars.; Nat. iod.; Nux v.; *Phyt.*; Quill.; Sal. ac.; *Sang.*; Sang. n.; Scilla; *Wyeth*.

Inflammation, catarrhal, acute, predisposition to—Alumen; *Bar. c.*; Graph.; Lach.; Sul.

Inflammation, catarrhal, chronic—Æsc.; *Alum.*; Am. br.; *Am. caust.*; Arg. iod.; *Arg. m.*; *Arg. n.*; Ars.; Arum; Aur.; Bar. c.; Brom.; Calc. p.; Can. ind.; Carbo v.; Caust.; Cinnab.; Cistus; *Coccus*; Cub.; Elaps; Ferr. p.; Graph.; Hep.; *Hydr.*; *Iod.*; *Kali bich.*; Kali c.; Kali chlor.; Lach.; *Lyc.*; Med.; Merc. c.; Merc. i. fl.; *Merc.*; Nat. c.; Nat. m.; Nux v.; Ox. ac.; Penthor.; Petrol.; Phos.; Puls.; *Rumex*; Sabad.; Sabal; *Sang.*; Sec.; Senega; *Sep.*; Stann.; Sumb.; Tab.; *Wyeth.*

Inflammation, follicular, acute—Æsc.; Apis; Bell.; Caps.; *Ferr. p.*; Iod.; Kali bich.; *Kali m.*; Merc.; *Phyt.*; Sang. n.; Wyeth.

Inflammation, follicular, chronic (clergymen's sore throat)—Æsc.; *Alum.*; Am. br.; *Arg. n.*; Arn.; Ars. iod.; *Arum*; Calc. fl.; Calc. p.; Caps.; Caust.; Cinnab.; Cistus; Dros.; Hep.; *Hydr.*; Ign.; *Kali bich.*; Kali m.; *Lach.*; Merc. cy.; *Merc. i. r.*; Nat. m.; Nux v.; Phos.; *Phyt.*; *Sang. n.*; Sticta; Still.; Sul.; *Wyeth.*

Inflammation, herpetic—*Apis*; Ars.; Bor.; Hydr.; Jacar.; *Kali bich.*; Kali chlor.; Lach.; Merc. i. fl.; Nat. s.; *Phyt.*; Sal. ac.

Inflammation, rheumatic—Acon.; Bry.; Colch.; Guaiac.; Phyt.; Rhus t.

Inflammation, septic—Am. c.; *Hep.*; Mur. ac.; *Sil.*

Inflammation, tubercular—Merc. i. r.

AGGRAVATIONS—From cold—*Cistus*; Fluor. ac.; Hep.; *Lyc.*

From drinks, warm or hot—*Lach.*; Merc. i. fl.; Phyt.

From menses—Lac c.

From pressure—Lach.; Merc. c.

From sleep—*Lach.*; Lyc.

From suppressed foot sweat—*Bar. c.*; Psor.; Sil.

From swallowing, empty—Antipyr.; *Bar. c.*; Crotal.; Dolichos; *Hep.*; Justicia; Lac c.; *Lach.*; Merc. i. fl.; Merc. i. r.; *Merc.*; Phyt.; Sabad.

From swallowing liquids—Bell.; Bry.; Ign.; *Lach.*

From swallowing solids—Bapt.; Merc. s.; Morph. See Deglutition.

From swallowing sweet things—Spong.

From warmth—Coccus; Iod.; Lach.; *Merc.*

In afternoon—Lach.

In bed—Merc. i. fl.; *Merc.*

In intervals of swallowing—Caps.; Ign.

On left side—*Lach.*; Merc. i. r.; Sabad.

On left to right—Lac c.; *Lach.*; Sabad.

On right side—Bar. c.; *Bell.*; Guaiac.; *Lyc.*; Mag. p.; Merc. i. fl.; Merc.; Niccol.; Phyt.; Pod.; Sang.; Sul.

AMELIORATIONS—From inspiring cold air:—Sang.

From swallowing—Gels.; *Ign.*

From swallowing liquids—Cistus.

From swallowing liquids, warm—Alum.; Ars.; Calc. fl.; *Lyc.*; Morph.; Sabad.

From swallowing solids—*Ign.*; Lach.

PAPULES—Hippoz.; Iod. See Follicular Pharyngitis.

Paralysis, neuroses—*Alum.*; Bar. m.; *Bell.*; Caust.; Cocc.; Con.; Cur.;

Gels.; Hep.; *Hyos.;* *Ign.;* *Lach.;* Lob. infl.; Lyc.; Merc.; Morph.; Nit. ac.; *Nux m.;* Plumb. m.; *Pop. c.;* Rhus t.; *Sil.;* Stram.; Sul.

Peristalsis reversed—Ambra; Asaf.

Plug or lump sensation—Alum.; Bar. c.; *Bell.;* Carbo v.; Graph.; *Hep.; Ign.; Lach.;* Lob. infl.; Merc. i. fl.; Nat. m.; *Nux v.;* Plumb. ac.; Phyt.; Puls.; Rumex; Sul.; Wyeth.

Pustules—Æth. See Ulceration.

Rawness, roughness, scraping—Acon.; *Æsc.;* Alum.; Am. c.; *Am. caust.;* Am. m.; *Arg. m.; Arg. n.;* Arum; Bar. c.; Bell.; *Bry.;* Brom.; Carbo v.; *Caust.;* Coccus; Con.; Cub.; *Dros.;* Fagop.; Gels.; *Hep.; Hepat.;* Homar.; Hydr.; Iod.; *Kali bich.;* Kali c.; Lact. ac.; Merc. cy.; Merc.; Nit. ac.; *Nux v.;* Onosm.; Penthor.; *Phos.; Phyt.; Pop. c.;* Puls.; *Rumex; Sang.;* Sang. n.; *Sep.;* Sticta; Sul.

Redness—Acon.; *Æsc.; Bell.;* Ferr. p.; Gins.; Merc. i. fl.; Merc. i. r.; Merc. nit.; Merc.; Sal. ac.; *Sul.*

Redness, dark, livid—*Ail.;* Alum.; *Am. c.;* Am. caust.; Amygd. pers.; *Apis;* Arag.; *Arg. n.;* Ars.; *Bapt.;* Bell.; Canth.; Caps.; Crot.; Diph.; *Gymnocl.; Lach.;* Merc. c.; Mur. ac.; *Naja;* Nat. ars.; Penthor.; *Phyt.;* Puls.; Wyeth.; Zinc. carb.

Redness, glossy, as if varnished—Alum.; *Apis;* Arag.; Bell.; Cistus; Hydr.; Kali bich.; *Lac c.;* Phos.

Relaxation—Æsc.; Alumen; *Alum.;* Am. m.; Bar. c.; *Calc. p.;* Eucal.; Penthor.

Sensitive, sore, tender—Acon.; *Æsc.;* Ail.; *Apis;* Arg. m.; *Arg. n.;* Arn.; *Arum;* Atrop.; Bar. c.; *Bell.;* Brom.; Bry.; Calc. p.; *Canth.; Caps.;* Carb. ac.; *Caust.;* Dolichos; Fagop.; Ferr. p.; Fluor. ac.; Graph.; *Gymnocl.; Hep.;* Homar.; Hydr.; Ign.; *Kali bich.;* Kali c.; Kali iod.; *Kali per.;* Lac c.; *Lach.;* Lachnanth.; Led.; Lyc.; Menthol; *Merc. c.;* Merc. cy.; *Merc. i. fl.; Merc. i. r.; Merc.;* Mur. ac.; Naja; Nit. ac.; *Nux v.;* Ox. ac.; Petrol.; *Phos.; Phyt.;* Pop. c.; Quill.; Rhus t.; Sabad.; *Sang.;* Sang. n.; Spong.; Sul.; Trifol.; Verbasc.; Wyeth.

Sore, irritable of smokers—Æsc.; Arg. n.; Caps.; Nat. m.; Nux v.

Spasm—Bell.; Canth.; *Sumb.* See Constriction.

Sticking, pricking, splinter-like pains, extending to ears, worse swallowing, yawning, etc.—Agar.; Alum.; *Arg. n.;* Dolichos; Ferr. iod.; Gels.; Guaiac.; *Hep.; Kali bich.; Kali c.;* Lac c.; *Nit ac.; Phyt.;* Psor.; Sil.; Staph.

Stiffness—Æsc.; Kali m.; Mag. p.; Mez.; Nux m.; Phyt.; *Rhus t.* See Constriction.

Swelling—Acon.; *Æsc.;* Ail.; *Apis;* Arg. n.; Arum; Bapt.; Bar. c.; *Bell.;* Canth.; *Caps.;* Crot.; Gymnocl.; *Hep.;* Kali bich.; Kali m.; *Kali per.;* Lac c.; *Lach.;* Merc. c.; *Merc. cy.; Merc. i. fl.; Merc. i. r.; Merc.;* Naja; Nat. ars.; *Phyt.;* Sabad.; Sang.; Vespa; Wyeth. See Inflammation.

Syphilis—*Aur.;* Bell.; Cinnab.; Fluor. ac.; Hydr.; *Kali bich.;* Kali iod.; Merc. c.; *Merc. i. fl.; Merc. i. r.;* Merc. nit.; Mez.; *Nit ac.; Phyt.;* Sul.

Tickling, as from hair—Æsc. gl.; Allium s.; Ambra; *Arg. n.;* Caust.; Dros.;

THROAT

Hepat.; *Kali bich.*; Lach.; Nat. m.; Nit. ac.; Nux v.; Pulex; *Sabad.*; Sang.; Sul.; *Val.*; Yucca.

Ulceration—Ail.; Am. c.; *Apis*; Aral.; Bapt.; *Cinnab.*; Hydr.; *Hydrast. mur.*; *Kali bich.*; Kali m.; *Lach.*; Merc. c.; Merc. cy.; Merc. i. fl.; Merc. i. r.; Merc.; Mur. ac.; *Nit. ac.*; *Phyt.*; Sang.; Vinca m.

Ulceration, aphthous—*Canth.*; Eucal.; *Hydrast. mur.*; Nit. ac.

Ulceration, gangrenous—Ail.; Am. c.; *Ars.*; Bapt.; Crot.; Echin.; Kali chlor.; Kali perm.; Kali n.; *Lach.*; *Merc. cy.*; Merc.; Mur. ac.; Sil.

Ulceration, mercurial—Hep.; Hydr.; Lyc.; Nit. ac.

Ulceration, syphilitic—Aur. m.; Calc. fl.; *Fluor. ac.*; Hippoz.; Jacor. gual.; *Kali bich.*; Kali iod.; Lach.; Lyc.; *Merc. c.*; Merc. i. fl.; Merc. i. r.; Merc.; *Nit. ac.*; Phyt.; Still.

Veins, varicose—*Æsc.*; Aloe; *Bar. m.*; Ham.; Phyt.; Puls.

TONSILS—Abscess (peritonsillar): Calc. s.

DEPOSITS ON—Creamy, extends over tonsils, uvula, soft palate:—Nat. p.

Dark, dry, wrinkled—Ars.

Dark, gangrenous—Bapt.

Grayish, dirty, like macerated skin, covering tonsils, uvula pharynx—Phyt.

Grayish, dirty, thick, with fiery red margins—Apis.

Grayish, extends to posterior nares, air passages, later purplish black—Echin.

Grayish patch on tonsils—Kali m.

Grayish, thick; shred-like borders, adherent or free—Merc. v.

Grayish-white, in crypts—Ign.

Grayish-yellow, slight; easily detached; worse on left—Merc. i. r.

Patchy on right tonsil and inflamed fauces, easily detached—Merc. i. fl.

Plugs of mucus constantly form in crypts—Calc. fl.

Shining, glazed white or yellow patch—Lac c.

Thick, brownish-yellow like wash leather, or firm, fibrinous, pearly, extends over tonsils, soft palate—Kali bich.

Thick, dark gray, or brownish black—Diph.

Thin, false; on yellowish red tonsils and fauces—Merc. s.

Thin, then dark, gangrenous—Merc. cy.

HYPERTROPHY—Induration: Alumen; Ars. iod.; Aur.; Bac.; *Bar. c.*; *Bar. iod.*; Bar. m.; Brom.; Calc. c.; Calc. fl.; *Calc. iod.*; *Calc. p.*; Ferr. p.; Hep.; *Iod.*; *Kali bich.*; Kali m.; Merc. i. fl.; *Merc. i. r.*; Plumb. iod.; Phyt.; Sil.; Sul. iod.; Thuya.

Hypertrophy, with hardness of hearing—*Bar. c.*; Calc. p.; *Hep.*; Lyc.; Plumb.; Psor.

Inflammation (tonsillitis): Acute Catarrhal and Follicular: Acon.; Ail.; Am. m.; Amyg. pers.; *Apis*; *Bapt.*; Bar. ac.; *Bar. c.*; Bar. m.; *Bell.*; Brom.; Caps.; Dulc.; Eucal.; Ferr. p.; Gels.; Gins.; *Guaiac.*; *Gymnocl.*; Hep.; *Ign.*; Iod.; Kali bich.; *Kali m.*; Lac c.; *Lach.*; Lyc.; *Merc. i. fl.*; *Merc. i. r.*; Merc. s.; Naja; Nat. s.; *Phyt.*; Rhus t.; Sabad.; *Sang.*; *Sil.*; Sul.

Inflammation, acute phlegmonous (quinsy): Acon.; Apis; *Bar. c.*; *Bar. iod.*; *Bell.*; Caps.; Cinnab.; Guaiac.; *Hep.*; Lac c.; Lach.; Lyc.;

THROAT 767

Merc. i. fl.; Merc. i. r.; *Merc. s.; Merc. v.; Phyt.; Psor.;* Sang.; Sang. n.; Sil.; *Tar. c.;* Vespa.

Inflammation, chronic tendency—*Bar. c.;* Calc. p.; Fucus; Hep.; Lach.; Lyc.; Psor.; *Sil.*

Redness, dark—Ail.; Amyg. am.; *Bapt.;* Brom.; Caps.; Diph.; Gymnocl.; *Lach.;* Merc.; *Phyt.*

Swelling—*Acon.;* Am. m.; *Apis;* Ars. iod.; Bar. ac.; *Bar. c.; Bell.;* Brom.; Calc. c.; Calc. p.; Caps.; Cinnab.; Cistus; Diph.; Ferr. p.; Gels.; Guaiac.; *Hep.;* Ign.; Iod.; Kali bich.; Kali m.; *Lach.;* Lyc.; Merc. c.; *Merc. i. fl.; Merc. i. r.; Merc.; Phyt.;* Psor.; *Sang. n.* See Tonsillitis.

Ulceration—*Ars.;* Bar. c.; Echin.; *Hep.;* Ign.; *Kali bich.;* Lach.; Lyc.; Merc. c.; Merc. i. fl.; Merc. i. r.; Merc. per.; Merc. s.; Nat. s.; Nit. ac.; Phyt.; *Sil.* See Follicular Tonsillitis.

Ulceration, gangrenous—Am. c.; Ars.; Bapt.; Crot.; *Lach.; Merc. cy.;* Mur. ac.

UVULA—Constricted feeling—Acon.

Edematous, sac-like—*Apis;* Ars.; Caps.; *Kali bich.;* Mur. ac.; *Nat. ars.;* Phos.; Phyt.; Rhus t.

Elongation, relaxation—*Alumen;* Alum.; Bar. c.; Bell.; Calc. fl.; Canth.; *Caps.;* Coccinel.; *Coccus;* Croc.; Fagop.; Hep.; *Hyos.; Kali bich.; Merc. c.;* Merc.; Nat. m.; Nux v.; *Phos.; Phyt.;* Rumex ac.; Sabad.; Wyeth.

Inflammation (uvulitis)—*Acon.;* Amygd. pers.; *Bell.;* Caps.; Cistus; Iod.; *Kali bich.; Kali per.; Merc. c.;* Merc.; Nat. s.; Nux v.; Puls.; Sul. iod.

Pain—Trifol.; Tussil.

Sore spot behind, better by eating—Am. m.

Ulceration—Indium; *Kali bich.;* Merc. c.

Whitened, shrivelled—Carb. ac.

White, tenacious, mucus—Am. caust.

STOMACH

APPETITE—Defective, lost (anorexia)—*Abies n.*; Alet.; Alfal.; Am. c.; *Ant. c.*; Arn.; *Ars.*; *Bapt.*; Bism.; But. ac.; Calc. c.; Calc. p.; Caps.; *Carb. ac.*; Carbo v.; Card. m.; *Chel.*; *Chin. ars.*; Chionanth.; *Cinch.*; Coca; Cocc.; Coff.; Colch.; Cycl.; Dig.; *Ferr. m.*; *Gent.*; Glycerin; Helon.; Hydr.; *Ign.*; *Ipec.*; Iris; Kali bich.; *Lecith.*; *Lyc.*; Merc. d.; Myr.; Niccol.; *Nux v.*; Phos. ac.; Phos.; Plat.; Prun. sp.; Prun. v.; Puls.; Raph.; *Rhus t.*; Sep.; Stront.; Strych. ars.; *Strych. p.*; Sul.; Symphor.; Tarax.

Appetite, increased, ravenous (bulimy)—Abies c.; *Abrot.*; Agar.; *Alfal.*; Allium s.; *Anac.*; Ars.; Ars. br.; Bell.; Brassica; Bry.; Cact.; *Calc. c.*; Calend.; *Chel.*; Cim.; *Cina*; Cinch.; Ferr. m.; Glycerin; Granat.; Graph.; Hep.; Ichth.; Ign.; *Iod.*; Kali c.; Lact. ac.; Lap. alb.; Lob. infl.; *Lyc.*; Merc.; Nat. c.; *Nat. m.*; *Nux v.*; Oleand.; Op.; *Petrol.*; Petros.; *Phos.*; *Psor.*; Rhus t.; Sec.; Stann.; *Sul.*; *Thyr.*; *Uran. n.*; Zinc. m.

Appetite, increased, hungry at night—Abies. n.; *Cina*; Cinch.; Ign.; Lyc.; Nat. c.; Petrol.; *Phos.*; *Psor.*; Selen.; *Sul.*

Appetite, increased, hungry before noon—Hep.; *Sul.*; Zinc. m.

Appetite, increased, hungry, even after a meal—*Alfal.*; Calc. c.; Casc.; *Cina*; Iod.; Indol; Lac c.; *Lyc.*; Med.; Phos.; Phyt.; *Psor.*; Staph.; Stront.; Sul.; Zinc.

Appetite, increased, yet loses flesh—Abrot.; Acet. ac.; *Iod.*; *Nat. m.*; Sanic.; Tub.; Uran. n.

Appetite, increased, yet quickly satiated—Am. c.; Arn.; Ars.; Bar. c.; Carbo v.; *Cinch.*; *Cycl.*; Ferr.; Lith. c.; *Lyc.*; Nat. m.; Nux v.; Petros.; Pod.; Prun. sp.; *Sep.*; *Sul.*

APPETITE PERVERTED—AVERSIONS: Alcoholic beverages:—Ign.; Sil.

Beer—Asaf.; Bell.; Cinch.; Nux v.; Puls.

Boiled food—Calc. c.

Brandy—Ign.; Lob. erin.

Bread—Chenop. gl.; Cycl.; Ign.; *Lyc.*; *Nat. m.*; Puls.; Sul.

Butter—Cycl.; Hep.; *Puls.*; Sang.

Coffee—*Cham.*; Fluor. ac.; *Nux v.*; Sul. ac.

Drinks in general—Bell.; *Canth.*; Cocc.; Ign.; Kali bich.; Lyssin; Nux v.; Stram. See Hydrophobia.

Drinks, warm and hot—Cham.; Kali s.; *Puls.*

Eggs—Ferr. m.

Fats—*Calc. c.*; Carbo an.; *Carbo v.*; *Cycl.*; Hep.; Nat. m.; Petrol.; *Puls.*; Sep.

Food cooked—Graph.; Sil.

Food in general—*Ant. c.*; *Ars.*; Canth.; Cocc.; Colch.; Dulc.; Ferr. m.; Ign.; *Ipec.*; Kali bich.; Kali c.; *Nux v.*; Pod.; Puls.; Rheum; Rhus t.; Sabad.; Yerba. See Anorexia.

Food, smell, sight of—Ant. c.; *Ars.;* Cocc.; *Colch.;* Dig.; *Nux v.;* Sep.; Sil.; Stann.; Symphor.
Food, warm, hot—Calc. c.; Ign.; Lyc.; Petrol.; *Puls.;* Sil.; Ver. a.
Meat—Aloe; *Alum.; Arn.;* Bell.; *Calc. c.; Carbo v.;* Card. m.; Chenop. gl.; Cinch.; Colch.; Crotal.; *Cycl.;* Ferr. p.; *Graph.;* Lyc.; Morph.; *Mur. ac.; Nit. ac.;* Petrol.; *Puls.; Sep.;* Sil.; Stront.; Sul.; Thuya.
Milk—Arn.; Bell.; *Carbo v.;* Ferr. p.; *Guaiac.;* Nat. c.; Pastin.; Puls.; Sep.; Sil.; *Sul.*
Potatoes—Alum.; Thuya.
Salt food—Graph.; Selen.
Sour things—Dros.; Ferr. m.; Sul.
Sweets—Bar. c.; Caust.; *Graph.;* Radium; Sul.
Tobacco—Arn.; Calc. c.; Canth.; Cocc.; *Lob. infl.;* Nat. m.; *Nux v.;* Plant.
Tobacco, odor of—Cascar.; *Ign.;* Lob. infl.
Wine—Sul.

APPETITE—PERVERTED CRAVINGS (pica): Acids, pickles, sour things: *Abies c.;* Alum.; Am. m.; *Ant. c.;* Ant. t.; Arn.; *Ars.;* Arundo; Calc. c.; Carbo an.; *Chel.; Cinch.;* Cod.; *Hep.;* Ign.; Jonosia; Kali bich.; Lact. v.; *Mag. c.;* Myr.; Nat. m.; *Phos ac.; Puls.;* Sec.; *Sep.;* Thea; *Ver. a.*
Alcoholic beverages—*Ars.; Asar.;* Calc. ars.; *Caps.; Carb. ac.;* Carbo v.; Cinch.; *Coca;* Cocc.; Ferr. p.; *Kali bich.;* Lach.; Lecith.; Med.; Mosch.; *Nux v.;* Phos.; Psor.; Puls.; *Selen.;* Staph.; Stront.; *Sul.; Sul. ac.; Syph.;* Tub.
Apples—Aloe; Ant. t.; Guaiac.; Tellur.
Beer, bitter—Aloe; Cocc.; *Kali bich.;* Nat. m.; Nux v.; Puls.
Bread—Ferr. m.; Stront.
Butter—Ferr. m.
Buttermilk—Elaps.
Charcoal coal, chalk, etc.—*Alum.; Calc. c.;* Cic.; Ign.; Nit. ac.; *Psor.*
Cheese—Arg. n.; Cistus.
Coffee—*Angust.;* Ars.; Con.; Lecith.; Mosch.
Drinks, cold—*Acon.;* Ant. t.; Asim.; *Ars.;* Bell.; *Bry.;* Calc. c.; Cocc.; *Cupr. m.;* Dulc.; *Merc.;* Nat. s.; Onosm.; Phos.; Rhus t.; *Ver. a.* See Thirst.
Drinks, hot—Angust.; Cascar.; Castan.; *Chel.; Lyc.;* Med.; Sabad.; Spig.
Effervescent beverages—Colch.
Eggs—Calc. c.
Farinaceous food—Calc. p.; Sabad.
Fats—Mez.; Nit. ac.; Nux v.; Sul.
Food, coarse, raw—*Abies c.;* Sil.
Food, cold—Bry.; Phos.; Puls.; Sil.
Food, fish—Sul. ac.
Food, warm, hot—Chel.; Cupr. m.; Sabad.
Fruits, juicy things—Aloe; *Ant. t.;* Cinch.; Mag. c.; Med.; *Phos. ac.;* Phos.; Ver. a.

STOMACH

Ham rind—Calc. p.
Lemonade—Am. m.; Cycl.; Puls.; Sab.; Sec.
Meat—*Abies c.*; *Calc. p.*; Lil. t.; *Mag. c.*; Menyanth.
Meat, salt, smoked—Calc. p.
Milk—Apis; Ars.; *Phos. ac.*; *Rhus t.*; Sabal; Sul.
Oysters—Lach.
Salt—Calc. c.; Carbo v.; *Caust.*; Con.; Med.; Nat. m.; Nit. ac.; *Phos.*; Sul.; Ver. a.
Spices—*Alum.*; *Cinch.*; Fluor. ac.; *Hep.*; Nux m.; *Nux v.*; Phos.; Sang.; Staph.
Sweets, candy—Alfal.; Am. c.; *Arg. n.*; Calc. c.; *Cina*; Coca; *Cocaine*; Crot.; Jonosia; *Kali c.*; *Lyc.*; Mag. m.; Med.; Sabad.; *Sul.*
Tea—Alum.; Hep.
Tobacco—*Asar.*; *Carb. ac.*; Carbo v.; Coca; Daphne; *Staph.*
Tonics—Puls.
Various things—Bry.; Cham.; *Cina*; *Cinch.*; Fluor. ac.; Rheum; Sang.
Vegetables—Abies c.; Mag. c.
Water, cold—*Acon.*; Agar. emet.; Ant. t.; Apoc.; *Ars.*; Asim.; Bell.; Bry.; *Colc. c.*; *Eup. perf.*; Onosm.; Op.; *Phos.*; Ver. a. See Thirst.

APPETITE—THINGS THAT DISAGREE—Beer:—Ferr. m.; *Kali bich.*
Bread—Ant. c.; *Hydr.*; Lyc.; *Nat. m.*; Nit. ac.; Puls.
Butter—Carbo an.; *Carbo v.*; Nat. m.; Puls.
Cabbage—Bry.; Carbo v.; Kali c.; Lyc.; Petrol.
Cheese—Col.
Coffee—Carbo v.; Lyc.; *Nux v.*
Drinks, cold—*Ars.*; Calad.; Dig.; Elaps; Kali iod.; *Ver. a.*
Drinks, warm, hot—Bry.; Graph.; *Phos.*; Puls.; Pyr.
Eggs—Colch.
Fats—Ant. c.; Calc. c.; Carbo v.; *Cycl.*; Lyc.; *Puls.*; Thuya.
Fish—Carbo v.
Food, cold—Kali iod.
Food of any kind—Alet.; Amyg. pers.; *Carbo v.*; Lach.; Mosch.; Nat. c.
Food, warm—Puls.
Meat—Ars.; Bor.; *Bry.*; Carbo v.; *Cinch.*; Mag. m.; Nat. m.; *Puls.*; Selen.; Sil.; Ver. a.
Meat in excess—Allium s.
Fruits—*Ars.*; Carbo v.; *Caust.*; Ferr. m.; Kali bich.; *Rumex.*
Melons—Zing.
Milk—Æth.; *Calc. c.*; *Carbo v.*; Cinch.; Kali iod.; Lact. v.; Mag. c.; *Mag. m.*; Niccol.; Ol. j. as.; Pod.; Rheum; Sep.; *Sul.*
Mushrooms, poisonous—Camph.
Odor of food nauseates—*Ars.*; Cocc.; *Colch.*; Dig.; *Sep.*
Onions—Brom.; Lyc.; Thuya.
Oysters—Carbo v.; Lyc.
Pastry—Ant. c.; Lyc.; *Puls.*
Pork—Ant. c.; Carbo v.; Cycl.; *Puls.*
Potatoes—*Alum.*; Sep.
Salt food—Carbo v.

STOMACH 771

Sausage—Acet. ac.; Ars.; Puls.
Soup—Kali c.
Sour foods, drinks—*Ant. c.;* Carbo v.; Dros.; Nat. m.; Phos. ac.
Starchy food—*Carbo v.;* Cinch.; Lyc.; *Nat. c.;* Nat. s.; Sul.
Strawberries—Ox. ac.
Sweets—*Arg. n.;* Ipec.; Lyc.; Sul.; Zinc.
Tea—*Cinch.;* Diosc.; Ferr. m.; Kali hypoph.; *Selen.;* Thuya.
Tobacco—*Ign.;* Kali bich.; Lob. infl.; Lyc.; Phos.; *Selen.;* Tab.
Vegetables—Hydr.
Vinegar—Ant. c.; Carbo v.
Water—*Ars.;* Chin. ars.
Water, impure—Zing.
Wine—Ant. c.; Zinc. m.

ATONY—(myasthenia): Bell.; Ign.; Podophylin; *Strych. p.*

BILIOUSNESS—Æsc.; Aloe; Aqua mar.; *Bapt.;* Berb. v.; *Bry.;* Card. m.; Cham.; *Chel.;* Chionanth.; *Cinch.;* Crot.; Diosc.; *Euonym.;* Eup. perf.; Ferr. m.; Gent.; *Hydr.;* Iris; Kali c.; *Lept.;* Lyc.; Mag. m.; *Merc.;* Myr.; *Nat. s.;* Nitro-mur. ac.; *Nux v.;* Pod.; Ptel.; *Puls.;* Sep.; Sul.; *Tarax.; Triost.;* Yucca. See Liver.

CANCER—Acet. ac.; Am. m.; Arg. n.; *Ars.; Bell.;* Bar. c.; Bism.; Cadm. s.; Calc. fl.; *Condur.;* Con.; Carbo v.; Graph.; *Hydr.; Kali bich.;* Kali c.; *Kreos.;* Mag. p.; Nux v.; *Ornithog.;* Phos.; Plumb. m.; Sec. See Generalities.

CARDIAC ORIFICE—**Contraction**: Alum.; *Bar. m.;* Bry.; Datura; Phos.; Plumb. m.

Pain (cardialgia)—*Agar.; Arg. n.;* Asaf.; Bar. c.; Bism.; Can. ind.; *Carbo v.;* Caul.; *Cupr. m.; Ferr. cy.;* Ferr. tart.; Formica; Ign.; Mag. m.; Nat. m.; Nit. ac.; *Nux v.; Oniscus;* Stront. c.; Thea. See Pain.

Spasmodic contraction, painful, cardio-spasm—Æth.; *Agar.;* Am. c.; *Arg. n.;* Ars.; *Bell.;* Calc. c.; Caul.; *Con.;* Hyos.; *Ign.;* Nat. m.; *Nux v.;* Phos.; Puls.; Rhus t.; Sep.; Sil.

Dilatation (gastroptosis)—Bism.; Graph.; *Hydrast. mur.;* Kali bich.; *Nux v.;* Phos.; Puls.; Xanthor.

GASTRALGIA—See Pain.

GASTRIC AFFECTIONS, better in open air—Adon.

GASTRIC AFFECTIONS, of cigar-makers—Ign.

HEMORRHAGE (hematemesis): Acet. ac.; Acon.; Arn.; *Ars.;* Bothrops; *Cact.;* Canth.; Carbo v.; *Cinch.; Cocaine;* Crot.; Cupr. m.; Erig.; Ferr. p.; Ficcus; *Geran.; Ham.;* Hyos.; *Ipec.;* Kreos.; Mangif. ind.; *Millef.;* Nit. ac.; Nux v.; *Phos.; Sec.;* Trill.; Zinc. m.

HICCOUGH—(**singultus**): Æth.; Agar.; Amyl; Ars.; Bell.; *Cajup.;* Caps.; Carbo an.; Carbo v.; *Cic.;* Cocaine; Cocc.; *Cupr. m.; Cycl.;* Diosc.; Eup. perf.; *Gins.;* Hep.; Hydroc. ac.; Hyos.; *Ign.;* Kali br.; Mag. p.; *Morph.; Mosch.;* Nat. m.; Niccol.; Nicot.; Nux m.; *Nux v.;* Ol. succin.; Ran. b.; Stram.; *Sul. ac.;* Tab.; Ver. a.; Ver. v.; Zinc. oxy.; *Zinc. v.*

STOMACH

Hiccough, after smoking—Ign.; Selen.

Hiccough, followed by spasm—Cupr. m.

Hiccough, with belching—Ant. c.; *Cajup.*; Cic.; Cinch.; *Diosc.*; *Nux v.*; Wyeth.

Hiccough, with hysterical, nervous symptoms—Gels.; *Ign.*; *Mosch.*; Nux m.; Zinc. v.

Hiccough, with pains in back, after eating, nursing—Teucr.

Hiccough, with retching, vomiting—Jatropha; Mag. p.; Merc.; *Nux v.*

Hiccough, with spasm of esophagus—Ver. v.

Hiccough, with yawning—Amyl; Carls.; *Cocc.*

HYPER-ACIDITY (hyperchlorhydria): Acet. ac.; Anac.; Ant. c.; *Arg. n.*; Atrop.; Bism.; Caffeine; *Calc. c.*; Calc. p.; Carbo v.; Cham.; Chin. ars.; Cinch.; Con.; Grind.; Hydr.; Ign.; *Iris*; Lob. infl.; Lyc.; Mag. c.; Mur. ac.; Nat. c.; Nat. p.; *Nux v.*; *Orexine tan.*; Petrol.; Phos.; Prun. v.; Puls.; Robin.; Sul.; *Sul. ac.*

Hyperæsthesia—*Arg. n.*; Ars.; Bism.; Chin. ars

Hyperperistalsis—Ars.; Fel. tauri; Hyos.; *Ign.*; Phos.

INDIGESTION—DYSPEPSIA—Remedies in general: Abies c.; *Abies n.*; Abrot.; Acet. ac.; Æsc.; Æth.; Agar.; Alet.; Alfal.; Allium s.; Alnus; Aloe; Alum.; Anac.; Ant. c.; Ant. t.; Apoc.; *Arg. n.*; Aristol.; Arn.; Ars.; Atrop.; Bapt.; Bar. c.; Bell.; *Bism.*; Brom.; *Bry.*; Calc. c.; Calc. chlor.; Caps.; Carb. ac.; Carbo v.; Card. m.; Cascara sag.; *Cham.*; Chel.; Cina; *Cinch.*; *Coca*; Cochlear.; *Colch.*; Col.; Corn. fl.; Cupr. ac.; *Cycl.*; *Diosc.*; Fel tauri; Ferr. m.; Gent.; *Graph.*; Hep.; Homar.; Hydr.; *Ign.*; Iod.; *Ipec.*; Iris; *Kali bich.*; Kali c.; Kali m.; Lach.; Lept.; *Lob. infl.*; Lyc.; Merc.; *Nat. c.*; Nat. m.; Nat. s.; Nit. ac.; *Nux m.*; *Nux v.*; Op.; Petrol.; Phos. ac.; *Phos.*; Picr. ac.; Pod.; Pop. tr.; Prun. sp.; Prun. v.; Ptel.; *Puls.*; *Robin.*; Sal. ac.; Sang.; *Sep.*; Stann.; *Strych. ferr. cit.*; *Sul.*; Sul. ac.; Uran. n.; Xerophyl.

CAUSE.—Abuse of drugs—Nux v.

Acids—*Ant. c.*; Ars.; Cinch.; Nat. m.

Aged, debilitated—Abies n.; Ars.; Bar. c.; *Carbo v.*; Cinch.; Fluor. ac.; Hydr.; Kali c.

Beer—Ant. t.; Bapt.; Bry.; *Kali bich.*; Lyc.; *Nux v.*

Bread—Ant. c.; Bry.; Lyc.; Nat. m.

Bright's disease—Apoc. See Urinary System.

Buckwheat cakes—Puls.

Cheese—Ars.; Carbo v.; Col.; Nux v.

Coffee—Cham.; Kali c.; Lyc.; *Nux v.*

Cold bathing—Ant. c.

Debauchery in general—Ant. t.; *Carbo v.*; Cinch.; Nat. s.; *Nux v.*

Decayed meat, fish—Ars.; Carbo v.

Dietetic indiscretions—Allium s.; *Ant. c.*; Bry.; *Carbo v.*; Cinch.; Coff.; *Ipec.*; Lyc.; Nat. c.; *Nux v.*; Puls.; Xanth.

Egg albumen—Nux v.

Excesses—Carbo v.; *Cinch.*; Kali c.; *Nux v.*

Fat food—Ant. c.; *Calc. c.*; Carbo v.; *Cycl.*; Ipec.; *Kali m.*; *Puls.*; Thuya.

STOMACH 773

Fatigue, brain fag, in children—Calc. fl.
Fevers, acute, after—Cinch.; Quass.
Flatulent food—Cinch.; Lyc.; Puls.
Fruits—Ars.; *Cinch.;* Elaps; *Puls.;* Ver. a.
Gastric juice, scanty—Alnus; *Alum.;* Lyc.
Gout—Ant. t.; Cinch.; *Colch.;* Nux m.; Thuya.
Hasty eating, drinking—Anac.; Coff.; *Oleand.*
Hot weather—Ant. c.; *Bry.*
Ice water, ices—Ars.; Carbo v.; Elaps; Ipec.; Kali c.; Nat. c.; *Puls.*
Lactation—*Cinch.;* Sinap. a.
Meats—*Caust.;* Ipec.; Puls.; Sil.
Melons—Ars.; Zing.
Menstruation—Arg. n.; Cop.; Sep. See Female Sexual System.
Milk—*Æth.;* Calc. c.; Carbo v.; Mag. c.; Mag. m.; Nit. ac.; Sul. ac.; Sul.
Nervous, from unpleasant emotions—Cham.; Nux m.; Nux v.
Night watching—Nux v.
Pastry—Ant. c.; Carbo v.; Ipec.; Kali m.; Lyc.; *Puls.*
Pork sausage—Cinch.; Puls.
Pregnancy—Sabad.; *Sinap a.;* Thea.
Salt, abuse of—Phos.
Sedentary life—Nux v.
Sweets—Ant. c.; *Arg. n.;* Ipec.; *Lyc.;* Zinc. m.
Tea—Abies n.; *Cinch.; Diosc.;* Puls.; Thea; Thuya.
Tobacco—Abies n.; *Nux v.;* Sep.
Urticaria—Cop.
Vegetables, tobacco—Ars.; Asclep t.; Nat. c.; Nux v.; *Sep.*
Water—Ars.
Wines, liquors—Ant. c.; Caps.; Carbo v.; Coff.; Nat. s.; *Nux v.;* Sul.; Sul. ac.; Zinc. m.

TYPE—Atonic, nervous, acid—Alet.; *Alfal.;* Alston.; Anac.; Angust.; *Arg. n.;* Calc. c.; Caps.; Carb. ac.; *Carbo v.;* Cinch.; Ferr.; Grind.; Hep.; *Ign.;* Jugl. c.; *Kali p.;* Lob. infl.; *Lyc.;* Mag. c.; Nat. c.; *Nux v.;* Phos.; *Ptel.;* Quass.; Ratanh.; Robin.; Sul. ac.; Sul.; Val.

Catarrhal—Abies c.; Abies n.; Ant. c.; *Arg. n.;* Bals. per.; Calc. c.; Carb. ac.; Carbo v.; Cinch.; Collins.; Coryd.; Geran.; *Hydr.;* Hydroc. ac.; Illic.; *Ipec.; Kali bich.;* Lyc.; Nux v.; Ox. ac.; *Puls.;* Sul. See Chronic Catarrhal Gastritis.

Latent or masked—Cact.; Carbo v.; Cinch.; Hydroc. ac.; *Nat. m.; Sep.;* Spig.; Tab.

SYMPTOMS AND CONDITIONS—Acidity: Arg. n.; *Calc. c.;* Carbo v.; Ign.; Lob. infl.; Lyc.; Nat. c.; *Nux v.;* Puls.; *Robin.;* Sul. See Hyperchlorhydria.

Cough—Lob. syph.; Taxus. See Respiratory System.

Digestion, weak, slow (bradypepsia)—Alston.; Anac.; *Ant. c.; Arg. n.;* Ars.; Asaf.; Bism.; *Bry.;* Caps.; *Carbo an.; Carbo v.;* Cinch.; Cochlear.; Coff.; Colch.; *Cycl.; Diosc.;* Eucal.; Granat.; *Graph.; Hydr.;* Ipec.;

STOMACH

Kali bich.; *Lyc.;* Merc.; *Nat. c.;* Nat. m.; *Nux v.;* Prun. v.; *Puls.;* Zing. See Indigestion.

Distress from simplest food—Alet.; Amyg. pers.; Ant. c.; Carbo an.; *Carbo v.;* Cinch.; Dig.; Hep.; Kali c.; Lach.; Nat. c.; Nux v.; Puls.

Drowsiness, sleepiness—Æth.; Ant. c.; Bism.; Carbo v.; Cinch.; *Epiph.;* Fel tauri; Graph.; Grat.; Kali c.; *Lyc.;* Nat. chlor.; Nat. m.; Nux m.; Nux v.; Phos. ac.; Phos.; Sarrac.; Staph.; Sul.

Eructations, belching—*Abies n.;* Acet. ac.; Agar.; Alum.; Anac.; Ant. c.; Arg. n.; Arn.; Asaf.; Bism.; Bry.; Cajup.; Calc. c.; Calc. p.; Caps.; Carb. ac.; Carbo an.; Carbo v.; Cham.; Cinch.; Cycl.; Diosc.; Fagop.; Ferr. m.; Ferr. p.; Glycerin; Graph.; Grat.; Hep.; Hydr.; Ind.; Iod.; Ipec.; Jugl. c.; Kali bich.; *Kali c.;* Lob. infl.; *Lyc.;* Mag. c.; *Mosch.;* Nat. c.; Nat. p.; Nat. m.; Nit. ac.; Nux m.; Nux v.; Petrol.; Phos.; Pod.; *Puls.;* Robin.; Rumex; Sal. ac.; Sang.; Sep.; Sil.; *Sul.;* Sul. ac.; Uran. n.; Val.

Eructations, odorless, tasteless, empty—*Agar.;* Aloe; Ambra; Am. m.; Anac.; Asar.; Bism.; Calad.; Calc. iod.; Coca; Cocc.; Hep.; Ign.; *Iod.;* Oleand.; Plat.

Eructations, rancid, putrid, foul—*Arn.;* Asaf.; Bism.; Calc. iod.; Carbo v.; Cham.; Cycl.; Diosc.; Graph.; Hydr.; Kali c.; Mag. m.; Mag. s.; Ornithog.; Plumb.; Psor.; *Puls.;* Raph.; Sang.; Sep.; Sul.; Thuya; Val.; Xerophyl.

Eructations, relieve temporarily—*Arg. n.;* Asaf.; Bar. c.; Bry.; Calc. p.; Carbo v.; Kali c.; Lach.; Mosch.; Nux m.; Nux v.; Ol. an.; Ox. ac.; Puls.

Eructations, sour, burning, acid, bitter—Acet. ac.; Ant. c.; Arg. n.; *Bry.;* Calc. c.; Calc. iod.; Calc. p.; Carb. ac.; Carbo an.; Carbo v.; Cham.; Cinch.; Diosc.; Ferr. p.; Fluor. ac.; Graph.; Ipec.; Hep.; *Hydr.;* Kali c.; Lact. ac.; Lact. v.; *Lyc.;* Mag. c.; Nat. c.; Nat. m.; Nat. nit.; Nat. p.; Nit. ac.; Nit. mur. ac.; Nux v.; Ox. ac.; Petrol.; Phos. ac.; Phos.; Pod.; Puls.; Raph.; Robin.; Sabal; Sal. ac.; Senec.; Sep.; Sil.; Sinap. n.; Sul. ac.; Sul.; Xerophyl.

Eructations, tasting of ingesta—Ant. c.; Carbo v.; Cinch.; Cycl.; *Ferr.;* Graph.; *Puls.;* Sep.; Sil.; Sul.

Fainting—Ars.; Cinch.; Mosch.; Nux m.; Nux v.; Phos. ac.

Flatulent distention of stomach drumlike—*Abies c.;* Agar.; Ant. c.; Apoc.; Arg. n.; Asaf.; Bry.; But. ac.; Cajup.; Calc. c.; Calc. fl.; Caps.; Carb. ac.; Carbo v.; Cinch.; Colch.; Cycl.; Diosc.; Ferr. magnet.; Graph.; Grat.; Hydr.; *Ign.;* Indol; Iod.; Jugl. c.; Kali bich.; Kali c.; *Lach.;* Lyc.; Mosch.; Nux m.; Nux v.; Ox. ac.; Phos. ac.; Phos.; Pop. tr.; Puls.; Sil.; Sul.; Thuya. See Sensation.

Headache—Arg. n.; *Bry.;* Carbo v.; Cinch.; Cycl.; Kali c.; Lach.; Lept.; *Ign.;* Nat. m.; Nux m.; *Nux v.;* Puls.; Robin.; Sang.; Tarax. See Head.

Heartburn, pyrosis—Am. c.; Ant. c.; Apomorph.; *Arg. n.;* Ars.; Bism.; Bry.; Cajup.; Calc. c.; Calend.; Caps.; Carb. ac.; Carbo v.; Chin. s.; Datura; Diosc.; Fagop.; Gall. ac.; Graph.; Iod.; Kali c.; Lach.; Lob. infl.; *Lyc.;* Mag. c.; Phos. ac.; Mag. m.; Nat. m.; Nit. ac.; Nux v.;

STOMACH

Nux m.; Ox. ac.; *Puls.*; Robin.; Sang.; Sinap.; Sinap. n.; *Sul. ac.*; Tab.

Hiccough—Bry.; Hyos.; Ign.; *Nux v.*; Paris; Sep.

Lassitude, weakness—Act. sp.; Ant. t.; *Ars.*; Can. s.; Caps.; Carbo an.; *Carbo v.*; Cinch.; Graph.; Grat.; Hydr.; *Lyc.*; *Nux v.*; Phos.; Puls.; Sep.

Mental depression, dullness—Anac.; Cinch.; Cycl.; Hydr.; Lyc.; Nat. c.; Nit. ac.; *Nux v.*; Puls.; Sep.; Tab. See Mind.

Nausea, vomiting—Æth.; *Ant. c.*; Ant. t.; *Arg. n.*; *Ars.*; Atrop.; Bism.; Bry.; *Carb. ac.*; Carbo v.; Cham.; Cocc.; Ferr. m.; Graph.; Ign.; *Ipec.*; *Kali bich.*; Kreos.; Lept.; Lob. infl.; Lyc.; Nat. c.; *Nux v.*; Petrol.; Phos.; *Puls.*; Rhus t.; Sang.; Sep.; Sil. See Vomiting.

Pain—*Abies n.*; Æsc.; Anis.; *Arg. n.*; Arn.; *Ars.*; Bry.; Calc. iod.; Calc. mur.; Carbo v.; Cinch.; Col.; Cupressus; Diosc.; Gamb.; *Hedeoma*; Homar.; Ipec.; Kali m.; Nat. m.; *Nux v.*; Paraf.; *Phos.*; Puls.; Scutel.; Sep.; Stann.; Thuya. See Pain.

Pain immediately after eating—*Abies n.*; Arn.; Ars.; Calc. c., *Carbo v.*; Cinch.; Cocc.; *Kali bich.*; Kali c.; Lyc.; *Nux m.*; Physost.

Pain several hours after eating—Æsc.; *Agar.*; Anac.; Bry., Calc. hypoph.; Con.; *Nux v.*; Ox. ac.; *Puls.*

Palpitation of the heart—Abies c.; *Arg. n.*; *Cact.*; *Carbo v.*; Hydroc. ac.; Lyc.; *Nat. m.*; *Nux v.*; *Puls.*; Sep.; *Spig.*; Tab. See Circulatory System.

Pressure as from a stone—*Abies n.*; Acon.; Æsc.; Anac.; *Arg. n.*; Arn.; Ars.; Bry.; *Calc. c.*; Calc. m.; Carbo v.; Cham.; Cinch.; Dig.; Ferr. m.; Graph.; Hep.; *Kali bich.*; Lob. infl.; *Lyc.*; *Nux v.*; Phos. ac.; *Phos.*; Puls.; Rhus t.; Rumex; Scilla; Sep.; Sul.

Pulsation in epigastrium—*Asaf.*; Eucal.; *Hydr.*; Nat. m.; *Puls.*; Selen.; Sep.

Pulsation in rectum—Aloe.

Regurgitation of food—Æth.; *Alum.*; Am. m.; *Ant. c.*; Asaf.; *Carbo v.*; Cham.; Cinch.; Ferr. iod.; Ferr.; Graph.; Ign.; *Ipec.*; Merc.; Nat. p.; *Nux v.*; Phos.; *Puls.*; Quass.; *Sul.*

Salivation—Cycl.; Lob. infl.; *Merc.*; Nat. m.; Puls.; Sang. See Mouth.

Sweating—Carbo v.; Nat. m.; Nit. ac.; Sep.

Toothache—Cham.; Kali c.; Lyc.; Nat. c.; Nit. ac.

Vertigo—Bry.; Carbo v.; Cinch.; Cycl.; *Grat.*; Ign.; *Nux v.*; Puls.; Rhus t. See Head.

Waterbrash—*Abies n.*; Acet. ac.; *Ant. c.*; Ars.; Bism.; *Bry.*; Calc. c.; *Carbo v.*; Diosc.; Fagop.; Graph.; Hep.; Hydr.; Kali c.; Lact. ac.; *Lyc.*; Mag. m.; Nat. m.; Nit. ac.; *Nux v.*; Pod.; *Puls.*; Sep.; Sul.; Symphor.; Ver. a.

INFLAMMATION (gastritis): acute: Acon.; Agar. emet.; *Ant. t.*; *Ars.*; Bell.; Bism.; Bry.; Canth.; Ferr. p.; Hedeoma; *Hydr.*; Hyos.; *Ipec.*; Iris; *Kali bich.*; Kali chlor.; Merc. c.; *Nux v.*; Ox. ac.; *Phos.*; Puls.; Santon.; Sinap. a.; Ver. a.; Zinc.

Inflammation, acute, from alcoholic abuse—Arg. n.; *Ars.*; Bism.; Crot.; Cupr.; *Gaulth.*; Lach.; *Nux v.*; Phos.

STOMACH

Inflammation, acute, with intestinal involvement (gastro-enteritis): Alumen; Arg. n.; Ars.; Bapt.; Bism.; Bry.; Cupr.; Merc. c.; Merc.; Rhus t.; Santon.; Zinc.

Inflammation, chronic (catarrh of stomach)—Alum.; Ant. c.; Ant. t.; Arg. n.; Arn.; Ars.; Bism.; Calc. c.; Calc. chlor.; Caps.; Carb. ac.; Carbo v.; Cinch.; Colch.; Dig.; Graph.; Hydr.; Hydroc. ac.; Illic.; Iod.; Ipec.; Kali bich.; Kali c.; Lyc.; Merc. c.; Nux v.; Op.; Ox. ac.; Phos.; Pod.; Puls.; Rumex; Sang.; Sep.; Sil.; Sul.; Ver. a.; Zinc.

NAUSEA—(qualmishness): Ant. c.; Ant. t.; Apoc.; Apomorph.; Arg. n.; Arn.; Ars.; Asar.; Bell.; Berb. v.; Bism.; Bry.; Cadm. s.; Carb. ac.; Carbo v.; Card. m.; Cascar.; Cham.; Chel.; Chionanth.; Cocc.; Colch.; Cupr. m.; Cycl.; Dig.; Eug. j.; Fagop.; Ferr. m.; Glon.; Hedeoma; Hyper.; Ichth.; Ipec.; Iris; Kali bich.; Kali c.; Kal.; Kreos.; Lach.; Lact. ac.; Lob. infl.; Merc. c.; Merc. s.; Morph.; Nat. c.; Nat. m.; Nux v.; Ostrya; Petrol.; Pod.; Puls.; Sabad.; Sang.; Sarcol.; ac.; Sep.; Spig.; Strych.; Symphor.; Tab.; Ther.; Ver. a.; Ver. v.

Nausea after abdominal operations—Staph.

Nausea after eating—Am. c.; Asar.; Cycl.; Graph.; Nux v.; Puls.; Sil.

Nausea before breakfast—Berb. v.; Gossyp.; Nux v.; Sep.

Nausea from beer—Kali bich.

Nausea from closing eyes—Lach.; Ther.; Thuya.

Nausea from coffee—Cham.

Nausea from fat—Nit. ac.

Nausea from ices, cold—Ars.

Nausea from pessaries—Nux m.

Nausea from looking at moving objects—Asar.; Cocc.; Ipec.; Jabor.

Nausea from immersing hands in warm water—Phos.

Nausea from nervousness, emotional excitement—Menthol.

Nausea from pregnancy—Cocc.; Con.; Lact. ac.; Lac. v. c.; Lob. infl.; Mag. c.; Mag. m.; Phos. ac.; Piloc.; Sep.; Staph.; Strych.; Sul. See Female Sexual System.

Nausea from riding in cars, boat—Arn.; Cocc.; Lac d.; Nux m.; Nux v.; Petrol.; Sanic.: Ther.

Nausea from smell or sight of food—Æth.; Ars.; Cocc.; Colch.; Nux v.; Puls.; Sep.; Stann.; Symphor.

Nausea from smoking—Euphras.; Ign.; Ipec.; Nux v.; Phos.; Tab.

Nausea from sweets—Graph.

Nausea from water—Apoc.; Ars.; Ver. a.

Nausea from water, aerated, champagne—Digitox.

With cramps—Triost.

With desire for stool—Dulc.

With diarrhoea, anxiety—Ant. t.

With drowsiness—Apoc.

With faintness—Bry.; Cocc.; Colch.; Hep.; Nux v.; Plat.; Puls.; Tab.; Val.

With headache—Aloe; Formica; Puls.

With hunger—Berb. aq.; Cocc.; Ign.; Val.

With menses—Cocc.; Crot.: Symphor.

STOMACH

With pain, coldness—Cadm. s.; Hep.
With pale, twitching face, no relief from vomiting—Ipec.
With pressure downward, in intestines—Agn.
With relief from eating—*Lact. ac.*; Mez.; Santon.; Sep.; Vip. op.
With relief from lemonade—Cycl.; Puls.
With relief from lying down—Echin.; *Kali c.*; Puls.
With relief from smoking—Eug. j.
With relief from swallow of cold water—Cupr. m.
With relief from uncovering abdomen; in open air—Tab.
With salivation—*Ipec.*; Petrol.; Sang.
With vertigo—*Cocc.*; Hyos.; Lach.; Puls.; Tab.; *Ther.*
With vision dim—Myg.
With weakness, anxiety, recurs periodically—Ars.
Worse after eating—Asar.; Berb. aq.; Dig.; *Ipec.*; Nux v.; Puls.
Worse from least sound or noise—Ther.
Worse from motion, rising—Ars.; *Bry.*; Cocc.; Symphor.; *Tab.*; Triost.; Ver. a.
Worse in morning—Anac.; Calc. c.; Fagop.; Carbo v.; *Graph.*; Lact. ac.; Nat. c.; *Nux v.*; Phos.; Puls.; *Sep.*; Sil.; Sul.

NERVOUS DISORDERS—*Agar.*; Bell.; Col.; *Mag. p.*; Nux v.; Sang. See Pain.

PAIN (gastrodynia): Type: Aching:—Æsc.; Anac.; *Hydr.*; Ruta.

Burning, as from ulcer—*Acet. ac.*; Agar. emet.; *Arg. n.*; Arn.; *Ars.*; Asaf.; Bism.; Cadm. br.; Canth.; *Carbo v.*; *Chin. ars.*; Colch.; *Condur.*; Con.; Datura; Formica; Graph.; *Iod.*; Iris; Kali iod.; Laburn.; *Lact. ac.*; Lapis alb.; Mancin.; Nat. m.; *Nux v.*; Ox. ac.; *Phos.*; Robin.; Sep.; *Sul.*; Uran. See Sensations.

Crampy, contractive, colicky, drawing—*Abies n.*; Act. sp.; *Agar. ph.*; *Arg. n.*; Bapt.; *Bell.*; Bism.; But. ac.; Cact.; Calc. c.; Calc. iod.; *Carbo v.*; *Cham.*; Cocaine; *Cocc.*; *Col.*; Con.; Cupr. m.; Datura; Granat.; *Graph.*; *Ign.*; Ipec.; Jatropha; Kali c.; Lob. infl.; *Mag. p.*; *Nux v.*; Petrol.; Phos.; Plat.; Ptel.; Sep.; Ver. v. See Sensations.

Cutting, lancinating, stitching, spasmodic, paroxysmal, darting, tearing, shooting—Acon.; Act. sp.; *Arg. n.*; *Atrop.*; *Bell.*; Bism.; *Bry.*; Carbo v.; Card. m.; Caust.; *Chin. ars.*; *Col.*; Con.; *Cupressus*; *Cupr. ac.*; Cupr. m.; *Diosc.*; Hydr.; Ign.; Iris; Kali c.; *Mag. p.*; *Nux v.*; Ox. ac.; Ratanh.; Sep.; Sul.; Thall.

Epigastric (pit of stomach)—*Abies c.*; *Abies n.*; Act. sp.; Æsc.; Aloe; Am. m.; Anac.; *Arg. n.*; Arn.; *Ars.*; Bar. m.; *Bell.*; Bism.; *Bry.*; Calc. c.; Calc. iod.; Carb. ac.; Carbo v.; Cina; Col.; Cupr.; *Diosc.*; Graph.; *Hydr.*; Jatropha; Kali bich.; Kali c.; Kal.; Lob. infl.; Lyc.; Nat. m.; *Nux v.*; Ox. ac.; Paraf.; *Phos.*; Sep.; Sang.; Ver. a.

Gnawing, hungry-like—*Abies c.*; Abrot.; Æsc.; Agar.; Am. m.; *Anac.*; *Arg. n.*; Asar.; Cina; Ign.; *Iod.*; Lach.; Phos.; *Puls.*; Ruta; Sep.; Uran. See Sensations.

Neuralgic (gastralgia)—Abies n.; Acet. ac.; Æsc.; Alum.; Anac.; *Arg. n.*; Ars.; *Atrop.*; *Bell.*; Bism.; *Bry.*; *Carbo v.*; Chel.; Cham.; *Chin. ars.*;

Cina; *Cocc.*; Cod.; Colch.; *Col.*; Condur.; *Cupr. ars.*; Dig.; *Diosc.*; Ferr. m.; Gels.; Glon.; *Graph.*; *Hydroc. ac.*; Ign.; *Ipec.*; Kali c.; Lob. infl.; *Mag. p.*; Menthol; Niccol.; Nux m.; *Nux v.*; *Ox. ac.*; Petrol.; Plumb.; Ptel.; Puls.; Quass.; Rham. c.; Ruta; Spig.; Stann.; *Stryck.*; Sul. ac.; Tab.; *Ver. a.*; Zinc.

Concomitants to gastralgia—With anemia—*Ferr.*; Glon.; Graph.

With backache, anxiety, despondency, sallow face—Nit. ac.

With chronic gastritis—Alum.; Atrop.; Bism.; Lyc.

With chronic ulcer—Arg. n.

With constipation—Bry.; Graph.; Nux v.; Physost.; *Plumb.*

With extension to sides, then to back—Cochlear.

With extension to shoulders—Niccol.

With gout—Colch.; Urt.

With hysteria—Asaf.; Ign.; Plat.

With lactation—Carbo v.; Cinch.

With menses—Arg. n.; Cocc.

With nervous depression—Arg. n.; Gaulth.; *Nux v.*

With pain in throat and spine alternately—Paraf.

With pregnancy—Petrol.

With recurrence—Graph.

With uterine disorder—Bor.

Sickening pain—Ostrya.

MODALITIES TO PAIN—Aggravation: At night: Anac.; Arg. n.; Ars.; Cham.; Cocc.; Ign.; Kali bich.

From beer—Bapt.; *Kali bich.*

From bending forward—Kal.

From coffee—Canth.; Cham.; Nux v.; Ox. ac.

From empty stomach—*Anac.*; Cina; Hydroc. ac.; *Petrol.*

From food—*Arg. n.*; Bell.; *Bry.*, Ign.; Kali bich.; *Nux v.*

From food, warm—Bar. c.

From jar—Aloe; *Bell.*; Bry.

From nursing—Æth.

From pressure—Arg. n.; Calc. c.; Cochlear.; Ign.

From touch—Bell.; Ign.; Nux v.; *Ox. ac.*

From walking, descending stairs—Bry.

From water, cold—Calc. c.

From worms—*Cina*; Granat.

AMELIORATION—From bending backward, standing erect: Bell.; *Diosc.*

From drinks, cold—Bism.

From drinks, warm—Graph.; Ver. v.

From eating—*Anac.*; Brom.; Calc. p.; *Chel.*; Graph.; *Hep.*; Homar.; Hydroc. ac.; Ign.; *Iod.*; Kreos.; Lach.; Nat. m.; *Petrol.*; Puls.; Sep.

From ice cream—Phos.

From pressure—Bry.; Fluor ac.; *Plumb.*

From sitting erect—Kal.

From vomiting—Hyos.; Plumb. m.

PYLORUS—Constriction—Can. ind.; *Cinch.*; Hep.; *Nux v.*; Phos.; Ornithog.; Sil.

STOMACH

Induration—Bism.; *Condur.;* Graph.; *Phos.;* Sep.; *Strych. p.*

Pain—Canth.; Cepa; *Hep.;* Lyc.; Merc.; *Ornithog.;* Tussil.; *Uran.* See Constriction.

SENSATION—Anxiety: Ars.; Kali c.; Nit. ac.; Phos.; Ver. a.

As if stomach were full of dry food—Calad.

As if stomach were pressed against spine—Arn.

As if stomach were swimming in water—Abrot.

Burning heat—Abies c.; Acet. ac.; *Acon.;* Agar.; Arg. n.; Ars.; Bism.; Calopt.; *Canth.;* Carb. ac.; *Carbo v.;* Caust.; Colch.; Col.; Ferr. m.; Glycerin; Graph.; Hep.; *Iris; Lact. ac.;* Merc. c.; Nat. m.; *Phos.;* Sang.; Sep.; *Sul.;* Tereb.

Coldness—Abrot.; Bov.; Calc. c.; Calc. sil.; Camph.; Cinch.; *Colch.;* Elaps; Hippom.; Kali c.; Kreos.; *Menyanth.;* Ol. an.; Ox. ac.; Pyrus; Sabad.; *Sul. ac.;* Tab.; *Ver. a.*

Distended, drumlike, tightness, clothing intolerable—*Abies c.;* Absinth.; Agar.; *Ambra; Anac.;* Ant. c.; *Apoc.; Arg. n.;* Ars.; Asaf.; But. ac.; *Cajup.;* Calc. c.; Calc. fl.; Calc. iod.; Calc. p.; *Caps.;* Carb. ac.; *Carbo v.;* Cham.; Chel.; *Cinch.;* Cocc.; *Colch.; Diosc.;* Euonym.; Fel tauri; Ferr. m.; *Graph.;* Grat.; Ign.; *Kali c.; Lach.;* Lecith.; Lob. infl.; *Lyc.;* Merc. c.; Mosch.; Nat. cholein; Nat. m.; Nit. ac.; *Nux m.; Nux v.;* Ornithog.; Pop. tr.; *Puls.;* Sul.

Empty, faint, sinking, "all gone" feeling—*Abies c.;* Anac.; Apoc.; Asaf.; Bapt.; *Bar. mur.;* Caps.; Carbo an.; *Carbo v.;* Cim.; Cocc.; *Dig.; Diosc.;* Gels.; Graph.; *Hydr.;* Hydroc. ac.; *Ign.;* Kali c.; Kali p.; Lac c.; Latrod.; *Lob. infl.;* Lyc.; *Merc. s.;* Morph.; Murex; Ornithog.; Petrol.; *Phos.;* Ptel.; *Puls.;* Radium; Sang.; *Sep.;* Stann.; *Sul.; Tab.;* Tellur.; Thea; Thuya; Trill.; Vib. op.

Empty feeling, aggravated 11 a. m., unable to wait for lunch—*Sul.;* Zinc. m.

Empty feeling, relieved by eating—Anac.; *Chel.;* Iod.; Nat. c.; Mur.; Phos.; *Sep.;* Sul.

Empty feeling, relieved by lying down, wine—Sep.

Heaviness, pressure, as from stone or lump—*Abies n.;* Acon.; *Arg. n.;* Arn.; *Ars.;* Bism.; *Bry.;* Calc. c.; *Carbo v.;* Cham.; *Cinch.;* Colch.; Dig.; Ferr. m.; *Graph.; Kali bich.;* Kali c.; Lob. infl.; *Lyc.; Nux v.;* Passifl.; *Phos.;* Piloc.; *Puls.;* Robin.; Sang.; Sep.; Spig.; *Sul.;* Xerophyl.; Zing.

Pulsations, throbbing—*Arg. n.;* Asaf.; *Cact.;* Cic.; *Crot.;* Eucal.; *Hydr.;* Iod.; *Kali c.;* Kali iod.; Lach.; *Nat. m.;* Oleand.; *Puls.;* Rheum.

Relaxed, hanging down feeling—Agar.; *Hydr.;* Ign.; *Ipec.; Staph.;* Sul. ac.; *Tab.*

Tenderness, to contact, pressure, jars—*Apis; Arg. n.;* Ars.; Bell.; Bov.; Bry.; *Calc. c.;* Calc. iod.; Canth.; Carbo v.; Card. m.; *Cinch.;* Colch.; Dig.; *Kali bich.;* Kali c.; *Lach.;* Lecith.; Lyc.; *Merc. c.; Merc. s.;* Nat. c.; Nat. m.; Nux m.; *Nux v.;* Phos.; Puls.; Sang.; Sil.; Spig.; Stann.; Sul.

Trembling—Arg. n.; Crot.

Softening (gastro-malacia)—Calc. c.; Kreos.; Merc. d.

THIRST—*Acet. ac.;* Acon.; Alfal.; Ant. c.; Ant. t.; Apoc.; Arn.; *Ars.;* Ars. iod.; Bell.; Berb. v.; Bism.; *Bry.;* Camph.; *Canth.;* Caps.; Cham.; Chin. ars.; Cinch.; Cocc.; Colch.; Crot.; Cupr. ars.; Dulc.; *Eup. perf.;* Helleb.; Helon.; Ichth.; Indol.; Iod.; Kali br.; Lact. ac.; Laur.; Lecith.; Mag. c.; Mag. p.; Med.; Merc. c.; *Merc.;* Morph.; *Nat. m.;* Nux v.; Op.; Petros.; Phos. ac.; *Phos.;* Pod.; Rhus ar.; *Rhus t.;* Sang.; Scilla; Sec.; Sep.; Stram.; *Sul.;* Tereb.; Thuya; Uran. n.; *Ver. a.;* Ver. v.

Constant sipping of cold water—*Acon.;* Ant. t.; *Ars.;* Hyos.; Onosm.; Sanic.

Drinks seldom, but much—*Bry.;* Helleb.; Pod.; *Sul.;* Ver. a.

Thirstlessness—*Æth.;* Ant. t.; *Apis;* Berb. v.; Cinch.; Coff.; Cycl.; *Gels.;* Helleb.; Menyanth.; Nux m.; *Puls.;* Sabad.; Sars.

ULCER OF STOMACH—*Arg. n.;* Ars.; Atrop.; Bell.; Bism.; Calc. ars.; Condur.; Crot.; Ferr. acet.; *Geran.;* Graph.; Grind.; Ham.; *Hydr.;* Iod.; Ipec.; *Kali bich.;* Kali iod.; Kreos.; Lyc.; *Merc. c.;* Merc.; Op.; *Ornithog.;* Petrol.; *Phos.;* Plumb. ac.; Ratanh.; Sinap. a.; Symphyt.; *Uran.*

VOMITING, retching—Remedies, in general: Abrot.; Acon.; *Æth.;* Agar. phal.; Alumen; Amyg. pers.; *Ant. c.; Ant. t.;* Apoc.; *Apomorph.; Arg. n.;* Ars.; Atrop.; *Bell.; Bism.; Bry.;* Cadm. s.; Calc. c.; Calc. m.; Camph. monobr.; Can. ind.; Canth.; Caps.; *Carb. ac.;* Card. m.; Cascarilla; *Cerium;* Cham.; Chel.; Cinch.; *Cocc.; Colch.; Cupr. ac.; Cupr. ars.;* Cupr. m.; Dros.; Eup. perf.; *Ferr. m.;* Ferr. mur.; Ferr. p.; Gaulth.; Geran.; Granat.; Graph.; Iod.; *Ipec.; Iris;* Jatropha; *Kali bich.;* Kali ox.; *Kreos.;* Lach.; Lact. ac.; *Lob. infl.; Mag. c.;* Merc. c.; *Morph.;* Nat. m.; Nat. p.; *Nux v.; Op.;* Petrol.; *Phos.;* Pix l.; Plumb.; *Puls.;* Ricin. com.; Sang.; Sarcol. ac.; *Sep.;* Stann.; Strych. et ferr. cit.; *Symphor.; Tab.;* Uran.; Val.; *Ver. a.;* Xerophyl.; Zinc

CAUSE—Anger in nursing mother, affecting milk—Val.

Anger, with indignation—Cham.; Col.; Staph.

Beer—Cupr.; Ipec.; *Kali bich.*

Bowels impacted—Op.; Plumb.; Pyr.

Cancer (hepatic, gastric, uterine)—Carb. ac.; Kreos.

Cerebral—Apomorph.; Bell.; Glon.; Plumb. m.

Clearing throat of mucus in morning—Bry.; Euphras.

Climacteric—Aquil.

Closing eyes—Ther.

Cyclic, in infants—Cupr. ars.; Ingluv.; Iris; Kreos.; Merc. d.

Drinks, cold, can only retain hot drinks—Apoc.; *Ars.;* Ars. iod.; Calad.; Cascar.; *Chel.;* Ver. a.

Drinks of any kind—Acon.; Apoc.; Ant. t.; *Ars.;* Bism.; *Canth.;* Dulc.; *Eup. perf.;* Ipec.; Sanic.; Sil.; *Ver. a.*

Drinks, warm—Bry.; Phos.; *Puls.;* Pyr.; Sanic.

Drunkards in morning—Ant. t.; Ars.; Carb. ac.; *Cupr. ars;* Cupr m.; Ipec.; Lob. infl.; *Nux v.*

Eating, drinking—Acet. ac.; *Ant. c.;* Ant. t.; *Ars.;* Bism.; *Bry.;* Calc.

STOMACH

mur.; Cina; Colch.; Crot.; *Ferr. m.;* Ferr. p.; Hyos.; Iod.; *Ipec.;* Lyc.; Nux v.; *Phos.;* Puls.; Sil.; Ver. a.; Ver. v.

Eruptions repercussed—Cupr. m.

Gastric irritation—Ant. c.; *Ars.;* Bism.; Ferr. m.; Ipec.; Nux v.; Phos.; Puls.; Ver. a.

Hysterical—*Aquil.;* Ign.; *Kreos.;* Plat.; Val.

Lying on any side, except right—Ant. t.

Lying on right side or back—Crot.

Menses, after—Crot. See Female Sexual System.

Milk—*Æth.;* Ars.; Calc. c.; Ferr.; Kreos.; Mag. c.; Mag. m.; Merc. d.; Merc. s.

Motion—*Bry.;* Cocc.; Colch.; Dig.; Nux v.; *Tab.;* Ther.; Ver. a.

Phthisis—Kali br.; Kreos.

Post-operative (laparotomy)—Æth.; *Bism.; Cepa; Nux v.;* Phos.; Staph.; *Strych.*

Pregnancy—Acet. ac.; Alet.; *Amyg. pers.;* Ant. t.; *Apomorph.;* Ars; Bism.; Carb. ac.; *Cerium;* Cocaine; *Cocc.; Cod.;* Cucurb.; *Cupr. ac.;* Ferr. m.; Gossyp.; Graph.; Ign.; Ingluv.; *Ipec.;* Iris; *Kreos.;* Lac d.; *Lact. ac.;* Lob. infl.; *Mag. c.; Nux v.;* Petrol.; Phos.; Psor.; Puls.; *Sep.;* Stront. br.; Strych.; Symphor.; *Tab.*

Pressure on spine and cervical region—Cim.

Raising head—Apomorph.; *Bry.;* Stram.

Reflex—Apomorph.; Cerium; Cocc.; *Ipec.;* Kreos.; *Val.*

Renal origin—Kreos.; Nux v.

Riding in cars—Arn.; *Cocc.;* Ipec.; Kreos.; Nux v.; Petrol.; Sanic.; S.

Scarlet fever—Ail.; *Bell.*

Sea-sickness; car sickness—*Apomorph.;* Ars.; Bor.; Carb. ac.; Cerium; Cocc.; Coff.; Glon.; Ipec.; *Kreos.;* Nicot.; *Nux v.;* Op.; *Petrol.; Sep.;* Staph.; Tab.; Ther.

Water, sight of, must close eyes while bathing—Lyssin; Phos.

TYPE—Acid, sour: Ant c.; Ars.; Bry.; Calad.; *Calc. c.;* Card. m.; Cham.; *Ferr. m.;* Ferr. p.; Iod.; *Iris;* Kali c.; Lac d.; Lact. ac.; *Lyc.;* Mag. c.; *Nat. p.; Nat. s.; Nux v.;* Puls.; *Robin.;* Sul.; Sul. ac.

Bilious (green, yellow)—*Acon.;* Æth.; Ant. c.; Ars.; Bell.; *Bry.;* Carb. ac ; *Card. m.; Cham.; Chel.;* Crot.; Eup. arom.; *Eup. perf.;* Grat.; Ipec.; *Iris;* Kali c.; Lept.; Nux v.; Nyctanth.; Petrol.; *Pod.;* Puls.; Robin.; *Sang.;* Sep.; Tart. ac.

Black—*Ars.; Cadm. s.; Crot.;* Mancin; Pix l.

Bloody—*Acon.;* Arg. n.; *Ars.;* Bothrops; Cadm. s.; *Canth.;* Crot.; Ferr. m.; *Ferr. p.;* Ficcus; *Geran.; Ham.; Ipec.;* Iris; Mez.; *Phos.;* Sec. See Hemetemesis.

Coffee-grounds, like—*Ars.;* Cadm. s.; *Crot.;* Lach.; *Merc. c.;* Ornithog.; Pyr.; Sec.

Fecal—Op.; Plumb.; Pyr.; Raph.

Food, undigested—*Ant. c.;* Apoc.; Atrop.; Bals. per.; Bism.; *Bry.;* Cerium; *Cinch.;* Colch.; Cupr.; *Ferr. m.;* Ferr. mur.; Ferr. p.; Graph.; *Ipec.;* Iris; Kreos.; Lac c.; Nux v.; Petrol.; Phos.; *Puls.;* Sang.; Strych. ferr. cit.; Ver. a.

Milk, coagula—*Æth.*; Ant. c.; *Calc. c.*; Ipec.; *Mag. c.*; Mag. m.; Merc. d.; Merc.; Pod.; Sanic.; *Val.*

Mucus slimy—Æth.; Ant. c.; *Ant. t.*; *Arg. n.*; Ars.; Bals. per.; Cadm. s.; Carbo v.; Colch.; *Ipec.*; Iris; Jatropha; *Kali bich.*; Kali m.; Kreos.; Merc. c.; Nux v.; Ox. ac.; Petrol.; *Puls.*; Ver. a.; Zinc.

Watery—Abrot.; *Ars.*; Bism.; Bry.; *Euphorbia*; Euphorb. cor.; Iod.; Iris; *Kreos.*; Lac c.; *Mag. c.*; Oleand.; Ver. a.

Yeast, like—Nat. c.; Nat. s.

CONCOMITANTS—With abdominal rumbling—Pod.

With appetite—Iod.; Lob. infl.

With bowels obstructed, impacted-Op.; Plumb.; Pyr.

With chilliness—Ars.; Dulc.; Puls.; Tab.

With cholera—*Ars.*; Camph. See Abdomen.

With chronic tendency—Lob. infl.

With clavus, fickle appetite, salivation, copious lemon colored urine—Ign.

With colic, cramps—Bism.; *Cupr. ars.*; *Cupr. m.*; Op.; Plumb.; Pix l.; Sarrac.; *Ver. a.* See Abdomen.

With collapse, weakness—Æth.; *Ant. t.*; *Ars.*; Cadm. s.; Crotal.; Euphorb. cor.; *Lob. infl.*; *Tab.*; *Ver. a.*; Ver. v.

With constipation—Nux v.; Op.; Plumb.

With depression of spirits—Nux v.

With diarrhoea—Ars.; Bism.; Calc. c.; Cham.; *Cupr. ars.*; Curp. m.; *Ipec.*; Iris; Kreos.; Merc. c.; Phos.; Pulex; Puls.; Resorc.; *Ver. a.* See Abdomen.

With drowsiness—*Æth.*; *Ant. t.*; Ipec.; Mag. c.

With fear, heat, thirst, profuse urine and sweat—Acon.

With fruitless, anxious retching—Ars.; Bism.; Cupr.; Pod.

With headache—Apomorph.; Iris; Petrol. See Head.

With heart, weak—Ars.; Camph.; *Dig.*

With intervals of days between attacks—Bism.

With midnight occurrence; can eat at once after emptying stomach—Ferr. m.

With nausea—Æth.; Amyg. pers.; Ant. t.; Bry.; *Ipec.*; Iris; *Lob. infl.*; Nux v.; Petrol.; *Puls.*; Sang.; Symphor.; Ver. a. See Nausea.

With relief of symptoms—Ant. t.; Puls.

With relief from eating, drinking—Anac.; Tab.

With relief from cold drinks—Cupr.; *Phos.*; Puls.

With relief from hot drinks—Ars.; Chel.

With relief from lying down—Bry.; Colch.; Nux v.; Symphor.

With relief from lying on right side—Ant. t.

With relief from uncovering abdomen; in fresh open air—Tab.

With salivation—Graph.; Ign.; *Ipec.*; Iris; Kreos.; Lact. ac.; *Lob. infl.*; Puls.; Tab.

With spasms—*Cupr. m.*; Hyos.; Op.

With tongue clean—Cina; Dig.; *Ipec.*

With vertigo—Cocc.; Ign.; *Nux v.*; *Tab.*

ABDOMEN

APPENDICITIS. See Typhlitis.

BURNING heat—Abies c.; *Acon.*; *Aloe;* Alston.; Ant. c.; *Apis;* Arg. n.; *Ars.;* *Bell.;* Bry.; Camph.; *Canth.;* Carbo v.; Colch.; Crot.; *Iris;* Kali bich.; *Limul.;* Lyc.; *Merc. c.;* Nat. s.; Nux v.; *Ox. ac.;* Phos. ac.; *Phos.;* Pod.; Rhus t.; Sang.; Sec.; Sep.; Sul.; Ver. a.

CÆCUM, affections of—Ars.; Lach.; Rhus v.; Ver. v. See Appendicitis, typhlitis.

COLDNESS—*Æth.;* Ambra; Aur. m.; Cadm. s.; *Calc c.;* Camph.; Caps.; *Cinch.;* *Colch.;* Elaps; Grat.; *Kali br.;* *Kali c.;* Lach.; *Menyanth.;* Phell.; Phos.; Sec.; Sep.; *Tab.;* Ver. a.

COLIC—PAIN—Remedies in general: *Acon.;* Adren.; Aloe; Alum.; *Arg. n.;* Arn.; *Ars.;* Bar. c.; *Bell.;* Bry.; Cajup.; *Calc. p.;* Carb. ac.; Carbo v.; *Cham.;* Chin. ars.; Cic.; *Cina;* *Cinch.;* *Cocc.;* Coff.; Collins.; *Colch.;* Col.; Crot. t.; Cupr. ac.; *Cupr. m.;* Cycl.; Dig.; *Diosc.;* Elat.; Filix m.; *Gamb.;* Grat.; *Ign.;* Illic.; *Ipec.;* Iris ten.; *Iris;* Jal.; Lept.; *Limul.;* Lyc.; *Mag. c.;* *Mag. p.;* Mentha; *Merc. c.;* Merc.; Morph.; Nat. s.; *Nux v.;* Oniscus; *Op.;* Ox. ac.; Paraf.; *Plat.;* Plumb. ac.; Plumb. chrom.; *Plumb. m.;* Pod.; Polyg.; *Puls.;* Raph.; *Rheum;* *Rhus t.;* Sab.; Samb.; Sars.; *Senna;* Sep.; *Sil.;* Sinap. n.; *Stann.;* Staph.; Strych.; Thuya; *Ver. a.;* *Vib. op.;* Zinc. m.

CAUSE AND NATURE—Alternates with vertigo: Col.; Spig.

Babies' colic—Æth.; Asaf.; Bell.; Calc. p.; Cataria; Cepa; *Cham.;* *Cina;* Col.; *Illic.;* Jal.; Kali br.; Lyc.; *Mag. p.;* Mentha pip.; Nepeta; Rheum, Senna; Staph.

Biliary, gall-stone colic—Atrop.; Bell.; *Berb. v.;* Bry.; *Calc. c.;* Card. m.; Cham.; Chionanth.; *Cinch.;* Col.; Diosc.; Ipec.; Iris; Lyc.; Mentha; Morph. acet.; Pod.; Ricin.; Tereb.; Triost. See Gall Bladder.

Chronic tendency—Lyc.; Staph.

Flatulent colic—Absinth; Agar.; Alfal.; *Aloe;* Anis.; *Arg. n.;* Asaf.; *Bell.;* But. ac.; Cajup.; Calc. p.; Carbon. s.; *Carbo v.;* *Cham.;* Cina; *Cinch.;* *Cocc.;* Col.; *Diosc.;* Hydroc. ac.; *Illic.;* Ipec.; Iris; *Lyc.,* *Mag. p.;* Mentha; *Nux v.;* Op.; Plumb. m.; *Polygon.;* Puls.; Radium; Raph.; Robin.; Sang.; *Senna;* Zinc.

From anger—*Cham.;* Col.; Staph.

From carriage riding—Carbo v.; Cocc.

From cold—Acon.; Cepa; *Cham.;* Col.; Nux v.

From eating cheese—Col.

From eating cucumber salad—Cepa.

From gastric disorder—Carbo v.; *Cinch.;* Col.; Diosc.; Ipec.; Lyc.; *Nux v.;* Puls.

From lithotomy, ovariotomy, attending abdominal section—Bism.; Hep.; Nux v.; Raph.; *Staph.*

From uncovering—Nux v.; Rheum.

ABDOMEN

From wet feet—Cepa; Cham.; Dolichos; Dulc.
From worms—Artem.; Bism.; *Cina;* Filix m.; Granat.; *Indigo;* Merc. s.; Nat. p.; Sabad.; Spig.
Hemorrhoidal—Æsc.; Cepa; Col.; *Nux v.;* Puls.; Sul.
Hysterical—Alet.; *Asaf.;* Cajup.; Cocc.; *Ign.;* Val.
Menstrual—Bell.; Castor.; Cham.; *Cocc.;* Col.; *Puls.* See Female Sexual Organs.
Neuralgic, enteralgic—Alumen; Ant. t.; Ars.; *Atrop.; Bell.;* Cham.; *Cocc.; Col.;* Cupr. ars.; Cupr. m.; *Diosc.;* Euphorb.; Hydroc. ac.; Hyos.; Kali c.; *Mag. p.; Nux v.;* Op.; Plumb. ac.; *Plumb. m.;* Santon.; Tab.; Ver. a.; Zinc. m. See Type of Pain.
Renal—*Berb. v.;* Calc. c.; Diosc.; Eryng.; *Lyc.; Morph. acet.;* Occin.; Sars.; *Tab.; Tereb.* See Urinary System.
Rheumatic—Caust.; Col.; Diosc.; Phyt.; Ver. a.
Toxic (lead, copper)—Alumen; *Alum.;* Bell.; Ferr.; Nat. s.; Nux m.; Nux v.; *Op.;* Plat.; Sul.; Ver. a.

LOCATION—Abdominal muscles—Acon.; *Arn.;* Bell.; *Bellis ; Cupr. m.;* Ham.; Mag. m.; Nat. nit.; Plumb. m.; *Rhus t.;* Strych.; Sul.
Abdominal ring—*Cocc.;* Graph.; Mez.; *Nat. m.;* Nux v.; Stront.
Ascending colon—Rhus t.
Groins—Alum.; Am. m.; Merc. c.; Pod.
Hypochondria—Carbo v.; *Cinch.;* Diosc.; *Nux v.;* Pyrus; Sep. See Type of Pain.
Hypogastrium—*Aloe; Bell.;* Bism.; Cepa; Cocc.; *Diosc.;* Eucal.; Ham.; Kali c.; *Lyc.;* Mag. c.; *Nux v.;* Pall.; Paraf.; Plat.; *Sab.;* Sep.; Sul.; Tromb.; Ver. v. See Sexual System.
Ileo-caecal—Aloe; Bell.; Bry.; Coff.; Ferr. p.; *Gamb.;* Iris ten.; Kali m.; Limul.; Mag. c.; *Merc. c.; Merc. s.;* Plumb.; Radium; Rhus t. See Appendicitis.
Inguinal—Am. m.; Ars.; Calc. c.; Graph.; Sep.
In small spots—Bry.; Col.; *Ox. ac.*
Transverse colon—*Bell.;* Cham.; Colch.; Merc. c.; Raph.
Umbilical (about navel)—*Aloe; Ben. ac.;* Berb. v.; *Bov.; Bry.;* Calc. p.; Carbo v.; *Cham.; Chel.;* Cina; *Col.; Diosc.; Dulc.; Gamb.; Granat.;* Hyper.; Indigo; *Kali bich.; Ipec.;* Lept.; Lyc.; *Nux m.;* Nux v.; Pelias; Plat.; *Plumb.;* Puls.; Raph.; *Rheum;* Senec.; *Spig.; Stann.;* Sul.; *Ver. a.;* Verbasc.

TYPE OF PAIN—Bruised: Æth.; Allium s.; *Apis;* Apoc.; *Arn.;* Ars.; *Bellis;* Bry.; Carbo v.; Col.; *Con.;* Eucal.; Ferr. m.; *Ham.; Merc. c.;* Nat. s.; Nit. ac.; *Nux v.;* Phyt.; Puls.; *Sul.*
Colicky, crampy, constricting, cutting, griping, pinching—Acon.; *Æsc.;* Agar.; *Aloe;* Ant. t.; Argem. mex.; Arg. cy.; *Arg. n.;* Arn.; Asaf.; *Bell.;* Bism.; Bry.; *Calc. p.;* Cataria; *Cham.; Cina; Cinch.; Cocc.; Col.;* Colch.; Con.; Crot. t.; *Cupr. ars.;* Cupr. m.; *Diosc.; Dulc.; Elat.;* Eup. perf.; Filix m.; *Gamb.;* Grat.; *Hyper.;* Ign.; Iod.; *Ipec.;* Iris; *Jal.; Jatropha;* Kali bich.; Kali c.; Lach.; Lept.; *Lyc.;* Mag. c.; *Mag. p.; Merc. c.;* Nat. s.; Niccol.; Nit. ac.; *Nux v.;* Phos.; Phyt.; *Plumb. ac.;* Plumb. chrom.; *Polyg.;* Puls.; Radium; Raph.; *Rheum;* Sab.;

ABDOMEN

Sec.; *Sep.;* Spig.; *Stann.;* Strych.; Sul ; Tromb.; *Ver. a.;* Vib. op.; Zinc.

Pressing, plug-like—*Aloe;* Alum.; *Anac.; Bell.;* Bry.; *Cocc* ; Hyos ; Kali c ; Mez.; Nux v.; Œnoth.; *Plat.;* Plumb. m.; Puls.; Ran s.; Sab ; *Sep.*

Pulsating, bubbling—Æth ; *Aloe;* Bar. m.; *Bell.: Berb v.;* Calc. c.; Ign.; Sang ; Selen ; Tarax.

Radiating, shooting, darting, tearing, spasmodic—*Acon ;* Argem. mex.; *Bell.; Bry.;* Calc. c.; *Cham ; Cocc.;* Cochlear ; *Col ;* Cupr. ac.; *Cupr. ars ; Diosc.;* Graph.; Ipec.; Kali c.; *Lyc.; Mag p ;* Merc.; Morph.; *Nux v.;* Ox. ac.; Paraf ; Plat.; *Plumb.;* Pod ; *Puls.; Sul.* See Enteralgia

Stitching—Agar.; Apis; Arn.; *Bell.; Bry.;* Chin ars.; Hep.; *Kali c.;* Lach.; Spig.

CONCOMITANTS—Abdomen retracted, as if drawn by string—Chel.; *Plumb. m.;* Pod ; Tab

Abdomen, retracted, tense, scanty urine, desire to stretch—Plumb. m.

Abdomen swollen, pad-like—*Bell.,* Raph.

Agitation, chill ascending from hypogastrium to cheeks—Col.

Alternates with coryza—Calc. c

Alternates with delirium and pain in atrophied limbs—Plumb. m.

Alternates with vertigo—Col ; Spig.

Backache—Cham.; *Lyc.;* Morph.; Puls.; Samb.

Cheeks red, hot sweat—Cham.

Chilliness—Nux v.; Puls.

Collapse—Æth.; Camph.; Cupr., *Ver. a.*

Constipation—Allium s.; *Aloe;* Alum.; Cocc.; Collins.; Grat.; Lyc.; Nux v.; Op.; *Plumb. ac.;* Sil.

Convulsions—Bell.; Cic.

Cramps in calves—Col.; *Cupr. ac.;* Plumb. m ; Pod.

Delirium alternating—Plumb. m

Diarrhoea—Ars.; Cham.; *Col.;* Mag. c.; Polyg.; Puls., Samb.; Ver. a.

Empty feeling, heat, faintness—*Cocc.;* Hydr.

Hands yellow, blue nails—Sil.

Hiccough, suffocative, in chest and stomach—Ver. a.

Hunger, yet refuses food—Bar. c.

Itching of nose, pale, bluish face—*Cina;* Filix m.

Nausea, frequent, watery, slimy stools—Cham.; Samb.

Pain and aching in thighs—Col.

Painful contraction in limbs following—Abrot.

Periodical recurrence—Aran.; *Cinch.;* Diosc.; Illic.; Kali br.

Pulsation in abdominal aorta, epigastric constriction—Dig.

Red urine—Bov.; Lyc.

Restlessness twitching and turning for relief—Col.

Rumbling of flatus, nausea, liquid feces—Polyg.

Scanty stools, flatus without relief—Cina.

Sour stools—Rheum.

Tenesmus (pelvic)—Staph.

Tossing about, anxiety, no relief from flatus—*Cham.;* Mag. p.
Urging to stool—*Aloe;* Cinch.; Lept.; Nat. s.; *Nux v.;* Op.
Urine suppressed—Acon.; Plumb. ac.
Vomiting—*Bell.;* Cadm. s.; Plumb. ac.
Vomiting, hiccough, belching, screaming—Hyos.
Yawning, spasmodic, drowsiness—Spiranth.

MODALITIES—Aggravation: About 4-5 P. M.: Col.; Kali br.; *Lyc.*
 After midnight—*Ars.;* Cocc.
 At night, after supper—Grat.
 At night—Cham.; Cinch.; Cocc.; Senna; Sul.
 From bending, coughing—Ars.; Bell.; *Bry.;* Nat. m.
 From bending forward—Ant. t.; *Diosc.;* Sinap. n.
 From bending forward, lying down, pressure—Acon.; *Diosc.*
 From drinking—Col.; Sul.
 From drinking cold water—Cupr. m.
 From eating—Bar. c.; *Calc. p.;* Cinch.; *Col.;* Kali bich.; *Nux v.;* Psor.; Zinc.
 From jar, pressure—Acon.; Aloe; *Bell.;* Plumb.
 From motion, relief from lying on side—Bry.; Cocc.
 From smoking—Menyanth.
 From sweets—Filix m.
 From touch, pressure, motion—Bry.
 From uncovering arm, leg; standing—Rheum.
 From warmth, at night—Cham.

AMELIORATION—From bending double—Bov.; Cinch.; *Col.; Mag. p.;* Pod.; Sep.; *Stann.;* Sul.; Ver. a.
 From eating—Bov.; Homar.
 From flatus voided per ano—Aloe; *Carbo v.; Cinch.;* Cocc.; *Col.;* Nat. s.; Sul.
 From hot applications or warmth—Ars.; Col.; *Mag. p.;* Pod.; Puls.; Sil.
 From lying with knees drawn up—Lach.
 From pressure—*Col.; Mag. p.;* Nit. ac.; Plumb.; Rhus t.; *Stann.*
 From rubbing—Plumb. m.
 From rubbing, warmth—Mag. p.
 From sitting erect—Sinap. n.
 From sitting, lying down—Nux v.
 From stool—Aloe; Col.; Tanac.; Ver. a.
 From straightening body backward or moving about—Diosc.
 From walking about—Cepa; Diosc.; Mag. p.; Puls.; *Rhus t.;* Ver. a.
 From walking bent over—Aloe; *Col.;* Nux v.; Rhus t.
 From warm soup—Acon.

FLATULENT—Distention, fulness, heaviness, meteorism, tympanites—*Abies n.; Abrot.;* Absinth.; Acet. ac.; Acon.; Agar.; Alfal.; *Aloe;* Ant. c.; Apis; *Arg. n.;* Ars.; *Asaf.;* Bar. c.; *Bell.;* Bov.; *Cajup.; Calc. c.;* Calc. iod.; Carb. ac.; *Carbo v.; Cham.;* Chel.; Cina; *Cinch.;* Cocc.; Colch.; Collins.; *Col.;* Cupr. m.; *Diosc.;* Graph.; Ign.; *Illic.;* Indol; Iris; *Kali c.; Lach.; Limul.; Lyc.; Mag. c.; Mag. p.;* Merc. c.; Merc.; Momord.; Mosch.; Mur. ac.; Naph.; Nat. c.; *Nat. n't.;* Nat. m.; *Nat.*

s.; *Nux m.*; *Nux v.*; Oniscus; *Op.*; *Opuntia*; *Ornithog.*; *Phos. ac.*; Pod.; *Poth.*; *Puls.*; Radium; *Raph.*; Rheum; Rhod.; *Rhus gl.*; Rhus t.; Sars.; *Senna*; *Sep.*; *Sil.*; Stront. c.; Sul.; Sumb.; *Tarax.*; *Tereb.*; Thea; *Thuya*; Uran. n.; Val.; Xanth.; Zing.

Flatulence, hysterical—Alet.; *Ambra*; Arg. n.; *Asaf.*; Cajup.; Cham.; Cocc.; *Ign.*; Kali p.; *Nux m.*; Plat.; Poth.; *Sumb.*; Tarax.; Thea; *Val.*

Flatulence, incarcerated in flexures—Am. c.; Aur.; Bell.; Calc. c.; Calc. p.; Carb. ac.; *Carbo v.*; *Cham.*; *Cinch.*; Colch.; *Col.*; *Graph.*; Hep.; Ign ; Kali c.; Limul.; *Lyc.*; *Momord.*; *Nux v.*; Pall.; Phos.; Plumb. m.; Puls.; *Raph.*; Rhus gl.; Robin.; Staph.; Sul.; Thuya.

Flatulence, offensive, per ano—*Aloe;* Arn.; Bry.; *Carbo v.*; Ferr. magnet.; Graph ; Oleand.; Sil.

Flatulence, post operative, no relief from passing it—Cinch.

Gurgling, rumbling, borborygmus—*Aloe;* Apoc.; Ars.; Bapt.; Bell.; Carbon. s ; Carbo v.; *Cham.*; Cina; *Cinch.*; Colch.; Col.; Conv.; Cupr. ars.; Crot. t.; *Diosc.*; *Gamb.*; Glycerin; *Graph.*; Grat.; Hep.; Ipec.; *Jatropha*; Kali c.; *Lyc.*; Merc.; *Nat. s.*; Nux v.; Oleand.; *Phos. ac.*; Pod.; Puls.; Ricin. com.; *Rumex*; Sanic.; Sep.; Sil.; Thea; Xerophyl.

Hardness—Abrot.; Anac.; *Bar. c.*; *Calc. c.*; Carbo v.; *Cina*; Cinch.; Cupr.; *Graph.*; *Lyc.*; Nat. c.; Nux v.; Op.; *Plumb. ac.*; *Raph.*; *Sil.*; Sul.; Thuya.

Jumping, as of living thing—Arundo; Brachygl.; Branca; *Croc.*; Cycl.; Nux m.; *Op.*; Sabad ; Sul.; *Thuya.*

Large, in girls at puberty—Calc. c.; *Graph.*; Lach.; Sul.

Large, pendulous in women who have borne many children—Aur. m.; Aur. mur.; Bell.; Frax. am.; *Helon.*; Phos.; *Sep.*

Large, pot-bellied, flabby—Am. m.; *Calc. c.*; *Calc. p.*; Mez.; Pod.; Sanic.; Sars ; *Sep.*; *Sil.*; Sul.; Thuya.

Large, protrudes here and there—Croc.; Nux m.; Sul.; Thuya.

Retracted, sunken, scow-shaped—*Calc p.*; Euphorb.; Iodof.; Kali bich.; *Kali br.*; *Plumb. ac.*; Plumb. chrom.; *Plumb. m.*; Pod.; Ptel.; Quass.; Zinc.

Sensitive, tender to touch, pressure—Acet. ac.; *Acon.*; Aloe; *Apis; Arg n.*; *Arn.*; Ars.; Bapt.; *Bell.*; *Bov.*; *Bry.*; Calc. c.; *Carbo v.*; Card. m.; Cinch.; Coff.; Col.; Con ; Cupr. m.; Euonym.; Ferr. m.; Gamb.; *Graph.*; *Ham.*; Hedeoma; Helleb.; Kali bich.; *Lach.*; *Lyc.*; *Merc. c.*; Mur. ac.; Nux v.; Pod.; *Ran. b.*; Rhus t.; *Sep.*; Sil.; *Sumb.*; Sul.; *Tereb.*; *Ver. a.*; Vib. op.

Spots, brown—Caul.; *Lyc.*; Phos.; *Sep.*; **Thuya.**

Spots, red—Hyos. See Skin.

Trembling in—Lil. t.

Weak, as if diarrhœa would ensue—*Aloe;* Ant. c.; Apium gr.; Bor.; Crot. t.; Eucal.; Ferr. m.; Formica; Nux v.; *Opuntia;* Ran. s. See Diarrhœa.

Weak, empty, sinking, relaxed feeling—Abrot.; Acet. ac.; *Arn.*; Alston.; Ant. c.; Cham.; Cocc.; Euphorb.; Glycerin; *Hydr.*; *Ign.*; *Opuntia;* Petrol.; Physost.; *Phos.*; Plumb. ac.; *Pod.*; Quass.; Sep.; Stann.; Staph.; Sulphon.; Sul. ac.; *Ver. a.*

ABDOMEN

ANUS—RECTUM—Abscess (peri-rectal): Calc. s.; Rhus t.; Sil.

Burning, smarting, heat—Abies c.; *Æsc.; Aloe;* Alumen; Alum.; Ambra; Am. m.; Ant. c.; *Ars.;* Bell.; Berb. v.; *Canth.; Caps.; Carbo v.;* Cepa; Chenop. gl.; *Collins.;* Con.; Eucal.; Euonym.; *Gamb.;* Graph.; Ham.; Hydr.; *Iris;* Jugl. c.; Jugl. r.; Kali c.; Merc.; *Nat. m.;* Nit. ac.; *Oleand.;* Pæonia; Prun. sp.; *Ratanh.;* Rheum; Sang. n.; Senna; *Sul.;* Tromb.

Burning before and during stool—Aloe; Am. m.; Ars.; Col.; Con.; *Hydr.; Iris;* Jugl. c.; Merc.; Ol. an.; Rheum.

Burning after stool—Æsc.; Alumen; Am. m.; *Ars.;* Aur.; Berb. v.; *Canth.; Caps.; Carbo v.;* Chenop. gl.; *Gamb.; Nat. m.;* Nit. ac.; Ol. an.; *Pæonia;* Prun. sp.; *Ratanh.;* Sil.; *Stront.;* Sul.

Congestion—*Æsc.; Aloe;* Alum.; *Collins.:* Hyper.; Nat. m.; Nit. ac.; Sab.; *Sep.;* Sul.

ERUPTIONS, growths—Cancer, scirrhus of, also sigmoid; intolerable pains: Alumen; Phyt.; Spig.

Condylomata—Benz. ac.; Kali br.; *Nit. ac.; Thuya.*

Eczema—Berb. v.; Graph.; *Merc. pr. rub.* See Skin.

Eminences, studding interior—Polyg.

Fissures, rhagades, excoriations, ulcerations, soreness, rawness—*Æsc.;* Agn.; *Aloe;* Apis; Arg. n.; *Ars.; Calc. fl.; Carbo v.;* Caust.; Cimex; *Condur.;* Graph.; Ham.; *Hydr.; Ign.;* Iris; Kali iod.; Lach.; Led.; Merc. d.; Merc.; Morph.; Mur. ac.; *Nat. m.; Nit. ac.;* Nit. mur. ac.; *Pæonia;* Petrol.; Phos.; Phyt.; Plat.; *Plumb.; Ratanh.;* Rhus t.; Sang. n.; Sanic.; *Sedum;* Sep.; *Sil.;* Sul.; Syph.; *Thuya;* Vib. op.

Fistula in ano—Aur. mur.; Bar. mur.; *Berb. v.; Calc. p.;* Calc. s.; Carbo v.; *Caust.; Fluor. ac.;* Graph.; Hydr.; Lach.; Myrist.; *Nit. ac.;* Nux v.; *Pæonia;* Phos.; Quercus; Ratanh.; *Sil.;* Sul.; Thuya.

Fistula in ano alternates with chest disorders—Berb. v.; Calc. p.; *Sil.*

Pockets—Polygon.

Rash, fiery red in babies—Med.

Hæmorrhage (enterrhagia)—Acal.; Acet. ac.; *Æsc.;* Aloe; *Alumen;* Alum.; Arn.; *Cact.; Carbo v.;* Cascar.; Cinch.; *Cinnam.;* Cob.; Cocaine; Crot.; Erig.; *Ham.;* Ign.; *Ipec.;* Kali c.; *Lach.;* Lycop.; Mangif. ind.; Merc. cy.; *Millef.;* Mur. ac.; Nat. m.; *Nit. ac.;* Phos. ac.; *Phos.;* Sedum; Sep.; Sul. ac.; Sul.; *Tereb.;* Thuya.

Haemorrhage during stool—*Alumen;* Alum.; Carbo v.; Ign.; Iod.; *Ipec.;* Kali c.; *Phos.;* Psor.; Sep.

Inflammation (proctitis)—*Æsc.;* Aloe; Alum.; Ambra; *Ant. c.;* Colch.; *Collins.;* Merc c.; *Merc.; Nit. ac.;* Pæonia; *Phos.; Pod.;* Ricin.; Sabal; Zing.

Inflammation, syphilitic—Bell.; Merc.; *Nit. ac.;* Sul.

Itching (pruritus)—Acon.; *Æsc.;* Aloe; *Alum.; Ambra;* Anac.; *Ant. c.; Bar. c.;* Bov.; Cadm. iod.; *Calc. c.;* Carbo v.; Cascar.; *Caust.; Cina; Collins.;* Cop.; *Ferr. iod.;* Ferr. m.; Granat.; Graph.; Homar.; *Ign.; Indigo; Lyc.; Med.; Pæonia;* Petrol.; Phos.; Pin. sylv.; Plat.; Polyg.; Radium; Ratanh.; Rumex; Sabad.; *Sacchar. of.;* Sang. n.; Sep.; *Spig.;* Staph.; *Sul.;* Tellur.; Tereb.; *Teucr.;* Uran.; Zinc.

ABDOMEN 789

Moisture—Aloe; Am. m.; *Anac.*; *Ant. c.*; Bar. c; *Calc. c.*; *Carbo v*; Caust.; Graph.; *Hep.*; Med.; Nit. ac.; Nit. mur. ac.; Pæonia; Phos.; Ratanh.; *Sep.*; *Sil*; Sul. ac.
Operations on, to be given preceding—Collins.

PAIN—Aching—*Æsc.*; Alet.; Alumen; Collins; Graph.; Lyc.; *Ratanh.*
Bearing down, pressing—*Aloe*; Alum.; Ars.; *Cact.*; Ceanoth.; Chenop. gl ; *Euphras.*; Hyper.; Kali c.; Lach.; *Lil. t.*; Med.; Op.; Prun. sp.; *Sep*; *Sul*; Sul. ac ; Xerophyl.
Contraction, spasmodic—Æsc. gl.; *Æsc.*; Anac.; Arg. n.; *Bell.*; Cact.; *Caust*; Collins; Ferr. m.; Grat.; Hydr.; *Ign.*; *Lach.*; Lyc.; *Med.*; Meli.; Merc.; Mez.; *Nat m.*; *Nit. ac.*; Nit. mur. ac.; *Nux v.*; *Plumb. ac.*; *Ratanh.*; Sanic.; Sedum; Sep ; *Syph.*; Tab.; Verbasc.
Lancinating, even after soft stool—*Alumen*; Nat. m.; *Nit. ac.*; Ratanh.
Long lasting, after stool—*Æsc.*; Aloe; Alumen; Am. m.; *Graph.*; *Hydr.*, *Ign.*; Merc. cy.; *Mur. ac.*; *Nat. m.*; *Nit. ac.*; Pæonia; *Ratanh.*; *Sedum*; Sep.; *Sil.*; Sul.; Thuya; Vib. op.
Neuralgic (proctalgia)—*Atrop.*; Bar. m.; *Bell.*; Colch.; *Crot. t.*; Ign.; Kali c.; Lach.; Lyc.; Ox. ac.; Phos.; Plumb.; *Strych.*; Tar. h.
Splinter-like, pricking, stinging, stitching, cutting, shooting—Acon.; *Æsc.*; Alum.; Am. m.; Bell.; Caust.; Cepa; *Collins.*; *Ign.*; Kali c.; *Lach.*; Lyc.; Merc.; Mez ; *Nat. m.*; *Nit. ac.*, Plat ; *Ratanh.*; Ruta; Sep.; Sil.; *Sul.*; Thuya.
Throbbing, pulsating—Aloe; *Bell.*; Caps.; Ham.; Lach.; *Meli.*; Merc.; Nat. m.

PARETIC—Condition of rectum and sphincters—*Aloe*; Alum.; *Caust.*; *Erig.*; Gels ; Graph.; Hyos.; Mur. ac.; Op.; Oxytr.; Phos. ac.; *Phos.*; Plumb. m.; Sil.; Sulphon.; Tab.
Paretic condition of rectum, feels plugged—*Aloe*; Anac.; Can. ind.; Kali bich.; Med.; Plat.; Plumb. m.; *Sep.*; Sul ac.
Paretic condition of rectum, with sense of insecurity of sphincters—*Aloe*; Alum.; Apoc.; Erig.; Ferr. m.; *Nux v.*; Sanic.; Sec.
Patulous anus—*Apis*; Phos.; Sec.; Solan. t.

PROLAPSUS ANI—*Æsc. gl.*; *Æsc.*; Aloe; Ant. c.; *Aral.*; *Arn.*; *Bell.*; Carbo v.; Caust.; Colch.; *Ferr. m.*; *Ferr. p.*; Gamb.; Ham.; Hydr.; *Ign.*; Kali c.; Mag. p.; *Mur. ac.*; Nux v.; *Phos.*; Plumb.; *Pod.*; Polypor.; *Ruta*; *Sep.*; Solan. tub.; *Sul.*; Tab.; Tromb.
Prolapsus after confinement, stooping—Pod.; Ruta.
Prolapsus from debility—Pod.
Prolapsus from sneezing—Pod.
Prolapsus from straining, overlifting—Ign.; Nit. ac.; Pod.; Ruta.
Prolapsus from urinating—Mur. ac.
Prolapsus in children—Bell.; Ferr. m.; *Ferr. p.*; Ign.; Mur. ac.; Nux v ; Pod.
Prolapsus, with diarrhæa, stool—*Æsc.*; *Aloe*; Carbo v.; Colch.; Crot. t.; Fluor. ac.; *Gamb.*; Ham.; *Ign.*; Kali c.; Mur. ac.; *Pod.*; Phos.; *Ruta*; Sul.
Prolapsus with piles, in alcoholics, leading sedentary life—Æsc. gl.
Prolapsus with stool, rectal spasm—Ign.

790 ABDOMEN

REDNESS—around—*Cham.*; Merc. cy.; Pæonia; *Sul.*; Zing. See Fissures Proctitis.

Stricture—*Bell.*; Coff.; Hydr.; Ign.; *Nit. ac.*; Phos.; *Sil.*; Tab.; Thiosin. See Pain.

Torn, bleeding, after stool—Lac d.; *Nat. m.*; *Nit. ac.* See Fissures.

CATARRH—Gastro-duodenal: Card. m.; *Cinch.*; Hydr.; Sang. See Stomach.

CHOLERA—ASIATICA: *Acon.*; Agar. phal.; *Ars.*; Bell.; Bry.; *Camph.*; *Canth.*; Carbo v.; Chin. s.; Cic.; Colch.; *Cupr. ac.*; *Cupr. ars.*; *Cupr. m.*; Dig.; Euphorb. cor.; Guaco; *Hydroc. ac.*; *Ipec.*; Jatropha; Kali bich.; Lach.; Merc. c.; Naja; Nux v.; Op.; *Phos. ac.*; Phos.; Quass.; Rhus t.; Sec.; Sul.; Tab.; Tereb.; *Ver. a.*; Zinc. m.

CHOLERA INFANTUM—Summer complaint: *Acon.*; *Æth.*; Ant. t.; *Apis*; Arg. n.; *Ars.*; Bell.; *Bism.*; Bry.; Cadm. s.; Calc. ac.; *Calc. c.*; *Calc. p.*; Camph.; Camph. monobr.; Canth.; Cham.; Cinch.; Col.; Crot. t.; *Cuphea*; Cupr. ac.; *Cupr. ars.*; Cupr. m.; Elat.; *Euphorb. cor.*; Ferr. p.; Graph.; Hydroc. ac.; Indol; *Iodof.*; *Ipec.*; Iris; *Kali br.*; Kreos.; *Laur.*; Merc.; Nat. m.; Ox. ac.; Passifl.; Phos.; Phyt.; Pod.; Psor.; Resorc.; Sec.; Sep.; *Sil.*; Sul.; Tab.; *Ver. a.*; Zinc. m.

CHOLERA MORBUS—Ant. *t.*; *Ars.*; Bism.; Camph.; Chloral.; Colch.; Col.; *Crot. t.*; *Cupr. ars.*; Cupr. m.; Elat.; Grat.; Hydroc. ac.; *Ipec.*; Iris; Operc.; Op.; *Pod.*; Sec.; *Ver. a.*

CHOLERINE—Ant. c.; Ars.; *Crot. t.*; *Cupr. ars.*; Diosc.; Elat.; Euphorb. cor.; *Grat.*; *Ipec.*; Iris; *Jatropha*; Nuphar; *Phos. ac.*; Sec.; *Ver. a.*

CONSTIPATION—Remedies in general: Abies n.; Acon.; *Æsc. gl.*; *Æsc.*; Agar.; Alet.; *Aloe*; *Alumen*; *Alum.*; Am. c.; *Am. m.*; *Anac.*; Apis; *Arn.*; Asar.; Berb. v.; *Bry.*; *Calc. c.*; Calc. fl.; Carb. ac.; *Casc. sag.*; *Caust.*; Chel.; Chionanth.; Cinch.; Coca; *Collins.*; Croc.; *Dolichos*; Eug. j.; Euonym.; *Euphras.*; Fel tauri; Ferr. m.; Gels.; *Glycerin*; *Graph.*; *Grat.*; Guaiac.; Hep.; *Hydr.*; Ign.; *Iris*; *Kali bich.*; Kali c.; Kali m.; Lac d.; Lach.; Lact. ac.; *Lyc.*; *Mag. m.*; Mez.; Morph.; Nabalus; *Nat. m.*; *Nit. ac.*; Nit. mur. ac.; *Nux v.*; Nyctanth.; *Op.*; *Paraf.*; *Phos.*; Physost.; Phyt.; *Plat.*; *Plumb. ac.*; Plumb. m.; *Pod.*; *Psor.*; Pyr.; Ratanh.; Rham. c.; Sanic.; *Selen.*; Senna; *Sep.*; *Sil.*; Sil. mar.; Spig.; *Staph.*; Strych.; *Sul.*; *Symphor.*; *Syph.*; Tab.; Tan. ac.; Tub.; *Ver. a.*; *Zinc. m.*; Zinc. mur.

CAUSE AND TYPE—Abuse of enemas—*Op.*

After confinement, hepatic and uterine inertia—Mez.

Alternating with diarrhæa—*Abrot.*; Am. m.; *Ant. c.*; Bry.; Calc. chlor.; Card. m.; Cascar.; *Chel.*; *Collins.*; Ferr. cy.; *Hydr.*; Iod.; *Nux v.*; Pod.; Ptel.; Radium; Ruta; *Sul.*; Ver. a.

From abuse of purgatives—*Aloe*; Hydr.; *Nux v.*; Sul.

From cheese—Col.

From gastric derangements—*Bry.*; Hydr.; *Nux v.*; Puls.

From going to sea—Bry.; Lyc.

From gouty acidity—Grat.

From haemorrhoids—*Æsc. gl.*; *Æsc.*; Caust.; *Collins.*; Hydr.; Nat. m.; *Nux v.*; Pod.; *Sul.* See Piles.

ABDOMEN

From impaction—Plumb. m ; Pyr.; Selen.
From lead poisoning—Op.; Plat.
From mechanical injuries—Arn.; Ruta.
From mental shock, nervous strain—Mag. c.
From peristaltic irregularity—Anac.; Nux v.
From travelling; in emigrants—Plat.
From torpor of rectum—Aloe; *Alum.;* *Anac.;* Caust.; Cinch.; Lach.; Lyc.; Nat. m.; *Op.;* Psor.; Selen.; *Sep.; Sil ;* Ver. a.
From torpor, inertia, dryness of intestines—Æsc.; Æth.; Alet.; Alumen; *Alum.; Bry.;* Caffeine; *Collins.;* Ferr. m.; Hydr.; *Lyc.;* Meli.; Mez.; *Nat. m.;* Nux v.; *Op.;* Physost.; *Plat.; Plumb. ac.;* Pyr.; Ruta; Sanic.; Selen.; *Sul.;* Ver. a.
Infants, bottle fed; artificial food—Alum.; Nux v.; Op.
Infants, children—Æsc.; *Alum.;* Apis; Bell.; *Bry.;* Calc. c.; Caust.; *Collins.;* Croc.; Hydr.; *Lyc.; Mag. m.; Nux v.;* Nyct. arb. tr.; *Paraf.;* Pod.; Psor.; Sanic.; *Sep.; Sil.;* Sul.; Ver. a.
In old people—Alum.; Ant. c.; Hydr.; Lyc.; Op.; Phyt.; *Selen.;* Sul.
In rheumatic subjects, flatulence, indigestion—Mag. p.
In women—Æsc.; Alet.; *Alum.;* Ambra; Anac.; Arn.; Asaf.; Bry.; Calc. c.; *Collins.;* Con.; *Graph.;* Hydr.; Ign.; Lach.; Lyc.; Mez.; *Nat. m.;* Nux v.; Op.; *Plat.; Plumb.;* Pod.: Puls.; *Sep.;* Sil.; Sul.

TYPE OF STOOL—**Dry, crumbling at verge of anus:** Am. m.; *Mag. m.; Nat. m.;* Sanic.; Zinc.
Dry, difficult, scanty, knotty, ball or dung-like—Æsc. gl.; Æsc.; *Alumen; Alum.;* Aster.; Bar. c.; *Card. m.;* Caust.; *Chel.;* Collins.; Glycerin; Graph.; Indol; *Lyc.; Mag. m.;* Morph.; Nit. ac.; *Nux v.;* Op.; Petrol.; *Plat.; Plumb.;* Pyr.; Sanic.; *Sep.; Sul.;* Thuya; Ver. a.; Verbasc.; Xerophyl.; Zinc.
Dry, large, painful—Æsc.; Alet.; Aloe; *Alum.; Bry.;* Calc. c.; Caust.; Glycerin; *Graph.; Kali c.;* Lac d.; Meli.; Nat. m.; Nux v.; Op.; Pyr.; Sanic.; *Selen.;* Sep.; *Sul.; Ver. a.;* Vib. op.
Dry, must be mechanically removed—Aloe; Alum.; Bry.; Calc. c.; Indol; *Op.; Plumb.;* Ruta; Sanic.; *Selen.;* Sep.; *Sil.;* Ver. a.
Dry, with frequent urging—Alumen; *Anac.;* Aster.; Carbo v.; *Caust.;* Con.; Ferr. m.; Glycerin; Granat.; *Ign.;* Iod.; Lac d.; *Lyc.;* Nit. ac.; Nit. mur. ac.; *Nux v.;* Paraf.; *Plat.; Phos.;* Pod.; Robin; Ruta; *Sil.;* Sep.; Spig.; *Sul.*
Dry, with partial expulsion and receding—Op.; Sanic.; *Sil.;* Thuya.
Frequent, ineffectual urging—Ambra; Anac.; Caust.; Ferr. m.; Graph.; Lyc.; Nat. m.; *Nux v.;* Plat.; Sul.
Hard—Æsc.; Aloe; *Am. m.;* Ant. c.; Bar. c.; *Bry.;* Calc. c.; *Chel.;* Con.; Glycerin; Indol; Iod.; Lac d.; *Luc.; Mag. m.; Nat. m.; Op.;* Phos.; *Plumb.;* Ratanh.; Sanic.; Selen.; *Sul.*
Hard, covered with mucus—Alum.; Am. m.; Cascar.; *Caust.; Collins.;* Cop.; *Graph.; Hydr.;* Nux v.; Sep.
Hard, then pasty liquid—Calc. c.; Lyc.
Large, black, carrion like—Pyr.
Light colored, grayish, chalky—Acon.; Alumen; *Calc. c.; Chel.;* Chionanth.;

ABDOMEN

Cinch.; Collins.; *Dig.*; Dolicnos; *Hep.*; Hydr.; Iberis; Indol; Kali m.; *Merc. d.*; *Pod.*; Sanic.; Steliar.

No desire or urging—*Alum.*; *Bry.*; Graph.; Hydr.; *Op.*

Pasty, tenacious, adhering to anus—Alum.; Chel.; Chionanth.; *Plat.*

Slender, quill-like—Arn.; *Caust.*; *Phos.*; Staph.

Soft stool even passed with difficulty—Agn.; Alum.; Anac.; Chel.; Chionanth.; *Plat.*; Ratanh.; Sil.

CONCOMITANTS—**Abdominal weakness, shuddering:** Plat.

Anus very sore—Graph.; Nat. m.; Nit. ac.; Sil.

Backache—*Æsc.*; Euonym.; *Ferr.*; Kali bich.; Sul. See Back.

Bleeding—Alum.; Am. m.; Anac.; Calc. p.; *Collins.*; Lac d.; Lamium; Morph.; Nat. m.; *Nit. ac.*; *Nux v.*; Phos.; Psor.; Sep.; Vib. op.

Colic, cramps—Collins.; *Cupr.*; Glon.; Op.; *Plumb. ac.*

Contraction, spasmodic of anus—Caust.; *Lach.*; *Lyc.*; *Nat. m.*; Nit. ac.; Plumb. ac.; Plumb. m.; Sil. See Rectum.

Enuresis—Caust.

Fainting—Ver. a.

Fetor oris—*Carb. ac.*; Op.; Psor.

Gall-stones, jaundice—Chionanth. See Gall Bladder.

Headache—Bry.; Gels.; *Hydr.*; Iris; Nux v.; Sep.; Ver. a. See Headache.

Heart weak—Phyt.; Spig.

Hernia, umbilical—Cocc.; Nux v.

Nervous, from presence of others, even nurse—Ambra.

Pain, compels child to desist from effort—Ign.; Lyc.; *Sul.*; Thuya.

Passes better leaning far back—Med.

Passes better standing—Caust.

Piles—*Æsc.*; *Aloe*; Alumen; *Calc. fl.*; Caust.; Collins.; Euonym.; Glon.; Graph.; Kali s.; Lyc.; Nit. ac.; *Nux v.*; Paraf.; *Ratanh.*; Sil.; *Sul.*; Wyeth. See Hæmorrhoids.

Prolapsus—*Æsc.*; Alum.; Ferr. m.; *Ign.*; Lyc.; Med.; *Pod.*; Ruta; Sep.; Sul. See Rectum.

Prolapsus uteri—Stann.

Prostate enlarged—Arn.; Sil. See Male Sexual System.

Prostatic fluid—Alum.; Hep.

Rectal pain, persistent—*Æsc.*; Aloe; Alumen; Caust.; Hydr.; *Ign.*; Lyc.; Mur. ac.; *Nat. m.*; *Nit. ac.*; Ratanh.; Sep.; Sul.; Thuya. See Rectum.

Sensation of lightheadedness—Indol.

Sensation of something remaining behind—Aloe; Alum.; Lyc.; Nat. m.; Nux v.; Sep.; Sil.; Sul.

Urging absent, no desire—*Alum.*; Bry.; Graph.; Hydr.; Indol; *Op.*; Sanic.; Sul.; Ver. a.

Urging felt in lower abdomen—Aloe. See Frequent Urging.

Urging felt in upper abdomen—Anac.; *Ign.*; Ver. a.

DIAPHRAGM—**Inflammation (diaphragmitis)**: Atrop.; Bell.; Bism.; *Bry.*; *Cact.*; *Cupr.*; Hep.; Hyos.; Ign.; *Nux v.*; Ran. b.; Stram.; Ver. v.

Pain—Asaf.; Bism.; *Bry.*; Cact.; *Cim.*; Nat. m.; Nux v.; Sec.; Spig.; Stann.; Sticta; *Strych.*; Ver. a.; Zinc. ox.

Rheumatism—Bry.; Cact.; *Cim.*; Spig.; Sticta.

ABDOMEN 793

DIARRHOEA—Enteritis: Acute: Acal.; Acet. ac.; *Acon.*; *Æth.*; Agar. pha!.; *Aloe;* *Alston.;* Andros.; *Ant. c.;* Ant. t.; *Apis;* Apoc.; *Arg. n.;* *Arn.;* *Ars.;* Ars. iod.; *Asaf.;* *Bapt.;* *Bell.;* Benz. ac.; *Bism.;* Bov.; *Bry.;* Cadm. s.; Calc. ac.; *Calc. c.;* *Calc. p.;* *Camph.;* *Canth.;* *Caps.;* Carb. ac.; *Carbo v.;* *Cham.;* *Chel.;* *Chin. ars.*, Cina; *Cinch.;* Colch.; Collins.; Col.; *Corn. c.;* *Crot. t.;* Cuphea; Cupr. ac.; *Cupr. ars.;* *Cycl.;* *Dulc.;* Echin.; *Elat.;* Epilop.; *Eucal.;* *Euphorb. cor.;* Ferr. m.; *Ferr. p.;* Fluor. ac.; Formica; *Gamb.;* *Gels.;* *Grat.;* Helleb.; Hep.; Hyos.; *Iod.;* *Ipec.;* *Iris;* Jal.; *Jatropha;* *Kali bich.;* Kali chlor.; Kali p.; Lept.; *Mag. c.;* *Merc. d.;* *Merc. s.;* *Merc. v.;* Morph.; Mur. ac.; Nat. m.; *Nat. s.;* Nit. ac.; *Nuphar;* *Nux v.;* Oleand.; *Op.;* Opuntia; Oreodaph.; Pæonia; *Petrol.;* *Phos. ac.;* *Phos.;* Physost.; *Pod.;* Polyg.; *Prun. sp.;* Psor.; *Puls.;* *Rheum;* *Rhus t.;* Rhus v.; Ricin. com.; *Rumex;* Santon.; *Sec.;* *Sep.;* *Sil.;* *Sul.;* Sul. ac.; Tab.; Tereb.; *Thuya;* Val.; *Ver. a.;* Zinc.; Zing.

Chronic—Acet. ac.; Allium s.; Aloe; Angust.; Ant. c.; *Arg. n.;* Arn.; *Ars.;* Ars. iod.; Bapt.; *Calc. c.;* Calc. p.; Cetraria; *Chaparro;* *Cinch.;* Coto; Crot. t.; *Cupr. ars.;* Elaps; *Ferr. m.;* Gamb.; *Graph.;* Hep.; *Iod.;* Iodof.; Ipec.; *Kali bich.;* Lach.; Lact. ac.; *Liatris;* Lyc.; Mag. m.; Merc. d.; *Merc.;* Nabalus; *Nat. s.;* Nit. ac.; Oleand.; *Phos. ac.*, *Phos.;* Pod.; Psor.; Puls.; Rhus ar.; Rhus t.; Rumex; Strych. ars.; Sul.; *Thuya;* Tub.; Urt.

CAUSE—OCCURRENCE—Alternates with headache: Aloe; Pod.

From acids—Aloe; *Ant. c.;* Phos. ac.; Sul.

From acute diseases—Carbo v.; Cinch.; Psor. See Typhoid Fever.

From alcoholic abuse—Ars.; Lach.; Nux v.

From anger—*Cham.;* Col.; Staph.

From bathing—*Ant. c.;* Pod.

From beer, ale—Aloe; Cinch.; Ipec.; *Kali bich.;* Mur. ac.; *Sul.*

From cabbage; saurkraut—Bry.; Petrol.

From camping—*Alston.;* Jugl. c.; Pod.

From catarrh, bronchial, suppressed—Sang.

From change of weather, draughts—*Acon.;* Bry.; Calc. s.; *Caps.;* Colch.: *Dulc.;* Ipec.; *Merc.;* *Nat. s.;* Psor.; Rhus t.; Sil.

From chilling cold drinks, ices—*Acon.;* Agraph.; *Ars.;* Bell.; *Bry.;* Camph.; Carbo v.; Caust.; Cham.; Grat.; Nux m.; *Puls.;* Staph.

From coffee—Cistus; *Cycl.;* Ox. ac.; Thuya.

From coryza ceasing—Sang.

From disorganization—Ars.

From eggs—Chin ars.

From emotional excitement, fright—*Acon.;* *Arg. n.;* *Gels.;* Hyos.; *Ign.;* Kali p.; *Op.;* *Phos. ac.;* Puls.; Ver. a.; Zinc.

From eruptions repelled—Ant. t.; Apis; *Bry.;* Dulc.; Petrol.; Psor.; *Sul.*

From fats—Cycl.; Kali m.; *Puls.;* Thuya.

From food, crude—Cham.

From fruits—Ars.; *Bry.;* Calc. p.; *Cinch.;* Cistus; Col.; Crot. t.; Ipec.; Pod.; *Puls.;* Ver. a.; Zing.

From gastric derangements—*Ant. c.;* Bry.; Cinch.; Col.; Ipec.; Lyc.; Nux v.; Puls.

From high game—Crot.; Pyr.
From hot weather—Acon.; Aloe; Ambros.; *Ant. c.*; Ars.; *Bry.*; Camph.; Caps.; *Cham.*; *Cinch.*; Crot. t.; *Cuphea*; Ferr. p.; Gamb.; *Ipec.*; Iris; Merc.; Nux m.; *Pod.*; Sil.; Ver. a.
From hydrocephalus acute—Helleb.
From hyperacidity—Cham.; Rheum; Robin.
From intestinal atony, debility—*Arg. n.*; Caps.; *Cinch.*; *Ferr.*; Œnanthe; Oreodaph.; *Sec.*
From jaundice—*Chionanth.*; Dig.; Nux v.
From meat putrescent—Ars.; Crot.
From milk—*Æth.*; Calc. c.; Cinch.; Lyc.; *Mag. c.*; *Mag. m.*; Nat. c.; Niccol.; *Sep.*; Sul.; Val.
From milk boiled—Nux m.
From motion—Apis; *Bry.*; Cinch.; Colch.; Nat. s.
From motion downward—Bor.; Cham.; Sanic.
From nephritis—Tereb.
From noxious effluvia—Bapt.; Carb. ac.; Crot.
From onions—Thuya.
From oysters—*Brom.*; Lyc.; Sul. ac.
From perspiration checked—*Acon.*; Cham.; Ferr. p.
From pork—Acon. lyc.; *Puls.*
From sweets—*Arg. n.*; Calc. s.; Crot .t.; *Gamb.*; Merc. v.
From tobacco—Cham.; Tab.
From tuberculosis—Acet. ac.; Arg. n.; *Arn.*; Ars.; *Ars. iod.*; *Bapt.*; Bism.; *Cinch.*; Coto; *Cupr. ars.*; Elaps; Ferr. m.; Iod.; Iodof.; Phos. ac.; *Phos.*; Puls.; Rumex. See Tuberculosis.
From typhoid fever—*Ars.*; *Bapt.*; Echin.; *Epilob.*; Eucal.; *Hyos.*; Lach.; *Mur. ac.*; Nuphar; Op.; Phos. ac.; *Rhus t.*; Stram. See Typhoid Fever.
From ulceration of intestines—Kali bich.; Merc. c.
From urination—Aloe; Alum.; Apis.
From vaccination—*Sil.*; Thuya.
From veal—Kali n.
From vegetables, melons—*Ars.*; *Bry.*; Petrol.; Zing.
From water polluted—*Alston.*; Camph.; Zing.
In infants, children—*Acon.*; *Æth.*; Apis; *Arg. n.*; *Ars.*; Arundo; Bapt.; *Bell.*; Benz. ac.; Bism.; *Bor.*; Calc. ac.; *Calc. c.*; *Calc. p.*; Camph.; *Cham.*; Cinch.; Cina; *Col.*; Colost.; *Crot. t.*; Dulc.; Ferr.; Grat.; *Helleb.*; Hep.; *Ipec.*; Jal.; Kali br.; *Kreos.*; Laur.; Lyc.; Lyssin; *Mag. c.*; *Merc. c.*; *Merc. d.*; Merc.; Nit. ac.; *Nux v.*; Paul.; Phos. ac.; Phos.; *Pod.*; *Psor.*; *Rheum*; Sabad.; Sep.; *Sil.*; *Sul.*; Val.; *Ver. a.*
Infants (dentition)—Acet. ac.; *Acon.*; *Æth.*; Arundo; *Bell.*; Benz. ac.; Bor.; Calc. ac.; *Calc. c.*; *Calc. p.*; *Cham.*; Ipec.; Jal.; *Kreos.*; *Mag. c.*; Merc. v.; Nux m.; Oleand.; *Phyt.*; *Pod.*; Psor.; Rheum; *Sil.*
In old people—*Ant. c.*; Bov.; *Carbo v.*; *Cinch.*; Gamb.; Op.; Phos.; *Sul.*
In women, before and during menses—Am. c.; *Am. m.*; *Bov.*; Ver. a. See Female Sexual System.
In women, lying-in period—*Cham.*; *Hyos.*; Psor.; *Sec.*; Stram.

TYPE OF STOOL—**Acrid, excoriating, burning**: *Ars.*; Bry.; Carbo v.; *Cham.*;

ABDOMEN

Cuphea; *Graph.*; Iris; Kreos.; *Merc. c.*; Merc. d.; Merc. sul.; Merc. v.; Pod.; *Sul.*; Tereb.

Bilious—Ant. t.; *Bry.*; Card. m.; *Cham.*; Cinch.; *Corn. c.*; Crot. t.; Fluor. ac.; Gamb.; *Ipec.*; *Iris*; Jugl. c.; *Lept.*; Lyc.; *Merc. d.*; Merc.; Nat. s.; Nyctanth.; *Pod.*; Puls.; Sang.; Tarax.; Yucca.

Black—*Ars.*; Brom.; Camph.; *Caps.*; *Carb. ac.*; Cinch.; *Crot.*; Echin.; *Lept.*; Morph.; *Op.*; *Psor.*; Pyr.; *Scilla*; Stram.; Sul. ac.; Ver. a.

Blood-streaked slime—Agar.; *Aloe*; Arg. n.; *Arn.*; Bell.; *Canth.*; *Caps.*; Col.; *Cupr. ars.*; Euphorbia; *Ipec.*; Lil. t.; Kreos.; Mag. c.; *Merc. c.*; Merc. d.; *Merc. v.*; *Nux v.*; Pod.; *Psor.*; *Rhus t.*; *Sul.*; Trill. See Dysentery.

Bloody—Æth.; Ail.; Aloe; Am. m.; *Arg. n.*; Arn.; *Ars.*; *Bapt.*; Bothrops; Cadm. s.; *Canth.*; *Caps.*; Carb. ac.; *Colch.*; Col.; Crot.; Cupr. ars.; Dulc.; Ferr. p.; Ham.; *Ipec.*; Kali bich.; Kreos.; Lach.; *Merc. c.*; Merc. d.; *Merc. v.*; *Nux v.*; *Phos.*; Pod.; *Sec.*; Senec.; *Sul.*; Tereb.; Tromb.; Val.

Brown, dark—Apis; Arn.; *Ars.*; Asaf.; *Bapt.*; *Bry.*; Cinch.; Col.; Corn. c.; Cupr. ac.; Cupr. ars.; Ferr. mur.; *Graph.*; Kali bich.; Kreos.; *Lept.*; Mur. ac.; Nux v.; Pod.; *Psor.*; Pyr.; *Raph.*; Rheum; Rumex; *Scilla*; Sec.; Senec.; Sul.; Tub.

Changeable—Am. m.; *Cham.*; Euonym.; Merc. v.; *Pod.*; Puls.; Sanic.; Sil.; *Sul.*

Clay-colored, chalk-like, light-colored—Aloe; *Bell.*; Benz. ac.; Berb. v.; *Calc. c.*; Chel.; *Dig.*; Euphorbia; Gels.; *Hep.*; Kali c.; *Merc. d.*; Merc. v.; Myr.; *Phos. ac.*; Phos.; Pod.; Sep.

Coffee-ground-like, mealy—Crotal.; Dig.; *Lach.*; Pod.; **Tart. ac.**

Colliquative (debilitating)—Acet. ac.; Angoph.; Arist.; *Ars.*; *Cinch.*; *Colch.*; Coto; *Cupr. ars.*; Diosc.; Elaps; Kali p.; Phell.; *Phos.*; *Sec.*; Sep.; *Tab.*; Tart. ac.; Upas; *Ver. a.*

Fatty, oily—Caust.; *Iod.*; Iris; Phos.

Fermented, flatulent, noisy, spluttering expulsion—Acal.; Agar.; Alfal.; *Aloe*; Apoc.; *Arg. n.*; Arn.; Benz. ac.; Bor.; *Calc .p.*; Cham.; *Cinch.*; Col.; Corn. c.; *Crot. t.*; *Elat.*; *Gamb.*; Graph.; *Grat.*; Gummi; Iod.; *Ipec.*; *Jatropha*; Kali bich.; *Mag. c.*; *Nat. sulphuros.*; *Nat. s.*; Op.; *Phos. ac.*; Phos.; Pod.; Puls.; Rheum; Rhus t.; Sanic.; Sec.; Sticta; *Sul.*; *Thuya*; Triost.; *Ver. a.*; Yucca.

Frequent—Acet. ac.; *Acon.*; Aloe; *Ars.*; Calc. ac.; Caps.; *Carbo v.*; *Cham.*; *Cinch.*; Crot. t.; Cuphea; *Cupr. ars.*; Elat.; Ipec.; Mag. c.; *Merc. c.*; Merc. v.; Nit. ac.; Nux v.; Phos. ac.; *Pod.*; Rheum; Rhus t.; Sil.; Sul.; Tereb.; *Ver. a.*

Frog spawn or scum-like—Helleb.; Mag. c.; *Phos.*; Sanic.

Gelatinous, jelly-like—*Aloe*; Cadm. s.; *Colch.*; *Col.*; Euphorbia; *Helleb.*; Kali bich.; Oxytr.; *Phos.*; Pod.; *Rhus t.*

Green—Acon.; Æth.; Ant. t.; *Apis*; Arg. n.; *Ars.*; *Bell.*; Bor.; Bry.; Calc. ac.; Calc. c.; *Calc. p.*; *Cham.*; Col.; Crot. t.; Dulc.; *Elat.*; Gamb.; *Gels.*; Grat.; Gummi; *Hep.*; Iodof.; *Ipec.*; Iris; Kreos.; Laur.; *Mag. c.*; Merc. c.; *Merc. d.*; *Merc. v.*; *Mez.*; *Paul*; Phos.; Pod.; Puls.; Sal. ac.; Sanic.; *Sec.*; Sul.; Tab.; Val.; *Ver. a.*

Green, turning to blue—Calc. p.; Phos.

ABDOMEN

Gurgling, gushing—Aloe; Apis; *Crot. t.;* Elat.: *Gamb.;* Grat.; Gummi; *Jatropha;* Kali bich.; Merc. s.; Nat. s.; *Petrol.; Phos.;* Pod.; Sang.; Sec.; *Thuya;* Tub.; Ver. a. See Fermented.

Hot—*Calc. p.; Cham.;* Diosc.; Ferr.; Merc. c.; Merc. sul.; Pod.; *Sul.* See Acrid.

Involuntary—*Aloe; Apis;* Apoc.; *Arn.;* Ars.; *Bapt.;* Camph.; Carb. ac.; *Carbo v.; Gels.;* Helleb.; *Hyos.;* Op.; *Phos. ac.; Phos.;* Pod.; Psor.; Pyr.; Rhus t.; *Sec.;* Strych.; Sul.; *Ver. a.;* Zinc.

Involuntary, as if anus were wide open—*Apis;* Apoc.; *Phos.;* Sec.; Tromb.

Involuntary, when passing flatus—*Aloe;* Calc. c.; Iod.; *Mur. ac.;* Nat. m.; Nat. s.; *Oleand.; Phos. ac.; Pod.;* Pyr.; Sanic.

Involuntary, when passing urine—*Aloe; Alum.;* Apis; Cic.; Hyos.; *Mur. ac.; Scilla;* Sul.; Ver. a.

Lumpy, hard—Aloe; Ant. c.; Bar. c.; Bell.; Bry.; Cham.; Cina; Con.; Cub.; Glon.; *Graph.; Mag. c.;* Petrol.; Phos.; *Pod.;* Senec.; Tromb.

Mucous, slimy—*Aloe;* Am. m.; *Ant. c.;* Apis; Arg. n.; *Arn.; Ars.; Bell.;* Bor.; Calc. ac.; *Calc. p.; Canth.; Caps.;* Carb. ac.; *Carbo v.; Cham.;* Cina; Cinch.; Cocc.; *Colch.; Col.; Cop.; Dulc.;* Ferr.; Graph.; Gummi; Helleb.; Hep.; *Ipec.;* Kali m.; Laur.; *Mag. c.; Merc. c.;* Merc. d.; *Merc. s.; Merc. v.;* Nit. ac.; *Nux v.;* Phos.; Pod.; Prun. sp.; *Puls.;* Rneum; Ricin. com.; Rhus t.; Ruta; Sep.; Spig.; *Sul.;* Tab.; Tereb.; Urt. See Dysentery.

Non-debilitating—Calc. c.; Graph.; *Phos. ac.;* Puls.

Offensive, cadaverous—Ail.; Ant. c.; *Arg. n.; Arn.;* Ars.; *Asaf.;* Asclep. t.; *Bapt.; Benz. ac.;* Bism.; *Bor.; Bry.;* Calc. c.; Calc. p.; Carb. ac.; *Carbo v.; Cham.;* Cinch.; Col.; Corn. c.; Crotal.; *Graph.;* Hep.; *Kali p.;* Kreos.; Lach.; *Lept.; Merc. c.;* Merc. d.; Merc. v.; Mur. ac.; Nit. ac.; Nux m.; Op.; Petrol.; Phos. ac.; *Phos.; Pod.; Psor.;* Pulex; Pyr.; *Rheum;* Rhus t.; Rumex; Sanic.; *Scilla; Sec.;* Sil.; Stram.; Sul. ac.; *Sul.; Tereb.;* Tub.

Painless—Alfal.; *Alston.;* Amanita; *Apis;* Ars.; *Bapt.;* Bellis; Bism.; Bor.; Chaparro; *Cinch.;* Colch.; Crot. t.; Dulc.; *Ferr. m.; Gels.; Graph.;* Grat.; Hep.; *Hyos.;* Ipec.; Nit. ac.; *Phos. ac.; Phos.; Pod.;* Psor.; *Puls.;* Pyr.; Rhus t.; Ricin.; Rumex; Scilla; Sec.; Sil.; *Sul.*

Papescent—Æsc.; Alfal.; Aloe; Ars.; Bism.; *Bor.; Bry.;* Chel.; *Cinch.;* Col.; *Cycl.;* Gamb.; Gels.; *Graph.; Lept.;* Mag. c.; *Merc. d.;* Merc.; Nit. ac.; Pæonia; *Pod.;* Rheum; Sep.; Sil.; *Sul.;* Val.; Zinc.

Profuse—Acet. ac.; Ant. c.; *Asaf.; Benz. ac.;* Bism.; Bry.; Calc. ac.; Calc. c.; Chel.; Cinch.; Coto; *Crot. t.; Elat.; Euonym.;* Euphor. c.; Gamb.; *Jatropha;* Lept.; Merc.; Nat. nit.; Operc.; Paul.; Phos.; Pod.; Psor.; Rhus t.; *Sec.;* Sticta; *Tereb.; Thuya; Ver. a.*

Purulent—Apis; Arn.; Calc. s.; *Hep.;* Merc.; Phos.; Sil.

Rice-water—*Ars.;* Camph.; *Jatropha;* Kali p.; Merc. s.; Ricin. com.; Ver. a.

Sago or tallow particles, like—Phos.

Scanty—Acon.; *Aloe;* Ars.; *Bell.;* Camph.; Canth.; Caps.; *Colch.;* Col.; *Merc. c.;* Merc. d.; *Merc. v.;* Nit. ac.; *Nux v.;* Oleand.: Sul. See Dysentery.

ABDOMEN

Shreddy, stringy, membranous, like scrapings of intestines—Aloe; *Arg. n.;* Ars.; Asar.; Bolet.; *Canth.; Carb. ac.; Colch.;* Kali bich.; Kali n.; *Merc. c.;* Merc.; Mur. ac.; *Nit. ac.;* Pod.; Puls.; Sul. ac.

Sour—Calc. ac.; *Calc. c.;* Colch.; Col.; *Colost.;* Graph.; *Hep.:* Jal.; *Mag. c.;* Merc. v.; Nit. ac.; *Pod.; Rheum;* Robin.; Sul.

Spinach chopped, like—Acon.; Arg. n.; Cham.

Sudden, imperative, cannot wait—*Aloe;* Cinch.; Cistus; *Crot. t.; Gamb.; Lil. t.;* Nat. c.; Pæonia; Pod.; *Psor.; Rumex; Sul.;* Tab.; Tromb.; Tub ; *Ver. a.*

Tenacious, glairy—*Asar.; Caps.;* Crot. t.; Helleb., *Kali bich.* See Mucous.

Undigested, lienteric—Abrot.; Æth.; *Ant. c.;* Arg. n.; *Ars.; Asar.; Bry.; Calc. c.; Calc. p.;* Cham.; *Cinch.;* Crot. t.; Ferr. ac.; *Ferr. m.;* Ferr. p.; *Graph.;* Hep.; Iodof.; *Mag. c.;* Nit. ac.; Nux m.; Nux v.; *Oleand.; Phos. ac.; Phos.; Pod.; Psor.; Puls.;* Sul.; Val.

Watery, like washing of meat—*Canth.;* Phos.; Rhus t.

Watery, thin—Acet. ac.; Acon.; Æth.; Aloe; *Alston.; Ant. c.;* Ant. t.; *Apis; Apoc.; Ars.;* Asaf.; *Bapt.; Benz. ac.;* Bism.; *Bor.; Bry.;* Calc. ac.; Calc. c.; *Calc. p.;* Carbo v.; *Cham.;* Chel.; *Cinch.;* Colch.; *Col.;* Crotal.; *Crot. t.;* Cuphea; *Cupr. ars.;* ·Cycl.; *Elat.;* Ferr. m.; *Gamb.;* Graph.; *Grat.;* Hep.; Hyos.; Iod.; Iodof.; Ipec.; *Iris;* Jal.; *Jatropha;* Kali bich.; Kali n.; Laur.; *Mag. c.;* Mur. ac.; Nat. s.; Oleand.; Operc.; Petrol.; *Phos. ac.;* Phos.; *Pod.; Psor.;* Puls.; *Rheum;* Rhus t.; Rumex; *Sec.; Senec.; Sul.;* Tab.; Tereb.; Thuya; Tromb.; Tub.; *Ver. a.;* Zinc.

White—Acon.; Ant. c.; *Bell.; Benz. ac.; Calc. c.;* Caust.; Cham.; Chel.; Cina; Cocc.; *Colch.;* Crot.; Cub.; *Dig.;* Dulc.; *Helleb.; Hep.;* Iod.; Ipec.; Kali m.; Mag. c.; *Merc. d.;* Merc.; Mez.; Nux m.; *Phos. ac.; Phos.; Pod.;* Puls.; Tromb.

Yellow—Æth.; Agar.; Alfal.; Aloe; *Apis; Ars.;* Asar.; *Bor.; Calc. c.; Card. m.;* Cham.; *Chel.; Cinch.;* Col.; *Crot. t.;* Cycl.; Dulc.; *Gamb.;* Gels.; Grat.; Gummi; *Hep.;* Hyos.; Ipec.; Merc.; *Nat. c.;* Nat. s.; *Nuphar;* Nux m.; Petrol.; Phos. ac.; *Pod.;* Puls.; Rheum; Rhus t.; Senna; Sep.; Sul.; Tab.; Thuya.

CONCOMITANTS—BEFORE STOOL: Chilliness: Ars.; Camph.; Elat.; Merc. v.; Phos.; Ver. a.

Colic, cramps—Æth.; *Aloe;* Alston.; *Bell.;* Bor.; Cascar.; *Cham.;* Cina; *Cinch.; Col.;* Crot. t.; *Cupr. ars.; Diosc.;* Dulc.; *Elat.;* Gamb.; Gummi; *Ipec.;* Iris; Lept.; *Mag. c.;* Merc. d.; Merc.; Nux v.; *Rheum;* Senna; Sul.; Tromb.; *Ver. a.* See Colic.

Flatulent rumbling—*Aloe;* Asaf.; Carbo v.; *Colch.;* Col.; *Gamb.;* Kali c.; Nat. s.; Oleand.; *Pod.;* Puls.

Nausea—*Bry.;* Chrom. ac.; *Colch.; Ipec.;* Merc. v.; Rhus t.; Sep.

Urging, painful—*Aloe;* Ars.; *Bell.;* Camph.; Cistus; Col.; Con.; *Crot. t.;* Formica; Gamb.; Grat.; Hep.; *Ign.;* Kali bich.; Lept.; *Merc. c.; Merc. d.;* Merc. v.; Nat. s.; *Nux v.:* Oleand.; Phos.; Pod.; Rheum; Sil.; *Stront.; Sul.; Ver. a.*

DURING STOOL—Backache: *Æsc.;* Caps.; Colch.; *Nux v.;* Puls.

Burning in anus—*Aloe;* Ars.; *Canth.;* Carbo v.; Chenop. gl.; Con.; *Iris;*

ABDOMEN

Jugl. c.; *Merc. d.*; *Mur. ac.*; Pod.; Prun. sp.; *Ratanh.*; Rheum; Tereb.; Tromb.; Ver. a. See Anus.

Chilliness—*Ars.*; Bell.; Colch.; Ipec.; *Jatropha*; *Merc. v.*; Rheum; Ricin. com.; *Sec.*; Tromb.; Ver. a.

Colic, cramps—*Aloe*; Alston.; *Ars.*; Bry.; Camph.; *Canth.*; Caps.; Ceanoth.; *Cham.*; Cinch.; *Col.*; Crot. t.; *Cupr. ars.*; *Cupr. m.*; Dulc.; *Elat.*; Gamb.; *Ipec.*; Iris; *Jatropha*; Lept.; *Merc. c.*; Merc. d.; *Merc. v.*; Pod.; Rheum; Ricin. com.; Sec.; Sil.; Sul.; Triost.; *Tromb.*; Ver. a.; Zing. See Colic.

Fainting—Aloe; *Ars.*; Crot.; *Merc. v.*; Nux m.; Sul.

Flatus, fetid, expelled—Agar.; *Aloe*; *Arg. n.*; *Calc. p.*; *Carbo v.*; Cinch.; Ign.; Jatropha; *Nat. s.*; Phos. ac.; Pod.; Thuya.

Hunger—Aloe; Ferr. m.; Sec.

Nausea, vomiting—Æth.; *Ant. t.*; *Ars.*; *Bism.*; Camph.; Carb. ac.; Chrom. ac.; *Colch.*; Crot t.; Cupr.; Filix m.; *Ipec.*; *Iris*; *Jatropha*; Merc.; Opuntia; Phos.; *Pod.*; Tab.; Triost.; Ver. a.

Pain tearing down posterior limbs—Rhus t.

Stinging pains—Caps.

Tenesmus of bladder—Canth.; Lil. t.; *Merc. c.*

Tenesmus, relieved by stool—Nux v.

Tenesmus, urging painful—Acon.; *Aloe*; Angoph.; Arn.; *Ars.*; *Bell.*; Calc. c.; *Canth.*; Caps.; Carb. ac.; *Colch.*; *Col.*; Crot. t.; Cuphea; Cupr. ac.; *Cupr. ars.*; *Ipec.*; Ign.; *Kali bich.*; Kali n.; Liatris; Mag. c.; *Merc. c.*; Merc. d.; *Merc. s.*; *Merc. v.*; Morph.; Nat. s.; Nit. ac.; *Nux v.*; Op.; Phos.; Plumb. ac.; *Pod.*; Rheum; Rhus t.; *Senec.*; Sil.; *Sul.*; Tab.; Tromb.; Ver. a.

Vomiting, hiccough, suffocative, in stomach and chest—Ver. a.

AFTER STOOL—**Anus burning:** Aloe; Apoc.; *Ars.*; Bry.; *Canth.*; Caps.; Carbo v.; Col.; *Gamb.*; Grat.; *Iris*; Kali c.; Merc. c.; Merc. s.; Merc. v.; Nit. ac.; Oleand.; Prun. sp.; *Ratanh.*; Sul.; Tromb.; Ver. a. See Anus.

Coldness—Aloe; *Ars.*; Camph.; *Canth.*; Caps.; Carbo v.; Formica; Ipec.; Merc. v.; *Sec.*; Tab.; *Ver. a.*

Debility, exhaustion—Acet. ac.; Æth.; *Ail.*; Aloe; Amanita; *Arg. n.*; Arn.; *Ars.*; Bism.; *Camph.*; *Cinch.*; *Colch.*; *Con.*; Crot. t.; Cupr. m.; Elat.; Ferr. m.; Iris; Jatropha; *Kali p.*; Mag. c.; Nit. ac.; *Phos.*; Pod.; *Rhus t.*; *Sec.*; Sep.; Sul. ac.; *Tab.*; *Tereb.*; Tromb.; Tub.; Upas; Ver. a.

Fainting—*Aloe*; Ars.; Con.; Crot. t.; *Merc.*; Nux m.; Pæonia; Sars.; *Tereb.*; Ver. a.

Hæmorrhoids—*Aloe*; Ham.; Mur. ac.; Sul. See Hæmorrhoids.

Pains persist in abdomen—Aloe; *Col.*; Crot. t.; Diosc.; *Gamb.*; Grat.; *Merc. c.*; Merc. v.; Rheum; Tromb.; Ver. a.

Palpitation, trembling in limbs—Ars.

Prolapsus ani—*Aloe*; Alum.; Calc. ac.; Carbo v.; Ham.; *Ign.*; Merc. v.; Nit. ac.; *Pod.*; Sul.; Tromb. See Rectum.

Sleep, as soon as tenesmus ceases—Colch.; *Sul.*

Stool natural in evening—Aloe; Pod.

ABDOMEN

Sweat—Acet. ac.; Aloe; Ant. t.; Ars.; Phos. ac.; Tab.; Tub.; *Ver. a.*
Tenesmus (never-get-done feeling)—Æth.; Aloe; Ars.; *Bell.; Canth.; Caps.;* Colch.; *Gamb.;* Ign.; Ipec.; Kali bich.; Mag. c.; *Merc. c.; Merc. d.; Merc. s.; Merc. v.;* Nit. ac.; Nux v.; *Pod.;* Rheum; Senna; Sil.; *Sul.;* Tromb.
Thirst—Acet. ac.; *Caps.;* Dulc.
Vomiting—Arg. n.; Colch.; Cupr.; *Ipec.; Iris; Nux v.;* Ver. a.
Weakness in abdomen and rectum—Pod.

MODALITIES—Aggravations: From eating, drinking: Aloe; *Alston.; Apis;* Apoc.; *Arg. n.;* Ars.; Bry.; Canth.; *Cinch.; Col.; Crot. t.; Ferr. m.;* Kali p.; Lyc.; Nux v.; *Phos.; Pod.;* Puls.; Rheum; Sanic.; Sul.; Tanac.; Thuya; *Tromb.; Ver. a.*
From motion—Aloe; Apis; *Bry.;* Cinch.; *Colch.;* Crot. t.; *Nat. s.;* Rheum; Ver. a.
From sundown to sunrise—Colch.
In afternoon—Bell.; Calc. c.; *Cinch.;* Corn. c.; *Lyc.*
In autumn—Cinch.; *Colch.; Merc.;* Nux m.; Ver. a.
In daytime only—Hep.; *Petrol.;* Piloc.
In evening, night—*Ars.;* Bellis; Bov.; Calc. c.; Chel.; *Cinch.;* Dulc.; *Ferr. m.;* Iris; *Merc.;* Nat. nit.; Nux m.; Pod.; *Puls.;* Psor.; *Rhus t.; Stront.;* Sul.; Wyeth.
In morning, early—Acet. ac.; *Aloe;* Ichthy.; Iris; Lil. t.; Med.; *Nat. s.;* Nit. ac.; *Nuphar; Nux v.;* Petrol.; Phos.; *Pod.; Psor.;* Rhus v.; *Rumex;* Sticta; *Sul.;* Thuya; Tromb.; Tub.
In morning—*Aloe; Apis;* Bov.; *Bry.;* Cact.; Cistus; Crot. t.; Ferr. m.; Graph.; *Kali bich.;* Lil. t.; Lyc.; Nux v.
In periodical attacks—Apis; Ars.; *Cinch.;* Euphorb. cor.; *Kali bich.;* Iris; Mag. c.; Thuya.

DUODENUM—Catarrhal inflammation (duodenitis): Ars.; Aur.; Berb. v.; Cham.; Chel.; *Cinch.; Hydr.; Kali bich.;* Lyc.; Merc. d.; Merc. s.; Nat. s.; Nux v.; *Pod.;* Ricin. com.; Sang.

Ulceration—*Kali bich.;* Symphyt.; Uran.

DYSENTERY—*Acon.; Aloe;* Alston.; Ambros.; Ant. t.; Apis; *Arg. n.;* Arn.; *Ars.;* Asclep. t.; *Bapt.;* Bell.; Calc. c.; *Canth.; Caps.;* Carb. ac.; Carbo v.; Chaparro; *Cinch.;* Colch.; Collins.; *Col.;* Cuphea; *Cupr. ars.;* Dulc.; Emetine; *Erig.;* Eucal.; Ferr. p.; Gamb.; Ham.; Hep.; *Ipec.;* Iris; *Kali bich.; Kali chlor.;* Kali m.; Kali p.; Lach.; Leonur.; Lept.; Lil. t.; Lyc.; *Mag. c.;* Merc. d.; Merc. s.; *Merc. v.;* Nit. ac.; *Nux v.;* Operc.; Op.; Phos. ac.; *Phos.;* Plumb. ac.; *Pod;* Puls.; Rheum; *Rhus t.;* Sec.; *Silph.; Sul.; Tanac.;* Trill.; *Tromb;* Xanth.; Vaccin.; Ver. a.; Zinc. s.
Abuse of local treatment; diphtheritic form—Nit. ac.
Chronic, intractable cases—Aloe; Arg. n.; *Ars.;* Cinch.; Cop.; *Dulc.;* Hep.; *Merc. c.; Nit. ac.; Nux v.;* Phos. ac.; Pod.; Rhus ars.; *Sul.*
Hemorrhoidal form—Aloe; Collins.; Ham.
In old people—Bapt.
In plethoric, nervous, climacteric females—Lil. t.
With nausea from straining pain; little thirst—Ipec.

ABDOMEN

With long intervals between—*Arn.;* Cinch.
With periodical recurrence in spring or early summer—Kali bich.
With rheumatic pains all over—Asclep. t.
With tearing down thighs—Rhus t.
Worse in autumn—Acon.; *Colch.;* Dulc.; *Ipec.;* Merc. c.; *Merc. v.;* Sul. See Diarrhœa.

ENTERITIS—See Diarrhœa.

ENTERO-COLITIS—See Diarrhœa.

GALL-BLADDER—BILIARY CALCULI (cholelithiasis)—Aur.; Bapt.; Berb. v.; Boldo; Bry.; *Calc. c.; Card. m.;* Chel.; *Chionanth.;* Cholest.; *Cinch.; Diosc.;* Fel tauri; Ferr. s.; Gels.; *Hydr.;* Jugl. c.; Lach.; Lept.; Myr.; *Nux v.;* Pichi; Pod.; Ptel.; Tarax.

Biliary colic—Ars.; Atrop. sul.; *Bell.;* Berb. v.; *Calc. c.; Card. m.;* Cham.; Chel.; Chionanth.; *Cinch.; Col.;* Dig.; *Diosc.;* Gels.; *Hydr.;* Ipec.; Lyc.; Morph. acet.; *Nux v.;* Op.; Tereb.

HÆMORRHOIDS—(piles): **Remedies in general:** Abrot.; *Acon.; Æsc. gl.; Æsc.; Aloe; Am. c.;* Am. m.; Apis; *Ars.;* Aur. m.; Bar. c.; *Bell.;* Brom.; *Calc. fl.; Caps.;* Carbo an.; *Carbo v ; Card. m.;* Caust.; Cham.; Chrom. ac.; *Collins.;* Cop.; Diosc.; Ferr. p.; *Fluor. ac.;* Grat.; Ham.; Hep.; Hydr.; *Hyper.;* Ign.; *Kali m.;* Kali s.; *Lach.; Lyc.;* Mag. m.; *Millef.; Mucuna;* Mur. ac.; Negundo; *Nit. ac.; Nux v.; Pæonia;* Pinus sylv.; *Pod.; Polyg.;* Puls.; Radium; *Ratanh.;* Sab.; Scrophul.; Sedum; Sep.; *Semperv. t.; Sul.;* Sul. ac.; Thuya; Verbasc.; *Wyeth.;* Zing.

Bleeding—Acon.; Æsc.; *Aloe; Am. c.;* Bell.; Calc. fl.; *Caps.;* Card. m.; Chrom. ac.; *Collins.;* Erig.; Ferr. p.; *Ficcus;* Ham.; Hydr.; Hyper.; Kali m.; Lept.; Lycop.; *Millef.;* Mur. ac.; Nit. ac.; *Nux v.;* Opere.; Phos.; *Sab.;* Scrophul.; Sep.; *Sul.;* Thlaspi.

Bleeding, dark, venous blood—Aloe; *Ham.;* Hydr., Kali m.; *Sul.*

Blind—*Æsc ;* Calc. fl.; Collins.; *Ign.;* Mucuna; *Nux v.;* Puls.; *Sul.;* Wyeth.

Bluish, purplish—Æsc. gl.; *Æsc.; Aloe;* Ars.; Caps.; Carbo v.; Ham.; Lach.; Lyc.; *Mur ac.*

Burning, smarting—*Æsc.;* Aloe; Am. m.; *Ars.;* Calc. c.; *Caps.;* Carbo an ; Carbo v.; Caust.; *Fluor. ac.;* Graph ; *Ign.;* Mag. m.; *Mucuna;* Negundo; *Nux v.;* Psor.; *Ratanh.; Sul.;* Sul. ac.

Inflamed—*Acon.;* Æsc.; Aloe; Bell.; Caust.; Cop.; Ferr. p.; Mur. ac.; Verbasc. See Sensitive.

Itching—*Æsc.; Aloe· Cips.;* Carbo v.; Caust.; Cop.; Glon.; *Ham.;* Mur. ac.; Nit. ac.; *Nux v.;* Petros.; Puls.; *Sul.*

Mucous piles, continually oozing—*Aloe;* Am. m.; *Ant. c.;* Caps.; Carbo v.; Caust.; Puls.; Sep ; Sul. ac.; Sul.

Protruding, grape-like, swollen—*Æsc.; Aloe; Am. c.;* Caps.; *Carbo v.; Caust.; Collins.; Diosc.;* Graph.; Ham.; Kali c.; Lach.; *Mur. ac.;* Nux m.; *Nux v.;* Ratanh.; Scrophul.; Sep.; Sul ; Thuya.

Protruding when urinating—Bar. c.; *Mur. ac.*

Sensitive, exquisitely painful—Æsc. gl.; *Æsc.; Aloe;* Ars.; *Bell.;* Cact.; *Caps.;* Carbo v ; *Caust.;* Cham.; Collins.; Ferr. p.; Graph.; *Ham.;*

ABDOMEN

Hyper.; **Kali c.;** *Lach.; Lyc.;* Mag. m.; *Mur. ac.;* Nat. m.; Nit. ac.; *Nux v.;* Plant.; Puls.; *Ratanh.;* Scrophul.; *Sedum;* Sep.; *Sil.;* Sul.; Thuya; Verbasc.; Zing.

White piles—Carbo v.

CONCOMITANTS—With abdominal plethora—Æsc.; *Aloe;* Collins.; Ham.; Negundo; Nux v.; Sep.; *Sul.*

With backache—Æsc. gl.; *Æsc.; Bell.;* Calc. fl.; Chrom. ac.; Euonym.; Ham.; Ign.; Nux v.; Sul. See Back.

With constipation—Æsc. gl.; *Æsc.;* Am. m.; Anac.; *Collins.;* Euonym.; Kali s.; *Nux v.;* Paraf.; Sil.; *Sul.;* Verbasc.

With debility—Ars.; Cinch.; Ham.; Hydr.; Mur. ac.

With epistaxis—Carbo v.

With fissures, soreness of anus—Caps.; Cham.; *Nit. ac.;* Ratanh.; *Sedum.*

With heart disease—Cact.; Collins.; Dig.

With hypochondriasis—Æsc.; Grat.; *Nux v.*

With pelvic congestion—*Aloe;* Collins.; Ham.; Hep.; Mucuna; *Pod.;* Nux v.; Sep.; *Sul.*

With prolapsus ani et uteri—Pod.

With spasm of sphincter—Lach.; Sil.

With stitches in rectum during cough—Ign.; *Kali c.;* Lach.; Nit. ac.

With sudden development in marantic children—Mur. ac.

With tenesmus, anal and visceral, diarrhoea—Caps.

With tenesmus, constriction, lancinating pains—Nux v.

With tenesmus, dysenteric stools—Aloe; Sul.

With tenesmus, in pregnant females—Collins.

With vicarious bleeding—Ham.; Millef.

AGGRAVATIONS—After confinement: Aloe; Apis. See Female Sexual System.

After stool for hours—Æsc.; Am. m.; Ign.; Ratanh.; Sul.

As rheumatic symptoms abate—Abrot.

During climacteric—Æsc.; Lach. See Female Sexual System.

During menses—Am. c.; Lach.

During sitting—Graph.; Ign.; *Thuya.*

From alcoholic abuse, in sedentary persons—Æsc. gl.; Nux v.

From coughing, sneezing—Caust.; *Kali c.;* Lach.

From leucorrhœa suppressed—Am. m.

From talking, thinking of them—Caust.

From walking—Caust.; Sep.

AMELIORATIONS—From cold water: *Aloe;* Nux v.; Ratanh.

From hot water—*Ars.;* Mur. ac.

From lying down—Am. c.

From walking—Ign.

HERNIA—Æsc.; Alum.; Am. c.; Aur.; Calc. c.; Calc. p.; *Cocc.;* Col.; Iris fact.; *Lyc.;* Mag. c.; *Nux v.;* Ox. ac.; Petrol.; Phos.; Picrot.; Sil.; Sul. ac.; Ver. a.; Zinc.

Incarcerated—Lob. infl.; *Millef.;* Nux v.; *Op.;* Plumb.

In children—*Calc. c.;* Lyc.; Nit. ac.; *Nux v.;* Sil.; Sul.

Scrotal, congenital—Mag. m.

ABDOMEN

Strangulated—Acon.; *Bell.*; Lyc.; Nux v.; *Op.*; Plumb.
Umbilical—Calc. c.; Cocc.; *Nux v.*; Plumb. m.

INTESTINES—Intussusception, obstruction: Acon.; Atrop.; *Bell.*; Colch.; Col.; *Merc. c.*; Nux v.; *Op.*; *Plumb.*; Thuya; Ver. a.
Obstruction, post-operative—Acon.; *Arn.*; Bell.; Merc. c.
Paralysis—Eser. sal.; Plumb. ac.
Ulceration—Arg. n.; Cupr.; *Kali bich.*; Merc. c.; Sul. ac.; Sul.; Tereb.; Uran.

JAUNDICE (icterus)—*Acon.*; Aloe; Am. m.; Arg. n.; Astacus; Ars.; *Aur. m. n.*; Aur.; *Berb. v.*; *Bry.*; *Card. m.*; Cascara sag.; *Ceanoth.*; *Cham.*; *Chel.*; Chelone; *Chionanth.*; Cholest.; *Cinch.*; Corn. c.; *Crot.*; *Dig.*; Dolichos; Eup. perf.; Hep.; *Hydr.*, Iod.; Jugl. c.; Kali bich.; Kali c.; Kali picr.; Lach.; *Lept.*; *Lyc.*; Merc. c.; *Merc. d.*; *Merc. s.*; *Myr.*; Nat. m.; *Nat. p.*; Nat. s.; Nit. ac.; *Nux v.*; Ostrya; *Phos.*; Picr. ac.; Plumb.; *Pod.*; Ptel.; Rumex; Ruta; Sep.; Still.; Sul.; *Tarax.*; *Yucca;* Veron.; *Vipera.*
Anemia; brain disease; pregnancy—Phos.
Chronic—Aur.; Chel.; *Con.*; Iod.; *Phos.*
Extension of catarrhal process—Am. m.; *Chel.*; Chionanth.; *Cinch.*; Dig.; *Hydr.*; Lob. infl.; Merc.; Nux v.; Pod.
From mental emotion—Bry.; *Cham.*; Lach.; Nux v.; Vipera.
Infantile—Cham.; *Lupul.*; Merc. d.; Merc. s.; Myr.
Malignant—Acon.; *Ars.*; Crot.; Lach.; Merc.; *Phos.*

HYPOCHONDRIA—Pain in left side: *Alum.*; Am. m.; Arg. n.; *Bapt. conf.*; Carbo v.; *Ceanoth.*; *Cim.*; Con.; Dig.; Grind.; Kali c.; Lyc.; Nat. c.; Nat. m.; Nit. ac.; Ox. ac.; Parth.; Polymn.; *Puls.*; Quercus; Scilla; Sep.; Urt. See Spleen.
Pain in right side—Æsc.; *Aloe;* Aur.; Bapt.; *Berb. v.;* Bolet.; *Bry.*; Calc. c.; Carbo v.; *Chel.*; *Cinch.*; Con.; *Diosc.*; Gins.; Jacar.; Jatropha; *Kali bich.*; Kali c.; Limul.; *Lyc.*; Merc.; *Nat. s.*; Nux v.; Ol. j. as.; Phyt.; *Pod.*; *Ptel.*; Quass.; Ran. s.; Sul.; Wyeth. See Liver.

LIVER—Abscess:—Ars.; *Bell.*; Boldo; Bry.; Chin. ars.; *Hep.*; Lach.; Merc.; Phos.; Raph.; Rhus t.; *Sil.*; Vipera.
Affections in general—Abies c.; *Æsc.*; *Aloe;* *Am. m.*; Ars. iod.; *Astacus;* Aur. m.; *Aur. m. n.*; *Berb. v.*; Brassica; *Bry.*; Calc. c.; *Card. m.*; *Ceanoth.*; *Cham.*; *Chel.*; Chelone; Chenop.; *Chionanth.*; Cholest.; *Cinch.*; Cob.; Con.; Corn. c.; Croc.; Crot.; Diosc.; Dolichos; *Eup. perf.;* Euonym.; *Ferr. picr.*; *Hep.*; Hydr.; Iod.; Iodof.; *Iris;* Kali c.; Kali iod.; Lach.; *Lept.*; Lyc.; *Mag. m.*; Mang. s.; Marrub.; *Merc. s.*; *Myr.*; Nat. s.; Nux v.; Phos.; Pichi; Plumb.; *Pod.*; *Ptel.*; Puls.; Querc.; Raph.; Selen.; *Sep.*; Stellar.; *Sul.*; *Tarax.*; Thlaspi; Uran.; Vanad.; Veron.
Atrophy, acute, yellow—Dig.; *Phos.*; Pod.
Atrophy (cirrhosis)—Abies c.; Apoc.; Ars.; *Ars. iod.*; Aur. m.; *Aur. mur.*; Calc. ars.; *Card. m.*; Cascara sag.; *Cinch.;* Fel tauri; Fluor. ac.; Graph.; Hydr.; *Iod.*; Kali bich.; Kali iod.; Lyc.; Merc. d.; *Merc.*; *Nasturt. aq.*; Nat. chlor.; Nit. ac.; Nit. mur. ac.; Nux v.; *Phos.*; Plumb.; Pod.; Quass.; Senec.

ABDOMEN

Cancer—Ars.; Chel.; *Cholest.;* Con.; Hydr.; Lach.; Nit. ac.; Phos.

CONGESTION (hyperemia, fullness, torpidity)—Abies c.; Æsc. gl.; *Æsc.;* Agar.; *Aloe;* Ars.; Berb. aq.; *Berb. v.;* Brassica; *Bry.;* *Card. m.;* Cham.; *Chel.;* Chelone; Chin. s.; *Cinch.;* Croc.; Dig.; Eup. perf.; Euonym.; *Hep.;* *Hydr.;* *Iris;* Kali bich.; *Kali m.;* *Lach.;* *Lept.;* *Lyc.;* *Mag. m.;* *Merc. d.;* *Merc.;* Mucuna; Nat. s.; Nit. ac.; Nit. mur. ac.; *Nux v.;* Phos.; Pier. ac.; *Pod.;* Quass.; Senna; *Sep.;* Stellar.; Still.; Sul.; Tromb.; *Vipera.*

Congestion, chronic—Am. m.; *Chel.;* *Cholest.;* Cinch.; Con.; *Hep.;* Hydr.; Iod.; *Kali c.;* Lept.; *Lyc.;* Mag. m.; Merc. d.; Merc. s.; Nat. s.; *Pod.;* Seler.; *Sep.;* Sul.; Vipera.

Enlargement (hypertrophy)—Æsc.; Agar.; *Ars.;* Calc. ars.; Card. m.; *Chel.;* Chin. ars.; *Chionanth.;* *Cinch.;* Col.; Con.; *Dig.;* Ferr. ars.; Ferr. iod.; Glycerin; Graph.; Iod.; Kali c.; Mag. m.; Mang. ac.; *Merc. d.;* *Merc.;* Nat. s.; *Nux v.;* Pod.; Sec.; *Selen.;* Stellar.; *Tarax.;* Vipera; Zinc. See Congestion.

Enlargements in drunkards—Absinth.; Am. m.; Ars.; Fluor. ac.; Lach.; Nux v.; Sul.

Fatty degeneration—Aur. m.; Chel.; Kali bich.; Phlorid.; Phos.; *Pier. ac.;* Vanad.

Induration—Abies c.; Ars.; *Aur.;* Cinch.; *Con.;* Fluor. ac.; *Graph.;* Lyc.; Mag. m.; Merc.; Nux v.; Sil.; *Tarax.;* Zinc. See Cirrhosis.

Inflammation (perihepatitis, hepatitis)—Acon.; Act. sp.; Ars.; Aur.; *Bry.;* Cham.; *Chel.;* Corn. c.; *Hep.;* Iod.; Kali iod.; *Lach.;* Merc. d.; *Merc.;* Nat. s.; *Phos.;* Psor.; Sil.; Stellar.; Sul.

Pain (hepatalgia)—Acon.; *Æsc.;* Aloe; Am. c.; Am. m.; Ars.; Bell.; Berb. v.; Boldo; *Bry.;* Calc. s.; Carbo v.; *Card. m.;* *Ceanoth.;* *Chel.;* Chelone; Cholest.; *Cinch.;* Cob.; Con.; Crot.; *Dig.;* *Diosc.;* Jatropha; Kali c.; Lach.; *Lept.;* *Lyc.;* *Mag. m.;* *Merc.;* Merc. d.; *Myr.;* *Nux v.;* Ol. j. as.; Parth.; *Pod.;* *Ptel.;* Ran. b.; *Ran. s.;* Sang.; Selen.; *Sep.;* Stann.; Sul.; Tarax.; Yucca.

Pain dragging, on turning on left side—Bry.; Ptel.

Pain, pressive—Anac.; Carbo an.; Cinch.; *Kali c.;* Lyc.; Mag. m.; Merc.

Pain, stitching—Acon.; *Agar.;* Am. m.; Bell.; Benz. ac.; *Berb. v.;* Bry.; Carbo v.; *Chel.;* Cinch.; Diosc.; Hep.; Jugl. c.; Kali bich.; *Kali c.;* Merc. c.; Merc.; Nat. m.; Nat. s.; *Nux v.;* Ox. ac.; Quass.; Ran. b.; Sep.; Stellar.; Sul.

Pain, relieved lying on painful side—Bry.; Ptel.; Sep.

Pain, relieved rubbing and shaking liver region—Pod.

Pains worse lying on left side—*Bry.;* Nat. s.; *Ptel.*

Pain worse lying on right side—Chel.; Diosc.; Kali c.; *Mag. m.;* *Merc.*

Pigmentary degeneration—Arg. n.

Sensitiveness to touch, pressure—*Æsc.;* *Aloe;* Bapt.; *Bell.;* *Berb. v.;* Bry.; Calc. c.; *Card. m.;* Chaparro; *Chel.;* Chelone; *Chionanth.;* *Cinch.;* *Dig.;* Eup. perf.; Fluor. ac.; Graph.; Hydr.; Iod.; *Iris;* *Kali c.;* *Lach.;* Lept.; *Lyc.;* *Mag. m.;* *Merc. d.;* Merc.; Nat. s.; *Nux v.;* Nyctanth.; Phos.; *Pod.;* *Ptel.;* *Ran. b.;* Sanic.; Senna; *Sep.;* Stellar.; Sul.; Tarax.; Zinc.

Syphilis—Aur. mur.; Kali iod.; Merc. i. r. See Male Sexual System.

Waxy liver—Calc. c.; *Kali iod.;* Phos.; Sil.

PANCREAS—Affections: Ars.; *Atrop.;* Bar. m.; Bell.; Calc. ars.; Carbo an.; Carbo v.; Chionanth.; *Iod.; Iris;* Jabor.; Kali iod.; *Merc.;* Nux v.; Pancreat.; *Phos.;* Piloc.; Puls.

PERINEUM—Ars.; Asaf.; Bell.; Bov.; Can. ind.; Carbo v.; *Chimaph.; Cycl.;* Kali bich.; Lyc.; Melastoma; Merc.; *Ol. an.; Pæonia; Sanic.;* Santal; Selen.; Tellur.

PERITONITIS—*Acon.; Apis;* Arn.; Ars.; Atrop.; *Bell.; Bry.;* Calc. c.; *Canth.;* Carbo v.; Cham.; Cim.; *Cinch.; Col.; Crot.;* Ferr. p.; Hep.; Ipec.; Kali chlor.; *Lach.;* Lyc.; *Merc. c.;* Merc. d.; *Merc.; Rhus t.;* Sang. n.; *Sinap. n.;* Solan. n.; Sul.; Tereb.; Ver. v.; *Wyeth.*

Chronic—Apis; *Lyc.;* Merc. d.; Sul.

Pseudo-peritonitis, hysterical—Bell.; Col.; Ver. a.

Tubercular—*Abrot.;* Ars.; Ars. iod.; Calc. c.; Carbo v.; *Cinch.;* Iod.; Psor.; Sul.; *Tub.*

PERITYPHLITIS—*Ars.;* Bell.; *Iris min.;* Iris ten.; *Lach.;* Merc. c.; Rhus t

SPLEEN—Atrophy, induration:—Agn.; Eucal.; *Iod.;* Phos.

Diseases, epidemic, in domestic animals—Anthrac.

Enlargement—Agar.; Agn.; Aran.; *Ars.;* Ars. iod.; Aur. mur.; Bellis; *Calc. ars.;* Caps.; Card. m.; *Ceanoth.;* Ced.; Chionanth.; *Chin. s.; Cinch.;* Ferr. ac.; *Ferr. ars.;* Ferr. iod.; Grind.; *Helianth.;* Iod.; Mag. m.; Malar.; Merc. i. r.; *Nat. m.;* Persicaria; Phos. ac.; Phos.; *Polym.; Querc.;* Succin.; Sul. ac.; Urt.

Inflammation (splenitis)—Aran.; Arn.; Iod.; *Ceanoth.; Chin. s.; Cinch.;* Ferr. p.; Iod.; Plumb. iod.; *Polym.;* Succin.; Ver. v. See Enlargement.

Pain—*Agar.;* Agn.; Am. m.; Arn.; *Ars.;* Ars. m.; Caps.; *Ceanoth.;* Cim.; *Cinch.;* Cobalt.; *Diosc.;* Grind.; *Helianth.; Helon.;* Ilex; Iod.; *Kali jod.; Lob. cer.; Nat. m.;* Parth.; Plumb.; *Polym. noed.;* Ptel.; Quass.; Querc.; Ran. b.; Rhus t.; Scilla; Sul.; Urt.

Pain, stitching—Agar.; Alston.; Am. m.; *Bellis;* Berb. v.; Carbo v.; *Ceanoth.;* Chel.; Cinch.; Con.; Kali bich.; Nat. m.; Ran. b.; Rhod.; Sul.; Tarax.; *Ther.*

TYPHLITIS, APPENDICITIS—Acon.; Arn.; *Ars.;* Bapt.; Bell.; *Bry.;* Canth.; Card. m.; Colch., Collins.; *Col.; Crot.; Diosc.; Echin.;* Ferr. p.; Gins.; Hep.; Iris ten.; Kali m.; *Lach.;* Lyc.; *Merc. c.;* Merc.; Nux v.; Op.; Plumb.; Rhamnus; *Rhus t.;* Sil.; Sul.; Ver. a.

UMBILICUS, Navel—Bleeding from, in newborn: Abrot.; *Calc. p.*

Bubbling sensation—Berb. v.

Burning—Acon.; Ars.

Eczema—Merc. pr. rub.

Pain, soreness about—Æsc.; *Aloe;* Anac.; Benz. ac.; *Bov.; Bry.; Calc. p.;* Carbo v.; Caust.; Cham.; Chel.; Chionanth.; *Cina;* Cocc.; *Col.;* Con.; Crot. t.; *Dulc.;* Euonym.; *Gamb.; Granat.;* Hyper.; *Ipec.;* Lept.; Lyc.; *Nux m.;* Nux v.; Oleand.; Ox. ac.; Paraf.; *Phos. ac.;* Plat.; *Plumb. m.;* Ran. sc.; Raph.; *Rheum;* Senec.; Sil.; *Spig.;* Stann.; Sul.; Taxus; Verbasc.; *Ver. a.;* Zinc. m.

ABDOMEN

Retraction—Calc. p.; *Plumb.*; Pod.
Ulcer, above—Ars.
Urine, oozing from—Hyos.
WORMS—**Remedies in general:** Æsc.; *Ambros.*; Apoc. andr.; *Ars.*; Bapt.; Bell.; Calad.; *Calc. c.*; *Chelone*; Cic.; *Cina*; Cupr. ac.; Cupr. oxy.; Ferr. mur.; Ferr. s.; *Filix m.*; *Granat.*; Ign.; Indigo; Ipec.; Kali m.; Kuosso; Lyc.; Merc. c.; *Naph.*; *Nat. p.*; Passifl.; Puls.; Quass.; *Ratanh.*; *Sabad.*; *Santon.*; Sil.; *Spig.*; *Stann.*; Sul.; Sumb.; Tereb.; *Teucr.*; Ver. a.; *Viola od.*
Ascaris lumbricoides—*Abrot.*: Æsc.; Ant. c.; Calc. c.; *Chelone*; *Cina*; Ferr. m.; Granat.; Helmintoch.; Ign.; Indigo; Kali chlor.; Lyc.; Merc. d.; Naph.; Pin. sylv.; *Sabad.*; *Santon.*; *Spig.*; Stann.; Sul.; Tereb.; *Teucr.*; Urt.
Oxyuris vermicularis—Ars.; Bapt.; *Chelone*; *Cina*; Ign.; Indigo; Lyc.; Merc. d.; Merc. s.; Nat. p.; Ratanh.; *Santon.*; Sil.; Sinap. n.; Spig.; Teucr.; Val.
Taenia—Argem. mex.; Carbo v.; Cucur.; Cupr. ac.; Cupr. oxy.; *Filix m.*; *Granat.*; Graph.; Kali iod.; Kamala; *Kuosso*; Mag. m.; Merc.; Pelletierine; Phos.; Puls.; Sabad.; Sab.; Santon.; Stann.; Sul.; Tereb.; Val.
Trichinæ—Ars.; Bapt.; Cupr. oxy.

URINARY SYSTEM

AFFECTIONS, in old men—Alfal.; Aloe; Cop.; Hep.; Phos.; *Pop. tr.*; Staph.; Sul. See Weakness.

BLADDER—Atony: *Ars.*; Dulc.; Hep.; Op.; *Plumb.*; Rhus ar.; Rhus t.; Scilla; Tereb. See Paralysis.

Cystocele—Staph.

ENURESIS—Incontinence: Remedies in general: Acon.; Agar.; Apis; *Arg. n.*; Arn.; Ars.; Atrop.; *Bell.*; *Benz. ac.*; Calc. c.; Canth.; *Caust.*; Cic.; Cim.; *Cina*; Con.; *Dulc.*; Equis.; Eryng. aq.; Eup. perf.; *Eup. purp.*; Ferr. m.; Ferr. p.; *Gels.*; Hydrang.; Hyos.; *Kali br.*; Kali n.; Kali p.; Kreos.; Linar.; *Lupul.*; Lyc.; Mag. p.; Med.; *Nux v.*; Op.; Petrol.; Phos. ac.; Physal.; Plant.; *Puls*; *Rhus ars.*; Rhus t.; *Sabal*; Sanic.; Santon.; Sec.; Senega; Sep.; Sil.; Stram.; *Sul.*; Tereb.; *Thyr.*; Thuya; Tritic.; Tub.; Uran.; Verbasc.; Zinc. m. See Flow.

TYPE—OCCURRENCE—Diurnal: Arg. n.; Bell.; Caust.; Equis.; Ferr. m.; Ferr. p.; Sec.

In old people—Aloe; Ammon. benz.; *Arg. n.*; *Benz. ac.*; Canth.; Equis.; Gels.; Nit. ac.; *Rhus ar.*; Sec.; Senega; *Turnera*.

Nocturnal—Am. c.; Arg. n.; Arn.; Ars.; *Bell.*; Benz. ac.; Calc. c.; *Caust.*; Cina; Coca; *Equis.*; Eup. purp.; Ferr. iod.; Ferr. p.; Gels.; Hep.; *Ign.*; Kali br.; Mag. p.; Med.; Physal.; *Plant.*; *Puls.*; Quass.; *Rhus ar.*; Santon ; Sec.; *Sil.*; *Sul.*; Thuya; *Thyr.*; Uran.; Verbasc.

CAUSE—Catheterization, after: Mag. p.

Digestive disturbances—Benz. ac.; *Nux v.*; Puls.

During first sleep: child aroused with difficulty—Caust.; Kreos.; Sep.

During full moon; intractable cases; eczematous history—Psor.

Habit the only ascertainable cause—Equis.

History of sycosis—Med.

Hysteria—Ign.; Val m.

Weak or paretic sphincter vesicae—Apoc.; *Bell.*; *Caust.*; Con.; Ferr. p.; Gels.; Nux v.; Rhus ar.; *Sabal*; Sec.; *Strych.* See Paralysis.

Worms—Cina; *Santon.*; Sul.

FEELING—As if ball or plug, in bladder—Anac.; Kali br.; Lach.; Santal.

Feeling, as if chill rising from, to back—Sars.

Feeling, as if distended—Anthem.; *Apoc.*; Ars.; Berb. v.; *Con.*; Conv.; Dig.; *Equis.*; Eup. perf.; Gels ; *Hyos.*; Mel cum sale; Pareira; *Puls.*; Ruta: Santon.; *Sars.*; Sep.; Staph.; *Sul.*; Uva.

Hæmorrhage—*Amyg. pers.*; Cact.; Carbo v.; Frig.; *Ham.*; Millef.; *Nit ac.*; Rhus ar.; *Sec.*; *Thlaspi.* See Hæmaturia.

Hypertrophy, concentric—Pichi.

INFLAMMATION (cystitis)—Acute: Acon.; Ant. t.; Apis; Ars.; Aspar.; *Bell.*; Benz. ac.; Berb. v.; *Camph.*; Camphor. ac.; *Can. s.*; *Canth.*; Caps.; Chimaph ; Con.; *Cop.*; Cub.; Dig.; *Dulc.*; Elat.; *Equis.*; Erig.; *Eucal.*; *Eup. purp.*; Ferr. ac.; *Ferr. p.*; Gels.; Helleb.; Hydrang.; Hyos.; Lach.; *Merc. c.*; Methyl. bl.; Nit. ac.; Nux v.; *Ol. sant.*; *Pareira*;

URINARY SYSTEM

Petros.; Pichi; Pip. m.; *Pop. tr.*; Prun. sp.; *Puls.*; Sabal; *Sab.*; Sars.; Saurur.; Sep.; *Stigm.*; Sul.; *Tereb.*; Tritic.; Uva; Vesic.

From abuse of cantharis—Apis; Camph.

From gonorrhoea—Bell.; Benz. ac.; *Canth.*; *Cop.*; Cub.; Merc. c.; Puls.; Sabal.

From operations, and in pregnancy—Pop. tr.

With fever, strangury—*Acon.*; Bell.; *Canth.*; Gels.; Hydrang.; Stigm.

Inflammation, chronic—*Ars.*; Bals. per.; Baros.; *Benz. ac.*; Berb. v.; *Buchu;* Can. s.; *Canth.*; Carbo v.; *Caust.*; *Chimaph.*; Coccus; Col.; *Cop.*; Cub.; *Dulc.*; *Epig.*; Eryng. aq.; Eucal.; *Eup. purp.*; *Fabiana;* Grind.; *Hydr.*; Iod.; Junip.; Kava; Lith. c.; *Lyc.*; *Merc. c.*; Nit. ac.; *Pareira;* Pichi; Pip. m.; *Pop. tr.*; Prun. sp.; *Puls.*; Rhus ar.; *Sabal;* Santon.; Senega; *Sep.*; Silph.; *Stigm.*; *Tereb.*; Thlaspi; Thuya; Tritic.; Tub.; *Uva;* Vesic.; Zea.

IRRITABILITY—Bladder and neck: *Acon.*; Alfal.; Aloe; *Apis;* Baros.; *Bell.*; *Benz. ac.*; *Berb. v.*; Buchu; Calc. c.; *Camph.*; Can. s.; *Canth.*; Caps.; Caust.; *Cop.*; Cub.; Dig.; *Equis.*; Erig.; Eryng. aq.; *Eup. purp.*; Ferr. ac.; Ferr. m.; *Ferr. p.*; Guaiac.; Hyos.; Kali br.; Mitchella; Nit. mur. ac.; *Nux v.*; Oxytr.; Pareira; *Petros.*; Prun. sp.; Rhus ar.; *Sabal; Senec.;* Senega; Sep.; Staph.; *Stigm.*; *Tereb.*; Thuya; *Tritic.*; Vesic.

Irritability in women—Berb. v.; Cop.; Cub.; *Eup. purp.*; Gels.; Hedeoma; Kreos.; Senec.; *Sep.*; Staph.

PAIN—*Acon.*; Ambra; *Bell.*; *Berb. v.*; Camph.; *Canth.*; Carbo v.; Caul.; *Caust.*; Coccus; *Cop.*; Dig.; *Dulc.*; *Equis.*; Erig.; *Eryng.*; Ign.; Lach.; *Lyc.*; Naph.; Nit. ac.; Op.; *Pareira;* Pichi; Piloc.; *Pop. tr.*; Prun. sp.; Pulex; *Puls.*; *Rhus ar.*; *Staph.*; Stigm.; Strych.; *Tereb.*; Thuya; Tritic.; Uran. n.; *Uva.* See Cystitis.

TYPE—Aching—Berb. v.; Conv.; *Equis.*; Eup. purp.; *Pop. tr.*; Sep.; Sticta; Tereb.

Burning—*Acon.*; Ars.; Baros.; *Berb. v.*; Camph.; *Canth.*; *Cop.*; *Ferr. picr.*; Staph.; *Tereb.*; Thuya; *Uva.*

Cramp-like, constricting—*Bell.*; *Berb. v.*; *Cact.*; Can. s.; Canth.; Caps.; Lyc.; Op.; *Polyg.*; Prun. sp.; *Sars.*; Tereb.

Cutting, stitching—*Acon.*; Æth.; *Bell.*; *Berb. v.*; *Canth.*; Coccus; Con.; *Lyc.*; Tereb.

Neuralgic, spasmodic—*Bell.*; *Berb. v.*; Canth.; Caul.; Lith. c.; *Lyc.*; Merc. c.; *Pareira;* Puls.; *Staph.*; Uva.

Pressing—Aloe; Brachygl.; *Cact.*; Carbo v.; Coccus; *Con.*; Dig.; *Dulc.*; *Equis.*; Lach.; Lil. t.; *Lyc.*; Mel cum sale; *Pop. tr.*; Pulex; *Puls.*; Ruta; Sep.; Staph.; Sul.; Tereb.; Verbasc.

Radiating to spermatic cord—Clem.; Lith. c.; Puls.; Spong.

MODALITIES—AGGRAVATIONS: After urination:—*Canth.*; Caust.; Epig.; *Equis.*; Pichi; Ruta. See Urination.

From drinking water—Canth.

From lithotomy—Staph.

From walking—Con.; Prun. sp.

AMELIORATIONS—From rest:—Con.
  From urination—Coccus.; Hedeoma.
  From walking—Ign.; Tereb.

PARALYSIS—Alum.; Apoc.; *Arn.; Ars.;* Aur.; Cact.; Camph.; Can. ind.; *Canth.; Caust.;* Con.; Dig.; Dulc.; Eucal.; *Equis.; Ferr. m.;* Ferr. p.; *Gels.;* Helleb.; *Hyos.;* Lach.; Morph.; *Nux v.; Op.; Plumb. m.;* Psor.; Puls.; *Sec.;* Strych.; Thuya.
  Paralysis of sphincter—Ars.; *Bell.; Caust.;* Cic.; *Dulc.; Hyos.;* Ign.; Lach.; Laur.; Nat. m.; Op.; Sul.; Thuya; Zinc.

POLYPI—Papilloma:—Ars.; *Calc. c.;* Thuya.
  Prolapsus—Hyos.; Pyrus; Staph.
  Sensitiveness, tenderness of vesical region—*Acon.; Bell.;* Berb. v.; *Canth.;* Coccus; *Equis.;* Eup. purp.; Merc. c.; Sars.; Sticta; *Tereb.* See Pain.
  Spasm (cystospasm)—Canth.; Gels.; *Hyos.;* Nux v.; Puls.
  Spasm following operations on orifice—*Bell.;* Col.; *Hyper.*

TENESMUS VESICAE—*Acon.: Apis;* Arn.; *Bell.;* Benz. ac.; Camph.; Can. s.; *Canth.; Caps.;* Cham.; Chimaph.; Coccus; *Col.; Cop.;* Cub.; Epig.; *Equis.;* Eryng.; *Eup. purp.;* Ferr. p.; Hydrang.; Hyos.; Ipec.; *Lil. t.;* Lith. c.; Lyc.; Med.; *Merc. c.;* Nit. ac.; *Nux v.; Oniscus;* Pichi; *Plumb. m.; Pop. tr.;* Prun. sp.; *Puls.;* Rham. c.; Rhus t.; *Sabal;* Sars.; *Senec.;* Staph.; *Stigm.; Tereb.;* Vesic.

WEAKNESS—Inability to retain urine, dribbling—Aloe; Ananth.; *Apoc.; Bell.; Benz. ac.;* Brachygl.; Camph., *Can. ind.; Caust.;* Clem.; Con., *Equis.;* Erig.; Euphras.; *Gels.;* Hep.; *Nux v.;* Petrol.; Picr. ac.; Pulex; Puls.; *Rhus ar.;* Santon.; Sabal; *Sars.;* Selen.; Solan. lyc.; *Staph.;* Tereb.; Thymol; Tribul.; Uva; *Verbasc.;* Vesic.; Xerophyl.
  Weakness in old men—Alum.; *Benz. ac.;* Carb. ac.; Clem.; Con.; *Pop. tr.;* Selen.; *Staph.* See Paralysis.

KIDNEYS—Abscess (perinephritic):—Arn.; Bell.; *Hep.;* Merc.; Ver. v.

CALCULI—GRAVEL (nephrolithiasis)—COLIC:—*Arg. n.; Bell.;* Benz. ac.. *Berb. v.;* Buchu; Calc. c.; Calc. ren.; *Canth.;* Cham.; Chin. s.; *Coccus:* Col.; *Diosc.; Epig.;* Erig.; Eryng.; *Eup. purp.;* Hedeoma; Hep.; Hydrang.; Ipomœa; *Lyc.;* Med.; *Nit. ac.; Nux v.; Ocimum;* Oniscus; Op.; Oxyden.; *Pareira; Pichi;* Piperaz.; Polygon.; *Sars.;* Sep.; *Solid.; Stigm.; Tab.;* Thlaspi; Urt.; Uva; Vesic.
  Colic, worse left side—*Berb. v.;* Canth.; Tab.
  Colic, worse right side—*Lyc.;* Nux v.; Ocimum; Sars.
  Inter-paroxysmal treatment—*Berb. v.; Calc. c.;* Chin. s.; Hydrang.; *Lyc..* Nux v.; *Sep.;* Urt.

CONGESTION, acute—*Acon.;* Arg. n.; Arn.; Aur.; *Bell.;* Benz. ac.; *Berb v.;* Bry.; Camph.; *Canth.;* Dig.; *Dulc.;* Eucal.; Eryng. aq.; *Helleb.; Helon.;* Hydroc. ac.; *Junip.;* Kali bich.; Merc. c.; *Ol. sant.;* Op.; Rhus t.; Senec.; Solid.; *Tereb.;* Ver. v. See Nephritis.
  Congestion, chronic (passive, from heart or kidney disease)—Acon.; Arn.; Bell.; *Caffeine; Conv.; Dig.;* Glon.; Phos.; *Stroph.;* Strych.; Ver. v. See Heart.

DEGENERATION, acute, amyloid, fatty—Apis; *Ars.; Aur. mur.;* Bell.;

URINARY SYSTEM

Cic.; *Cupr. ac.*; Ferr. mur.; Hydroc. ac.; *Kali iod.*; Lyc.; *Nit. ac.*; Phos. ac.; *Phos.*; Rhus t.; Tereb. See Nephritis.

FLOATING KIDNEY (nephroptosis) reflex symptoms:—*Bell.*; Cham.; Col.; Gels.; *Ign.*; Lach.; Puls.; *Strych. ars.*; Sul.; Zinc.

INFLAMMATION (nephritis)—Bright's disease:

ACUTE AND SUBACUTE PARENCHYMATOUS NEPHRITIS—Acon.; Ant. t.; *Apis*; Apoc.; Ars.; *Aur. mur.*; Bell.; Berb. v.; *Can. s.*; *Canth.*; Chel.; Chimaph.; *Chin. s.*; Colch.; Conv.; *Cupr. ars.*; Dig.; Dulc.; Eucal.; Eup. perf.; Ferr. iod.; Fuschina; Glon.; *Helleb.*; Helon.; Hep.; Hydrocot.; Irid.; Junip.; Kali bich.; *Kali chlor.*; Kali citr.; Kal.; Koch's lymph; Lach.; Merc. s.; Methyl. bl.; Nit. ac;; *Ol. Sant.*; Phos. ac.; *Phos.*; Pichi; Picr. ac.; Plumb. ac.; Ploygon.; Rhus t.; *Sab.*; *Samb.*; Scilla; Sec.; Senec.; Serum ang.; *Tereb.*; Ver. a.; Ver. v.; Zing.

CAUSE—From cold, or wet exposure—Acon.; Ant. t.; Apis; Canth.; *Dulc.*; Rhus t.; Tereb.

From influenza—Eucal.

From malaria—*Ars.*; Eup. perf.; Tereb.

From pregnancy—Apis; Apoc.; *Cupr. ars.*; Helon.; Kal.; Merc. c.; Sab. See Female Sexual System.

From scarlet fever, diphtheria—Acon.; *Apis*; Ars.; Bell.; *Canth.*; Conv.; Cop.; Dig.; Ferr. iod.; *Helleb.*; Hep.; Kal.; Lach.; Merc. c.; Methyl. bl.; Nat. s.; Nit. sp. d.; *Rhus t.*; Sec.; Tereb.

From suppurations—Apoc.; Chin. s.; Hep.; Phos.; Plumb. c.; Sil.; Tereb.

CONCOMITANTS—Dropsy:—Acon.; Adon. v.; Ant. t.; *Apis; Apoc.*; Ars.; Aur. mur.; Canth.; Colch.; Cop.; *Dig.*; *Helleb.*; Merc. c.; Piloc.; Samb.; Scilla; Senec.; Tereb. See Dropsy (Generalities).

Heart failure—Adon. v.; Ars.; *Caffeine*; *Dig.*; Glon.; Spart.; Stroph.; Ver. v.

Pneumonia—Chel.; Phos.

Uraemic symptoms—Æth.; Am. c.; Ars.; Bell.; Can. ind.; *Carb. ac.*; Cic.; *Cupr. ars.*; Helleb.; Hyos.; Morph.; Op.; Piloc.; Stram.; Urea.

ACUTE, SUPPURATIVE NEPHRITIS—Acon.; Arn.; Bell.; Camph.; Calc. s.; *Can. s.*; Canth.; *Chin. s.*; Eucal.; Hekla; Hep.; Kali n.; Merc. c.; Naph.; Sil.; Ver. v.

CHRONIC, INTERSTITIAL NEPHRITIS—Apis; *Ars.*; *Aur. mur.*; Aur. m. n.; Cact.; *Chin. s.*; Colch.; Conv.; *Dig.*; Ferr. m.; *Ferr. mur.*; *Glon.*; Iod.; Kali c.; *Kali iod.*; Koch's lymph; Lith. ac.; Lith. benz.; Lith. c.; Merc. d.; *Nat. iod.*; *Nit ac.*; Nux v.; Op.; Phos. ac.; Phos.; Plumb. c.; *Plumb. iod.*; *Plumb. m.*; Sang.; Zinc. picr. See Arteriosclerosis (Circulatory System).

CHRONIC, PARENCHYMATOUS NEPHRITIS—Am. benz.; *Apis*; *Ars.*; Aur. mur.; Aur. m. n.; Benz. ac.; Berb v.; *Brachygl.*; Calc. ars.; Calc. p.; Can. ind.; *Canth.*; Chin. ars; Conv.; Dig.; Eup. purp.; *Euonym.*; Ferr. ars.; Ferr. cit.; *Ferr. mur.*; Ferr. p.; Form. ac.; Glon.; *Helon.*; Hydroc. ac.; Junip.; Kali ars.; *Kali chlor.*; Kali cit.; *Kali iod.*; *Kali m.*; Kal.; Koch's lymph; Lonic.; *Lyc.*; *Merc. c.*; Nat. chlor.; *Nit. ac.*; Piloc.; Plumb.; Senec.; Solania; *Solid.*; Spart.; Tereb.; Urea; Vesic.

SYMPTOMS—URAEMIA: In general:—*Am. c.;* Apis; Apoc.; Ars.; Asclep. c.; *Bell.;* Can. ind.; *Canth.;* Carb. ac.; Cic.; Cupr. ac.; *Cupr. ars.;* Glon.; Helleb.; Hydroc. ac.; Hyos.; Kali br.; *Morph.;* Op.; Phos.; Picr. ac.; Piloc.; Quebracho; Serum ang.; Stram.; *Tereb.;* Urea; Urt.; Ver. v.

Coma—*Am. c.;* Bell.; Bry.; *Carb. ac.;* Cupr. ars.; *Helleb.;* Merc. c.; *Morph.;* Op.; Ver. v.

Convulsions—Bell.; Carb. ac.; Chloral.; *Cic.;* Cupr. ac.; *Cupr. ars.;* Glon.; *Hydroc. ac.;* Kali br.; Merc. c.; Op.; Piloc.; Plumb.; Ver. v. See Convulsions (Nervous System).

Headache—Arn.; Can. ind.; Carb. ac.; Cupr. ars.; *Glon.;* Hyper.; Sang.; Zinc. picr. See Head.

Vomiting—*Ars.;* Iod.; Kreos.; Nux v. See Stomach.

PAIN IN RENAL REGION—Burning:—*Acon.;* Ars.; Aur.; Berb. v.; But. ac.; *Canth.;* Hedeoma; *Helon.;* Kali iod.; Lach.; *Lyc.;* Merc. c.; *Phos.;* Sab.; *Sul.;* Tereb. See Back.

Cutting, digging, boring—Arn.; *Berb. v.; Canth.;* Eup. purp.; Ipec.; *Lyc.;* Rhus t.; Tereb.

Drawing, tensive—*Berb. v.;* Can. s.; *Canth.;* Chel.; Coccus; *Colch.;* Dulc.; Lach.; *Lyc.;* Nit. ac.; Solid.; *Tereb.*

Neuralgic, radiating (nephralgia), tearing, lancinating—*Arg. n.;* Arn.; *Bell.; Berb. v.;* Calc. c.; *Canth.;* Chel.; Chin. s.; *Coccinel; Coccus; Diosc.;* Eryng. aq.; Ferr. mur.; *Hedeoma; Hydrang.;* Lach.; *Lyc.;* Kali iod.; Nit. ac.; *Nux v.; Ocimum;* Oxytr.; Pareira; Phos.; Sab.; *Sars.;* Scrophul.; *Solid.; Tab.;* Tereb.; Thlaspi; Vespa. See Nephrolithiasis.

Pressing—Arg. n.; *Arn.;* Aur. mur.; *Berb. v.; Canth.;* Chin. s.; *Lyc.;* Nit. ac.; *Ocimum;* Petrol.; *Phos. ac.; Sep.; Tereb.;* Uva; Xerophyl.

Stitching—Berb. v.; *Canth.;* Colch.; *Kali c.;* Pareira.

Throbbing—Act. sp.; *Berb. v.;* Chimaph.; Med.; Sab.

Weariness, aching, lameness—*Acon.;* Alum.; Am. br.; Apis; *Arg. n.; Benz. ac.; Berb. v.;* Can. ind.; *Canth.;* Chel.; Cina; Conv.; Cop.; *Eup. purp.; Hedeoma; Helon.;* Hydrang.; Junip.; Kali bich.; Lyc.; Nat. chlor.; *Nux v.; Ol. sant.; Phyt.; Pier. ac.;* Pin. sylv.; *Sab.; Sep.;* Solid.; Stellar.; Tereb.; Ustil.; *Uva;* Vespa. See Back.

MODALITIES—AGGRAVATIONS: At 2 P. M.: Kal.

From lifting, sudden effort—Calc. p.

From lying down—Conv.

From motion—*Berb. v.; Canth.;* Chel.; Kali iod.

From pressure—*Berb. v.;* Canth.; Colch.; *Solid.*

From sitting—*Berb. v.;* Ferr. mur.

From stooping, lying down—Berb. v.

From stretching legs—Colch.

From wine—Benz. ac.

On left side—Æsc.; Berb. v.; *Hedeoma;* Hydrang.; Tab.; Uva.

On right side—Am. benz.; Can. ind.; *Chel.;* Equis.; Lith. c.; *Lyc.;* Ocimum; Phyt.; Picr. ac.; *Sars.;* Tereb.

AMELIORATIONS—From lying on back: Cahinca.

From lying on back, legs drawn up—Colch.

URINARY SYSTEM

From standing—Berb. v.
From urination—Lyc.; Med.
From walking—Ferr. mur.

PERI-NEPHRITIS—Acon.; Bry.; Chin. s.; Hep.; Merc.; Sil.

PYELITIS—Inflammation of pelvis: Acute: Acon.; *Ars.*; Aur.; *Bell.*; *Benz. ac.*; Berb. v.; Bry.; *Can. s.*; *Canth.*; Cinch.; *Cop.*; *Cupr. ars.*; Epig.; *Ferr. mur.*; Hekla; Hep.; Kali bich.; *Merc. c.*; Nit. ac.; *Puls.*; *Rhus t.*; Stigm.; *Tereb.*; Thuya; *Tritic.*; *Uva*; *Ver. v.*
Calculous—Hep.; *Hydrang.*; Lyc.; *Piparaz.*; Sil.; Uva. See Nephrolithiasis.
Chronic—Ars.; *Benz. ac.*; Berb. v.; *Buchu*; *Chimaph.*; Chin. s.; Cinch.; *Cop.*; Hep.; Hydrast. mur.; Hydrast. s.; *Junip.*; *Kali bich.*; *Ol. sant.*; Pareira; Puls.; Sep.; Sil.; Sul.; Stigm.; *Uva.*

SENSITIVENESS, tenderness—*Acon.*; Apis; *Berb. v.*; Calc. ars.; Can. s.; *Canth.*; Equis.; *Helon.*; Phyt.; *Solid.*; *Tereb.* See Pain.

SYPHILIS—Aur.; Kali iod.; Merc. c. See Male Sexual System.
Traumatisms—Acon.; *Arn.*; Bell.; Ver. v.

TUBERCULOSIS—*Ars. iod.*; Bac.; Calc. c.; Calc. hypoph.; *Calc. iod.*; *Chin. ars.*; Chin. s.; Hekla; Kali iod.; Kreos. See Tuberculosis (Respiratory System).

URETHRA—Burning, smarting, heat—*Acon.*; Apis; *Arg. n.*; *Berb. v.*; Cahinca; Calc. c.; *Can. ind.*; *Can. s.*; *Canth.*; *Caps.*; Chimaph.; *Clem.*; Con.; Cop.; Dig.; Gels.; *Hydrang.*; *Merc. c.*; *Merc.*; Mez.; Nat. c.; Nit. mur. ac.; Oniscus; Petrol.; *Petros.*; Phos.; Selen.; Staph.; *Sul.*; *Tereb.*; *Thuya*; *Uran.*; Zing.
Burning between acts of urination—Berb. v.; Can. s.; Staph.
Caruncle—Can. s.; *Eucal.*; Teucr.; *Thuya.*
Discharge, mucous—Hep.; Merc. c.; Nat. m.
Hæmorrhage—Calc. c.; Lyc.
Inflammation (urethritis)—*Acon.*; Apis; *Arg. n.*; Camph.; *Can. s.*; *Canth.*; Caps.; Caust.; *Cop.*; *Cub.*; *Doryph.*; *Gels.*; Kali bich.; Kali iod.; Merc. c.; Nux v.; Petrol.; Sab.; Sul.; *Thuya*; Yohimb. See Male Sexual System.
Itching—Acon.; Alum.; Ambra; *Arg. n.*; Canth.; Caust.; Col.; *Ferr. iod.*; Ferr. m.; Gins.; Lyc.; *Merc.*; Mez.; *Nit. ac.*; Ol. an.; Pareira; Petrol.; *Petros.*; Staph.; *Sul.*; Thuya; Tussil.

MEATUS—Burning: Acon.; Ambra; Bor.; Can. s.; *Canth.*; *Caps.*; Clem.; Gels.; Menthol; *Petros.*; Selen.; *Sul.*; Zing.
Eruptions around—Caps.
Itching—Alum.; *Ambra*; Caust.; Col.; Gins.; *Petros.*
Ulcers around—Eucal.
Swelling—Acon.; Arg. n.; *Can. s.*; *Canth.*; Cop.; Gels.; *Merc.*; *Ol. sant.*; Sul. See Urethritis.
Membranous-prostatic involvement—Sabal.

PAIN IN URETHRA—Constricting: *Arg. n.*; *Can. s.*; Caps.; *Clem.*; Ferr. iod.; Ol. sant.; *Petros.*
Cutting—Alum.; Ant. c.; *Berb. v.*; *Canth.*; Nat. m.; Oniscus; *Petros.*

Soreness, tenderness irritation—Agn.; Anag.; *Arg. n.*; *Berb. v.*; Brachygl.; *Can. s.*; *Canth.*; Caust.; Clem.; *Cop.*; Cub.; Ferr. picr.; Gels.; Kali iod.; Tussil.

Stitching, stinging—Agar.; *Apis*; *Arg. n.*; Aspar.; *Berb. v.*; Can. ind.; *Can. s.*; Caps.; Carbo v.; *Clem.*; Merc. c.; Merc.; Nit. ac.; Petros.; *Thuya*.

SENSIBILITY—Diminished—Kali br.

STRICTURE, organic—Acon.; Arg. n.; Arn.; Calc. iod.; *Canth.*; *Clem.*; Eucal.; Lob. infl.; Phos.; Puls.; *Sil.*; *Sul. iod*.

Stricture, spasmodic—*Acon.*; Bell.; *Camph.*; Canth.; Eryng.; Hydrang.; Nux v.; Petros.

URINARY FLOW—DESIRE—Constant desire: Absinth.; *Acon.*; Ananth.; *Bell.*; Berb. v.; Cact.; *Can. s.*; *Canth.*; Carbo v.; Caust.; Ceanoth.; Coccus; *Cop.*; Dig.; Dulc.; Equis.; *Eup. purp.*; *Ferr. mur.*; Gels.; Guaiac.; Kreos.; *Lil. t.*; Lyssin; *Murex*; Op.; *Pareira*; Ruta; *Sabal*; Senec.; Sep.; *Staph.*; Sulphon.; *Sul.*; *Thuya*; *Tritic.*; Zing. See Cystitis.

Constant after labor—Op.; *Staph*.

Constant at night—Dig.; *Sabal*.

Constant from prolapsus uteri—Lil. t.

Constant, on seeing running water—Canth.; Lyssin; Sul.

DIABETES INSIPIDUS—Copious, profuse; polyuria; diuresis: *Acet. ac.*; Acon.; *Alfal.*; Am. acet.; Apoc.; *Arg. m.*; Arg. mur.; Ars.; *Aur. mur.*; *Bell.*; Bry.; Cahinca; *Can. ind.*; Caust.; Cepa; Chin. s.; Chionanth.; Cina; *Cod.*; Conv.; Dulc.; Equis.; *Eup. purp.*; *Ferr. mur.*; Ferr. n.; Gels.; Glycerin; *Glon.*; Gnaph.; Guaco; *Helleb.*; *Helon.*; *Ign.*; Indol; Kali c.; Kali iod.; *Kali n.*; *Kreos.*; Lact. ac.; Led.; *Lil. t.*; Lith. c.; *Lyc.*; Mag. p.; Merc. c.; Mosch.; *Murex*; *Nat. m.*; Niccol. s.; *Nit. ac.*; Nux v.; *Ol. an.*; Oxytr.; *Phos. ac.*; Phos.; Physal.; Picr. ac.; Plat. m. n.; Puls.; Quass.; *Rhus ar.*; *Samb.*; Sang.; Santon.; Sars.; *Scilla*; *Sinap. n.*; Spart.; Staph.; *Stroph.*; *Sul.*; Tarax.; Tereb.; Thymol; *Thyr.*; *Uran.*; Verbasc.; Ver. v. See Diabetes.

Copious at night—Ambra; Kali iod.; *Lyc.*; *Murex*; Petrol.; *Phos. ac.*; Quass.; *Scilla*.

DYSURIA—Difficult, slow, painful: *Acon.*; *Alum.*; Ant. t.; *Apis*; Apoc.; *Arg. n.*; Arn.; *Ars.*; *Bell.*; *Benz. ac.*; Camph.; *Can. ind.*; *Can. s.*; *Canth.*; Caps.; Cascara; *Caust.*; Chimaph.; *Clem.*; Coccus; *Con.*; Cop.; Cucurb. cit.; Dig.; Dulc.; *Epig.*; Equis.; *Eup. purp.*; *Fabiana*; Ferr. p.; *Hep.*; Hydrang.; Hyper.; Hyos.; Kreos.; Lith. c.; *Lyc.*; Med.; Merc. c.; *Morph.*; Mur. ac.; *Nat. m.*; Nit. ac.; Nux v.; Ocimum; *Ol. sant.*; Op.; *Pareira*; Petros.; Pichi; *Plumb.*; Pop. tr.; Puls.; Rhus t.; Ruta; *Sabal*; *Santon.*; *Sars.*; Selen.; *Sep.*; *Solid.*; Staph.; Stigm.; Taxus; Thlaspi; *Tritic.*; *Uva*; Verbasc.; Vib. op.; Zinc. See Scanty.

Difficult, in pregnancy, and afer confinement—Equis.

Difficult, in presence of others—Ambra; Hep.; Mur. ac.; *Nat. m.*

Difficult, in young, married women—Staph

Difficult, must lie down—Kreos.

Difficult, must sit bent backwards—Zinc.

URINARY SYSTEM

Difficult, must stand with feet wide apart, body inclined forward—Chimaph.
Difficult, must strain—Acon.; Alum.; Can. ind.; Chimaph.; Equis.; Hyos.; Kali c.; Kreos.; Lyc.; Mag. m.; Nux v.; Op.; Papaya; Pareira; Prun. s.; Sabal; Zinc. See Bladder.
Difficult, with prolapsus ani—Mur. ac.
Difficult, with prostatic or uterine diseases—Con.; Staph.
Divided stream—Anag.; Arg. n.; Can. s.; Canth.
Feeble stream—Cham.; Clem.; Helleb.; Hep.; Merc.; Sars.

FREQUENT desire—Acon.; Agar.; Agn.; Alfal.; Aloe; Alum.; Ant. c.; Apis; Arg. n.; Aspar.; Aur. mur.; Bar. c.; Bell.; Benz. ac.; Berb. v.; Bor. ac.; Calc. ars.; Calc. c.; Can. s.; Canth.; Caps.; Carls.; Caust.; Chimaph.; Clem.; Coccus; Colch.; Col.; Conv.; Cub.; Dig.; Equis.; Ferr. p.; Fer. picr.; Formica; Gels.; Glycerin; Helleb.; Helon.; Hydrang.; Ign.; Indol; Jatropha; Kali c.; Kal.; Kreos.; Lact. ac.; Lil. t.; Lith. benz.; Lith. c.; Lyc.; Merc. c.; Merc. v.; Nat. c.; Nit. ac.; Nux v.; Ocimum; Ol. sant.; Ox. ac.; Phos. ac.; Piloc.; Plumb.; Prun. sp.; Pulex; Puls.; Sabal; Sab.; Samb.; Santon.; Sars.; Scilla; Sec.; Sep.; Sil.; Staph.; Sul.; Tritic.; Uva; Vespa; Zing.
Frequent desire at night—Alum.; Aur. mur.; Bor.; Calc. c.; Carb. ac.; Caust.; Coccus; Con.; Ferr.; Ferr. picr.; Glycerin; Graph.; Kali c.; Kreos.; Murex; Nat. m.; Phos. ac.; Physal.; Picr. ac.; Puls.; Sang.; Sars.; Scilla; Sep.; Solan. lyc.; Sul.; Tereb.; Thuya; Xerophyl.
Imperative, irresistible, sudden desire—Acon.; Agar.; Aloe; Apis; Arg. n.; Bor.; Can. s.; Canth.; Carls.; Equis.; Hedeoma; Ign.; Kreos.; Lathyr.; Merc. c.; Merc.; Murex; Naph.; Ol. an.; Pareira; Petros.; Pop. tr.; Prun. sp.; Puls.; Quass.; Ruta; Santon.; Scutel.; Sul.; Thuya.
Intermittent, interrupted flow—Agar.; Can. ind.; Caps.; Clem.; Con.; Gels.; Hep.; Mag. s.; Pulex; Puls.; Sabal; Sars.; Sedum; Thuya; Zinc. m.

INVOLUNTARY—Alum.; Arg. n.; Arn.; Ars.; Bell.; Calc. c.; Caust.; Cina; Dulc.; Echin.; Equis.; Ferr. m.; Gels.; Hyos.; Kali br.; Kreos.; Op.; Petrol.; Puls.; Rhus ar.; Rhus t.; Ruta; Sabal; Saponin; Sars.; Selen.; Senega; Sil.; Solan. lyc.; Sul.; Uva; Xerophyl. See Bladder.
Involuntary, at night—Ars.; Bell.; Calc. c.; Caust.; Cina; Kali br.; Kreos.; Plant.; Puls.; Rhus t.; Senega; Sep.; Sil.; Sul.; Uva. See Enuresis.
Involuntary, during first sleep—Kreos.; Sep.
Involuntary, when coughing, sneezing, walking, laughing—Bell.; Calc. c.; Canth.; Caps.; Caust.; Ferr. m.; Ferr. mur.; Ferr. p.; Ign.; Kali c.; Nat. m.; Puls.; Scilla; Selen.; Sul.; Vib. op.; Xerophyl.; Zinc.
Involuntary, when dreaming of act—Equis.; Kreos.
Involuntary, without consciousness of—Apoc.; Arg. n.; Caust.; Sars.

RETENTION (ischuria)—Acon.; Apis; Apium gr.; Arn.; Ars.; Bell.; Camph.; Can. ind.; Can. s.; Canth.; Caust.; Chimaph.; Cic.; Cop.; Dulc.; Equis.; Eup. purp.; Hyos.; Ign.; Lyc.; Merc. c.; Morph.; Nux v.; Op.; Plumb. m.; Puls.; Rhus t.; Sars.; Stigm.; Strych.; Sul.; Tereb.; Zinc. m.
From atony of fundus—Tereb.
From cold or wet exposure—Acon.; Dulc.; Gels.; Rhus t.
From fever, acute illness—Ferr. p.; Op.

From fright—*Acon.;* Op.
From hysteria—Ign.; Zinc.
From inflammation—*Acon.;* Can. ind.; *Canth.;* Nux v.; Puls.
From overexertion—Arn.
From paralysis—*Caust.;* Dulc.; Hyos.; Nux v.; *Op.; Plumb. m.;* Strych.
From post partum—Hyos.; Op.
From prostatic hypertrophy—Chimaph.; Dig.; Morph.; Zinc. See Male Sexual System.
From spasmodic constriction of neck of bladder—*Bell.;* Cact.; Camph.; Canth.; *Hyos.;* Lyc.; *Nux v.;* Op.; Puls.; Rhus t.; Stram.; Thlaspi.
From suppressed discharges or eruptions—Camph.
From surgical operations—Caust.

SCANTY FLOW—*Acon.;* Adon. v.; *Alfal.;* Apis; Apoc.; *Arg. n.;* Ars.; Aur. mur.; *Bell.; Benz. ac.; Berb. v.;* Bry.; Camph.; Can. s.; *Canth.;* Carb. ac.; Carbo v.; *Chimaph.;* Clem.; *Colch.;* Col.; Conv.; Cupr. ars.; *Dig.;* Dulc.; Equis.; Eup. purp.; Fluor. ac.; Graph.; *Helleb.; Junip.;* Kali bich.; Kali chlor.; Kali iod.; Kreos.; Lach.; Lecith.; Lil. t.; Lith. c.; Lyc.; Lyssin; Menthol; *Merc. c.;* Merc. cy.; *Nit. ac.; Nux v.;* Op.; Phos.; Picr. ac.; *Piloc.; Plumb.;* Prun. sp.; Pulex; Puls.; Ruta; *Sab.; Sars.; Scilla;* Selen.; Senec.; Senega; Sep.; Serum ang.; *Solid.; Stroph.;* Sul.; Sul. ac.; Sulphon.; *Tereb.; Uva;* Zing.

Scanty, drop by drop—*Acon.;* Æsc.; *Apis;* Arn.; *Bell.;* Bor.; *Canth.;* Caps.; Caust.; Clem.; Colch.; *Cop.;* Dig.; Equis.; Inula; *Lyc.; Merc. c.;* Merc.; Nux v.; Plumb.; *Puls.;* Rhus t.; *Sabal;* Staph.; Sul.

STRANGURY—*Acon.;* Ant. t.; *Apis;* Apoc.; *Ars.; Bell.; Camph.;* Can. s.; *Canth.; Caps.;* Col.; Con.; *Cop.;* Dulc.; Eryng.; *Eup. purp.;* Hydrang.; Juncus; Junip.; Junip. v.; Lyc.; *Merc. c.;* Morph.; Nux m.; *Nux v.; Pareira; Petros;* Prun. sp.; Puls.; Sab.; Sars.; Senna; Stigm.; *Tereb.;* Thlaspi; *Tritic.; Urt.;* Verbasc.; Zing.

In children—Bor.; Lyc.; Sars.
In females—Apis; Caps.; *Cop.;* Dig.; Eup. purp.; Lil. t.; *Sab.;* Staph.; Ver. v.; Vib. op.
Nervous type—Apis; Bell.; Caps.; *Eryng.;* Morph.; Petros.

SUPPRESSION (anuria)—*Acon.;* Agar. ph.; Alfal.; *Apis;* Apoc.; *Ars.;* Ars. hyd.; *Bell.;* Bry.; Camph.; Canth.; Coff.; Colch.; Cupr. ac.; *Dig.;* Formal.; *Helleb.;* Junip.; Kali bich.; Kali chlor.; Lyc.; *Merc. c.;* Merc. cy.; Nit. ac.; Op.; *Oxyden.;* Petrol.; Phyt.; Picr. ac.; Puls.; Sec.; *Solid.;* Stigm.; Stram.; *Tereb.;* Ver. a.; Zing.

URINATION—COMPLAINTS BEFORE ACT: Anxiety, agony: Acon.; Bor.; *Canth.;* Phos. ac.

Burning—Ars.; *Berb. v.;* Camph.; *Can. s.; Canth.;* Cochlear.; Cop. See Urethra.
Leucorrhœa, yellow—Kreos.
Pain—*Acon.; Berb. v.;* Bor.; *Canth.;* Can. s.; Erig.; Kali c.; Lith. c.; Lyc.; Piloc.; Rhus ar.; Sanic.; Sars.; Senega; Sep. See Pain (bladder, kidneys, urethra).

COMPLAINTS DURING ACT—Burning, smarting: *Acon.;* Ambra; Anac.; Anag.; *Apis;* Apoc.; *Arg. n.;* Ars.; *Berb. v.;* Bor. ac.; *Bor.;* Camph.;

URINARY SYSTEM

Can. ind.; *Can. s.*; *Canth.*; Caps.; Carbo v.; Cepa; Chimaph.; *Cop.*; Cub.; Dig.; Epig.; *Equis.*; Erig.; Eryng. aq.; *Eup. purp.*; Gels.; Glycerin; Helleb.; *Kreos.*; *Lyc.*; *Merc. c.*; Merc. s.; Nit. ac.; Nux v.; Ocimum; *Ol. sant.*; Ox. ac.; *Pareira*; Phos.; Puls.; Rhus ar.; *Sep.*; Staph.; *Sul.*; *Tereb.*; Thuya; Uva; Verbasc.; *Vespa.*

Chill—*Acon.*; Sars.; Sep.

Meatus, agglutination—Anag.; Can. s.

Meatus, burning (also prepuce)—Calad.; Calc. c.; *Can. s.*; Gels.; Menthol; *Merc. c.*; Puls.

Meatus, itching—Ambra; Cop.; Lyc.; Nux v.

PAINS IN GENERAL—*Acon.*; Apis; *Arg. n.*; Berb. aq.; *Berb. v.*; Blatta am.; Bor. ac.; Camph.; *Can. s.*; *Canth.*; *Caps.*; *Chimaph.*; *Col.*; Dig.; Doryph.; *Equis.*; Erig.; Graph.; Hedeoma; *Lith. c.*; *Lyc.*; Merc.; Nit. ac.; *Nux v.*; *Pareira*; *Petrol.*; Phos.; Puls.; *Rhus ar.*; Sabal; *Sars.*; Sep.

Cutting, stinging, stitching—*Acon.*; Ant. c.; Apis; Berb. aq.; *Berb. v.*; Bor.; Camph.; *Can. s.*; *Canth.*; Cochlear.; Col.; Con.; Hydrang.; Nux v.; *Pareira*; Puls.

Drawing, radiating to labia—Eupion.

Drawing, radiating to chest and shoulders—Glycerin.

Drawing, radiating to perineum—Lyc.; Sep.

Drawing, radiating to sacrum, coccyx—Graph.

Drawing, radiating to testicles—*Berb. v.*; Cahinca; Erig.

Drawing, radiating to thighs—Berb. v.; Pareira.

Pressive—Camph.; Cop.; Lyc.; *Sep.*

Pressive in heart—Lith. c.

Spasmodic, toward end of act—*Arg. n.*; Bor. ac.; Puls.

Stool, involuntary—Sul.

Sweating—Merc. c.

COMPLAINTS AFTER ACT—Burning, smarting: *Acon.*; Anac.; Apis; *Arg. n.*; Bell.; *Berb. v.*; Camph.; *Can. s.*; *Canth.*; *Caps.*; Chimaph.; Cochlear.; Cub.; *Kreos.*; Lyc.; Mag. s.; *Merc. c.*; Nat. c.; *Nat. m.*; Phos. ac.; *Pichi*; Puls.; Rhus t.; Senega; Staph.; *Sul.*; *Thuya*; Uva.

Dribbling—*Arg. n.*; Benz. ac.; Calc. c.; Camph.; Can. ind.; Caust.; *Clem.*; Con.; Lyc.; *Pareira*; *Selen.*; Thuya; Zing. See Bladder.

Emission, seminal—Calad.; Hep.; Phos. ac.

Exhaustion—Ars.; Berb. v.

Hæmorrhoids—Bar. c.

Meatus, and urethra, tingling—Clem.; Thuya.

Meatus, burning—Caps.; Puls.

PAINS—Aching, bruised: *Berb. v.*; Equis.; Sul.

Cutting, tearing, stitching—*Berb. v.*; Bov.; Camph.; *Can. s.*; *Canth.*; *Caps.*; Cochlear.; *Cub.*; Guaiac.; Mag. s.; Merc. acet.; *Nat. m.*; Nux v.; Petros.; Prun. sp.; *Sars.*; *Thuya*; Uva.

Pressive, in perineum—Am. m.; Lyc.

Sensation as if urine remained behind—Alum.; *Berb. v.*; Dig.; Eup. purp.; Eryng. aq.; Gels.; *Hep.*; *Kali bich.*; Ruta; Sec.; Sil.; Staph.; *Thuya.*

Severe, at close, and after act—Apis; *Berb. v.*; *Canth.*; Echin.; *Equis.*;

816 URINARY SYSTEM

Lith. c.; Med.; Merc. acet.; *Nat. m.*; Petros.; Puls.; Ruta; *Sars.*; Staph.; *Thuya.*

Spasmodic—*Nat. m.*; Nux v.; Puls.

Perspiration—Merc. c.

Tenesmus, urging, straining—Arg. n.; *Camph.*; *Canth.*; Chimaph.; Epig.; *Equis.*; Eryng. aq.; Lith. c.; Nit. ac.; Pichi; *Pop. tr.*; *Puls.*; Ruta; Sabal; Sars.; *Staph.*; Stigm.; Sul.

URINE—TYPE: Acid: Acon.; *Benz. ac.*; Canth.; Chin. s.; Euonym.; Lith. c.; *Lyc.*; *Merc. c.*; Mur. ac.; *Nit. ac.*; Nit. mur. ac.; Nux v.; Ocimum; Puls.; Sars.; Sep.; *Sul.*; *Uva.* See Burning.

ALBUMINURIA—Albuminous: Acetan.; Adon. v.; *Am. benz.*; Ant. t.; *Apis*; Ars.; Aur. mur.; Bell.; Berb. v.; Calc. ars.; Can. s.; *Canth.*; Carb. ac.; Chin. s.; *Colch.*; Conv.; Cop.; Cupr. ac.; Cupr. ars.; *Dig.*; Equis.; Euonym.; *Eup. purp.*; Ferr. ars.; *Ferr. mur.*; Ferr. picr.; Formica; Fuschina; Glon.; *Helleb.*; Helon.; Kali chlor.; *Kal.*; Lach.; Lecith.; Lith. c.; *Lyc.*; *Merc. c.*; Merc. cy.; Methyl. bl.; Mur. ac.; Nit. ac.; Ocimum; Ol. sant.; *Osm.*; Phos. ac.; *Phos.*; *Plumb. c.*; Plumb. m.; Radium; Sab.; Scilla; *Sec.*; Sil.; *Solid.*; Stroph.; *Tereb.*; Thyr.; Uran. n.; Viscum a.

Alkaline—Am. c.; Benz. ac.; *Kali acet.*; Mag. p.; Med.; *Phos. ac.* See Nephritis.

BLOOD (hæmaturia)—*Acon.*; Ant. t.; Apis; *Arn.*; Ars.; Ars. hydrog.; Bell.; Berb. v.; Cact.; Camph.; *Can. s.*; *Canth.*; *Carb. ac.*; Chin. s.; Cina; Cinch.; *Coccus*; Colch.; *Cop.*; *Crot.*; Dulc.; Epig.; Equis.; Erig.; Eucal.; Ferr. p.; Ficcus; Gall. ac.; Geran.; *Ham.*; Hep.; *Ipec.*; Kali chlor.; Kreos.; *Lach.*; *Lyc.*; Mangif. ind.; Merc. c.; Merc.; *Millef.*; *Nit. ac.*; *Nux v.*; Ocimum; Ol. sant.; *Pareira*; *Phos.*; Pichi; Picr. ac.; Plumb.; *Rhus ar.*; Sab.; Santon.; *Sars.*; Scilla; Sec.; *Senec.*; *Solid.*; Stigm.; *Tereb.*; *Thlaspi*; *Uva.*

Burning, scalding, hot—*Acon.*; Apis; Bell.; Benz. ac.; *Bor.*; Camph.; *Can. s.*; *Canth.*; Coccus; Conv.; Hep.; Kali bich.; *Kal.*; *Lyc.*; Merc. c.; Nit. ac.; Phos.; Pichi; Pop. tr.; Sars.; *Sul.* See Acid.

Cold feeling—Nit. ac.

Heavy feeling—Thlaspi.

Oily pellicle—Adon. v.; *Crot. t.*; Hep.; Lyc.; *Iod.*; Petrol.; Phos.; Sumbul.

Viscid, gluey—*Col.*; Pareira; *Phos. ac.* See Deposit.

COLOR—APPEARANCE—Black, inky: *Apis*; Arn.; *Benz. din.*; *Benz. ac.*; Canth.; Carb. ac.; Colch.; Dig.; *Helleb.*; Kreos.; Lach.; Merc. c.; Naph.; Nit. ac.; Pareira; *Tereb.*

Brown, dark—*Apis*; Apoc.; Arg. n.; Arn.; Ars.; *Bell.*; *Benz. ac.*; *Bry.*; Canth.; Carb. ac.; Carbo v.; *Chel.*; Chin. s.; Coccus; *Colch.*; Crot.; *Dig.*; Fluor. ac.; Helleb.; Kali c.; Kali chlor.; Lach.; *Lyc.*; Merc. c.; Myr.; Nat. c.; Nat. chlor.; *Nit. ac.*; *Nux v.*; Phos. ac.; Phos.; Phyt.; Picr. ac.; Plumb.; Prun. sp.; *Rhus t.*; *Sep.*; Solid.; Staph.; Sulphon.; *Tereb.*

Cloudy, turbid—*Ambra*; Am. c.; Apoc.; *Arg. m.*; Ars.; *Aur. mur.*; Bell.; Benz. ac.; Berb. v.; Camph.; *Can. s.*; *Canth.*; Card. m.; Caust.; Chel.;

URINARY SYSTEM

Chimaph.; Chin. s.; Cina; Colch.; Col.; Con.; *Cop.;* Crot. t.; Daphne; *Dig.;* Dulc.; Graph.; Helleb.; Helon.; *Hep.;* Kali c.; Kreos.; Lith. c.; *Lyc.;* Lyssin; Nit. ac.; Nit. mur. ac.; *Ocimum;* Petrol.; *Phos. ac.; Phos.; Plumb.; Puls.;* Raph.; Rhus t.; *Sars.; Sep.;* Solid.; Sul.; *Tereb.;* Thuya; Zing.

Deep—*Bell.;* Calc. c.; Dig.; Helleb.; Lach.; *Lyc.;* Merc.; Nit. ac.; *Sep.*

Frothy—Apis; *Berb. v.;* Cop.; Crot. t.; Cub.; *Lach.;* Myr.; Raph.; Sars.

Greenish—Ars.; *Berb. v.;* Camph.; Can. ind.; *Carb. ac.; Ceanoth.;* Chimaph.; Cop.; Laburn.; Mag. s.; Ol. an.; Ruta; *Santon.;* Uva.

Milky—Chel.; *Cina;* Col.; Con.; Dulc.; Eup. purp.; Iod.; Lil. t.; Merc.; *Phos. ac.;* Phos.; Raph.; Still.; Uva; *Viola od.*

Pale, clear, limpid—*Acet. ac.;* Berb. v.; Caust.; Crot. t.; Equis.; *Gels.;* Helon.; *Ign.;* Kreos.; Lycop.; Mag. m.; Mosch.; *Nat. m.;* Nit. ac.; Nux v.; *Phos. ac.; Phos.;* Puls.; Staph.; *Sul.* See Polyuria.

Pink—Sulphon.

Red, dark—*Acon.; Apis;* Bell.; Benz. ac.; *Bry.;* Canth.; Carbo v.; Coccus; Cupr. ac.; *Dig.;* Hep.; *Kali bich.;* Lob. infl.; Merc. c.; Merc. d.; Nux v.; Petrol.; Phyt.; Scilla; Selen.; Solid.

Red, fiery, high colored—*Acon.;* Ant. c.; *Apis;* Apoc.; Arg. n.; Ars.; *Bell.; Benz. ac.; Berb. v.; Bry.;* Camph.; Can. s.; *Canth.;* Carb. ac.; Cepa; Chel.; Chimaph.; Cupr. ac.; *Equis.;* Euonym.; Glon.; *Helleb.; Hep.;* Kali bich.; *Lith. c.; Lyc.;* Merc. d.; *Myr.;* Nit .ac.; Ocimum; Phyt.; Picr. ac.; Puls.; Rheum; *Rhus t.;* Sab.; *Sars.;* Selen.; Senec.; Sul.; *Tereb.;* Thuya; Uva; Ver. v.

Smoky—Am. benz.; *Benz. ac.;* Helleb.; *Tereb.* See Bloody.

Thick—Ammon. benz.; Ananth.; *Benz. ac.;* Camph.; Cina; Coccus; *Col.;* Con.; Daphne; Dig.; *Dulc.; Hep.;* Iod.; *Merc. c.;* Ocimum; *Phos.;* Still.; Sep.; Zing.

Yellow—Absinth.; Bell.; Berb. v.; *Card. m.;* Ceanoth.; Cinch.; Dahpne; Hydr.; Ign.; Kal.; Lact. ac.; Ocimum; Op.; Plumb. m.; Solid.; Uva.

Yellow, dark—Bov.; Bry.; Camph.; *Chel.;* Chenop.; Crot. t.; *Iod.; Kali p.;* Myr.; Petrol.; *Picr. ac.;* Pod.

ODOR—Fetid, foul: *Am. benz.;* Am. c.; Apis; Ars.; *Aspar.; Bapt.; Benz. ac.;* Berb. v.; *Calc. c.;* Camph.; Carbo an.; *Chimaph.;* Col.; Conv.; Cupr. ars.; Daphne; *Dulc.; Graph.;* Hydr.; Indium; Kali bich.; Kreos.; Lach.; *Lyc.;* Merc.; Naph.; *Nit ac.;* Ocimum; Petrol.; *Phos.;* Physal.; Pulex; *Sep.;* Solid.; Stront. br.; Sul.; Tropæol.; Uran. n.

Fish-like—Uran. n.

Garlicky—Cupr. ars.

Musk-like—Ocimum.

Pungent, ammoniacal—*Bor.;* Cahinca; Cop.; Dig.; Naph.; *Nit. ac.; Pareira;* Petrol.; Solid.; Stigm.

Sharp, intensely strong—*Absinth.;* Am. benz.; Arg. n.; *Benz. ac.; Bor.; Calc. c.;* Carbo v.; *Chin. s.;* Erig.; *Lyc.;* Picr. ac.; Pin. sylv.; *Sul.;* Viola od.; Zing.

Sharp, like cat's urine—Cajup.; Viola tr.

Sharp, like horse's urine—Benz. ac.; *Nit. ac.*

Sour—Calc. c.; *Graph.;* Nat. c.; Petrol.; Sep.; Solid.

URINARY SYSTEM

Sweet, violaceous—Arg. m.; *Cop.*; Cub.; Eucal.; Ferr. iod!; Inula; *Junip.*; Phos.; Primula; Salol; *Tereb.*; Thyr.
Valerian, like—Murex.

SEDIMENT—TYPE: Aceton (azoturia): Ars.; Aur. mur.; *Calc. mur.*; Carb. ac.; *Caust.*; Colch.; Cupr. ars.; *Euonym.*; Nat. sal.; Phos.; Senna.

Bile—Ceanoth.; Chionanth.; *Chel.*; Kali chlor.; Myr.; Nat. s.; Sep. See Liver.

Blood—Ars.; *Berb. v.*; Cact.; *Can. s.*; *Canth.*; *Carb. ac.*; Colch.; Dulc.; Ham.; Hep.; Lyc.; *Nit. ac.*; Pareira; *Phos.*; Tereb. See Bloody.

Casts—*Apis*; *Ars.*; Aur. mur.; Brachygl.; *Canth.*; *Carb. ac.*; Chel.; Crot.; Kali chlor.; Merc. c.; Nat. chlor.; *Phos.*; Picr. ac.; Pichi; *Plumb.*; Radium; Sulphon.; Tereb. See Nephritis.

Cells, debris—Arg. n.; *Ars.*; *Berb. v.*; Brachygl.; Cact.; *Canth.*; *Carb. ac.*; Chel.; Crot.; Hep.; Kali bich.; *Merc. c.*; *Phos.*; Picr. ac.; Solid.; Tereb. See Nephritis.

Chlorides, diminished—Bar. m.; Chel.; Col.

Chlorides, increased—Chin. s.; Radium; Senna.

Chyluria—Col.; Iod.; *Kali bich.*; *Phos. ac.*; Uva. See Milky Urine.

Coffee-ground like—Dig.; *Helleb.*; Tereb.

Flocculent, flaky—*Berb. v.*; Caust.; Phos.; Sars.

Gelatinous, gluey, viscid—Berb. v.; *Cina*; *Col.*; *Ocimum*; *Phos. ac.*; Puls. See Mucous.

Grayish-white, granular—Berb. v.; Calc. c.; Canth.; *Graph.*; Sars.; Sep.

Hæmatoporphyrinuria—*Sulphon.*; Trion.

Hæmoglobinuria—*Ars. hydrog.*; Carb. ac.; Chin. ars.; Chin. s.; Ferr. p.; Kali bich.; *Kali chlor.*; Nat. nit.; Phos.; Picr. ac.; Santon.

Indican—Alfal.; Indol; Nux m.; Picr. ac.

Lithic acid, uric acid, gravel, brick dust—Arg. n.; Arn.; *Aspar.*; Baros.; *Bar. m.*; Bell.; *Benz. ac.*; *Berb. v.*; Calc. ren.; Can. s.; *Canth.*; Caust.; Chel.; *Chin. s.*; *Cinch.*; Coccin. sept.; Cochlear.; *Coccus*; Colch.; Col.; Dig.; Diosc.; *Epig.*; *Eup. ar.*; *Eup. purp.*; Eryng.; Ferr. mur.; Galium; Graph.; *Hedeoma*; *Hydrang.*; *Kali c.*; Kali iod.; Kreos.; *Lith. benz.*; *Lith. c.*; Lob. infl.; *Lyc.*; Merc. c.; Nat. m.; Nat. s.; *Nit. ac.*; Nit. mur. ac.; *Nux v.*; *Ocimum*; Pareira; Pariet.; Phos. ac.; Phos.; Physal.; Pichi; Piperaz.; Plumb. iod.; Puls.; Sars.; Selen.; Senna; Sep.; Skook. ch.; *Solid.*; Stigm.; *Thlaspi*; Tritic.; Urt.; Vesic. See Calculi.

Mucus, slime—Apoc.; Ars.; Aspar.; Bals. per.; *Baros.*; *Benz. ac.*; *Berb. v.*; Brachygl.; Calc. c.; *Can. s.*; *Canth.*; *Chimaph.*; Chin. s.; Cina; *Cub.*; Dulc.; Epig.; *Equis.*; Eup. purp.; *Hep.*; Hydrang.; *Kali bich.*; *Lyc.*; Menthol; Merc. c.; Nit. ac.; Nux v.; *Pareira*; Pichi; *Pop. tr.*; *Puls.*; Sars.; Senega; Sep.; *Solid.*; Stigm.; Sul.; *Tritic.*; *Uva.* See Cystitis.

Oxalates (oxaluria)—*Berb. v.*; Brachygl.; *Kali s.*; Lysidin; Nat. p.; Nit. ac.; *Nit. mur. ac.*; Ox. ac.; Senna.

Phosphates (phosphaturia)—*Alfal.*; Arn.; Avena; Bell.; Benz. ac.; Brachygl.; Calc. c.; *Calc. p.*; Can. s.; Chel.; Chin. s.; Graph.; Guaco; Guaiac.; Helon.; Hydrang.; Kali chlor.; Lecith.; Nit. ac.; *Phos. ac.*; *Picr. ac.*; Sang.; Senna; *Solid.*; Thlaspi; Uran. n.

Pus (pyuria)—*Ars.*; Aspar.; Baros.; *Benz. ac.*; Berb. v.; Bry.; Calc. c.;

Can. s.; Canth.; Chimaph.; Cop.; Dulc.; Epig.; Eucal.; Hep.; Hyos.; Kali bich.; Lith. c.; Lyc.; Merc. c.; Nit. ac.; Nux v.; Ocimum; Phos.; Pichi; Pop. tr.; Sars.; Sep.; Stigm.; Sul-; Tereb.; Thlaspi; Tritic.; Uva.

Rose colored—Am. phos.

DIABETES—Sugar: Acet. ac.; Adren.; Am. acet.; Arg. m.; Arg. n.; Aristol.; Arn.; Ars. br.; Ars. iod.; Ars.; Asclep. vinc.; Aur.; Aur. mur.; Bell.; Bor. ac.; Bov.; Bry.; Caps.; Carb. ac.; Ceanoth.; Cham.; Chel.; Chimaph.; Chionanth.; Coca; Cod.; Colch.; Crot.; Cupr. ars.; Cur.; Eup. purp.; Fel tauri; Ferr. iod.; Ferr. mur.; Fluor. ac.; Glon.; Glycerin; Grind.; Helleb.; Helon.; Iod.; Iris; Kali acet.; Kali br.; Kreos.; Lach.; Lact. ac.; Lecith.; Lycop.; Lyc.; Lyssin; Morph.; Mosch.; Murex; Nat. m.; Nat. s.; Nit. ac.; Nux v.; Op.; Pancreat.; Phaseol.; Phos. ac.; Phos.; Phlorid.; Picr. ac.; Plumb. iod.; Plumb.; Pod.; Rhus ar.; Scilla; Sec.; Sil.; Sizyg.; Strych. ars.; Sul.; Tar. h.; Tarax.; Tereb.; Uran. n.; Urea; Vanad.

Assimilative disorders—Uran. n.

Gastro-hepatic origin—Ars. iod.; Ars.; Bry.; Calc. c.; Cham.; Chel.; Kreos.; Lact. ac.; Lept.; Lyc.; Nux v.; Uran. n.

Nervous origin—Ars.; Aur. mur.; Calc. c.; Ign.; Phos. ac.; Strych. ars.

Pancreatic origin—Iris; Pancreat.; Phos.

With debility—Acet. ac.; Op.

With gangrene, boils, carbuncles, diarrhœa—Ars.

With gouty symptoms—Lact. ac.; Nat. s.

With impotency—Coca; Mosch.

With melancholia, emaciation, thirst, restlessness—Helon.

With motor paralysis—Cur.

With rapid course—Cur.; Morph.

With ulceration—Sizyg.

MALE SEXUAL SYSTEM

BUBO—Acon.; Angust.; Apis; Aur. mur.; Bad.; *Bell.;* Calend.; *Carbo an.;* Carbo v.; Caust.; *Cinnab.;* Hep.; Jacar.; *Kali iod.;* Merc. i. r.; Merc. pr. rub.; *Merc. s.; Nit. ac.;* Phos. ac.; *Phyt.;* Sil.; Sul.; Syph.; **Tar. c.**
 Bubo, chancroidal—Ars. iod.; Merc. c.; *Merc. i. r.; Merc. s.;* Sil.
 Bubo, indurated—Alum.; Bad.; *Carbo an.;* Merc. s.
 Bubo, phagedenic—*Ars.;* Graph.; Hydr.; *Kali iod.;* Lach.; *Merc. i. r.; Merc. s.; Nit. ac.;* Sil.; Sul.

CHANCROID—Coral.; *Jacar.;* Kali bich.; Merc. pr. rub.; *Merc. s.;* Nit. ac.; Thuya.
 Chancroid, complications—*Ars.;* Hekla; *Hep.;* Lach.; *Sil.;* Sul.; Thuya.

COITUS—Aversion to: Arn.; Graph.; Lyc. See Desire.
 Coitus, followed by backache—*Can. ind.;* Kali c.
 Coitus, followed by irritability—Selen.
 Coitus, followed by nausea, vomiting—Mosch.
 Coitus, followed by pain in perineum—Alum.
 Coitus, followed by pain in urethra—Canth.
 Coitus, followed by prostration—Agar.; Calc. c.; *Cinch.;* Con.; Dig.; *Kali c.;* Kali p.; Nat. c.; Selen.; Thaspium. See Impotence.
 Coitus, followed by pollution, increased desire—Nat. m.; Phos. ac.
 Coitus, followed by toothache—Daphne.
 Coitus, followed by urging to urinate—Staph.
 Coitus, followed by vertigo—Bov.; Sep.
 Coitus, followed by vomiting—Mosch.
 Coitus, followed by weak vision—Kali c.
 Coitus, painful—Arg. n.; Calc. c.; Sabal. See Impotence.

CONDYLOMATA—Aur. mur.; *Cinnab.;* Euphras.; Kali iod.; *Lyc.;* Merc.; Nat. s.; *Nit. ac.; Sab.;* Staph.; *Thuya.* See Syphilis.

CONTUSIONS—Of genitals: Arn.; Con.

DESIRE—Diminished, lost: *Agn.; Arg. n.;* Bar. c.; Berb. v.; *Calc. c.;* Caps.; Con.; Hep.; Ign.; Iod.; Kali br.; *Kali c.;* Lecith.; *Lyc.;* Nit. ac.; Nuph.; Onosm.; Oxytr.; Phos. ac.; *Sabal; Selen.;* Sil.; Sul.; X-ray. See Impotence.
 Desire increased (erethism, satyriasis)—Alum.; Anac.; Bov.; Calad.; Camph.; *Can. ind.;* Can. s.; *Canth.;* Dulc.; Fluor. ac.; *Gins.;* Graph.; Hippom.; *Hyos.;* Ign.; Kali br.; Lach.; Lyc.; Lyssin; *Mosch.;* Nat. m.; Nux v.; Ol. an.; Onosm.; *Orig.; Phos.;* Pier. ac.; *Plat.;* Sab.; *Salix n.;* Stram.; Tar. h.; Thaspium; Thymol; Upas; Ver. a.; *Zinc. p.*
 Desire increased in old men but impotent—Lyc.; Selen.
 Desire perverted—Agn.; Nux v.; Plat.; Staph.
 Desire suppressed, ill effect from—Con.

GENITALS—Burning, heat: Spong.; Sil. See Gonorrhœa.
 Genitals, itching (pruritus)—Agar.; *Ambra;* Anac.; *Calad.;* Crot. t.; *Fagop.;* Rhus d.; *Rhus t.;* Sep.; Sul.; Tar. c. See Skin.

MALE SEXUAL SYSTEM

Genitals, relaxed, flabby, cold, weak—Absinth.; *Agn.;* *Calad.;* Caps.; *Cinch.;* Con.; *Diosc.;* Gels.; Ham.; *Lyc.;* Nuph.; *Phos. ac.;* Phos.; *Selen.;* Sep.; Staph.; Sul.; Uran. See Impotence.

GONORRHOEA—(specific urethritis) **Remedies in general:** *Acon.;* Agn.; Apis; *Arg. n.;* Baros.; Benz. ac.; *Camph.;* Can. s.; *Canth.;* Caps.; *Clem.;* Cop.; Cub.; Dig.; *Doryph.;* Echin.; Equis.; Erig.; Eucal.; Euphorb. pil.; Fabiana; Ferr.; *Gels.;* Hep.; *Hydr.;* Ichthy.; Jacar.; *Kali bich.;* Kali s.; Kreos.; Med.; *Merc. c.;* Merc. pr. rub.; *Merc. s.; Merc. v.;* Methyl. bl.; Naph.; Nat. s.; *Nit. ac.;* Nux v.; *Ol. sant.;* Pareira; *Petros.;* Pichi; Pin. c.; *Puls.;* Sabal; Sab. ; Salix n.; *Sep.;* Sil.; Stigm.; *Sul.;* Tereb.; *Thuya;* Tritic.; *Tussil.;* Zing.

Acute, inflammatory stage—*Acon.;* Arg. n.; Atrop.; *Can. s.; Canth.;* Caps.; *Gels.;* Petros.

Adenitis, lymphangitis—Acon.; Apis; *Bell.;* Hep.; *Merc.*

Chordee—Acon.; *Agave;* Anac.; Arg. n.; Bell.; Berb. v.; *Camph. monobr.; Can. ind.;* Can. s.; *Canth.;* Caps.; Clem.; Cop.; Gels.; Hyos.; Jacar.; Kali br.; *Lupul.;* Merc.; Œnanthe; Ol. sant.; Phos.; *Picr. ac.;* Pip. m.; Salix n.; Tereb.; Tussil.; Yohimb.: Zinc.; picr.

Chronic, subacute stage—Arg. n.; Can. s.; *Cop.;* Cub.; Erig.; *Hep.; Hydr.; Kali s.;* Merc. c.; Merc. i. r.; Merc.; Naph.; *Nat. s.; Ol. sant.;* Pin. c.; Psor.; *Puls.;* Rhod.; *Sabal;* Sep.; Sil.; Stigm.; *Sul.; Thuya.* See Gleet.

Cowperitis—Acon.; *Can. s.;* Gels.; *Hep.;* Merc. c.; Petros.; Pichi; Sabal; Sil. See Bladder.

DISCHARGE—Acrid, corroding: Cop.; Gels.; *Hydr.; Merc. c.;* Thuya.

Bloody—Arg. n.; *Canth.;* Cub.; *Merc. c.;* Millef.

Milky, glairy, mucus—Can. ind.; *Can. s.;* Cop.; Cupr. ars.; Graph.; *Hydr.; Kali bich.; Nat. m.; Petros.;* Puls.; Sep. See Gleet.

Muco-purulent, yellowish-green—Agn.; Alum.; *Arg. n.;* Baros.; *Can. s.;* Canth.; Caps.; Cob.; *Cop.;* Cub.; Dig.; *Hep.; Hydr.;* Jacar.; Kali iod.; *Kali s.; Merc. c.; Merc. s.;* Nat. m.; *Nat. s.;* Ol. sant.; *Puls.;* Sab.; Sep.; Sil.; Sul.; *Thuya;* Tussil.; Zing. See Gleet.

Watery—*Can. s.;* Fluor. ac.; Mez.; Millef.; *Nat. m.;* Sep.; Sul.; Thuya.

Folliculitis—Caps.; Hep.; Merc. s.; Sep.; Sil.

GLEET—Abies c.; *Agn.;* Arg. n.; Calad.; Calc. p.; *Can. s.; Canth.;* Caps.; Chimaph.; *Cinnab.;* Clem.; *Cub.;* Dorpyh.; Erig.; Graph.; *Hydr.;* Kali bich.; Kali iod.; *Kali s.;* Matico; Med.; Merc.; *Naph.; Nat. m.;* Nat. s.; *Nit. ac.;* Nux v.; *Ol. sant..;* Petros.; Pip. m.; Pop. tr.; *Puls.; Sabal;* Selen.; *Sep.;* Sil.; *Thuya;* Zinc. mur.

Ophthalmia—*Acon.;* Apis; Arg. n.; *Bell.;* Ipec.; Merc. c.

Orchitis, epididymitis—Aur. m.; Clem.; Gels.; Ham.; Puls.; Rhod.; *Spong.*

Prostatic involvement—Caps.; Cub.; Pareira; *Thuya.* See Prostatitis.

Rheumatism—*Acon.;* Arg. n.; Clem.; Cop.; *Daphne;* Gels.; Guaiac.; Iod.; *Irisin;* Kali iod.; *Med.; Merc.;* Nat. s.; *Phyt.; Puls.; Sars.;* Sul.; *Thuya.*

Stricture, organic—Acon.; *Arg. n.;* Calc. iod.; Canth.; Caps.; *Clem.;* Cop.; *Fluor. ac.;* Iod.; *Kali iod.;* Merc. pr. rub.; *Merc.;* Nux v.; Ol.

sant.; Pareira; Petros.; Puls.; Sep.; *Sil.*; Sul.; Sul. iod.; *Thiosin.*; *Thuya.*

Suppression ill effects—*Agn.*; Ant. t.; Benz. ac.; *Clem.*; Kali iod.; *Med.*; Nat. s.; *Puls.*; Sars.; *Thuya*; X-ray.

IMPOTENCE—*Agn.*; *Anac.*; Ant. c.; *Arg. n.*; Arn.; Ars.; Avena; Bar. c.; Berb. v.; *Calad.*; Calc. c.; Camph.; Carbon. s.; Chin. s.; *Cinch.*; *Cob.*; Con.; Damiana; Dig.; *Diosc.*; *Gels.*; Glycerin; Graph.; Hyper.; Ign.; Iod.; Kali br.; Kali iod.; Lecith.; *Lyc.*; Nat. m.; Nit .ac.; Nuph.; *Nux v.*; Onosm.; *Phos. ac.*; *Phos.*; Picr. ac.; Plumb. m.; *Sabal*; *Salix n.*; *Selen.*; Sep.; Sil.; Staph.; *Strych.*; Sul.; Thuya; Tribul.; *Yohimb.*; Zinc.; Zinc. p. See Spermatorrhœa.

MASTURBATION—**Ill effects:** Agn.; *Anac.*; Apis; Arg. m.; Bellis; *Calad.*; Calc. c.; *Calc. p.*; *Cinch.*; Con.; *Diosc.*; *Gels.*; Graph.; Grat.; *Kali br.*; *Lyc.*; Nat. m.; *Nux v.*; *Phos. ac.*; *Picr. ac.*; Plat.; *Salix n.*; *Staph.*; Still.; *Sul.*; Tab.; Thuya; Tribul.; Ustil.; Zinc. m.; Zinc. oxyd.

PENIS—**Atrophy:** Ant. c.; Arg. m.; Staph.

Glans: Epithelioma: Arg. n.; *Ars.*; Con.; Thuya.

Gangrene—Canth.; Lach.

Itching—*Acon.*; Ars.; Bell.; *Calad.*; *Canth.*; Caps.; Cinch.; Cinnab.; Coccus; *Con.*; Cop.; Coral.; *Crot. t.*; Graph.; Ham.; *Hep.*; Ign.; Kali bich.; Lyc.; *Merc.*; Nat. m.; Nux v.; *Puls.*; Selen.; Sep.; Staph.; *Sul.*; Thuya; *Viola tr.*

PAINS—**Burning, sore:** Anac.; *Ars.*; Bell.; *Can. s.*; *Canth.*; *Caps.*; Cinch.; Cinnab.; Con.; Cop.; Coral.; Crot. t.; *Gels.*; Ign.; Lyc.; *Merc. c.*; Mez.; *Nit. ac.*; Nuph.; Nux v.; Puls.; Rhus t.; Sep.; *Sul.*; *Thuya*; Viola tr.

Cutting, stitching, tearing—*Acon.*; Apis; *Arg. n.*; Calad.; *Can. s.*; *Canth.*; Caps.; Con.; *Hep.*; *Lyc.*; Naph.; Nat. m.; *Nit. ac.*; Papaya; *Pareira*; Petrol.; Phos. ac.; *Phyt.*; Prun. sp.; *Sars.*; Staph.; Sul.

Pressive, pinching—*Canth.*; Caps.; Graph.; Kali bich.; *Nit. ac.*; Puls.; *Rhod.*

Throbbing—Coccus; Ham.; Lith. c.; Nat. m.; *Nit. ac.*

Priapism—See Chordee.

Pustules—*Ars. hydr.*; Coccus; Hep.; *Kali bich.*; Merc.

Rash and spots—Antipyr.; *Bell.*; Bry.; Calad.; Can. s.; Caust.; *Cinnab.*; Gels.; Lach.; *Merc.*; Nat. m.; Petrol.; *Rhus t.*; Sep.; *Sul.*; Thuya.

Swollen, inflamed glans—*Acon.*; Antipyr.; *Apis*; *Arg. n.*; Arn.; Ars.; Calad.; *Can. s.*; *Canth.*; *Cop.*; Coral.; *Cub.*; Dig.; *Gels.*; Ham.; *Merc. c.*; Merc. s.; *Nit. ac.*; Phos. ac.; *Rhus t.*; Sars.; *Thuya.* See Gonorrhœa.

Ulcers, excoriations—*Ars.*; Can. s.; *Caust.*; Cop.; *Coral.*; Crot. t.; *Hep.*; *Merc. c.*; *Merc.*; Mez.; *Nit. ac.*; Osm.; Sep.; *Thuya.*

PREPUCE—**Constriction (paraphimosis, phimosis):** Acon.; *Apis*; Arn.; Bell.; Can. s.; *Canth.*; Caps.; Dig.; Euphras.; Ham.; *Merc. c.*; *Merc. s.*; *Nit. ac.*; Ol. sant.; Phos. ac.; *Rhus t.*; Sab.; Sul.; *Thuya.*

Herpes—Ars.; Carbo v.; Caust.; *Crot. t.*; Graph.; *Hep.*; Jugl. r.; *Merc.*; Mez.; *Nit. ac.*; Petrol.; Phos. ac.; *Rhus t.*; Sars.; *Thuya.*

Inflammation (balanitis, balano-postitis)—*Acon.*; Apis; Calad.; *Can. s.*;

MALE SEXUAL SYSTEM

Canth.; Cinnab.; Coccus; Con.; Crot. t.; Dig.; *Gels.; Jacar.;* Lyc.; Merc. c.; *Merc. s.; Nit. ac.;* Ol. sant.; *Rhus t.;* Sul.; *Thuya;* Viola tr.

Itching—Ars.; *Canth.; Caps.;* Cinnab.; *Con.;* Graph.; Ign.; Lyc.; *Merc. s.;* Nit. ac.; Nux v.; Puls.; *Rhus t.;* Sil.; *Sul.;* Thuya; Zing.

Pains—Acon.; Bell.; *Berb. v.;* Calad.; *Can. s.; Canth.;* Cinnab.; Coccus; Con.; *Cop.;* Coral.; Ign.; Merc. c.; *Merc.; Nit. ac.;* Nux v.; *Rhus t.;* Sep.; Sul.; *Thuya.*

Ulcers, excoriations—*Ars.;* Can. s.; *Caust.;* Cop.; *Coral.;* Hep.; Ign.; Merc.; *Nit. ac.;* Nux v.; Phos. ac.; Phyt.; Sep.; *Sil.; Thuya.*

Varices—Ham.; Lach.

Warts, condylomata—Apis; *Cinnab.;* Hep.; Kreos.; Lyc.; Nat. m.; *Nit. ac.;* Phos. ac.; *Sab.;* Sep.; Staph.; *Thuya.*

PROSTATE GLAND—**Affections in general:** Æsc.; Aloe; Baros.; Caust.; *Ferr. picr.;* Hep.; *Hydrang.;* Iod.; Kali iod.; *Melast.;* Merc. s.; Pareira; Phyt.; Pichi; Picr. ac.; Pop. tr.; *Sabal; Solid.;* Staph.; Sul. iod.; *Thuya;* Turnera.

Congestion—Acon.; *Aloe;* Arn.; Bell.; *Canth.;* Con.; Cop.; Cub.; Ferr. p.; Gels.; Kali br.; Kali iod.; Lith. c.; *Ol. sant.;* Puls.; *Sabal;* Thuya.

Hypertrophy—Alfal.; *Aloe;* Am. m.; *Arg. n.; Bar. c.;* Benz. ac.; Calc. fl.; Calc. iod.; *Chimaph.;* Chrom. s.; *Cim.;* Con.; Eup. purp.; *Ferr. picr.; Gels.;* Graph.; Hep.; *Hydrang.;* Ikshug.; Iod.; Kali bich.; Kali br.; Lyc.; Med.; Ol. sant.; Oxyden.; Pareira; Picr. ac.; Pip. m.; *Pop. t.;* Puls.; Rhus ar.; *Sabal;* Sars.; *Senec.; Solid.;* Staph.; *Sul.; Thiosin.; Thuya;* Thyr.; Tritic.

Inflammation (prostatitis): Acute: Acon.; Æsc.; Aloe; Apis; *Bell.;* Bry.; Canth.; *Chimaph.;* Colch.; *Cop.;* Cub.; Dig.; Ferr. p.; *Gels.;* Hep.; *Iod.;* Kali br.; Kali iod.; Merc. c.; *Merc. d.; Nit. ac.;* Nitrum; Ol. sant.; *Pichi;* Picr. ac.; *Puls.;* Sabad.; *Sabal;* Salix n.; Selen.; *Sil.;* Solid.; Staph.; *Thuya;* Tritic.; *Ver. v.;* Vesic.

Inflammation, chronic—Alum.; *Aur.;* Bar. c.; Brachygl.; Calad.; Carbon. s.; Caust.; Clem.; *Con.; Ferr. picr.;* Graph.; Hep.; Hydrocot.; Iod.; *Lyc.; Merc. c.; Merc.; Nit. ac.;* Nux v.; Phyt.; *Puls.;* Sabad.; *Sabal; Selen.;* Sep.; Sil.; Solid.; Staph.; Sul.; *Thuya; Tribul.* See Prostatitis.

Weakness (prostatorrhœa); discharge during stool, urination, straining: Acet. ac.; Æsc.; *Agn.; Alum.;* Anac.; *Arg. n. Can. s.;* Caust.; *Chimaph.;* Con.; Cub.; Eryng.; Hep.; Junip.; Kali bich.; Lyc.; Nit. ac.; Nuph.; Nux v.; Petrol.; *Phos. ac.;* Phos.; Puls.; Sabal; *Selen.;* Sil.; *Sul.;* Tereb.; Thuya; Thymol; *Turnera;* Zinc. m.

PUBIC HAIR—**Loss:** Merc.; Nit. ac.; Selen.; Zinc.

SCROTUM—**Cancer, epithelioma:** Ars.; Fuligo; Thuya.

Cold, relaxed—*Agn.;* Calad.; Calc. c.; *Caps.;* Gels.; Lyc.; Merc.; *Phos. ac.;* Sep.; Staph.; Sul. See Impotence.

Eczema—Alumen; Ant. c.; Canth.; *Crot. t.; Graph.;* Hep.; Cleand.; Petrol.; Phos. ac.; *Rhus t.;* Sanic.; Sul.

HYDROCELE—**Œdema:** Abrot.; Ampel.; *Apis;* Ars.; *Aur.;* Bry.; Calad.; *Calc. c.;* Calc. fl.; Calc. p.; Canth.; Chel.; Cinch.; *Con.;* Dig.; Dulc.; *Fluor. ac.; Graph.;* Helleb.; *Iod.;* Kali iod.; Merc.; *Puls.; Rhod.;* Rhus t.; Samb.; Scilla; *Selen.;* Sil.; *Spong.;* Sul.

MALE SEXUAL SYSTEM

Induration—Calad.; Rhus t.
Inflammation—*Apis*; Ars.; Crot. t.; Euphorb.; *Ham.*; Rhus t.; Ver. v.
Itching—*Ambra;* Carbo v.; Caust.; *Crot. t.*; Euphorb.; *Graph.*; *Hep.*; Nit. ac.; Nux v.; Petrol.; Phos. ac.; Rhus t.; *Sars.*; Selen.; Sil.; Thuya; Urt. See Skin.
Hæmatocele, acute—Acon.; *Arn.*; Con.; Erig.; Ham.; Nux v.; *Puls.*; Sul.
Hæmatocele, chronic—Iod.; *Kali iod.*; Sul.
Nodules, hard, suppurating—Nit. ac. See Skin.
Numbness—*Ambra;* Am. c.; Sep. See Itching.
Pain—Am. c.; Berb. v.; *Clem.*; Iod.; Kali c.; *Merc.*; Nux v.; *Thuya.* See Inflammation.
Prurigo—*Ant. c.*; Aur.; **Graph.**; **Mur. ac.**; **Nat. s.**; *Nit. ac.*; Nux v.; *Rhus t.*; Staph.
Retraction—Plumb. m.
Spots, brown—Con.
Sweat—Bell.; *Calad.*; Calc. **c.**; Coral.; Cupr. ars.; *Diosc.*; Fagop.; Nat. m.; Petrol.; Sep.; *Sil.*; *Sul.*; Thuya; Uran. n.
Swelling—*Apis;* Ars.; Bell.; Brom.; *Canth.*; *Clem.*; Con.; Ign.; Nit. ac.; *Puls.*; Rhus d.; *Rhus t.*; Sep. See Inflammation.
Tubercles—Con.; *Iod.*; Sil.; Sul.; Teucr.

VARICOCELE—Acon.; *Arn.*; Ferr. *p.*; *Ham.*; Lach.; Nux v.; Plumb.; *Puls.*; Ruta; Sul.

SEMINAL VESICULITIS—Acute: Acon.; Æsc.; Aloe; *Bell.*; Canth.; Cub.; Ferr. *p.*; Hep.; Kali br.; *Merc.*; *Phyt.*; *Puls.*; Selen.; Sil.; ver. v.
Chronic—*Agn.*; *Arg. n.*; Aur.; Bar. c.; Calad.; *Can. s.*; Cinch.; Clem.; Con.; Cub.; Ferr. picr.; Graph.; *Hep.*; *Iod.*; Kali br.; *Lyc.*; Merc.; Nux v.; Ox. ac.; Phos. ac.; Phyt.; *Puls.*; *Selen.*; Sep.; *Sil.*; Staph.; Sul.; Tribul.; Zinc. See Prostatitis.

SEXUAL EXCESSES—Ill effects: Agar.; *Agn.*; Anac.; Avena; Calad.; Calc. c.; *Cinch.*; Con.; Digitaline; *Gels.*; Graph.; Kali br.; Kali p.; Lyc.; Lyssin; Nat. m.; *Nux v.*; *Phos. ac.*; Phos.; Samb.; Selen.; Sil.; Staph.; Tribul. See Impotence, Spermatorrhœa.

SPERMATIC CORD—Pain in general: Anthem.; *Arg. n.*; Arundo; Aur.; *Bell.*; Berb. v.; Calc. c.; Cahinca; *Can. s.*; Caps.; *Clem.*; Cinch.; Con.; Diosc.; *Ham.*; Indium; Kali c.; Lith. c.; *Merc. i. r.*; Morph.; *Nit. ac.*; Nux v.; Ol. an.; Osm.; Ox. ac.; Oxytr.; Phyt.; Picr. ac.; *Puls.*; Sars.; Senec.; Sil.; *Spong.*; Staph.; Sul.; *Thlaspi*; *Thuya*; Tussil.; Ver. v.
Drawing—*Cahinca;* Calc. c.; *Clem.*; Con.; Ham.; Indium; Ol. an.; *Puls.*; Rhod.; Senec.; *Staph.*; Zinc. m.
Neuralgic—*Arg. n.*; Aur.; *Bell.*; Berb. v.; Clem.; Ham.; Menthol; Nit. ac.; Nux v.; *Ox. ac.*; Phyt.; *Spong.*
Swelling—Anthem.; *Can. s.*; Cinch.; *Ham.*; Kali c.; *Puls.*; *Spong.*
Tenderness—*Bell.*; *Clem.*; Ham.; Merc. i. r.; *Ox. ac.*; Phyt.; Rhod.; *Spong.*; Tussil.

SPERMATORRHOEA—(sexual debility, deficient physical power, nocturnal pollutions):—Absinth.; *Agn.*; *Anac.*; Arg. m.; *Arg. n.*; Arn.; Ars.;

MALE SEXUAL SYSTEM

Aur.; *Avena;* Bar. c.; *Calad.; Calc. c.; Calc. p.;* Camph. monobr.; Can. ind.; *Canth.;* Carbon. s.; Carbo v.; Chlorum; Cim.; *Cinch.; Cob.;* Coca; Cocc.; *Con.;* Cupr. m.; *Dig.; Digitaline; Diosc.;* Eryng.; *Ferr. br.;* Formica; *Gels.; Gins.; Graph.;* Hyper.; Ikshug.; Iod.; Iris; *Kali br.; Kali c.; Kali p.;* Lyc.; Lyssin; *Lupul.; Med.;* Mosch.; *Nat. m.;* Nit. ac.; *Nuph.; Nux v.; Onosm.;* Orchit; *Phos. ac.; Phos.; Picr. ac.;* Plumb. phos.; *Sabal;. Salix n.;* Scutel.; *Selen.; Sep.; Sil.; Staph.; Strych.; Sul.;* Sul. ac.; Sumb.; Thuya; *Thymol;* Titan.; Turnera; Upas.; Ustil.; *Yohimb.; Zinc. picr.;* Viola tr.

With brain fag, mental torpidity—Phos. ac.

With debility, backache, weak legs—Aur.; Calc. c.; Calc. p.; *Cinch.; Cob.;* Con.; Cupr. m.; Dig.; *Diosc.;* Eryng.; Formica; Gels.; *Kali c.;* Lyc.; Med.; Nat. p.; *Nux v.; Phos. ac.; Picr. ac.;* Sars.; Selen.; *Staph.; Sul.;* Turnera; Zinc. m.

With dreams absent—Anac.; *Arg. n.;* Dig.; Gels.; Hep.; Nat. p.; *Picr. ac,* See Sleep.

With dreams amorous—Ambra; *Calad.;* Can. ind.; Cob.; Con.; Diosc.; Lyc.; *Nux v.; Phos.;* Sars.; Selen.; Senec.; Staph.; Thymol; Ustil.; Viola tr. See Sleep.

With emission and orgasm absent—Calad.; Calc. c.; Selen.

With emissions bloody—Ambra; *Canth.;* Led.; *Merc.;* Petrol.; Sars.

With emissions diurnal, straining at stool—*Alum.;* Canth.; Cim.; *Cinch.;* Digitaline; Gels.; Kali br.; *Nuph.; Phos. ac.;* Phos.; Picr. ac.; *Selen.;* Tribul. See Prostatorrhœa.

With emissions, premature—*Agn.;* Bar. c.; *Calad.; Calc. c.;* Carbo v.; *Cinch.; Cob.;* Con.; *Graph.; Lyc.;* Ol. an.; Onosm.; *Phos. ac.;* Phos.; *Selen.;* Sep.; Sul.; Titan.; Zinc. m.

With emissions profuse, frequent; after coitus—Phos. ac.

With emissions too slow—Calc. c.; Lyc.; Nat. m.; Zinc. m.

With erections deficient—Agar.; *Agn.;* Arg. m.; Arg. n.; Calad.; Calc. c.; Caust.; *Con.;* Graph.; Hep.; Kali c.; *Lyc.;* Mag. c.; Nit. ac.; Nuph.; *Phos. ac.;* Phos.; *Selen.;* Sul.; Zinc. m.

With erections painful—Can. ind.; *Canth.;* Ign.; Merc.; Mosch.; *Nit. ac.;* Nux v.; Picr. ac.; Puls.; Sabad.; Thuya.

With irritability, despondency—*Aur.; Calc. c.;* Calad.; Cim.; *Cinch.;* Con.; Diosc.; Kali br.; *Nux v.;* Phos. ac.; Phos.; *Selen.; Staph.*

With masturbatic tendency—Ustil.

With rheumatic pains—Gins.

With vision weak—Kali c.

With wasting of testes—*Iod.;* Sabal.

SYPHILIS—**Remedies in general:** *Æthiops;* Alnus; Anac.; Ant. c.; Arg. iod.; Ars.; Ars. br.; Ars. iod.; *Ars. m.;* Ars. s. fl.; Asaf.; Aur. ars.; Aur. iod.; Aur.; Aur. m. n.; Aur. mur.; Bad.; Bapt.; *Bèrb. aq.;* Calc. fl.; *Calop.; Carbo an.;* Carbo v.; Caust.; Chin. ars.; Cinnab.; Condur.; *Coryd.;* Echin.; *Fluor. ac.;* Francisca; Gels.; Graph.; Guaiac.; *Guaco;* Hekla; *Hep.;* Hippoz.; Hydrocot.; *Iod.;* Jacar.; *Kali bich.; Kali iod.;* Kali m.; *Kreos.;* Lach.; Lonic.; Lyc.; *Merc. aur.;* Merc. br.; *Merc. c.;* Merc. d.; *Merc. i. fl.; Merc. i. r.; Merc. nit.; Merc. pr. rub.; Merc. s.;*

Merc. tan.; *Merc. v.*; *Mez.*; *Nit ac.*; Osm.; Phos. ac.; Phos.; *Phyt.*; Plat.; *Plat. mur.*; Psor.; Rhus gl.; Sars.; Staph.; *Still.*; Sul.; *Syph.*; *Thuya*.

Abuse of mercury—Angust.; *Aur.*; Calop.; Carbo an.; Fluor. ac.; Hep.; Kali iod.; *Nit. ac.*; Rhus gl.; Sul.

Adenopathy—*Bad.*; Carbo an.; Graph.; *Hep.*; Iod.; *Merc. i. fl.*; *Merc. i. r.*; Merc. s.; Phyt. See Glands (Generalities).

Alopecia—*Ars.*; Aur.; Carbo v.; Cinnab.; *Fluor. ac.*; Graph.; *Hep.*; Kali iod.; Lyc.; Merc. i. fl.; *Merc. v.*; *Nit. ac.*; *Phos.*; Sul. See Scalp.

Bone and cartilage lesions—Arg. m.; *Asaf.*; *Aur.*; Aur. mur.; Calc. fl.; Carbo v.; *Fluor. ac.*; Hep.; *Kali bich.*; *Kali iod.*; Lach.; *Merc.*; *Mez.*; *Nit. ac.*; Phos. ac.; *Phos.*; Phyt.; Sars.; *Sil.*; Staph; Still.; Sul. See Bones (Generalities).

Cachexia, anæmia, emaciation—*Ars.*; *Aur.*; Calop.; Carbo an.; Carbo v.; Ferr. iod.; Ferr. lact.; *Iod.*; Merc.; Sars.

Chancre and primary lesions—Ananth.; Apis; Arg. n.; Ars.; Asaf.; *Cinnab.*; Coral.; Hep.; *Jacar.*; Kali bich.; *Kali iod.*; Lyc.; *Merc. c.*; *Merc. i. fl.*; *Merc. i. r.*; *Merc. s.*; *Merc. v.*; *Nit. ac.*; Phos. ac.; Phos.; Plat.; Plat. mur.; Sil.; Sul.

Chancre, gangrenous—Ars.; Lach.

Chancre, hard—Carbo an.; Kali iod.; Merc. i. fl.; *Merc. i. r.*; Merc. s.

Chancre, indurated, with lardaceous base; deep, round, penetrating; painful, bleeding; raw, everted edges—Merc. s.

Chancre, phagedenic—Ars.; *Cinnab.*; Hydr.; Lach.; *Merc. c.*; *Nit. ac.*; Sil.

Chancre, soft—Coral.; Merc. s.; Nit. ac.; Thuya.

Condylomata—Aur. mur.; *Cinnab.*; Euphras.; Kali iod.; Mercuries; Plat. mur.; Nat. s.; *Nit. ac.*; *Sab.*; Staph.; *Thuya*.

CONGENITAL, infantile—*Æthiops*; Ars. iod.; Ars. m.; *Aur.*; Calc. fl.; *Calc. iod.*; Coral.; Kali iod.; *Kreos.*; *Merc. d.*; *Merc. s.*; *Merc. v.*; *Nit. ac.*; Psor.; Syph.

Exotoses—*Calc. fl.*; Fluor. ac.; *Hekla*; Merc. phos.; Phos. See Bones.

Fever—Bapt.; *Chin. s.*; Cinch.; Gels.; *Merc.*; Phyt.

Gummata, nodes—Asaf.; *Aur.*; Berb. aq.; *Calc. fl.*; Carbo an.; Condur.; *Coryd.*; *Fluor. ac.*; Iod.; *Kali bich.*; *Kali iod.*; Merc.; Mez.; Nit. ac.; *Phyt.*; Sil.; Staph.; *Still.*; Sul.; Thuya.

Headache—*Kali iod.*; Merc.; Sars.; Still.; *Syph.* See Head.

Mucous patches—*Asaf.*; Aur.; Calc. fl.; Calop.; *Cinnab* ; *Condur.*; Fluor. ac.; *Hep.*; Iod.; *Kali bich.*; Kali iod.; Kali m.; *Merc. c.*; Merc. d.; *Merc. nit.*; *Merc. pr. rub.*; *Merc. s.*; *Nit. ac.*; Phyt.; Sang.; Staph.; Still.; *Thuya*.

Onychia, paronychia—*Ant. c.*; Ars.; Graph.; Kali iod.; *Mercuries*. See Whitlow (Skin).

Ozæna—*Aur.*; Kali bich.; Still. See Nose.

Nervous lesions—Anac.; Asaf.; *Aur.*; Iod.; *Kali iod.*; Lyc.; Merc. nit.; *Merc. phos.*; Mez.; Phos.

Nocturnal pains (osteocopic)—Asaf.; *Aur.*; Calc. fl.; Cinnab.; *Coryd.*; *Eup. perf.*; Fluor. ac.; Hep.; *Kali bich.*; *Kali iod.*; Lach.; Lyc.; Merc.; Mez.; Phos.; *Phyt.*; Sars.; Still.

MALE SEXUAL SYSTEM

Rheumatism—*Guaiac.;* Hekla; Hep.; *Kali bich.;* Kali iod.; *Merc.;* Nit. mur. ac.; *Phyt.;* Still. See Locomotor System.

Secondary stage—*Aur.;* Berb. aq.; Calop.; *Cinnab.;* Fluor. ac.; *Graph.;* Guaiac.; Iod.; *Kali bich.; Kali iod.;* Lyc.; Merc. br.; Merc. c.; *Merc. i. fl.; Merc. i. r.;* Merc. s.; *Merc. v.; Nit. ac.;* Osm.; Phos.; Phyt.; Rhus gl.; Sars.; *Still.;* Thuya.

Stomatitis, mercurial—Nit. ac.

SYPHILIDES—Bullæ:—Kali iod.; Syph.

Eczematous—*Ars.; Graph.;* Kreos.; Merc. s.; Petrol.; Phyt.; *Sars.* See Skin.

Papular—*Calop.;* Kali iod.; Lach.; Merc. c.; *Merc. i. r.;* Merc. s.

Pigmentary—Calc. s.; Nit. ac.

Psoriasis—Asaf.; *Graph.; Kali bich.;* Nit. ac.; Phos.

Pustular—*Ant. t.;* Asaf.; *Calop.;* Fluor. ac.; *Hep.;* Ign.; *Kali bich.;* Kali iod.; Lach.; *Merc. nit.;* Mez.; *Nit. ac.*

Roseolæ—Kali iod.; Merc. c.; Merc. i. r.; *Merc. s.;* Phos.; Phyt.

Rupia—Ars.; *Berb. aq.;* Kali iod.; *Merc.; Nit. ac.;* Phyt.; Syph.

Spots, copper-colored—*Carbo an.;* Carbo v.; *Coral.;* Kali iod.; Lyc.; Merc.; Nit. ac.; Sul.

Squamous—*Ars.;* Ars. iod.; *Ars. s. fl.;* Bor.; *Cinnab.;* Fluor. ac.; Kali iod.; Merc. c.; Merc. i. fl.; Merc. nit.; *Merc. pr. rub.;* Merc. s.; Merc. tan.; *Nit. ac.;* Phos.; Phyt.; Sars.; Sul.

Tubercular—*Ars.;* Aur.; *Carbo an.;* Fluor. ac.; Hydrocot.; *Kali iod.;* Merc. i. r.; Still.; Thuya.

Ulcerations—Ars.; *Asaf.;* Aur.; *Aur. mur.;* Carbo v.; *Cinnab.;* Cistus; Condur.; *Coral.; Fluor. ac.;* Graph.; *Hep.;* Iod.; *Kali bich.;* Kali iod.; Lach.; Lyc.; *Merc. c.;* Merc. cy.; Merc. d.; *Merc. pr. rub.;* Merc. v.; Mez.; *Nit. ac.; Phyt.;* Sil.; Staph.; Still.; Sul.; *Thuya.* See Mucous Patches.

Vesicular—*Cinnab.;* Merc. c.; *Merc. i. r.;* Thuya.

Tertiary stage—Ars. iod.; *Aur.;* Aur. mur.; Calcareas; Carbo v.; Cinnab.; *Fluor. ac.;* Graph.; Guaiac.; Hoang n.; Iod.; *Kali bich.; Kali iod.;* Lyc.; *Mercuries; Mez.; Nit. ac.;* Phos. ac.; *Phos.; Phyt.;* Psor.; Staph.; Sul.; Thuya.

Throat symptoms—Bor.; Calc. fl.; *Cinnab.;* Fluor. ac.; Kali bich.; Lyc.; *Merc. c.;* Merc. d.; Merc. i. fl.; Merc. i. r.; Merc.; *Nit. ac.; Phyt.;* Still.

Visceral symptoms—*Ars.;* Ars. iod.; Aur.; Ceanoth.; Hep.; *Kali bich.;* Kali iod.; Merc. aur.; *Merc. c.;* Merc. i. r.; *Merc. s.;* Merc. tan.; *Nux v.*

TESTICLES—Abscess:—Hep.; Merc.; Still.

Atrophy—Agn.; Ant. c.; *Arg. n.; Aur.;* Caps.; Carbon. s.; Cereus serf.; *Iod.;* Kali br.; Lyssin; *Rhod.;* Sabal.

Coldness—*Agn.;* Berb. v.; *Diosc.;* Merc.; Sil. See Impotence.

Cysts—*Apis;* Con.; *Graph.;* Sep.; Sul.

Hernia—Ars.; *Bar. c.;* Calc. c.; Carbo v.; Hep.; *Merc.;* **Nit. ac.;** *Sil.;* Thuya.

Hypertrophy—Bar. c.; *Berb. v.;* Cinnab.; Con.; *Ham.; Iod.;* Merc. i. r.; *Merc.;* Puls.; Stigm. See Inflammatory.

Induration, hard—Acon.; *Agn.;* Arg. n.; Arn.; *Aur.; Bar. c.;* Bell.;

MALE SEXUAL SYSTEM

Brom.; Calc. fl.; Carbo v.; *Clem.; Con.;* Cop.; *Iod.;* Kali c.; Merc.; Ox. ac.; *Phyt.;* Plumb.; *Rhod.; Sil.; Spong.;* Sul. See Inflammation.

Inflammation of epididymis (epididymitis)—*Acon.;* Apis; Arg. n.; *Bell.;* Can. s.; Cinch.; *Clem.; Gels.; Ham.; Merc.;* Phyt.; *Puls.; Rhod.; Sabal; Spong.;* Sul.; Teucr. scor.; Thuya.

Inflammation of testes (orchitis)—Acute:—*Acon.;* Ant. t.; Arg. m.; Arg. n.; *Bell.;* Brom.; Cham.; Chin. s.; Cinch.; *Clem.;* Cub.; Gels.; *Ham.;* Kali s.; *Merc.;* Nit. ac.; Nux v.; *Phyt.;* Polyg.; *Puls.; Rhod.; Spong.;* Teucr. scor.; Ver. v.

Inflammation, chronic—Agn.; *Aur.;* Bar. c.; *Calc. iod.;* Cinch.; *Clem.; Con.;* Gels.; *Hep.;* Hyper.; Iod.; *Kali iod.;* Lyc.; Merc.; Nit. ac.; Phyt.; *Puls.;* Rhod.; Rhus t.; *Spong.;* Sul.

Inflammation, metastatic—*Puls.;* Staph.

Inflammation, syphilitic—Aur.; *Kali iod.;* Merc. i. r.

PAINS—In general: *Acon.;* Agn.; *Apis;* Arg. m.; *Arg. n.; Aur.; Bell.;* Berb. v.; *Brom.;* Cahinca; *Can. s.;* Caps.; Cereus bon.; Cham.; *Clem.; Con.;* Eriod.; Gins.; *Ham.;* Hydr.; Ign.; Iod.; Kali c.; *Lycop.;* Lyc.; Merc. i. r.; Merc.; Nit. ac.; Nux v.; *Ox. ac.; Oxytr.;* Papaya; Phos. ac.; Picr. ac.; *Puls.; Rhod.;* Salix n.; Sep.; *Spong.;* Staph.; Sul.; *Thuya.*

Aching, dragging, relaxed—Apis; *Aur.;* Can. s.; *Clem.; Con.;* Iod.; Nit. ac.; Nux .v; Phos. ac.; *Puls.; Spong.;* Staph.; Sul.; *Thuya.*

Bruised, crushed, squeezed, contractive pain—*Acon.; Arg. m.; Arg. n.; Aur.;* Cham.; Carbo v.; *Clem.; Con.;* Gins.; *Ham.;* Kali c.; Nit. ac.; *Ol. an.;* Ox. ac.; *Puls.; Rhod.;* Sep.; *Spong.;* Staph.

Neuralgic (testalgia)—Arg. n.; *Aur.;* Bell.; *Berb. v.; Clem.; Col.;* Con.: Euphras.; *Ham.;* Ign.; *Mag. p.;* Merc.; Nux v.; Ol. an.; *Ox. ac.;* Oxytr.; *Puls.;* Spong.; Ver. v.; Zinc. m.

Sensitive, sore, tender—*Acon.;* Apis; *Bell.;* Berb. v.; Brom.; *Clem.; Con.,* Cop.; *Ham.;* Indium; Merc. i. r.; *Phos. ac.; Puls.; Rhod.;* Sep.; *Spong.;* Staph.

RETRACTION—Arg. n.; *Aur.;* Bell.; Brom.; Camph.; Cinch.; *Clem.;* Col.; Euphras.; Nit. ac.; *Ol. an.;* Puls.; *Rhod.;* Zinc.

Swelling—*Acon.;* Agn.; *Apis;* Arg. m.; *Arg. n.;* Arn.; Ars.; *Aur.;* Aur. m. n.; *Bell.; Brom.;* Calc. p.; Carbo v.; *Clem.; Con.;* Cop.; Dig.; Graph.; *Ham.; Iod.; Kali c.;* Lyc.; *Merc. c.;* Merc.; Millef.; Ocimum; Phos. ac.; *Puls.; Rhod.; Spong.;* Staph.; Tussil.; *Ver. v.;* Zinc. See Inflammation.

TUBERCULOSIS—*Aur.;* Bac. test.; *Merc.;* Scrophul.; Spong.; *Teucr. scor.*

Tuberculosis, pseudo—*Aur.;* Calc. c.; Hep.; *Merc. i. r.; Sil.;* Spong.; Sul.

Tumors (sarcocele)—*Aur.; Calc. c.;* Clem.; Merc. i. r.; **Puls.; Rhod.;** Sil.; *Spong.;* Tub. See Hypertrophy.

Undescended testicle in boys—Thyr.

FEMALE SEXUAL SYSTEM

COITION—Fainting during: Murex; Orig.; *Plat.*

Coition, hæmorrhage after—*Arg.* n.; Kreos.; Nit. ac.; Sep.

Coition, painful—Apis; Arg. n.; Bell.; *Berb. v.*; Ferr.; Kreos.; Lyc.; Lyssin; Plat.; Sep.; *Staph.*; Thuya. See Vaginismus.

CONCEPTION, difficult (sterility)—*Agn.*; Alet.; Am. c.; Aur. m.; *Bar. m.*; *Bor.*; Calc. c.; Can. ind.; Caul.; *Con.*; Eup. purp.; Gossyp.; *Graph.*; Helon.; *Iod.*; Lecith.; *Med.*; Nat. c.; *Nat. m.*; Nat. p.; Phos.; *Plat.*; Sabal.

Conception easy—Merc.; Nat. m.

DESIRE, diminished or lost—*Agn.*; Am. c.; Berb. v.; Caust.; Ferr. mur.; Graph.; *Helon.*; *Ign.*; Nat. m.; Onosm.; Plumb.; *Sep.*

Desire, increased (nymphomania)—Ambra; *Aster.*; Arundo; Bufo; Calc. c.; *Calc. p.*; Camph.; *Canth.*; Cim.; Cinch.; Coca; Dulc.; *Ferrula*; *Grat.*; *Hyos.*; Kali br.; *Kali p.*; Kreos.; Lach.; Mosch.; *Murex*; Nux v.; *Orig.*; Phos.; Picr. ac.; *Plat.*; Raph.; R*o*bin.; Sab.; Sil.; *Stram.*; Strych.; Tar. h.; *Ver. a.*; Xerophyl.; Zinc.

Desire increased, must keep busy to repress it—Lil. t.

Desire, suppressed, ill effects—*Con.*; Sabal.

GONORRHOEA—*Acon.*; Alumen; Apis; Arg. n.; *Can. s.*; *Canth.*; *Cop.*; *Cub.*; Jacar.; Kreos.; Med.; Merc. c.; *Merc.*; Ol. sant.; Petros.; *Puls.*; Sep.; Sul.; *Thuya.* See Leucorrhœa, Vaginitis, Vulvitis.

LEUCORRHOEA—Remedies in general: Agar.; *Agn.*; *Alet.*; Alnus; Al*u*m.; Ambra; Am. c.; *Am. m.*; Arg. n.; *Ars.*; Asaf.; Aur. mur.; *Aur. m. n.*; Baros.; Bar. mur.; Bell.; *Bor.*; *Bov.*; Calc. c.; Calc. p.; *Canth.*; Carbo v.; *Caul.*; Caust.; Cham.; Cim.; *Cinch.*; Cocc.; *Con.*; *Cop.*; Dictam.; *Eucal.*; Eupion; Ferr. iod.; *Frax. am.*; Gels.; *Graph.*; Hedeoma; Helon.; Helonin; Hep.; *Hydr.*; Hydrocot.; Ign.; Iod.; Jacar.; Jonosia; Kali bich.; *Kali c.*; Kali m.; *Kali s.*; *Kreos.*; Lil. t.; *Lyc.*; Mag. c.; *Mag. m.*; Merc. pr. rub.; *Merc.*; Mez.; Murex; Naja; *Nat. m.*; *Nat. s.*; *Nit. ac.*; Nux v.; Orig.; Ova t.; Pall.; Picr. ac.; *Psor.*; Pulex; *Puls.*; Sab.; Sec.; Sil.; Spiranth.; *Stann.*; Sul.; Sul. ac.; Thlaspi; *Thuya*; Tilia; Trill.; Vib. op.; *Xanth.*; Zinc. m.

TYPE—Acrid, corroding, burning:—Æsc.; *Alum.*; Am. c.; Aral.; *Ars.*; Ars. iod.; Aur.; Aur. mur.; *Bor.*; *Bov.*; Calc. c.; Calc. iod.; Carb. ac.; Carbo an.; Carbo v.; Caul.; *Cham.*; Con.; *Cop.*; Eucal.; Ferr. br.; *Graph.*; Guaco; Helonin; Hep.; *Hydr.*; Ign.; *Iod.*; *Kreos.*; Lach.; Lil. t.; *Lyc.*; Med.; *Merc.*; Nat. m.; Nit. ac.; Phos.; Puls.; Sab.; *Sep.*; Sil.; *Sul.*; Sul. ac.; Thasp.

Albuminous, slimy, mucous—*Agn.*; *Alum.*; Ambra; Am. m.; Berb. v.; *Bor.*; Bov.; Calc. c.; *Calc. p.*; Ferr. iod.; Graph.; Hematox; Hydr.; Inula; Iod.; Kali m.; *Kali s.*; Kreos.; Mag. c.; Mez.; Plat.; *Puls.*; Sul. ac.; *Thuya*; Tilia.

Blackish—*Cinch.*; Thlaspi.

Bland—Bor.; Calc. p.; Eupion; *Frax. am.*; Kali m.; Puls.; Stann.

Bloody—Arg. n.; Ars.; Bufo; Calc. ars.; Carbo v.; *Cinch.*; Cocc.; Con.; Kreos.; Merc. c.; *Merc.*; Murex; Nit. ac.; Nux m.; *Sep.*; *Spiranth.*; Sul. ac.; *Thlaspi.*

Brown—Æsc.; Am. m.; Kreos.; *Lil. t.*; Nit. ac.; *Sec.*; *Sep.*

Flesh colored, like washing of meat, non-offensive—*Nit. ac.*

Greenish—*Bov.*; Carb. ac.; Carbo v.; *Kali s.*; Lach.; *Merc.*; *Murex*; Nat. s.; Nit. ac.; Phos.; Pulex; *Puls.*; Sec.; *Sep.*; Sul.; Thuya.

Gushing—Cocc.; *Eupion*; *Graph.*; *Sep.* See Profuse.

Intermittent—Con.; Sul.

Itching—*Ambra*; Anac.; Calc. c.; *Calc. iod.*; Carb. ac.; *Cinch.*; Hedeoma; Helonin; Hydr.; *Kreos.*; *Merc.*; *Sep.* See Pruritus.

Lumpy—Ant. c.; Hydr.; Psor.

Milky, white—Aur.; Bell.; *Bor.*; Calc. c.; *Calc. iod.*; Calc. p.; Canth.; Carbo v.; *Con.*; *Cop.*; Ferr. m.; *Graph.*; Hematox.; Iod.; *Kali m.*; Naja; Ova t.; Paraf.; *Puls.*; *Sep.*; *Sil.*; *Stann.*; Sul.

Offensive—Aral.; Ars.; Bufo; *Carb. ac.*; Cinch.; Eucal.; Guaco; *Helon.*; *Hep.*; *Kreos.*; *Merc.*; Med.; Nit. ac.; Nux v.; *Psor.*; Pulex; Robin.; Sab.; Sang.; Sanic.; Sec.; Sep.; Thlaspi; Ustil.

Painful—Mag. m.; Sil.; Sul. See Concomitants.

Painless—Am. m.; Puls.

Profuse—*Alum.*; Ambra; Am. c.; *Arg. n.*; Ars.; Aur.; Bor.; *Calc. c.*; Calc. p.; Carb. ac.; *Caul.*; Caust.; Con.; Fluor. ac.; *Graph.*; Guaco; Helonin; *Hydr.*; Hydrocot.; Iod.; Kreos.; Lil. t.; Mag. s.; *Merc.*; Nat. m.; Ova t.; Phos.; Pulex; *Puls.*; *Sep.*; Sil.; *Stann.*; *Syph.*; Thasp.; *Thuya*; Tilia; Trill.

Purulent, staining, yellow—Æsc.; *Agn.*; Alumen; Arg. n.; *Ars.*; Aur. mur.; *Bov.*; Calc. c.; *Can. s.*; Carbo an.; Ceanoth.; Cham.; *Cinch.*; Eupion; *Fagop.*; Helonin; *Hydr.*; Ign.; Iod.; *Kali bich.*; *Kali s.*; Kreos.; Lach.; Lil. t.; Lyc.; Merc. i. fl.; *Merc.*; Nat. s.; Pulex; *Puls.*; *Sep.*; Stann.; Sul.; Trill.; Ustil.

Thick—Æsc.; Aur.; *Bov.*; Canth.; Carbo v.; Con.; Helonin; *Hydr.*; *Iod.*; Kali m.; Kreos.; Mag. s.; Merc.; Murex; Nit. ac.; *Puls.*; Sab.; *Sep.*; Thuya.

Thin, watery—*Am. c.*; *Ars.*; Bell.; Bufo; Cham.; Frax. am.; *Graph.*; *Kali s.*; Kreos.; Lil. t.; *Merc. c.*; Merc.; Naja; Nat. m.; *Nit. ac.*; Plat.; Puls.; *Sep.*; *Syph.*; Sul.

Viscid, stringy, tough—*Æsc.*; *Alum.*; Asar.; Bov.; Dictam.; Ferr. br.; Graph.; *Hydr.*; Iris; *Kali bich.*; *Kali m.*; Nit. ac.; *Pall.*; Phyt.; Sab.; Trill.

OCCURRENCE—MODALITIES—After coitus: Nat. c.

After menses and between periods—Æsc.; *Alum.*; Bor.; *Bov.*; Calc. c.; Cocc.; Con.; *Eupion*; *Graph.*; Hydr.; *Iod.*; Kal.; *Kreos.*; *Nit. ac.*; Phos. ac.; *Puls.*; Sab.; *Sep.*; Thlaspi; *Xanth.*

After stool—Mag. m.

After urination—*Am. m.*; Con.; *Kreos.*; Mag. m.; Niccol.; Plat.; *Sep.*; Sil.

At climaxis—Psor.; Sang.

At night—Ambra; Caust.; Merc.; **Nit. ac.**

Before menses—*Alum.;* Bar. c.; Bor.; *Bov.; Calc. c.*, Calc. p.; Carbo v.; Con.; *Graph.;* Kreos.; Picr. ac.; *Puls.; Sep.;* Thlaspi.

Better from washing with cold water—Alum.

From motion, walking—*Bov.;* Carbo an.; Euphorb. pil.; Graph.; Helonin; *Mag. m.;* Tilia.

From rest—Fagop.

From sitting, relieved by walking—Cact.; *Cocc.;* Cycl.

From urine, contact of—Kreos.; *Merc.;* Sul.

In daytime—Alum.; Plat.

In infants, little girls—*Asperula; Calc. c.;* Can. s.; Carb. ac.; *Caul.; Cina; Cub.;* Hydr.; Merc. i. fl.; Merc.; *Millef.; Puls.; Sep.;* Syph.

In old, weak women—Ars.; *Helon.;* Nit. ac.; Sec.

In pregnant women—Cocc.; Kali c.; Sep.

Instead of menses—*Cocc.;* Graph.; *Iod.; Nux m.:* Phos.; Puls.; Senec.; *Sep.;* Xanth.

CONCOMITANTS—**Abdominal pain, colic preceding and attending:** *Am. m.;* Aral.; *Ars.;* Bell.; Calc. c.; *Con.;* Graph.; Ham.; Hematox.; Ign.; Lyc.; *Mag. m.;* Nat. c.; *Sep.;* Sil.; *Sul.;* Syph.

Backache and weak feeling, preceding and attending—*Æsc.; Eupion;* Graph.; *Helon.;* Kali bich.; Kreos.; Mag. s.; *Murex;* Nat. chlor.; *Nat. m.;* Ova t.; Psor.; *Stann.*

Cervical erosion, bleeding easily—Alum.; *Alnus;* Arg. n.; Dictam.; *Hydr.;* Hydrocot.; *Kali bich.*

Debility, weakness—*Alet.; Alum.;* Calc. c.; Carbo an.; *Caul.;* Caust.; Cinch.; *Cocc.;* Con.; Guaco; *Helon.;* Helonin; Hydr.; *Kreos.;* Onosm.; Phos.; *Psor.;* Puls.; Sep.; *Stann.*

Diarrhœa—Puls.

Feeling, as if warm water running—Bor.

Feeling of fulness, heat, relieved by cold water—Acon.

Hæmorrhage, obstinate, intermittent—Kreos.

Hepatic derangement, costiveness—Hydr.

History of abortion—Alet.; Caul.; *Sab.;* Sep.

Hysterical spasm in uterus and abdomen—Mag. m.

Mental symptoms—Murex.

Moth spots on forehead—Caul.; Sep.

Metorrhagia following—Mag. m.

Pruritus vulvæ—Agar.; Alum.; *Ambra; Anac.;* Calc. c.; *Fagop.; Helon.;* Hydr.; Kreos.; Merc.; *Sep.;* Sul.

Relaxation of genitals—Agn.; *Caul.;* Sec.; Sep.

Spasmodic contraction of vagina—Aur. m. n.

Urinary irritation—Berb. v.; *Erig.;* Kreos.; Sep.

MAMMAE—**Abscess:** Bry.; Crot. t.; Graph.; *Hep.; Phos.;* Phyt.; *Sil.;* Sul. See Mastitis.

Atrophy—Chimaph.; *Con.; Iod.;* Kali iod.; Nit. ac.; Onosm.; *Sabal.*

Cancer—*Arg. n.;* Ars. iod.; *Ars.; Aster.;* Bad.; Bapt.; Bar. iod.; Brom.; Bry.; Calc. iod.; *Carbo an.;* Carcinos.; Cic.; Clem.; *Condur.; Con.; Galium;* Graph.; Hep.; Hoang nan.; *Hydr.; Kali iod.;* Kreos.; Lach.;

FEMALE SEXUAL SYSTEM

Phos.; *Plumb. iod.;* Psor.; Sang.; *Scirrhin.;* Semperv. t.; Sil.; Sul.; Tar. c.; *Thuya.* See Tumors.

Cancer, bleeding—Hoang nan.; Kreos.; Lach.; *Phos.;* Sang.; Thuya.

Cancer, scirrhous—Ars.; Carbo an.; Condur.; *Con.;* Hydr.; Kreos.; Lapis alb.; Phyt.; *Scirrhin.; Sil.*

Induration, hardness—Alumen; Ananth.; *Aster.;* Bar. iod.; Bell.; *Bry.;* Bufo; *Calc. fl.; Carbo an.;* Carbo v.; Cham.; Cistus; Clem.; *Con.; Graph.; Iod.;* Kreos.; Lac c.; *Lapis alb.;* Merc.; Nit. ac.; *Phyt.; Plumb. iod.; Plumb. m.*

Inflammation (mastitis)—*Acon.;* Ant. t.; Apis; Arn.; Ars.; *Bell.; Bry.;* Calc. c.; *Cham.;* Cistus; *Con.; Crot. t.;* Ferr. p.; Galega; Graph.; *Hep.; Lac c.;* Lach.; *Merc.; Phell.; Phos.; Phyt.;* Plant.; *Puls.;* Sabad.; *Sil.;* Sul. See Pain, Swelling.

NIPPLES—Burning, itching: *Agar.;* Arundo; *Ars.;* Castor.; *Crot. t.;* Lyc.; Onosm.; Orig.; Petrol.; Puls.; Sil.; *Sul.*

Cracks, fissures, ulcerations—Ananth.; *Arn.;* Ars.; *Aur. sul.;* Calc. ox.; Calend.; Carbo v.; *Castor.;* Caust.; *Cham.; Condur.; Con.; Crot. t.; Eup. ar.;* Galium; Geran.; *Graph.;* Ham.; Hep.; Hippom.; Merc.; Nit. ac.; *Pæonia; Phell.;* Phos.; *Phyt.; Ratanh.; Sep.; Sil.;* Sul. See Soreness.

Inflamed, tender to touch—*Cham.;* Helon.; *Phyt.*

Retraction—Carbo an.; Hydr.; Lapis alb.; Nux m.; *Sars.;* Sil.

Soreness, tenderness—Apium gr.; *Arn.;* Bor.; Calend.; *Castor.; Cham.;* Cistus; *Con.; Crot. t.; Eup. ar.; Graph.;* Ham.; Helon.; *Hep.;* Hydr.; Lac c.; Med.; Ocimum; Orig.; Paraf.; *Phell.;* Phos.; *Phyt.; Ratanh.;* Sang.; Sil.; Sul.; Zinc.

PAIN IN BREASTS (mastodynia)—Acon.; Allium s.; Apis; Arg. n.; *Aster.;* Aur. sul.; *Bell.;* Brom.; *Bry.; Calc. c.;* Carbo an.; Cham.; *Chimaph.; Cim.; Con.;* Cotyled.; Croc.; *Crot. t.; Hep.;* Hydr.; Hyper.; Lac c.; Lach.; *Lact. ac.; Lapis alb.;* Lepid.; Med.; Merc. per.; *Merc.;* Murex; Nat. m.; Onosm.; Pall.; *Phell.; Phos.; Phyt.; Plumb. iod.;* Plumb. m.; Polyg.; Prun. sp.; Psor.; Puls.; *Sang.;* Sil.; Sumb.; Zinc.

Pain, inframammary—*Cim.;* Puls.; *Ran. b.;* Raph.; Sumb.; Ustil.; Zinc. m.

Pain relieved by supporting heavy mammæ—*Bry.; Lac c.;* Phyt.

Pain worse from jar, toward evening—Lac c.

SWELLING—Allium s.; Ananth.; *Asaf.; Aster.;* Aur. sul.; *Bell.;* Bellis; *Bry.;* Castor.; Dulc.; *Graph.;* Helon.; Lac c.; Merc. per.; *Merc.;* Onosm.; Phos.; *Phyt.;* Psor.; Puls.; Solan. ol.; Urt. See Mastitis.

Tenderness, soreness—Arg. n.; *Aster.; Bell.; Bry.;* Calc. c.; Carbo an.; *Cham.;* Clem.; *Con.;* Dulc.; *Helon.; Hep.;* Iod.; Kali m.; *Lac c.;* Lach.; *Med.;* Merc.; Onosm.; *Phyt.;* Plumb.; Radium; Sabal; Syph. See Pain.

TUMORS, nodosities—Ars. iod.; *Aster.; Bell.;* Berb. aq.; *Brom.;* Bry.; Calend.; Calc. c.; *Calc. fl.; Calc. iod.;* Carbo an.; Cham.; *Chimaph.;* Clem.; Condur.; *Con.;* Ferr. iod.; Gnaph.; *Graph.;* Hekla; *Hydr.; Iod.;* Lach.; Lapis alb.; Lyc.; *Merc. i. fl.;* Murex; Nit. ac.; Phos.;

FEMALE SEXUAL SYSTEM

Phyt.; Plumb. iod.; Psor.; *Puls.;* Sab.; Sang.; *Scirrin.; Scrophul.; Sil.;* Thuya; *Thyr.;* Tub. See Cancer, Swelling, Inflammation.

Ulceration—Aster.; Calend.; Clem.; *Hep.; Merc.;* Pæonia; Phos.; *Phyt.; Sil.*

MASTURBATION—In children, due to pruritus vulvæ: Calad.; *Orig.;* Zinc. m.

MENOPAUSE—Climacteric period; change of life; Remedies in general: Acon.; Agar.; Alet.; *Amyl;* Aquil.; Arg. n.; *Bell.; Bellis;* Bor. ac.; *Cact.;* Calc. ars.; Calc. c.; Caps.; Carbo v.; *Caul.; Cim.;* Cocc.; Coff.; Con.; Cycl.; Ferr.; *Gels.; Glon.;* Graph.; Helon.; *Ign.; Jabor.;* Kali br.; *Kali c.; Kreos.; Lach.;* Mag. c.; *Mancin.; Murex; Nux m.; Nux v.;* Oophor.; Plumb.; *Puls.; Sang.;* Semperv. t.; *Sep.; Sul.;* Sul. ac.; Ther.; *Ustil.;* Val.; Vipera; Viscum; Zinc. v.

Anxiety—Acon.; *Amyl;* Sep.

Breasts enlarged, painful—Sang.

Burning in vertex—*Lach.;* Nux v.; Sang.; *Sul.*

Burning of palms and soles—Sang.; *Sul.*

Congestions—Acon.; *Amyl;* Calc. c.; *Glon.;* Lach.; Sang.; Sep.; *Sul.; Ustil.*

Cough, burning in chest, periodical neuralgia—Sang.

Earache—Sang.

Fainting spells—Cim.; Crotal.; Ferr.; *Glon.; Lach.;* Nux m.; Sep.; *Sul.;* Trill.

Falling of hair—Sep.

Fatigue, persistent tiredness, fagged womb—Bellis.

Fatigue without cause, muscular weakness, chilliness—Calc. c.

Flooding—Aloe; Amyl; Apoc.; *Arg. m.;* Arg. n.; Aur. mur.; Calc. c.; Caps.; *Cim.;* Cinch.; Ferr.; Hydrastinin; Kali br.; Lach.; Med.; Nit. ac.; Plumb.; Sab.; Sanguisorba.; *Sedum;* Sep.; Thlaspi; *Trill.; Ustil.;* Vinca. See Metrorrhagia.

Flushings—Acon.; *Amyl;* Bell.; Bor. ac.; Calc. c.; *Cim.;* Crotal.; Dig.; Ferr.; *Glon.; Ign.; Jabor.;* Kali br.; Kali c.; *Lach.; Mang. ac.;* Niccol. s.; Nux v.; Oophor.; Phos. ac.; Piloc.; *Sang.;* Sedum; Sep.; Stront.; *Sul.;* Sul. ac.; *Sumbul;* Tub.; *Ustil.;* Val.; Ver. v.; Vespa; Vinca; Zinc. v.

Globus hystericus—Amyl; *Lach.;* Val.; Zinc. v.

Headache—*Amyl;* Cact.; *Cim.;* Cinch.; Croc.; *Cyprip.;* Ferr.; *Glon.;* Ign.; Lach.; *Sang.; Sep.;* Stront. c.

Hysterical tendencies—*Ign.;* Val.; Zinc. v.

Inframammary pains—Cim.

Liver disorders—Card. m.

Mental depression or irritability—*Cim.;* Ign.; Kali br.; *Lach.;* Mancin.; Psor.; Val.; Zinc. v.

Nervous erethism—Absinth.; Arg. n.; *Cim.;* Coff.; Dig.; *Ign.;* Kali br.; *Lach.;* Oophor.; *Ther.;* Val.; Zinc. v.

Pains in uterus—Agar.; *Cim.;* Cocc.; Lach.; Puls.; Sep.

Palpitation—*Amyl;* Calc. ars.; Ferr.; Glon.; Kali br.; *Lach.;* Sep.; Trill.; Val.

Perspiration, profuse—Amyl; Bell.; Crotal.; Hep.; *Jabor.*; Lach.; Nux v.; Sep.; Tilia; Val.
Pruritus—Calad.
Salivation—Jabor.
Sexual excitement—Mancin.; *Murex*.
Sinking at stomach—Cim.; Crotal.; Dig.; Hydroc. ac.; *Ign.*; *Sep.*; Trill.
Ulcers, superficial, sores, on lower limbs—Polyg.
Vertigo, tinnitus—Glon.; Lach.; Trill.; Ustil.
Weakness—Dig.; Helon.; Lach.; Sep.

MENSTRUATION—TYPE: AMENORRHOEA: Remedies in general:
Acon.; Alet.; Alnus; *Apis*; Apoc.; Ars.; Avena; Bell.; Bry.; *Calc. c.*; Can. s.; *Caul.*; Caust.; *Cim.*; Con.; *Cycl.*; Dulc.; *Euphras.*; Ferr. ars.; *Ferr. m.*; Ferr. red.; Gels.; *Glon.*; Graph.; Hedeoma; *Helleb.*; Helon.; Jonosia; *Kali c.*; *Kali perm.*; Lil. t.; Mang. ac.; *Merc. per.*; *Nat. m.*; Nux v.; Op.; Ova t.; Parth.; Phos. ac.; Pinus lamb.; *Plat.*; Plumb.; *Polyg.*; *Puls.*; Sec.; *Senec.*; *Sep.*; Spong.; *Sul.*; Tanac.; Thyr.; Ustil.; *Xanth*.

Before the proper age—*Calc. c.*; Calc. p.; Carbo v.; Cinch.; Cocc.; *Sab.*; Sil.; Ver. a.

Delayed, first menses—Calc. c.; Calc. p.; Ferr.; Graph.; *Kali c.*; Kali per.; Polyg.; *Puls.*; Senec.; Sep.; Turnera.

Delayed, tardy flow—Acon.; Alet.; *Caust.*; *Cim.*; Con.; Cupr. m.; Dulc; Euphras.; *Ferr. cit. strych.*; Gels.; Glon.; Gossyp.; *Graph.*; Hell o.; Iod.; Jonosia; *Kali c.*; Kali m.; Kali p.; Kali s.; Lac d.; *Mag. c.*; *Nat. m.*; Nux m.; Phos.; Pulex; *Puls.*; Radium; Sabad.; *Senec.*; *Sep.*; *Sul.*; Thasp.; Val.; *Vib. op.*; Zinc.

Intermittent—Coccus; Ferr. m.; Kreos.; *Lac c.*; Mag. s.; *Meli.*; Murex; Nux v.; Phos.; *Puls.*; Sabad.; *Sep.*; Sul.; Xanth.

Irregular—Ambra; Caul.; *Cim.*; *Cocc.*; *Cycl.*; *Graph.*; Iod.; Jonosia; Lil. t.; *Nux m.*; *Nux v.*; Phos.; Piscidia; *Puls.*; Radium; Sec.; Senec.; *Sep.*; Sul.

Protracted—Acon.; Calc. s.; Caust.; *Con.*; Crot.; Cupr. m.; Ferr.; Graph.; Iod.; Kreos.; *Lyc.*; Nat. m.; Nux m.; Nux v.; *Phos.*; Rhus t.

Scanty flow—Alet.; *Alum.*; Apis; Berb. v.; *Bor.*; Canth.; *Caul.*; Caust.; *Cim.*; *Cocc.*; *Con.*; Cycl.; Dulc.; *Euphras.*; Ferr. cit. ctrych.; Gels.; *Graph.*; Ign.; *Kali c.*; *Kali p.*; Kali s.; Lach.; Lamina; Lil t.; *Mag. c.*; Mang. ac.; *Meli.*; Merc. per.; *Nat. m.*; Nux v.; *Ol. an.*; Phos.; Plat.; *Puls.*; Sang.; *Senec.*; *Sep.*; Sil.; *Sul.*; Val.; *Vib. op.*; Xanth. See Dysmenorrhœa.

Suppressed—*Acon.*; Apis; Bell.; *Bry.*; Calc. c.; Ceanoth.; Cham.; Chionanth.; *Cim.*; *Con.*; Croc.; Cupr.; *Cycl.*; *Dulc.*; Ferr.; Gels.; *Glon.*; Graph.; Helon.; Ign.; Kali c.; *Kali m.*; Lach.; Leonorus; Nat. m.; Nux m.; *Op.*; Pod.; *Puls.*; *Puls. nut.*; *Senec.*; Sep.; Sul.; *Tanac.*; Taxus; Tub.; Ver. v.; Zinc.

Suppressed, from anæmic conditions—Ars. iod.; Ars.; Caust.; Ferr. ars.; *Ferr. cit. stry*; Ferr. red.; Graph.; *Kali c.*; Kali perm.; Kali p.; Mag. ac.; Nat. m.; Ova t.; *Puls.*; Senec.

Suppressed from anger with indignation—Cham.; Col.; Staph.

FEMALE SEXUAL SYSTEM

Suppressed, from cold water, exposure, chilling—*Acon.;* Ant. c.; Bell.; Calc. c.; Cham.; Cim.; Con.; Dulc.; Graph.; Lac c.; *Lac d.;* Phos.; Puls.; Rhus t.; Sul.; Ver. v.; Xanth.

Suppressed, from disappointed love—Helleb.

Suppressed, from fright, vexation—Act. sp.; *Acon.;* Cim.; Col.; Lyc.; Op.; Ver. a.

Suppressed, from transient, localized, uterine congestion, followed by chronic anæmic state—Sabai.

Suppressed, in emigrants—Bry.; Plat.

Suppressed, with asthma—Spong.

Suppressed, with cerebral congestion—*Acon.;* Apis; *Bell.;* Bry.; Calc. c. Cim.; *Gels.;* Glon.; Lach.; Psor.; Sep.; Sul.; *Ver. v.*

Suppressed, with congestion to chest—Acon.; Calc. c.; Sep.

Suppressed, with cramps to chest—Cupr. m.

Suppressed, with delirium, mania—Stram.

Suppressed, with dropsy—Apis; Apoc.; Kali c.

Suppressed, with fainting spells, drowsiness—Kali c.; *Nux m.;* Op.

Suppressed, with gastralgia or spasms—Cocc.

Suppressed, with jaundice—Chionanth.

Suppressed, with neuralgic pains about head, face—*Gels.*

Suppressed, with ophthalmia—Puls.

Suppressed, with ovaritis—*Acon.;* Cim.

Suppressed, with pelvic pressure, ovarian tenderness—Ant. c.; Bell.

Suppressed, with pelvic tenesmus—Pod.

Suppressed, with rheumatic pains—Bry.; Cim.; Rhus t.

Suppressed, with vicarious bleeding—*Bry.;* Crot.; Dig.; Erig.; Eupion; Ferr.; *Ham.;* Ipec.; Kali c.; Lach.; Millef.; Nat. s.; *Phos.;* Puls.; Sabad.; Sang.; Senec.; Sil.; Sul.; Trill.; Ustil.

DYSMENORRHŒA—Remedies in general: Acetan.; Acon.; Am. acet.; *Apioline;* Apis; Apium gr.; Aquil.; Atrop.; Avena; *Bell.;* Bor.; Bov.; Brom.; Bry.; *Cact.;* Calc. c.; Canth.; Castoreum; *Caul.; Cham.;* Cim.; Cocc.; *Coff.;* Collins.; *Col.;* Croc.; Cupr. m.; Dulc.; Epiph.; Ferr.; Ferr. p.; *Gels.;* Glon.; *Gnaph.;* Gossyp.; Graph.; *Guaiac.; Ham.;* Helon.; Hyos.; Ign.; *Kali perm.;* Lach.; Lil. t.; *Macrot.; Mag. c.;* Mag. m.; *Mag. p.;* Merc.; Millef.; Morph.; Nux m.; Nux v.; Op.; Plat.; *Puls.;* Rhus t.; Sab.; Sang.; Santon.; *Sec.; Senec.;* Sep.; Stram.; Thyr.; Tub.; Ustil.; *Ver. a.;* Ver. v.; *Vib. op.;* Vib. pr.; *Xanth.;* Zinc.

TYPE—Irregular, every two weeks, or so: Bor.; *Bov.; Calc. c.;* Calc. p.; Croc.; Ferr. p.; *Helon.;* Ign.; Mag. s.; Mez.; Murex; Nit. ac.; Nux v.; Phos. ac.; Phyt.; Sab.; Sec.; Thlaspi; *Trill.;* Ust.

Irregular—Am. c.; *Bell.;* Bry.; *Calc. c.; Caul.;* Cim.; Cocc.; *Cycl.;* Guaiac.; Inula; Mag. s.; Murex; *Nat. m.;* Nux v.; Physost.; *Puls.;* Sec.; Senec.; Sep. See Amenorrhœa.

Membranous—Ars.; Bell.; *Bor.; Brom.;* Bry.; *Calc. acet.;* Calc. c.; Cham.; Collins.; Con.; Cycl.; Guaiac.; Heliotr.; Lac c.; *Mag. p.;* Merc.; Rhus t.; *Sul.;* Ustil.; *Vib. op.*

Nonobstructive, from ovarian irritation—*Apis;* Bell.; Ham.; Xanth.

Nonobstructive, from uterine irritation—*Cham.;* Coff.; Nit. ac.; Xanth.

Premature—Am. c.; *Calc. c.*; Caust.; Cocc.; Con.; Cycl.; Ign.; *Kali c.*; Lamina; Lil. t.; *Mag. p.*; Nat. m.; *Nux v.*; Ol. an.; Phos.; Sab.; Sep.; Sinap. n.; Sil.; *Sul.*; *Xanth.* See Irregular.

Rheumatic—Caul.; Caust.; *Cim.*; Cocc.; Guaiac.; Rham. c.

Spasmodic, neuralgic—Acon.; Agar.; *Bell.*; *Caul.*; Cham.; *Cim.*; Coff.; Collins.; *Gels.*; Glon.; Gnaph.; Mag. m.; *Mag. p.*; *Nux v.*; *Puls.*; Sab.; Santon.; *Sec.*; Senec.; Sep.; Ver. v.; *Vib. op.*; Xanth.

Spasmodic, with uterine congestion—Acon.; *Bell.*; Cim.; Collins.; Gels.; Puls.; *Sab.*; Sep.; Ver. v.

MENORRHAGIA—(**profuse, premature flow**): **Remedies in general:** Achill.; Agar.; *Alet.*; Aloe; Ambra; *Am. c.*; Apoc.; *Aran.*; Arn.; *Ars.*; *Bell.*; Bor.; Bov.; Bry.; *Cact.*; *Calc. c.*; Calc. p.; *Can. ind.*; *Canth.*; Carbo v.; Caul.; Ceanoth.; *Cham.*; Chin. s.; Cim.; *Cinch.*; *Cinnam.*; Collins.; Col.; *Croc.*; *Cycl.*; Dig.; *Erig.*; Ferr. m.; *Ferr. p.*; Ferr. red.; Ficcus; *Geran.*; Glycerin; *Ham.*; *Helon.*; Hydr.; Ign.; Jonosia; *Kali c.*; *Kali m.*; *Kreos.*; Lac c.; Lach.; Led.; Lil. t.; Mag. c.; Mez.; *Millef.*; Murex; *Nit. ac.*; *Nux v.*; Pall.; Paraf.; Phos. ac.; *Phos.*; Phyt.; *Plat.*; *Plumb.*; Ruta; *Sab.*; *Sec.*; Sedum; *Sep.*; Sil.; *Stann.*; Sul. ac.; Sul.; Thlaspi; *Trill.*; Ustil.; Vinca; *Xanth.*

After miscarriage, parturition—Apis; *Cim.*; Cinch.; Helon.; Kali c.; *Nit. ac.*; *Sab.*; Sep.; Sul.; Thlaspi; *Ustil.*; Vib. op.

Every alternate period, profuse—Thlaspi.

Protracted, premature, profuse—*Aloe*; Asar.; *Bell.*; *Calc. c.*; Cal. iod.; Carbo an.; *Cinnam.*; Coff.; Ferr. ac.; Ferr. m.; Fluor. ac.; Glycerin; Grat.; Ign.; Kreos.; *Millef.*; Murex; *Nux v.*; Onosm.; *Plat.*; Raph.; Rhus t.; *Sab.*; Sanguisorba; *Sec.*; Sul.; *Thlaspi*; *Trill.*; Tub.; Xanth.

TYPE OF MENSTRUAL BLOOD—**Acrid, corroding**: Am. c.; Kali c.; Lach.; Mag. c.; Nat. s.; Nit. ac.; *Rhus t.*; Sab.; Sil.; *Sul.*

Bright-red—Acon.; *Bell.*; Brom.; Calc. p.; *Cinnam.*; *Erig.*; Glycerin; Ferr. p.; *Ipec.*; Lac c.; *Millef.*; Sab.; Sang.; *Trill.*; Ustil.

Changeable—Puls.

Coagulated—Am. m.; *Bell.*; Bov.; *Cham.*; Cim.; *Cinch.*; Cocc.; *Coccus;* Coff.; *Croc.*; *Cycl.*; Glycerin; Helon.; Jugl. r.; *Kali m.*; Lil. t.; Mag. m.; Med.; Murex; Nux v.; *Plat.*; Plumb.; *Puls.*; *Sab.*; Sang.; Sul.; *Thlaspi*; Trill.; Ustil.

Dark, blackish—Apis; *Asar.*; Bov.; Calc. p.; Canth.; Caul.; Cham.; *Cim.*, *Cinch.*; Cocc.; *Coccus;* Coff.; *Croc.*; *Cycl.*; Elaps; *Ham.*; Helon.; *Ign.*; Kali m.; *Kali n.*; Kreos.; Lach.; *Lil. t.*; Mag. c.; Mag. m.; Mag. p.; Med.; Nit. ac.; Nux v.; *Plat.*; Plumb.; *Puls.*; Sab.; Sec.; Sep.; *Thlaspi*; Trill.; *Ustil.*; *Xanth.*

Hot—Bell.

Membranous, shreddy, like meat washings—Brom.; *Cycl.*; Ferr. m.; Nat. c.; *Nit. ac.* See Coagulated.

Offensive—*Bell.*; Carbo v.; Cim.; Cop.; Helon.; *Kali c.*; Kali p.; *Lil. t.*; Mag. c.; *Med.*; Plat.; *Psor.*; Pyr.; *Sab.*; Sang.; *Sec.*; Sul.; Vib. op.

Pale—*Alum.*; Ars.; *Carbo v.*; Ferr. m.; *Graph.*; *Kali c.*; Nat. p.; *Puls.*; Sul. See Watery.

Partly fluid, partly clotted—*Ferr.*; Ham.; Plumb.; *Sab.*; Sec.

FEMALE SEXUAL SYSTEM

Pitch-like—Cact.; Cocc.; *Croc.*; Kali m.; *Mag. c.*; Med.; *Plat.*
Stringy, glairy, viscid, thick—Arg. n.; Coccus; *Croc.*; *Kali m.*; Kreos.; Lac c.; Mag. c.; Mag. p.; *Nit. ac.*; Nux m.; *Plat.*; Puls.; Sul.; *Trill.*; *Ust.*; *Xanth.*
Watery, thin—Æth.; Alumen; Eupion; Ferr. ac.; *Ferr. m.*; Gossyp.; Kali p.; Nat. p.; Phos.; *Sab.*; *Sec.*
COMPLAINTS, PRECEDING AND ATTENDING FLOW—**Abdomen distended:** Apoc.; Aran.; Cham.; *Cinch.*; Cocc.; Kali c.; Kreos.; Nux v. See Abdomen.
Abdomen sore—Ham.; Sep. See Abdomen.
Abdomen, weight—Aloe; Bell.; Glycerin; Kali s.; Puls.; *Sep.*
Anus, sore—Ars.; *Mur. ac.* See Anus.
Aphonia—*Gels.*; Graph.
Asthmatic seizures awaken her from sleep—Cupr.; *Iod.*; *Lach.*; Spong.
Axillæ, itching—Sang.
Backache, general bad feelings—Kali c.
Blindness—Cycl.; Puls.
Breasts, icy cold—Med.
Breasts, milk in them, in place of menses—Merc. v.
Breasts, tender, swollen—Bry.; Calc. c.; Canth.; *Con.*; Graph.; *Helon.*; Kali c.; *Lac c.*; Mag. c.; Merc.; *Murex*; *Phyt.*; Puls.; Sang.
Burning in hands and soles—Carbo v.
Catalepsy—Mosch.
Chilliness, coldness—Am. c.; Apis; Calc. c.; Cham.; Glycerin; Graph.; Nux v.; Plat.; *Puls.*; Sec.; Sep.; *Sil.*; Ver. a.
Cholera-like symptoms—*Am. c.*; Bov.; Ver. a.
Colds—Mag. c.; Sep.
Constipation—Am. c.; Collins.; Graph.; Nat. m.; Nux v.; Plat.; *Plumb.*; Sep.; *Sil.*; Sul.
Cough—*Graph.*; Lac c.; *Sul.*
Deafness, tinnitus—Kreos.
Diarrhœa—Am. c.; *Am. m.*; Ars.; Bov.; Cham.; Kreos.; Phos.; Puls.; Ver. a.
Epistaxis—Acon.; Bry.; Dig.; Gels.; Nat. s.; Sep.; Sul.
Eruptions—Allium s.; *Bell.*; Bellis; Calc. c.; *Cim.*; Con.; *Dulc.*; Eug. j.; *Graph.*; *Kali ars.*; Kali c.; Mag. m.; Mang. ac.; *Med.*; Psor.; Sang.; Sars.; Sil.; Thuya; Ver. a.
Eyes, blindness or fiery spots—Cycl.; Sep.
Eyes, burning—Niccol.
Eyes, diplopia—Gels.
Eyes, ophthalmia—Puls.
Face flushed—*Bell.*; Calc. p.; Ferr. m.; *Ferr. p.*; Gels.; *Sang.*
Face pale, eyes sunken—Cycl.; Ipec.; Ver. a.
Feet and cheeks swollen—Apis; Graph.
Feet cold, damp—Calc. c.
Feet, pain in—Am. m.
Feet, swollen—Graph.; Lyc.; Puls.
Flushes of heat—Ferr.; Glon.; *Lach.*; *Sang.*; Sul.
Frenzy—Acon.

FEMALE SEXUAL SYSTEM

Genitals, sensitive—Am. c.; Cocc.; *Lach.;* Kali c.; *Plat.* See Vaginismus.

Headache, congestive symptoms—Aster.; *Bell.;* Bry.; Cim.; Cocc.; Croc.; *Cycl.;* Ferr. m.; Ferr. p.; Gels.; Glon.; Graph.; Kali p.; Kreos.; Lac c.; Lach.; Nat. c.; *Nat. m.; Nux v.;* Puls.; *Sang.; Sep.; Sul.; Ustil.;* Ver. v.; Xanth.

Heart, pain, palpitation, etc.—*Cact.;* Crot.; Eupion; Lach.; *Lith. c.;* Sep.; Spong.

Hoarseness, coryza, sweats—Graph.

Hunger—Spong.

Hysterical symptoms—Caul.; *Cim.;* Gels.; *Ign.; Mag. m.;* Nux v.; Plat.; Puls.; Senec.; Vib. op.

Inflammation of throat, chest, bladder—Senec.

Insomnia—Agar.; Senec.

Irritability—*Cham.;* Cocc.; Eupion; Kreos.; Lil. t.; Lyc.; Mag. m.; *Nux v.*

Joint pains—Caul.; Sab.

Labia burning—Calc. c.

Lachrymation, catarrhal state of eyes, nose—Euphras.

Leucorrhæa—Bar. c.; Bor.; *Calc. c.;* Carbo v.; Caust.; Graph.; Iod.; *Nat. m.;* Puls.

Leucorrhæa, acrid—Lach.; Sep.

Mania, chorea—Cim.

Mania, sexual—Can. ind.; *Dulc.;* Plat.; Stram.; Ver. a.

Morning sickness, nausea, vomiting—*Am. m.;* Bor.; Cocc.; Cycl.; Graph.; Ichth.; *Ipec.;* Kreos.; Meli.; Nat. m.; Nux v.; Puls.; Sep.; Thlaspi; Ver. a.

Mouth sore, swelling of gums, cheeks; bleeding ulcer—Phos.

Mouth, tongue, throat dry, especially during sleep—Nux m.; Tar. h.

Nervous disturbance, restlessness—Acon.; *Cham.;* Caul.; *Cim.;* Ign.; Kreos.; *Lach.;* Mag. m.; *Mag. p.;* Nit. ac.; Puls.; *Salix n.;* Senec.; Sep.; Trill.; Vib. op.; Xanth.

Nipples and breasts icy cold—Med.

Old symptoms aggravated—Nux v.

Pain, burning in left ovarian region, on motion—Croc.; *Thuya;* Ustil.

Pain, colicky, labor-like, spasmodic—*Alet.;* Aloe; *Am. c.;* Am. m.; Apis; *Bell.;* Bor.; *Bov.;* Brom.; Calc. c.; *Caul.; Cham.;* Cim.; Cinch.; Cocc.; *Coff.;* Col.; Cupr. m.; *Cycl.;* Ferr. m.; Ferr. p.; Gels.; Graph.; Helon. Hematox; Ign.; Jonosia; Kali c.; Kreos.; Lil. t.; *Mag. c.; Mag. m.; Mag. p.;* Med.; Meli.; Nat. m.; Nit. ac.; Nux m.; *Nux v.;* Plat.; Puls.; Sab.; Sec.; Sep.; Stann.; Thlaspi; *Ver. a.;* Ver. v.; Vespa; Vib. op.; Xanth.

Pain, extending around pelvis, from sacrum to groin—Plat.; Puls.; Sep.; Vib. op.

Pain extending down hips, thighs, legs—*Am. m.;* Berb. v.; Bry.; Castor.; *Caul.;* Cham.; *Cim.;* Coff.; Col.; Con.; *Gels.;* Graph.; Lil. t.; Mag. c.; Mag. m.; Nit. ac.; Plat.; Sep.; Trill.; *Vib. op.;* Xanth.

Pain, extending through pelvis antero-posteriorly or laterally—Bell.

Pain, extending to back (sacrum, coccyx)—*Am. c.;* Am. m.; Asar.; Bell.; Bor.; Calc. c.; *Calc. p.;* Caust.; *Cham.;* Cic.; *Cim.;* Cupr. m.; Cycl.; *Gels.;* Graph.; *Helon.; Kali c.;* Kreos.; Mag. m.; Nit. ac.; *Nux v.*

Phos.; Plat.; Pod : *Puls.*; Radium; Sab.; *Senec.*; *Sep.*; Spong.; Vib. op.; *Xanth.*

Pain, extending to chest—Caul.; Cham.; Cim.; *Cupr. m.*

Pain, extending to groins—Bor.; *Caul.*; Kali c.; Lil. t.; Plat.; **Tanac.**; *Ustil.*

Pain, extending to liver—Phos. ac.

Pain, extending to pubes—Alnus; Bov.; Col.; Cycl.; Radium; *Sab.*; Sep.: Vib. op.

Pain, extending to rectum—*Aloe;* Xerophyl.

Pain in feet—Am. m.

Pain in malar bones—Stann.

Pain in ovaries—*Apis;* Bell.; Bry.; Cact.; Canth.; *Cim.*; Col.; Ham.; Iod.; Jonosia; Kali n.; *Lach.; Lil. t.;* Picr. ac.; Salix n.; Tar. h.; *Thuya;* Vib. op.

Pruritus—Calc. c.; *Graph.;* Hep.; Inula; Kali c.; *Sil.;* Sul.

Rectal and vesical irritation—Sab.

Sadness—Am. c.; Aur.; Brom.; Caust.; *Cim.;* Cocc.; Ferr.; Helleb.; Helon.; *Ign.;* Lyc.; Nat. c.; *Nat. m.*: Nit. ac.; Phos.; Plat.; *Puls.;* Sep.; Stann.; Vespa.

Salivation—Pulex.

Sexual excitement—Plat.

Sore throat—Canth.; *Lac c.;* Mag. c.

Spasms—Artem.; *Bufo;* Calc. s.; Caul.; *Cim.;* Cupr. m.; Gels.; *Hyos.; Ign.;* Kali br.; Lach.; Mag. m.; Œnanthe; *Plat.;* Tar. h.

Stomach disturbances—Arg. n.; Ars.; Bry.; Kali c.; Lach.; *Lyc.;* Nux m.; *Nux v.;* Puls.; Sep.; Sul.

Stretching, yawning—Am. c.; Puls.

Syncope—Ars.; Cinch.; Ign.; *Mosch.;* Nux m.; *Nux v.;* Ver. a.

Tinnitus—*Ferr.;* Kreos.

Toothache—Am. c.; Calc. c.; Cham.; Mag. c.; *Puls.;* Sep.

Urinary symptoms—Calc. p.; *Canth.;* Coccus; *Gels.;* Hyos.; Mag. p.; Med.; Nux v.; Plat.; Pulex; Puls.; *Senec.;* Sep.; Ver. v.; Vib. op.

Vertigo—Calc. c.; Cycl.; Nux v.

Weakness—*Alum.;* Am. c.; Carbo an.; *Cinch.;* Cocc.; Ferr. m.; Glycerin; Graph.; *Helon.;* Hematox.; Ign.; Iod.; Niccol.; Puls.; *Ver. a.*

COMPLAINTS FOLLOWING MENSES—**Diarrhœa**: Graph.; Puls.

Erethism, neuralgic pains, inframammary pains, insomnia—Cim.

Eruption—Kreos.

Headache—Croc.; Lach.; Lil. t.; Puls.; Sep.

Headache, throbbing, with sore eyes—Nat. m.

Hemorrhoids—Cocc.

Hysterical symptoms—Ferr. m.

Leucorrhœa—Æsc.; Alum.; Graph.; *Kreos.:* Nit. ac. See **Leucorrhœa.**

Mammæ swollen, milky secretion—Cycl.

Old symptoms aggravated—Nux v.

Ovarian pain—Zinc. m.

Pains (intermenstrual)—*Bry.;* Ham.; Iod.; Kreos.; *Sep.*

Pruritus—Con.; Lyc.; *Tar. h.*

FEMALE SEXUAL SYSTEM

Show occasional, every few days—Bor.; Bov.

Vomiting—Croc.

Weakness, profound—*Alum.*; Am. c.; Am. m.; *Ars.*; Calc. c.; *Carbo an.*; Carbo v.; Cim.; *Cinch.*; *Cocc.*; Ferr.; Glycerin; Graph.; Iod.; Ipec.; Kali c.; Mag. c.; Phos.; Thlaspi; *Trill.*; *Ver. a.*; Vinca.

MODALITIES—AGGRAVATION: At night: Am. c.; *Am. m.*; Bor.; Bov.; Coccus; *Mag. c.*; Mag. m.; Zinc.

During flow—*Cim.*; Ham.; Kreos.; *Puls.*; *Tub.*

From excitement—*Calc. c.*; *Sul.*; Tub.

From lying down, rest—Am. c.; Am. m.; Bov.; Cycl.; Kreos.; Mag. c.; Zinc.

From motion—Bov.; Bry.; Canth.; Caust.; Erig.; *Lil. t.*; Mag. p.; *Sab.*; Sec.; Thlaspi; *Trill.*

From sleep—Mag. c

In morning, daytime—Bor.; Cact.; Carbo an.; *Caust.*; Cycl.; *Lil. t.*; Puls.; Sep.

AMELIORATION—From establishment of flow: Aster.; Cereum ox.; Cycl.; Eupion; *Lach.*; Mag. p.; Senec.; Zinc.

From cold drinks—Kreos.

From hot applications—Mag. p.

From lying down—Bov.; Cact.; Caust.; Lil. t.

From motion—Am. m.; *Cycl.*; Kreos.; *Mag. c.*; Sab.

NYMPHOMANIA—Ambra; Aster.; Bar. mur.; Calc. p.; Camph.; *Canth.*; Coca; Dulc.; *Ferrula gl.*; Fluor. ac.; *Grat.*; *Hyos.*; Kali br.; Lach.; Lil. t.; *Murex*; Orig.; Phos.; Plat.; Raph.; *Robin.*; Salix n.; Stram.; Strych.; *Tar. h.*; Val.; *Ver. a.*

OVARIES—Abscess: Cinch.; *Hep.*; Lach.; *Merc.*; Phos. ac.; Pyr.; Sil.

Atrophy—*Iod.*; Oophor.; Orchit.

Complaints attending, or following, ovariotomy—Ars.; *Bell.*; *Bry.*; Cinch.; Coff.; *Col.*; Hyper.; Ipec.; Lyc.; Naja; Nux v.; *Oophor.*; Orchit.; Staph.

Congestion—Acon.; Æsc.; Aloe; Am. br.; *Apis*; Arg. n.; *Bell.*; Bry.; Canth.; *Cim.*; Col.; Con.; *Gels.*; Ham.; Iod.; *Lil. t.*; Merc.; Naja; *Nat. chlor.*; Sep.; Tar. h.; Ustil.; *Vib. op.* See Inflammation.

CYSTS, DROPSY—*Apis*; Apoc.; Arn.; Ars.; *Aur. iod.*; Aur. m. n.; Bell.; Bov.; Bry.; Cinch.; *Col.*; Con.; Ferr. iod.; Graph.; *Iod.*; Kali br.; Lach.; Lil. t.; *Lyc.*; Med.; Oophor.; Rhod.; Sab.; Tereb.; Zinc.

Induration—Aur.; Aur. m. n.; Carbo an.; *Con.*; Graph.; *Iod.*; Lach.; Pall.; Plat.; Ustil.

Inflammation (ovaritis)–Acute: Acon.; Am. br.; *Apis*; *Bell.*; *Bry.*; Cact.; *Canth.*; *Cim.*; *Col.*; Con.; Ferr. p.; Guaiac.; *Ham.*; Iod.; *Lach.*; Lil. t.; *Merc. c.*; Merc.; Phos. ac.; Plat.; *Puls.*; Sab.; Thuya; Viscum.

Acute, with peritoneal involvement—*Acon.*; Apis; Ars.; *Bell.*; Bry.; Canth.; Chin. s.; Cinch.; Col.; *Hep.*; *Merc. c.*; Sil.

Inflammation, chronic, with induration—*Con.*; Graph.; *Iod.*; Lach.; Pall.; Plat.; Sabal; Sep.; *Thuya.*

FEMALE SEXUAL SYSTEM

PAIN—Boring: *Col.*; Zinc. m.

Burning—*Apis*; Ars.; Bufo; Canth.; Con.; Eupion; *Fagop.*; Kali n.; Lil. t.; Plat.; Thuya; Ustil.; Zinc. *x*.

Crampy, constrictive—*Cact.*; Col.; Naja.

Cutting, darting, tearing—Absinth.; Acon.; *Bell.*; *Bry.*; Caps.; *Col.*; Con.; Croc.; *Lil. t.*; Naja; Puls.

Cutting, extending to thighs, legs—*Bry.*; Cim.; Croc.; Lil. t.; Phos.; Pod.; Wyeth.; *Xanth.*; Zinc. v.

Dull, constant—Aur. br.; Hydrocot.; Niccol.; Sep.

Dull, numb, aching—Pod.

Dull, wedge-like in uterus—Iod.

Neuralgic (ovaralgia)—Am. br.; *Apis*; Apium gr.; *Atrop.*; *Bell.*; Berb. v.; Bry.; *Cact.*; Canth.; *Caul.*; *Cim.*; *Col.*; *Con.*; Ferr.; Ferr. p.; *Gels.*; Gossyp.; Graph.; Ham.; Hyper.; Kali br.; *Lach.*; *Lil. t.*; *Mag. p.*; Meli; Merc. c.; Merc.; *Naja*; Phyt.; *Plat.*; Pod.; Puls.; *Sabal*; Salix n.; Sumb.; *Staph.*; Thea; Ustil.; *Vib. op.*; Xanth.; *Zinc. v.*

Neuralgic, intermittent—*Gossyp.*; Thaspium; Zizia.

Stinging—*Apis*; Canth.; Con.; Lil. t.; Merc.

Throbbing—Bell.; Brachygl.; Branca; *Cact.*; Hep.

Pain, in left ovary—Am. br.; Apis; Apium gr.; *Arg. m.*; Caps.; Carb. ac.; *Cim.*; *Col.*; Erig.; Eup. purp.; Frax. am.; Graph.; Iod.; *Lach.*; *Lil. t.*; Med.; Murex; *Naja*; Ov. g. pell.; Phos.; Picr. ac.; Thaspium; Thea; *Thuya*; Ustil.; *Vespa*; Wyeth.; *Xanth.*; Zinc.

Pain, in right ovary—Absinth.; *Apis*; Ars.; *Bell.*; Branca; Bry.; Col.; Eupion; Fagop.; Graph.; Iod.; Lach.; Lil. t.; *Lyc.*; *Pall.*; Phyt.; Pod.; Ustil.

Pain, with aggravation, from deep breathing—Bry.

Pain, with aggravation, from walking, riding, relieved by lying down—Carb. ac.; Pod.; Sep.; *Thuya*; Ustil.

Pain, with frequent urination—Vespa.

Pain, with numbness, shifting gases in ascending colon—Pod.

Pain, with relief, by drawing up leg—Apium gr.; Col.

Pain, with relief by flow—Lach.; Zinc. m.

Pain, with relief from pressure, tight bandage—Col.

Pain, with restlessness, can't keep still—Kali br.; Vib. op.; *Zinc*.

Pain, with sympathetic heart symptoms—Cim.; *Lil. t.*; Naja.

Swelling—Am. br.; Apis; Bell.; Brom.; Graph.; Ham.; *Lach.*; Pall.; Tar. h.; Ustil. See Congestion, Inflammation.

Tenderness, to touch, motion—Ant. c.; Apis; Bell.; Bry.; Canth.; Carbo an.; *Cim.*; Ham.; Hep.; Iod.; *Lach.*; Lil. t.; *Plat.*; Sabal; Tar. h.; Thea; Thuya; Ustil.; Zinc. v.

Traumatic conditions—Arn.; Ham.; Psor.

Tumors—*Apis*; Aur. m. n.; Bov.; Col.; Con.; Graph.; *Iod.*; Kali br.; Lach.; Oophor.; Pod.; *Sec.* See Cysts.

PELVIC—Abscess: Apis; Calc. c.; Hep.; Merc. c.; Pall.; Sil.

Pelvic cellulitis—Acon.; *Apis*; Ars.; Bell.; Bry.; Calc. c.; Canth.; *Cim.*; Hep.; Med.; *Merc. i. r.*; Merc. s.; Pyr.; *Rhus t.*; Sil.; Tereb.; Tilia; Ver. v.

842   FEMALE SEXUAL SYSTEM

Pelvic hæmatocele—Acon.; Apis; *Arn.*; Ars.; Bell.; Canth.; Cinch.; Col.; Dig.; *Ferr.*; *Ham.*; Ipec.; *Kali iod.*; Lach.; *Merc.*; Millef.; Nit. ac.; Phos.; Sab.; Sec.; Sul.; Tereb.; Thlaspi.

Pelvic peritonitis—*Acon.*; *Apis*; Arn.; Ars.; *Bell.*; *Bry.*; *Canth.*; Chin. s.; Cim.; Cinch.; *Col.*; Gels.; *Hep.*; Hyos.; *Lach.*; *Merc. c.*; Op.; Pall.; Rhus t.; Sab.; Sec.; *Sil.*; Tereb.; Ver. v. See Cellulitis, Metritis.

Pelvic peritonitis, with menorrhagia—Ars.; Ham.; Sab.; Thlaspi.

PREGNANCY AND LABOR—ABORTION: Remedies in general: Acon.; *Alet.*; Arn.; Bell.; Calc. fl.; *Caul.*; Cham.; *Cim.*; Cinnam.; Cinch.; Coff.; Croc.; Gossyp.; *Helon.*; Hyos.; Ipec.; *Kali c.*; Millef.; Nit. ac.; Nux v.; Op.; *Pinus lamb.*; Pyr.; Rhus t.; *Sab.*; *Sec.*; *Sep.*; Tanac.; Thlaspi; Trill.; *Vib. op.*

Abortion from debility—*Alet.*; Caul.; Chin. s.; Cinch.; *Helon.*; Sec.

From fatty degeneration of placenta—Phos.

From fright, emotions—*Acon.*; Cham.; Cim.; Op.

From mental depression, shock, watching, low fever—Bapt.

From ovarian disease—Apis.

From syphilitic taint—Aur.; Kali iod.; Merc. c.

From traumatism—Arn.; Cinnam.

With blood dark, fluid; formication—Sec.

With blood intermittent, pains spasmodic, excites suffocation, fainting; craves fresh air—Puls.

With blood light, fluid; painless—Millef.

With hæmorrhage persisting—Nit. ac.; Thlaspi.

With pains, frequent, labor-like; no discharge—Sec.

With pains, from small of back, around to abdomen, ending in crampy, squeezing, bearing down, tearing down thighs—Vib. op.

With pains, from small of back, to pubes, worse from motion; blood partly clotted—Sab.

With pains from small of back to thighs; weak back; pains worse from motion; also subsequent debility and sweat—Kali c.

With pains, flying across abdomen, doubling her up; chills; pricking in breasts; pains in loins—Cim.

With pains, irregular, feeble, tormenting; scanty flow, or long continued, passive oozing; backache, weakness, internal trembling—Caul.

With retained secundines—Cinch.; Pyr.

With septicæmia—Pyr.

With sequelæ—Kali c.; Sab.; Sul.

Tendency to abort—*Alet.*; Apis; Aur.; Bac.; Calc. c.; *Caul.*; *Cim.*; *Helon*; Kali c.; Kali iod.; Merc. c.; Merc.; Plumb.; Puls.; *Sab.*; *Sec.*; *Sep.*; Sil.; Sul.; Syph.; *Vib. op.*; *Vib. pr.*; Zinc. m.

Tendency to abort at second or third month—*Cim.*; Kali c.; Sab.; Sec.; Vib. op.

Threatened—*Acon.*; Arn.; *Bapt.*; Bell.; *Caul.*; Cham.; Cim.; Cinch.; Coff.; Croc.; Eup. purp.; Ferr. m.; *Helon.*; Millef.; Plumb. m.; Puls.; Sab.; Sec.; Trill.; *Vib. op.*; Vib. pr.

COMPLAINTS DURING PREGNANCY—Abdomen, must lie on, during early months: Acet. ac.; Pod.

FEMALE SEXUAL SYSTEM

Acne—*Bell.;* Sab.; Sep. See Skin.
Albuminuria—*Apis;* Ars.; Aur. mur.; *Cupr. ars.;* Gels.; Glon.; *Helon.;* Indium; *Kali chlor.;* Kal.; *Merc. c.;* Phos.; Sab.; Thlaspi; Thyr.; Ver. v. See Kidneys (Urinary System).
Arms hot, sore, painful—Zing.
Backache—*Æsc.;* Kali c. See Locomotor System.
Bilious complications—Chel.
Bladder disturbances, tenesmus—*Bell.;* Canth.; *Caust.;* Equis.; Ferr.; Nux v.; Pop. tr.; *Puls.;* Staph.
Breasts, painful, inflammatory—*Bell.;* Bry.
Breasts, painful, neuralgic—*Con.;* Puls.
Congestion of brain—*Glon.* See Head.
Constipation—Alum.; *Collins.;* Lyc.; Nux v.; Op.; *Plat.;* Plumb., Sep. See Abdomen.
Convulsions, spasms—Amyl; Cupr. m.; *Glon.;* Hyos.; Lyssin; Œnanthe. See Nervous System.
Cough—Acon.; *Apoc.;* Bell.; Bry.; *Cham.;* Caust.; *Con.;* Coral.; *Dros.;* Glon.; *Hyos.;* Kali br.; Ipec.; Nux v.; Vib. op.
Cramps, in calves—Cham.; *Cupr.;* Mag. p.; Nux v.; Ver. a.
Cravings, abnormal—*Alum.;* Calc. c.; Carbo v.; *Sep.* See Stomach.
Diarrhœa—Ferr. m.; Helleb.; Nux m.; Petrol.; Phos. ac.; *Puls.;* Sec.; Sul.
Discharge bloody—Erig.; Kali c.; Phos.; Rhus t. See Abortion.
Dyspepsia (heartburn, acidity)—Acet. ac.; Anac.; Calc. c.; Canth.; Caps.; Diosc.; *Nux v.;* Puls. See Stomach.
Dyspnœa—Apoc.; Lyc.; Nux v.; Puls.; *Viola od.* See Respiratory System.
False pregnancy—*Caul.;* Croc.; Nux v.; *Thuya.*
Gastralgia—Petrol.
Goitre—Hydr.
Hæmorrhoids—Collins.; Pod.; Sul. See Abdomen.
Herpes—Sep.
Hiccough—Cycl. See Stomach.
Insanity—Hyos. See Mind.
Mental symptoms—*Acon.;* Cham.; *Cim.;* Puls. See Mind.
Metrorrhagia—Cinch.; Cinnam.; Ipec.; Nit. ac.; Sec.; Trill. See Uterus.
Morning sickness (nausea, vomiting)—Acet. ac.; Acon.; Alet.; *Amyg. pers.;* Anac.; Ant. t.; *Apomorph.;* Arg. n.; *Ars.;* Bry.; Carb. ac.; *Cereum ox.; Cim.;* Cocc.; Colch.; *Cucurb.;* Cupr. ae.; Cycl.; Gnaph.; *Gossyp.;* Ingluv.; *Ipec.;* Iris; Kali m.; *Kreos.;* Lac d.; Lact. ac.; *Lob. infl.;* Mag. c.; Merc.; Nat. p.; Nux m.; *Nux v.;* Petrol.; Phos.; Piloc.; Psor.; *Puls.;* Sep.; Staph.; *Symphor.;* Tab.; Ther.; *Thyr.* See Stomach.
Mouth, sore—Hydr.; Sinap. a. See Mouth.
Nervous sensitiveness, extreme—Acon.; Asar.; Cim.; *Ther.*
Pain, false labor—*Caul.;* Cham.; *Cim.;* Gels.; *Puls.;* Sec.
Pain in abdomen, as if strained, left side—Am. m.
Pain, in lumbar region, dragging, distressful—Arn.; *Bell.; Kali c.;* Nux v.; Puls.; Rhus t.
Pain, rheumatic—Acon.; Alet.; *Cim.;* Op.; Rhus t.
Plethora—Acon.

844 FEMALE SEXUAL SYSTEM

Pruritus, vulvæ et vaginæ—Acon.; *Ambra;* Ant. c.; Bor.; *Calad.; Collins.;* Ichth.; *Sep.;* Tab. See Vulva.

Retinitis—Gels.

Salivation—Acet. ac.; Ars.; *Iod.; Jabor.;* Kreos.; Lact. ac.; *Merc. s.;* Nat. m.; *Piloc.;* Sul.

Sexual excitement—Plat. See Nymphomania.

Sleeplessness—*Acon.;* Cim.; *Coff.;* Nux v.; Puls.; Sul.

Toothache—Acon.; Bell.; *Calc. fl.; Cham.;* Coff.; *Kreos.; Mag. c.;* Nux v.; Ratanh.; Sep.; *Staph.;* Tab.

Toxæmic conditions—Kali chlor.

Uterine and abdominal soreness—Ham.; Puls.

Varicose veins—Arn.; Bellis; Calc. c.; Carbo v.; Ham.; Lyc.; Millef.; Sul.; Zinc. m.

Vertigo—Bell.; Cocc.; Nux v.

Weariness in limbs, cannot walk—Bellis.

PARTURITION—LABOR: CONVULSIONS (eclampsia): Acon.; Æth.; Amyl; Arn.; *Bell.;* Canth.; Cham.; *Chloral;* Cic.; Cim.; Coff.; *Cupr. ars.;* Cupr. m.; Gels.; Glon.; *Hydroc. ac.; Hyos.;* Ign.; Ipec.; Kali br.; Merc. c.; Merc. d.; *Œnanthe;* Op.; Piloc.; Plat.; Solan. n.; Spiræa; Stram.; *Ver. v.;* Zinc. m.

PAINS—Backache violent, wants it pressed—Caust.; *Kali c.*

Excessive—Bell.; Coff.

False labor pains—Bell.; Cham.; *Caul.; Cim.;* Gels.; Nux v.; *Puls.;* Sec.; Vib. op.

Hour glass contraction—Bell.; Sec.

Labor delayed—Kali p.; Pituitrin.

Labor premature—Sab.

Needle-like prickings in cervix—Caul.

Shifting, across abdomen, doubling her up; pricking in mammæ; shivers during first stage—Cim.

Shifting, all over, exhaustion; fretful; shivering—Caul.

Shifting, from back to rectum, with urging to stool, or urination—Nux v.

Shifting, from loins down legs—Aloe; *Bufo;* Carbo v.; Caul.; Cham.; *Nux v.*

Shifting upwards—*Cham.;* Gels.

Spasmodic, irregular, intermittent, ineffectual, fleeting—Arn.; Artem.; *Bell.;* Bor.; *Caul.;* Caust.; *Cham.;* Chloral; *Cim.;* Cinnam.; *Cinch.;* Coff.; *Gels.;* Kali c.; Kali p.; Nat. m.; *Nux v.;* Op.; Pituitrin; *Puls.;* Sacchar. of.; Sec.

With dyspnœa from constriction of middle of chest arresting pains—Lob. infl.

With hypersensitiveness to pain—*Acon.;* Bell.; *Caul.;* Caust.; *Cham.; Cim.;* Cinch.; *Coff.; Gels.;* Hyos.; Ign.; *Nux v.;* Puls.

With relief from pressure in back—Caust.; *Kali c.*

With syncope—Cim.; Nux v.; Puls.; Sec.

PLACENTA—Retained: Arn.; Canth.; Caul.; Cim.; Cinch.; Ergotin; Gossyp.; *Hydr.; Ign.;* Puls.; Sab.; Sec.; Viscum.

RIGID OS—Acon.; *Bell.; Caul.;* Cham.; Cim.; *Gels.;* Lob. infl.; *Ver. v.*

FEMALE SEXUAL SYSTEM

PUERPERIUM—(Lying-in period): After-pains: *Acon.;* Amyl; *Arn.; Bell.;* Calc. c.; *Caul.;* Carbo v.; *Cham.; Cim.;* Cocc.; *Coff.;* Cupr. ars.; Cupr. m.; *Gels.;* Ign.; Kali c.; Lach.; Nux v.; *Puls.;* Pyr.; Rhus t.; *Sab.; Sec.;* Sep.; Vib. op.; *Vib. pr.; Xanth.*

After pains, across lower abdomen, into groins—Caul.; Cim.

After pains, extending into shins—Carbo v.; Cocc.

After pains severe, distressing, in calves and soles—Cupr. m.

Backache, debility, sweat—Kali c.

Complications prevented—*Arn.;* Calend.

Constipation—*Bry.; Collins.;* Nux v.; Ver. a.; Zinc. m.

Diarrhœa—*Cham.;* Hyos.; Puls.

Hemorrhage (flooding, post-partum)—*Acet. ac.;* Am. m.; Amyl; Arn.; Ars.; *Bell.;* Caul.; Cham.; *Cinch.; Cinnam.;* Croc.; Cycl.; Ferr.; Geran.; *Ham.;* Hyos.; Ign.; *Ipec.;* Kali c.; *Millef.;* Nit. ac.; Puls.; *Sab.; Sec.;* Trill.; Ustil.

With bright red fluid; painless flow—Millef.

With bright red, hot, profuse flow in gushes—Bell.

With bright red, hot, profuse flow; collapsic symptoms—Ipec.

With collicky, bearing-down pains, relieved by gush of blood—Cycl.

With dark, thick, paroxysmal flow; debility—Cinch.

With habitual tendency; profuse, dark, clotted—Trill.

With pain from back to pubes; dark, clotted, painless flow—Sab.

With passive, dark, fluid blood, worse from motion; thin females; relaxed uterus; formication—Sec.

With uterine inertia—Am. m.; Caul.; Puls.; Sec.

Hæmorrhoids—Acon.; *Aloe;* Bell.; Ign.; Puls.

LOCHIA—Acrid: Bapt.; Kreos.; *Nit. ac.;* Pyr.

Lochia bloody—Chrom. ac.; *Trill.*

Lochia bloody, dark—Caul.; Cham.; Kreos.; Nit. ac.; Pyr.; *Sec.*

Lochia bloody, in gushes, worse from motion—Erig.

Lochia hot, scanty—Bell.

Lochia intermittent—Con.; Kreos.; Pyr.; Rhus t.; Sul.

Lochia offensive—Bapt.; *Bell.;* Carb. ac.; *Carbo an.;* Carbo v.; Chrom. ac.; Crot. t.; Erig.; *Kreos.;* Nit. ac.; Pyr.; Rhus t.; *Sec.;* Sep.; Sul.

Lochia prolonged—Calc. c.; *Caul.;* Cinch.; Helon.; Millef.; Rhus t.; Sab.; *Sec.;* Trill.; *Ustil.*

Lochia scanty—Bell.; Cham.; Puls.

Lochia suppressed—*Acon.;* Aral.; Bell.; *Bry.;* Cham.; Echin.; Hyos.; Leonorus; Op.; Puls.; Pyr.; *Sec.; Sul.;* Zinc.

Nymphomania—Cinch.; *Plat.;* Ver. a.

Panaritium—Cepa.

Prolapsus recti—Ruta. See Abdomen.

Puerperal cellulitis—Hep.; *Rhus t.;* Ver. v.

Puerperal fever (milk fever)—Acon.; Bry.; *Calc. c.;* Cham.

Puerperal fever, septic (septicæmia)—*Acon.;* Ail.; Arn.; Ars.; Bapt.; *Bell.;* Bry.; Calc. c.; *Carb. ac.;* Canth.; Cham.; *Chin. s.;* Cim.; Crot.; Echin.; *Hydroc. ac.;* Hyos.; Kali c.; Kali p.; Lach.; Lyc.; *Merc. c.;* Merc. s.; Nux v.; *Puls.; Pyr.;* Rhus t.; Sec.; Sep.; Tereb.; *Ver. v.* See Pyæmia (Generalities).

Puerperal mania—Bell.; *Can. ind.*; Cim.; *Hyos.*; Pla..; Senec.; *Stram.*; Ver. v.; Zinc. See Mind.
Puerperal melancholia—*Agn.*; Aur.; *Cim.*; Plat.; Puls. See Mind.
Puerperal metritis—Bell.; *Canth.*; Lach.; Nux v.; Tilia. See Uterus.
Puerperal peritonitis—Acon.; *Bell.*; Bry.; Merc. c.; Pyr.; Sul.; Tereb. See Abdomen.
Puerperal phlebitis after forceps delivery—Cepa.
Puerperal tympany—Tereb.
Sweating—Cham.; Samb.; Stram.
Urinary incontinence—Arn.; Bell.; Caust.; Hyos.; Trill.
Urinary retention, suppression—Acon.; Arn.; *Bell.*; Equis.; *Hyos.*; Op.; Staph.; Stram.

COMPLAINTS AFTER PUERPERIUM—Acne on chin: Sep.
Constipation—Lil. t.; *Lyc.*; Mez.; Ver. a. See Abdomen.
Hair falls out—Carbo v.; Nat. m.; *Sep.*
Hæmorrhoids—Ham. See Abdomen.

LACTATION—Discharge from vagina, bloody during nursing: Sil.
Excitement, sexual, during nursing—Calc. p.
Menses during—Calc. c.; Pall.
Milk, absent, or scanty, tardy (agalactea)—Acon.; *Agn.*; *Asaf.*; Bry.; *Calc. c.*; Caust.; Cham.; Chel.; Formica; Fragar.; *Lac c.*; Lac d.; *Phos. ac.*; Phos.; Phyt.; Piloc.; *Puls.*; *Ricinus*; Sec.; *Sil.*; Sticta; *Thyr.*; Urt.; X-ray.
Milk, bloody—Bufo.
Milk, bluish, transparent, sour, impoverished, or faulty, so child rejects it—Acet. ac.; Calc. c.; *Calc. p.*; Merc.; *Phos. ac.*; Sabal; *Sil.*; Sul.
Milk suppressed—*Acon.*; Agn.; Bell.; *Bry.*; Camph. monobr.; Cham.; Phyt.; *Puls.*; Sec.; Zinc. m.
Milk, too profuse (galactorrhœa)—Bell.; Bor.; *Calc. c.*; Cham.; Chimaph.; Con.; Erig.; Iod.; Lac c.; Lact. v.; *Medusa*; Parth.; Phos.; Phyt.; Pip. m.; Rheum; Ricinus; Sabal; *Salvia*; Sec.; *Solan. olec.*; Spiranth.; Ustil.
Milk, too profuse (to dry up during weaning)—Asaf.; Bry.; *Calc. c.*; Con.; Lac c.; *Puls.*; Urt.
Pain, drawing from nipple, all over body, during nursing—Phyt.; Puls.; Sil.
Pain, drawing from nipple through to back, during nursing; nipple very sore—Crot. t.
Pain, intolerable, between nursings—Phell.
Pain, in opposite breast—Bor.
Prolonged nursing, with anæmia, debility—*Acet. ac.*; Calc. p.; Carbo an.; Cinch.; Phos. ac.
Menorrhagia—*Calc. c.*; Phos.; *Sil.*
Milk leg (phlegmasia alba dolens)—Acon.; Apis; Ars.; Bell.; Bism.; Bry.; Bufo; Crot.; Ham.; Lach.; *Puls.*; Rhus t.; Sul.; Urt.
Nipples fissured from nursing—Graph.; Ratanh.; Sep.
Prolapsus uteri—Pod. See Uterus.
Sore mouth—Hydr.; Sinap. a.
Sub-involution—*Aur. m. n.*; Calc. c.; Caul.; Cim.; Croc.; *Epiph.*; Ferr.

FEMALE SEXUAL SYSTEM 847

iod.; *Frax. am.*; *Helon.*; Hydr.; *Kali b*.; *Lil. t.*; Mer. c. sale; Nat. hypochl.; Pod.; *Sec.*; *Sep.*; Ustil.

Weakness—Chin. s.; Cinch.; Kali c.

Weaning, ill effects—Bry.; Cycl.; Fragar.; Puls.

PUBIC HAIR—Falls out: Nat. m.; Nit. ac.; Zinc. m.

TUBES, FALLOPIAN—Inflammation (salpingitis): Acon.; Apis; *Ars.*; Bry.; Canth.; Chin. s.; *Col.*; Eupion; Hep.; *Merc. c.*; Sabal. See Metritis, Peritonitis.

UTERUS—Atony, weakness, relaxation: Abies c.; *Alet.*; Aloe; Alston.; Alum; Bellis; *Caul.*; *Cinch.*; Ferr. iod.; *Helon.*; Lappa; *Lil. t.*; Puls.; Rhus ar.; *Sab.*; *Sec.*; *Sep.*; *Trill.*; Ustil. See Displacements.

CERVIX—Induration of, and os: Alumen; *Aur. m.*; *Aur. mur.*; Aur. m. n.; Carbo an.; Con.; Helon.; *Kali cy.*; *Iod.*; Kal.; Mag. m.; Nat. c.; *Plat.*; Sep.

Cervix, inflammation (endocervicitis)—Ant. t.; Arg. n.; *Ars.*; *Bell.*; Calend.; Hydr.; Lyc.; *Merc. c.*; Merc.; Nit. ac.; Sep. See Ulceration.

Cervix, redness—Hydrocot.; Mitchella.

Cervix, swelling, scirrhus-like—Ananth.

Cervix, swelling, with urinary symptoms—Canth.

Cervix, tenesmus—Bell.; Ferr. m.

Cervix, tumors, cancerous—Carbo an.; Iod.; Kreos.; Thuya.

Cervix, ulceration—Alnus; Arg. m.; Arg. n.; Ars.; Aur. m. n.; Bufo; *Carb. ac.*; Carbo ar ; Fluor. ac.; *Hydr.*; *Hydrocot.*; Kali ars.; *Kreos.*; Lyc.; *Merc. c.*; Merc.; Murex; Phyt.; *Sep.*; Sul. ac.; Thuya; *Ustil.*; *Vespa.*

Cervix, ulceration, bleeding easily—Alnus; Arg. n.; Carbo an.; Kreos.

Cervix, ulceration, deep—Merc. c.

Cervix, ulceration, in aged—Sul. ac.

Cervix, ulceration, spongy—Arg. n.; Kreos.

Cervix, ulceration, superficial—*Hydr.*; Merc.

Cervix, ulceration, with fetid, acrid discharge—Ars.; Carb. ac.

Cervix, ulceration, with fetid, ichorous, bloody discharge—Carbo an.; Kreos.

CONGESTION—Acon.; *Aloe*; Aur.; *Bell.*; Bellis; *Caul.*; Cim.; *Collins.*; Croc.; *Frax. am.*; Gels.; Iod.; *Lit. t.*; Mag. p.; Mitchella; Murex; Puls.; Sabal; *Sep.*; Stroph.; Sul.; Tar. h.; *Ver. v.* See Inflammation.

Congestion, chronic or passive—Æsc.; *Aur.*; Calc. c.; Cim.; *Collins.* Helon.; Lach.; *Polymnia*; Sep.; Stann.; Sul.; Ustil.

Consciousness of a womb; very tender to jars—*Helon.*; Lyc.; Lyssin; *Med.*; Murex.

Disorders, with reflex heart symptoms—Cim.; Lil. t.

Disorders, with toothache, headache, salivation, neuralgia—Sep.

DISPLACEMENTS (flexions, versions)—*Abies c.*; Æsc.; *Bell.*; Carb. ac.; *Eupion*; *Ferr. iod.*; Ferr. m.; *Frax. am.*; Heliotr.; *Helon.*; Lappa; *Lil. t.*; Mel c. sale; Murex; Pall.; *Puls.*; Sabal; Sec.; Senec.; *Sep.*; Stann.

Displacements, prolapsus—Abies c.; Æsc.; Agar.; *Alet.*; Aloe; Arg. m.; Asperula; *Aur. m. n.*; *Bell.*; Benz. ac.; Calc. c.; Calc. p.; Calc. sil.; Caul.; *Collins.*; Con.; Ferr. br.; *Ferr. iod.*; Ferr. m.; *Frax. am.*; Graph.;

Helon.; Ign.; Kali bich.; Kreos.; Lach.; *Lil. t.;* Lyssin; *Mel c. sale;* Murex; Nat. chlor.; Nat. m.; Nux m.; *Nux v.;* Onosm.; Pall.; Plat.; Pod.; Puls.; *Rhus t.;* Sec.; Senec.; *Sep.;* Stann.; Staph.; Tilia; Trill.; Zinc. v.

HÆMORRHAGE (Metrorrhagia): Remedies in general—Acet. ac.; Achill.; Agar.; *Ambra;* Apis; Arg. n.; Arg. oxy.; *Arn.; Ars.;* Aur. mur. kali; *Bell.; Bov.;* Bry.; *Cact.; Calc. c.;* Canth.; *Caul.; Cham.;* Cim.; Cina; *Cinch.; Cinnam.;* Collins.; *Croc.;* Crot. casc.; Crot.; Dictam.; Elaps; *Erig.; Ferr. ac.;* Ferr. m.; *Ferr. p.;* Fuligo; *Ham.;* Helon.; Hydrast.; Iod.; *Ipec.;* Jonosia; Junip. v.; *Kali n.;* Kreos.; *Lach.;* Lil. t.; Mag. m.; Mangif. ind.; Millef.; Mitchella; Nat. chlor.; *Nit. ac.;* Nux v.; *Phos.;* Plat.; Plumb.; Puls.; *Pyr.; Rhus ar.;* Robin.; *Sab.; Sec.; Sep.;* Sul. ac.; Sul.; *Stram.;* Tereb.; *Thlaspi; Trill.;* Ustil.; *Vinca;* Viscum; Xanth.

From chlorosis; climacteric; cancer uteri—Med.; Phos.; Thlaspi; Ust.

From currettage—Nit. ac.

From fibroids—Calc. c.; Nit. ac.; *Phos.;* Sab.; Sec.; Sul. ac.; *Thlaspi; Trill.;* Vinca.

From mechanical injury, straining, undue exertion—*Ambra;* Arn.; *Cinnam.;* Ham.

From parturition, abortion—Caul.; Cham.; Cinch.; Croc.; Ipec.; Millef.; Nit. ac.; *Sab.; Sec.;* Thlaspi. See Pregnancy.

From retained placenta—Sab.; Sec.; Stram.

From uterine atony, malarial cases—Cinch.

Inter-menstrual—*Ambra;* Arg. n.; *Bov.; Calc. c.;* Cham.; Elaps; *Ham.; Ipec.;* Mag. s.; *Phos.;* Rhus t.; Robin.; *Sab.;* Vinca.

With backache, relieved by pressure, sitting—Kali c.

With blood, black—Caul.; *Croc.;* Elaps; Mag. c.; *Plat.*

With blood, bright red, profuse, gushing, from least motion—Acal.; *Bell.;* Bov.; Cham.; Erig.; *Ipec.;* Med.; *Millef.;* Mitchella; Phos.; Sab.; Sec.; *Trill.;* Ustil.; Viscum.

With blood, clotted or partly clotted—Acal.; *Bell.;* Cham.; *Cinch.;* Cocc.; Croc.; Cycl.; Erig.; *Ipec.;* Kali c.; Lach.; *Plat.; Plumb.;* Puls.; Rhus t.; *Sab.;* Thlaspi; Trill.; Ustil.; Viscum.

With blood clotted or fluid; paroxysmal or continual flow; nausea, vomiting; palpitation, pulse quick, feeble when moved; vital depression; fainting on raising head from pillow—Apoc.

With blood dark, fluid, offensive—Crot.

With blood, profuse, painless—Millef.; Nit. ac.

With blood, profuse, painless, dark, venous—*Ham.;* Mangif. ind.

With blood, profuse, passive, obstinate—Caul.; Cinnam.

With blood, profuse, passive, thin, fetid; in cachectic females—Sec.

With blood, profuse, very dark, thick, tarry; dragging, downward, pressing in pelvis and groins, followed by sacral pain; unnatural genital sensibility and irritability—Plat.

With blood thin; painless flow—Carbo an.; Cinch.; Sec.

With congestive headache—Bell.; Glon.

With fainting—Apis; *Cinch.;* Ferr. m.; *Trill.*

FEMALE SEXUAL SYSTEM

With faintness in stomach—Crot.; Trill.

With feeling, as if back and hips were falling to pieces, relieved by bandaging; fainting—Trill.

With feeling of enlarged head—Bad.

With flow in paroxysms, bright red; joint pains—Sab.

With flow in paroxysms, thin, light blood, firm coagula; severe labor-like pains—Cham.

With heavy abdomen, faintness, stinging pains—Apis.

With hysteria—Caul.; Cim.; Mag. m.

With labor-like pains—*Caul.; Cham.; Cim.;* Ham.; Sab.; Sec.; Thlaspi; Viscum.

With nausea—Apoc.; Caps.; *Ipec.*

With nervous erethism at menopause—Arg. n.; *Lach.*

With painful micturition; pallor; violent irritation of rectum, bladder; prolapsus—Erig.

With pain extending to navel; dyspnœa—Ipec.

With pain passing around pelvis, from sacrum to groin—Puls.; Sep.

With pain passing from sacrum to pubes—Sab.

With pain passing through pelvis, antero-posteriorly or laterally—Bell.

With septic fever—Pyr.

With sexual excitement—Ambra; Plat.; Sab.

With uterine congestion, inflammation—Sab.

With weak heart—Am. m.; Dig.

HYDROMETRA—Nat. hypochlor.; Sep.

   Induration—Aur.; Aur. m. kali; *Aur. m. n.;* Carbo an.; *Con.;* Graph.; *Iod.;* Kal.; Kreos.; Mag. m.; Plat.; *Sep.*

INFLAMMATION (endometritis, metritis)—*Acute:* Acon.; Ant. iod.; *Apis;* Arn.; *Ars.;* Bell.; Bry.; Canth.; Cham.; *Cim.;* Cinch.; Con.; Gels.; Hep.; Hyos.; *Iod.;* Kali c.; Kali iod.; Lach.; Lil. t.; *Mel c. sale;* Merc. c.; Nux v.; Op.; Phos. ac.; Plat.; *Puls.;* Rhus t.; *Sab.;* Sec.; *Sep.; Sil.;* Stram.; Sul.; Tereb.; Tilia; *Ver. v.*

   Inflammation, chronic—Alet.; Aloe; *Ars.; Aur. m.; Aur. m. n.;* Bor.; *Calc. c.; Carb. ac.;* Caul.; Chin. ars.; *Cim.; Con.;* Graph.; *Helon.; Hydr.;* Hydrocot.; Inula.; *Iod.; Kali bich.;* Kali c.; Kali s.; Kreos.; Lach.; *Mag. m.; Mel c. sale;* Merc.; *Murex;* Nat. m.; Nit. ac.; *Nux v.; Phos. ac.;* Phos.; Plumb.; *Puls.;* Rhus t.; *Sab.; Sec.; Sep.;* Sil.; Stram.; *Sul.*

   Inflammation, chronic, follicular—*Hydr.;* Hydrocot.; Iod.; Merc.

   Inflammation, chronic, with arterial congestion—Bell.; Lil. t.; *Sab.*

   Inflammation, chronic, with venous congestion—Aloe; *Collins.;* Mag. m.; Murex; *Sep.*

   Inflammation, hæmorrhagic cases—Ars.; Ham.; Led.; Phos.; *Sec.; Thlaspi.*

   Inflammation, peri or para metritis—Acon.; *Bell.;* Canth.; Col.; Hep.; *Merc. c.;* Sil.

IRRITABLE uterus (hysteralgia)—Bell.; Caul.; *Cim.;* Ign.; *Lil. t.; Mag. m.;* Murex; Tar. h. See Pain.

MOLES, foreign bodies, promote expulsion—Canth.; Sab.

PAIN—Bruised, broken feeling, of pelvic bones:—*Æsc.;* Arn.; Bellis; Lappa; *Trill.*

Burning—Acon.; *Ars.;* *Bell.;* Bufo; Calc. ars.; *Canth.;* Carbo an.; Con.; Hep.; Kreos.; Lapis alb.; Murex; Pall.; *Sec.;* *Tereb.;* Xanth.

Colicky, cramps, labor-like, bearing down—*Agar.;* Apis; Arg. m.; Calad.; Calc. c.; Can. ind.; *Caul.;* Caust.; Cham.; *Cim.;* *Cocc.;* *Col.;* Con.; *Cupr.;* Diosc.; Ferr. iod.; Ferr.; *Gels.;* *Gossyp.;* Hedeoma; *Ign.;* Inula; *Ipec.;* *Lach.;* Mag. p.; Nat. m.; *Nux v.;* Onosm.; Op.; Plat.; *Puls.;* *Sab.;* *Sec.;* Sil.; Thlaspi; Tilia; *Vib. op.;* Xanth. See Labor.

Constricting, squeezing—*Bellis;* *Cact.;* Cham.; Cinch.; *Gels.;* *Mag. p.;* Nux v.; Polygon.; *Sep.;* Ustil.

Neuralgic, lancinating, spasmodic, tearing, shooting, cutting, stitching—Acon.; *Agar.;* Apis; *Aran.;* *Bell.;* Bry.; Bufo; Calc. c.; *Cim.;* Cinch.; *Col.;* *Con.;* Crot. casc.; Cupr. ars.; *Diosc.;* Ferr.; Graph.; Kali p.; Lach.; *Lil. t.;* Mag. m.; *Mag. p.;* Merc.; *Murex;* Op.; *Plat.;* Puls.; Sec.; Tar. h.; *Vib. op.;* Viscum. See Dysmenorrhœa.

Neuralgic, from back, circumferentially—Plat.; Sep.

Neuralgic, from back to abdomen—Sep.; Viscum.

Neuralgic, from back to pubes—Bell.; Sab.

Neuralgic, from back to thighs, legs—Bufo; Carb. ac.; Cham.; *Cim.;* Puls.; *Sab.*

Neuralgic, from hip to hip—*Bell.;* Calc. c.; *Cim.;* Cinch.; *Col.;* Pall.

Neuralgic, from navel to uterus—Ipec.

Neuralgic, radiating to chest—Lach.; Murex; Vespa.

Neuralgic, right side, upward across body, thence to left mamma—Murex.

Pressing, as if viscera would protrude from vagina—*Agar.;* *Bell.;* Cim.; Cinnam.; Crot.; *Ferr. iod.;* Ferr. m.; *Frax. am.;* Gossyp.; Heliotr.; Kali ferrocy.; *Kreos.;* Lac c.; *Lil. t.;* Lyc.; Mosch.; *Murex;* Nat. c.; Nat. chlor.; Nat. m.; *Nux v.;* Onosm.; Ova g. pell.; Pall.; *Pod.;* *Puls.;* Sanic.; *Sep.;* *Stann.;* *Sul.;* Tilia; Trill.; Vib. op.; Xanth.; Xeroph.

Pressing, heaviness, fullness, dragging in pelvis—Agar.; Alet.; *Aloe;* Ant. c.; *Aur. m. n.;* *Bell.;* Calc. c.; Calend.; Carb. ac.; *Cim.;* Cinch.; *Cocc.;* Collins.; Con.; Ferr. br.; Frax. am.; Glycerin; Gnaph.; *Gossyp.;* Helon.; Kali bich.; Lappa; *Lil. t.;* Mag. c.; *Mag. m.;* Merc.; Murex; Nat. c.; Nat. chlor.; *Nux v.;* *Plat.;* Plumb.; *Pod.;* Polygon.; *Sep.;* Sul.; Trill.; Wyeth. v.; Zinc. v.

Pressing in back—Agar.; *Bell.;* Carb. ac.; Cham.; *Cim.;* *Gels.;* Gossyp.; Hedeoma; *Helon.;* Inula; *Kali c.;* Kreos.; Nat. m.; Onosm.; Trill.; Vespa; Vib. op.

Pulsating, throbbing—*Æsc.;* Bell.; *Cact.;* Hep.; Murex.

Splinter-like when walking or riding—Arg. n.

Ulcerative, between anus and perineum, when walking or sitting—Cycl.

HYSOMETRA—Bell.; Bry.; *Brom.;* Lac c.; *Lyc.;* Nux v.; Phos. ac.; Sang.

Soreness, tenderness of uterus—Abies c.; Acon.; *Apis;* Arg. m.; Arn.; *Bell.;* Bellis; Bry.; *Cim.;* Conv.; *Helon.;* Kreos.; *Lach.;* Lappa; *Lil. t.;* Lyssin; Mag. m.; *Mel c. sale;* Merc.; *Murex;* Plat.; Sanic.; *Sep.;* Thlaspi; Tilia.

FEMALE SEXUAL SYSTEM

TUMORS—Cancer, malignant disease: *Arg. m.*; *Ars. iod.*: Ars.; *Aur. m. n.*; Bell.; Bov.; Calc. ars.; Calc. s.; *Caltha*; *Carbo an.*; Carcinos; Cham.; Cinch.; Con.; *Graph.*; *Hydr.*; Iod.; Irid.; *Kali bich.*; Kali p.; Kali s.; *Kreos.*; Lach.; *Lapis alb.*; Mag. p.; Med.; Murex; Ova t.; *Phos.*; Phyt.; Rhus t.; *Sec.*; Sep.; *Sil.*; Staph.; Sul.; Tar. c.; Thlaspi; *Thuya*; Trill.; Zinc. m.

Cancer, hæmorrhage—Bell.; Crotal.; Kreos.; Lach.; Sab.; *Thlaspi*; Ustil.

Fibroids, polypi, myo-fibromata—*Aur. iod.*; *Aur. mur.*; Bell.; *Calc. c.*; *Calc. iod.*; Calc. p.; *Calend.*; Cinch.; Con.; Erod.; Ferr.; *Frax. am.*; Ham.; Hydr.; *Hydrocot.*; Iod.; Ipec.; *Kali iod.*; Lach.; Led.; Lyc.; Merc. c.; *Merc. i. r.*; *Nit. ac.*; *Phos.*; Plat.; Plumb.; Puls.; Sabal; Sab.; Sang.; Sec.; Sep.; Sil.; Solid.; Staph.; Sul.; *Thlaspi*; *Thuya*; *Thyr.*; Trill.

VAGINA—Aphthous patches, ulcers, erosions—Alumen; *Arg. n.*; Carbo v.; *Caul.*; *Graph.*; *Helon.*; *Hydr.*; Ign.; Kreos.; Lyc.; Lyssin; Merc.; Nat-m.; *Nit. ac.*; Rhus t.; Robin.; *Sep.*; Thuya.

Burning, heat—*Acon.*; Alum.; Antipyr.; Aur. mur.; *Bell.*; *Berb. v.*; Bov.; *Canth.*; Carbo an.; Carbo v.; Ferr. p.; *Hydrocot.*; Kali bich.; Kali c.; *Kreos.*; Lyc.; Lyssin; *Merc. c.*; Merc.; Nat. m.; *Nit. ac.*; Pop. c.; Pulex; *Sep.*; Spiranth.; *Sul.*

Burning, heat, after coitus—Lyc.; Lyssin.

Coldness—Bor. ac.

Cysts—Lyc.; Puls.; *Rhod.*; Sil.

Dryness—Acon.; Apis; *Bell.*; Ferr. p.; *Lyc.*; Lyssin; *Nat. m.*; Spiranth. See Inflammation.

Flatus, emission—*Brom.*; Lac c.; *Lyc.*; Nux m.; Sang.

Inflammation (vaginitis)—Acute:—*Acon.*; *Apis*; Arn.; Ars.; *Bell.*; Can. s.; *Canth.*; Cim.; Con.; *Crot. t.*; Gels.; *Helon.*; *Hydr.*; Kali c.; Kali m.; *Kreos.*; *Merc. c.*; Rhus t.; *Sep.*; Sul.; Thuya.

Inflammation, chronic—Ars.; Bor.; *Calc. c.*; Grind.; Hydr.; Iod.; *Kreos.*; Kali m.; *Merc.*; Nit. ac.; *Puls.*; *Sep.*; Sul. See Vulvitis.

Itching—Antipyr.; Arundo; Aur. mur.; *Calad.*; *Canth.*; *Con.*; *Helon.*; Hydrocot.; Hydr.; *Kreos.*; Merc.; Scrophul.; *Sep.*; Sil.; *Sul.* See Pruritus Vulvæ.

Pain, pressing—*Bell.*; Calc. c.; Chimaph.; Cinnab.; *Ferr. iod.*; Stann.

Pain, stinging, stitching, shooting, tearing—*Apis*; Cimex; Cim.; Col.; Kreos.; *Rhus t.*; Sab.; Sep.

Pain, throbbing—Bell.

Prolapsus vaginæ—Alum.; *Bell.*; Ferr.; Granat.; Kreos.; Lach.; *Lappa*; Nux m.; Nux v.; Ocimum; *Sep.*; *Stann.*; Staph.; Sul. ac.

Sensitiveness (vaginismus)—*Acon.*; Aur.; *Bell.*; *Berb. v.*; *Cact.*; *Caul.*; Caust.; Carbo v.; *Cim.*; *Oocc.*; *Coff.*; Con.; Ferr. iod.; Ferr. m.; Ferr. p.; *Gels.*; Ham.; *Ign.*; Kreos.; Lac c.; Lyssin; *Mag. p.*; *Murex*; Mur. ac.; Nit. ac.; Nux v.; Orig.; *Plat.*; *Plumb.*; Sil.; *Staph.*; Tar. h.; *Thuya*.

VULVA-LABIA—Abscess (vulvo-vaginal): *Apis*; Bell.; Bor.; Hep.; Kreos.; Iod.; Lach.; *Merc.*; Puls.; Rhus t.; Sep.; *Sil.*; Sul.

Burning—Acon.; Am. c.; Aur.; Bov.; *Canth.*; Carbo v.; *Graph.*: Helon.;

Kreos.; Lyc.; *Merc.*; Puls.; *Rhus t.*; Sep.; Sil.; *Sul.*; **Thuya.** See **Pain.**
Cancer—*Ars.*; Con.; Thuya.
Dryness—*Acon.*; *Bell.*; Calc. c.; Lyc.; Tar. h. See Vulvitis.
Eczema—Rhus t.
Erysipelas, with edema—*Apis.*
Hair falling out—Merc.; Nit. ac.
Hyperæsthesia, soreness—Acon.; *Bell.*; *Cim.*; Cocc.; *Coff.*; Ferr. iod.; *Gels.*; Hep.; *Ign.*; Kali br.; *Kreos.*; Mag. p.; *Merc.*; *Murex*; *Nit. ac.*; Nux v.; Petrol.; *Plat.*; *Sep.*; Sul.; *Thuya*; Tilia; Zinc. m.
Inflammation (vulvitis)—*Acon.*; Ambra; *Apis*; Ars.; *Bell.*; Brom.; *Calc. c.*; *Canth.*; *Carbo v.*; Chimaph.; Coccus; Collins; *Cop.*; Eupion; Gossyp.; *Graph.*; Ham.; *Helon.*; *Hydr.*; *Kreos.*; Lyc.; Mag. p.; *Merc. c.*; *Merc.*; Ocimum; Plat.; Puls.; Rhus divers.; *Rhus t.*; *Sep.*; Sil.; Sul.; *Thuya.*
Vulvitis, follicular, herpetic—Ars.; Crot. t.; *Dulc.*; Merc.; Nat. m.; Robin.; *Sep.*; Spiranth.; Thuya; *Xerophyl.*
Itching (pruritus)—Agar.; *Ambra*; Apis; *Ars.*; Arundo; Berb. v.; Bov.; Calad.; *Calc. c.*; *Canth.*; Carb. ac.; *Carbo v.*; Caust.; Coff.; *Collins.*; Con.; Conv.; Cop.; Crot. t.; Dulc.; *Fagop.*; Ferr. iod.; *Graph.*; Grind.; Guaco; *Helon.*; Hydr.; Kali bich.; Kali br.; Kali c.; *Kreos.*; Lil. t.; *Lyc.*; *Merc.*; Mez.; Nat. m.; Nit. ac.; *Orig.*; Petrol.; Picr. ac.; *Plat.*; *Radium*; Rhus div.; *Rhus t.*; Rhus v.; Scrophul.; *Sep.*; Spiranth.; Staph.; *Sul.*; Tar. c.; *Tar. h.*; Thuya; *Urt.*; Xerophyl.; Zinc. m.
Pain—Apis; Ars.; *Bell.*; Berb. v.; *Calc. c.*; *Can. s.*; Con.; Ferr.; Kali c.; *Kreos.*; Lyc.; Meli.; *Merc. c.*; *Phos.*; Plat.; Sab.; *Sep.*; Sul. See Vulvitis.
Papules, pustules—*Carb. ac.*; Graph.; *Sep.*; Sul.
Polypi—Bell.; Calc. c.; *Phos.*; Teucr.; *Thuya.*
Sensation, as if wet—Eup. purp.; Petrol.
Soreness, tenderness—*Acon.*; Ambra; *Bell.*; Caust.; Conv.; *Graph.*; Helon.; Hep.; *Kreos.*; Ova g. pell.; *Plat.*; *Sep.*; Sul.; Tar. h.; Urt.
Soreness, with ulcers—Arg. n.; *Hep.*; Merc.; *Nit. ac.*; Thuya.
Sweat, offensive—*Calc. c.*; Fagop.; Lyc.; *Merc.*; Petrol.; *Sul.*; Thuya.
Ulcers—*Ars.*; *Aur. m. n.*; Graph.; Mur. ac.; *Nit. ac.*; Sep.; Syph.
Varices—Calc. c.; Carbo v.; Lyc.
Warts—Aur. mur.; Med.; *Thuya.*

CIRCULATORY SYSTEM

ARTERIES—AORTA—Inflamed, acute (aortitis): Acon.; Apis; Glon.; Tub.

Aorta, inflamed, chronically (aortitis chronica)—Adon. v.; *Adren.*; *Ant. ars.*; *Ars. iod.*; Aur. ars.; Aur.; *Cact.*; Chin. s.; Crat.; Cupr.; Glon.; Kali iod.; Lyc.; *Nat. iod.*; Spig.; Stroph.

Aortitis, ulcerative—Acon.; Ars.; Chin. s.

Aorta, pain—Adren.; Strych. See Angina Pectoris.

Arteritis—Ars.; Carbo v.; Echin.; *Kali iod.*; Lach.; *Nat. iod.*; Sec.

Atheroma of arteries (arterio-sclerosis)—Adren.; *Am. iod.*; Am. vanad.; Ant. ars.; Arn.; Ars.; *Ars. iod.*; *Aur. iod.*; Aur.; Aur. m. n.; Bar. c.; Bar. m.; Cact.; Calc. fl.; Chin. s.; Con.; Crat.; Ergotin; *Glon.*; Iodothyr.; *Kali iod.*; Kali sal.; Lach.; Lith. c.; *Nat. iod.*; Phos.; *Plumb. iod.*; Plumb. m.; *Polygon. av.*; Sec.; Stront. c.; *Stront. iod.*; Stroph.; Sumb.; *Vanad.* See Interstitial Nephritis.

Carotids, pulsate—*Acon.*; Amyl; *Bell.*; *Cact.*; Cinch.; Fagop.; *Glon.*; Lil. t.; Sab.; *Ver. v.* See Pulse.

Circulation, sluggish—Æth.; Calc. c.; *Calc. p.*; Carbo an.; *Carbo v.*; Cim.; Cinnam.; Ferr. p.; *Gels.*; Led.; Nat. m.; *Rhus t.*; Sil. See Heart.

Congestion of blood (local)—*Acon.*; Æsc.; Ambra; *Amyl*; Aur.; *Bell.*; *Cact.*; Calc. c.; Centaur.; Cupr. m.; Ferr. m.; *Ferr. p.*; Gadus mor.; *Glon.*; Kali iod.; Lil. t.; Lonic.; *Meli.*; Millef.; Phos.; *Sang.*; Sep.; Sil.; Spong.; Stellar.; *Sul.*; *Ver. v.*

Degeneration, fatty—Phos. See Heart.

Dilatation-Aneurism—Acon.; Ars. iod.; *Bar. c.*; *Bar. m.*; Cact.; Calc. fl.; Calc. p.; Glon.; Iod.; *Kali iod.*; Kal.; Lach.; Lith. c.; *Lyc.*; Lycop.; Morph.; *Nat. iod.*; Plumb.; Puls.; Spig.; Spong.; *Ver. v.*

Aneurism, capillary—*Calc. fl.*; Fluor. ac.; Tub.

Aneurism, pain—Cact. See Angina Pectoris.

RUPTURE of artery (apoplexy)—*Acon.*; Apis; *Arn.*; Aster.; Bar. c.; *Bell.*; Cact.; Camph.; Caust.; Chenop.; Cinch.; Croc.; Crotal.; Cupr. m.; Formica; *Glon.*; Hydroc. ac.; Hyos.; Junip. v.; Kali br.; Kali iod.; Lach.; Laur.; Nux v.; Op.; Phos.; Sep.; Stram.; Sul.; Ver. a.; *Ver. v.*

Rupture of artery; post-hemiplegia—*Arn.*; Ars.; Bar. c.; Bell.; Bothrops; *Caust.*; *Cocc.*; Cupr. m.; Cur.; Lach.; Nux v.; Phos.; *Plumb.*; Rhus t.; Vipera; Zinc. m.

Rupture of artery: predisposition to, or threatened—*Acon.*; Arn.; Ars.; Bar. c.; *Bell.*; Calc. fl.; *Gels.*; *Glon.*; Guaco; Hyos.; *Lach.*; Laur.; Nux v.; Op.; Phos.; Stront. c.

HEART—Action tumultuous, violent, labored: Abies c.; Absinth.; *Acon.*; Æsc.; *Agar.*; Ammon.; *Amyl*; Ars.; *Aur.*; *Bell.*; Bry.; *Cact.*; Carb. ac.; Cim.; Colch.; Conv.; Ephedra; Gels.; *Glon.*; Helod.; Iberis; Kal.; *Lil. t.*; Lycop.; *Nat. m.*; Physost.; Prun. sp.; Pyr.; *Spig.*; Spong.; *Ver. v.* See Pulse.

AFFECTIONS in general—*Acon.*; Adon. v.; Am. c.; Am. m.; *Amyl*; Apoc.; Arn.; *Ars. iod.*; Ars.; Aur. m.; Aur. mur.; Bar. c.; Bell.; Benz. ac.;

Bry.; *Cact.*; *Calc. ars.*; Calc. fl.; Carbo v.; Cim.; Cinch.; Coca; Colch.; *Collins.*; *Conv.*; Coronilla; *Crat.*; *Crot.*; *Digitaline*; *Dig.*; Ferr. m.; Fer. p.; Gels.; *Glon.*; Grind.; *Hydroc. ac.*; *Iberis*; Ign.; Iod.; Kali c.; Kali chlor.; *Kal.*; *Lach.*; Laur.; Lepid.; *Lil. t.*; Lith. c.; *Lycop.*; Merc. c.; Mosch.; *Naja*; Nat. iod.; Nat. m.; Nux v.; *Ox. ac.*; *Phaseol.*; *Phos.*; Piloc.; Scilla; *Spart.*; *Spig.*; *Spong.*; *Stroph.*; *Strych.*; Sumb.; Thyr.; Val.; Ver. v. See Separate Diseases of Heart.

Affections, rheumatic—Acon.; Aur.; Benz. ac.; *Bry.*; Cact.; Caust.; Cim.; Colch.; Ign.; *Kal.*; Led.; Lith. c.; Lycop.; Naja; Phyt.; *Rhus t.*; *Spig.*; Ver. v.

Affections, with hæmorrhoids—Cact.; *Collins.*; Dig.

CYANOSIS—Acetan.; Am. c.; *Ant. ars.*; *Ant. t.*; *Ars.*; Benz. nit.; Carbo an.; *Carbo v.*; Crot.; Cupr.; *Dig.*; Hydroc. ac.; Lach.; *Laur.*; Lycop.; Merc. cy.; Nat. nit.; Phos.; Piloc.; Psor.; *Rhus t.*; Samb.; Tab.; Zinc. m.

DEBILITY, weakness—Acetan.; Acet. ac.; *Adon. v.*; Adren.; *Am. c.*; *Am. m.*; Ant. ars.; *Ars.*; *Ars. iod.*; Aur.; *Cact.*; *Calc. ars.*; Camph.; Carb. ac.; *Carbo v.*; Chin. ars.; Cinch.; *Conv.*; *Crat.*; *Dig.*; Diosc.; Eel serum; Euphorbia; Ferr.; Grind.; Helod.; *Hydroc. ac.*; *Iberis*; Kali c.; Kal.; Lach.; Lil. t.; Lycop.; Morph.; Mosch.; Nerium; Nit. ac.; Nux m.; Phaseol.; Plumb.; Prun. sp.; Psor.; Pyr.; Sarcol. ac.; Scilla; *Spart.*; Spig.; *Stroph.*; Tab.; Thyr.; *Ver. a.*

Debility, weakness, muscular, "heart failure"—Adon. v.; Adren.; Agaricin; *Alcohol*; Amyl; Ant. t.; Atrop.; *Caffeine*; Camphorated oil; Cocaine; Conv.; Crat.; *Digitaline*; *Dig.*; Ether; *Glon.*; Oxygen inhalation; Sacchar. of.; Saline infusion; Serum ang.; Spart.; Stroph.; *Strych. s.*; Ver. a.

Debility, weakness, nervous—Adren.; *Cact.*; *Iberis*; Ign.; *Lil. t.*; Lith. c.; *Mosch.*; *Naja*; Piloc.; Prun. v.; Spart.; *Spig.*; Tab.; *Val.*

Debility, weakness, with dropsy—*Acetan.*; *Adon. v.*; *Apoc.*; Ars. iod.; *Ars.*; Asclep. syr.; Cact.; *Caffeine*; Collins.; *Conv.*; *Dig.*; Iberis; Lach.; Lycop.; Oleand.; Scilla; Spart.; *Stroph.* See Generalities.

DEGENERATION, fatty—Adon. æst.; Adon. v.; Arn.; Ars. iod.; *Ars.*; *Aur.*; *Bar. c.*; Cim.; Crat.; Cupr. ac.; Fucus; *Kali c.*; Kali feroc.; Kal.; Phos. ac.; *Phos.*; Physost.; *Phyt.*; Sacchar. of.; Stroph.; Strych. ars.; Strych. p.; *Vanad.*

DILATATION—Adon. v.; Am. c.; Ars. iod.; *Ars.*; *Bar. c.*; *Cact.*; Cim.; Conv.; *Crat.*; *Dig.*; Gels.; Iberis; *Naja*; *Phaseol.*; Phos.; Physost.; Prun. sp.; Spart. s.; *Spig.*; Stroph.; Tab.; Ver. v. See Debility, muscular.

DYSPNOEA (cardiac)—*Acon. fer.*; Acon.; Adon. v.; *Adren.*; Am. c.; Apis; Arn.; Ars.; Ars. iod.; Aur. m.; *Cact.*; *Calc. ars.*; Carbo v.; *Chin. ars.*; Cim.; Collins.; Conv.; *Dig.*; *Glon.*; *Iberis*; Kali n.; Kal.; Lach.; Laur.; Lycop.; Magnol.; Naja; Ox. ac.; Op.; *Quebracho*; Spig.; Spong.; Stroph.; Strych. ars.; Sumb.; Viscum. See Respiratory System.

Hydropericardium—Apis; Apoc.; Ant. ars.; Ars.; Iod.; Lach.

HYPERTROPHY—Acon.; *Arn.*; Ars.; Aur.; Bell.; *Brom.*; *Cact.*; Caffeine; *Caust.*; Cereus; *Conv.*; *Crat.*; *Dig.*; Glon.; *Iberis*; Iod.; Kal.; Lil. t.;

CIRCULATORY SYSTEM 855

Lycop.; *Naja;* Phos.; Phyt.; *Rhus t.:* Spig.; *Spong.;* Stroph.; Strych. ars.; *Ver. v.;* Viscum.

Hypertrophy uncomplicated, of athletes—Arn.; Brom.; Caust.; *Rhus t.*

Inflammation (ENDOCARDITIS)—Acute: Acon.; Ars.; Bell.; *Cact.;* Colch.; Conv.; Dig.; *Lach.;* Magnol.; *Naja;* Phos.; *Spig.;* Spong.; Tab.; Ver. v. See Pericarditis.

Endocarditis, malignant—Acon.; Ars.; *Chin. s.;* Crot.; Lach.; Vipera.

Endocarditis, rheumatic—Acon.; Adon. v.; Bell.; *Bry.;* Colch.; Kali c.; Kal.; Rhus t.; *Spig.*

MYOCARDITIS—Acon.; Adon. v.; *Ars. iod.;* Aur. mur.; Cact.; Chin. ars.; Crat.; *Dig.;* Galanth.; Iod.; Lach.; Phos.; Stroph.; *Vipera.* See Weakness, Degeneration.

PERICARDITIS, acute—*Acon.;* Adon. v.; Ant. ars.; *Apis; Ars.;* Asclep. t.; Bell.; *Bry.;* Cact.; Can. s.; *Canth.;* Colch.; Dig.; Iod.; Kali c.; *Kali iod.;* Kal.; Magnol.; Merc. c.; *Merc.;* Naja; Nat. m.; Phaseol.; Scilla; *Spig.; Spong.;* Sul.; Ver. a.; Ver. v.

Pericarditis, chronic—Apis; *Aur. iod.;* Calc. fl.; Kali c.; Scilla; Spig.; Sul.

Pericarditis, rheumatic—Acon.; Anac.; Bry.; *Colchicine;* Colch.; Crat.; Kal.; Rhus t.; *Spig.*

NEUROSES—*Acon.;* Adren.; Cact.; Cham.; Cinch.; *Coff.;* Ferr.; *Gels.; Iber.; Ign.;* Lach.; *Lil. t.;* Lycop.; *Mosch.;* Nux v.; Prun. v.; Scutel.; Sep.; *Spig.; Tab.;* Ver. a.; Zinc. m.

Neuroses, irritable from influenza—Iberis; Spart. s.

Neuroses, irritable from tea, coffee—Agaricine.

Neuroses, irritable from tobacco—*Agaricine;* Agn.; Ars.; Calad.; *Conv.;* Dig.; *Kal.;* Lycop.; Nux v.; *Phos.; Spig.;* Staph.; *Stroph.;* Tab.; Ver. a.

Neuroses, irritable from suppressed hæmorrhoids—Collins.

Neuroses, irritable from utero-ovarian disease—Cim.; Lil. t.

Neuroses, irritable tremulousness, from scarlet fever—Lach.

PAIN—Abies n.; *Acon.; Adon. v.; Amyl;* Apis; Arn.; *Ars.;* Aster.; *Bry.; Cact.;* Calc. fl.; *Canth.;* Cereus; Cereus serp.; *Cim.;* Coff.; *Colch.;* Conv.; Crat.; Daphne; *Dig.;* Diosc.; *Ferr. tart.; Hematox.; Hydroc. ac.;* Iberis; *Kal.;* Lach.; *Latrod.;* Lepid.; *Lil. t.; Lith. c.;* Lob. infl.; Lycop.; Magnol.; Med.; *Naja;* Onosm.; *Ox. ac.;* Ov. g. p.; *Pæonia;* Pip. nig.; Ptel.; *Spig.; Spong.; Stroph.;* Syph.; Tab.; *Ther.;* Thyr.; *Ver. v.;* Zinc. v.

Pain at apex—Lil. t.

Pain at base—Lob. infl.

Pain constricting, as if squeezed in vise—*Acon.;* Adon. v.; Amyl; Arn.; Ars.; *Cact.;* Cadm. s.; Calc. ars.; Coccus; Colch.; Iodof.; *Iod.;* Kali c.; Lach.; Laur.; *Lil. t.;* Lycop.; Mag. p.; Magnol.; Nux m.; Ptel.; Spong.; Thyr.

Neuralgic—ANGINA PECTORIS—*Acon.;* Adren.; *Amyl;* Arg. cy.; Arg. n.; *Arn.;* Ars. iod.; *Ars.;* Aur. mur.; Bism.; *Cact.;* Camph.; Cereus; Chin. ars.; *Cim.; Cocaine;* Conv.; *Crat.;* Crot.; *Cupr. ac.; Cupr. m.;* Dig.; Diosc.; *Glon.; Hematox.; Hydroc. ac.;* Kali c.; Kali iod.; Kal.; *Latrod · Lil. t.;* Lith. c.; Lob. infl.; *Mag. p.;* Magnol.; Morph.; *Naja;*

Nat. iod.; Nat. ʟit.; *Nux v.;* Oleand.; *Ox. ac.;* Phos.; Phyt.; Pip. nig.; Prun. sp.; Samb.; Spart.; *Spig.; Spong.;* Staph.; Stront. c.; Stront. iod.; *Tab.;* Thyr.; Ver. v.; Zinc. v.

From abuse of coffee—Coff.

From abuse of stimulants—Nux v.; Spig.

From muscular origin—Cupr.; Hydroc. ac.

From organic heart disease—*Ars. iod.; Cact.;* Calc. fl.; Crat.; Kal.; Nat. iod.; Stront. iod.; Tab.

From rheumatism—Cim.; Lith. c.

From straining, overlifting—*Arn.;* Carbo an.; Caust.

From tobacco—Kal.; Lil. t.; Nux v.; Spig.; Staph.; Tab.

Pseudo-angina pectoris—Aconitine; Cact.; *Lil. t.; Mosch.;* Nux v.; Tar. h. See Pain.

Præcordial oppression, anxiety, heaviness—Acon.; Adon. v.; Adren.; Æsc.; Agar.; Am. c.; Amyl; Apis; Ars.; *Ars. iod.;* Aspar.; Aur.; Brom.; Bry.; *Cact.;* Calc. ars.; Calc. c.; *Camph.;* Carbo v.; Cereus; Cim.; Colch.; Collins.; Cotyled.; *Crat.;* Cupr.; *Dig.;* Diosc.; Ferr.; Glon.; Hematox.; *Hydroc. ac.;* Iberis; Ign.; *Iod.;* Ipec.; Kal.; *Lach.; Latrod.;* Laur.; *Lil. t.;* Lith. c.; *Lycop.;* Magnol.; Menyanth.; *Naja;* Nat. ars.; Primula v.; *Puls.;* Sapon.; *Spig.; Spong.;* Tab.; *Thea;* Thyr.; Vanad.; Ver. v.

Shooting, down left shoulder, arm to fingers—*Acon.;* Arn.; Asper.; Bism.; *Cact.;* Cim.; Crot.; *Kal.; Latrod.;* Lepid.; Naja; *Ox. ac.; Rhus t.; Spig.;* Tab.

Shooting, from apex to base—Med.

Shooting, from base to apex at night—Syph.

Shooting from back to clavicle, shoulder—Spig.

Shooting, lancinating, tearing—Ars.; Bell.; *Cact.;* Cereus; Cim.; Colch.; Daphne; Glon.; *Iberis; Kal.; Latrod.;* Lil. t.; Lith. c.; Magnol.; Menthol; *Ox. ac.;* Pæonia; Phyt.; *Spig.;* Syph.; Tab. See Neuralgia.

Stitching, cutting—Abies n.; *Acon.;* Anac.; Ars.; Asclep. t.; *Bry.; Cact.;* Can. ind.; Caust.; Cereus; Dig.; Iberis; *Kali c.;* Kali n.; Lith. c.; Naja; Spig.

PALPITATION—*Abies c.;* Acon.; Adon. v.; Agar.; Agaricine; Amyl; Apis; *Arg. n.;* Ars.; Asaf.; *Aur. m.;* Aur. mur.; Bar. c.; *Bell.; Cact.;* Calc. ars.; Calc. c.; Camph.; Canth.; Can. ind.; Carbo v.; Chin. ars.; *Cim.;* Cinch.; *Coca; Cocc.; Coff.;* Colch.; Con.; *Conv.;* Crat.; Cupr.; Digitaline; *Dig.;* Fagop.; Ferrum; Ferr. p.; *Gels.; Glon.;* Hydr.; *Hydroc. ac.; Iberis; Ign.; Iod.; Kali c.;* Kali ferr. cy.; *Kal.; Lach.;* Laur.; *Lil. t.;* Lob. infl.; *Lycop.; Mosch.;* Naja; *Nat. m.;* Nerium; Nux m.; *Nux v.;* Oleand.; Ol. j. as.; Ox. ac.; *Phaseol.;* Phos. ac.; *Phos.;* Plat.; *Puls.; Pyr.;* Sec.; Sep.; *Spig.; Spong.; Sul.; Sumb.; Tab.;* Thea; Thyr.; Val.; Ver. v.; Zinc.

CAUSE—Anæmia, vital drains: Ars.; *Cinch.;* Dig.; *Ferr. red.;* Kali c.; Kali ferrocy.; Nat. m.; *Phos. ac.;* Phos.; Puls.; Spig.; Ver. a.

Children, growing too fast—Phos. ac.

Dyspepsia—Abies c.; *Abies n.;* Arg. n.; Cact.; *Carbo v.; Cinch.;* Coca;

Coff.; Collins.; Diosc.; Hydroc. ac.; Lyc.; *Nux v.;* *Puls.;* Prun. v.; Sep.; Spig.; Tab.

Emotional causes—*Acon.;* Ambra; Am. val.; Anac.; Cact.; *Calc. ars.;* Cham.; *Coff.;* Gels.; Hydroc. ac.; *Ign.;* Iod.; Lach.; Lith. c.; *Mosch.;* Nux m.; Nux v.; Op.; Plat.; Sep.; Tar. h.

Eruption suppressed—Calc. c.

Exertion, even slightest—Bell.; Brom.; Cim.; Coca; Conv.; *Dig.; Iberis; Iod.;* Nat. m.; Sarcol. ac.; *Thyr.*

Grief—*Ign.;* Phos. ac.

Heart-strain—*Arn.;* Bor.; *Caust.;* Coca.

Nervous irritation—Atrop.; Cact.; *Coff.; Glon.;* Hydroc. ac.; Hyos.; Ign., Kali c.; Kali p.; Lil. t.; Lycop.; Mag. p.; Mosch.; Naja; Sep.; Spig.; Sumb.

Prolonged brain work, sexual excesses—Coca.

Tea drinking—Cinch.

Tobacco—Agar.; Ars.; Cact.; Gels.; Nux v.; Stroph.

Uterine disease—Conv.; Lil. t.

Worms—Spig.

CONCOMITANTS—With anguish, restlessness: Acon.; Æth.; Ars.; Calc. c.; Coff.; Ign.; Lach.; Nat. m.; Phaseol.; *Phos.; Puls.;* Sapon.; Spig.; *Spong.;* Ver. a.: Zinc. m.

With burning at heart—Kali c.

With choking in throat—Iberis; Lach.; Naja.

With dim vision—Puls.

With dyspnœa—Am. c.; *Cact.;* Dig.; *Glon.;* Glycerin; Lach.; Oleand.; Naja; Ox. ac.; *Phos.;* Spig.; *Spong.;* Ver. a.; Zinc. m.

With face red—Agar.; Aur.; Bell.; Glon.

With fainting—Acon.; *Cham.; Lach.;* Nat. m.; *Nux m.;* Petrol.; *Tab.*

With fetor oris—Spig.

With flatulence—*Arg. n.;* Cact.; Carbo v.; *Nux v.*

With headache—Æth.; Bell.; Lith. c.

With heart-labored, reverberates in head—Aur.; Bell.; Glon.; Spig.; Spong.

With heart weak—Coca; Dig.

With hot feeling, uncomfortable—Ant. t.; Calc. c.; Kali c.; Petrol.

With pain, præcordial—*Acon.;* Ars.; *Cact.;* Cham.; Caust.; *Coff.;* Hydroc. ac.; Laur.; Mag. m.; Naja; *Spig.;* Spong.

With piles or suppressed menses alternating—Collins.

With sleeplessness—Cim.; Coca; *Ign.;* Spig.

With stomach, heavy feeling in—Upas.

With stomach, sinking in—Cim.

With tinnitus, mental depression, anorexia, chest oppression—Coca.

With trembling—Asaf.; Lach.; Rhus t.; *Sul. ac.*

With urination copious—Coff.

With uterine soreness—Conv.

With vertigo—Adon. v.; Æth.; Cact.; Coronilla; *Iberis;* Spig.

With weakness, empty feeling in chest—Oleand.

AGGRAVATION—After eating: Calc. c.; Lil. t.; Lyc.; Nat. m.; *Nux v.;* Puls.

At approach of menses—*Cact.*; Crot.; Spong.
At night—*Ars.*; Cact.; Calc. c.; Iberis; Ign.; Lil. t.; Lyc.; Nat. m.; Phos.; Tab.
During sleep—Alston.; Am. c.; *Can. ind.*; Iberis; Phos. ac.; Spong.
From least motion—Acon.; Bell.; *Cact.*; *Calc. ars.*; Cim.; *Dig.*; Ferr.; Iberis; *Lil. t.*; Nat. m.; *Spig.*
From lying down—*Ars.*; Kali c.; Lach.; Lil. t.; Nat. m.; Nux v.; Sep.; Spig.; Thyr.
From lying on left side—Bar. c.; *Cact.*; Lac c.; *Lach.*; Lyc.; Nat. m.; Phos.; Puls.; *Tab.*; Thea.
From lying on right side—*Alumen*; Arg. n.
From mental exertion—Calc. ars.
From rising—Cact.
From sitting—Mag. m.; Phos.; Rhus t.
From sitting bent forward—Kal.
From stooping forward—Spig.
From thinking of it—Bar. c.; Gels.; Ox. ac.
In morning on waking—Kali c.; Nux v.

AMELIORATION—Lying on right side: Lac c.; Tab.
Motion—Ferr. m.; Gels.; *Mag. m.*

PULSE—Full, round, bounding, strong, felt all over: Acon.; Æsc.; Am. m.; Amyl; Antipyr.; Arn.; *Aur.*; Bar. c.; *Bell.*; Bry.; *Cact.*; Calc. c.; Canth.; Coff.; Cupr.; Fagop.; Ferr. m.; *Glon.*; *Iod.*; Lil. t.; Lycop.; Onosm.; Op.; Physost.; Piloc.; Poth.; Puls.; Sab.; Spig.; Spong.; Ver. v.
Intermittent—Acon.; Apoc.; Bapt.; *Cact.*; *Carbo v.*; Cinch.; Colch.; Conv.; Crat.; *Dig.*; Ferr. mur.; *Iberis*; Ign.; Kali c.; Kal.; Lil. t.; Lycop.; Merc. c.; Merc. cy.; Nat. m.; Nux m.; Phos. ac.; Pip. nig.; Rhus t.; Sec.; Sep.; Spig.; Stroph.; Tab.; Tereb.; Thea; Ver. a.; *Ver. v.*; Zinc. m.
Intermittent, every third to seventh beat—Dig.; Mur. ac.
Iregular—Acetan.; Acon.; Adon. v.; Adren.; *Agaricine*; Antipyr.; Apoc.; Arn.; *Ars.*; Ars. iod.; *Aur.*; Bell.; *Cact.*; Caffeine; Camph.; Cim.; Cinch.; Conv.; Crat.; *Dig.*; Eel serum; Ferr. m.; Gels.; *Glon.*; *Hydroc. ac.*; *Iberis*; Ign.; Kali c.; Kal.; Lach.; Laur.; Lil. t.; Lycop.; Mur. ac.; Naja; Nat. m.; Nux m.; Phaseol.; Phos. ac.; Piloc.; Puls.; Rhus t.; Sang.; Sec.; Serum ang.; Spart.; Spig.; Stroph.; Strych. ars.; Strych. p.; Sumb.; *Tab.*; Thea; Ver. a.; *Ver. v.*; Zinc. m.
Rapid (tachycardia)—*Abies n.*; Acon.; Adon. v.; Adren.; *Agn.*; Am. val.; Ant. ars.; Ant. c.; *Ant. t.*; Antipyr.; Apoc.; Arn.; Ars. iod.; *Bell.*; Bry.; *Cact.*; Canth.; Carbo v.; Coff.; Colch.; Collins.; Conv.; Crat.; Dig.; Diph.; Eel serum; Ferr. p.; *Gels.*; Glon.; *Iberis*; Kal.; Kali chlor.; Lach.; Latrod.; Led.; *Lil. t.*; Lycop.; Merc. c.; Morph.; Mur. ac.; *Naja*; Nat. m.; Phaseol.; *Phos.*; Phyt.; Piloc.; Pyr.; Rhod.; Rhus t.; Sec.; Sep.; Spong.; Stroph.; Strych. p.; Tab.; Tereb.; Thea; *Thyr.*; Ver. a.; Ver. v. See Weak.
Rapid in morning—Ars.; Sul.
Rapid, out of all proportion to temperature—Lil. t.; Pyr.

CIRCULATORY SYSTEM

Slow (brachycardia)—*Abies n.*; Adon. v.; Adren.; Æsc.; Apoc.; Cact.; Camph.; Can. ind.; Canth.; Caust.; Colch.; Cupr.; *Dig.*; Eserine; *Gels.*; Helod.; Helleb.; Kal.; Latrod.; Lupul.; Lycopers.; Morph.; Myr.; Naja; Op.; Pip. nig.; Rhus t.; Spig.; Tab.; Ver. a.; *Ver. v.* See Weak.

Slow, alternating with rapid—Cinch.; Dig.; *Gels.*; Iod.; Morph.

Soft, compressible—Acal.; *Ars.*; Bapt.; *Caffeine;* Conv.; Ferr. m.; Ferr. p.; *Gels.*; Kali c.; *Phos.*; Plumb.; Ver. a.; Ver. v. See Weak.

Weak, fluttering, almost imperceptible—Acetan.; Acon.; *Adon. v.;* Adren.; Æth.; *Agaricine;* Ail.; Am. m.; Ant. ars.; Ant. t.; Apis; Arn.; *Ars.;* Ars. iod.; Aur.; Aspar.; Bar. m.; *Cact.*; *Caffeine;* Camph.; Carb. ac.; Carbo v.; Cim.; Colch.; Collins.; *Conv.*; Crat.; Crot.; *Dig.*; Diph.; Eel serum; *Ferr. m.*; *Gels.*; *Hydroc. ac.*; Hysocin. hydrobr.; Iod.; *Kali c.*; Kali chlor.; *Kali n.*; Kal.; Lach.; *Latrod.*; Laur.; Lycop.; Merc. c.; *Merc. cy.*; Morph.; *Mur. ac.*; Naja; Op.; Ox. ac.; *Phaseol.*; Phos. ac.; *Phos.*; Physost.; Plumb.; Pyr.; Rhus t.; Sang.; *Sapon.*; Sec.; Spart.; *Spig.*; Sul.; *Tab.*; Tereb.; *Thyr.*; Ver. a.; *Ver. v.*; Viscum; Zinc. m.

SENSATIONS—As if drops were falling from heart: Can. s.

As if heart were burning—Kali c.; Op.; Tar. h.

As if heart were ceasing its beat—Antipyr.; Chin. ars., Cim.; Crat.; *Dig.*, Lob. infl.; *Phaseol.*; Trifol.

As if heart were ceasing its beat, then started suddenly—*Aur.*; Conv.; Lil. t.; Sep.

As if heart were ceasing its beat when moving about, must keep still—Cocaine; *Dig.*

As if heart were ceasing its beat when resting, must move about—Gels.; Trifol.

As if heart were cold—Calc. c.; *Carbo an.*; Graph.; Helod.; Kali bich.; Kali m.; Kali n.; Lil. t.; *Nat. m.*; Petrol.

As if heart were fluttering—Absinth.; Acon.; Amyl; Apoc.; Asaf.; *Cact.*; Cim.; Conv.; Crot.; Ferr.; Glon.; *Iberis;* Kal.; Lach.; *Lil. t.*; Lith. c.; *Mosch.*; Naja; *Nat. m.*; Nux m.; *Phaseol.*; Phos. ac.; *Physost.*; Pyr.; *Spig.*; Sul. ac.; Thea. See Palpitation.

As if heart were purring—Pyr.; Spig.

As if heart were squeezed by iron hand—Arn.; *Cact.*; Iod.; *Lil. t.*; Sul.; Vanad.; Viscum.

As if heart were suspended by thread—Kali c.; Lach.

As if heart were too full, bursting—*Æsc.*; Amyl; Aur. m.; *Bell.*; Bufo; *Cact.*; Cenchris; Collins.; Conv.; *Glon.*; Glycerin; Iberis; Lact.; *Lil. t.*; Pyr.; *Spig.*; Stroph.; *Sul.*; Vanad.

As if heart were tired—Pyr.

As if heart were twisted—*Lach.*; Tar. h.

Soreness, tenderness of heart—*Arn.*; *Cact.*; Camph.; Gels.; Hematox.; Lith. c.; Lycop.; *Naja;* Sec.; *Spig.*

SYNCOPE—(fainting): Acetan.; Acet. ac.; *Acon.*; Alet.; Amyl; Apis; *Ars.*; Cact.; Canth.; Carbo v.; Cham.; Cim.; *Cinch.*; Collins.; Croc.; Cupr.; *Dig.*; Ferr.; Glon.; *Ign.*; Ipec.; Lach.; Lil. t.; *Linar.*; Mag. m.; Magnol.; *Mosch.*; Nux m.; Nux v.; Op.; Phaseol.; Phos. ac.; Phos.; Puls.;

Sep.; *Spig.;* Spong.; *Sul.; Sumb.;* Tab.; Thyr.; *Trill.; Ver. a.;* Zinc.
Syncope from odors, in morning, after eating—Nux v.
Syncope, lipothymia, hysterical—*Acon.;* Apium v.; Asaf.; Cham.; Cocc.; Cupr.; *Ign.;* Lach.; *Mosch.;* Nux m.

VALVULAR DISEASE—Acon.; *Adon. v.;* Apoc.; *Ars.; Ars. iod.;* Aur. br.; Aur. iod.; Aur. m.; *Cact.;* Calc. fl.; Camph.; *Conv.; Crat.;* Dig.; Ferr.; Galanth.; *Glon.;* Iod.; Kal.; Lach.; Laur.; Lith. c.; *Lycop.; Naja;* Ox. ac.; Phos.; Plumb.; Rhus t.; Sang.; Serum ang.; *Spig.; Spong.;* Stigm.; *Stroph.;* Thyr.; Viscum.

VEINS—Engorged, distended (plethora): Adon. v.; *Æsc.; Aloe;* Arn.; Ars.; Aur.; Bellis; Calc. c.; Calc. hypoph.; Camph.; *Carbo an.; Carbo v.;* Chin. s.; *Collins.;* Conv.; *Dig.;* Fluor. ac.; *Ham.;* Lept.; Lyc.; *Nux v.;* Op.; Plumb.; *Puls.; Sep.;* Spong.; Stellar.; *Sul.;* Verb.
Veins engorged (pelvic)—*Aloe;* Collins.; *Sep.;* Sul.
Veins engorged (portal)—Æsc.; *Aloe; Collins.;* Lept.; Lyc.; Nux v.; Sul.
Veins inflamed (phlebitis)—Acon.; Agar.; *Apis;* Arn.; *Ars.;* Bell.; Crot.; *Ham.;* Kali c.; *Lach.;* Lyc.; Merc.; Phos.; *Puls.;* Stront. c.; Vipera.
Veins inflamed, chronic—Arn.; Merc.; *Puls.;* Ruta.
Veins varicosed—Acet. ac.; *Æsc.;* Alumen; Apis; Ars.; Bellis; Calc. c.; *Calc. fl.; Calc. iod.;* Carbo v.; *Card. m.;* Caust.; Collins.; Ferr. p.; *Fluor. ac.;* Graph.; *Ham.;* Kali ars.; Lach.; *Lyc.;* Magnif.; Mur. ac.; Nat. m.; Pæonia; Plumb.; Polyg.; *Puls.;* Ran. s.; Ruta; Scirrhin; Sep.; *Staph.;* Stront. c.; *Sul.;* Sul. ac.; *Vipera;* Zinc. m.

LOCOMOTOR SYSTEM

AXILLAE—Abscess: Hep.; Irid.; Jugl. r.
Acne—Carbo v.
Eczema—Elaps; Nat. m.
Herpes—Carbo an.
Pain, in muscles, right side—Prim. v.
Pain, with, or without swelling—Jugl. c.
Sweat, profuse, offensive—Bov.; Calc. c.; Hep.; Kali c.; Lyc.; Nit. ac.; Osm.; Petrol.; Sep.; Sil.; Strych. p.; Sul.; Tellur.; Thuya.

BACK—Bent, arch-like, opisthotonos: Angust.; Cic.; Nat. s.; Nicot.; Op.; Phyt.; Strych. See Convulsions (Nervous System.)
Burning between scapulæ—Glon.; Lyc.; Phos.; Sul.
Burning—Alum.; Ars.; Aur. mur.; Berb. v.; Calc. fl.; Carbo an.; Helod.; Helon.; Kali p.; Lyc.; Med.; Nit. ac.; Phos.; Picr. ac.; Sep.; Tereb.; Ustil.; Xerophyl.
Burning in small spots—Agar.; Phos.; Ran. b.; Sul.
Coldness between scapulæ—Abies c.; Am. m.; Helod.; Lachnanth.; Sep.
Coldness—Abies c.; Acon.; Ars.; Benz. ac.; Gels.; Gins.; Quass.; Raph.; Sep.; Strych.; Ver. a.
Curvature (scoliosis)—Bar. c.; Calc. c.; Phos. ac.; Phos.; Sil.; Sul.
Eruption—Sep.
Lameness, stiffness—Abrot.; Acon.; Æsc.; Agar.; Am. m.; Bell.; Berb. v.; Bry.; Calc. c.; Camph. monobr.; Caust.; Cim.; Cupr. ars.; Diosc.; Dulc.; Gettysburg Water; Gins.; Helon.; Hyper.; Kali c.; Kali p.; Kal.; Lachnanth.; Led.; Lyc.; Nicot.; Physost.; Phyt.; Rhus t.; Ruta; Sarcol. ac.; Sep.; Spong.; Staph.; Strych.; Sul. ac.; Sul.; Zing.
Numbness—Acon.; Berb. v.; Calc. p.; Ox. ac.; Oxytr.; Sec.; Sil.
PAIN in general—Abrot.; Acon.; Æsc.; Agar.; Alum.; Am. c.; Angust.; Ant. t.; Apis; Arg. m.; Arg. n.; Arn.; Bar. c.; Bell.; Berb. v.; Bry.; Calc. c.; Calc. p.; Can. ind.; Carb. ac.; Caul.; Caust.; Cham.; Chin. s.; Cic.; Cim.; Cinch.; Cob.; Cocc.; Colch.; Col.; Dulc.; Eup. perf.; Graph.; Guaco; Ham.; Helon.; Homar.; Kali bich.; Kali c.; Kali m.; Lach.; Lil. t.; Lyc.; Mag. m.; Mag. s.; Med.; Merc.; Mez.; Mormord.; Nat. c.; Nat. m.; Nit. ac.; Nux v.; Ox. ac.; Paraf.; Petrol.; Phos. ac.; Picr. ac.; Puls.; Radium; Ran. ac.; Rhod.; Rhus t.; Ruta; Sao.; Sang.; Sarrac.; Scolop.; Sec.; Selen.; Sep.; Sil.; Staph.; Stellar.; Strych.; Sul.; Tar. h.; Tellur.; Ther.; Triost.; Upas; Variol.; Wyeth.; Xerophyl.; Zinc. m.
Aching, as if it would break and give out—Æsc.; Æth.; Am. m.; Bell.; Can. ind.; Cham.; Chel.; Dulc.; Eup. perf.; Eupion; Graph.; Ham.; Kali bich.; Kal.; Kreos.; Nat. m.; Ol. an.; Ova t.; Phos.; Plat.; Puls.; Rhus t.; Sarcol. ac.; Sanic.; Senega; Sil.; Trill.
Aching, dull, constant (backache)—Abies n.; Æsc.; Agar.; Aloe; Am. m.; Ant. t.; Apoc.; Arg. m.; Arg. n.; Arn.; Bapt.; Bellis; Berb. v.; But. ac.; Calc. c.; Calc. fl.; Canth.; Cim.; Cob.; Coccinel.; Cocc.; Colch.; Con.; Conv.; Cupr. ars.; Dulc.; Euonym.; Eupion; Ferr. p.; Gels.;

Glycerin; *Helon.;* Hyper.; Inula; Ipomœa; *Kali c.;* Kali iod.; *Kal.;* Kreos.; Lach.; Lith. benz.; Lycoper.; *Lyc.;* Morph.; *Nat. m.; Nux v.;* Ol. an.; *Ol. j. as.; Ox. ac.;* Pall.; Petrol.; Phos. ac.; *Phyt.;* Picr. ac.; Piscidia; *Pulex; Puls.; Radium; Rhus t.;* Ruta; *Sabal;* Sab.; Senec.; *Sep.;* Solan. lyc.; Solid.; *Staph.; Still.; Sul.;* Symphyt.; *Tereb.;* Upas; *Vib. op.;* Viscum; Zinc. m.

Between scapulæ—*Acon.;* Apomorph.; Asclep. t.; Bar. c.; *Calc. c.;* **Can.** ind.; Con.; Guaco; Guaiac.; Jugl. c.; Kali c.; Med.; *Pod.;* Radium; *Rhus t.;* Sep.; Sul.; Zinc. m.

Bruised—*Acon.;* Æsc.; Agar.; Ant. t.; *Arn.;* Bar. c.; *Berb. v.;* Bry.; Cina; *Dulc.;* Gins.; Graph.; *Ham.;* Mag. s.; *Merc.;* Nat. m.; *Nux v.;* Phos. ac.; *Phyt.; Rhus t.; Ruta;* Sil.; Sul.; Tellur.

Crampy—*Bell.;* Cim.; Cinch.; *Col.;* Graph.; Iris; Mag. p.; Ova t.; Sep.

Digging, cutting—Sep.

Drawing—Anac.; Carbo v.; *Caust.; Kali c.;* Lyc.; Nux v.; Rhus t.; *Sab.;* Sul.

Falling apart sensation, involving small of back, Sacro-iliac synchondroses; relieved by bandaging tightly—Trill.

Heaviness, dragging, weight—Æsc.; *Aloe; Am. m.;* Anac.; Ant. c.; Benz. ac.; *Berb. v.;* Bov.; Colch.; *Eup. purp.; Helon.;* Hydr.; Kali c.; *Kreos.; Lil. t.;* Nat. s.; Picr. ac.; *Sep.* See Female Sexual System.

Lancinating, drawing, tearing—Alum.; Asclep. t.; *Berb. v.;* Colch.; *Col.;* Kali m.; Lyc.; Mimosa; Nux v.; *Scolop.;* Sep.; Sil.; Stellar.; *Strych.*

Lancinating, extends down thighs, legs—*Æsc.;* Aur. mur.; Bapt.; *Berb. v.;* Carb. ac.; Cocc.; *Col.;* Cur.; Ham.; *Helon.;* Kali c.; Kali m.; Lac c.; *Ox. ac.;* Phyt.; *Scolop.; Stellar.;* Tellur.; Xerophyl.

Lancinating, extends to pelvis—*Arg. n.;* Aur. mur.; Berb. v.; Cham.; *Cim.;* Eupion; Ham.; Sil.; *Variol.;* Viscum.

Lancinating, extends to pubes—*Sab.;* Vib. op.; Xanth.

Lancinating, extends upwards—Aspar.; *Gels.*

Paralytic—Cocc.; Kali p.; Nat. m.; Sil.

Pressing, plug-like—*Æsc.; Agar.; Anac.;* Aur. mur.; Benz. ac.; *Berb. v.;* Colch.; Hyper.; Nat. m.; *Nux v.;* Sep.; Tellur.

Sensitiveness extreme of sacrum—Lob. infl.

Stitching, piercing, pricking—Agar.; Aloe; Alum.; Apis; *Berb. v.;* Bry.; Guaiac., Hyper.; *Kali c.;* Merc.; Nat. s.; Sul.; Tellur.; Ther.

MODALITIES—AGGRAVATION: After emission: Cob.

After masturbation—Nux v.; Phos. ac.; Staph.

At night—Aloe; Calc. c.; Lyc.; *Merc.;* Mez.; Nat. m.; *Staph.;* Viscum.

From cold exposure—Acon.; Bry.; *Rhod.;* Sul.

From damp exposure—Dulc.; Phyt.; *Rhus t.*

From eating—Kali c.

From exertion—Agar.; *Berb. v.;* Cocc.; Hyper.; Kali c.; Kali p.; Ox. ac.; Sul. See Motion.

From jar, touch—*Acon.;* Berb. v.; *Bry.;* Kali bich.; *Lob. infl.;* Mez.; Sil.; *Tellur.*

From lying down—Bell.; *Berb. v.;* Niccol. s.; Nux v.; Rhus t.

From motion, beginning—Lac c.; *Rhus t.*

LOCOMOTOR SYSTEM

From motion, walking—*Æsc.;* Aloe; *Ant. t.;* Bell.; *Bry.; Caust.;* Chel.; Cinch.; *Colch.;* Kali bich.; *Kali c.* Mez.; *Nux v.;* Ox. ac.; Parat.; Petrol.; Phyt.; Ran. ac.; Sep.; *Sul.*

From resting, sitting—*Agar.;* Alum.; Ant. t.; Bell.; *Berb. v.;* Can. ind.; Cob.; Ferr. mur.; Kali p.; Kreos.; *Lac c.;* Merc.; Nux v.; Puls.; *Rhus t.;* Sep.; Sul.; *Zinc. m.*

From standing—*Æsc.;* Bell.; Nux v.; Sarcol. ac.; Sep.

From stooping—*Æsc.;* Berb. v.; Diosc.; Guaco; Tellur.

From warmth—*Kali s.;* Puls.; Sul.

In morning—Agar.; *Berb. v.;* Bry.; Conv.; Kali c.; Nat. m.; Nux v.; Petrol.; Phyt.; Ruta; Selen.; *Staph.*

When rising from seat—Æsc.; Arg. n.; *Berb. v.; Caust.;* Kali p.; *Lach.;* Sil.; Sul.; Tellur.

AMELIORATION—After rising: Kali c.; Ruta; Staph.

From bending backward—Rhus t.

From bending forward—Lob. infl.

From emission—Zinc. m.

From lying on abdomen—Acet. ac.

From lying on back—Æsc.; *Cob.;* Gnaph.; Nat. m.; Rhus t.; Ruta.

From lying on something hard, or firm support—Eupion; *Nat. m.; Rhus t.;* Sep.

From lying, sitting—Sep.

From motion, walking—Arg. n.; Bell.; Caust.; *Cob.;* Ferr. mur.; *Helon.;* Kali m.; Kreos.; Merc.; *Puls.;* Radium; *Rhus t.;* Sep.; Staph.; *Sul.;* Zinc. m.

From rest—*Æsc.;* Colch.; Nux v.; Sil.

From sitting—Bell.

From standing—Arg. n.; Caust.; Sul.

From urination—*Lyc.;* Med.

WEAKNESS—Of back: Abrot.; *Æsc. gl.; Æsc.;* Alum.; Ant. t.; Arn.; Berb. v.; But. ac.; Calc. c.; *Calc. p.;* Cinch.; *Cocc.;* Glycerin; Graph.; Guaco; *Helon.;* Ign.; Irid.; Jacar.; *Kali c.;* Merc.; Nat. m.; Nux v.; Ox. ac.; Petrol.; Phos. ac.; Phos.; *Picr. ac.;* Pod.; *Sarrac.;* Sep.; Sil.; Staph.; *Zins. m.*

BODY—Bruised, sore feeling, all over: Abrot.; Ampel.; Apis; *Arn.;* Bapt.; Bellis; Caust.; Cic.; Cim.; *Cinch.; Eup. perf.; Gels.;* Ham.; Hep.; Iberis; Lil. t.; *Mang. ac.;* Med.; Morph.; Nux m.; *Phyt.;* Psor.; *Pyr.; Radium; Rhus t.;* Ruta; Sarcol. ac.; Solan. lyc.; Staph.; Tellur.; *Thuya;* Wyeth.

Burning, in various parts—Acon.; *Agar.;* Apis; *Ars.; Canth.;* Caps.; *Carbo an.;* Phos. ac.; *Phos.;* Sul.

Coldness—Acon.; *Æth.;* Ant. t.; Ars.; Atham.; *Bar. m.; Bor. ac.;* Cadm. s.; *Camph.;* Camph. monobr.; *Chloral;* Cupr.; *Helod.; Jatropha;* Lachnanth.; Luffa; *Sec.;* Tab.; *Ver. a.;* Zinc .m.

Constriction, as if caged—Cact.; Med.

Numbness—*Acon.;* Ars.; Cic.; Con.; *Ox. ac.; Phos.;* Plumb. m.; *Sec.*

Swelling—*Apis;* Doryph.; Frag. See Dropsy (Generalities).

Trembling—*Agar.*; Cod.; Con.; *Gels.*; Hyos.; Iberis; Lonic.; *Myg.*; Phos.; Sarcol. ac.

COCCYX—Burning on touch: Carbo an.
Itching—Bov.; Graph.
Neuralgia, worse rising from sitting posture—Lach.
Numbness—Plat.
Pain (coccygodynia)—Ant. t.; Arn.; *Bell.*; *Bry.*; *Calc. caust.*; Castorea; *Caust.*; *Cic.*; *Cim.*; Cistus; Con.; Ferr. p.; Fluor. ac.; *Graph.*; *Hyper.*; Kali bich.; Kali c.; Kali iod.; *Kreos.*; Lac c.; *Lach.*; Lobel. infl.; Mag. c.; *Mag. p.*; Merc.; *Paris*; Petrol.; Phos.; Rhus t.; Sil.; *Tar. h.*; Tetradym.; Xanth.; Zinc. m.
Bruised—Am. m.; Arn.; Caust.; Ruta; Sul.
Bruised from injury—Hyper.
Dragging, drawing—Ant. t.; *Caust.*; Graph.; Kreos.
Tearing, lancinating—*Bell.*; Canth.; *Cic.*; Kali bich.; *Mag. p.*; Merc.
Ulcer—Pæonia.

EXTREMITIES—Coldness: Acon.; Agar.; *Agar. ph.*; *Bell.*; *Calc. c.*; Calc. hypoph.; *Calc. p.*; *Camph.*; *Coccinel.*; Crat.; Dulc.; Ferr. m.; Hedeoma; *Helod.*; Hydroc. ac.; Ign.; Kal.; Lol. tem.; Lonic.; Meli.; Merc.; *Mur. ac.*; Nat. m.; Nux m.; Oleand.; Op.; *Phyt.*; Quass.; Sang.; *Sec.*; Sulphon.; Trill.; *Ver. a.*; Zinc. m.
Itching—*Arundo*; Kali c.; Lyc.; Pall.; *Phos.*; Prun. v.; Val.
Lameness, stiffness—*Agar.*; Agaricine; Aloe; *Calc. p.*; Carbo v.; *Cocc.*; *Eucal.*; Gins.; Ipec.; Kali p.; *Lith. c.*; *Rhus t.*; Triost.; Xerophyl.; Zinc. m.
Numbness, tingling, fall asleep—Absinth.; Acon.; Alum.; Aran.; *Arg. n.*; Avena; Bar. c.; Calc. c.; *Calc. p.*; Camph.; *Carbo v.*; *Caust.*; Cham.; Cic.; Cinch.; *Cocc.*; Gels.; Helod.; *Kali c.*; Kal.; Lonic.; *Morph.*; Nat. m.; *Onosm.*; Op.; Ox. ac.; Phos.; Picr. ac.; *Plat.*; Plumb. m.; *Sec.*; Sil.; Solan. n.; Sul.; *Thall.*; Ver. a.; Zinc. m.

PAIN—Aching: Æsc.; Apis; *Arn.*; Ars.; Azadir.; *Bry.*; Calc. c.; Carbo v.; Caust.; Cepa; *Cim.*; Cinch.; *Con.*; Cur.; Cycl.; Echin.; Eucal.; *Gels.*; Hedeoma; Kal.; Merc.; Myr.; Pyr.; Quass.; *Radium*; Ran. sc.; *Rhod.*; Rhus t.; Sec.; Sil.; Staph.; *Stellar.*; Strych. p.; Thyr.
Bone-pains—Aran.; Aur.; Calc. p.; *Eup. perf.*; Gels.; *Kali bich.*; Kali iod.; Mag. mur.; Mang. ac.; *Mere.*; *Mez.*; Phos. ac.; Ran. sc.; Rhus ven.; Ruta; *Sang.*; Sars.; *Still.*; Stront. c.; Triost.
Cramp-like, constricting—Abrot.; Alumen; Ant. t.; Antipyr.; *Asaf.*; Calc. c.; Canth.; Carbon. s.; *Cocc.*; *Col.*; Croc.; *Cupr. m.*; Gins.; Mag. p.; Menyanth.; *Plat.*; Sec.; Sil.; *Strych.*; Ver. a.
Drawing—Camph.; Caust.; Graph.; Hep.; Kali c.; Lyc.; Nat. m.; Rhus t.
Erratic, fly about—*Caul.*; Iris; Kali bich.; *Kali s.*; Kal.; *Lac c.*; Magnol.; *Mang. ac.*; Phyt.; *Puls.*; Rhod.; Sal. ac.; *Stellar.*
Growing pains—Apium gr.; Calc. p.; *Guaiac.*; Hippom.; Phos. ac. See Bones (Generalities).
Hysterical contractures—Bell.; *Cocc.*; *Cupr.*; Hyos.; *Ign.*; Lyc.; Merc.; Nux v.; Stram.; Zinc. m.
Neuralgic, lancinating, tearing, shooting—Absinth.; Acon.; Alum.; Bell.;

Branca; *Carbon. s.;* Caul.; *Cham.;* Daphne; Elat.; Eucal.; Gels.; Guaiac.; Kali c.; Kal.; Lyc.; *Mag. p.;* Magnol.; *Mimosa;* Nit. ac.; Ox. ac.; Phos.; Phyt.; *Rhod.;* Rhus t.; Sars.; Sil.; Strych.

Rheumatico-gouty—*Acon.;* Anag.; Ant. t.; Apis; *Arn.;* Aspar.; Bell.; Branca; *Bry.;* Calc. c.; *Calc. p.;* Caul.; Caust.; Cham.; *Colch.;* Dulc.; Eucal.; Guaiac.; Iod.; Kali c.; *Kal.;* Lac c.; Lyc.; *Merc.;* Prun. v.; *Radium; Rhod.; Rhus t.;* Sang.; *Stellar.;* Sticta.

Shock-like, paralytic—Cina; Colch.; *Phyt.; Thall.;* Veratrin; Ver. v.; Xanth.

Sprained, dislocated feeling—*Arn.;* Bellis; Calc. c.; Carbo v.; *Cinch.;* Rhus t.; *Ruta.* See Joints.

Paralysis—*Acon.;* Alum.; *Bar. ac.; Caust.; Cocc.; Con.;* Cur.; Dub.; *Dulc.;* Hedeoma; Kal.; *Lol. tem.;* Nux v.; Oleand.; Op.; *Phos.;* Picr. ac.; Rhus t.; Sec.; Sil. See Nervous System.

Sprains, chronic—Graph.; Petrol.; *Stront. c.* See Generalities.

Stretching continually—Alum.; Amyl; Angust.; *Ars.;* Cinch.; Quass.; Sep.

Trembling, twitching, jerking—Acon.; *Agar.;* Alum.; Apis; *Arg. n.;* Ars.; Bell.; Calc. p.; Carbo v.; Caust.; *Cim.;* Cinch.; *Cina; Cocc.; Con.;* Cupr. ars.; *Cupr. m.; Gels.;* Helod.; *Hyper.; Hyos.; Ign.;* Kali c.; Lach.; *Lol. tem.;* Lonic.; Lyc.; Mag. p.; *Merc.;* Morph.; *Myg.;* Op.; Phos. ac.; *Phos.;* Physost.; Rhus t.; *Sec.;* Sep.; Sil.; Stram.; *Strych.;* Sulphon.; Sul.; *Tar. h.;* Thall.; *Val.;* Viola od.; Xerophyl.; Zinc. m.; Zinc. s. See Weakness.

Weakness, debility—Æth.; Agar.; *Alum.; Am. caust.;* Am. m.; Anac.; Apis; Arg. n.; *Ars.;* Asar.; Bellis; Bism.; *Calc. c.; Caust.; Cinch.; Cocc.; Con.;* Cupr. m.; Cur.; Cyprip.; Dig.; Eucal.; *Gels.;* Gins.; Helon.; Hippom.; *Kali bich.;* Kal.; Lecith.; Lyc.; Mag. p.; Med.; Merc.; *Mur. ac.;* Myr.; Nat. c.; Nat. m.; Niccol. s.; Nux v.; *Onosm.;* Ox. ac.; *Phos. ac.; Phos.; Picr. ac.; Plat.;* Prim. v.; Puls.; *Sarcol. ac.;* Scutel.; Selen.; Sep.; Sil.; *Stann.;* Strych. p.; Sulphon.; *Thall.;* Thuya; Ver. a.; *Zinc. m.* See Neurasthenia (Nervous System).

UPPER EXTREMITIES—ARM: See Extremities in general.

Coldness—Apis; Carbo v.; Raph.; Ver. a.

Eruptions—Arundo; Caust.; Phos. ac.; Sul.

Gangrenous ulceration—Ran. flam.

Heaviness—*Acon.; Alum.;* Can. ind.; Cim.; *Cur.;* Ham.; Hep.; *Latrod.;* Lyc.; Nat. m.; Ver. a.

Intolerant of band around—Ov. g. p.

Itching—Fagop.

Jerking, involuntary motion—*Agar.;* Ant. c.; *Cic.;* Cina; Cocc.; *Ipec.;* Lact. v.; Lyc.; Op.; Tar. h.; *Thlasp.*

Jerking, or involuntary motion, of one arm, and leg—Apoc.; Bry.; *Helleb.; Myg.;* Zinc. m.

Lameness, stiffness—*Acon.;* Am. c.; Bapt.; Can. ind.; *Caust.;* Paris; Rhus ven.; Thasp.; Ver. a.

Nodules—Hippoz.

Numbness, fail asleep—*Acon.;* Ambra; Aran.; Aster.; Bar. c.; *Cact.;* Cham.; Cim.; *Cocc.;* Dig.; *Graph.;* Iberis; Ign.; Kali c.; *Latrod.;*

Lil. t.; Lyc.; *Mag. m.*; Magnol.; *Nux v.*; Paris; Phos.; *Rhus t.*; Sep.; Sil.; Xanth.

Numbness, left arm—Acon.; Dig.; Kal.; Puls.; *Rhus t.*; Sumb.

Numbness, right arm—Phyt.

PAINS—Æsc.; *Alum.*; *Anag.*; Calc. c.; *Caust.*; Cepa; Cic.; Cinnab.; *Eup. perf.*; Ferr. picr.; Gels.; Guaco; *Guaiac.*; Indium; Mag. m.; Nat. m.; Phos.; *Phyt.*; *Rhus t.*; *Sang.*; Solan. lyc.; *Stellar.*; Sticta; *Sul.*; Wyeth.; *Zinc. m.*

Pain in left arm—Acon.; Agar.; Aster.; *Cact.*; *Cim.*; Colch.; Crot.; Iberis; Kal.; *Latrod.*; Magnol.; Mag. s.; *Rhus t.*; *Spig.*; Tab.; Xanth.

Pain in right arm—*Ferr. mur.*; Ferr. picr.; Pip. m.; Rhus v.; *Sang.*; Solan. lyc.; Viola od.; Wyeth.

Aching—Bapt.; Berb. v.; *Caust.*; Gels.; Jal.; Lith. c.; Nat. ars.; Ol. j. as.; Sarrac.

Aching, weakness, when singing, using voice—Stann.

Bruised, cramp-like—Acon.; Arg. n.; *Cocc.*; Cupr. m.; Oleand.; *Phos. ac.*; Sec.; Sul. ac.; Ver. v.; *Zinc. s.*

Drawing—Calc. c.; *Caust.*; Lyc.; *Mag. m.*; Mur. ac.; Oleand.; Sep.; Sil.; Zinc. m.

Neuralgic (brachyalgia)—*Acon. rad.*; Alum.; Bry.; *Hyper.*; Kali c.; *Kal.*; Lyc.; Merc.; *Nux v.*; Pip. m.; *Puls.*; *Rhus t.*; Scutel.; Sul.; Teucr.; Ver. a.; Viscum.

Paralysis—Cocc.; Ferr.; Gels.; Nux v.; Rhus t.

Sensibility, diminished—Carbon. s.; Phos.

Tearing, stitching—Calc. c.; Ferr.; Hep.; Phos.; Sep.; Sil.

Trembling—Cod.; Cocc.; *Gels.*; Kali br.; *Phos.*; Sil. See Weakness.

Weakness—*Alumen*; Anac.; *Cur.*; Dig.; Iod.; Kali c.; Lach.; Lyc.; Mag. p.; Med.; Nat. m.; Sarcol. ac.; Sep.; *Sil.*; *Stann.*; Sul.

FOREARM—See Extremities.

Coldness—Arn.; Brom.; Med.

Pain—Anac.; Cinnab.; *Eup. perf.*; Ferr. mur.; Ferr. picr.; Gels.; Guaco; *Hyper.*; Kali c.; *Kal.*; Phyt.; *Rhus t.*; Sep.; Stann.

Paralysis—Arg. n.; Nux v.; Plumb.; Sil. See Nervous System.

Soreness of flexor carpi ulnaris—Brachygl.

Unsteadiness of muscles of forearm, hands—Caust.

HAND—**Automatic motion of hand and head**—Apoc.; Bry.; Helleb.; Zinc. m.

Blueness, distended veins: Am. c.; Amyl; *Ant. t.*; *Carbo an.*; Dig.; Elaps; Laur.; *Nit. ac.*; Oleand.; Samb.; Stront. c.; *Ver. a.* See Cyanosis (Circulatory System).

Burning, heat—*Acon.*; Agar.; Carbo v.; Cocc.; *Lach.*; Lyc.; *Med.*; Ol. j. as.; *Phos.*; Sang.; Sil.

Chapping—Alum.; *Calc. c.*; Castor.; Cistus; *Graph.*; Lyc.; Mag. c.; Nat. ars.; Nat. c.; *Petrol.*; Sars.; Sulphurous ac.

Coldness—Abies c.; Acon.; *Ant. t.*; Apis; Ars.; Cact.; Calc. c.; *Camph.*; Carbon. ox.; Cic.; *Cinch.*; Con.; Cupr.; *Dig.*; Iod.; *Menyanth.*; Nat. m.; Nit. ac.; Scilla; *Tab.*; Thuya; Trifol.; Ver. a.

Coldness of one, warmth of the other—Cinch.; Dig.; Ipec.; Puls.

Cramps—Bell.; Calc. c.; *Sec.*; Sil.

LOCOMOTOR SYSTEM

Cramps (writers'); piano or violin players, typists—Ambra; *Arg. m.; Arg. n.;* Brachygl.; *Caust.; Cim.;* Cupr.; Cycl.; *Gels.;* Graph.; Hep.; *Mag. p.;* Ruta; *Stann.;* Sul. ac.; Sul. See Nervous System.

Dryness—Lyc.; Zinc. m.

Enlarged feeling—*Aran.;* Caust.; *Cocc.;* Gins.; Kali n.

Eruption—Bor.; Cistus; Pedic.; *Pix l.* See Skin.

Fidgety—*Kali br.; Myg.;* Tar. h.; Zinc. m.

Hypothenar eminences bright red—Acon.

Itching—Agar.; Tellur.

Nodotities, gouty, on dorsum—*Am. phos.;* Eucal.; Med. See Fingers.

Numbness, go asleep—*Acon.;* Arg. n.; Ars.; Bor.; Can. ind.; *Caust.; Cocc.;* Cod.; *Colch.;* Graph.; *Hyper.;* Iberis; Laburn.; Lach.; Lil. t.; Lyc.; Mag. p.; Nat. c.; Nux v.; *Phos.;* Physost.; Pyr.; Raph.; Sec.; Tela ar.

Pains—Bruised: *Ruta;* Ver. a.

Lancinating—*Cepa;* Lappa; Selen.; Sul.

Rheumatic—Ambra; Berb. v.; *Caul.; Caust.;* Chel.; Guaiac.; Led.; *Puls.; Rhus t.; Ruta;* Sang.; Solan. lyc.

Paralysis—Ferr.; Laburn.; Merc.; Plumb. ac.; Ruta; Sil.

PALMS—Blisters: Bufo.

Burning—*Azadir.;* Bolet.; Ferr. m.; Ferr. p.; Gadus; *Lach.;* Lachnanth.; Limul.; Nat. m.; *Ol. j. as.;* Petrol.; *Phos.;* Prim. v.; Puls. nut.; *Sang.;* Sep.; *Sul.*

Chapping, fissuring—Calc. fl.; *Ran. b.*

Cramps—*Cupr. m.;* Scrophul.; Zing.

Desquamation—Elaps.

Eruption, dry, bran-like, itching—Anag.; *Ars.;* X-ray.

Injury with intolerable pain—Hyper.

Itching—Ant. s. a.; *Fagop.; Granat.;* Limulus; Ran. b.; Tub.

Pains—Azadir.; Trifol.

Stiffness of hands while writing—Kali m.

Sweating—*Calc. c.;* Cocc.; Con.; Dulc.; Fagop.; *Fluor. ac.;* Nat. m.; Picr. ac.; Sep.; *Sil.;* Strych. p.; *Sul.;* Wyeth.

Swelling—Æsc.; Agar.; *Apis;* Arg. n.; Ars.; Arundo; Bry.; *Cact.;* Calc. c.; Crot.; Elaps; Ferr. p.; Nat. chlor.; *Rhus div.* See Dropsy (Generalities).

Twitching, trembling, weakness—Act. sp.; Anac.; Ant. c.; Ant. t.; *Arg. n.;* Arn.; Avena; Calc. c.; *Cic.; Cina;* Cocc.; *Con.; Cur.; Gels.;* Hippom.; Lach.; Lact. v.; Lol. tem.; *Mag. p.; Merc.; Phos.;* Sars.; *Sarcol. ac.;* Sil.; *Stann.; Stram.;* Sul.; Tab.; Zinc. m.

Warts—*Anac.;* Ant. c.; Calc. c.; *Dulc.;* Ferr. mag.; *Ferr. picr.;* Nat. c.; Nat. m.; *Ruta.*

Yellow color—Chel.; Sep. See Skin.

FINGERS—Blueness, coldness: Chel.; Crat.; Cupr. m.; Ver. a. See Hands

Blue, numb, shrivelled, spread apart, or bent backward—Sec.

Burning—*Azadir.;* Gin.; Oleand.; Sars.; *Sul.*

Chapped tips, cracks, fissures—Alum.; *Graph.;* Nat. m.; *Petrol.; Ran. b.;* Sanic.; Sars.

Cramp-like, contracted, clenching—*Æth.*; Ambra; Anag.; *Arg. n.*; Bism.; Brachygl.; Can. s.; Caust.; *Cic.*; Cina; Cocc.; Colchicine; *Cupr. ac.*; *Cupr. m.*; Cycl.; Diosc.; *Helleb.*; Kali bich.; Laur.; Lyc.; Paris; Ruta; Sec.; Solan. t.; Stann.; *Sul. ac.*

Crooked—Kali c.; Lyc.

Crushed, mashed tips—Hyper.

Eruptions—Alnus; Anac.; *Bov.*; Graph.; Limul.; *Lob. er.*; Nat. c.; Nit. ac.; *Petrol.:* Prim. far.; *Rhus t.*; Sars.; Selen.; Veronal. See Skin.

Exostoses—Calc. fl.; *Hekla.*

Fidgety, must move constantly—Kali br.

Hypertrophy—Aur. mur.

Impression deep, from scissors—Bov.

Itching between—Phos. ac. See Skin.

Jerking, when holding pen—*Caust.*; Cina; Cycl.; Kali c.; *Stann.*; Sul. ac.

Joints, inflamed, painful—*Benz. ac.*; Berb. v.; *Bry.*; Fluor. ac.; Lyc.; Med.; *Nat. p.*; Pip. m.; Prim. sylv.; Puls.; *Rhus t.*; Staph.; *Stellar.* See Rheumatism.

Joints, nodosities on—*Am. phos.*; *Benz. ac.*; Benzoin; Calc. c.; Calc. fl.; Caul.; *Colch.*; Graph.; Led.; Lith. c.; *Lyc.*; Med.; Staph.; Stellar. See Joints.

Joints, pain in—Bry.; Graph.; Led.; Lyc.; Sil.; Sul.

Joints, stiff—Carbo v.; *Caul.*; Lyc.; Prim. sylv.; Puls. See Joints.

Numbness, tingling of fingers—*Acon.*; Æsc.; Ambra; Apis; Ars.; Aster.; Bar. c.; Calc. c.; *Cocaine;* Con.; *Dig.*; Lathyrus; Lyc.; Mag. p.; Mag. s.; Nat. m.; Nit. ac.; *Ox. ac.*; Paris; Phos.; Propyl.; Sarcol. ac.; Sec.; Sil.; *Thall.*; Thuya; Upas; Verbasc.; Zinc. m.

Pains, at root of nails—Berb. v.; Bism.; *Cepa;* Myrist. seb.

Pains in general—Abrot.; Azadir.; Lil. t.; Sec.

Pains in tips—Am. m.; Bor.; Chel.; *Hyper.*; Kali c.; *Sec.*; Sil.; Teucr.

Pains, rheumatic—*Act. sp.*; *Ant. c.*; Berb. v.; *Caul.*; Colch.; Fagop.; Granat.; Graph.; Guaco; Hyper.; Lappa; *Led.*; Lith. c.; Lyc.; Med.; Pæonia; Puls.; Ran. sc.; *Rhus t.* See Rheumatism.

Pains, tearing—*Act. sp.*; Am. m.; *Caul.*; Caust.; Ced.; Led.; Lyc.; *Puls.*; Rhus t.

Pains, throbbing—Amyl; Bor.

Panaritium—Alum.; Am. c.; Diosc.; Myrist. seb.; Sil.

Sensibility, diminished—*Carbon. s.*; Pop. c.; Sec.

Sensitive to cold—*Cistus;* Hep.

Skin, dry, shrivelled—Æth. See Skin.

Skin peels off—Elaps. See Skin.

Soreness between—Nat. ars. See Skin.

Stiffness, rigidity—Am. c.; Carbon. s.; *Caul.*; Cocc.; Lyc.; Oleand.; Puls.; Sil. See Joints.

Swelling—*Am. c.*; Bry.; Carbon. s.; Cinnam.; Hep.; Kali m.; Lith. c. Mang.; Oleand.; Puls.; *Thuya.*

Thick, horny tips—*Ant. c.*; Pop. c.

Trembling—Bry.; Iod.; Kali br.; Lolium; Merc.; Oleand.; Rhus t.; Zinc. m.

Ulcers—Alum.; Arundo; Ars.; Bor.; Sep.

LOCOMOTOR SYSTEM 869

Weariness—Bov.; Calc. c.; *Cur.*; *Gels.*; Hippom.; Phos.; Sil. See Hand.
LOWER EXTREMITIES—BUTTOCKS (glutei): Cold feeling: Daphne.
   Cold feeling, fall asleep—Calc. p.
   Cramp—Graph.
   Emaciation—Lathyr.
   Pain to hips, small of back—Staph.
   Pricking—Guaiac.
   Swelling—Phos. ac.
LOINS—LUMBAGO: Acon.; Act. sp.; *Æsc.*; Agar.; *Aloe*; Ant. t.; Arn.; Bell.; Berb. v.; Bry.; Calc. fl.; Calc. p.; Carb. ac.; Carbon. s.; Caul.; Cham.; Chel.; Cim.; Cina; Colch.; Col.; Diosc.; Dulc.; Eup. perf.; Ferr. m.; Gins.; Gnaph.; Guaiac.; Hydr.; *Hymosa;* Ipomoea; Kali bich.; Kali c.; Kali iod.; Kali ox.; Lathyr.; Led.; Lith. benz.; Lyc.; Macrot.; Merc. s.; Nat. m.; Nux v.; Pampin.; Picr. ac.; Phyt.; Puls.; Radium; Rham. c.; Rhod.; Rhus t.; Ruta; Sabal; Senec.; Sep.; Spiranth.; Sul.; Tereb.; Vib. op.
   Alternates, with headache, piles—Aloe.
   With aggravation in open air—Agar.
   With aggravation on beginning to move—Anac.; Con.; Glycerin; Rhus t.
   With aggravation, on beginning to move, relieved by continued motion—Calc. fl.; Rhus t.
   With aggravation on exertion; during day; while sitting—Agar.
   With aggravation on lying down—Bell.; Murex.
   With chronic tendency—Æsc.; Berb. v.; Calc. fl.; Rhus t.; Sil.
   With masturbatic origin; sexual weakness—Nux v.
   With numbness, in lower part of back, weight in pelvis—Gnaph.
   With relief from lying down—Euonym.; Sep.
   With relief, from slow walking—Ferr. m.
   With retching, cold, clammy sweat, from least motion—Lathyr.
   With sciatica—Rhus t.
THIGS-LEGS—Blue, painful, swollen, if hanging down: Lathyr.
   Burning—*Ars.*; Arundo; Bar. c.; Kali c.; Led.; Lyc.; Mez.; Still.
   Coldness—Acon.; Alum.; Astrag.; Berb. v.; Bism.; Calc. c.; Calc. p.; Carbo an.; Carbo v.; Colch.; Crot.; Lact. ac.; Lact. v.; *Laur.*; Lyc.; Merc.; Mez.; Nat. m.; Nit. ac.; Ox. ac.; Sep.; Sil.; Tab.; Ver. a.; Zinc. m.
   Contractions of hamstrings, tendons—Am. m.; Caust.; Cimex; Col.; Graph.; Guaiac.; Lach.; Med.; Nat. m.; Ruta; Sul.
   Curved limbs, cannot be straightened, and vice versa—Cic.
   Emaciation—*Abrot.*; Acet. ac.; Kali iod.; Lathyr.; Pin. sylv.
   Enlargement of femur, in rachitic infants—Calc. fl.
   Eruptions—Calc. c.; Chrysar.; Gins.; Graph.; Mag. c.; Petrol.; Sul. See Skin.
   Erysipelas—Sul. See Skin.
   Excoriation, itching over tibia—Bism.
   Heaviness—Alum.; Bry.; Calc. c.; Can. ind.; Cim.; Con.; Gins.; Guaco; Helleb.; Med.; Nux v.; Pall.; Picr. ac.; Sep.; Sulphon.; Sul.; Verbasc.; Vib. op.

LOCOMOTOR SYSTEM

Itching—Bellis; Bov.; *Fagop.;* Nit. ac.; *Rumex;* Stellar.

Motion involuntary—Bry.; Helleb.; Lyc.; *Myg.;* Tar. h. See Trembling.

Numbness, formication, "going asleep"—*Agar.; Alum.;* Aran.; Calc. c.; *Calc. p.; Caust.;* Carbon. s.; *Cocc.;* Col.; Crot.; *Gnaph.;* Graph.; Kali c.; Kali iod.; Lact. v.; Mez.; *Nux v.;* Onosm.; *Phos.; Rhus t.;* Sarcol. ac.; *Sec.;* Sep.; *Sul.;* Tar. h.; Tela ar.; *Triost.;* Zinc. m.

PAINS—In general: Agar.; Can. ind.; *Caps.; Carbon. s.;* Carbo an.; Chel.; Cic.; Diad.; *Diosc.;* Euphorb.; Ferr. m.; *Gels.; Gnaph.;* Helod.; Illic.; Indigo; Iod.; Irid.; *Kali c.; Kal.;* Lach.; Mag. m.; Mang. ac.; Mang. ox.; Menisp.; Murex; Nat. s.; Nit. ac.; Phos. ac.; *Phos.;* Picr. ac.; *Plumb. m.;* Puls.; *Rhus t.;* Sab.; Sil.; Tongo; Trifol.; Vib. op.; *Vipera.*

Aching, bruised—Arg. n.; *Arn.; Bapt.;* Calc. c.; *Cim.;* Cocc.; *Colch.;* Diosc.; *Eup. perf.; Gels.;* Guaiac.; Laur.; Lil. t.; Mag. c.; Med.; *Phos. ac.; Pyr.;* Sab.; Sarcol. ac.; Sep.; Solan. lyc.; Staph.; Ulnus; *Variol.*

Cramps, contractions—Abrot.; Æsc. gl.; Agar.; Ambra; Am. br.; *Am. m.;* Anac.; *Arn.;* Bapt.; Bar. c.; *Calc. c.; Camph.;* Carb. ac.; Carbo an.; Carbo v.; *Caust.;* Cholas ter.; *Cimex;* Cim.; Cinch.; *Cocc.;* Colch.; Col.; Con.; *Cupr. ars.; Cupr. m.;* Eupion; Ferr. m.; *Gels.;* Hyper.; Hyos.; Irid.; Jatropha; Lathyrus; Lol. tem.; *Lyc.; Mag. p.;* Med.; Nit. ac.; *Nux v.;* Ox. ac.; Pin. sylv.; Plumb. m.; Puls.; *Rhus t.;* Sarcol. ac.; *Sec.;* Sep.; *Sil.;* Solan. t.; *Sul.;* Ustil.; *Ver. a.;* Vipera; Zinc. s.

Cramps (tailor's)—Anac.; Anag.; Mag. p.

Pains in tibia—Ars.; Bad.; Carbo an.; *Dulc.;* Ferr. m.; *Kali bich.; Lach.;* Mang. ox.; *Mez.; Phos.;* Sep.

Rending, tearing, lancinating—*Am. m.;* Ars.; Bapt.; Bar. ac.; *Bell.;* Bellis; Cob.; Col.; *Diosc.; Hyper.;* Kali bich.; Kali c.; *Kal.;* Lyc.; Nit. ac.; *Plumb. m.;* Puls.; *Rhus t.;* Sep.; *Sul.;* Teucr.; Viscum.

Rheumatic—Berb. v.; *Bry.;* Chel.; Colch.; Daphne; *Dulc.;* Led.; *Phyt.;* Merc.; *Rhus t.;* Sang.; Stellar.; Val. See Rheumatism.

Paralysis—*Agar.;* Alum.; Bry.; *Can. ind.;* Chel.; *Cocc.;* Crot.; Dulc.; Gels.; *Guaco;* Kali iod.; Kali tart.; *Lathyr.;* Nux v.; Oleand.; *Plumb. m.; Rhus t.;* Sec.; Sulphon.; Tab.; *Thall.;* Ver. a.; Zinc. m. See Nervous System.

Restless, fidgety—Ars.; Carbo v.; *Caust.;* Cim.; Cinch.; Con.; Crot.; Graph.; Kali br.; Lil. t.; Lyc.; *Med.; Menyanth.;* Merc. c.; Myg.; Nit. ac.; *Phos.; Rhus t.;* Ruta; Scutel.; *Sep.;* Sulphon.; Tar. h.; *Tarax.;* Thasp.; *Zinc. m.;* Zinc. v.

Rigidity, stiffness, lameness—Alum.; Angust.; *Arg. n.;* Bapt.; Bar. m.; Calc. c.; *Cic.;* Colch.; *Con.;* Diosc.; *Eup. perf.;* Guaiac.; *Lathyr.;* Physost.; Plat.; *Rhus t.;* Sarcol. ac.; Sep.; *Strych.;* Xerophyl.

Sensibility, diminished—Ox. ac.; Phos. See Nervous System.

Sensibility, increased—Lach.; Lathyr. See Nervous System.

Spots on, red—Calc. c.; Sul.

Stretching—Am. c.; *Amyl;* Helleb.; Helod. See Fever.

Sweat, cold, clammy, at P. M.—Calc. c.; Merc.

Sweat extending below knees in A. M.—Sul.

Sweat on thighs, exhausting at P. M.—Carbo an.

Swelling—*Acet. ac.; Apis;* Ars.; Aur.; *Cact.;* Chel.; Colch.; *Dig.;* **Eup.**

perf.; *Ferr. m.;* Fluor. ac.; Graph.; Kali c.; Lathyr.; *Lyc.;* Merc.; Phos.; *Rhus t.;* Samb.; Sep.; Stront. c.; *Stroph.;* Sul.; Thyr.; Viscum. See Dropsy (Generalities).

Trembling—Æsc. gl.; Arg. m.; *Cob.; Cocc.;* Cod.; Colch.; *Con.;* Cur.; Doryph.; *Gels.;* Lol. tem.; *Mimosa;* Nit. ac.; Phos. ac.; Phos.; Tab.; Zinc. m.

Trickling, as from drops of water—Acon.

Ulcers—*Ars.;* Calc. c.; Carbo v.; Cistus; Echin.; Lyc.; Phos. ac.; Rhus t.; Sacchar. of.; *Sil.;* Trifol. See Generalities.

Weakness, easily fatigued—Æsc.; *Alumen; Alum.;* Am. c.; Arg. m.; Arg. n.; Bar. m.; Berb. v.; *Calc. p.; Can. ind.;* Cim.; Cob.; *Cocc.;* Colch.; *Con.;* Cupr. m.; Cur.; Dig.; Ferr m.; *Formica; Gels.;* Ham.; Kali c.; Kal.; Lach.; Med.; *Nat. m.; Nux v.; Oleand.;* Onosm.; Pœonia; Phell.; *Phos. ac.; Phos.; Picr. ac.;* Rhus t.; Ruta; Sarrac.; *Sarcol. ac.;* Sil.; Stann.; Sul.; Vib. op.

FEET—**Affections of ball, and dorsum of toes:** Can. s.

Bunions—Agar.; *Benz. ac.;* Hyper.; *Kali iod.;* Rhod.; *Sil.;* Ver. v. See Skin.

Burning—Agar.; Am. c.; *Apis;* Azadir.; Branca; Bor.; Graph.; Helod.; Kali c.; *Lach.;* Led.; *Med.;* Nat. m.; Phos. ac.; *Phos.;* Puls.; Sec.; Sep.; Sil.; *Sul.*

Chilblains—*Abrot.;* Agar.; Petrol.; Sul.; Tamus; Zinc. m. See Skin.

Coldness—*Acon.;* Alum.; *Ars.;* Calc. c.; Camph.; Carbo an.; *Carbo v.;* Caust.; Chel.; Cistus; Con.; Dig.; *Dulc.;* Elaps, Helod.; Kali c.; *Lach.;* Lyc.; Menyanth.; *Mur. ac.;* Oleand.; Petrol.; Picr. ac.; Plat.; Puls.; Samb.; Scilla; *Sec.;* Sep.; *Sil.;* Sul. ac.; Sul.; Trifol.; *Ver. a*

Coldness, clammy—Bar. c.; *Calc. c.;* Laur.; *Sep.;* Strych. p.

Coldness during day, burning soles at night—Sul.

Coldness of one, warmth of other—Chel.; *Cinch.;* Dig.; Ipec.; *Lyc.*

Enlarged feeling—Apis.

Eruptions—Bism.; Elaps; Graph.; *Petrol.* See Skin.

Fidgety—*Cina;* Kali p.; *Med.;* Sul.; Tar. h.; *Zinc. m.; Zinc. v.*

Itching, worse from scratching, warmth of bed—Led.; Puls.; Rhus t.

Spasmodic motion of left foot—Cina.

Tender feet with shop girls—Scilla.

HEELS—**Blisters:** Scilla.

Burning—Cycl.; Graph. See Feet.

Numbness—*Alum.;* Ign.

Os Calcis, pain—Aran.

Purring sensation, extending to right toes—Astrag.

PAINS—**In general**—*Agar.;* Am. c.; *Am. m.;* Brom.; *Calc. caust.; Caul.; Caust.;* Colch.; *Cycl.;* Ferr. m.; *Graph.;* Kali iod.; *Led.; Mang. ac.;* Nat. ars.; Nit. ac.; *Phos. ac.; Phyt.;* Ran. b.; *Rhus t.;* Sab.; Sep.; *Sil.;* Tetradyn.; Thuya; Upas; *Val.;* Zinc. m.

Aching, bruised—Agar.; Arn.; Laur.; Led.; *Phyt.; Rhus t.*

Soreness—Agar.; Ant. c.; Caust.; Cepa; *Cycl.;* Jal.; Kali bich.; Med.; Phos. ac.; Phyt.; Val.

Soreness, as if stepping on pebbles—Hep.; Lyc.

Tendo-Achilles, pain—Aristol.; *Benz. ac.;* Calc. caust.; Caust.; *Cim.;* Ign.; Med.; *Mur. ac.;* Nat. ars.; Ruta; Tetradyn.; Thuya; Upas; *Val.*

Ulcerative—Am. m.; Berb. v.; *Phos. ac.;* Puls.; *Ran. b.*

Ulcers on heels—Ars.; Arundo; Cepa; Lamium.

Itching of feet—*Agar.;* Am. m.; Ant. s. a.; *Bov.;* Caust.; Magnol.; Nat. s.; Sul.; *Tellur.*

Itching, worse on scratching, warmth of bed—Led.; *Puls.;* Rhus t.

Joints, gouty, enlarged—Eucal.; Puls. nut.; Tar. c.; *Zinc. m.* See Joints.

Numbness, formication, go asleep—Æth.; Am. m.; Ars.; Calc. c.; *Carbo v.;* Cob.; *Cocc.;* Cod.; Colch.; *Con.;* Fagop.; Gels.; *Hyper.;* Lact. v.; Mag. s.; Mez.; Nux v.; Onosm., *Physost.;* Phos.; Pyr.; *Sec.;* Sil.; Ulnus; Upas; Viola od.; *Zinc. m.*

PAINS—Aching, bruised: *Am. m.;* Arn.; Azadir.; Brom.; Dros.; Euonym.; Prun. sp.; *Ver. a.*

Cramps—Bism.; Cholas ter.; Cinch.; *Colch.;* Cupr. m.; Frax. am.; Jatropha; Lyc.; Nat. c.; *Sec.;* Sep.; Verbasc.; Zinc. m.

Lancinating—Abrot.; *Act. sp.;* Apis; Ced.; Led.; Lyc.; Nat. c.; Sep.

Rheumatic—*Act. sp.;* Apis; Berb. v.; *Caul.;* Caust.; *Colch.;* Graph.; Led.; *Lith. c.;* Mang. ac.; Myr.; Phyt.; *Puls.;* Ran. b.; *Rhus t.;* Ruta.

Sensibility, diminished—Carbon. s.

SOLES—Blistered: Bufo; Calc. c.; Cepa.

Burning—Anac.; Apoc. andr.; Arundo; Calc. c.; *Calc. s.;* Canth.; *Cham.;* Cupr.; Ferr. m.; Graph.; Ign.; Kreos.; *Lach.;* Lachnanth.; Limul.; Lyc.; Mang.; *Med.;* Niccol. s.; Petrol.; Phos. ac.; Puls.; *Sang.;* Sanic.; Sul.

Callosities—Anac. oc.; Ant. c.; Lyc.; Ran. b.; Sil. See Skin.

Injury, with intolerable pain—Hyper.

Itching—*Agar.;* Ananth.; Anthem.; *Calc. s.;* *Hydrocot.;* Indium; Nat. s.; Sil.

Numbness—*Cocc.;* Limul.; Raph.; Sep.

PAINS—In general: *Apoc. andr.;* Bor.; Can. ind.; Ferr.; *Guaco;* Kali iod.; Led.; Limul.; Mur. ac.; Nat. c.; Petrol.; Phos. ac.; *Puls.;* Verbasc.

Aching—Limul.; Puls.

Cramps—Agar.; Am. c.; Apoc. andr.; Carbo v.; *Colch.;* Cupr.; Med.; Nux v.; Stront.; Sul.; Verbasc.; Zinc.

Cramps, worse at P. M.—Cupr.; Eug. j.; Zing.

Pains, when walking—*Aloe;* Caust.; Graph.; Lyc.; Mur. ac.; *Petrol.;* Phos. ac.

Ulcerative, unable to walk—Canth.; Ign.; Phos.

Rawness, soreness, tenderness—Æsc.; Alum.; Ant. c.; Arn.; Bar. c.; Calc. c.; *Graph.;* Kali c.; Led.; Lyc.; *Med.;* Nat. c.; Nit. ac.; *Petrol.;* Phos. ac.; *Ruta;* Sanic.; Sil.

Swelling—Agar.; Alum.; Arundo; Calc. c.; Led.; Lyc.; Petrol. See Feet.

Ulcer—Ars.

Weakness—Hippom. See Feet.

SWEATING OF FEET—Alum.; Am c.; *Am. m.;* Ananth.; Apoc. andr.; Arundo; Bar. ac.; Bar. c.; *Calc. c.;* Carbo v.; Cob.; *Graph.;* Iod.; Lact.

ac.; *Lyc.*; Mag. m.; *Nit. ac.*; Ol. an.; *Petrol.*; Phos. ac.; *Psor.*; Rhus t.; Sal. ac.; *Sanic.*; Sep.; *Sil.*; *Sul.*; *Tellur.*; Thuya; Zinc. m.

Sweating, fetid—Alum.; Am. m.; Bar. c.; *But. ac.*; Calc. c.; Graph.; Kali c.; Nit. ac.; Petrol.; *Psor.*; *Sanic.*; *Sil.*; Zinc. m.

Sweating, suppressed—*Cupr.*; Sep.; Sil.; *Sul.*; Zinc. m.

Sweating, suppressed, then throat affections—Bar. c.; Graph.; Psor.; Sanic.; Sil.

Sweating, with soreness of toes—Bar. c.; Iod.; Lyc.; Nit. ac.; *Petrol.*; Sanic.; *Sil.*; Zinc. m

Swelling—*Acet. ac.*; Æsc.; Am. c.; *Apis; Ars.*; Arundo; Bry.; *Caci.*; Caust.; Cinch.; Colch.; *Dig.*; Ferr.; *Graph.*; *Ham.*; Helod.; Led.; Lyc.; *Merc. c.*; Merc.; Nat. m.; Nat. s.; Phos. ac.; Plumb. m., *Prun. sp.*; Puls.; Sacchar. of.; Samb.; Sep.; Sil.; *Stroph.*: Ver. a. See Dropsy (Generalities).

Tenderness, soreness—*Ant. c.*; Arn.; Bar. c.; Cepa; Led.; Petrol.; Phos. ac.; *Sil.*; Zinc. See Pain.

Trembling—*Gels.*; Phos.; Sars.; Sep.; Stram.

Ulcer—Bar. c.

Varices—*Ferr. acet.*; Ham. See Generalities.

Weakness—Acon.; Æsc.; Ant. c.; Ars.; Bov.; Can. s.; *Gels.*; Hippom.; Ign.; Lyc.; Mag. c.; Ran. rep.

TOES—Bunion on big toe—Agar.; *Benz. ac.*; Bor.; Hyper.; Iod.; Kali iod.; Rhod.; Sang.; Sars.; *Sil.*; Ver. v See Skin.

Burning—Alum.; Sars.

Callosities—Acet. ac.; Ant. c.; Calc. c.; Cur.; *Ferr. picr.*; Graph.; Hyper.; Lyc.; Nit. ac.; *Ran. b.*; Ran. sc.; Semperv. t.; Sep.; *Sil.*; Sul. ac. See Skin.

Chilblains—*Nit. ac.*; Sal. ac. See Skin.

Coldness—Sul.

Cracks of skin—Eug. j.; *Graph.*; *Petrol.*; Sabad.; Sars.

Crooked—Graph.

Crushed, with intolerable pain—Hyper.

Festering—Graph.

Itching—*Agar.*; Kali c.; Maland.

Joints inflamed—Am. c.; *Benz. ac.*; Bor.; Bothrops; Carbo v.; *Colch.*; Daphne; *Led.*; *Rhod.*; Teucr. See Joints.

Nails, deformed, thick—Ant. c.; Graph.; Sil.

Nails, inflamed—Sabad.

Nails, ingrowing—*Caust.*; *Graph.*; Hep.; Mag. p.; *Mag. pol. aust.*; *Nit. ac.*; *Sil.*; Staph.; Teucr.; Thuya.

Nails, pain around—Ant. c.; *Fluor. ac.*; Hep.; Nit. ac.; Teucr.

Numbness—Con.; Nat. m.; Phos.; Sil.; Sul.; Thall.

PAINS—Big toe—Am. c.; Ars.; Bar. c.; Calc. c.; Elat.; Eup. perf.; Kali c.; Led.; Plumb. m.; Prim. c.; Sep.; Sil.

Cramps—*Cupr. ac.*; Cupr. m.; Dig.; *Diosc.*; Hyos.; Lyc.; Rhus t.; Sec.; Sep.; Sul.

Rheumatic—*Act. sp.*; Apoc. andr.; *Benz. ac.*; Bor.; Bothrops; *Caul.*;

Caust.; *Colch.*; Daphne; *Gnaph.*; Hyper.; Kali c.; *Led.*; *Lith. c.*; Nit. ac.; Pæonia; Phos. ac.; *Puls.*; Sab.; *Sil.* See Gout.

Rheumatic, in big toe—Am. benz.; Arn.; *Benz. ac.*; Bor.; Bothrops; *Colch.*; Conv.; Gnaph.; Kali c.; *Led.*; Rhod.; Sil.

Rheumatic, in tips of toes—Am. m.; *Hyper.*; Kali c.; *Sil.*; Syph.

Tearing—*Act. sp.*; Am. m.; Benz. ac.; Brom.; *Caul.*; *Colch.*; Pall.; Sil.; Syph.

Soreness—Bar. c.; Brom.; Nat. ars.; Phos. ac. See Feet.

Stiffness—*Caul.*; Graph.; Led.; Sec. See Joints.

Ulcer of big toe—Sil.

Ulcer, pemphigus—*Ars.*; Graph.; Petrol.; Sep.

Wheals, eroding—Sul.

GAIT—Agility: Coff.

Ataxic—*Arg. n.*; Bell.; Helod.; Ign.; Nux v.; *Sec.*; *Sulphon.* See Locomotor Ataxia (Nervous System).

Sluggish, slow—Gels.; Phos. ac.; Phos.

Spastic; knees knock against each other when walking—Lathyr.

Staggering, unsteady, difficult walking—Acon.; *Agar.*; Agrost.; Angust.; *Arg. n.*; Asar.; Aster.; Astrag.; *Bell.*; Calc. p.; *Carbon. s.*; *Caust.*; Cocc.; Colch.; *Con.*; Dub.; *Gels.*; Helod.; Ign.; Lact. ac.; *Lathyr.*; Lil. t.; Lol.; Mang. ac.; Merc.; Morph.; Mur. ac.; *Myg.*; Nat. c.; Nux m.; *Nux v.*; Onosm.; Oxytr.; Pæonia; Phos. ac.; *Phos.*; Rhus t.; *Sec.*; Sep.; Stram.; Sulphon.; Tab.; Trion.; Zinc. m.

Staggering, unsteady, when unobserved—Arg. n.

Staggering, unsteady, when walking in dark, or with eyes closed—*Alum.*; *Arg. n.*; Carbon. s.; Dub.; *Gels.*; Iodof.; *Stram.*

Staggering, unsteady, with muscular inco-ordination—Alum.; Arag.; Arg. n.; Aster.; Astrag.; *Bar. m.*; Bell.; Cocc.; *Gels.*; Kali br.; Med.; Onosm.; Phos. ac.; *Physost.*; Picr. ac.; Plumb.; Sec.; Sil.; Trion.; Zinc. m.

Walking backward—Oxytr.

Walking backward, on metacarpo-phalangeal joint—Mang. ac.

Walking, child slow to learn—Bar. c.; Calc. c.; Calc. p.; Caust.; Nat. m.; Sil.

When walking, drags feet—*Myg.*; Nux v.; Tab.

When walking, foot shoots out, or turns—Acon.

When walking, heels do not touch ground—Lathyr.

When walking, joints feel painfully tense, as from ham-strings shortened—Am. m.; Caust.; Cimex.

When walking, legs feel heavy as lead—Med.

When walking, legs feel as if made of wood, or glass—Thuya.

When walking, legs involuntarily thrown forward—Merc.

When walking, lifts feet higher than usual, and brings them down hard—Helod.

When walking, limps involuntarily—Bell.

When walking, must stoop—Arn.; *Lathyr.*; Mang. ac.; Phos.; Sul.

When walking on uneven ground, very difficult—Lil. t.

When walking or standing, suddenly falling to ground—Mag. c.

When walking, seems to be walking on air—Dub.; Lac c.

LOCOMOTOR SYSTEM

When walking, stumbles easily, makes missteps—Agar.; Phos. ac.
When walking, tendency to fall forward; falls when walking backward—Mang. ac.
When walking, trembles all over—Lact. ac.

JOINTS—Burning:—Apis; Ars.; *Caust.*; Colch.; Mang. ac.; Merc.; *Rhus t.*; Sul.

Bursæ—Benz. ac.; Kali m.; *Ruta*; Sil.

Contraction, painful, of tendons, hamstrings—Abrot.; *Am. m.; Caust.; Cimex;* Col.; Formica; *Guaiac.;* Kali iod.; *Nat. m.; Tellur.*

Cracking, on motion—Acon.; Angust.; *Benz. ac.;* Calc. fl.; Camph.; *Caust.;* Cocc.; Gins.; *Graph.;* Kali bich.; Kali m.; Led.; Nat. m.; *Nat. p.; Nit. ac.; Petrol.;* Thuya; Zinc. m.

Dropsy (hydarthrosis)—*Apis;* Bov.; Canth.; Chin. s.; Cinch.; Iod.

Hysterical joints—*Arg. n.;* Cham.; Cotyled.; Hyper.; *Ign.;* Zinc. m.

Inflammation (ARTHRITIS)—Acute: Abrot.; *Acon.;* Arbut.; Benz. ac.; Berb. v.; *Bry.;* Caust.; Cim.; Cinch.; *Colch.;* Gnaph.; *Guaiac.;* Iod.; Kali bich.; Kali iod.; Kal.; *Led.;* Lil. t.; Lith. c.; Mang. ac.; *Merc.;* Nat. sil.; Nit. ac.; Phyt.; *Puls.;* Radium; Rhod.; *Rhus t.;* Sab.; Sal. ac.; Solid.; *Stellar.;* Sul. tereb.; Viola tr. See Rheumatism.

Inflammation, chronic (arthritis deformans)—Am. phos.; Ant. c.; Arbut.; Arn.; *Ars.;* Benz. ac.; Calc. c.; Calc. ren.; Caul.; *Caust.; Cim.; Cinch.;* Colch.; Colchicine; Ferr. iod.; Ferr. picr.; *Guaiac.; Iod.; Kali br.; Kali iod.;* Lact. ac.; Led.; Lyc.; Merc. c.; Nat. br.; Nat. p.; Nat. s.; *Piperaz.; Puls.;* Radium; Sab.; Sal. ac.; Sep.; Sul.; *Sul. tereb.;* Thyr.

Inflammation—GOUT—Abrot ; *Acon.; Am. benz.;* Apis; *Arn.;* Ars.; Aur. mur.; Aur. m. n.; Bell.; *Benz. ac.;* Berb. v.; *Bry.;* Cajup.; Calc. c.; Carls.; Cham.; *Chin. s.; Cinch.; Colch.; Colchicine;* Cupr.; Daphne; Dulc.; Ferr. picr.; Formica; *Guaiac.;* Irid.; Jabor.; Kali bich.; Kali iod.; Kal.; *Led.; Lith. c.; Lyc.;* Mang. ac.; Med.; *Merc. s.;* Nat. lact.; Nat. m.; Nat. sal.; Nux v ; Ox. ac.; Pancreat.; Phyt.; *Puls.;* Querc.; Rhod.; Rhus t.; *Sab.;* Sil.; Spig.; Stellar.; *Sul.;* Taxus; Uric ac.; Urt.

Debility after attack—Bellis; Cyprip.

Gout of chest—Colch.

Gout of eyes—Nux v.

Gout of hands, feet, little swelling, subacute—Led.

Gout of heart—Aur. mur.; Cact.; Conv.; Cupr. m.; Kal.

Gout of nerves (neuralgia)—*Colch.;* Col.; Sul.

Gout of stomach—Hydroc. ac.; Nux m.; Nux v.; Puls.

Gout of throat—Colch.; Merc. s.

Metastases to heart—Colch.; Kal.

Metastases to stomach—Ant. c.; Nux v.

Nervous restlessness—Ign.

Retrocedent or suppressed—*Cajup.;* Nat. m.; Ox. ac.; Rhus t.

Sub-acute—Guaiac.; *Led.;* Puls.

Uterine disorders—Sab.

Inflammation-SYNOVITIS—Acute: *Acon.; Apis;* Arn.; *Bell.;* Berb. v.; *Bry.;* Canth.; Fluor. ac.; *Hep.; Iod.;* Led.; *Puls.; Rhus t.;* Ruta; Sab.; *Sil.;* Slag; Sticta.

Inflammation, chronic—Am. phos.; Benz. ac.; Berb. v.; Calc. c.; Calc. fl.; Calc. p.; Caust.; Hep.; Iod.; Kali iod.; Merc. s.; Phyt.; Puls.; Rhus t.; Ruta; Sil.; Staph.; Stellar.; Sul.; Tub.

Itching in bends of joints—Phos. ac.

Lameness—Abrot.; Cepa; Rhus t.; Ruta; Sul. See Stiffness.

NODOSITIES, tophi—Agn.; Am. benz.; Am. phos.; Ant. t.; Aur.; Benz. ac.; Berb. v.; Calc. c.; Calc. ren.; Caul.; Caust.; Cim.; Colch.; Elat.; Eucal.; Eup. perf.; Formica; Graph.; Guaiac.; Hekla; Iod.; Kali ars.; Kali iod.; Kali sil.; Led.; Lith. c.; Lyc.; Med.; Nat. lact.; Nat. ureat.; Piperaz.; Rhod.; Ruta; Sab.; Staph.; Sul.; Urea; Uric ac.

PAINS—In general: Am. c.; Am. m.; Arg. m.; Bar. c.; Bry.; Calc. p.; Ced.; Diosc.; Dros.; Euonym.; Iod.; Kreos.; Lappa; Mang.; Sil.; Sul.; Zinc. m.

Bruised—Arn.; Bry.; Hyper.; Kal.; Mez.; Rhus t.; Ruta.

Cutting—Acon.; Bry.; Caul.; Cim.; Kal.

Digging at P. M.—Kali iod.; Mang. ac.; Merc. s.

Drawing, tensive—Aloe; Am. c.; Am. m.; Apoc. andr.; Caust.; Cimex; Cinch.; Colch.; Gins.; Mez.; Puls.; Rhus t.; Sul.

Neuralgic—Arg. m.; Ced.; Col.; Plumb.; Zinc. m.

Rheumatic—Abrot.; Acon.; Asclep. t.; Benz. ac.; Berb. v.; Bry.; Caul.; Caust.; Cim.; Cinch.; Colch.; Dig.; Diosc.; Ferr.; Formica; Guaiac.; Iod.; Kali bich.; Kal.; Lact. ac.; Led.; Merc. s.; Pinus sylv.; Puls.; Radium; Rham. c.; Rhod.; Rhus t.; Ruta; Sab.; Salol; Staph.; Stront. See Rheumatism.

Soreness, tenderness—Acon.; Am. m.; Apis; Arn.; Bell.; Bellis; Bry.; Colch.; Guaiac.; Ham.; Hep.; Kal.; Led.; Lith. c.; Meli.; Phyt.; Puls.; Rhus t.; Sab.; Sticta; Ver. a.; Verbasc.

Stitching, tearing, shifting, erratic—Apis; Benz. ac.; Bry.; Caust.; Cim.; Cinch.; Colch.; Guaiac.; Kali iod.; Kal.; Led.; Lith. c.; Magnol.; Merc. s.; Phos. ac.; Puls.; Rhus t.; Sul.; Ver. v.

Stiffness—Abrot.; Angust.; Apis; Apoc. andr.; Arn.; Asclep. t.; Bar. m.; Bry.; Caul.; Caust.; Colch.; Col.; Diosc.; Formica; Gins.; Guaiac.; Iod.; Kali iod.; Lyc.; Magnol.; Med.; Merc. s.; Mez.; Nux v.; Ol. j. as.; Petrol.; Phyt.; Pinus sylv.; Rhus t.; Sep.; Stellar.; Strych.; Sul.; Thiosin.; Triost.; Verbasc.

Swelling—Abrot.; Acon.; Act. sp.; Anag.; Apis; Ars.; Bell.; Benz. ac.; Bry.; Caust.; Cinch.; Colch.; Dig.; Guaiac.; Iod.; Kali m.; Kal.; Led.; Lith. c.; Mang. ac.; Med.; Merc. s.; Phyt.; Puls.; Rham. c.; Rhod.; Rhus t.; Sab.; Stellar.; Sticta.

Swelling, dark red—Bry.; Kal.; Rhus t.

Swelling, pale, white—Apis; Aur.; Bry.; Calc. c.; Calc. p.; Cistus; Colch.; Con.; Dig.; Iod.; Led.; Merc. c.; Merc. s.; Phos. ac.; Phos.; Puls.; Rhod.; Sil.; Sul.; Symphyt.; Tub. See Knee.

Swelling, shining—Acon.; Apis; Bell.; Bry.; Dig.; Mang. ac.; Sab.

Ulceration of cartilages—Merc. c.

Weakness—Acon.; Bar. m.; Bov.; Carbo an.; Caust.; Cinch.; Euphorb.; Hippom.; Led.; Phos.; Psor.; Mez.; Rhus t.; Zing.

Weakness, sprained easily—Carbo an.; Hep.; Led.

LOCOMOTOR SYSTEM

ANKLES—Itching: Puls.; Rhus t.; Selen.
  Itching, worse from scratching, warmth of bed—Led.
  Pain in general—Abrot.; Alum.; Am. c.; But. ac.; Caust.; Euonym.; Lappa; Lathyr.; Nat. m.; Sil.; Tetradyn.; Verbasc.; *Viscum.*
  Bruised, dislocated feeling—Bry.; Led.; Prun. sp.; *Ruta*; Sil.; Sul.
  Rheumatic—Abrot.; *Act. sp.;* Caul.; Caust.; Colch.; Guaco; Guaiac.; Led.; Mang. ac.; Mang. mur.; Med.; *Prophyl.; Puls.;* Radium; *Rhod.; Ruta;* Sil.; Stellar.; Sul.; Urt.
  Sprains—Carbo an.; *Led.;* Nat. ars.; *Nat. c.; Ruta;* Stront. c.
  Sprains, chronic—Bov.; *Stront. c.*
  Stiffness—Kali c.; Med.; Sep.; Sul.; Zinc. m.
  Swelling—Apis; *Arg. n.;* Ferr.; Ham.; *Led.;* Lyc.; Med.; Mimosa; Plumb.; Stann.; Stront. c. See Dropsy.
  Ulcer, itching—Sul.
  Weakness, "foot turns under"—Calc. c.; *Calc. p.; Carbo an.; Caust.;* Cham.; Ham.; Led.; Mang. ac.; Mang. mur.; Med.; *Nat. ars.; Nat. c.;* Nat. m.; Phos.; *Pinus sylv.; Ruta;* Sil.; Sul.

ELBOWS—Numbness: Puls.
  Pains—Ant. c.; *Arg. m.;* Ars.; *Caust.;* Cinnab.; Colch.; *Ferr. mur.;* Guaco; Kali c.; *Kal.;* Lyc.; *Menisp.;* Ol. j. as.; Phos.; Solan. lyc.; Sul.; *Viscum;* Zinc. ox.

HIPS—Morbus Coxarius: Diseases of: Acon.; *Arg. m.;* Ars.; Ars. iod.; Calc. c.; Calc. hyphos.; Calc. iod.; *Calc. p.; Caust.;* Cinch.; *Cistus;* Col.; Ferr. m.; Ferr. p.; Fluor. ac.; Hep.; Hippoz.; Hyper.; Iod.; *Kali c.; Kali iod.;* Merc. i. r.; Merc.; *Phos. ac.;* Phos.; Rhus t.; *Sil.;* Staph.; Still.; *Sul.;* Tub. See Coxalgia.
  Luxation—Col.
  Pain (coxalgia)—*Æsc.;* Allium s.; Arg. m.; *Ars.;* Berb. v.; *Bry.;* Calc. c.; *Calc. p.;* Carbo an.; Caust.; Cham.; Chel.; Cistus; Colch.; *Col.;* Con.; Dros.; Elat.; Ferr. m.; Formica; *Gels.;* Glycerin; Guaco; *Hyper.;* Kali c.; *Kali iod.;* Led.; Lil. t.; Limul.; Lyc.; Mag. mur.; Mez.; Murex; Nat. m.; Nat. s.; Nux m.; *Puls.;* Radium; Solan. n.; *Stram.;* Thuya; Tongo; Tromb.
  Pain, as if broken; as if pelvis was falling apart—Æsc.; *Trill.*
  Pain, as if sprained—*Æsc.;* Am. m.; *Calc. p.;* Caust.; *Col.;* Laur.; Nat. m.; *Puls.;* Rhus t.; Sarrac.
  Pain, in left hip—Am. m.; Col.; Irid; Ov. g. p.; Sang.; Solan. n.; *Stram.*
  Pain, in right hip—Agar.; Ant. t.; *Chel.;* Graph.; Kali c.; Led.; *Lil. t.;* Limul.; Nux m.; Pall.; Stram.

KNEES—Coldness—Agn.; Apis; Calc. c.; *Carbo v.;* Nat. c. See Extremities.
  Cracking, on motion—*Benz. ac.;* Caust.; *Cocc.;* Croc.; Diosc.; Nat. ars.; Nux v.
  Dislocation of patella, on going upstairs—Can. s.
  Dropsy—Caust.; Ced.; Iod.
  Herpes—Carbo v.; Graph.; Petrol.
  Hygroma patella—Arn.; Calc. p.; *Iod.*
  Inflammation (synovitis, bursitis: housemaid's knee): Acute: *Acon.; Apis;* Arn.; Bell.; *Bry.;* Canth.; Cistus; Helleb.; *Hep.;* Iod.; Kali

c.; *Kali iod.;* Phos.; *Puls.;* Rhus t.; Ruta; *Sil.;* *Slag;* *Sticta;* Sul. See Swelling.

Inflammation, chronic—Ant. t.; Benz. ac.; Berb. v.; *Calc. fl.;* Calc. p.; Hep.; *Iod.; Kali iod.; Merc. s.;* Phyt.; Rhus t.; Ruta; *Sil.;* Tub.

Numbness—Carbo v.; Meli.

Numbness, extends to scrotum, relieved by sitting—Bar. c.

PAINS—In general: Angust.; *Apis;* Bell.; Benz. ac.; *Berb. v.;* Calc. c.; Can. ind.; Diosc.; *Elaps;* Kali iod.; Keros.; Lappa; Mag. m.; *Meli.;* Mez.; Mur. ac.; Phos.; Sul.; Xerophyl.

Aching—Anac.; Con.; Led.; *Meli.;* Ol. j. as.

Boring, relieved by walking—Indigo.

Bruised—Ars.; *Berb. v.;* Bry.; Sarrac.

Digging, in left knee—Aur.; Caust.; Col.; Rhus t.; Spig.; Tarax.

Drawing—Calc. c.; Mag. m.; Mur. ac.; Phos.; Sul.

Rheumatic—Arg. m.; *Benz. ac.;* Berb. v.; Bry.; *Cinch.;* Cop.; Daphne; Elaps; Diosc.; *Dulc.;* Guaiac.; Jacar.; *Kali c.; Kali iod.; Lact. ac.; Led.; Mang. ac.:* Meli.; *Merc.;* Nat. p.; *Puls.;* Puls. nut.; Radium; Sab.; Sticta; Viscum.

Tearing—Calc. c.; *Caust.;* Col.; Granat.; Lyc.; *Merc.;* Petrol.; Sticta; Tarax.; Tongo; Ver. v.

Tensive, crampy—Anac.; Caps.; Lathyr.; Pæonia; *Puls.;* Sil.; *Verbasc.*

POPLITEAL SPACE, Itching—Lyc.; Sep.

Popliteal space, pain—Caust.; Lyc.; Physost.; Radium.

Popliteal space, prurigo—Ars.

REFLEXES—Diminished, lost: Cur.; Oxytr.; Plumb. m.; *Sec.;* Sulphon.

Reflexes increased—Anhal.; Can. ind.; Lathyr.; Mang. ac. See Nervous System.

Stiffness of knees—*Berb. v.;* Bry.; Lyc.; Mimosa; Petrol.; Sep.; Sul.

Swelling—*Apis;* Arn.; Bell.; Benz. ac.; Berb. v.; *Bry.;* Calc. c.; *Cinch.,* Cocc.; *Kali iod.;* Lyc.; Mag. c.; *Rhod.;* Sal. ac.; Sil.

Swelling, white—Acon.; *Apis;* Arn.; Calc. c.; Calc. p.; *Cistus; Kali iod.;* Led.; Phos. ac.; Phos.; *Puls.;* Rhus t.; Sil.; Slag; *Sticta;* Sul.; Tub.

Tenderness—Apis; Berb. v.; *Bry.;* Cinch.; Rhus t. See Joints.

Ulceration of cartilage—Merc. d.

Weakness—Acon.; Anac.; Aur.; *Cob.; Cocc.;* Diosc.; Hippom.; Lact. ac.; Nat. m.; Nit. ac.; Sul.

SHOULDERS-SCAPULÆ—Deltoid, pain, rheumatism: Ferr. p.; Glycerin; Lycopers.; Med.; Nux m.; Ox. ac.; Rhus t.; *Sang.;* Sticta; *Syph.; Urt.;* Viola od.; Zinc. ox.; Zing.

PAINS—In general: Alum.; *Am. phos.;* Anag.; Arn.; Azadir.; Bar. c.; *Can. ind.;* Chel.; Cocc.; Con.; *Fagop.;* Jugl. r.; Kreos.; Lyc.; Menisp.; *Myr.;* Nat ars.; Nat. c.; Nit. ac.; *Ran. b.;* Sep.; Ver. a.; Viscum.

Pain, between scapulæ—Æsc.; Ars.; Bry.; Camph.; *Chenop.;* Euonym.; *Granat.;* Guaiac.; Mag. s.

Pain burning, in small spots—Agar.; *Phos.;* Ran. b.; *Sul.*

Pain, drawing—Ars.; Berb. v.; Cham.; Col.; Sul.

Pain, in left—Acon.; *Æsc.; Agar.;* Ant. t.; *Aspar.;* Cham.; Chenop. gl.;

Col.; Eup. purp.; Ferr. m.; Led.; Lob. syph.; Nux m.; *Onosm.*; Rhodium; Stram.; Sul.

Pain, in left, lower angle—*Chenop. gl.*; Cupr. ars.; Ran. b.

Pain, in right—Abies c.; Am. m.; Bry.; *Chel.*; Chenop. gl.; *Col.*; Ferr. p.; Ferr. mur.; *Guaco*; Ichthy.; Ipomœa; Jugl. c.; *Kali c.*; Kal.; Mag. c.; Pall.; Phyt.; Puls. nut.; Ran. b.; *Sang.*; Solan. lyc.; *Sticta*; Stront.; Urt.

Pain, in right, lower angle—*Chel.*; Chenop. anth.; Kali c.; *Merc.*; Pod.

Pains, rheumatic—Acon.; Am. caust.; Berb. v.; Bry.; Colch.; Ferr. mur.; *Ferr. p.*; Guaiac.; Ham.; *Kali c.*; Kal.; Lact. ac.; *Led.*; Lith. c.; *Lith. lact.*; Med.; Ol. an.; Pall.; *Phyt.*; Prim.; Radium; *Ran. b.*; Rhod.; *Rhus t.*; Sang.; Stellar.; *Sticta*; Stront.; Sul.; Syph.; Urt.; Viola od.

Pains, worse singing, using voice—Stann.

Stitches, tearing—Am. m.; Bry.; Hyper.; Kali c.; Lyc.; Mag. c.; Nit. ac.

Stiffness—Cocc.; *Dulc.*; Granat.; Indium; *Phyt.*; Prim. v.; *Sang.*; Senec. jac.

WRISTS—Ganglion, on back: Benz. ac.; Calc. fl.; Phos.; Rhus t.; *Ruta*; Sil.; Thuya.

Gouty deposits—Calc. c.; Ruta.

PAINS—In general: Abrot.; Act. sp.; Am. c.; Bism.; Carbo an.; Caul.; Chel.; *Hippom.*; Kali c.; Nat. p.; *Pæonia*; Prophyl.; Rhod.; *Ruta*; Sep.; Sil.; Sul.; Urt.; *Viola od.*

Cramps, spasms, painful (writer's cramp)—*Arg. m.*; Arn.; Bell.; Bellis; *Caust.*; Con.; Cupr.; Cycl.; Ferr. iod.; *Gels.*; Mag. p.; Nux v.; Picr. ac.; Ran. b.; *Ruta*; Sec.; Sil.; *Stann.*; Staph.; Strych.; Sul. ac.; Viola od.; Zinc. m.

Rheumatic—Abrot.; *Act. sp.*; Benz. ac.; Calc. c.; *Caul.*; Caust.; Colch.; Hippom.; Lact. ac.; Lyc.; Prophyl.; *Rhod.*; Rhus t.; Rhus v.; *Ruta*; Sab.; Sep.; Solan. lyc.; Stellar.; Ulnus; Variol.; *Viola od.*; Wyeth.

Sprained, dislocated feeling—Bry.; Cistus; *Eup. perf.*; Hippom.; Ox. ac.; Rhus t.; *Ruta*; Ulnus.

Paralysis—Con.; Cur.; Hippom.; *Plumb. ac.*; Plumb. m.; Picr. ac.; Ruta; Stann. See Nervous System.

NECK—Burning: Guaco.

Cracking of cervical vertebræ, on motion—Aloe; Cocc.; *Nat. c.*; Niccol.; Ol. an.; Thuya.

Emaciation—Nat. m. See Generalities.

Eruption—Anac.; Clem.; Lyc.; Nat. m.; Petrol.; Sep.

Fullness, must loosen collar—*Amyl*; Fel tauri; *Glon.*; Lach.; Pyr.; Sep.

Itching—Ant. c.

Muscles, cervical, contraction, rigidity—*Cic.*; Cim.; Nicot.; *Strych.*

Muscles, cervical, shooting—Sul. ac.

Muscles, cervical, twitching—Agar.

Muscles, sterno-cleido-mastoid—*Gels.*; Rhod.; Tarax.; Trifol. See Torticollis.

NAPE OF NECK: PAINS—In general: Acon.; Æsc.; Am. c.; *Bell.*; Chin. ars.; *Cim.*; Col.; Fel tauri; Ferr. picr.; *Gels.*; Graph.; Hyper.; Jugl.

c.; Lach.; Lyc.; Myr.; *Nat. cholein;* Nat. s.; Paris; Ver. a.; Vib. op.; X-ray; Zinc. v.

Aching—Adon. v.; Æsc.; Angust.; Bapt.; Caust.; *Con.; Gels.; Guaiac.; Paris;* Radium; Ver. v.; Ver. v.; Zinc. m.

Dislocated, bruised feeling—Bell.; Caust.; Fagop.; Lachnanth.

Rheumatic—Acon.; *Bry.;* Calc. p.; Caust.; *Cim.;* Colch.; *Dulc.; Guaiac.;* Iod.; Kali iod.; *Lachnanth.;* Petrol.; Puls.; Radium; Rhod.; *Rhus t.;* Sang.; Stellar.; Sticta.

Tearing, shooting, stitching—*Acon.;* Asar.; Bad.; Bar. c.; Bell.; *Berb. v.; Bry.;* Chin. ars.; Colch.; Ferr. picr.; *Mag. p.;* Nux v.; *Strych.;* Xanth.

Tension—Con.; Sep.; Sul.; Tub.

Tensive numbness—Plat.

Stiffness—*Acon.;* Ant. t.; Bell.; *Bry.;* Calc. c.; Calc. caust.; Calc. p.; *Caust.;* Cham.; Chel.; *Cim.;* Cocc.; Colch.; *Dulc.;* Ferr. p.; Gels.; Guaiac.; Hyper.; Jugl. c.; Kali c.; Lac c.; *Lachnanth.;* Lyc.; Mag. c.; Med.; Menthol; *Merc. i. r.;* Nicot.; Nit. ac.; Nux v.; Pampin.; Petrol.; Phos.; Phyt.; *Puls.;* Radium; Rhodium; Rhod.; Rhus v.; Sep.; Stellar.; *Sticta;* Sul.; Trifol.; Vinca m.; X-ray.

Swelling—Calc. c.; Iod.; Lyc.; Phos.; Sil.

Tenderness—Amyl; *Bry.;* Cim.; Kali perm.; *Lach.;* Tarax.

Tumor, fatty—Bar. c.

Veins, swollen—Op.

Weakness, unable to hold head up—*Abrot.;* Æth.; Colch.; Fagop.; Kali c.; Sil. See Head.

Wry neck (torticollis)—*Acon.;* Agar.; Atrop.; *Bell.; Bry.; Cim.;* Colch.; Guaiac.; Hyos.; Ign.; *Lachnanth.;* Lyc.; Mag. p.; Myg.; Nux v.; Strych.; Thuya.

RHEUMATISM: TYPE—Articular, acute, RHEUMATIC FEVER: *Acon.;* Agar.; Am. benz.; Am. caust.; Ant. t.; *Apis; Arn.;* Ars.; *Bell.;* Benz. ac.; Berb. v.; *Bry.; Cact.; Calc. c.;* Calc. p.; Camph.; *Cascara;* Cham.; Chin. s.; *Cim.;* Cinch.; Clem.; *Colch.; Colchicine;* Col.; *Dulc.; Eup. perf.; Ferr. p.;* Formica; Franciscea; Gaulth.; Gels.; Gins.; *Guaiac.;* Ham.; Hymosa; *Kali bich.;* Kali c.; Kali iod.; Kali m.; Kal.; *Led.;* Lyc.; Macrot.; Merc. s.; *Merc. v.;* Methyl. sal.; Nat. lact.; Nat. sal.; Nux v.; Nyctanth.; Ox. ac.; Petrol.; Phyt.; *Prophyl.; Puls.;* Ran. b.; *Rham. c.;* Rhod.; *Rhus t.;* Ruta; *Sal. ac.;* Sang.; Spig.; *Stellar.;* Sticta; Still.; Strych.; *Sul.;* Syph.; Thuya; Tilia; Ver. a.; *Ver. v.; Viola od.*

Ascending pains—Arn.; *Led.*

Descending pains—Cact.; *Kal.*

Erratic, wandering pains—Apoc. andr.; *Caul.;* Cim.; Colch.; Kali bich.; Kal.; Kali s.; *Lac c.;* Mang.; Phyt.; *Puls.;* Puls. nut.; Rhod.; *Stellar.;* Sul.

Fibrous tissues (sheaths, tendons)—Arn.; Formic acid; Gettysburg Water; Phyt.; Rhod.; *Rhus t.*

Joints, large—*Acon.;* Arbut.; Arg. m.; Asclep. s.; *Bry.;* Dros.; *Merc.;* Mimosa; Rhus t.; Sticta; Ver. v.

Joints, small—*Act. sp.*; Benz. ac.; Bry.; *Caul.*; *Colch.*; Kali bich.; Lact. ac.; *Led.*; Lith. c.; Lith. lact.; *Puls.*; Rhod.; Ruta; *Sab.*; Viola od.

Mono-articular—Acon.; Apis; *Bry.*; Caust.; Cinch.; Cop.; *Merc.* See Joints.

Poly-articular—Arn.; *Bry.*; Guaiac.; *Puls.* See Erratic Pains.

CONCOMITANTS—Alternates with diarrhœa, dysentery: Abrot.; *Dulc.*; Gnaph.; *Kali bich.*

Alternates, with indigestion—Kali bich.

Alternates, with urticaria—Urt.

Auricular fibrillation following—Dig.

Debility—*Ars.*; Calc. p.; Chin. s.; *Cinch.*; *Colch.*; Ferr. carb.; Sul.

Fever, adynamic—Bry.; *Rhus t.*

Fever, remittent—Chin. s.

Metastases, to brain—Bell.; Op.

Metastases, to heart—Adon. v.; Avena; Cact.; *Kal.*; Lith. c.; Prophyl.; Spig.

Mild cases, in nervous persons—Viola od.

Nervousness, intense pains—Cham.; Coff.; Rhus t.

Numbness—Acon.; Cham.; Led.; *Rhus t.*

Restlessness—*Acon.*; Caust.; Cim.; Puls.; *Rhus t.*

Secretions checked—Abrot.

Sensitiveness to cold—Led.; *Merc.*

Sleeplessness—Bell.; Calc. c.; Coff.; Ign.

Skin diseases, acute, after—Dulc.

Sweating—*Calc. c.*; Hep.; Lact. ac.; *Merc.*; Rham. c.; Sal. ac.; Tilia.

Urticarial eruption—Urt.

AGGRAVATIONS—At night:—*Acon.*; Arn.; Cham.; *Cim.*; *Colch.*; Eucal.; *Kali iod.*; Kali m.; *Kal.*; Lact. ac.; Led.; *Merc.*; Phyt.; *Puls.*; Rhod.; Rhus t.; Sars.; Sil.; *Sul.*

Before storm—Puls.; *Rhod.*; Rhus t.

Colchicum, abuse—Led.

Crosswise, side to side—Lac c.

Every other day—Cinch.

From cold, dry weather—*Acon.*; Bry.; Caust.; Nux m.; *Rhod.*

From damp, wet weather—Arn.; Ars.; Calc. p.; Cim.; *Colch.*; *Dulc.*; Kali iod.; *Merc.*; Nat. s.; Nux m.; *Phyt.*; Ran. b.; *Rhod.*; *Rhus t.*; Sars.; Ver. a.

From melting snow—Calc. p.

From motion—Act. sp.; Apis; *Arn.*; *Bry.*; *Calc. c.*; Cim.; Clem.; *Cinch.*, Colch.; Formica; Gettysburg Water; Guaiac.; Iod.; *Kali m.*; Kal.; Lac c.; Led.; *Merc.*; Nux v.; Phyt.; Ran. b.; Sal. ac.; *Stellar.*

From rest—Euphorb.; Puls.; Rhod.; *Rhus t.*

From sweating—Hep.; *Merc.*; Tilia.

From touch—Act. sp.; Acon.; Apis; *Arn.*; *Bry.*; *Cinch.*; *Colch.*; Iod.; Lac c.; Ran. b.; Rhus t.; Sal. ac.

From warmth—Cham.; Kali m.; *Led.*; *Merc.*; Puls.

AMELIORATIONS—From motion, walking:—Cham.; Cinch.; Dulc.; Ferr. m.; Lyc.; *Puls.*; Rhod.; *Rhus t.*; Ver. a.

From pressure—Bry.; Formica.

From rest—Bry.; Gettysburg Water.

From warmth—*Ars.*; Bry.; Caust.; Kali bich.; Nux m.; Rhus t.; *Sil.*

From water, cold to feet—*Led.*; Sec.

In damp weather—Caust.

In open air—Kali m.; Puls.

ARTICULAR, CHRONIC—*Am. phos.*; Ant. c.; Anthrok.; Benz. ac.; Berb. v.; *Bry.*; Calc. c.; *Calc. caust.*; Carbon. s.; Caul.; *Caust.*; Cim.; Colch.; *Dulc.*; Euonym.; Ferr.; Guaiac.; Hep.; Iod.; Kali bich.; Kali c.; *Kali iod.*; Led.; *Lith. c.*; Lyc.; Med.; Merc.; Mez.; *Ol. j. as.*; Petrol.; Phyt.; *Puls.*; Rhod.; Rhus t.; Ruta; Sil.; *Stellar.*; Still.; *Sul.*; Sul. tereb.; Taxus. See Joints.

ARTHRITIS DEFORMANS—Arbut.; *Arn.*; *Ars.*; Benz. ac ; Calc. c.; Caps.; Caul.; *Caust.*; *Cim.*; *Colch.*; Colchicine; *Dulc.*; Ferr. iod.; Ferr. picr.; *Guaiac.*; *Iod.*; Kali c.; *Kali iod.*; Lact. ac.; Led.; Lyc.; Mang. ac.; Methyl. bl.; *Merc. c.*; Nat. p.; Pip. menth.; *Puls.*; Rhod.; *Sab.*; Sal. ac.; Sep.; *Sul.*; Sul. tereb.; Thymus Ext.; Thyr. See Joints.

Chronic, secondary to uterine disorder—Caul.; *Cim.*; *Puls.*; Sab.

Gonorrhœal—Acon.; *Arg. m.*; Arn.; Bry.; Caust.; Cim.; Clem.; Cop.; *Daphne*; Guaiac.; Iod.; *Irisin*; Jacar.; Kali bich.; Kali iod.; Kal.; *Med.*; Merc.; Nat. s.; Phyt.; *Puls.*; Rhus t.; *Sars.*; Sul.; *Thuya*.

Intercostal—Arn.; *Cim.*; Phyt.; *Ran. b.*; Rhus t.

Muscular (myalgia)—*Acon.*; Ant. t.; Apis; Arn.; *Bry.*; Calc. c.; *Cascara*; Caust.; Chin. s.; *Cim.*; Cinch.; Colch.; Dulc.; *Ferr.*; Gels.; Glycerin; Gnaph.; Ham.; Hyper.; Jacar.; Lyc.; *Macrot.*; Merc.; Phos.; **Phyt.**; *Ran. b.*; Rhod.; Rhus t.; Sang.; Sil.; Sul.; Syph.; Ver. v.

Paralytic—*Caust.*; Lathyr.; Phos. See Chronic.

Periosteal—Bell.; Cham.; Colch.; Cycl.; Guaiac.; *Kali bich.*; Kali iod.; Merc.; *Mez.*; Phos.; Phyt.; Sars.; Sil.

Subacute—Dulc.; *Led.*; Merc.; *Puls.*; Rhus t.

Syphilitic—See Periosteal.

RESPIRATORY SYSTEM

BRONCHIAL TUBES—ASTHMA: Remedies in general: *Acon.;* Alumen; Ambros.; Amyl; Ant. ars.; *Ant. t.;* Apis; *Aral.; Ars.;* Ars. iod.; Atrop.; *Bac.;* Bell.; *Blatta orient.;* Brom.; Bry.; Cinch.; Coff.; *Carbo v.;* Chin. ars.; Chlorum; Cic.; *Coca;* Cocaine; *Crot. t.; Cupr. ac.;* Cupr. ars.; Dros.; Dulc.; Egg Vaccine; Glon.; *Grind.;* Hep.; *Hydroc. ac.;* Illic.; Iod.: *Ipec.; Kali bich.; Kali c.;* Kali chlor.; *Kali iod.; Kali n.;* Kali p.; Lach.; Led.; *Lob. infl.;* Lyc.; Magnolia; Meph.; Morph.; Naja; *Naph.; Nat. s.; Nux v.; Passifl.; Pothos;* Psor.; *Ptel.;* Puls.; Quebr.; Sabad.; *Samb.;* Sang.; Scilla; Scrophul.; Silph.; *Stercul.;* Stram.; Strych.; *Sul.;* Syph.; Tab.; Tela ar.; *Thuya;* Tub.; Ver. a.; Ver. v.; *Viscum;* Zinc. m.; *Zing.*

TYPE—OCCURRENCE—Alternates with eruptions: Calad.; Caust.; Rhus t.; *Sul.*

Alternates, with itching rash—Calad.

Alternates, with spasmodic vomiting—Cupr. m.; Ipec.

Anger, from—Cham.; Nux v.

Cardiac—*Cact.;* Digitaline; Grind. sq.; Stroph. See Heart.

Epiglottis, spasm or weakness—Med.

Eruptions, suppressed, from—Ars.; Hep.; Psor.; *Sul.*

Foot sweat, suppressed, from—Ol. an.

Hay asthma—Aral.; *Arc.;* Ars. iod.; Chin. ars.; *Ipec.; Lob. infl.;* Naph.; Nat. s.; Nux v.; *Sabad.;* Sang.; Sticta; Sul. iod. See Rhinitis (Nose).

Hebdomadal—Cinch.; Ign.

Humid—Acon.; *Ant. iod.;* Ars.; *Bac.;* Bry.; *Can. ind.;* Cochlear.; Cupr.; *Dulc.;* Eucal.; Euphorb. pil.; Grind.; Hyper.; Iod.: *Kali bich.; Nat. s.;* Pulmo v.; Sabal; *Senega;* Stann.; *Sul.;* Thuya.

Humid, in children—*Nat. s.;* Samb.; Thuya.

Millar's—Arum drac.; *Arundo;* Coral.; Cupr.; Guarea; Hep.; Ipec.; Lach.; Lob. infl.; Mosch.; Poth.; *Samb.* See Laryngismus stridulus.

Miner's—Card. m.; Nat. ars.

Nervous—Acon.; Ambra; Amyl; *Asaf.;* Chin. s.; Cina; Coff.; *Cupr.;* Grind.; *Hydroc. ac.; Ipec.;* Kali p.; Lob. infl.; *Mosch.;* Nux m.; *Nux v.;* Sumb.; Tela ar.; Thymus; *Val.;* Ver. a.

Periodical—*Ars.;* Chin. ars.; *Cinch.;* Ipec.

Preceded by coryza—Aral.; Naja; Nux v.

Preceded by formication—Cistus; Lob. infl.

Preceded by rose cold—Sang.

Recent, uncomplicated cases—Hydroc. ac.

Sailors on shore—Brom.

Senile cases—Bar. m.

Tetter recedes with attack—Sul.

CONCOMITANTS—With bronchial catarrh:—Acon.; *Ant. t.; Ars.;* Blatta am.; *Bry.;* Cupr. ac.; *Eriod.;* Eucal.; *Grind.; Ipec.;* Kali iod.; Lob. infl.; Nat. s.; Oniscus; Sabal; Sul. See Humid.

With burning in throat and chest—Aral.

With constriction of throat—Cham.; Dros.; *Hydroc. ac.*; Lob. infl.; *Mosch.*
With cramp, muscular spasm of various parts—Cupr. m.
With cyanosis—Ars.; Cupr.; Samb.
With despondency, thinks he will die—*Ars.*; Psor.
With diarrhœa following—Nat. s.
With dysuria, nocturnal—Solid.
With every fresh cold—Nat. s.
With gastric derangement—Arg. n.; *Bry.*; Carbo v.; Ipec.; Kali m.; *Lob. infl.*; Lyc.; *Nux v.*; Puls.; Sang.; Ver. v.; Zing.
With gout, rheumatism—Led.; Sul.; *Viscum.*
With hæmorrhoids—Juncus; Nux v.
With hydrothorax—Colch.
With insomnia—Chloral; Telea ar.
With nausea, cardiac weakness, vertigo, vomiting, weak stomach, cold knees—Lob. infl.
With palpitation—Ars.; Cact.; Eucal.; Puls.
With thirst, nausea, stitches, burning in chest—Kali n.
With urine supersaturated with solids—Nat. nit.

MODALITIES—AGGRAVATION: After sleep: Aral.; Grind.; *Lach.*; Samb.
At night, lying down—*Aral.*; Ars.; Cistus, Con.; Ferr. ac.; *Grind.*; Lach.; Merc. pr. rub.; Naja; Puls.; *Samb.*; Sul.
From cold, damp weather—Ars.; *Dulc.*; *Nat. s.* See Humid.
From cold, dry weather—Acon.; Caust.; Hep.
From falling asleep—Am. c.; *Grind.*; Lac c.; *Lach.*; *Merc. pr. rub.*; Op.
From food—Kali p.; *Nux v.*; Puls.
From inhaling dust—*Ipec.*; Kali c.; Pothos.
From odors—Sang.
From sitting up—Ferr. ac.; Laur.; Psor.
From talking—Dros.; Meph.
In early A. M.—Am. c.; Ant. t.; *Ars.*; Grind.; Kali bich.; *Kali c.*; Nat. s.; Nux v.; Zing.
In spring—Aral.
In summer—Syph.

AMELIORATION—At sea: Brom.
From bending forward, rocking—Kali c.
From eructation—*Carbo v.*; Nux v.
From expectoration—Aral.; *Eriod.*; Grind.; Hyper.; *Ipec.*; Kali bich.; Zinc. m.
From lying down, keeping arms spread apart—Psor.
From lying on face, protruding tongue—Med.
From motion—Ferr. m.; Lob. infl.
From sitting up—Ars.; Kali c.; Merc. pr. rub.; Nux v.; *Puls.*
From sitting up, with head bent backward—Hep.
From stool—Pothos.
From vomiting—Cupr. m.
In damp weather—Caust.; Hep.
In open air—Naph.

BRONCHIECTASIS: BRONCHORRHOEA—Dilatation, with profuse, fetid,

purulent sputum: Acet. ac.; Allium s.; Alumen; Ant. t.; *Bac.; Bals. per.;* Benz. ac.; *Calc. c.;* Eucal.; Ferr. iod.; Grind.; *Hep.;* Ichth.; *Kali bich.; Kali c.;* Kreos.; Lyc.; Myos.; Myrt. c¹.; *Puls.;* Sang.; *Sil.; Stann.;* Sul.; Tub. See Chronic Bronchitis.

BRONCHITIS—Inflammation, acute:—*Acon.;* Am. c.; Am. iod.; Am. phos.; Ant. ars.; Ant. iod.; *Ant. t.;* Ars. iod.; Ars.; Asclep. t.; Aviare; *Bell.;* Blatta or.; *Brom.; Bry.; Caust.;* Cham.; Cinch.; Colch.; Cop.; *Dulc.;* Eup. perf.; Euphras.; *Ferr. p.;* Geis.; Grind.; *Hep.;* Hyos.; *Ipec.; Kali bich.;* Lob. infl.; Mang. ac.; *Merc. s.;* Naph.; Nat. ars.; Nit. ac.; *Phos.;* Piloc.; *Puls.;* Rhus t.; *Rumex; Sang.; Sang. n.;* Scilla; Solid.; Spong.; *Sticta; Sul.;* Sul. ac.; Thuya; Tub.; Ver. a.; Ver. v.; Zinc. m.

Capillary—Am. c.; Am. iod.; Ant. ars.; *Ant. t.;* Ars.; Bac.; *Bell.;* Bry.; Calc. c.; Camph.; *Carbo v.;* Chel.; Cupr. ac.; *Ferr. p.; Ipec.;* Kali c.; Kali iod.; *Kaolin;* Nit. ac.; Phos. ac.; Phos.; *Senega; Solanine;* Sul.; *Tereb.;* Ver. a.

Chronic (winter catarrhs)—Alumen; Alum.; *Ammon.; Am. c.;* Am. caust.; Am. iod.; Am. m.; Ant. ars.; Ant. iod.; *Ant. s. a.; Ant. t.; Ars. iod.; Ars.;* Bac.; *Bals. per.;* Bar. c.; *Bar. m.; Calc. c.;* Calc. iod.; Calc. sil.; Canth.; Carbo an.; *Carbo v.;* Ceanoth.; Chel.; *Cinch.;* Coccus; Con.; *Cop.;* Cub.; Dig.; Dros.; *Dulc.;* Eriod.; Eucal.; Grind.; *Hep.;* Hydr.; Hyos.; Ichth.; Iod.; *Ipec.; Kali bich.;* Kali c.; Kali hypophos.; *Kali iod.;* Kali s.; Kreos.; Lach.; *Lyc.; Merc. s.;* Myos.; Myrt. ch.; Nat. m.; Nat. s.; *Nit. ac.;* Nux v.; Phos.; Pix l.; *Puls.;* Rumex; Sabal; Sang.; *Scilla;* Sec.; *Senega;* Sep.; *Sil.;* Silph.; Spong.; *Stann.;* Strych.; *Sul.;* Taxus; Tereb.; Tub.; Ver. a.

Fibrinous—*Calc. acet.;* Bry.; Brom.; *Kali bich.;* Phos.

Toxemic—Am. c.; Ant. t.; Bry.; Colch.; Diphtherotox.; *Merc. c.*

Irritation of tubes—Acet. ac.; *Acon.;* Alumen; Ambros.; Brom.; *Bry.;* Chlorum; Ferr. p.; *Hep.; Phos.;* Piloc.; *Rumex;* Sang. n.; Spong. See Bronchitis.

Sensitiveness, to cold air—Allium s.; *Aral.;* Bac.; Calc. sil.; *Cham.;* Cinch.; *Coral.; Dulc.; Hep.;* Iod.; Kali c.; Mang. ac.; *Merc. s.;* Naja; *Psor.; Sil.;* Tub.

CHEST—Affections, after brain fag—Phos. ac.

Affections, after operations, for fistulæ—Berb. v.; Calc. p.; Sil.

Affections, after operations, for hydrothorax, empyema—Abrot.

Affections, after suppressed skin eruptions—Hep.

Affections, in circumscribed spots, persistent after inflammation—Senega.

Affections, in stone cutters with adynamia—Sil.

Burning—Acet. ac.; *Acon.;* Am. c.; Am. m.; Ant. t.; Apis; Aral.; *Ars.;* Bell.; *Brom.;* Bry.; *Calc. c.; Carbo v.;* Cic.; Euphorb.; Kreos.; Lyc.; Mag. m.; Mang. ac.; *Merc.;* Merc. sul.; Mez.; Myrtis; Ol. j. as.; Op.; *Phos.;* Primula; Ran. sc.; *Sang.;* Sang. n.; *Spong.; Sul.;* Wyeth.; Zinc. m.

Coldness—Abies c.; *Am. m.; Brom.;* Carbo an.; Cistus; *Coral; Elaps;* Helod.; *Kali c.;* Lith. c.

Eruptions on—Arundo; Jugl. c.; Kali br.; Lyc.; Petrol.

Inability to lie down (orthopnœa)—Acon. fer.; *Ars.*; *Conv.*; Dig.; Grind.; Lach.; Mag. p.; Puls.; Viscum. See Respiration.

Inability, to lie on left side—*Phos.*; Puls.

Inability, to lie on right side—Merc.

Injury followed by phthisis—Millef.; Ruta.

Itching, extending to nares—Coccus; Con.; Iod.; *Ipec.*; Puls.

Lightness, emptiness, eviscerated feeling—Cocc.; Nat. s.; *Phos.*; *Stann.*

PAINS—In general: Abrot.; Acal.; *Acon.*; *Apis*; Arg. n.; *Arn.*; Ars.; *Bell.*; Bor.; Brom.; Bry.; *Cact.*; Calc. c.; Caul.; *Caust.*; Chel.; *Cim.*; Collins.; Commocl.; Crot. t.; Dig.; Elaps; Eriod.; Gadus; *Hydroc. ac.*; Jugl. c.; *Kali c.*; Kali n.; *Kreos.*; Med.; Morph.; Myrtis; *Ox. ac.*; *Phos.*; Pothos.; Psor.; *Puls.*; *Ran. b.*; *Rumex*; *Sang.*; Solan. lyc.; Sticta; Strych. p.; Succin.; Sul.

Bruised, ulcerative—Ampel.; *Arn.*; Calc. c.; Eup. perf.; Kreos.; Lyc.; Phaseol.; *Psor.*; *Puls.*; *Ran. b.*; Ran. sc.; Sang.

Constriction, must frequently breathe deeply to expand lungs—Adon. v.; Asaf.; *Bry.*; *Dig.*; Ign.; Iod.; Lach.; Meli.; Millef.; *Mosch.*; Nat. s.; *Phos.*; Scilla; Xanth.

Constriction, spasmodic, tightness, fullness, oppression—Abies n.; *Acon.*; Adren.; Ambros.; Am. c.; *Ant. t.*; Apis; *Apoc.*; *Apium gr.*; Aral.; Arg. n.; *Ars.*; Asaf.; *Bac.*; Bell.; Brom.; *Bry.*; *Cact.*; Calc. ars.; *Calc. c.*; *Caps.*; Carbo v.; Cham.; *Chlorum*; Cic.; Coca; Cocc.; Coff.; *Cupr. ac.*; Cupr. m.; *Dig.*; Diosc.; Dulc.; *Ferr. m.*; Ferr. p.; Glon.; Glycerin; Grind.; Hematox.; Hep.; *Hydroc. ac.*; *Ipec.*; *Justicia*; Kali bich.; *Kali c.*; *Kali n.*; *Kreos.*; Lach.; Lact. v.; Laur.; *Lob. infl.*; Lyc.; Magnol.; Med.; Morph.; *Mosch.*; Naja; Naph.; *Nat. ars.*; *Nat. s.*; *Nit. sp. d.*; *Nux v.*; Ornothog.; Ox. ac.; *Phos.*; *Puls.*; Ran. b.; Ruta; Samb.; Sang.; Senega; Sep.; Sil.; Silph.; Solan. n.; Spig.; Spong.; Stram.; Strych.; Sul. ac.; *Sul.*; Ver. v.

Cutting—*Bry.*; Kali c.; Kali n.; Sul.; Zinc. m.

Pressing, heaviness, weight—*Abies n.*; Abrot.; Acon.; Am. c.; *Anac.*; Arg. n.; Arn.; *Ars.*; Aur.; Bry.; *Cact.*; *Calc. c.*; Cham.; Chel.; Ferr. iod.; Hematox.; Ipec.; Kali n.; *Kreos.*; *Lil. t.*; *Lob. infl.*; Lyc.; Phos. ac.; *Phos.*; Prun. pad.; Ptel.; *Puls.*; Ran. b.; Ruta; Samb.; Sang. n.; Senega; Sil.; *Spong.*; *Sul.*; Ver. v.

Stitching, tearing, darting, shooting—*Acon.*; Agar.; Allium s.; Am. c.; Ant. t.; Apium gr.; Ars.; *Asclep. t.*; Bell.; Berb. v.; *Bor.*; Brom.; *Bry.*; Calc. c.; Canth.; Caps.; *Carbo an.*; Carbo v.; *Caust.*; *Chel.*; Cim.; *Cinch.*; Coccus; Colch.; Crot. t.; *Elaps*; Formica; *Guaiac.*; Hematox.; Inula; *Kali c.*; Kali iod.; Kal.; *Lob. card.*; Lyc.; Menthol; Merc. c.; Merc.; Myrtis; *Nat. s.*; Nit. ac.; Nux v.; Ol. an.; Ol. j. as.; Pæonia; Phell.; *Phos.*; *Ran. b.*; Rhod.; Rhus t.; Rhus r.; Rumex; Sang.; *Scilla*; Sep.; *Sil.*; Spig.; Stann.; *Sticta*; *Sul.*; *Ther.*; Thuya; Trill.; Zing.

LOCATION—Cartilages, costal: Perichondritis: Arg. m.; Bell.; Cham.; *Cim.*; Guaiac.; Oleand.; Plumb.; Ruta.

Infra-mammary—*Cim.*; Puls.; Ran. b.; Ustil. See Female Sexual System.

Intercostal (pleurodynia)—Acon.; Am. c.; Aristol.; *Arn.*; Ars.; Asclep. t.; Azadir.; Bor.; *Bry.*; Caust.; Chel.; *Cim.*; Colch.; Echin.; Gaulth.;

Guaiac.; *Kali c.*; *Nux v.*; Ox. ac.; *Phos.*; **Puls.**; *Ran. b.*; Rham. c.; Rhod.; Rhus r.; *Rhus t.*; Rumex; Senega; Sinap. n.; Sul. ac.

Lung, left: Apex and middle portion—Acon.; Am. c.; *Anis.*; Ant. s. a.; Crot. t.; Illic.; *Lob. card.*; *Myrtis*; Pæonia; Phos.; *Pix l.*; Puls.; Ran. b.; Rumex; Sil.; Spig.; Stann.; Sticta; *Sul.*; *Ther.*; Tub.; Ustil.

Lower portion—Agar.; Ampel.; Asclep. t.; Calc. p.; Cim.; *Lob. syph.*; Lyc.; Myos.; *Nat. s.*; *Ox. ac.*; *Rumex*; Scilla; Sil.

Lung, right: Apex and middle portion—Abies c.; *Ars.*; Bor.; *Calc. c.*; Commocl.; Crot. t.; *Elaps*; Eriod.; *Illic.*; Iodof.; *Phell.*; Sang.; Upas.

Lower portion—Am. m.; Berb. v.; Bry.; Cact.; Card. m.; *Chel.*; Diosc.; Kali c.; Lyc.; Merc.

Substernal—Apium gr.; Ars.; Asclep. t.; Aster.; Aur.; Azadir.; *Bry.*; Card. m.; *Caust.*; Chel.; Con.; *Diosc.*; Jugl. r.; Kali n.; Kal.; *Kreos.*; Lact. v.; Morph.; Nit. ac.; Nit. sp. d.; Osm.; Phell.; Phos. ac.; Phos.; Psor.; Puls.; *Ran. b.*; Ran. sc.; *Rumex*; Ruta; Samb.; *Sang.*; Sang. n.; Sep.; Sil.; Spig.; Sul.; Trill.

MODALITIES—AGGRAVATIONS: From ascending: Ars.; Sep.

From bending forward—Sul.

From breathing, coughing—Am. m.; Arn.; *Bry.*; Colch.; Menthol; Nat. m.; Phos.; *Ran. b.*; Senega; Sep.; Sil.; Sul.

From cold drinks—Thuya.

From cold weather—Petrol.; Phos.

From damp weather—Ran. b.; Rhus t.; Spig.

From lying down, at night—Calc. c.; Sep.

From lying on affected side—Nux v.; Phos.; Stann.

From lying on left side—Phos.

From lying on right side—Kali c.; *Merc.*

From motion—Arn.; Ars.; Bry.; Calc. c.; Card. m.; Jugl. r.; Kali c.; Mag. c.; Phos.; Ran. b.; Senega; Sep.; Spig.; Sul.

From pressure—Arn.; Ars.; *Bry.*; Colch.; Nux v.; *Phos.*; *Ran. b.*

From spinal irritation—Agar.; Ran. b.

From talking—Alum.; Hep.; *Stann.*

From working—Am. m.; Lyc.; Sep.

AMELIORATIONS—From bending forward: Asclep. t.; **Hyos.**

From eructation—Bar. c.

From lying down—Psor.

From lying on affected side—Bry.; Puls.

From motion—Ign.; Puls.

From rapid walking—Lob. infl.

From rest—Bry.

In open air—Anac.; *Puls.*

Snesitiveness, tenderness, rawness of chest—Ant. t.; Aral.; *Arn.*; Ars.; Asclep. t.; *Bry.*; Calc. c.; Calc. p.; Calc. sil.; *Carbo v.*; *Caust.*; Cim.; Cur.; *Eup. perf.*; Ferr. p.; Ham.; *Iod.*; Kali c.; *Kaolin*; *Merc.*; Naph.; *Nat. s.*; *Nit. ac.*; *Ol. j. as.*; *Phos.*; Pop. c.; Puls.; *Ran. b.*; *Ran. sc.*; *Rumex*; *Sang.*; *Senega*; Sep.; Spong.; Stann.; Sul.

Spots on, brown—Sep.

Spots on, yellow—Phos.

Weakness, from least exertion, even talking, laughing, singing—Alumen; Am. c.; *Arg. m.*; *Calc. c.*; Canth.; *Carbo v.*; Cocc.; *Dig.*; Iod.; Kali c.; Lob. infl.; *Phos. ac.*; Phos.; Psor.; Ran. sc.; Rhus t.; Ruta; Spong.; *Stann.*; *Sul.*

COUGH—Remedies in general: *Acal.*; *Acet. ac.*; *Acon.*; *Allium s.*; *Alum.*; *Ambra*; Am. br.; *Am. c.*; Am. caust.; Am. m.; Ant. ars.; Ant. s. a.; *Ant. t.*; Aral.; Arn.; *Ars.*; *Ars. iod.*; Asclep. t.; Bals. per.; *Bell.*; *Bism.*; *Brom.*; *Bry.*; *Calc. c.*; *Canth.*; *Caps.*; Carb. ac.; *Carbo v.*; Caust.; *Cepa*; Cham.; Chel.; *Cim.*; Cina; Coccus; Cod.; Con.; Coral.; *Crot.*; Cupr. ac.; Cupr. m.; *Dros.*; Dulc.; *Eup. perf.*; Euphras.; Ferr. p.; *Hep.*; Hydroc. ac.; *Hyos.*; Hyosc. hydrobr.; Ign.; *Iod.*; *Ipec.*; *Kali bich.*; *Kali c.*; Kali chlor.; *Lach.*; *Lact. v.*; *Laur.*; *Lob. infl.*; *Lyc.*; *Mag. p.*; Mang. ac.; *Mentha*; Meph.; Merc. s.; *Merc. v.*; Myrtis; *Naja*; Nat. m.; *Nit. ac.*; *Nux v.*; Op.; *Osm.*; Phell.; *Phos.*; Pop. c.; *Puls.*; Rhus t.; *Rumex*; *Samb.*; *Sang.*; Santon.; *Scilla*; Senega; *Sil.*; Spong.; *Stann. iod.*; Stann.; *Sticta*; *Sul.*; Trifol.; Tub.; *Verbas. Viola od.*; Wyeth.

CAUSE, OCCURRENCE, AGGRAVATION—Abdomen, irritation from: Sep.

After anger in children—Anac.; Ant. t.

After anger, vexation, cleaning teeth—Staph.

After diarrhœa—Abrot.

After falling asleep, especially, in children, constant tickling cough without waking—*Acon.*; Agar.; *Aral.*; *Cham.*; Cycl.; Lach.; Nit. ac.; Sul.; Tub.; Verbasc. See Evening.

After sleep—Brom.; Lach.; Spong.

Afternoon, in—Am. m.; Lyc.; Thuya.

Air, hot—Kali s.

Arsenical wall paper—Calc. c.

Ascending—Am. c.

Bathing—Nux m.

Catarrh—Am. m.; Caust.; *Ipec.*; Kreos.; *Scilla*; Sticta.

Catarrh, post-nasal, in children and adults—Hydr.; Pop. c.; Spig.

Chest, feeling as if lump in—Abies n.

Cold air—*Acon.*; Alum.; Am. c.; Ars.; Bar. c.; Brom.; Calc. sil.; *Carbo v.*; *Cepa*; *Hep.*; Lach.; *Mentha*; Nit. ac.; *Phos.*; Rhus t.; *Rumex*; Scilla; Senega; *Spong.*; Trifol.

Cold air, to warm—Ant. c.; *Bry.*; Ipec.; *Nat. c.*; Scilla; Ver. a.

Condiments, vinegar, wine—Alum.

Dampness—Ant. t.; Calc. c.; *Dulc.*; *Nat. s.*; Nux m.

Daytime only—*Euphras.*; *Ferr.*; Nat. m.; Stann.; Staph.; Viola od.

Drinking—Ars.; *Bry.*; *Carbo v.*; Dros.; Hyos.; Lyc.; Phos.; Staph.

Drinking, cold—*Carbo v.*; *Hep.*; Merc.; Rhus t.; Scilla; Sil.; *Spong.*; Ver. a.

Eating—Anac.; Ant. ars.; Ant. t.; *Bry.*; *Calc. c.*; *Carbo v.*; *Cinch.*; Hyos.; Kali bich.; *Lach.*; *Mez.*; Myos.; *Nux v.*; Phos.; Staph.; Taxus; Zinc. m.

Eczema or itch suppressed—Psor.

Entering, warm room—Acon.; *Ant. c.*; Anthem.; *Bry.*; *Caust.*; Cham.; Merc.; *Nat. c.*; *Puls.*; Ran. b.; Ver. a.

RESPIRATORY SYSTEM

Evening, night—Acal.; *Acon.*; *Am. br.*; Am. c.; Ant. t.; Arn.; *Ars.*; *Bell.*; Bry.; *Calc. c.*; Caps.; *Carbo v.*; *Caust.*; *Cim.*; *Cod.*; *Colch.*; *Con.*; *Dros.*; Eup. perf.; Hep.; Hydroc. ac.; *Hyos.*; Kali br.; Ign.; Laur.; Lyc.; Mentha; Meph.; *Merc.*; Nit. ac.; Op.; Passifl.; Phos.; Prun. v.; Psor.; *Puls.*; *Rhus t.*; Rumex; Samb.; Sang.; Sanic.; Santon.; Sep.; Sil.; *Spong.*; Stann.; Sticta; Sul.; Tub.; Verbasc.

Before midnight—Aral.; *Bell.*; Carbo v.; Mag. m.; Phos.; Samb.; *Spong.*; Stann.

After midnight, early A. M.—*Acon.*; Am. br.; Am. c.; *Ars.*; Cupr. m.; Dros.; Hep.; Kali c.; Nux v.; Phell.; Rhus t.

Constriction in larynx, trachea—Ign.

Excitement—Ambra; Coral.; Ign.; Spong.; Tar. h. See Nervous.

Expiration—*Acon.*; *Caust.*; Nux v.

Exposure even of hand from under cover—Bar. c.; Hep.; Rhus t.

Heart disease—Arn.; Hydroc. ac.; Lach.; Laur.; Lycop.; *Naja*; *Spong.*

Influenza—Cepa; *Eriod.*; Hyos.; *Kali bich.*; Kali s.; *Kreos.*; *Pix l.*; Sang.; Senega; Stann.; Strych.

Injuries—Arn.; Millef.

Inspiration—Acet. ac.; Acon.; *Bell.*; Brom.; Bry.; Cina; Iod.; *Ipec.*; Kali bich.; Lach.; Mentha; Nat. m.; Phos.; Rumex; Scilla.; *Spong.*; Sticta.

Intermittent, suppressed—Eup. perf.

Liver affections—Am. m.

Lying down—Ant. ars.; *Aral.*; Ars.; *Bell.*; Bry.; *Caust.*; Cochlear.; Con.; Croc.; Crot. t.; Dros.; Dulc.; Hyos.; Ign.; Inula; Lith. c.; Meph.; Nit. ac.; Nux v.; Petrol.; *Phos.*; *Prun. v.*; Psor.; *Puls.*; Rumex; Sabad.; Sang.; Sil.; Sticta; Tub.; Verbasc.

Lying on back—Am. m.; Ars.; Iod.; Nux v.; Phos.

Lying on left side—Dros.; Phos.; Ptel.; Rumex; Stann.

Lying on right side—Am. m.; Benz. ac.; Merc.

Lying with head low—Am. m.; *Spong.*

Measles—Dros.; Dulc.; Eup. perf.; Euphras.; Ipec.; Kali bich.; *Puls.*; Sang.; Scilla; Sticta. See Skin.

Menses, or piles, suppressed—Millef.

Mental exertion—Nux v.

Morning—Acal.; Allium s.; *Alum.*; Ambra; Calc. c.; Cina; Coccus; Hep.; Iod.; Kali bich.; Kali iod.; Kali n.; Lyc.; Nat. m.; Nit. ac.; Puls.; Rhus t.; Selen.; Sep.; Sticta; Sil.; Tab.

Morning, early—Am. br.; Am. c.; Ars.; Caust.; Cupr. m.; Hep.; Kali c.; Nux v.; Phell.; Puls.; Sul.

Morning, on waking—Alum.; Ambra; Bry.; Coccus; Kali bich.; Psor.; Rhus t.

Motion—Ars.; Bell.; Bry.; Cina; Hep.; Iod.; Ipec.; Nux v.; Puls.; Senega; Spong.; Ver. a.

Odors strong; presence of strangers—Phos.

Old people—Ant. iod.; Ant. t.; Bar. c.; Bar. m.; Carbo v.; Hyos.; Kreos.; Myrtis; Rhus t.; Senega; Sil.; Sticta.

Operations for fistulæ, after—Berb. v.; Calc. p.; Sil.

Periodic, recurring in spring, autumn—Cina.
Pertussis after; from least cold—Caust.; Sang.
Physical exhaustion—Scilla; *Sticta*.
Pregnancy—*Apoc.*; Bry.; Caust.; *Con.*; *Kali br.*; Nux m.; Vib. op.
Reading, laughing, singing, talking—Alum.; *Ambra*; Anac.; *Arg. m.*; *Arg. n.*; Arum; Carbo v.; *Caust.*; Cim.; Collins.; *Con.*; *Dros.*; *Hep.*; Hyos.; Iridium; Lach.; *Mang. ac.*; Mentha; Nux v.; *Phos.*; *Rumex*; Sil.; Spong.; *Stann.*; Sul.
Reflex—Ambra; Apis; Phos.
Sciatica in summer alternating—Staph.
Standing still during a walk—Astac.; Ign.
Stomach, irritation, from—Bism.; *Bry.*; Calad.; Cereum ox.; Kali m.; *Lob. infl.*; Nat. m.; Nit. ac.; Nux v.; Phos.; *Sang.*; *Sep.*; Sul.; Ver. a.
Swallowing, from—Spong.
Sweets—Med.; *Spong.*; Zinc. m.
Tickling, as from dust, feather—Am. c.; Ars.; *Bell.*; *Calc. c.*; Caps.; Caust.; *Carbo v.*; Cina; *Dros.*; Euphorb. dath.; *Ign.*; Lac c.; Lach.; *Lact. v.*; Nat. m.; Nux v.; Paris; Phos.; *Rumex*; Sep.
Tickling, in chest (substernal, suprasternal fossa)—*Ambra*; Am. br.; *Ant. c.*; Apis; Arn.; Ars.; Brom.; *Bry.*; *Calc. c.*; Caps.; *Carbo v.*; *Caust.*; Cham.; Coccus; *Con.*; Ferr. ac.; *Ign.*; *Iod.*; Ipec.; Kali bich.; Kreos.; *Lach.*; *Mentha*; Myrtis; *Nux v.*; Osm.; Paris; Phos. ac.; *Phos.*; Puls.; Radium; Rhus t.; *Rumex*; Sang.; Sep.; *Sil.*; Spong.; *Stann.*; Sul.; Ver. a.
Tickling, in larynx—Alum.; *Arg. m.*; *Bell.*; Brom.; *Calc. c.*; Caps.; *Carbo v.*; Caust.; *Cepa*; Cochlear.; *Coccus*; *Con.*; Crot.; *Dros.*; Dulc.; Eryng.; Hep.; *Ign.*; Iod.; Ipec.; Kreos.; *Lach.*; Menthol; Nit. ac.; Phos.; Puls.; *Rumex*; Sang.; *Sil.*; Spong.; Sul.
Tickling, in throat—Alum.; Ambra; Am. c.; *Aral.*; *Arg. n.*; Bell.; *Calc. c.*; *Caps.*; Cham.; Cim.; Cina; *Con.*; *Dros.*; *Hep.*; Hepat.; Hyos.; *Ign.*; *Iod.*; Kali c.; Lact. v.; *Lob. infl.*; Meli.; Menthol; Nux v.; *Phos.*; Rumex; Stann. iod.; Sul.; Wyeth.
Tobacco smoke—Mentha; Merc.; Spong.; Staph.
Tonsils, enlarged—Bar. c.; Lach.
Touch, pressure—Lach.; *Rumex*.
Undressing, or uncovering body—Bar. c.; *Hep.*; Kali bich.; *Rhus t.*; Rumex.
Uvula, relaxed—Bar. c.; *Hyos.*; Kali c.; Merc. i. r.
Warmth—*Ant. c.*; *Bry.*; Caust.; Dros.; Dulc.; Ipec.; *Merc.*; Nat. c.; Nux m.; Puls.; Scilla.
Weeping—Arn.
Winter—Aloe; *Ant. s. a.*; Bry.; Cham.; Ipec.; Kreos.; Lippia; Psor. See Chronic Bronchitis.
Worms—Cina; Tereb.
Young, phthisical persons with constant, distressing night cough—Dros.

TYPE—Barking: Acon.; Ambra; *Bell.*; Coral.; *Dros.*; Hep.; Iod.; *Kali bich.*; Phos.; Samb.; Sinap. n.; *Spong.*; Ver. a. See Dry; Hoarse; Spasmodic.

RESPIRATORY SYSTEM

Chronic (phthisical)—*Allium s.;* Ant. *t.;* Ars. iod.; Bar. c.; Bry.; Calc. iod.; Calc. p.; Cham.; *Cod.;* Crot.; *Dros.;* Dulc.; Eup. perf.; Hyos. hydrobr.; Kreos.; Laur.; Lob. infl.; Lyc.; Mang.; Merc.; Naja; *Nit. ac.;* Phell.; Psor.; Puls.; Rumex; *Sang.;* Scilla; Sil.; *Spong.;* Sticta; Sul. See Tuberculosis.

Croupy—*Acon.;* Brom.; Gels.; *Hep.;* Iod.; *Kali bich.;* Nit. ac.; Phos.; *Spong.;* Staph. See Croup.

Dry, hard, racking, hacking, short, tight, tickling—*Acal.;* Acon.; Alumen; *Alum.;* Am. br.; Am. c.; Ant. s. a.; *Ars.;* Ars. iod.; *Arum;* Asclep. t.; Aviare; *Bell.;* Brom.; Bry.; *Calc. c.;* Calc. iod.; Canth.; *Caps.;* Carb. ac.; Carbo v.; *Caust.;* Cepa; *Cham.;* Cim.; *Cina;* Cochlear.; Cod.; Coff.; Con.; Coral.; Dig.; Dros.; Euphras.; Ferr. p.; Glycerin; *Hep.; Hydroc. ac.; Hyos.;* Hyosc. hydrobr.; *Ign.;* Iod.; Justicia; *Kali bich.; Kali br.; Kali c.;* Kali m.; Kreos.; *Lach.; Laur.; Lob. infl.;* Lyc.; Lycop.; Lycopers.; Mang.; Med.; *Mentha;* Menthol; Merc.; *Morph.; Naja;* Nat. m.; *Nit. ac.; Nux v.;* Ol. j. as.; *Onosm.;* Op.; *Osm.;* Petrol.; *Phos.;* Puls.; *Rhus t.; Rumex;* Salvia; Samb.; Sang.; *Sang. n.;* Scilla; *Senega; Sep.; Sil.; Spong.;* Stann.; *Sticta;* Sul.; Sul. ac.; Tela ar.; Tub.; Vanad.; Ver. a.; *Verbasc.;* Wyeth.

Explosive, noisy—*Caps.;* Dros.; *Osm.;* Solan. lyc.; Strych. See Spasmodic.

Fatiguing, exhausting, irritating—*Acon.;* Am. c.; Ant. iod.; *Ars.; Arum;* Aviare; Bals. per.; *Bell.;* Bry.; Calc. c.; *Caust.;* Cham.; Chel.; *Cod.;* Collins.; Con.; *Coral.;* Dros.; Eucal.; Hep.; *Hyos.;* Hydroc. ac.; *Ign.;* Iod.; *Ipec.;* Kali br.; Kreos.; Lact. v.; Laur.; *Lob. infl.;* Lyc.; *Mentha;* Menthol; Merc.; Myrtis; *Naja;* Nit. ac.; Op.; Phell.; *Phos.;* Psor.; Rumex as.; Rumex; *Sang; Scilla; Senega; Sep.; Sil.;* Silph. cyr.; *Sticta;* Strych.; Tela ar. See Spasmodic.

Hoarse, hollow, deep, metallic—*Acon.; Ambra;* Am. phos.; Ant. t.; Apoc.; Ars. iod.; *Arum;* Bell.; Brom.; Bry.; *Carbo v.; Caust.; Cina; Dros.;* Dulc.; Euphorb.; Euphras.; *Hep.;* Ign.; Iod.; Irid.; *Kali bich.;* Lippia; Lyc.; Mang.; Med.; Meph.; Myrtis; Nit. ac.; *Phos.;* Samb.; *Spong.;* Stann.; Ver. a.; *Verbasc.* See Spasmodic.

Laryngeal, nervous—Acon.; *Ambra;* Asar.; *Bell.;* Brom.; Caps.; Carbo v.; *Caust.;* Cina; *Coral.; Cupr.;* Dros.; Gels.; *Hep.;* Hydroc. ac.; *Hyos.; Ign.;* Ipec.; Kali br.; Kali m.; Lach.; Med.; Merc.; *Nit. ac.;* Nux v.; *Phos.;* Puls.; *Rumex; Santon.; Spong.;* Sul.; Tar. h.; Terebene; Ver. a.; Viola od.

Loose, rattling, gagging, choking, strangling—Am. br.; Am. m.; Ant. s.; *Ant. t.;* Ars.; Asclep. t.; Bals. per.; *Brom.; Calc. ac.; Calc. c.; Chel.;* Cina; Coccus; Cupr. m.; Dros.; *Dulc.;* Eup. perf.; *Hep.; Ipec.;* Kali bich.; *Kali c.;* Kali m.; Kali s.; Lyc.; *Merc.; Nat. s.;* Nit. ac.; Phos.; Puls.; *Rhus t.;* Samb.; Sang.; Scilla; *Senec.;* Senega; Sep.; Sil.; Stann.; Sticta; Sul.; Tereb.; Ver. a.

Spasmodic, paroxysmal, nervous, violent, suffocative—*Acon.;* Agar.; *Ambra; Am. br.;* Ant. ars.; Ant. t.; Aral.; *Arn.;* Ars.; Asar.; *Bell.;* Brom.; Bry.; Caps.; Carb. ac.; *Carbo v.; Caust.;* Cham.; *Chel.; Cina;* Coccus; Con.; *Coral.;* Crot. t.; *Cupr. ac.; Cupr. m.;* Dros.; Dulc.; Gels.; Glycerin; *Hep.; Hydroc. ac.; Hyos.; Ign.;* Iod.; *Ipec.; Justicia; Kali br. Kali c.; Kreos.; Lach.; Lact. v.;* Laur.; Led.; Lyc.; *Mag. p.;* Meph.;

RESPIRATORY SYSTEM

Merc.; Naph.; *Nat. m.*; *Nit. ac.*; Nux m.; *Nux v.*; Op.; *Osm.*: Pertussin; *Phos.*; Radium; *Rumex*; Samb.; Sang.; Santon.; *Scilla*; Sep.; *Sil.*; *Spong.*; Stann.; Sticta; *Sul.*; Trifol.; Ver. a.; *Viola od.*

Successive, in two paroxysms—Merc.; Puls.

Successive, in three paroxysms—Cupr. m.; Stann.

Wheezing, asthmatic—Ambros.; Ant. t.; *Ars.*; Benz. ac.; Croc.; Hep.; Iod.; *Ipec.*; Kali bich.; *Lob. infl.*; Meph.; Nit. ac.; Rhodium; Samb.; *Sang.*; Senega; *Spong.* See Spasmodic.

WHOOPING (pertussis)—*Acon.*; Alumen; Ambra; *Ambros.*; Am. br.; Am. m.; Am. picr.; Ant. c.; *Ant. t.*; *Arn.*; Bal.; *Bell.*; Bry.; Brom.; Caps; Carb. ac.; Carbo v.; Caust.; *Castanea*; Cereum ox.; *Chel.*; *Cina*; Cinch.; Cocaine; *Coccus*; Con.; *Coral.*; Coquel.; *Cupr. ac.*; *Cupr. m.*; *Dros.*; *Dulc.*; Eucal.; Euphorb. dath.; Euphras.; *Formal.*; Grind.; Hep.; *Hydroc. ac.*; *Hyos.*; Ipec.; *Justicia*; *Kali bich.*; Kali br.; *Kali c.*; *Kali m.*; Kali p.; Kali s.; Led.; *Lob. infl.*; Lob. m.; *Mag. p.*; *Meph.*; Merc.; *Naph.*; Nit. ac.; Ol. j. as.; Op.; Passifl.; Pertussin; Phos.; Pod.; *Puls.*; Samb.; Sang. n.; *Sep.*; Sil.; Solan. c.; Sticta; Sul.; Thymus; Tongo; *Trifol.*; *Ver. a.*; Viola od. See Spasmodic.

Whooping at night, "minute gun" during day—Coral.

Whooping, convulsions—*Bell.*; Cina; *Cupr. ac.*; Cupr. m.; Hydroc. ac.; Hyos.; Kali br.; Mag. p.; Narcissus; *Solan. c.*

Whooping, early stage (spasmodic)—*Acon.*; *Bell.*; Carb. ac.; Carbo v.; *Castanea*; Chel.; *Cina*; Coccus; Coral.; Cupr.; *Dros.*; Hyos.; Ipec.; Mag. p.; Meph.; Naph.; Narcissus; Samb.; Stann.; Thymus.

Whooping, hæmorrhage—*Arn.*; *Cereum ox.*; Coral.; Cupr.; *Dros.*; Ind.; *Ipec.*; Merc.

Whooping, later stages (catarrhal)—*Ant. t.*; Cinch.; Hep.; *Ipec.*; Puls.

Whooping, vomiting—Ant. t.; Bell.; Carbo v.; *Cereum ox.*; *Coccus*; *Cupr. m.*; *Dros.*; *Ipec.*; Lob. infl.; Ver. a.

Whooping—Concomitants: Body stiff, rigid, cyanosis: Am. c.; *Ant. t.*; Carbo v.; Cina; Coral.; *Cupr. ac.*; *Cupr. m.*; Iod.; *Ipec.*; Mag. p.; Meph.; Op.; Samb.; *Ver. a.*

Coryza—Alum.; Lyc.; Nat. c.

Crowing inspiration absent—Ambra.

Crying—*Arn.*; Bry.; *Caps.*; Samb.

Diarrhœa—Ant. t.; *Cupr. ars.*; Euphorb. dath.; Ipec.; *Rumex*; Ver. a.

Dyspnœa—Ambra; Am. c.; *Ant. t.*; Bell.; Brom.; *Carbo v.*; Cina; Coral.; *Cupr. m.*; *Dros.*; Euphorb.; Hep.; Hippoz.; Iod.; *Ipec.*; Kali bich.; *Lob. infl.*; *Meph.*; Naph.; Op.; *Samb.*; Senec.; *Ver. a.*; *Viola od* See Respiration.

Epistaxis, bleedings—*Arn.*; Bell.; Cereum ox.; Coral.; *Cupr.*; *Dros.*; Ind.; *Iod.*; Ipec.; Merc.

Paroxysms follow each other rapidly and violently—Dros.

Paroxysms wakes child at 6-7 A. M., vomiting of ropy mucus—Coccus.

Paroxysms with flow of tears—Nat. m.

Spasm of glottis—Cupr.; Meph.; Mosch.

Sublingual ulcer—Nit. ac.

Vomiting of solid food after regaining consciousness—Cupr. m.

With every cold, severe cough returns—Sang.

RESPIRATORY SYSTEM. 893

EXPECTORATION: TYPE—Acid: Carbo an.; Nit. ac.; Puls.
  Albuminous, clear, white—*Arg. m.*; Ars.; Bry.; Coccus; Eucal.; Kali m.; Scilla; *Selen.*; Sul.
  Bitter—Bry.; Calc. c.; Cham.; Dros.; Kali n.; Nit. ac.; *Puls.*
  Bloody, blood streaked—*Acon.*; Arg. n.; *Arn.*; *Ars.*; *Bell.*; Bry.; Calc. c.; Can. s.; Canth.; *Cetrar.*; Coral.; Crot.; *Dig.*; Dros.; Dulc.; *Elaps*; Ferr. p.; Hep.; Hyos.; Iod.; Ipec.; Kali c.; *Kali n.*; Laur.; Led.; Lyc.; Merc. c.; Merc.; *Millef.*; Nit. ac.; Nitrum; Nux v.; Op.; *Phos.*; Puls.; *Rhus t.*; Selen.; Sil.; Sul.; Trill.
  Casts—*Calc. ac.*; Kali bich.
  Daytime—Ambra; Bry.; Calc. c.; Hyos.; Stann.
  Easy, raising—*Arg. m.*; Carbo v.; Dulc.; Eriod.; Kali s.; *Nat. s.*; Puls.; Scilla; *Stann.*; Tub.
  Fetid, offensive—Ars.; Bor.; *Calc. c.*; *Caps.*; Carbo v.; Cop.; Euphras.; Kali c.; *Kali hypophos.*; Lyc.; Nit. ac.; *Phell.*; Phos. ac.; *Pix l.*; Psor.; *Sang.*; Sep.; *Sil.*; *Stann.*; Sul.
  Globular, lumpy—*Agar.*; Arg. m.; Am. m.; Ant. t.; *Bad.*; Calc. c.; Calc. fl.; *Chel.*; *Kali c.*; Mang.; Nat. selen.; Rhus t.; *Sil.*
  Gray, greenish, mucus—Am. phos.; Ant. s. a.; Ars.; *Benz. ac.*; Calc. c.; Calc. iod.; Calc. p.; Calend.; Can. s.; *Carbo v.*; *Cop.*; Dros.; Dulc.; Ferr. ac.; *Kali iod.*; Kali m.; Kali s.; Kaolin; *Lyc.*; Nat. c.; *Nat. s.*; *Paris*; Phos.; Psor.; *Puls.*; Senega; Sep.; Silph.; Spong.; *Stann.*; Sul.; Thuya.
  Herby taste—Bor.
  Liver-colored—Graph.; Lyc.; Puls.; Sep.; Stann.
  Profuse—Allium s.; *Ammon.*; *Am. m.*; Ant. ars.; *Ant. iod.*; Ant. t.; <u>Arg. m.</u>; *Ars. iod.*; Asclep. t.; *Bals. per.*; Calc. c.; Calc. sil.; Canth.; *Carbo v.*; Ceanoth.; Chel.; Cinch.; *Coccus*; Cop.; Dros.; *Dulc.*; Eucal.; Grind.; *Hep.*; Hepat.; Hydr.; Ipec.; *Kali bich.*; Kali c.; Kali iod.; *Kreos.*; Laur.; *Lyc.*; Merc.; Myos.; Myrt. ch.; Nat. ars.; Nat. s.; Phell.; Phos. ac.; Piloc.; *Puls.*; Ruta; Sang.; *Scilla; Senega*; Sep.; Sil.; Silph.; *Stann.*; *Sul.*; Tereb.; Trill.; Zing.
  Purulent, muco-purulent—Ammon.; Ant. iod.; Ars. iod.; Asclep. t.; *Bac.*; *Bals. per.*; *Calc. c.*; Calc. p.; Calc. sil.; Calc. s.; *Carbo v.*; Cinch.; Cop.; Dros.; Eucal.; *Eryng.*; *Hep.*; Hepat.; *Hydr.*; Iod.; *Kali bich.*; Kali c.; Kali iod.; *Kali p.*; Kali s.; *Kreos.*; Laur.; *Lyc.*; Merc.; Myos.; Myrtis; Myrt. ch.; Nat. c.; Nit. ac.; Phos. ac.; *Phos.*; *Pix l.*; Psor.; Ruta; Sang. n.; Sang.; Scilla; Sep.; *Sil.*; Solan. n.; *Stann.*; Sul.; Tereb.; Tereb. scor.; Trill.
  Rust-colored—*Bry.*; Ferr. p.; *Phos.*; Rhus t.; *Sang.*
  Salty—Ambra; Ars.; Calc. c.; *Kali iod.*; Lyc.; *Mag. c.*; Nat. c.; Nat. m.; Phos. ac.; Phos.; Psor.; Puls.; Scilla; *Sep.*; Sil.; Stann.
  Scanty—Alum.; Am. m.; *Ant. t.*; *Ars.*; Asclep. t.; Brom.; Bry.; *Caust.*; Cim.; Kali c.; Kali hypophos.; Ign.; Lach.; Morph.; Nit. ac.; *Nux v.*; Op.; *Phos.*; Rumex; Sang.; Scilla; Spong.; Zinc. m. See Viscid.
  Serous, frothy, watery—*Acon.*; Am. c.; *Ant. ars.*; *Ars.*; Bry.; Carbo v.; Croc.; Ferr. p.; Grind.; *Kali iod.*; Lach.; Merc.; Nat. m.; Œnanthe; Phos.; Piloc.; Silph.; *Tanac.*

Slips back, or must be swallowed—Arn.; *Caust.;* Con.; Iod.; *Kali e.;* Lach.; Nux m.; Spong.

Soapy—Caust.

Sour—Calc. c.; Iris; Lach.; Nit. ac.; Nux v.; Phos. ac.; Phos.; Stann.; Zinc.

Sweetish—Hepat.; Phos.; Sang. n.; *Stann.;* Sul.

Viscid, tenacious, difficult of raising—Allium s.; *Alum.;* Ammon.; *Am. c.; Am. m.;* Ant. iod.; Ant. s. a.; *Ant. t.;* Aral.; *Ars.;* Asclep. t.; Bals. per.; Bar. c.; Bar. m.; Bell.; Bov.; *Bry.;* Calc. c.; Can. s.; *Canth.;* Carbo v.; *Caust.;* Chel.; Cinch.; *Coccus;* Cupr. m.; Dulc.; Eucal.; Grind.; *Hydr.; Ipec.; Kali bich.;* Kali c.; *Kali hypophos.;* Kali m.; *Lach.;* Laur.; Lyc.; Mang. ac.; Merc.; Morph.; Myrtis; Naph.; Nat. s.; Nux v.; Osm.; *Paris;* Phos.; Psor.; Quill.; Rumex; *Sang.;* Sang. n.; Scilla; *Senega; Sep.; Sil.;* Silph.; Sul.; Stann.

EMPTY FEELING IN CHEST—Phos. ac.; *Stann.*

Eructations—Ambra; Caps.

Faintness—Sep.

Gaping, alternates with cough—Ant. t.

Grasps genitals—Zinc. m.

Grasps throat—Acon.; *Cepa; Iod.;* Lob. infl.

Gurgling, from throat to stomach—Cina.

Herpes facialis—Arn. See Skin.

Hiccough—Tab.

Hoarseness—Ambra; Am. c.; *Brom.;* Calc. c.; Calend.; Carbo v.; *Caust.; Dros.; Eup. perf.; Hep.;* Iod.; Lach.; Meph.; *Merc.; Phos.;* Sil.; *Spong.;* Sul.

Hyperesthesia of mucosæ—*Bell.;* Con.; *Hyos.;* Lach.; Phos.; *Rumex;* Sticta.

Lachrymation—Caps.; *Cepa;* Cina; *Euphras.;* Nat. m.; *Scilla.*

Left breast, feels cold—Nat. c.

PAIN—Chest: Abies n.; Ars.; *Bell.;* Brom.; *Bry.;* Caps.; Carbo v.; *Caust.;* Chel.; Cinch.; Cina; Commocl.; *Dros.,* Dulc.; Elaps; *Eup. perf.;* Euphorb.; Ign.; *Iod.;* Justicia; Kali bich.; *Kali c.;* Kali iod.; Kali n.; *Kreos.; Lact. v.;* Lyc.; Meph.; *Merc.;* Myrtis; Nat. c.; *Nat. s.; Niccol.;* Nux v.; Phell.; *Phos.;* Phyt.; *Rumex;* Senega; Sil.; Spong.; *Sticta; Sul.;* Thasp.

Distant parts—Agar.; Am. c.; Bell.; *Bry.; Caps.; Caust.;* Chel.; Lach.; Nat. m.; Senega.

Head—Æth.; Anac.; Asclep. t.; Bell.; *Bry.;* Carbo v.; Eup. perf.; Ferr. m.; Formica; Lyc.; *Nat. m.; Nux v.;* Sep.; Sul.

Head, he places hands to it—*Bry.;* Caps.; Nat. m.; Nat. s.

Larynx—Acon.; Ant. t.; Arg. m.; Arum; Asclep. t.; *Bell.;* Caust.; *Cepa,* Hep.; Inula; *Iod.;* Nit. ac.; *Phos.;* Rumex; *Spong.*

Stomach, abdomen—Asclep. t.; *Bry.;* Calc. c.; *Nux v.;* Puls.; Sep.; Sil.; Sul.; Thuya.

Throat—*Bell.; Lach.;* Merc. i. r.; Sil.

RESPIRATORY SYSTEM

POLYURIA—Scilla.

Prostration—Am. c.; *Ant. t.*; *Ars.*; Coral.; *Cupr. m.*; Cur.; Hep.; Iod.; *Ipec.*; Meph.; Nit. ac.; Phos. ac.; Rumex; *Ver. a.*

Rawness, soreness of chest—Amyg. am.; Ant. s. a.; *Ars.*; *Bry.*; Calc. c.; Carbo v.; *Caust.*; Coral.; Dig.; *Eup. perf.*; Ferr. p.; Gels.; Graph.; Mag. m.; Meph.; *Merc.*; *Phos.*; Rhus t.; *Rumex*; Selen.; Senega; *Stann.*

Rubs face, with fists—Scilla.

Sleepiness, between attacks—Euphorb. dath.

Sneezing, at end—Agar.; Bell.; Cina; Dros.; *Justicia*; *Scilla*; Senega.

Spasms—*Bell.*; Cina; *Cupr. ac.*; *Cupr. m.*; Hydroc. ac.; Œnanthe; *Solan. c.*

Spasm of chest—Samb.

Tingling, in chest—Acon.

Urine, involuntary, spurting—Alum.; Caps.; *Caust.*; Colch.; *Ferr.*; *Ferr. mur.*; Ferr. p.; Nat. m.; *Puls.*; Rumex; *Scilla*; Ver. a.; Verbasc.; *Yerba*; Zinc. m.

Vomiting; retching, gagging—Alumen; Anac.; *Ant. t.*; *Bry.*; Carbo v.; Coccus; *Cupr. ac.*; Cupr. ars.; Cupr. m.; Cur.; *Dros.*; Euphorb. dath.; Euphras.; *Ferr. m.*; *Hep.*; *Ipec.*; *Kali c.*; Kreos.; Meph.; Myos.; Nit. ac.; *Nux v.*; Phos.; Puls.; Sep.; *Sil.*; Ver. a.

AMELIORATIONS—From drinking, cold things: *Caust.*; *Cupr. m.*; Phos.; Tab.

From drinking, warm things—Spong.

From eating—Anac.; Bism.; Ferr.; *Spong.*

From eructations—Ambra; Angust.; Sang.

From expectoration—Zinc. m.

From lying down—Calc. p.; Ferr. m.; *Mang. ac.*; Sinap.

From lying on right side—Ant. t.

From lying on stomach—Med.

From placing hands, on chest—*Bry.*; Caps.; Cina; Dros.; *Eup. perf.*; Lact. v.; *Nat. s.*

From resolute suppression of cough—Ign.

From resting, on hands and feet—Eup. perf.

From resting, with hands on thighs—Niccol.

From sitting up—*Bry.*; Crot. t.; *Dros.*; Hep.; Hyos.; Nat. s.; Phell.; *Puls.*; Sang.

From warming air by covering head with bedclothes—Hep.; Rhus t.; *Rumex.*

From warmth—Bad.

LARYNX—Anesthesia: Kali br.

Burning—Am. caust.; Am. m.; Arg. m.; *Ars.*; Canth.; Mang.; *Merc.*; Mez.; *Paris*; Phos.; *Rumex*; *Sang.*; Spong.; Zing. See Pain.

Cancer—Nit. ac.; Thuya.

Coldness—*Brom.*; Rhus t.; Sul.

Constricted feeling—Acon.; *Bell.*; Brom.; Calad.; *Chlorum*; *Cupr.*; Dros.; Guaco; Hydroc. ac.; *Iod.*; Mang. ac.; Med.; *Mosch.*; Naja; Ox. ac.; Phos.; *Spong.*; Still.; Ver. a. See Spasms.

Dryness—Ars.; *Bell.;* Carbo v.; Caust.; Dros.; Dub.; Hep.; Iod.; **Kali bich.;** Kali iod.; Lemna; *Mang. ac.;* Mez.; *Phos.;* Pop. c.; *Sang.;* Senega; *Spong.* See Inflammation.

Edema of glottis—*Apis;* Ars.; Bell.; Chin. ars.; Chorum; *Kali iod.;* Lach.; Merc.; Piloc.; *Sang.;* Stram.; *Vipera.*

Epiglottis, affections—Cepa; Chlorum; Hepat.; Wyeth.

INFLAMMATION—LARYNGITIS—Acute, catarrhal: *Acon.; Æsc.;* Ant. t.; Apis; Arg. m.; Ars. iod.; *Arum; Bell.;* Brom.; Bry.; Canth.; Carbo v.; *Caust.; Cepa;* Cub.; Dros.; *Dulc.;* Eup. perf.; *Ferr. p.;* Guaiac.; *Hep.;* Iod.; Ipec.; *Kali bich.;* Kali iod.; *Merc.;* Menthol; Osm.; *Phos.; Rhus t.; Rumex; Samb.; Sang.; Spong.;* Sticta; Sul.

Inflammation, atrophic—Am. m.; *Kali bich.;* Kali iod.; Lach.; Mang. ac.; Phos.; Sang.

Inflammation, chronic, catarrhal—Am. br.; Am. iod.; Ant. s. a.; Ant. t.; *Arg. m.; Arg. n.;* Bar. c.; Bar. m.; Calc. c.; Calc. iod.; *Carbo v.; Caust.;* Coccus; Cotyled.; *Dros.; Hep.;* Iod.; Irid.; *Kali bich.;* Kali c.; *Kali iod.; Lach.; Mang. ac.;* Merc. c.; *Merc.;* Nat. m.; Nat. selen.; Nit. ac.; *Nux v.; Paris; Phos.; Puls.;* Rhus t.; Sang. n.; *Selen.; Senega; Stann.;* Still.; *Sul.;* Thuya.

Inflammation, follicular—Arg. n.; Hep.; *Iod.;* Kali iod.; Selen.; *Sul.*

Inflammation, membranous exudate—MEMBRANOUS CROUP—*Acet. ac.;* Acon.; Ammon.; *Am. caust.;* Ant. t.; Ars.; Ars. iod.; Bell.; *Brom.;* Calc. iod.; Con.; Dros.; Ferr. p.; Hep.; *Iod.; Kali bich.;* Kali chlor.; *Kali m.;* Kali n.; *Kaolin;* Lach.; Merc. cy.; *Merc.;* Phos.; Samb.; *Sang.; Spong.* See Diphtheria (Throat).

Inflammation—SPASMODIC CROUP—*Acon.;* Ant. t.; Ars.; Bell.; Benzoin; *Brom.;* Bry.; *Calc. fl.; Calc. iod.; Chlorum;* Cupr.; Euphorb.; Ferr. p.; *Hep.;* Ign.; *Iod.;* Ipec.; *Kali bich.;* Kali br.; *Kali n.;* Kaolin; Lach.; Meph.; Merc. i. fl.; Mosch.; Naja; Petrol.; *Phos.;* Poth.; Samb.; Sang.; *Spong.;* Ver. v.

Inflammation, syphilitic, associated with, secondary symptoms—Merc. c.; Merc. s.; Nit. ac.

Inflammation, syphilitic, associated with, tertiary symptoms—*Aur.;* Cinnab.; Iod.; *Kali bich.; Kali iod.;* Lach.; *Merc. c.;* Merc. i. fl.; Merc. i. r.; Mez.; *Nit. ac.;* Sang.; Thuya. See Syphilis (Male Sexual System).

Inflammation, syphilitic, hereditary—*Aur.;* Fluor. ac.; *Hep.;* Kreos.; Merc. i. fl.; *Merc. i. r.;* Merc.; *Nit. ac.; Phyt.;* Sul.; Thuya.

Inflammation, tuberculous—*Arg. n.;* Ars.; *Ars. iod.;* Atrop.; Bapt.; Brom.; *Calc. c.;* Calc. p.; Canth.; Carbo v.; *Caust.;* Chrom. oxy.; Cistus; *Dros.;* Ferr. p.; Hep.; *Iod.;* Ipec.; Jabor.; Kali c.; Kali m.; Kreos.; Lyc.; *Mang. ac.;* Merc. nit.; Naja; *Nat. selen.;* Nit. ac.; *Phos.; Selen.;* Spong.; *Stann.;* Sul.

Irritation—*Arg. m.;* Bar. c.; Caust.; Chlorum; *Hep.;* Kali bich.; Kali iod.; Kali perm.; *Lach.;* Mang. ac.; Nux v.; *Phos.* See Rawness.

Motion, up and down, violent—*Sul. ac.*

Mucus—Ant. t.; *Arg. m.;* Arg. n.; *Brom.; Bry.;* Canth.; Dros.; Hep.; *Kali bich.;* Kali c.; Lach.; *Mang. ac.;* Ox. ac.; Paris; Phos.; Rumex; *Samb.;* Sang.; Selen.; Senega; Stann. See Inflammation.

Pains—Acon.; Alum.; Arg. n.; Arum; *Bell.*; Bry.; *Cepa*; *Hep.*; *Iod.*; Justicia; Kreos.; Lach.; *Mang. ac.*; Med.; Merc. c.; Nit. ac.; *Osm.*; *Phos.*; Sang.; *Spong.* See Inflammation.

Polypus—Berb. v.; Psor.; Sang.; *Sang. n.*; *Teucr.*; Thuya.

Rawness, roughness, soreness, sensitiveness—Acon.; Alum.; Am. caust.; *Arg. m.*; Arn.; *Arum*; *Bar. c.*; *Bell.*; Benzoin; Brom.; Bry.; *Caust.*; Cham.; Cistus; Dros.; Eup. perf.; *Hep.*; Iod.; Kali bich.; *Kali iod.*; Kali perm.; Kaolin; *Lach.*; Lyc.; *Mag. p.*; *Mang. ac.*; Med.; *Merc.*; Nux v.; Osm.; Phos. ac.; *Phos.*; Puls.; Rhus t.; *Rumex*; Sang.; *Spong.*; *Sul.*; Zinc. m.

Spasm (laryngismus stridulus)—*Acon.*; Agar.; Am. caust.; Ars. iod.; Arum; *Bell.*; Brom.; *Calc. c.*; Calc. iod.; Calc. p.; Chel.; *Chlorum*; Chloral; Cic.; Cinch.; *Coral.*; *Cupr. ac.*; *Cupr. m.*; *Formal.*; Gels.; Granat.; Ign.; *Iod.*; *Ipec.*; Kali br.; *Lach.*; Meph.; *Mosch.*; Phos.; Samb.; Spong.; Stram.; *Strych.*; Vespa; Zinc. m.

Suffocative catarrh—Ambra; Ars.; Calc. c.; Coff.; Sang.; Spong.

Tickling—Alum.; *Ambra*; Ant. s. a.; *Bell.*; Calc. c.; Caps.; Carbo v.; Cepa; *Coccus*; Cop.; Dros.; Dulc.; *Iod.*; Kali bich.; *Phos.* See Cough.

Tumors, benign—Caust.; Kali bich.; Sang.; Thuya.

Tumors, malignant—*Ars.*; Ars. iod.; Bell.; Carbo an.; *Clem.*; *Con.*; Hydr.; Iod.; Kreos.; Lach.; Morph.; *Phyt.*; Sang.; Thuya.

Vocal cords, ulceration—Aur. iod.; Iod.; Lyc.; Merc. nit.

Vocal cords, weak—*Carbo v.*; *Caust.*; Coca; Dros.; Graph.; Penthor.; Phos. See Voice.

VOICE—Deep, bass—Brom.; Camph.; Carbo v.; *Caust.*; *Dros.*; Phos.; Pop. c.; Sang. n.; Stann.; Sul.; *Verbasc.*

High, piping—*Bell.*

Hoarse, aphonia—*Acon.*; Alumen; Alum.; Am. c.; *Am. caust.*; *Am. m.*; Ant. c.; Antipyr.; Arg. iod.; *Arg. m.*; *Arg. n.*; Arn.; Ars. iod.; *Arum*; Asclep. t.; Bar. c.; *Bell.*; Benzoin; Brom.; Bry.; *Calc. c.*; Calc. caust.; Camph.; *Carbo v.*; *Caust.*; Cham.; Chlorum; Cina; *Coca*; Cochlear.; Coccus; Cub.; *Dros.*; Dub.; *Dulc.*; *Eup. perf.*; Ferr. p.; Gels.; Graph.; *Hep.*; Hyos.; Ign.; Iod.; *Ipec.*; Justicia; *Kali bich.*; *Kali c.*; Kali chrom.; Kreos.; Mag. p.; *Mang. ac.*; Merc.; *Nit. ac.*; Nux m.; *Nux v.*; Op.; Osm.; *Ox. ac.*; Paris; Penthor.; Petrol.; *Phos.*; Plat.; *Pop. c.*; *Puls.*; Rhus t.; *Rumex*; *Samb.*; Sang.; Sang. n.; *Selen.*; Senega; Sep.; Sil.; *Spong.*; Stann.; Sticta; *Still.*; *Sul.*; Thuya; Ver. v.; *Verbasc.*; Vio'a od.

Hoarseness, capricious—Hep.; Puls.

Hoarseness, chronic—Ampelop.; *Arg. n.*; Bar. c.; Calc. c.; *Carbo v.*; *Caust.*; Graph.; *Mang. ac.*; *Phos.*; Sul.

Hoarseness, croupy—Acon.; Ail.; Brom.; Caust.; Cepa; Hep.; Kali s.; Spong.

Hoarseness, from cold weather—Carbo v.; Caust.; Rumex; Sul.

Hoarseness, from overheating—Ant. c.; Ant. t.; Brom.

Hoarseness, from overusing voice, especially public speakers, professional singers—Alum.; *Arg. m.*; *Arg. n.*; Arn.; *Arum*; Carbo v.; *Caust.*; Coca; Ferr. p.; Ferr. picr.; *Hep.*; Iod.; Mang. ac.; Med.; Merc. cy.;

RESPIRATORY SYSTEM

Merc. s.; Nat. selen.; Phos.; *Rhus t.*; *Selen.*; Spong.; Still.; Sul.; Tab.; Terebene.

Hoarseness, hysterical—Cocc.; Gels.; *Ign.*; Nux m.; Plat.

Hoarseness, painless—Bell.; *Calc. c.*; Carbo v.; Paris.

Hoarseness, paretic—Am. caust.; Bell.; *Caust.*; *Gels.*; Lach.; *Ox. ac.*; Phos.; Rumex; Sil.

Hoarseness, relieved temporarily by coughing or expectoration—Stann.

Hoarseness, worse, at end of cold—Ipec.

Hoarseness, worse, in A. M.—*Arum;* Benz. ac.; Calc. c.; *Caust.;* Eup. perf.; Hep.; *Mang.;* Nit. ac.; *Nux v.;* Sul.

Hoarseness, worse, in P. M.—Carbo v.; Kali bich.; Phos.; *Rumex.*

Hoarseness, worse, in damp weather—Carbo v.

Hoarseness, worse talking, singing, swallowing—Spong.

Hoarseness, worse, walking against wind—Acon.; Arum; *Euphras.*; Hep.; *Nux m.*

Hoarseness, worse when crying—Acon.; *Bell.*; Phos.; Spong.

Menstrual—Gels.

Nervous aphonia with cardiac disorder—Coca; Hydroc. ac.; Nux m.; Ox. ac.

Timbre, varies continually—Ant. c.; Arg. m.; *Arum;* Bell.; Carbo v.; Caust.; Dros.; Lach.; Rumex.

Voice producer, instantaneous—Arum; Caust.; *Coca;* Ferr. p.; *Pop. c.*

Voice, low, monotonous; economical speech—Mang. ac.; Mang. oxy.

Whispering, weak voice—Arg. m.; Camph.; Canth.; Carbo v.; *Caust.*; Dub.; *Phos.*; *Pop. c.*; Primula; Puls.; Ver. a.

LUNGS—Abscess: Acon.; *Ars. iod.*; Bell.; Caps.; Chin. ars.; *Cinch.*; Hep.; Iod.; Kali c.; Merc.; Sil.

Congestion—*Acon.*; Adren.; Ars. iod.; *Bell.*; Bothrops; *Cact.*; Conv.; Ferr. p.; Iod.; Kali n.; Lyc.; Nux v.; Op.; Phos.; Stroph.; Sulphon.; Upas; *Ver. v.* See Inflammation.

Congestion, passive—Carbo v.; *Dig.*; Ferr. m.; Hydroc. ac.; Nux v.; Phos.; Sul.

Dilation of cells (emphysema)—*Am. c.*; *Ant. ars.*; Ant. t.; *Ars.*; *Aur. mur.*; Bell.; Bry.; Calc. c.; *Calc. p.*; Carbo v.; Chin ars.; Cinch.; Dig.; Dros.; Eucal.; Glon.; Grind.; Hep.; Ipec.; Kali c.; *Lob. infl.*; *Lyc.*; Myrtis; Naph.; Nux v.; Phell.; *Phos.*; Puls.; Sep.; Spong.; *Strych.*; Sul. See Asthma.

Distended feeling—Tereb.

Edema—*Am. c.*; Am. iod.; *Ant. t.*; *Apis*; *Ars.*; Cochlear.; *Kali c.*; Kali iod.; Lach.; *Phos.*; Piloc.; Pulmo v.; *Sang.*; Senec.; Stroph.; Tub.

Gangrene—Arn.; *Ars.*; *Caps.*; Carbo an.; *Carbo v.*; *Crot.*; Eucal.; Dulc.; Hep.; Kreos.; *Lach.*; Lyc.; *Sec.*; Sil.

HAEMORRHAGE (hæmoptysis)—*Acal.*; Acet. ac.; *Achillea;* Acon.; *Allium s.*; *Arn.*; *Cact.*; Carbo v.; Chin. ars.; *Cinch.*; Cinnam.; Dig.; Erecht.; Ergot.; *Erig.*; Ferr. ac.; Ferr. m.; *Ferr. p.*; Gelat.; *Geran.*; Ham.; Helix t.; *Hydrast. mur.*; *Ipec.*; Kali c.; Kreos.; *Lamina;* Led.; Mangif.

ind.; Meli.; *Millef.;* Nat. nit.; *Phos.;* Rhus t.; Sang.; Stroph.; *Sul. ac.;* Tereb.; *Trill.; Ver. v.*

Hæmorrhage, bright, red, blood—Acal.; *Acon.;* Aran.; Cact.; Ferr. ac.; *Ferr. p.;* Geran.; Led.; *Millef.;* Nit. ac.; Rhus t.; Trill.

Hæmorrhage, dark, clotted blood—Arn.; Crot.; *Elaps;* Ferr. mur.; *Ham.;* Sul. ac.

Hæmorrhage, during menopause—Lach.

Hæmorrhage, hæmorrhoidal—Mez.; Nux v.

Hæmorrhage, in drunkards—Hyos.; *Led.;* Nux v.; *Op.*

Hæmorrhage, in periodical attacks—Kreos.

Hæmorrhage, in puerperal fevers—Ham.

Hæmorrhage, traumatic—Millef.

Hæmorrhage, tubercular—Acal.; Ferr. p.; Millef.; Nux v.; Trill.

Hæmorrhage, vicarious—Bry.; Ham.; Phos.

Hæmorrhage, with cough—*Acon.;* Acal.; *Ferr. ac.;* Ferr. p.; *Ipec.; Led.;* Phos. See Cough.

Hæmorrhage, without cough, or effort—*Acon.; Ham.;* Millef.; Sul. ac.

Hæmorrhage, with valvular disease—Cact.; Lycop.

Hot feeling—Acon. See Congestion.

Inflammation—BRONCHO-PNEUMONIA—*Acon.;* Am. iod.; Ant. ars.; *Ant. t.;* Ars.; *Ars. iod.;* Bell.; Bry.; *Chel.;* Ferr. p.; Glycerin; Iod.; *Ipec.;* Kali c.; *Koch's lymph; Phos.;* Puls.; *Scilla;* Solania; *Tub.*

Inflammation—CROUPOUS PNEUMONIA—*Acon.;* Agar.; Am. iod.; Ant. ars.; Ant. iod.; Ant. s. a.; *Ant. t.;* Apomorph.; Arn.; Ars.; *Bell.; Brom.; Bry.;* Caffeine; Camph.; Carb. ac.; Carbo v.; *Chel.;* Cinch.; Dig.; *Ferr. p.;* Gels.; Hep.; *Iod.;* Ipec.; Kali bich.; *Kali c.;* Kali iod.; Lach.; *Lyc.; Merc.;* Millef.; Nat. s.; Nit. ac.; Op.; Ox. ac.; *Phos.;* Puromococcin; Pneumotoxin; Pyr.; Ran. b.; Rhus t.; *Sang.;* Scilla; Senega; Strych.; *Sul.;* Tub.; Ver. a.; *Ver. v.*

Stages of pneumonia—Congestive: *Acon.;* Æsc.; Bell.; Bry.; *Ferr. p.; Iod.;* Sang.; *Ver. v.*

Consolidation—Ant. t.; *Bry.; Iod.;* Kali iod.; Kali m.; *Phos.;* Sang.; Sul.

Resolution—*Ant. t.;* Ant. s. a.; Ars.; Ars. iod.; Carbo v.; *Hep.;* Iod.. *Kali iod.;* Kali s.; *Lyc.;* Nat. s.; *Phos.; Sang.;* Sil.; Stann. iod.; *Sul.*

Type—Bilious—Ant. t.; *Chel.;* Lept.; Merc.; Phos.; Pod.

Latent—Chel.; Phos.; *Sul.*

Neglected, lingering, cases—Am. c.; Ant. iod.; Ant. s. a.; *Ant. t.;* Ars. iod.; Bry.; *Carbo v.;* Cinch.; Hep.; Kali iod.; Lach.; *Lyc.;* Phos.; Plumb.; Sul.

Secondary—Ant. ars.; *Ant. t.;* Ferr. p.; Phos.

Senile—Ant. ars.; *Ant. t.;* Dig.; Ferr. p.

Sycotic—Nat. s.

Typhoid—*Hyos.;* Lach.; Laur.; Merc. cy.; Op.; Phos.; *Rhus t.;* Sang.; Sul.

PARALYSIS of lungs—Am. c.; *Ant. ars.; Ant. t.;* Arn.; Bac.; Carbo v.; Cur.; Diphtherotox.; Dulc.; *Grind.;* Hydroc. ac.; Ipec.; Lach.; *Laur.; Lob. purp.;* Lyc.; Merc. cy.; Morph.; Mosch.; Phos.; *Solania.*

Tired feeling—Ail.; Arum.

TUBERCULOSIS (phthisis pulmonalis)—Acal.; Acon.; Agaricin; *Allium s.;* Ant. ars.; *Ant. iod.;* Ars.; *Ars. iod.;* Aur. ars.; Atrop.; Aviare; Bac.; Bals. per.; Bapt.; Bell.; Blatta or.; *Bry.;* Calc. ars.; *Calc. c.;* Calc. chlor.; Calc. hypophos.; *Calc. iod.; Calc. p.;* Calop.; Can. s.; Cetrar.; *Chin. ars.;* Cim.; Coccus; Cod.; *Crot.;* Cupr. ars.; *Dros.;* Dulc.; Eriod.; Ferr. ac.; *Ferr. ars.;* Ferr. iod.; Ferr. m.; *Ferr. p.;* Form. ac.; Formica; *Gall. ac.;* Guaiacol; Guaiac.; Ham.; Hep.; Helix; Hippoz.; Hydr.; Hyosc. hydrobr.; Hysterion; Ichth.; *Iod.;* Iodof.; Ipec.; Kalag.; Kali bich.; *Kali c.;* Kali n.; *Kreos.;* Lach.; *Lachnanth.;* Lact. ac.; Laur.; Lecith.; *Lyc.;* Mang. ac.; Med.; Millef.; *Myos.;* Myrtis; Naph.; *Nat. cacodyl.; Nat. selen.;* Nat. s.; *Nit. ac.;* Nux v.; Ox. ac.; *Phell.;* Phos. ac.; *Phos.;* Piloc.; Pineal gland ext.; *Polygon. av.;* Puls.; Rumex; Ruta; Salvia; *Sang.;* Sep.; *Sil.;* Silph. cyr.; *Spong.; Stann.;* Stann. iod.; Sticta; Succin.; *Sul.;* Teucr. scor.; Thea; Ther.; *Tub.;* Urea; Vanad.; Yerba.

Acute (phthisis florida)—Ant. t.; *Ars.;* Calc. c.; Calc. iod.; Ferr. ac.; Ferr. m.; Ferr. mur.; *Iod.; Phos.;* Piloc. mur.; *Sang.;* Ther.; Tub.

Cough—Allium s.; Ars.; *Ars. iod.;* Aviare; Bapt.; *Bell.;* Calc. c.; Caust.; Cinch.; *Cod.;* Con.; *Coral.;* Crot.; *Dros.;* Ferr. ac.; *Hep.; Hyos.;* Ipec.; *Kali c.;* Lach.; Laur.; Lob. infl.; Myos.; *Nit. ac.; Phos.;* Rumex; Sang.; *Sil.;* Silph. cyr.; Spong.; *Stann.;* Sticta.

Debility—Acal.; Ars.; *Ars. iod.;* Aviare; *Chin. ars.;* Phos.; Sil. See Nervous System.

Diarrhœa—Acet. ac.; Arg. n.; Arn.; *Ars.;* Ars. iod.; Calc. c.; *Cinch.;* Coto; Iod.; Iodof.; *Phos. ac.; Phos.;* Sil. See Abdomen.

Digestive disorders—Ars.; Aviare; Calc. c.; Carbo v.; *Cupr. ars.;* Ferr. ac.; Ferr. ars.; Gall. ac.; *Hydr.;* Kreos.; *Nux v.;* Strych. See Stomach.

Dyspnœa—Carbo v.; Ipec.; Phos.

Emaciation—Allium s.; Ars.; *Ars. iod.;* Calc. p.; Eriod.; *Ica.;* Myos.; Phos.; Sil.; Silph. cyr.; Tub. See Generalities.

Fever—Acon.; Allium s.; Ars.; Ars. iod.; Bapt.; Calc. iod.; *Chin. ars.;* Chin. s.; Cinch.; *Ferr. p.;* Iod.; Lyc.; Nit. ac.; Phos.; Sang.; Sil.; Stann.

Fibroid—Bry.; Calc. c.; Sang.; *Sil.*

Hemoptysis—Acal.; Achillea; Acon.; Calc. ars.; *Ferr. ac.;* Ferr. m.; *Ferr. p.; Ham.; Ipec.;* Millef.; Nit. ac.; *Phos.;* Piloc. mur.; *Trill.* See Hemoptysis.

Incipient—Acal.; Agar.; Ars. iod.; Calc. c.; Calc. iod.; Calc. p.; Dros.; *Ferr. p.;* Iod.; Kali c.; Kali iod.; Lachnanth.; Mang. ac.; Med.; Myrtis; Ol. j. as.; *Phos.;* Polygon.; Puls.; Sang.; Sec.; Succin.; Sul.; Trill.; *Tub.;* Vanad.

Insomnia—Allium s.; *Coff.;* Dig.; Sil. See Nervous System.

Liver disturbance—Chel.

Mechanical injury, after—Millef.; Ruta.

Night sweats—*Acet. ac.; Agaricin;* Ars.; Ars. iod.; Atrop.; *Cinch.;* Eriod.; Gall. ac.; Hep.; *Jabor.;* Kali iod.; Lyc.; Myos.; *Phos. ac.; Phos.;* Piloc.; Piloc. mur.; Salvia; Samb.; Sep.; *Sil.;* Silph. cyr.; Stann.; Yerba. See Fever.

Pains in chest—*Acon.*; *Bry.*; Calc. c.; Cim.; Guaiac.; *Kali c.*; Myrtis Phos.; Pix liq. See Chest.

Sore mouth—Lach.

PLEURÆ—EMPYEMA: Arn.; *Ars.*; Calc. c.; *Calc. s.*; Cinch.; Echin Ferr. m.; *Hep.*; Ipec.; Kali c.; *Merc.*; Nat. s.; Phos.; *Sil.*

Hydrothorax—*Adon. v.*; Ant. t.; *Apis*; Apoc.; *Ars.*; *Ars. iod.*; Canth. Carbo v.; Cinch.; Colch.; *Dig.*; Fluor. ac.; Helleb.; *Iod.*; *Kali c.*, Kali iod.; *Lact. v.*; Lyc.; *Merc. sul.*; Phaseol.; Phos.; Piloc.; *Ran. b.*; Scilla; *Senega*; *Sul.*

PLEURISY—Abrot.; *Acon.*; Ant. ars.; Ant. t.; *Apis*; Arn.; *Ars.*; *Asclep. t.*; Bell.; Bor.; *Bry.*; *Canth.*; Carbo an.; Cinch.; *Dig.*; Eriod.; Ferr. mur.; *Ferr. p.*; Formica; *Guaiac.*; Hep.; *Iod.*; *Kali c.*; Kali iod.; Led. Lob. card.; *Merc.*; Nat. s.; Op.; Phos.; Ran. b.; Rhus t.; Sabad.; *Scilla*; *Senega*; Sep.; Sil.; Spig.; *Sul.*; Tub.

Adhesions—Abrot.; Carbo an.; Hep.; Ran. b.; Sul.

Chronic—Ars. iod.; *Hep.*; *Iod.*; Kali iod.; Scilla; *Sul.*

Diaphragmatic—Acon.; *Bry.*; Cact.; Cupr.; Mosch.; *Ran. b.*

Rheumatic—Acon.; Arn.; *Bry.*; Ran. b.; Rhod.; Rhus t.

Tuberculosis—Ars. iod.; Bry.; Hep.; *Iod.*; Iodof.; Kali c.

With Bright's disease—Ars.; *Merc. c.* See Urinary System.

RESPIRATION—Arrested (apnœa): Ars.; Bov.; Camph.; Hydroc. ac.; Latrod.; Lyssin; Upas.

Arrested, on falling asleep—*Am. c.*; Dig.; *Grind.*; *Lach.*; Lac c.; Merc. pr. rub.; Op.; *Samb.*

Cheyne-Stokes—*Acon. fer.*; Antipyr.; Atrop.; Bell.; Carbo v.; Cocaine; *Grind.*; Kali cy.; *Morph.*; *Op.*; Parth.; *Spart. s.*

DYSPNŒA (difficult, embarrassed, oppressed, anxious): Acet. ac.; *Acon. fer.*; *Acon.*; Adren.; *Am. c.*; Amyl; *Ant. ars.*; Ant. iod.; *Ant. t.*; *Apis*, Apoc.; *Aral.*; *Ars.*; Ars. iod.; Aur.; *Bac.*; Bell.; *Blatta or.*; *Brom.*; Bry.; *Cact.*; Cajup.; *Calc. ars.*; *Calc. c.*; Canth.; Caps.; *Carbo v.*; Caust.; *Cepa*; Cham.; Chel.; *Chlorum*; Cinch.; *Coca*; Collins.; *Conv.*; *Crat.*; *Cupr. ac.*; Cupr. m.; *Cur.*; *Dig.*; Diósc.; Dros.; Ferr. m.; Ferr. p.; Fluor. ac.; *Formal.*; Glon.; *Grind.*; Hep.; Hydroc. ac.; Ign.; Iod.; *Ipec.*; *Justicia*; Kali bich.; *Kali c.*; Kali n.; *Lach.*; Laur.; Lob. infl.; Lyc.; Merc. c.; *Merc. sul.*; Mosch.; *Naph.*; Nat. ars.; *Nat. s.*; *Nux v.*; Op.; *Phos.*; Phyt.; Pothos; *Puls.*; Pulmo v.; *Quebracho*; Ran. b.; Ruta; *Samb.*; Sang.; *Scilla*; Senec.; *Senega*; Serum ang.; *Sil.*; Spig.; *Spong.*; Stann.; *Stroph.*; Strych.; *Sul.*; Tab.; Ver. a.; Ver. v.; *Viola od.*; Zinc. m. See Asthma.

Dyspnœa, aggravated at P. M.—Act. spic.; *Ars.*; Aur.; Cahinca; Calc. c.; Carbo v.; *Dig.*; Phos.; Puls.; *Samb.*; Sep.; *Sul.*; Trifol.

Dyspnœa, aggravated during damp, cloudy weather—Nat. s.

Dyspnœa, aggravated from ascending stairs—Am. c.; Ars.; Bor.; Calc. c.; Chin. ars.; Iod.; Ipec.; Lob. infl.; Nat. m.; Sep.

Dyspnœa, aggravated from exposure to cold air—Act. spic.; Lob. infl.

Dyspnœa, aggravated from foreign bodies—Ant. t.; Sil.

Dyspnœa, aggravated from least thing coming near mouth or nose—Lach.

Dyspnœa, aggravated from lying down—Abies n.; Act. spic.; Aral.; *Ars.*;

Cahinca; Dig.; Grind.; Lach.; Merc. sul.; Puls.; Sep.; Strych. ars.; Sul.

Dyspnœa, aggravated from lying on left side—Naja; Spig.; Tab.; Viscum.
Dyspnœa, aggravated from lying on right side—Viscum.
Dyspnœa, aggravated from lying with head low—Cinch.; Nitrum; Spong.
Dyspnœa, aggravated from myocardial disease—Sarcol. ac.
Dyspnœa, aggravated from nervous causes—Ambra; Arg. n.; Ars.; Asaf.; *Cajup.; Mosch.;* Nux m.; Puls.; *Val.:* Viola od.
Dyspnœa, aggravated from rest—Sil.
Dyspnœa, aggravated from sinking sensation in abdomen—Acet. ac.
Dyspnœa, aggravated from sitting up—Carbo v.; Laur.; Psor.; Sep.
Dyspnœa, aggravated from sleep—Dig.; *Lach.;* Samb.; Sep.; Spong.
Dyspnœa, aggravted from sleep; sitting indoors; relieved by rapid motion—Sep.
Dyspnœa, aggravated from stooping—Calc. c.; Sil.
Dyspnœa, aggravated from walking—*Acon.;* Am. c.; Carbo v.; Con.; *Ipec.;* Kali c.; Nat. m.; Sep.; Sil.
Dyspnœa, aggravated from working—Am. m.; Calc. c.; Lyc.; Nat. m.; Nit. ac.; Sep.; Sil.; Sumb.
Dyspnœa, aggravated in aged, alcoholics, athletics—Coca.
Dyspnœa, aggravated in children—Lyc.; Samb.
Dyspnœa, aggravated in lower chest—Lob. syph.; Nux v.
Dyspnœa, aggravated in morning—Ant. t.; Con.; Kali bich.; Kali c.; Nat. s.
Dyspnœa, aggravated in warm room—Am. c.; Puls.; Sep.
Dyspnœa, relieved from bending forward—Ars.; Kali c.
Dyspnœa, relieved from bending shoulders backwards—Calc. c.
Dyspnœa, relieved from eructating—Ambra; Ant. t.
Dyspnœa, relieved from expectoration—*Ant. t.;* Ars.; Kali bich.; Zinc. m.
Dyspnœa, relieved from fanning rapidly—Carbo v.
Dyspnœa, relieved from fanning slowly and at a distance—Lach.
Dyspnœa, relieved from lying down—Kali bich.; *Psor.*
Dyspnœa, relieved from lying on right side—Ant. t.
Dyspnœa, relieved from lying on right side, head high—Cact.; Spig.; Spong.
Dyspnœa, relieved from motion—Lob. infl.; Sep.
Dyspnœa, relieved from sitting up—Acon. fer.; Ant. t.; *Ars.;* Dig.; Laur.; Merc. sul.; Nat. s.; *Samb.;* Sul.; Tereb.
Dyspnœa, relieved from standing up—Can. s.
Dyspnœa, relieved from stretching arms apart—Psor.
Dyspnœa, relieved in open air—Calc. c.; Lach.; *Sul.*
Gasping—Brom.; Hydroc. ac.; *Ipec.;* Phos.; Samb.
Hoarse, hissing—Acet. ac.
Inspiration difficult—Brom.; Cact.; Chel.; Iod.; Nicot.; Ox. ac. See Dyspnœa.
Inspiration free, expiration impeded—*Chlorum;* Med.; Meph.; *Samb.*
Irregular—Ail.; Ant. t.; Bell.; Crat.; *Dig.;* Helleb.; Hippoz.; *Hydroc. ac.;* Op.; Trill.
Rapid, short, superficial—*Acon. fer.;* Acon.; Am. c.; *Ant. t.;* Apis; Apoc.; Aral.; *Ars.;* Bell.; *Bry.;* Calc. c.; Carbo v.; Cupr. ac.; Cupr.; Cur.; *Ferr. p.;* Hippoz.; Kali bich.; Lach.; Lob. purp.; Lyc.; Mag. p.; Merc.

cy.; Merc. sul.; Nat. s.; *Nux v.;* Ox. ac.; Phos. ac.; *Phos.;* Prun. sp.; Senega; Sil.; *Spong.;* Stann.; Sul. ac.

Rattling—Allium s.; *Ammon.;* Am. c.; Am. caust.; Am. m.; *Ant. ars.; Ant. t.;* Bals. per.; Bar. c.; Bar. m.; *Brom.;* Calc. ac.; Calc. c.; Can. s.; Carbo v.; Cham.; *Chel.;* Chlorum; *Cinch.;* Cupr. m.; Dulc.; Ferr. p.; Grind.; *Hep.; Ipec.;* Kali bich.; Kali c.; Kali m.; Kali n.; *Kali s.;* Lyc.; Meph.; *Nat. s.;* Œnanthe; *Op.;* Phos.; Pix l.; *Puls.;* Scilla; *Senega;* Sil.; *Stann.;* Sul.; Ver. a.

Sawing—Brom.; Iod.; Samb.; *Spong.*

Sighing—Ail.; Apoc.; Cact.; *Calc. p.;* Carb. ac.; Cereus bon.; *Dig.;* Gels.; Granat.; Helleb.; *Ign.; Lach.;* Led.; Naph.; Nat. p.; *Op.;* Phaseol.; Piloc.; Samb.; Sec.; Sulphon.

Slow, deep—Am. c.; Aur.; Benz. din.; Cact.; Can. ind.; Cinch.; Dig.; Gadus; Gels.; *Helleb.; Hydroc. ac.;* Laur.; Lob. purp.; *Op.;* Phaseol.; Piloc.; *Ver. v.*

Stertorous—Acon.; Am. c.; Arn.; Bell.; Bry.; Can. ind.; *Cinch.;* Euphorb. dath.; Helleb.; Hippoz.; *Hydroc. ac.;* Lob. purp.; Naja; Nat. sal.; *Œnanthe; Op.;* Phaseol.; Phos.; Piloc.; Sec.; *Sulphon.;* Tanac.; Trion.; Ver. v.; Viscum.

Suffocative—*Acon. fer.; Ant. t.; Apis; Ars.;* Bell.; Brom.; Cact.; *Calc. c.;* Camph.; *Chlorum; Cinch.;* Coral.; Cupr. m.; *Dig.;* Graph.; Grind.; *Guaiac.;* Hep.; Hydroc. ac.; Iod.; *Ipec.;* Kali bich.; Kali iod.; *Lach.; Latrod.;* Led.; Lil. t.; Lob. infl.; Lyc.; Meli.; Meph.; Merc. cy.; *Merc. pr. rub.;* Morph.; Mosch.; Naja; Puls.; *Samb.; Spong.; Sul.;* Tub.; Trifol.; Ver. a.; Viscum.

Wheezing—Alum.; Am. c.; Ant. iod.; *Ant. t.;* Aral.; *Ars.;* Can. s.; Carbo v.; Card. m.; Eriod.; *Grind.; Hep.;* Iod.; Iodof.; *Ipec.;* Justicia; Kali bich.; *Kali c.;* Lob. infl.; Lycop.; Nux v.; Prun. sp.; Samb.; Senega; *Spong.* See Asthma.

Whistling—Ars.; Ipec.; Samb.

TRACHEA—**Burning:** *Ars.;* Kali bich.; Sang. See Irritation.

Catarrh—Alum.; Ant. t.; Arg. n.; Ars.; *Bry.;* Calc. c.; Can. s.; Carbo v.; *Caust.;* Coccus; Conv.; Cotyled.; Ferr. iod.; Hep.; Iberis; Illic.; *Kali bich.;* Mang.; *Merc.;* Naph.; Nat. m.; Nux v.; Paris; *Rumex;* Sil.; *Stann.;* Sticta; Sul.; Tab.

Constricted feeling—Brom.; Cistus; Guaco; *Mosch.; Nux v.;* Xerophyl.

Dryness—Ars.; Bell.; Carbo v.; *Rumex;* Sang.; Spong. See Irritation.

Irritation, rawness, hypersensitiveness—Acet. ac.; Æsc.; Ambros.; Apis; Arg. m.; Arg. n.; Ars.; *Bell.;* Brom.; *Bry.;* Can. s.; Carbo an.; Carbo v.; *Caust.;* Ferr. p.; *Hyos.;* Kali bich.; Kaolin; *Lach.;* Mentha. Osm.; *Phos.; Rumex;* Sang.; Stann.; Still.; Sul.; Syph.; Xerophyl.

Tickling—Ambros.; Brom.; Calc. c.; Caps.; *Carbo v.;* Cop.; Ipec.; *Lach.;* Nux v.; *Phos.; Rumex.* See Cough.

SKIN

ACNE ROSACEA—Agar.; Ars.; *Ars. br.*; Ars. iod.; Bell.; *Carbo an.*; Caust.; Chrysar.; Eug. j.; *Hydrocot.*; Kali br.; Kali iod.; Kreos.; Nux v.; Oophor.; Petrol.; Psor.; Radium; Rhus r.; Rhus t.; Sep.; Sul.; *Sul. iod.*; Sulphurous ac.

ACNE SIMPLEX—*Ant. c.*; Ant. s. a.; *Ant. t.*; Ars.; *Ars. br.*; Ars. iod.; Ars. sul. rub.; Asimina; *Aster.*; *Bell.*; Bellis; Berb. aq.; *Bov.*; Calc. picr.; Calc. sil.; *Calc. s.*; Carb. ac.; *Carbo an.*; *Carbo v.*; Cic.; Cim.; Cob.; Ecl.in.; *Eug. j.*; Granat.; Graph.; *Hep.*; Hydrocot.; Jugl. c.; *Jugl. r.*; *Kali br.*; Kali bich.; *Kali iod.*; Kali m.; Lappa; *Led.*; *Lyc.*; Nabul. s.; Nat. br.; Nat. m.; Nit. ac.; *Nux v.*; Oleand.; Phos. ac.; Psor.; Puls.; Radium; Selen.; Sep.; Sil.; Staph.; *Sul.*; *Sul. iod.*; Sumb.; Thuya.

From abuse of KI—Aur.

From abuse of mercury—Kali iod.; Mez.; Nit. ac.

From cheese—Nux v.

From cosmetics—Bov.

From syphilis—Aur.; *Kali iod.*; Merc. s.; Nit. ac. See Male Sexual System.

In anaemic girls at puberty, with vertex headache, flatulent dyspepsia, better by eating—Calc. p.

In drunkards—Ant. c.; Bar. c.; *Led.*; *Nux v.*; Rhus t.

In fleshy young people, with coarse habits; bluish red, pustules on face, chest, shoulders—Kali br.

In scrofulous—Bar. c.; Brom.; *Calc. c.*; Calc. p.; Con.; Iod.; Merc. s.; Mez.; Sil.; *Sul.*

In tubercular children—Tub.

With cachexia—Ars.; Carbo v.; Nat. m.; Sil.

With gastric derangements—*Ant. c.*; *Carbo v.*; Cim.; Lyc.; *Nux v.*; Puls.; Robin.

With glandular swellings—Brom.; Calc. s.; Merc. s.

With indurated papules—Agar.; Arn.; Ars. iod.; Berb. v.; Bov.; Brom.; *Carbo an.*; Cob.; Con.; *Eug. j.*; Iod.; *Kali br.*; *Kali iod.*; Nat. br.; Nit. ac.; Robin.; *Sul.*; Thuya.

With menstrual irregularities—Aur. m. n.; Bell.; Bellis; *Berb. aq.*; Berb. v.; Calc. c.; *Cim.*; Con.; Eug. j.; *Graph.*; Kali br.; Kali c.; Kreos.; Nat. m.; Psor.; *Puls.*; *Sang.*; Sars.; Thuya; Ver. a.

With pregnancy—Bell.; Sab.; Sars.; Sep.

With rheumatism—Led.; Rhus t.

With sexual excesses—*Aur.*; Calc. c.; Kali br.; *Phos. ac.*; Rhus t.; Sep.; Thuya.

With scars unsightly—Carbo an.; Kali br.

With symmetrical distribution—Arn.

ACTINOMYCOSIS—Hekla; Hippoz.; Kali iod.; Nit. ac.

ALOPECIA—Alum.; Anthrok.; *Ars.*; Calc. s.; *Fluor. ac.*; Mancin.; *Nat. m.*; *Phos. ac.*; Phos.; Piloc.; *Pix l.*; Selen.; *Sep.*; Tub.; Vinca. See Scalp (Head).

SKIN

ANIDROSIS (deficient sweat, dry skin)—Acet. ac.; Acon.; *Æth.;* Alum.; Apoc.; Arg. n.; Ars.; *Bell.;* Berb. aq.; Crot. t.; *Graph.;* Iod.; *Kali ars.; Kali c.;* Kali iod.; Lach.; Mag. c.; *Malandr.;* Nat. c.; *Nux m.;* Op.; *Petrol.;* Phos.; Plumb. m.; *Psor.;* Sanic.; Sars.; Sec.; *Sul.;* Thyr.

ARTHRAX—Carbuncle; Malignant pustule: Acon.; *Anthrac.; Apis;* Arct. l.; Arn.; *Ars.;* Bell.; Bothrops; Bry.; Bufo; Calc. chlor.; *Carb. ac.;* Carbo v.; *Cinch.;* Crot.; Cupr. ars.; *Echin.;* Euphorb.; Hep.; Hippoz.; Lach.; Led.; Mur. ac.; Nit. ac.; Phyt.; Pyr.; Rhus t.; *Scolop.;* Sec.; *Sil.;* Sul.; Sul. ac.; *Tar. c.*

ATROPHY—of skin:—Ars.; Cocc.; Graph.; Sabad.; Sul.

BLISTERS, small—Apis; *Canth.;* Nat. m.; *Rhus t.;* Sec.

BLOOD BOILS—*Anthrac.;* Arn.; Ars.; Crot.; *Lach.;* Phos. ac.; Pyr.; Sec.

BLUENESS—Lividity: Agar.; *Ail.; Ant. t.;* Arn.; *Ars.;* Cadm. s.; Camph.; *Carbo an.; Carbo v.;* Cinch.; Crat.; Crot.; *Cupr.; Dig.;* Helleb.; Ipec.; Kali iod.; *Lach.; Laur.; Morph.;* Mur. ac.; *Sec.;* Sul. ac.; *Tar. c.; Ver. a.;* Vipera. See Face.

BROMIDROSIS (offensive sweat)—Art. v.; *Bapt.;* Bry.; Carbo an.; Cinch.; Con.; Graph.; *Hep.; Lyc.; Merc. s.; Nit. ac.;* Osm.; *Petrol.;* Phos.; *Psor.;* Pulex; Sep.; *Sil.;* Stann.; *Staph.;* Sul.; *Tellur.;* Thuya; Variol. **Bromidrosis, sour odor of body**—*Calc. c.;* Cham.; Colost.; Graph.; *Hep.;* Kreos.; Lac d.; *Mag. c.; Rheum; Sul. ac.;* Sul.

BURNING—Acet. ac.; *Acon.; Agar.;* Anac.; *Apis;* Ars.; Bapt.; *Bell.;* Bry.; *Canth.;* Caps.; Caust.; Dulc.; Euphorb.; *Formica;* Grind.; Kali c.; Kreos.; Medusa; *Nux v.;* Phos.; Radium; *Ran. b.; Rhus t.;* Sang.; Sec.; Sul.; Vespa. See Pruritus.

CALLOSITIES (corns)—*Ant. c.;* Elaeis; *Ferr. picr.; Graph.;* Hydr.; Lyc.; *Nit. ac.;* Petrol.; *Ran. b.;* Rhus t.; Sal. ac.; Sars.; Sep.; Sil.: *Thuya.* See Feet (Locomotor System).

CHILBLAINS. *Abrot.; Agar.;* Apis; Ars.; Bor.; Calc. c.; Calend.; *Canth.;* Carbo an.; Crot. t.; Cycl.; Ferr. p.; Fragar.; Ham.; *Hep.;* Lach.; Led.; Merc.; *Mur. ac.; Nit. ac.; Petrol.:* Plant.; *Puls.; Rhus t.;* Sil.; Sul. ac.; *Sul.; Tamus; Tereb.;* Thyr.; Ver. v.; Zinc. m.

CHLOASMA—Liver spots, moth patches: *Arg. n.;* Aur.; Cadm. s.; Card. m.; Caul.; Cob.; Cur.; Guar.; Laur.; *Lyc.; Nat. hyposul.;* Paul.; Petrol.; Plumb. m.; *Sep.;* Sul.; Thuya. See Spots, copper-colored.

CICATRICES—Affections:—*Caust.; Fluor. ac.; Graph.; Iod.;* Nit. ac.; Phyt.; Sil.; Sul. ac.; *Thiosin.*

COLDNESS—Abies c.; *Acet. ac.;* Acon.; Agar.; *Ail.;* Ant. chlor.; Ant. c.; *Ant. t.;* Ars.; Bothrops; Calc. c.; *Camph.; Carbo v.;* Chel.; Chin. ars.; Cinch.; Crat.; *Crot.;* Dig.; Ipec.; *Jatropha;* Lach.; *Latrod.; Laur.;* Med.; Pyr.; Rhus t.; *Sec.; Tab.; Ver. a.* (See Collapse Nervous System.) Coldness (Fever).

COMEDO—*Abrot.;* Bar. c.; Bell.; Calc. sil.; Cic.; *Dig.;* Eug. j.; Mez.; *Nit. ac.;* Sab.; *Selen.;* Sep.; *Sul.;* Sumb.

DECUBITUS (bed sores)—Arg. n.; *Arn.;* Bapt.; Carb. ac.; Carbo v.; Cinch.;

Echin.; *Fluor. ac.*; Hippoz.; *Lach.*; *Mur. ac.*; Nux m.; Pæonia; Petrol.; Pyr.; Sil.; *Sul. ac.*; Vipera. See Ulcer.

DERMAL (trophic lesions)—Thallium.

DERMATALGIA (pain, sensitiveness, soreness)—Agar.; Apis; Ars.; *Bad.*; Bell.; Bellis; Bov.; Chin. s.; *Cinch.*; Con.; Crot. t.; *Dolich.*; Euphorb.; Fagop.; *Hep.*; *Kali c.*; *Lach.*; Lyc.; Nux m.; *Oleand.*; Osm.; Pæonia; Petrol.; Phos.; *Psor.*; Ran. s.; Rhus d.; *Rhus t.*; Rumex; Semperv. t.; Sep.; *Sil.*; *Sul.*; Tar. c.; *Ther.*; *Vinca*; Xerophyl.

DRYNESS—*Acon.*; *Alum.*; *Ars.*; *Bell.*; Calc. c.; *Graph.*; Hydrocot.; Iod.; Lyc.; Nat. c.; Nit. ac.; *Nux m.*; Piloc.; *Plumb.*; *Psor.*; Sabad.; Sars.; Sec.

ECCHYMOSES—Æth.; *Arn.*; Ars.; Bellis; Bothrops; Carbo v.; Chloral; *Crot.*; *Ham.*; Kreos.; *Led.*; *Phos.*; Rhus t.; Sec.; *Sul. ac.*; Supraren. ex.; Tereb.

ECHTHYMA—Ant. c.; *Ant. t.*; *Ars.*; Bell.; *Cic.*; Cistus; Crot. t.; Hydr.; Jugl. c.; *Jugl. r.*; Kali bich.; Kreos.; *Lach.*; *Merc. s.*; Nit. ac.; Petrol.; Rhus t.; *Sec.*; Sil.; Sul.; Thuya.

ECZEMA—*Æthiops*; Alnus; Alum.; *Anac.*; Anthrok.; *Ant. c.*; Arbut.; Ars.; Ars. iod.; Berb. aq.; *Berb. v.*; Bor.; *Bov.*; *Calc. c.*; *Canth.*; Caps.; *Carb. ac.*; Carbo v.; Castor eq.; Caust.; Chrysar.; *Cic.*; *Clem.*; Commocl.; Con.; *Crot. t.*; Dulc.; Euphorb.; Fluor. ac.; Frax. am.; Fuligo; *Graph.*; *Hep.*; Hippoz.; Hydrocot.; Jugl. c.; *Kali ars.*; Kali m.; Kreos.; Lyc.; *Mang. ac.*; Merc. c.; Merc. d.; Merc. pr. rub.; *Merc. s.*; *Mez.*; Mur. ac.; Nat. ars.; Nat. m.; Nux v.; *Oleand.*; Persicaria; *Petrol.*; Piloc.; *Plumb.*; Pod.; Prim. v.; *Psor.*; *Rhus t.*; *Rhus v.*; Sars.; Sep.; Skook. ch.; *Sul.*; *Sul. iod.*; Thuya; Tub.; Ustil.; *Vinca*; *Viola tr.*; Xerophyl.; X-ray.

Acute form—Acon.; Anac.; Bell.; Canth.; *Chin. s.*; *Crot. t.*; Mez.; *Rhus t.*; Sep.

Eczema, behind ears—Ars.; Arundo; Bov.; Chrysarob.; *Graph.*; *Hep.*; Jugl. r.; Kali m.; Lyc.; *Mez.*; *Oleand.*; *Petrol.*; Psor.; Rhus t.; Sanic.; Scrophul.; Sep.; Staph.; Tub. See Ears.

Eczema, of face—Anac.; Ant. c.; Bac.; Calc. c.; *Carb. ac.*; Cic.; Col.; Cornus c.; *Crot. t.*; Hyper.; Kali ars.; Led.; Merc. pr. rub.; Psor.; Rhus t.; Sep.; Staph.; *Sul.*; *Sul. iod.*; *Vinca.* See Face.

Eczema, of flexures of joints—*Æth.*; Am. c.; Caust.; *Graph.*; Hep.; Kali ars.; Lyc.; *Mang. ac.*; *Nat. m.*; Psor.; *Sep.*; Sul.

Eczema, of hands—Anag.; Bar. c.; *Berb. v.*; *Bov.*; Calc. c.; *Graph.*; *Hep.*; Hyper.; Jugl. c.; Kreos.; Malandr.; *Petrol.*; Plumb.; Rhus v.; Sanic.; Selen.; Sep.; Still. See Hands (Locomotor System).

Eczema, of neurasthenic persons—*Anac.*; Ars.; Phos.; *Strych. ars.*; Strych. p.; Viola tr.; Zinc. p.

Eczema, of pudendum—Am. c.; Ant. c.; Ars.; Canth.; *Crot. t.*; Hep.; Plumb. m.; Rhus t.; Sanic.; Sep. See Female Sexual System.

Eczema, of rheumatico-gouty persons—Alum.; Arbut.; Lact. ac.; *Rhus t.*; Uric. ac.; Urea.

Eczema, of scalp—Astac.; Berb. aq.; *Calc. c.*; Cic.; Clem.; Fluor. ac.;

SKIN 907

Hep.; Kali m.; Lyc.; Mez.; Nat. m.; *Oleand.;* Petrol.; Psor.; Sep.; *Selen.;* Staph.; Sul.; Tub.; *Vinca;* Viola od. See Head.
Eczema, of strumous persons—*Æthiops; Ars. iod.;* Calc. c.; *Calc. iod.;* Calc. p.; Caust.; Cistus; Crot. t.; *Hep.;* Merc. c.; Merc. s.; Rumex; Sep.; Sil.; Tub.
Eczema, of whole body—Crot. t.; Rhus t.
Eczema, madidans—Cic.; Con.; Dulc.; Graph.; Hep.; Kali m.; Merc. c.; Merc. pr. rub.; Mez.; Sep.; Staph.; Tub.; Viola tr.
Eczema, with pigmentation in circumscribed areas following—Berb. v.
Eczema, with urinary, gastric, hepatic disorders—Lyc.
Eczema, worse after vaccination—Mez.
Eczema, worse at menstrual period, menopause—Mang. ac.
Eczema, worse at seashore, ocean voyage, excess of salt—Nat. m.
ELEPHANTIASIS—Anac. or.; *Ars.;* Calop.; Card. m.; *Elaeis;* Graph.; Ham.; *Hydrocot.;* Iod.; Lyc.; *Myrist. s.;* Sil.
EPHELIS (sunburn)—Bufo; Canth.; Kali c.; Robin.; Ver. a.
EPITHELIOMA—Acet. ac.; Alumen; *Ars* ; Ars. iod.; Cic.; *Condur.;* Con.; Euphorb.; Fuligo; *Hoang. n.;* Hydr.; Jequir.; Kali ars.; Kali s.; Lapis alb.; Lob. erin.; Lyc.; Nat. cacodyl.; Radium; Scrophul.; *Sep.;* Sil.; *Thuya.* See Face.
ERUPTIONS—Copper-colored: Ars.; Calc. iod.; *Carbo an.;* Kreos.; Nit. ac.
Eruptions, dry, scaly—Alumen; *Anag.;* Ant. c.; *Ars.;* Ars. iod.; *Berb. aq.;* Bov.; Cadm. s.; Canth.; Corydal.; Euphorb. d.; Graph.; *Hydrocot.; Iod.; Kali ars.;* Kali m.; Kali s.; Lith. c.; Lyc.; *Malandr.;* Merc. s.; Nat. m.; Nit. ac.; *Petrol.;* Phos.; Phyt.; Pip. m.; Pix l.; *Psor.; Sars.;* Selen.; Sep.; *Sul.;* Tub.; Xerophyl.
Eruptions, humid, moist—*Æthiops;* Ant. c.; Ant. t.; Bar. c.; Bov.; Caust.; Chrysarob.; *Clem.;* Crot. t.; *Dulc.;* Graph.; *Hep.;* Lyc.; Mancin.; Merc. s.; *Mez.;* Nat. m.; *Oleand.;* Petrol.; *Psor.; Rhus t.;* Sep.; Staph.; Stront.; Variol.; Viola tr.
Eruptions, pustular—Alnus; Ant. c.; *Ant. t.;* Bell.; *Berb. v.;* Bufo; Chel.; Cic.; *Crot. t.;* Echin.; Euphorb.; *Hep.;* Hippoz.; Iris; Jugl. r.; *Kali bich.;* Kali iod.; Kreos.; Lach.; Merc. c.; *Merc. s.;* Nit. ac.; Phyt.; *Psor.;* Ran. b.; Rhus v.; Sep.; *Sil.;* Sul.; Sul. iod.; Taxus; Variol.
Eruptions, scabby—Ant. c.; Ars.; Calc. c.; Chrysarob.; *Cic.;* Dulc.; Graph.; *Hep.; Lyc.;* Merc.; *Mez.;* Mur. ac.; Nat. m.; Petrol.; Staph.; *Sul.;* Viola tr.; Vinca.
Eruptions, better in winter—Kali bich.; Sars.
Eruptions, worse in spring—Nat. s.; Psor.; Sang.; *Sars.*
Eruptions, worse in winter—Aloe; *Alum.;* Ars.; *Petrol.; Psor.;* Sabad.
ERYSIPELAS—*Acon.;* Anac. oc.; Ananth.; *Apis; Arn.;* Ars.; Atrop.; Aur.; *Bell.;* Camph.; *Canth.;* Carb. ac.; Carbo v.; *Cinch.;* Commocl.; Cop.; Crot.; *Crot. t.; Echin.; Euphorb.; Graph.;* Hep.; Jugl. r.; *Lach.;* Led.; Nat. m.; Nat. s.; Prim. ob.; Ran. c.; *Rhus t.; Rhus v.;* Samb.; Sul.; Taxus; Ver. v.; *Xerophyl.*
Afebrile—*Graph.;* Hep.; Lyc.
Biliary, catarrhal duodenal symptoms—Hydr.
Constitutional tendency—Calend.; *Graph.;* Lach.; Psor.; Sul.

SKIN

Edema, persisting—*Apis;* Ars.; Aur.; Graph.; Hep.; Lyc.; Sul.

Facial—Apis; Arn.; *Bell.;* Bor.; Canth.; Carbo an.; *Euphorb.; Graph.;* Hep.; *Rhus t.;* Solan. n.; Sul.

Leg, below knee—Sul.

Mammæ—Carbo v.; Sul.

Neonatorum—Bell.; Camph.

Phlegmonous—Acon.; Anthrac.; Arn.; *Ars.;* Bell.; Bothrops; Crot.; Ferr. p.; Graph.; *Hep.;* Hippoz.; *Lach.;* Merc.; *Rhus t.;* Sil.; *Tar. c.;* Ver. v.

Recurrent and chronic—Ferr. p.; *Graph.;* Nat. m.; *Rhus t.; Sul.*

Repercussion—Cupr. ac.

Senile—*Am. c.;* Carbo an.

Swelling marked, burning, itching, stinging—Rhus t.

Traumatic—Calend.; Psor.

Traumatic: umbilical, of new born—Apis.

Vesicular—Anac. oc.; Arn.; *Canth.;* Carb. ac.; Caust.; Crot. t.; *Euphorb.;* Mez.; *Rhus t.; Rhus v.;* Tereb.; Urt.; Verb.; Ver. v.

Wandering—Apis; *Ars.;* Cinch.; *Graph.;* Hep.; Hydr.; Puls.; Sul.

ERYTHEMA—Intertrigo (chafing): *Æth.;* Agn.; Ars.; Bell.; Bor.; Calc. c.; *Caust.; Cham.;* Fagop.; *Graph.;* Jugl. r.; Kali br.; *Lyc.; Merc. s.,* Mez.; Oleand.; Ox. ac.; *Petrol.;* Psor.; Sul. ac.; *Sul.;* Tub.

Erythema multiforme—Antipyr.; Bor. ac.; Cop.; Vespa.

Erythema nodosum—Acon.; Ant. c.; *Apis;* Arn.; Ars.; Chin. ars.; *Chin. s.;* Cinch.; Ferr.; Led.; Nat. c.; Ptel.; *Rhus t.; Rhus v.*

Erythema simplex—*Acon.; Antipyr.;* Apis; *Arn.;* Ars. iod.; *Bell.;* Bufo; *Canth.;* Chloral.; Echin.; *Euphorb. d.;* Gaulth.; Grind.; Kali c.; Lact. ac.; *Merc.; Mez.;* Narcissus; Nux v.; Plumb. chrom.; *Rhus t.;* Robin.; Tereb.; Urt.; Ustil.; Ver. v.; Xerophyl.

Fibroma—Calc. ars.; *Con.; Iod.;* Kali br.; Lyc.; Sec.; Thuya.

FISSURES—Rhagades, chaps: *Alum.;* Anthrok.; Ars. s. fl.; Bad.; Bar. c.; Cact. fl.; *Cistus; Condur.;* Eug. j.; *Graph.; Hep.;* Kali ars.; Led.; *Lyc.; Malandr.;* Mang. ac.; Merc. i. r.; Merc. pr. rub.; *Nat. m.;* Nit. ac.; Oleand.; *Petrol.;* Pix l.; Ran. b.; Ratanh.; Rhus t.; *Sars.; Sil.;* Sul.; Xerophyl.; X-ray.

FLABBINESS—Non-tonicity: *Abrot.;* Aster.; Bar. c.; Ars.; Calc. c.; Chel.; *Hep.;* Ipec.; *Merc. v.;* Morph.: Op.; Nat. m.; Sanic.; Sars.; Salvia; Thyr.; Ver. a.

FOREIGN BODIES—To promote expulsion of fish bones, splinters, needles: Anag.; Hep.; Sil.

FORMICATION—Tingling, numbness: *Acon.;* Ambra; Apium gr.; Arundo; Calend.; *Cocaine;* Cod.; Medusa; *Mez.; Morph.;* Oleand.; Phos. ac.; Plat.; Rumex; Sec.; *Selen.;* Sil.; Staph.; *Sul. ac.;* Val.; Zinc. m.

FUNGUS HEMATODES—*Ars.;* Lach.; Lyc.; Mancin.; *Phos.; Thuya.*

FURUNCLE (boil)—Abrot.; Æth.; Ananth.; Anthrac.; Ant. c.; *Arn.;* Ars.; *Bell.; Bellis;* Calc. hypophos.; *Calc. picr.;* Calc. s.; Carbo v.; Echin.; Ferr. iod.; Gels.; *Hep.;* Hippoz.; *Ichth.;* Lach.; Lyc.; *Med.; Merc. s.;*

SKIN

Ol. myr.; Operc.; *Phos. ac.*; *Phyt.*; Picr. ac.; Rhus r.; Sec.; *Sil.*; *Sul.*; Sul. iod.; Sul. ac.; *Tar. c.*; Tub.; Zinc. ox.

Furuncle, recurrent tendency—*Arn.*; Ars.; Berb. v.; Calc. c.; *Calc. mur.*; Calc. p.; *Calc. picr.*; Echin.; Hep.; *Sul.*; Tub.

GANGRENE—Ail.; Anthrac.; Ant. c.; Apis; *Ars.*; Bothrops; Brass.; Brom.; Calend.; Canth.; Carb. ac.; Carbo an.; *Carbo v.*; Chlorum; Chrom. oxy.; Cinch.; Crot.; Cupr. ars.; *Echin.*; *Euphorb.*; Ferr. p.; Kali chlor.; Kali p.; Kreos.; *Lach.*; *Polygon. pers.*; Ran. ac.; Sal. ac.; *Sec.*; *Sul. ac.*; Tar. c.

Gangrene, senile—Am. c.; Ars.; Cepa; Sec.; Sul. ac.

Gangrene, traumatic—Arn.; Lach.; Sul. ac.

HERPES (tetter)—Acon.; Æthiops; Alnus; Anac.; Ananth.; Anthrok.; Apis; Arn.; *Ars.*; Bar. c.; Bor.; Bry.; Bufo; Calc. c.; *Canth.*; *Carb. ac.*; Caust.; Chrysarob.; Cistus; Clem.; Commocl.; *Crot. t.*; *Dulc.*; Eucal.; *Graph.*; *Kali bich.*; Lith. c.; *Merc. s.*; Mez.; Nat. c.; *Nat. m.*; *Nit. ac.*; Petrol.; Phos. ac.; Psor.; Ran. b.; Ran. sc.; *Rhus t.*; *Sars.*; *Sep.*; Sil.; *Sul.*; Tellur.; Variol.; Xerophyl.

Herpes, between fingers—Nit. ac.

Herpes, chronic—Alnus.

Herpes, Circinatus, tonsurans—Ars. s. fl.; Bar. c.; Calc. ac.; Calc. c.; Chrysar.; Equis. arv.; Hep.; Nat. c.; Nat. m.; Sep.; *Tellur.*; Tub. See Trichophytosis.

Herpes, Circinatus, in isolated spots—Sep.

Herpes, Circinatus, in intersecting rings—Tellur.

Herpes, dry—Bov.; Fluor. ac.; Mang.; Sep.; Sil.

Herpes, of chest, nape of neck—Nat. m.; Petrol.

Herpes, of chin—Ars.; Caust.; Graph.; Mez.; Sil.

Herpes, of face—Apis; *Ars.*; Calc. fl.; Caps.; Caust.; Clem.; Con.; Lach.; Limulus; *Nat. m.*; Ran. b.; *Rhus t.*; Sep.; Sul. See Face.

Herpes, of flexures of knees—Graph.; Hep.; *Nat. m.*; Sep.; Xerophyl.

Herpes, of genitals—Aur. mur.; Calc. c.; *Caust.*; Crot. t.; Dulc.; Hep.; Jugl. r.; *Merc. s.*; *Nit. ac.*; Petrol.; Phos. ac.; *Sars.*; Tereb. See Male Sexual System.

Herpes, of hands—Cistus; Dulc.; *Limul.*; Lith. c.; Nit. ac.

Herpes, of knees—Carbo v.; Petrol.

Herpes, of thigh—Graph.; Petrol.

Herpes, neuralgia after—Kal.; *Mez.*; Ran. b.; Still.; Variol.

Herpes, with glandular swelling—Dulc.

Herpes, with pimples or pustules surrounding; spread by coalescing—Hep.

HERPES ZOSTER—Zona; shingles—Apis; Arg. n.; *Ars.*; Aster.; *Canth.*; Carbon. ox.; *Caust.*; Ced.; *Cistus*; Commocl.; Crot. t.; *Dolich.*; Dulc.; Graph.; Grind.; Hyper.; Iris; Kali ars.; Kali m.; Kal.; Merc. s.; *Mez.*; Morph.; Pip. m.; *Prun. sp.*; *Ran. b.*; Ran. sc.; *Rhus t.*; Sal. ac.; Semperv. t.; Staph.; Strych. ars.; Sul.; Thuya; Variol.; Zinc. p.; Zinc. v

Chronic—Ars.; Semperv. t.

Neuralgia, persisting—Ars.; Dolich.; *Kal.*; *Mez.*; Ran. b.; Still.; Zinc. m.

HYDROA—Kali iod.; Kreos.; Mag. c.; *Nat. m.*; Rhus v. See Herpes.

HYPERIDROSIS (excessive sweating)—*Acet. ac.*; Æth.; *Agaricin*; Am. c.; Ant. t.; Ars. iod.; *Bapt.*; Bell.; Bolet.; *Calc. c.*, Cham.; *Cinch.*; Eser.; Ferr.; Graph.; *Jabor.*; Lact. ac.; *Merc. s.*; Nat. c.; Nit. ac.; Nux v.; Op.; *Phos. ac.*; Phos.; Piloc.; *Samb.*; Sanic.; Selen.; *Sep.*; *Sil.*; Sul. ac.; Sul.; Thuya; Ver. a. See Fever.

ICHTHYOSIS (fish skin disease)—*Ars.*; *Ars. iod.*; Aur.; Clem.; Graph.; *Hydrocot.*; Iod.; Kali iod.; Merc. s.; Nat. c.; Œnanthe; Phos.; Platanus; Plumb. m.; *Syph.*; Sul.; Thuya; *Thyr.*

IMPETIGO—Alnus; Ant. c.; Ant. s. a.; *Ant. t.*; *Ars.*; Arum.; Calc. mur.; Cic.; Clem.; *Dulc.*; Euphorb.; Graph.; Hep.; Iris; Jugl. c.; *Kali bich.*; Kali n.; Lyc.; *Mez.*; *Rhus t.*; Rhus v.; Sep.; Sil.; Sul.; Thuya; Viola tr.

KELOID—*Fluor. ac.*; *Graph.*; Nit. ac.; Sab.; Sil.

LENTIGO (freckles)—Am. c.; Bad.; Calc. c.; Graph.; *Kali c.*; *Lyc.*; Mur. ac.; Nat. c.; *Nit. ac.*; Petrol.; Phos.; *Sep.*; *Sul.*; Tab.

LEPRA, leprosy—Anac.; *Ars.*; *Bad.*; Calopt.; Carb. ac.; *Chaulmugra*; Conmod.; Cupr. ac.; Cur.; *Dipterocarpus*; Elaeis; Graph.; Guano; *Gynocardia*; *Hoang n.*; Hura; *Hydrocot.*; Jatropha goss.; Lach.; Merc. s.; Œnanthe; Phos.; *Pip. m.*; Sec.; Sep.; Sil.; Thyr.

LEUCODERMA—*Ars. s. fl.*; Nat. m.; Nit. ac.; Sumb.; Zinc. p. See Face, pale.

LICHEN PLANUS—Agar.; Anac.; *Ant. c.*; Apis; *Ars.*; *Ars. iod.*; Chin. ars.; Iod.; *Jugl. c.*; *Kali bich.*; Kali iod.; Led.; Merc.; Sars.; Staph.; *Sul. iod.*

LICHEN SIMPLEX—Alum.; Am. m.; *Ananth.*; *Ant. c.*; Apis; *Ars.*; *Bell.*; Bov.; Bry.; *Calad.*; Castan.; Dulc.; *Jugl. c.*; Kali ars.; *Kreos.*; Led.; *Lyc.*; Merc. s.; Nabul. s.; Nat. c.; *Plant.*; *Phyt.*; *Rumex*; Sep.; *Sul.*; Sul. iod.; Tilia. See Acne.

LUPUS ERYTHEMATOSUM—Apis; Cistus; Guarana; *Hydrocot.*; *Iod.*; *Kali bich.*; *Phos.*; Sep.; *Thyr.*

LUPUS VULGARIS—Apis; *Ars.*; *Ars. iod.*; *Aur. ars.*; Aur. iod.; *Aur. mur.*; Calc. c.; Calc. iod.; Calc. s.; *Cistus*; Condur.; Ferr. picr.; Form. ac.; Formica; Graph.; Guarana; *Hep.*; *Hydr.*; *Hydrocot.*; Irid.; Jequir.; *Kali bich.*; Kali iod.; Lyc.; Nit. ac.; Phyt.; Staph.; *Sul.*; Thiosin.; Thuya; *Tub.*; Urea; X-ray.

MILIARIA (prickly heat)—*Acon.*; Am. m.; Ars.; *Bry.*; Cact.; Centaurea; Hura; *Jabor.*; Led.; Raph.; Syzigium· Urt.

MILIUM—*Calc. iod.*; Staph.; Tab. See Acne.

MOLLUSCUM—*Brom.*; Bry.; *Calc. ars.*; Calc. c.; Kali iod.; Lyc.; Merc· s. Nat. m.; *Sil.*; Sul.; Teucr.

MORBUS SUDATORIUS—Acon.; Ars.; Carbo v.; Jabor.; Merc.

MORPHÆA—Ars.; *Phos.*; Sil. See Scleroderma.

NÆVUS—Acet. ac.; Calc. c.; *Carbo v.*; Condur.; *Fluor. ac.*; Lyc.; Phos.; Radium; *Thuya*.

SKIN

NAILS—Affections in general: Alum.; *Ant. c.;* Castor eq.; *Graph.;* Hyper.; Nit. ac.; *Sil.;* Upas; X-ray.

Affections of pulp, nails recede, leave raw surface—Sec.

Atrophy—Sil.

Biting of—Am. br.; Arum.

Blueness—Dig.; Ox. ac. See Cyanosis (Circulatory System).

Deformed—brittle, thickened (onchogryposis)—Alum.; Ananth.; *Ant. c.; Ars.;* Caust.; Diosc.; Fluor. ac.; *Graph.;* Merc.; Nat. m ; Sabad.; Sec.; Senec.; Sep.; *Sil.;* Thuya; X-ray.

Eruptions—Around nails: Graph.; Psor.; Stann. mur.

Falling off—Brass.; But. ac.; Helleb. fort.; Helleb.

Hangnails—*Nat. m.;* Sul.; Upas.

Hypertrophy (onychauxis)—Graph.

Inflammation—Around root (paronychia): Alum.; Bufo; Calc. s.; *Diosc.;* Graph.; Hep.; *Nat. s.* See Felon.

Inflammation of pulp (onychia)—Arn.; Calend.; *Fluor. ac.;* Graph.; Phos.; Psor.; Sars.; Sil.; Upas.

Inflammation, under toe nail—Sabad.

Ingrowing toe nail—Caust.; Magnet. aust.; Nit. ac.; *Sil.;* Staph.; Teucr.; Tetradyn.

Injury to matrix—Hyper.

Irritable feeling under finger nails, relieved by biting them—Am. brom.

Itching—About roof of: Upas.

Pains—Burning under: Sars.

Pains, gnawing, beneath finger nails—Alum.; Sars.; Sep.

Pains, neuralgic, beneath finger nails—Berb. v.

Pains, neuralgic—Alum.; *Cepa;* Colch.

Pains, smarting at roots—Sul.

Pains, splinter-like, beneath toe nails—Fluor. ac.

Pains, ulcerative, beneath toe nails—Ant. c.; Graph.; Teucr.

Skin around, dry, cracked—Graph.; Nat. m.; Petrol.

Skin around, pigmented—Naph.

Softening—Plumb.; Thuya.

Spots, white on—Alum.; Nit. ac.

Trophic changes—Radium.

Ulceration—Alum.; Graph.; Merc.; *Phos.;* Psor.; Sang.; Sars.; Sil.; Teucr.; Tetradyn.

Yellow color—Con.

ŒDEMA, SWELLING—Acal.; *Acet. ac* ; Acon.; *Agar.; Anac.; Apis; Ars.;* Bell.; Bellis; Bothrops; Bry.; *Dig.;* Elat.; Euphorb.; Ferr. m.; *Helleb.;* Hippoz.; Lach.; Lyc.; Nat. c.; Nat. sal.; Oleand.; Prim. ob.; *Prun. sp.;* Rhus t.; Samb.; *Thyr.*

ŒDEMA, ANGIONEUROTIC—Agar.; Antipyr.; Helleb.

OILY—Skin: Bry.; *Merc.; Nat. m.;* Plumb. m.; Psor.; Raph.; Sanic. See Seborrhœa.

PELLAGRA—*Ars.;* Ars. sul. rub.; Bov.; Cinch.; Gels.; Pedic.; Plumb. iod.; Psor.; Sec.; *Sedinha;* Sul.

Pellagra, cachexia—Ars.; Sec.

SKIN

Pellagra, fissures, desquamation, skin eruptions—Graph.; *Hep.*; Ign.; Phos.; Puls.; Sep.

PEMPHIGUS—Anac.; Antipyr.; *Ars.*; Arum tr.; Bufo; Caltha; *Canth.*; Carbon. ox.; Caust.; Dulc.; *Jugl. c.*; *Lach.*; *Mancin.*; *Merc. c.*; Merc. pr. rub.; Merc. s.; Nat. sal.; Phos. ac.; Phos. ; *Ran. b.*; *Ran. sc.*; Raph.; *Rhus t.*; Sep.; Thuya.

PETICHIÆ—*Arn.*; Ars.; Calc. c.; Cur.; Mur. ac.; *Phos.*; Sec.; *Sul. ac.* See Ecchymosis.

PHTHIRIASIS—Bac.; Cocc.; Merc.; *Nat. m.*; Oleand.; Psor.; *Sabad.*; *Staph.*

PITYRIASIS (dermatitis exfoliativa)—*Ars.*; Ars. iod.; Bac.; Berb. aq.; Calc. c.; Carb. ac.; Clem.; *Colch.*; *Fluor. ac.*; *Graph.*; *Kali ars.*; Mang. ac.; Merc. pr. rub.; *Mez.*; Nat. ars.; Phos.; Pip. m.; *Sep.*; Staph.; *Sul.*; Sul. iod.; *Sulphur. ac.*; Tellur.; Tereb.; Thyr.

PRAIRIE ITCH—Led.; Rhus t.; Rumex; Sul.

PRURIGO—Acon.; Alnus; *Ambra*; Anthrok.; *Ars.*; *Ars. iod.*; Ars. sul.; Carb. ac.; *Chloral.*; *Dolich.*; Diosc.; Kali bich.; *Lyc.*; *Merc.*; *Mez.*; *Nit. ac.*; *Oleand.*; Oophor.; Pedic.; *Rhus t.*; *Rhus v.*; *Rumex*; Sil.; *Sul.*; Tereb.

PRURITUS (itching of skin)—Acon.; *Agar.*; Alum.; *Ambra*; Anac. oc.; *Anac.*; Anag.; *Antipyr.*; Apis; *Ars.*; Calad.; Calc. c.; Canth.; *Carb. ac.*; Chloral.; Chrysar.; *Clem.*; *Crot. t.*; *Dolich.*; Dulc.; Elaeis; *Fagop.*; *Fluor. ac.*; Formica; Glon.; *Graph.*; Granat.; Grind.; Guano; Hep.; *Hydrocot.*; Hyper.; Ichth.; Ign.; *Lyc.*; Kreos.; Mag. c.; Malandr.; Mang. ac.; Med.; *Merc.*; *Mez.*; *Morph.*; Niccol.; Nux v.; Oleand.; Op.; Petrol.; *Pix l.*; Prim. ob.; Psor.; Pulex; *Radium*; Ran. b.; *Rhus t.*; *Rhus v.*; *Rumex*; *Sep.*; Staph.; *Sul.*; Sul. ac.; Syzgium Tar. c.; *Urt.*; Vespa; Xerophyl.

Pruritus of aged—Bar. ac.

Pruritus, of ankles—Nat. p.; Selen.; Sep.

Pruritus, of bends of elbows, knees—Selen.; Sep.

Pruritus, of chest, upper limbs—Arundo.

Pruritus, of ears, nose, arms, urethra—Sul. iod.

Pruritus, of face, hands, scalp—Clem.

Pruritus, of face, shoulders, chest—Kali br.

Pruritus, of feet, ankles—Led.

Pruritus, of feet, legs—Bov.

Pruritus, of feet, soles of—Ananth.; Hydrocot.

Pruritus, of genitals—*Ambra*; Ars. iod.; Bor.; *Calad.*; Carb. ac.; Carbo v.; Colch.; Collins.; Crot. t.; Dulc.; Fuligo; Guano; Helon.; Kreos.; Mez.; Nit. ac.; Rhus t.; Rhus v.; *Sep.*; Sil.; Tar. c. See Female Sexual System.

Pruritus, of hands, arms—Pip. m.; Selen.

Pruritus, of joints, abdomen—Pinus sylv.

Pruritus, of knees, elbows, hairy parts—Dolich.; Fagop.

Pruritus, of nose—Morph.; Strych.

Pruritus, of orifices—Fluor. ac.

SKIN

Pruritus, of thighs, bends of knees—Zinc. m.
Pruritus, of webs of fingers, bends of joints—Hep.; *Psor.*; Selen.; Sep.
Pruritus, ameliorated from cold—Berb. v.; Fagop.; Graph.; Mez.
Pruritus, ameliorated from hot water—Rhus v.
Pruritus, ameliorated from rubbing gently—Crot. t.
Pruritus, ameliorated from scratching—Asaf.; Cadm. s.; Mang. ac.; Merc. s.; *Oleand.; Rhus t.*
Pruritus, ameliorated from warmth—Ars.; Petrol.; Rumex.
Pruritus, followed by bleeding, pains, burning—Alum.; *Ars.; Crot. t.;* Murex; Pix l.; Psor.; Sep.; *Sul.;* Tilia.
Pruritus, followed by, change of site of itching—Mez.; Staph.
Pruritus, without eruption—Dolichos.
Pruritus, worse from contact—Ran. b.
Pruritus, worse from exposure, cold air—Dulc.; *Hep.;* Nat. s.; Oleand.; Petrol.; Rhus t.; *Rumex.*
Pruritus, worse from scratching—Ars.; Berb. v.; Crot. t.; Led.; *Mez.* Sep.; Sul.
Pruritus, worse from undressing; warmth of bed; at P. M—*Alum.;* Ant. c.; *Ars.;* Asimina; Bellis; Bov.; Carbo v.; Card. **m.**; Cistus; Dulc.; *Jugl. c.; Kali ars.;* Kreos.; Led.; Lyc.; *Menisp.; Mcrc.;* Merc. i. fl.; *Mez.; Nat. s.;* Oleand.; Psor.; Puls.; Rhus t.; *Rumex;* Sang.; Sep.; *Sul.;* Tub.
Pruritus, worse from washing, with cold water—Clem.; Tub.

PSORIASIS—Ant. t.; *Ars.; Ars. iod.;* Aster.; Aur. m. n.; Berb. aq.; *Bor.; Carb. ac.; Chrysar.;* Cic.; Coral.; Cupr. ac.; Fluor. ac.; *Graph.;* Hep.; Hydrocot.; Iris; *Kali ars.; Kali br.;* Kali s.; *Lyc.; Mang. ac.;* Merc. aur.; *Merc. s.;* Mur. ac.; Naph.; Nat. ars.; Nat. m.; Nit. ac.; Nit. mur. ac.; *Petrol.; Phos.;* Platanus; *Sep.;* Strych. ars.; Strych. p.; Stellar.; *Sul.;* Tereb.; Thuya; *Thyr.;* Tub.; Ustil.
Psoriasis, of palms—Calc. c.; Coral.; *Graph.; Hep.; Lyc.;* Med.; Petrol.; Phos.; Selen.
Psoriasis, of prepuce, nails—Graph.; *Sep.*
Psoriasis, of tongue—Graph.; Mur. ac.; Sep. See Tongue (Mouth).

PURPURA—Acon.; *Arn.; Ars.;* Bapt.; Bell.; Bry.; Carbo v.; Chin. s.; Chloral; *Crot.; Ham.;* Jugl. r.; Kali iod.; *Lach.;* Merc. s.; Phos. ac.; *Phos.;* Rhus t.; Rhus v.; Sec.; Sal. ac.; *Sul. ac.;* Sulphur.; Tereb.; Ver. v.
With colic—Bov.; Col.; Cupr.; Merc. c.; Thuya.
With debility—Arn.; *Ars.;* Carbo v.; Lach.; Merc. s.; *Sul. ac.*

PURPURA HÆMORRHAGICA—Alnus; *Arn.; Ars.;* Bothrops; Bry.; *Crot.;* Ferr. picr.; *Ham.;* Iod.; Ipec.; *Lach.;* Led.; Merc. c.; Merc. s.; Millef.; Naja; Nat. nit.; *Phos. ac.; Phos.;* Rhus v.; Sec.; *Sul. ac.; Tereb ;* Thlaspi.

PURPURA RHEUMATICA—Acon.; Ars.; *Bry.;* Merc. s.; *Rhus t.;* Rhus v.

RAYNAUD'S DISEASE—See Gangrene.

RHINO-SCLEROMA—Aur. m. n.; *Calc. p.;* Guarana; Rhus r.

ROSEOLA (rose-rash)—*Acon.;* Bell.; Cub.

RUPIA—Æthiops; Ant. t.; *Ars.;* Berb. aq.; Clem.; Graph.; Hydr.; *Kali iod.;* Lach.; Merc. i. r.; Nit. ac.; *Phyt.;* Sec.; Syph.; Thyr. See Syphilis (Male Sexual System).

SARCOMA CUTIS—Calc. p.; *Condur.;* Nit. ac.; Sil.

SCABIES (itch)—Aloe; Anthrok.; Caust.; *Crot. t.; Hep.;* Lyc.; Merc.; Nux v.; *Psor.;* Rhus v.; Selen.; *Sep.; Sul.*

SCLERODERMA—scleriasis (hidebound skin): Alum.; *Ant. c.;* Arg. n.; Ars.; Berb. aq.; *Bry.;* Caust.; *Crot. t.;* Echin.; *Elaeis; Hydrocot.;* Lyc.; Petrol.; Phos.; Ran. b.; Rhus r.; Sars.; Sil.; Still.; Sul.; Thiosin.; *Thyr.*

SCROFULODERMA—Calc. iod.; *Calc. s.;* Petrol.; Scroful.; Ther. See Separate Diseases.

SEBACEOUS CYSTS (wen)—*Bar. c.;* Benz. ac.; Brom.; Calc. sil.; *Con.;* Graph.; Hep.; Kali br.; *Kali iod.;* Nit. ac.; Phyt.; Thuya. See Scalp (Head).

SEBORRHŒA—*Am. m.;* Ars.; *Bry.;* Bufo; *Calc. c.;* Cinch.; Graph.; *Iod.;* Kali br.; *Kali c.;* Kali s.; Lyc.; Merc. s.; Mez.; *Nat. m.; Phos.; Plumb. m.;* Psor.; *Raph.;* Rhus t.; Sars.; *Selen.;* Sep.; Staph.; Sul. Thuya; *Vinca.* See Scalp (Head).

SENSIBILITY OF SKIN—**Diminished, or lost (analgesia, anæsthesia)**: Acet. ac.; *Acon.;* Ars.; Aur.; Bufo; *Can. ind.; Carbon. ox.;* Carbon. s.; Elaeis; Hyos.; *Ign.;* Kali br.; Merc.; *Nux v.; Plumb. m.;* Pop. c.; Sec.; Zinc. m.

Sensibility of skin increased to atmospheric changes—Dulc.; Hep.; Kali c.; Psor.; *Sul.*

SPOTS—**Blue**: Ars.; Led.; Sul. ac.

Spots, brown—Bac.; Card. m.; Con.; Iod.; Phos.; *Sep.;* Thuya.

Spots, circumscribed pigmentation following eczematous inflammation—Berb. v.; Lach.; *Lyc.;* Med.; Merc. d.; Merc.; *Nit. ac.;* Sil.; Sul.; Ustil.

Spots, copper-colored—*Carbo an.;* Carbo v.; *Coral.;* Syph.

Spots, livid—Agave; *Ail.; Bapt.;* Bothrops; *Morph.;* Ox. ac.; Sec.; *Sul. ac.*

Spots, red—Agar.; Bell.; Calc. c.; Con.; Kali c.; Sul.; Veronal.

Spots, white—Graph.; Sul.

Spots, yellow—Nat. p.; Phos.; Plumb. m.; Sep.; Sul.

Spots, yellow turning green—Con.

STROPHULUS (tooth rash)—Apis; *Bor.;* Calc. c.; *Cham.;* Cic.; Led.; Rhus t.; *Spiranth.;* Sumb.

SUDAMINÆ—Am. m.; Bry.; Urt.

SYCOSIS (barber's itch)—Anthrok.; *Ant. t.;* Ars.; Aur. m.; *Calc. c.;* Calc. s.; Chrysar.; *Cic.;* Cinnab.; Cocc.; Cypressus; *Graph.; Kali bich.;* Kali m.; Lith. c.; *Lyc.;* Med.; *Merc. pr. rub.;* Nat. s.; *Nit. ac.;* Petrol.; Plant.; *Plat.;* Sab.; Sep.; Sil.; *Staph.;* Stront. c.; Sul.; *Sul. iod.;* Tellur.; *Thuya.*

SYPHILIDÆ—See Syphilis (Male Sexual System).

TINEA FAVOSA—favus: Agar.; Ars. iod.; *Brom.*; Calc. c.; Dulc.; Graph.; Hep.; Jugl. r.; *Kali c.*; Lappa; *Lyc.*; Med.; *Mez.*; Oleand.; Phos.; *Sep.*; Sulphur. ac.; Sul.; Ustil.; Vinca; *Viola tr.* See Scalp (Head).

TINEA VERSICOLOR (chromophytosis)—Bac.; Chrysar.; Mez.; *Nat. ars.*; *Sep.*; Sul.; Tellur.

TRICHOPHYTOSIS—ringworm: Ant. c.; Ant. t.; *Ars.*; *Bac.*; Calc. c.; Calc. iod.; *Chrysar.*; *Graph.*; Hep.; Jugl. c.; Jugl. r.; Kali s.; Lyc.; Mez.; Psor.; Rhus t., Semperv. t.; *Sep.*; Sul.; *Tellur.*; Tub.; Viola tr. See Scalp (Head).

Trichophytosis, in intersecting rings over great portion of body; fever; great constitutional disturbances—Tellur.

Trichophytosis, in isolated spots on upper part of body—Sep.

ULCERS—Anac. oc.; *Ananth.*; *Anthrac.*; Arn.; *Ars.*; Aster.; Bals. per.; Bell.; *Calc. c.*; *Calc. p.*; *Calc. sil.*; *Calc. s.*; Calend.; *Carb. ac.*; Carbo an.; *Carbo v.*; Carbon. s.; Caust.; Cistus; *Clem.*; Commocl.; Con.; Crot.; Cupr. ars.; *Echin.*; *Fluor. ac.*; Galium ap.; *Geran.*; Graph.; Ham.; *Hep.*; Hippoz.; *Hydr.*; Iod.; Jugl. r.; Kali ars.; *Kali bich.*; Kali iod.; *Lach.*; Merc. c.; *Merc. s.*; *Mez.*; Nat. s.; *Nit. ac.*; *Pæonia*; Petrol.; Phos. ac.; Phos.; *Phyt.*; Psor.; Radium; Ran. ac.; Scrophul.; Sep.; *Sil.*; Sul. ac.; Sul.; *Syph.*; Tar. c.; Thuya; Trychnos.

Bleeding, easily, when touched—Ars.; Carbo v.; Dulc.; Hep.; Kreos.; *Lach.*; Merc.; Mez.; *Nit. ac.*; *Petrol.*; *Phos.*

Burning—Alumen; *Anthrac.*; Ars.; Carbo v.; Hep.; Kreos.; Mez.; Thuya.

Cancerous, malignant—Anthrac.; *Ars.*; *Aster.*; Carbo an.; Chimaph.; Clem.; Condur.; Fuligo; *Galium ap.*; Hydr.; Kreos.; Lach.; Tar. c.; Thuya.

Deep—Asaf.; Commocl.; *Kali bich.*; Kali iod.; Mur. ac.; *Nit. ac.*; Tar. c.

Eroding, of face—Con.

Fistulous—*Calc. fl.*; Calend.; Kali iod.; Nit. ac.; Phyt.; *Sil.*; Thuya.

Indolent, torpid—*Anag.*; Aster.; Bar. c.; Calc. fl.; *Calc. iod.*; *Calc. p.*; Carbo v.; Chel.; Con.; Cupr.; Eucal.; Euphorb.; Fluor. ac.; Fuligo; Geran.; Graph.; Hydr.; Kali bich.; *Kali iod.*; Lach.; Lyc.; *Merc. s.*; Nit. ac.; Pæonia; Phyt.; *Psor.*; Pyr.; *Sil.*; *Sul.*; Syph.; Syzyg.

Inflamed—*Ars.*; *Bell.*; Calend.; Carbo an.; Phyt. See Sensitive.

Phagedenic—*Ars.*; Carbo v.; *Crot.*; Kali ars.; Merc. c.; Merc. d.; Merc.; *Nit. ac.* See Gangrenous.

Scrofulous—*Calcareas*; Cinch.; Hep.; Iodides; Mercuries; Nit. ac.; *Sil.*; Sul.

Sensitive—Angust.; Arn.; Ars.; Asaf.; Calend.; Dulc.; Graph.; Hep.; Lach.; Mez.; *Nit. ac.*; Pæonia; Sil.; Tar. c.

Smooth, pale, shallow, on scalp, penis—Merc.

Superficial, flat—Ars.; Coral.; Lach.; Nit. ac.; Thuya.

Superficial, serpiginous—Chel.; Merc. c.; *Merc. s.*; Phos. ac.

Syphilitic—Ars.; Asaf.; Carbo v.; *Cinnab.*; Cistus; Coral.; *Fluor. ac.*; Graph.; Hep · *Iod.*; *Kali bich.*; *Kali iod.*; Lach.; Lyc.; *Merc. c.*; *Merc. i. r.*; Merc. s.; *Nit. ac.*; Phyt.; Sars.; Still.

Traumatic—Arn.; Con.

Varicose—Calc. fl.; Calend.; *Card. m.;* *Carbo v.;* Clem. vit.; Condur.; Eucal.; *Fluor. ac.;* *Ham.;* Lach.; Phyt.; Psor.; Pyr.; *Sec.*

Verrucous, on cheek—Ars.

Ulcers, from pemphigus blisters on toes, with ulcerated borders, moist, red, flat surface—Petrol.

Ulcers, from scarlet fever—Cham.

Ulcers, with base. blue or black—*Ars.;* Calc. fl.; Carbo an.; Lach.; Mur. ac.; Tar. c.

With base, dry, lardaceous—Phyt.

With base, indurated—*Alumen;* *Calc. fl.;* Commocl.; Con.

With base, lardaceous, surrounded with dark halo; dirty, unhealthy look; apt to coalesce—Merc. v.

With base, like raw flesh—Ars.; Merc. s.; *Nit. ac.*

With discharge, fetid, purulent, sloughing—*Ananth.;* *Anthrac.;* Ars.; Asaf.; Bapt.; Calc. fl.; Calend.; *Carb. ac.;* *Carbo v.;* Con.; Crot. t.; *Echin.;* Eucal.; Fluor. ac.; Gels.; *Geran.;* Hep.; Lach.; Merc. c.; *Merc. s.;* *Mez.;* Mur. ac.; *Nit. ac.:* Pæonia; Phos. ac.; Psor.; Pyr.; Puls.; Sil.; Sul.; *Thuya.*

With discharge, glutinous—*Graph.;* Kali bich.

With discharge, ichorous—Aster.; Carbo v.; *Carb. ac.;* Coral.; *Mez.*

With discharge, ichorous, foul—Anthrac.; *Ars.;* Asaf.; Mez.

With discharge, thin, acrid, foul—*Ars.;* Asaf.; Kali iod.; Nit. ac.

With edges, deep, regular, "punched out"—Kali bich.; Phos.

With edges, eczematous, copper-colored—Kali bich.

With edges, gangrenous—Anthrac.; *Ars.;* *Carbo v.;* Kreos.; Lach.; Nit. ac.; Sec.; *Sul. ac.;* Tar. c.

With edges, indurated—Calc. fl.; Carbo an.; Commocl.; Nit. ac.; Pæonia; Phos. ac.

With edges, irregular, undefined—*Merc. s.;* Nit. ac.

With edges, raised—Ars.; Calend.; Nit. ac.; Phos. ac.; *Sil.* See Granulations.

With fungous growths—Mur. ac.

With glazed, shining appearance—Lac c.

With granulations, exuberant—Apium gr.; *Ars.;* Carbo an.; *Caust.;* Fluor. ac.; *Nit. ac.;* Petrol.; Phos. ac.; *Sil.;* Thuya.

With itching—Mez.; Phos. ac.; Sil.

Without pain or redness; uneven, jagged base, dirty pus—Phos. ac.

With pain, in small spot, lightning-like; worse from warmth—Fluor. ac.

With pain, splinter-like—Ham.; Hep.; *Nit. ac.*

With pimples surrounding it—Grind.; *Hep.;* Lach.; Merc. s.

With small ulcers, surrounding it—Phos.; Sil.

With stupor, low delirium, prostration—Bapt.

With vesicles, surrounding it; red shining areolæ—Fluor. ac.; Hep.; *Mez.*

UNHEALTHY SKIN—**Every scratch festers, or heals with difficulty**—*Bor.;* Bufo; Calc. c.; Calc. s.; Calend.; Carbon. s.; Cham.; *Graph.;* *Hep.;* Hydr.; Lyc.; *Merc. s.;* *Petrol.;* Pip. m.; Psor.; *Pur.;* *Sil.;* *Sul.*

URTICARIA (hives, nettle rash)—Acon.; Anac.; Anthrok.; *Ant. c.;* *Antipyr.;* Apium gr.; *Apis;* Ars.; Astac.; Berb. v.; *Bombyx;* *Bov.;* Calc. c.;

Camph.; Chin. s.; *Chloral*; *Cim.*; Cina; Condu...; Con.; *Cop.*; Crot. t.; *Dulc.*; Fagop.; *Fragar.*; Hep.; Homar. fl.; *Ichth.*; Ign.; Ipec.; Kali c.; Kali chlor.; Medusa; Nat. m.; *Nat. p.*; Nit. ac.; Nux v.; Petrol.; *Puls.*; *Rhus t.*; Rhus v.; Robin.; Sanic.; Sep.; Stann.; Stroph.; Strych. p.; *Sul.*; Tereb.; Tetradyn.; *Triost.*; *Urt.*; Ustil.; Vespa.

Chronic—*Anac.*; *Ant. c.*; Antipyr.; *Ars.*; Astac.; *Bov.*; Calc. c.; *Chloral*; Condur.; *Cop.*; *Dulc.*; Hep.; Ichth.; *Lyc.*; Nat. m.; *Rhus t.*; Sep.; Stroph.; *Sul.*; Urt.

Nodosa—Bov.; Urt.

Tuberosa—*Anac.*; Bolet. lur.

CAUSE—CONCOMITANTS—From emotion: Anac.; Bov.; Ign.; Kali br.
From exertion, excessive—Con.; Nat. m.
From exposure—Chloral.; *Dulc.*; Rhus t.
From gastric derangement—*Ant. c.*; Ars.; Carbo v.; Cop.; Dulc.; Nux v.; Puls.; Robin.; Triost.
From menstrual conditions—Bell.; *Cim.*; *Dulc.*; Kali c.; Mag. c.; Puls.; Ustil.
From shellfish, roe—Camph.
From suppressed malaria—Elat.
From sweat—Apis.
With catarrh—Cepa; Dulc.
With chill, of intermittents—Ign.; Nat. m.
With constipation, fever—Cop.
With croup, alternating—Ars.
With diarrhœa—Apis; Bov.; *Puls.*
With edema—*Apis*; Vespa.
With erosion, on toes—Sul.
With itching, burning after scratching; no fever—Dulc.
With liver disturbance—Astac.
With petechial disturbance, or erysipelatous eruption—Fragar.
With rheumatic lameness, palpitation, diarrhœa—*Bov.*; Dulc.
With rheumatism, alternating—Urt.
With sequelæ, from suppressed hives—Apis; Urt
With sudden coming and going—Antipyr.
With sudden, violent onset; syncope—Camph.

MODALITIES-AGGRAVATIONS: At climacteric: Morph.; Ustil.
At menstrual period—*Cim.*; *Dulc.*; Kali c.; Mag. c.
At night—Ant. c.; Ars.
From bathing, walking in A. M.—Bov.
From cold—Ars.; Dulc.; Rhus t.; Rumex; Sep.
From exertion, exercise—Apis; Calc. c.; Hep.; Nat. m.; P. or.; Sanic.; Urt.
From fruit, pork, buckwheat—Puls.
From open air—Nit. ac.; Sep.
From spirituous drinks—Chloral.
From warmth—Apis; Dulc.; Kali c.; Lyc.; Sul.
In children—Cop.
Periodically, every year—Urt.

AMELIORATIONS—From cold water: Apis; Dulc.

From hot drinks—Chloral.
From open air—Calc. c.
From warmth—Ars.; Chloral; Sep.

VACCINIA—*Acon.*; Ant. t.; Apis; *Bell.*; Merc. s.; Phos.; *Sil.*; Sul.; *Thuya;* Vac.

VERUCCA (warts)—Acet. ac.; Am. c.; Anac. oc.; Anag.; *Ant. c.*; Ant. t.; Ars. br.; Aur. m. n.; Bar. c.; *Calc. c.*; Castorea; *Cast. eq.*; *Caust.*; Chrom. oxy.; Cinnab.; *Dulc.*; Ferr. picr.; Kali m.; Kali perm.; Lyc.; *Mag. s.*; *Nat. c.*; Nat. m.; Nat. s.; *Nit. ac.*; Ran. b.; Semperv. t.; Sep.; *Sil.*; Staph.; Sul.; Sul. ac.; *Thuya;* X-ray.

Bleed easily—Cinnab.

Bleed easily, jagged, large—Caust.; *Nit. ac.*

Condylomata, fig warts—Calc. c.; *Cinnab.*; Euphras.; Kali iod.; *Lyc.*; Med.; Merc. c.; Merc. s.; Nat. s.; *Nit. ac.*; Phos. ac.; *Sab.*; Sep.; Sil.; *Staph.*; *Thuya.*

Cracked, ragged, with furfuraceous areola—Lyc.

Flat, smooth, sore—Ruta.

Horny, broad—Rhus t.

Large, seedy—Thuya.

Large, smooth, fleshy, on back of hands—Dulc.

Lupoid—Ferr. picr.

Moist, itching, flat, broad—Thuya.

Moist, oozing—Nit. ac.

Painful, hard, stiff, shining—Sil.

Painful, sticking—*Nit. ac.*; Staph.; Thuya.

Pedunculated—Caust.; Lyc.; *Nit. ac.*; Sab.; Staph.; *Thuya.*

Situated, on body, general—Nat. s.; Sep.

Situated, on breast—Castor.

Situated, on face, hands—Calc. c.; Caust.; Carbo an.; Dulc.; Kali c.

Situated, on forehead—Castorea.

Situated, on genito-anal surface—Nit. ac.; Thuya.

Situated, on hands—Anac.; *Bufo;* Ferr. magnet.; Kali m.; Lach.; Nat c.; *Nat. m.;* Rhus t.; Ruta.

Situated, on neck, arms, hands, soft, smooth—Ant. c.

Situated, on nose, finger tips, eye brows—Caust.

Situated, on prepuce—Cinnab.; Phos. ac.; Sab.

Small, all over body—Caust.

Smooth—Calc. c.; Ruta.

Sycotic, syphilitic—Nit. ac.

WHITLOW—**felon, panaritium:** Alum.; Am. c.; *Anthrac.*; Apis; Bell.; *Bry.*; Bufo; Calc. fl.; Calc. s.; Calend.; Cepa; Crot.; *Diosc.*; *Fluor. ac.*; *Hep.*; Hyper.; Led.; Merc. s.; Myrist. seb.; Nat. s.; Ol. myrist.; Phos.; *Sil.*; Tar. c.

Malignant tendency—Anthrac.; *Ars.*; Carb. ac.; *Lach.*

Predisposition to—Diosc.; Hep.

Recurrence—Sil.

Traumatic—Led.

FEVER

CHILLINESS, coldness—Abies c.; *Acon.*; Æth.; *Agar.*; Alum.; *Ant. t.*; Apis; *Aran.*; Arn.; *Ars.*; *Ars. iod.*; Asar.; Astac.; Bapt.; Berb. v.: Bry.; *Calc. ars.*; *Calc. c.*; *Calc. sil.*; Calend.; *Camph.*; Canth.; *Caps.*; *Carbo v.*; Castor.; Caust.; Ced.; Cimex; Cocaine; *Colch.*; Corn. fl.; Crat.; Dulc.; Echin.; Eup. purp.; Ferr. m.; Gels.; Graph.; Helod.; Hep.; Ipec.; Jatropha; *Kali c.*; Lac d.; *Laur.*; Led.; Lob. purp.; Lyc.; *Mag. p.*; *Menyanth.*; *Merc. s.*; Morph.; Mosch.; *Nat. m.*; *Nux v.*; Op.; Phos.; Pimpin.; Plat.; *Puls.*; Pyrus; Radium; Sabad.; *Sec.*; Sil.; Sul.; *Tab.*; Tela ar.; Val.; Ver. a.

Chilliness, after epileptic fit—Cupr. m.

Chilliness, in abdomen, legs—Menyanth.

Chilliness, in arms—Raph.

Chilliness, in back and feet—Bell.; Canth.

Chilliness, in back, between shoulder blades—*Am. m.*; Castor.; *Lachnanth.*; Pyr.; Tub.

Chilliness, in back, hips, to legs—Ham.

Chilliness, in body and feet, head and face hot—Arn.

Chilliness, in body, with face and breath hot—Cham.

Chilliness, in bones, extremities; severe, general—Pyr.

Chilliness, in chest, on walking in open air—Ran. b.

Chilliness, in forearms—Carbo v.; Med.

Chilliness, in hands—Dros.

Chilliness, in hands and back—Cact.

Chilliness, in hands, back, feet and knees—Benz. ac.; *Chin. ars.*

Chilliness, in hands, body warm—Tab.

Chilliness, in head and limbs—Calc. c.; Ferr. m.

Chilliness, in knees—*Carbo v.*; Cimex; Phos.

Chilliness, in lower limbs—Calc. c.; Cocc.

Chilliness, in lumbar region—Agar.

Chilliness, in single parts—*Asar.*; Calad.; *Calc. c.*; Kali bich.; Paris; Puls.

Chilliness, in waves, along spine—Abies c.; *Acon.*; Æsc.; *Ars.* Bolet.; Calend.; Conv.; Dulc.; Echin.; Frax. am.; *Gels.*; Helod.; *Mag. p.*; Med.; Raph.; Strych.; Tub.; Zinc. m.

Chilliness, with aching in shoulders, joints, small of back; yawning, stretching—Bolet.

Chilliness, with catarrh—Merc. s.

Chilliness, with cough, dry, fatiguing—Rhus t.

Chilliness, with deficient, animal heat—Alu. Bar. c.; Calc. c.; Calc. p.; Calc. sil.; Led.; Lyc.; Psor.; Sep.; Sil.; h.; Thuya; Ver. a.

Chilliness, with desire to uncover abdomen—Tab.

Chilliness, with evening pains of whatever kind; in warm room—Puls.

Chilliness, with face, head, palms hot—Ferr. m.

Chilliness, with face hot—Dros.; Ign.

Chilliness, with flatulent colic, nausea, vertigo, hot skin, sweat, heat of head—Cocc.

Chilliness, with headache—Conv.

FEVER

Chilliness, with headache, extending to parietal region, red eyes—Ced.
Chilliness, with heat and desire to stretch—Rhus t.
Chilliness, with heat, alternately—Abies n.; Acon.; *Apis;* Ars.; Bapt.; Bell.; Bolet.; Bry.; *Cham.;* Dig.; Laur.; Mag. s.; Merc. c.; *Merc. s.;* Phyt.; Puls.; Solan. n.; Solid.
Chilliness, with ill numor—Caps.
Chilliness, with loquacity—Pod.
Chilliness, with nausea—Echin.; *Ipec.*
Chilliness, with nervousness—*Asar.;* Cim.; Croc.; *Gels.;* Gossyp.; Nat. m.
Chilliness, with no relief from warmth—Aran.; *Cadm. s.;* Caust.; Chin. s.; Dros.; Laur.; Mag. p.; *Merc. s.;* Pulex; Puls.; Sil.
Chilliness, with pain—Coff.; Dulc.; *Puls.;* Sil.
Chilliness, with pain, racking in limbs, anxious restlessness—Ars.
Chilliness, with pallor—Cocaine.
Chilliness, with pruritus—Mez.
Chilliness, with rheumatic pain, and soreness—Bapt.; Homar.; Rhus t.
Chilliness, with septic symptoms—*Pyr.;* Tar. c.
Chilliness, with suffocative feeling—Arg. n.; Mag. p.
Chilliness, with thirst—Acon.; *Ars.;* Caps.; Carbo v.; Conv.; Dulc.; Ign.; Sec.; Sep.; Ver. a.
Chilliness, with thirstlessness—Dros.; Gels.; Nux m.; *Puls.*
Chilliness, worse after anger—Aur.; *Bry.;* Cham.
Chilliness, worse after dinner—Mag. p.
Chilliness, worse after drinking—Caps.
Chilliness, worse after eating A. M.—Puls.
Chilliness, worse from dampness, rain, not relieved by warmth—Aran.
Chilliness, worse from least exposure, "air goes right through"—*Acon.;* Ag Agraph.; Am. phos.; Arg. n.; *Ars.;* Ars. iod.; Astac.; *Calc. c.; Calc. p.;* Calend.; Canchal.; Caps.; Cinch.; *Hep.; Kali c.;* Merc. c.; *Merc. s.;* Mez.; *Nux v.;* Psor.; Sep.; *Sil.;* Tub.
Chilliness, worse from least motion—Ars.; *Nux v.;* Spig.
Chilliness, worse from touch—Acon.; *Kali c.; Sil.;* Spig.
Chilliness, worse from warmth, covering—*Camph.;* Hep.; Med.; Sanic.; Sec.; Sul.
Chilliness, worse in morning—Calc. c.
Chilliness, worse toward evening and night—Acon.; Alum.; Am. c.; *Ars.;* Ced.; Dulc.; Mag. c.; Mag. p.; Menthol; *Merc. s.;* Ol. j. as.; *Phos.; Puls.;* Sep.

FEBRILE HEAT—Abies n.; Acet. ac.; *Acon.; Æsc.;* Æth.; Agar.; Agrost.; Allium s.; Ant. c.; Arn.; *Bapt.; Bell.; Bry.;* Calop.; Camph.; Canth.; Carbo v.; *Cham.;* Chin. ars.; *Cim.;* Cinch.; Dulc.; Eucal.; *Ferr. p.; Gels.;* Glon.; Ign.; Iod.; *Merc.;* Millef.; Morph.; Nit. ac.; Nux m.; *Nux v.;* Op.; Phyt.; Pulex; *Puls.; Rhus t.; Samb.;* Sep.; Sil.; Spiræa; *Spiranth.;* Stram.; Tereb.; Thuya; Val.; *Ver. v.*
Febrile heat, ascends from pelvic organs—Sep.
Febrile heat, from anger—Cham.; Cocc.; Sep.
Febrile heat, in evening; falls asleep during, awakens when it ceases—Calad.

Febrile heat, in flashes, ebullitions—Acet. ac.; *Amyl;* Antipyr.; *Ars.;* Ars. iod.; Bolet.; Calc. c.; *Carls.;* Chimaph.; *Dig.;* Erech.; Fer. red.; Frax. am.; Hep.; Ign.; Indigo; Iod.; Jabor.; *Kali c.;* Lach.; Lyc.; Med.; Merc. s.; *Niccol.;* Petrol.; *Phos.;* Puls.; *Sang.;* Sep.; *Sul.;* *Sul. ac.;* Urt.; Val.; Viscum; Yohimb.

Febrile heat, in lower part of back, hip, thighs—Berb. v.

Febrile heat, in palms of hands—Chenop. gl.

Febrile heat, in soles of feet—Canth.

Febrile heat, in spots—Agar.; Apis.

Febrile heat, in whole body, face red, hot; yet chilly from least motion or uncovering—Nux v.

Febrile heat, with chill predominant—Bry.

Febrile heat, with colic—Ver. a.

Febrile heat, with decline towards A. M., without sweat—Gels.

Febrile heat, with delirium; headache—Agar.; Bell.

Febrile heat, with drowsy stupefaction; agonized tossing about, in search of a cool place; must be uncovered; vomiting, diarrhœa; convulsions—Op.

Febrile heat, with dryness, during sleep or on falling asleep; deep, dry, cough—Samb.

Febrile heat, with dryness, no sweat—Alum.; *Nux m.*

Febrile heat, with excitement, nervous agitation—*Acon.;* Tela ar.

Febrile heat, with external coldness—Ars.; Canth.

Febrile heat, with faintness, sweat—*Dig.;* Sep.; *Sul.;* Sul. ac.

Febrile heat, with flatulence, bowel movement—Radium.

Febrile heat, with headache—Astac.

Febrile heat, with headache as from thousand hammers—Nat. m

Febrile heat, with hot face, back chilly, feet cold—Puls.

Febrile heat, with hot face, cold hands and feet—Stram.

Febrile heat, with hot face, cool body, asthenic states—Arn.; Phyt.

Febrile heat, with hot face, unquenchable thirst, taste of bile, nausea, anxiety, restlessness, dry tongue; after anger—Cham.

Febrile heat, with hunger, for days preceding—Staph.

Febrile heat, with itching eyes, tearing in limbs, numbness of body, headache—Ced.

Febrile heat, with lassitude, in afternoon; throbs all over—Lil. t.

Febrile heat, with night sweats—*Acet. ac.;* Hep.

Febrile heat, with palpitation, precordial anguish—Calc. c.

Febrile heat, with prostration—Ant. t.; *Chin. ars.;* Phyt.

Febrile heat, with pulsations—*Bell.;* *Lil. t.;* Puls.; Thuya.

Febrile heat, with pulsations, and distended veins—*Puls.;* Thuya.

Febrile heat, with red spot on left cheek—Acet. ac.

Febrile heat, with restlessness, cheeks red, apathy—Iod.

Febrile heat, with restless sleep—Calc. c.

Febrile heat, with skin dry, hot; face red or red and pale alternately; arterial excitement; anguish, restlessness, tossing about—Acon.

Febrile heat, with skin dry, pungent; arterial excitement; distended, superficial vessels—Bell.

Febrile heat, with slow, nervous, insidious course; vertigo—Cocc.

922 FEVER

Febrile heat, smothered feeling, if covered—Arg. n.
Febrile heat, with soreness of body—*Arn.;* Franc.; Phyt.; *Rhus t.*
Febrile heat, with spasms—Acetan.; *Bell.*
Febrile heat, with stretching of limbs—Rhus t.
Febrile heat, with sudden onset; dry, burning skin; rapid, small, wiry pulse—Pyr.
Febrile heat, with tendency to cover up—Ign.; *Nux v.;* Samb.; Stann.
Febrile heat, with thirst—*Acon.;* Ant. c.; Bry.; Laur.; Puls.; Tereb.
Febrile heat, with thirstlessness—*Acet. ac.;* Æth.; Bell.; Gels.; *Ign.;* Mur. ac.; *Nux m.; Puls.;* Samb.
Febrile heat, worse at night—Acon.; Æsc.; Ant. c.; Ars.; Bell.; Calad.; *Calc. c.;* Gels.; *Hep.;* Kali s.; Mag. c.; *Petrol.;* Phos.; *Puls.;* Sil.; Stann.; Urt.
Febrile heat, worse during menses—Calc. c.; Thuya.
Febrile heat, worse during sleep—Acon.; Calad.; *Samb.*
Febrile heat, worse covering up—Ign.
Febrile heat, worse from motion, then chilly—Nux v.
Febrile heat, worse from uncovering—*Merc. s.; Nux v.;* Samb.; Stront.
Febrile heat, worse in afternoon—Azadir.; Bell.; Ferr.
Febrile heat, worse in morning in bed—Kali c.
Febrile heat, worse on awaking—Laur.
Febrile heat, worse when sitting, walking in open air—Sep.

SWEAT: TYPE—Bloody: *Crot.;* Lach.; Lyc.; Nux m.; Nux v.
Cold, clammy—Abies c.; *Acet. ac.;* Æth.; *Amyl;* Ant. ars.; *Ant. t.;* Ars.; Benz. ac.; Cact.; *Calc. c.;* Calc. p.; *Camph.;* Canth.; *Carbo v.;* Cinch.; Corn. fl.; Crot.; *Cupr. ars.;* Dig.; Dulc.; Elaps; Euphorb. d.; Formal.; Ign.; Ipec.; Lach.; Laur.; Lob. infl.; Lupul.; Lyc.; Med.; Merc. c.; Merc. cy.; *Merc. s.;* Nat. c.; Pyr.; Sanic.; Sec.; Sul. ac.; *Tab.;* Tela ar.; *Tereb.; Ver a.;* Ver. v.
Greasy, oily—Bry.; Carbo v.; Cinch.; Lupul.; Mag. c.; *Merc. s.*
Hot—Æsc.; Carbo v.; *Cham.;* Chenop. gl.; *Lach.; Op.;* Tilia; Ver. v.

LOCALIZED, in general—Bry.; *Calc. c.;* Cinch.; *Fluor. ac.;* Hep.; *Petrol.;* Phos.; Plectranth.; *Puls.;* Selen.; *Sil.;* Sul.
Localized, in anterior part of body—Selen.
Localized, in axillæ—Calc. c.; Nit. ac.; Osm.; Petrol.; Sep.; Sil. See Locomotor System.
Localized, on chest—*Calc. c.;* Cocc.; Euphras.; *Phos.;* Stann.; Strych.
Localized, on covered parts—Bell.
Localized, on extremities, upper right—Formal.
Localized, on face, forehead—*Acet. ac.;* Benz. ac.; *Calc. c.;* Cina; Euphorb. d.; *Lob. infl.;* Phos.; Rheum; Sinap.; Stann.; Sul.; Val.; *Ver. a.*
Localized, on feet—Calc c.; *Graph.;* Lact. ac.; Merc. s.; *Petrol.;* Phos.; Sep.; Sil. See Feet (Locomotor System).
Localized, on genitals—Calc. c.; Petrol.; Phos. ac.; Thuya. See Male Sexual System.
Localized, on hands—Calc. c.; Cina; Con.; Fluor. ac.; Nit. ac.; *Phos.;* Sil. See Locomotor System.
Localized, on head, nape of neck—Bell.; *Calc. c.;* Phos.; Puls.; Rheum; Samb.; Sanic.; Sil.; Stann.; Strych.; Ver. a.

FEVER

Localized, on lower body—Croc.; Ran. ac.; Sanic.
Localized, on part lain on—Acon.
Localized, on parts in contact with each other—Niccoi. s.
Localized, on posterior part of body—Sep.
Localized, on side not reclined upon—Benz.; Thuya.
Localized, on uncovered parts—Thuya.
Localized, on upper body—Azadir.; Calc. c.; Cham.; Kali c.; Nux v.; Sil.
Localized, unilaterally—Jabor.; Nux v.; Puls.

ODOR—Fetid, offensive: Art. v.; Bapt.; But. ac.; Calc. c.; Carbo an.; Cimex; Con.; Daphne; Fluor. ac.; Hep.; Kali iod.; Lyc.; Merc. s.; Nit. ac.; Ol. an.; Osm.; Petrol.; Phos.; Psor.; Puls.; Sep.; Sil.; Solan. t.; Stann.; Staph.; Sul.; Taxus; Thuya; Variol. See Bromidrosis (Skin).
Odor, musty, mouldy—Stann.
Odor, sour, acid—Arn.; Bry.; Calc. c.; Cham.; Fluor. ac.; Graph.; Hep.; Kreos.; Lac d.; Mag. c.; Merc.; Nux v.; Pyr.; Rheum; Robin.; Sanic.; Sep.; Sil.; Sul.; Sul. ac.; Thuya.
Odor, sweetish—Calad.; Thuya.
Odor, urinous—Eryng. aq.; Nit. ac.

PROFUSE sweat (hyperidrosis)—Acet. ac.; Acon.; Æsc.; Agaricin; Am. acet.; Ant. t.; Ars.; Ars. iod.; Bapt.; Bell.; Bolet.; Bry.; Calc. c.; Canth.; Cham.; Cinch.; Cocc.; Con.; Croc.; Eser.; Ferr. iod.; Ferr. m.; Fluor. ac.; Graph.; Hep.; Hyper.; Iod.; Jabor.; Kali c.; Lact. ac.; Lob. infl.; Merc. s.; Morph.; Nit. ac.; Nux v.; Op.; Phos. ac.; Phos.; Piloc.; Polyp.; Psor.; Puls.; Sal. ac.; Samb.; Sanic.; Selen.; Sep.; Sil.; Stann.; Sul.; Sul. ac.; Thuya; Tilia; Ver. a.; Zinc. m.
Profuse, debilitating (colliquative)—Acet. ac.; Camph.; Carbo an.; Carbo v.; Castor.; Chrysanth.; Cinch.; Eup. perf.; Ferr. m.; Gels.; Merc. v.; Nit. ac.; Nitrum; Op.; Phell.; Phos. ac.; Phos.; Pyr.; Rhus gl.; Salvia; Samb.; Stann.; Sul. ac.

SCANTY—Apis; Conv.; Lach.; Nux m.
Viscid—Abies c.; Fluor. ac.; Hep.; Lyc.; Merc. s.; Phallus; Phos.
Yellow, staining—Ars.; Carbo an.; Lach.; Lyc.; Merc. s.

OCCURRENCE—After acute diseases: Psor.
After eating, drinking—Carbo v.; Cham.; Kali c.
At end of fever, or only at beginning of sleep—Ars.
During climacteric—Hep.; Jabor.; Tilia. See Female Sexual System.
During exertion, motion—Asar.; But. ac.; Calc. c.; Carbo an.; Cinch.; Eup. purp.; Eupion; Graph.; Hep.; Iod.; Kali c.; Lyc.; Merc. c.; Merc. s.; Nat. c.; Nat. m.; Phos. ac.; Psor.; Sep.; Sil.; Sul.
During morning, day time—Bry.; Carbo an.; Carbo v.; Hep.; Lyc.; Nat. m.; Nux v.; Phos.; Sep.; Sil.; Sul.; Zinc. m.
During morning, early—Stann.
During sleep (night sweats)—Acet. ac.; Agar.; Agaricin; Aral.; Ars. iod.; Bar. c.; Bell.; Bolet.; Calc. c.; Carbo an.; Carbo v.; Cham.; Chrysanth.; Cinch.; Con.; Corn. fl.; Euphras.; Ferr. p.; Hep.; Iod.; Ipec.; Jabor.; Kali c.; Kali iod.; Lyc.; Merc. s.; Myos.; Nat. tell.; Nit. ac.; Nux v.; Op.; Petrol.; Phos. ac.; Phos.; Phyt.; Picrot.; Piloc.; Pop. tr.; Psor.;

Salvia; Sang.; Sanic.; Sep.; *Sil.;* Stann.; Staph.; Stront. c.; Sul.; *Tarax.;* Thall.; *Thuya;* Tilia; Zinc. m.

During waking hours—Con.; Hep.; Merc.; Phos. ac.; Phos.; *Samb.*

From nervous depression, phthisis; convalescence, from acute disease—Jabor.

From nervous shock; sitting quietly—Anac.; Sep.

Sweat, affords no relief, or aggravates symptoms—Ant. t.; Bell.; Bolet.; Chin. s.; Ferr. m.; Formica; *Hep.; Merc. s.;* Phos. ac.; Pyr.; Sep.; Stram.

Sweat, affords relief, to symptoms—*Acon.; Ars.;* Calad.; Cupr. m.; Eup. perf.; Franc.; *Nat. m.; Psor.;* Senega; *Ver. a.*

TYPE OF FEVER: BILIOUS—*Bapt.;* Bry.; *Cham.;* Cinch.; Col.; Crot.; Euonym.; *Eup. perf.;* Gels.; Ipec.; Lept.; *Merc. c.; Merc. s.;* Nux v.; Nyct.; Pod.; Rhus t.; Tarax.

CATHETER—*Acon.;* Camph. ac.; Petros.

DENGUE—*Acon.;* Ars.; Bell.; Bry.; Canth.; Cinch.; *Eup. perf.; Gels.;* Ipec.; Nux v.; *Rhus t.;* Rhus v.

DYSENTERIC—Nux v.

ENTERIC—TYPHOID FEVER—Agar.; Agaricin; *Ail.; Apis;* Arg. n.; Arn.; Ars.; Arum tr.; Bapt.; *Bell.;* Bry.; Calc. c.; *Carbo v.;* Cina; Cinch.; Colch.; Crot.; Cupr. ars.; Echin.; *Eucal.; Gels.;* Glon.; *Helleb.;* Hydr.; *Hyos.;* Hyosc. hydrobr.; Iod.; Ipec.; Kali p.; *Lach.;* Laur.; *Lyc.;* Merc. cy.; *Merc. s.;* Methyl. bl.; Mosch.; *Mur. ac.; Nit. ac.; Nux m.; Op.; Phos. ac.; Phos.; Pyr.; Rhus t.;* Selen.; *Stram.;* Strych.; Sul. ac.; Sumb.; *Tereb.;* Vaccin. myr.; Val.; Ver. a.; Xerophyl.; Zinc. m.

CONCOMITANTS—Biliousness: *Bry.;* Chel.; Hydr.; Lept.; *Merc. s.;* Nux v.

Carriers; after inoculation with anti-typhoid serum—Bapt.

Constipation—*Bry.;* Hydr.; Nux v.; Op.

Decubitus—Arn.; *Ars.;* Bapt.; Carbo v.; *Lach.;* Mur. ac.; Pyr.; *Sec.*

Delirium—Agar.; *Agaricin;* Ars.; Bapt.; *Bell.;* Can. ind.; *Hyos.; Hyosc hydrobr.;* Lach.; Methyl. bl.; Op.; Phos. ac.; Phos.; Rhus t.; *Stram.,* Tereb.; Val.

Diarrhœa—Arn.; *Ars.;* Bapt.; Crot.; *Cupr. ars.; Epilob.;* Lach.; *Merc. s.;* Phos. ac.; Rhus t.

Diarrhœa, involuntary—Apis; *Arn.;* Ars.; Hyos.; Mur. ac.; *Phos. ac.*

Ecchymoses—*Arn.; Ars.;* Carbo v.; Mur. ac.

Epistaxis—*Acon.;* Bry.; Croc.; *Ham.; Ipec.;* Meli.; Phos. ac.; Rhus t.

Fever—Ars.; Bapt.; *Bell.;* Gels.; Methyl. bl.; Rhus t.; Stram.

Gastric symptoms—*Bry.;* Canth.; Carbo v.; *Hydr.;* Merc. s.; Nux v.; Puls.

Headache—Acetan.; *Bell.;* Bry.; Gels.; Hyos.; Nux v.; Rhus t.

Hæmorrhage—*Alumen;* Alum., Ars.; *Bapt.;* Carbo v.; Cinch.; *Crot.:* Elaps; *Ham.;* Hydrastin. sul.; Ipec.; Kreos.; Lach.; *Millef.; Mur. ac.; Nit. ac.;* Nux m.; *Phos. ac.;* Sec.; *Tereb.*

Insomnia—Bell.; *Coff.;* Gels.; *Hyosc. hydrobr.; Hyos.;* Op.; Rhus t.

Laryngeal affections—Apis; Merc. c.
Multiple abscesses—Ars.; Hep.; Sil.
Myocarditis—Pineal gland ext.
Nervous symptoms, adynamia—Agar.; *Agaricin;* Apis; *Ars.;* Bapt.; *Bell.;* Bry.; Cocc.; Colch.; Gels.; Helleb.; *Hyos.; Hyosc. hydrobr.; Ign.;* Lach.; Lyc.; *Mur. ac.; Phos. ac.; Phos.;* Rhus t.; *Stram.;* Sumb.; Val.; Zinc. m.
Nervous symptoms, collapse—*Ars.;* Camph.; Carbo v.; Cinch.; Hyosc. hydrobr.; *Laur.;* Mur. ac.; Sec.; Ver. a.
Peritonitis—Ars.; *Bell.;* Carbo v.; Col.; *Merc. c.;* Rhus t.; Tereb.
Pneumonia, bronchial symptoms—*Ant. t.;* Ars.; Bell.; *Bry.;* Hyos.; *Ipec.;* Lach.; *Phos.;* Puls.; Rhus t.; *Sang.;* Sul.; Tereb.
Putrescent pneumonia—Ars.; Mur. ac.
Soreness, muscular—*Arn.;* Bapt.; Bry.; Gels.; *Rhus t.*
Stage of convalescence—Ars. iod.; Carbo v.; *Cinch.;* Cocc.; Hydr.; Kali p.; Nux v.; *Psor.;* Sul.; Tarax.
Tympanites—*Asaf.; Ars.;* Bapt.; *Carbo v.;* Cinch.; Cocc.; Colch.; Lyc.; Mehtyl. bl.; Millef.; Mur. ac.; *Nux m.; Phos. ac.;* Rhus t.; *Tereb.*
Ulcer, corneal—Apis; Ipec.
Urination, profuse—Gels.; Mur. ac.; *Phos. ac.*
Urination, scanty, painful—Apis; Ars.; *Canth.*

EXANTHEMATA: ERUPTIVE FEVER: RUBELLA—(rotheln, German measles): Acon.; Bell.; Cop. See Rubeola (Measles).

RUBEOLA—**MEASLES**—*Acon.;* Ail.; Ant. t.; *Ars.; Ars. iod.;* Bell.; *Bry.;* Camph.; Coff.; Dulc.; Eup. perf.; *Euphras.;* Ferr. p.; *Gels.;* Ipec.; *Kali bich.;* Kali m.; Lach.; Merc. c.; Merc. pr. rub.; Merc. s.; Op.; Puls.; Rhus t.; Scilla; Spong.; *Sticta;* Stram.; Sul.; Ver. v.; Viola od.

CONCOMITANTS: Adenitis—Kali bich.; Merc. i. r.
Bronchial and pulmonary symptoms—*Ant. t.;* Bell.; *Bry.;* Chel.; Ferr. p.; *Ipec.;* Kali bich.; *Phos.;* Rumex; *Sticta;* Ver. v.; Viola iod.
Bronchial and pulmonary symptoms persisting—Calc. c.; Iod.; Kali c.; Sil.; Sul.
Catarrhal symptoms—Ars.; Cepa; Dulc.; *Euphras.;* Gels.; Kali bich.; Merc. s.; *Puls.;* Sabad.; *Sticta.*
Cerebral and convulsive symptoms—Æth.; Apis; *Bell.;* Camph.; Coff.; *Cupr. ac.;* Stram.; Ver. v.; Viola od.; Zinc. m.
Cough, croupy—Acon.; Coff.; Dros.; Euphras.; Gels.; Hep.; Kali bich.; Spong.; Sticta.
Diarrhœa—Ars.; Cinch.; *Ipec.;* Merc. s.; *Puls.;* Ver. a.
Diphtheritic symptoms—Lach.; Merc. cy.
Epistaxis—Acon.; Bry.; Ipec.
Eye symptoms—Ars.; *Euphras.;* Kali bich.; Puls.
Gangrene of mouth, vulva—Ars.; Kali chlor.; Lach.
Insomnia, cough—Calc. c.; Coff.
Laryngitis—Dros.; Gels.; *Kali bich.;* Viola od.
Low fever, toxemia—*Ail.; Ars.;* Bapt.; Carbo v.; Crot.; *Lach.; Mur. ac.; Rhus t.;* Sul.
Malignant types (black or epidemic)—Ail.; *Ars.;* Crot.; Lach.

Otalgia, rheumatoid symptoms—Puls.

Rash, retrocedent, or suppressed—Ant. t.; Apis; *Bry.;* Camph.; *Cupr. ac.; Ipec.; Lach.; Stram.*

Rash, tardy development—Ant. t.; Apis; *Bry.;* Cupr. m.; Dulc.; Gels.; Ipec.; *Stram.;* Sul.; Tub.; Ver. v.; *Zinc. m.*

Sequelæ—Am. c.; *Ars.;* Bry.; Camph.; Coff.; *Cupr. ac.;* Dros.; Kali c.; Merc. c.; Merc. s.; Op.; *Puls.;* Sang.; Sticta; *Sul.; Tub.;* Zinc. m.

SCARLET FEVER—*Acon.; Ail.;* Am. c.; *Apis; Ars.;* Arum; *Asimina; Bell.;* Bry.; Canth.; *Carb. ac.;* Chin. ars.; Commoel.; *Crot.;* Cupr. ac.; Cupr. m.; Dub.; Echin.; Eucal.; *Gels.;* Hep.; Hyos.; Ipec.; Kali chlor.; Kali s.; Lac c.; *Lach.;* Lyc.; Merc. s.; Merc. i. r.; *Mur. ac.;* Op.; Phyt.; *Rhus t.;* Sang.; Sil.; Solan. n.; Spig.; *Stram.;* Tereb.; Zinc. m.

CONCOMITANTS: Adenitis, cervical—Ail.; Am. c.; Asimina; *Bell.; Carb. ac.;* Crot.; Hep.; Lach.; *Merc. i. r.;* Merc. s.; *Rhus t.*

Adenitis, parotid—Am. c.; Phyt.; Rhus t.

Albuminuria and dropsy—Acon.; Am. c.; *Apis;* Apoc.; *Ars.; Canth.;* Colch.; *Dig.; Helleb.;* Hep.; Kali chlor.; Lach.; Nat. s.; *Tereb.* See Nephritis (Urinary System).

Anginosa (sore throat)—Acon.; *Ail.; Apis;* Ars.; *Asimina; Bar. c.; Bell.;* Brom.; Kali perm.; Lac c.; *Lach.;* Merc.; Mur. ac.; *Phyt.;* Rhus t.

Anginosa, ulcerativa—*Am. c.; Apis; Ars.;* Arum; Bar. c.; Crot.; Hep.; *Lach.; Merc. cy.;* Merc. i. r.; *Mur. ac.;* Nit. ac.

Cellulitis—Ail.; Am. c.; *Apis;* Lach.; *Rhus t.*

Chronic tendencies aroused—Calc. c.; Hep.; Rhus t.

Diarrhœa—Ail.; Ars.; Asimina; Phos.; Rhus t.

Edema of glottis—*Apis;* Apium v.; Chin. s.; Merc. c.

Edema of lungs—*Ant. t.;* Can. s.; Phos.; Scilla.

Fever—Acon.; *Apis;* Asimina; Bapt.; *Bell.;* Gels.; Rhus t.

Laryngitis—Brom.; Spong.

Malignant tendency, adynamia—*Ail.;* Am. c.; *Apis; Ars.;* Arum; Bapt.; *Carb. ac.;* Carbo v.; *Crot.;* Cupr. ac.; Echin.; Hydroc. ac.; *Lach.;* Merc. cy.; *Mur. ac.;* Phos.; *Rhus t.;* Tab.; Zinc. m.

Miliary type—*Acon.; Ail.;* Am. c.; Apis; Ars.; Bry.; *Coff.;* Kali ars.; Lach.; Rhus t.

Nervous, convulsive, cerebral symptoms—Æth.; Ail.; Am. c.; Apis; Ars.; *Bell.;* Camph.; *Cupr. ac.;* Cupr. m.; *Hyos.;* Rhus t.; *Stram.;* Sul.; Zinc. m.

Rash, delayed development—Apis; Ars.; *Bry.;* Lach.; Rhus t.; Zinc. m.

Rash, hæmorrhage in—Crot.; *Lach.;* Mur. ac.; Phos.

Rash, livid—*Ail.; Lach.;* Mur. ac.; Solan. n.

Rash, livid, partial, patchy—Ail.

Rash, retrocedent, threatened brain paralysis—*Ail.;* Am. c.; *Cupr. ac.;* Sul.; Tub.; *Zinc. m.*

Rash, retrocession of—Am. c.; *Apis;* Ars.; Bry.; Calc. c.; *Camph.; Cupr. ac.;* Cupr. m.; *Stram.;* Sul.; Ver. a.; *Zinc. m.*

Raw, bloody, itching, painful, surfaces; must pick and bore into them—Arum.

Rheumatic symptoms—Bry.; *Rhus t.;* Spig.

FEVER

SEQUELAE: Adenitis—Brom.; Hep.; Lach.; *Merc. i. r.;* Phyt.
Deafness; sore, bleeding nose—Mur. ac.
Desquamation, in large flakes, several times—Arum.
Ear disorders—Bell.; Carb. ac.; Carbo v.; Gels.; *Hep.;* *Merc. s.;* Sil.; Sul.
Nephritis (post-scarlatinal)—Apis; Ars.; Arum; Canth.; Helleb. See Urinary System.
Nose disorders—Arum; Aur. mur.; Mur. ac.; Sul.
Stomatitis ulcerative—Arum; Mur. ac.
Typhoidal symptoms—Ail.; Arum; *Hyos.;* Lach.; *Rhus t.;* Stram. See Malignant.
Vomiting—Ail.; Asimina; *Bell.;* Cupr. m.

VARICELLA—CHICKENPOX—*Acon.; Ant. t.;* Apis; Bry.; *Dulc.;* Kali m.; Led.; *Merc. s.;* Rhus d.; *Rhus t.;* Urt.; Variol.

VARIOLA—SMALLPOX—Acon.; Am. c.; Anac.; *Ant. t.;* Apis; Ars.; *Bapt.; Bry.; Carb. ac.;* Chin. s.; Cim.; Crot.; Cupr. ac.; Gels.; *Hep.;* Hydr.; *Kali bich.;* Lach.; *Merc. s.;* Millef.; Op.; Phos.; *Rhus t.;* Sarrac.; Sinap.; Sul.; Thuya; *Variol.;* Ver. v.

TYPE—Confluent: Ars.; Hippoz.; *Merc. s.;* Phos.; Sul.; Variol.
Discrete—*Ant. t.; Bapt.;* Bell.; Gels.; Sul.
Hæmorrhage—Ars.; *Crot.; Ham.; Lach.; Phos.;* Nat. nit.; *Sec.;* Sul.
Malignant—Am. c.; Ant. t.; *Ars.;* Bapt.; *Carb. ac.; Crot.;* Lach.; *Mur. ac.;* Phos. ac.; Phos.; *Rhus t.;* Sec.; Sul.; Variol.

COMPLICATIONS—Adenitis: *Merc. i. r.;* Rhus t.
Boils—*Hep.;* Phos.; Sul.
Collapsic symptoms—*Ars.;* Carbo v.; Lach.; *Mur. ac.;* Phos. ac.
Delirium—*Bell.;* Stram.; Ver. v.
Dropsical swellings—*Apis;* Ars.; Canth.
Fever, initial—*Acon.;* Ant. t.; *Bapt.; Bell.;* Gels.; Variol.; *Ver. v.*
Fever suppurative—Acon.; Bell.; Merc.; *Rhus t.*
Ophthalmia—Merc. s.; Sul.
Pulmonary symptoms—Acon.; *Ant. t.;* Bry.; *Phos.;* Sul.; Ver. v.
Repercussion of eruption—Ars.; *Camph.;* Cupr. m.; Sul.; Zinc. m.

FEBRICULA (simple, continued fever)—*Acon.;* Arn.; *Ars.; Bapt.;* Bell.; Bry.; Camph.; *Ferr. p.;* Gels.; Ipec.; Kal.; Merc. s.; Nux v.; Puls.; *Rhus t.*

GASTRIC—Acon.; *Ant. c.; Ars.; Bapt.; Bry.;* Calc. c.; Cinch.; Hydr.; *Ipec.;* Lyc.; Merc. s.; Nux v.; Phos. ac.; *Puls.;* Rhus t.; Santon.

HECTIC—Abrot.; *Acet. ac.;* Acon.; Arg. m.; *Ars.;* Ars. iod.; *Bals. per.; Bapt.;* Calc. c.; Calc. iod.; Calc. s.; Carbo v.; *Chin. ars.; Cinch.; Ferr. m.;* Gels.; *Hep.;* Iod.; Lyc.; Med.; *Merc. s.;* Nit. ac.; Ol. j. as.; Phell.; Phos. ac.; *Phos.;* Pyr.; *Sang.;* Sil.; Stann.; Sul.

INFLAMMATORY—Acon.; Bell.; Bry.

INFLUENZA (grippe)—*Acon.;* Æsc.; Ant. ars.; Ant. iod.; Ant. t.; Arn.; *Ars.; Ars. iod.;* Ars. s. r.; Asclep. t.; *Bapt.; Bell.;* Brom.; *Bry.;* Calc. c.; Camph.; Canchal.; *Carb. ac.;* Card. m.; Caust.; *Cepa; Chin. s.;* Cinch.; Cupr. ars.; Cycl.; Dros.; *Dulc.;* Eryng.; *Eucal.; Eup. perf.;* Euphorbia; Euphras.; Ferr. p.; *Gels.;* Glon.; Glycerin; Gymnocl.;

Influenzin; Iod.; Ipec.; Kali bich.; Kali c.; **Kali iod.**; Kali s.; **Lach.**; Lob. cer.; *Lob. purp.*; Lyc.; Merc. s.; *Nat. sal.*; *Nux v.*; Phos.; Phyt.; Pod.; Psor.; Puls.; Pyr.; Rhus r.; *Rhus t.*; Rumex; Sabad.; Sal. ac.; Sang.; *Sang. n.*; Sarcol. ac.; Senega; Silph.; Spig.; Spong.; *Sticta*; Sul.; *Sul. rub.*; Triost.; Ver. a.

Influenza, debility of—Abrot.; Adon. v.; *Ars. iod.*; *Avena*; Carb. ac.; *Chin. ars.*; Chin. s.; *Cinch.*; Con.; Eup. perf.; Gels.; *Iberis*; Lac c.; Lathyr.; Phos.; Psor.; Sal. ac.; Sarcol. ac.

Influenza, pain remaining—Lycopers.

INTERMITTENT FEVER (ague, malarial)—Acon.; *Alston.*; Am. m.; *Am. picr.*; *Amyl*; Ant. c.; Ant. t.; *Apis*; *Aran.*; Arn.; *Ars.*; Ars. br.; Azadir.; Baja; Bapt.; Bell.; Bolet.; Bry.; Cact.; *Camph. monobr.*; Canchal.; *Caps.*; Carb. ac.; *Carbo v.*; Ceanoth.; *Ced.*; Centaur.; *Chin. ars.*; Chin. mur.; Chin. s.; Chionanth.; Cimex; *Cina*; *Cinch.*; *Corn. fl.*; Crot.; *Echin.*; Elat.; Eucal.; *Eup. perf.*; *Eup. purp.*; Ferr. m.; Ferr. p.; *Gels.*; *Helianth.*; Hep.; Hydr.; *Ign.*; *Ipec.*; *Lach.*; Laur.; Lyc.; Malland.; *Menyanth.*; Methyl. bl.; *Nat. m.*; Nat. s.; Nitrum; *Nux v.*; Op.; Ostrya; Pambot.; Parth.; Petros.; Phell.; *Phos. ac.*; Pod.; Polyp.; Puls.; Rhus t.; Sabad.; Spig.; Sul.; Tarax.; *Tela ar.*; Thuya; Urt.; Verb.; *Ver. a.*; Ver. v.

TYPE—Abuse of quinine, cachexia: Am. m.; Aran.; Arn.; *Ars.*; Ars. iod.; *Calc. ars.*; Carbo v.; Ceanoth.; Chelone; *Chin. ars.*; Eucal.; Eup. perf.; Ferr. m.; *Hydr.*; *Ipec.*; *Lach.*; Malar. off.; Malland.; *Nat. m.*; *Polymia*; Puls.; Sul.; Ver. a.

Chronic, inveterate cases—Abies n.; Am. m.; Aran.; *Ars.*; Ars. br.; Calc. ars.; Canchal.; Carbo v.; Corn. c.; Corn. fl.; *Helianth.*; Ign.; *Nat. m.*, Puls.; Pyr.; Querc.; Tela ar. See Abuse of Quinine.

Congestive—Camph.; *Op.*; Ver. a

Dumb ague—*Ars.*; Ced.; Chelone; Chin. s.; *Gels.*; *Ipec.*; Malland.; Nux v.

Impure cases, in non-malarial regions—Ipec.; Nux v.

Nervo-hysterical persons—Aran.; Cocc.; Ign.; Tar. h.

Pernicious cases—*Ars.*; Camph.; Chin. hydrobr.; *Chin. s.*; Crot.; *Ver. a.*

Recent cases—Acon.; Aran.; Ars.; Chin. s.; Cinch.; Ipec.; Tar. h.

Stages, partial, irregular—Aran.; *Ars.*; Cact.; *Carbo v.*; Eup. perf.; Eup. purp.; *Ipec.*; Nat. m.

Stages, regular, well defined—*Chin. s.*; Cinch.

CHILL: OCCURRENCE—TYPE—Afternoon: 1 P. M. daily: Ferr. p.

Afternoon, 2 P. M.—Calc. c.; Lach.

Afternoon, 3 P. M.—Apis; Chin. s.

Afternoon, 3-4 P. M.—Lyc.; Thuya

Afternoon, 4-8 P. M.—Lyc.

Afternoon, 4 P. M.—Æsc.

Afternoon, 5 P. M.—Cinch.

Afternoon, late, evening, night—Aran.; Bolet.; Ced.; Ipec.; Petrol.; Tar. h.

Anticipating—*Chin. s.*; Cinch.; Nux v.

Forenoon—Cinch.; Formal.; Nux v.

Hebdomadal—Cinch.

FEVER

Midday—Gels.
Midnight—Ars.; Nux v.
Mingled, with heat—Ant. t.; Apis; *Ars.;* Cinch.; *Nux v.;* Tar. h.; Ver.
a. See Chilliness.
Morning—Chin. s.
Morning, 1-2 A. M.—Ars.
3 A. M.—Thuya.
4 A. M.—Ferr. m.
5 A. M.—Cinch.
6-7 A. M.—Pod.
7-9 A. M.; at noon following day—Eup. perf.
9-11 A. M.—Bapt.; Bolet.; Mag. s.; *Nat. m.;* Wyeth.
11 A. M. and 11 P. M.—Cact.
Periodical—Aran.; A**r**s.; Bolet.; Cact.; *Ced.; Chin. s.;* Cina; Cinch.; *Eucal.;* Ipec.
Periodical, every 7 or 14 days; never at night—Cinch.
Periodical, every spring—Carbo v.; *Lach.;* Sul.
Prolonged—Aran.; Bolet.; Cact.; Canchal.; *Caps.; Chin. s.;* Eup. purp.; Ipec.; Menyanth.; Nat. m.; *Nux v.;* Plumb.; Pod.; Puls.; Pyr.; *Sabad.; Ver. a.;* Ver. v.
Quartan—Baja; *Chin. s.;* Cinch.; Helleb.
Quotidian—Ars.; Bolet.; Chin. s.; Ign.; Lob. infl.; Nitrum; Nux v.; Plumb.; Tar. h.
Slight—Ars.; Azar.; Carbo v.; Cina; Cinch.; Eup. perf.; Eup. purp.; *Ipec.*
Tertian—Calc. c.; *Chin. s.;* Cinch.; Ipec.; Lyc.

LOCATION—Abdomen:—*Apis; Calc. c.;* Menyanth.
Back—Apis; Bolet.; Conv.; Dulc.; *Eup. perf.;* Eup. purp.; *Gels.; Lach.;* Mag. s.; *Nat. m.;* Pyr.
Back, between scapulæ—Am. m.; *Caps.;* Pyr.; Sep.
Back, dorsal region—Eup. perf.; Lach.
Back, lumbar region—Eup. perf.; Nat. m.
Breast—Cinch.
Feet—Gels.; Lach.; Nat. m.; Sabad.
Hand, left—Carbo v.; Nux m.
Nose, tip of—Menyanth.
Thigh—Rhus t.; *Thuya.*

CONCOMITANTS—Anxiety, exhaustion, hypochrondriacal ideas, mental confusion, vertigo, tension of stomach, no relief from warmth—Nux. v.
Anxiety, palpitation, nausea, canine hunger, pressing pain in hypogastrium, congestive headache, distended painful veins—Chin. s.; Cinch.
Blue lips, nails—Eup. perf.; Eup. purp.; Menyanth.; Nat. m.; *Nux v.;* Ver. a.
Cardiac region, pain in—Cact.; Tar. h.
Collapsic symptoms; skin icy cold; pallor, cold sweat on forehead—Ver. a.
Cough, dry, teasing—Rhus t.
Diarrhœa—Caps.; Elat.; Ver. a.
Face and hands bloated—Lyc.

Face red—Ferr. m.; Ign.; Nux v.

Forehead, cold sweat on—Ipec.; Ver. a.

Gastric symptoms—Ant. c.; Arg n.; Ars.; Bolet.; Canchal.; Eup. perf.; Ipec.; Lyc.; Nux v.; Puls.

Hands, feel dead—Apis; Nux v.

Headache—Bolet.; Chin. s.; Cinch.; Conv.; Eup. perf.; Eup. purp.; Nat. m.; Nux v.

Headache, vertigo, yawning, stretching, general discomfort—Ars.

Heart symptoms, enterrhagia—Cact.

Hæmorrhoidal symptoms—Caps.

Hyperæsthesia—Ign.

Hyperæsthesia of spine—Chin. s.

Loquacity—Pod.

Nausea before chill—Ipec.

No two chills alike—Puls.

Pain in bones, limbs, soreness—Aran.; Bolet.; Canchal.; Caps.; Chin. s.; Cinch.; Eup. perf.; Eup. purp.; Formal.; Gels.; Nat. m.; Nux v.; Phell.

Pains, in joints—Cinch.

Pains, in knees, ankles, wrists, hypogastrium—Pod.

Restlessness—Ars.; Eup. perf.; Rhus t.

Sighing—Ign.

Thirst—Apis; Ars.; Caps.; Carbo v.; Cina; Cinch.; Conv.; Dulc.; Eup. perf.; Ign.; Nat. m.; Nux v.; Nyctanth.; Ver. a.; Wyeth.

Thirst, after chill—Ars.

Thirst, before chill—Chin. s.; Cinch.; Eup. perf.; Gels.; Menyanth.; Nyctanth.

Thirstlessness—Chin. s.; Cimex; Cinch.; Eup. purp.; Gels.; Nat. m.

Vehemence, rage, preceding—Cimex.

Vomiting, bilious—Eup. perf.; Ipec.; Lyc.; Nat. m.; Nux v.; Nyxtanth.

Yawning, somnolency, accelerated breathing—Nat. m.

Yawning, stretching—Ars.; Elat.; Lyc.; Nux v.

MODALITIES—Aggravated from acids: Lach.

Aggravated, from drink—Caps.

Aggravated, from exposure—Nux v.

Aggravated, from exposure, lying down—Cimex.

Aggravated, from motion—Apis.

Aggravated, from warmth—Apis; Canchal.; Chin. s.; Cinch.; Nux v.

Ameliorated from warmth—Caps.; Ign.

FEVER PAROXYSM—Afternoon, glowing heat, in face, hands, feet—Azadir.

Anxiety, restlessness, lipothymia, oppression—Ars.

Backache—Eup. perf.; Nat. m.

Chill, intermingled—Ars.; Chin. s.; Cinch.; Nux v.; Tar. h

Chilliness, after heat of face—Calc. c.

Congestion of head, drowsiness, costiveness, rectal and vesical tenesmus; chilled from uncovering—Nux v.

Delirium—Ars.; Pod.; Sabad.

Desire to be covered—Nux v.

Desire to be uncovered—Ign.; Ipec.

FEVER

Diarrhœa—Ant. c.; *Ipec.*; Ver. a.
Dyspnœa—Apis; Ars.; Conv.; Ipec.
Face, hot, feet cold—Cinch.; Petrol.
Face pale, insomnia—Ant. t.
Gastric symptoms—Ars.; Eup. perf.; *Ipec.*; Nux v.; Puls.
Hands warm, face cold—Cina.
Headache—Apis; Ars.; *Bell.*; Ced.; Cinch.; Eup. perf.; *Nat. m.*; Nux v.; Wyeth.
Headache, yellowish tongue, nausea, faintness in epigastrium, costiveness—Polyp.
Heat, burning—Apis; *Ars.*; Caps.; *Eup. perf.*; Formal.; *Ipec.*; Lach.; Nux v.
Hunger—Cina; Cinch.
Hydroa—Hep.; *Nat. m.*; Rhus t.
Lachrymation—Sabad.
Loquacity—Pod.
Mental confusion—Formal.
Nettle rash—Apis; Ign.; Rhus t.
Night—Ars.
Pain, colicky—Cina.
Pain, in head, back, limbs—Nux v.
Pain in the vertebræ, dorsal—Chin. s.
Pain, spasms, paralysis—Ars.
Paroysms, frequent, transient—Carbo v.
Prolonged heat—Ars.; Bolet.; Ign.
Prostration, fainting, cold sweat—Ver. a.
Pupils, immobile, pain in abdomen, sopor, tension throughout body—Op.
Sighing—Ign.
Sleepiness—Ant. t.; Apis; Corn. fl.; Gels.; Op.
Thirst—*Ars.*; Chin. s.; Cinch.; *Eup. perf.*; Nat. m.; Nux v.; Nyxtanth.; Op.; Ver. a.
Thirstlessness—Apis; Caps.; Chin. s.; Cimex; Cinch.; *Ign.*; Nat. m.; Puls.; Sabad.; Wyeth.
Tongue clean—Ars.; Cina.
Trembling of limbs, slow pulse—Chin. s.; Op.
Unconsciousness—Nat. m.
Vomiting—Ars.; Cim.; Cina; Eup. perf.; *Ipec.*; Ver. a.
Sweat—Ant. c.; Aran.; Azadir.; *Bolet.*; Bry.; *Chin. s.*; Cimex.; Cina; *Cinch.*; Conv.; Eup. perf.; Lyc.; Nat. m.; Nux v.; Op.; *Phos. ac.*; *Ver. a.*; Wyeth. See Sweat.
Sweat scanty or absent—*Apis;* Ars.; Carbo v.; Eup. perf.; Nux v.
Sweat, with coldness—Plumb.
Sweat, with covering up—Cinch.; Hep.
Sweat, with relief of pains—Nat. m.
Sweat, with sleep—Cinch.; Con.; Pod.; Thuya.
Sweat, with thirst—Ars.; *Chin. s.;* Nux v.

APYREXIA—Adynamia, gastro-intestinal pains, sallow face, dropsical swellings, enlarged liver and spleen, restlessness, sleeplessness, spams, diarœa, albur inaria—Ars.

FEVER

Adynamia hydræmia, chlorosis—Cinch.; Puls.

Adynamia, morning headache, depression, costiveness, amenorrhœa, enlarged liver, desire for quiet, sallow face—Nat. m.

Gastro-enteric symptoms—Cinch.; Hydr.; *Ipec.*; *Nux v.*; Puls.

Jaundice—Ars.; Bolet.; Card. m.; Nux v.; Pod.

Nervous symptoms—Gels.

Pains—Led.

Relapses from dietetic errors—Ipec.

Spleen enlarged—Ars.; *Ceanoth.*; **Chin. s.**; **Cinch.**; **Ferr. m.**; **Nat. m.**

Thirst—Ars.; Cimex; Ign.

Vomiting—Ipec.

Vomiting, abdominal griping, pain in back, loins—Ver. a.

LOW FEVERS—*Ail.*; *Arn.*; *Ars.*; Bapt.; Camph.; Cocc.; Crot.; Eup. ar.; *Lach.*; *Mur. ac.*; Nit. sp. d.; *Phos. ac.*; Phos.; Pyr.; *Rhus t.*; Tereb.; Urt. See Typhus.

MEDITERRANEAN FEVER—Bapt.; Bry.; *Colch.*; Merc. s.; Rhus t.

PUERPERAL FEVER—Acon.; Pyr.; Ver. a. See Female Sexual System.

REFLEX, from local irritation—*Cham.*; *Cina*; Gels.; Ign.; Ipec.; Merc.; Nux v.; Sang.; Sul.; Ver. v.

RELAPSING FEVER—Acon.; Ars.; Bapt.; Bry.; Cim.; *Eucal.*; Eup. perf.; Rhus t.

REMITTENT FEVER—Acon.; Ant. c.; *Ars.*; Bell.; Bry.; **Chin. s.**; *Cina*; Cinch.; Crot.; *Gels.*; Hyos.; *Ipec.*; Merc. s.; Nit. ac.; Nux v.; Nyctanth.; Puls.; Rhus t.; Sul.

Remittent, bilious, low—Bry.; Crot.; Eup. perf.; Gels.; Ipec.; Merc. d.; Nyctanth.; Pod.

Remittent, in children—Ant. c.; Cina; *Gels.*; Lept.; Puls.; Santon.

SEPTIC FEVER—Ail.; Anthrac.; *Ars.*; Crot.; Echin.; *Pyr.*; Ver. v. See Pyemia (Generalities).

SYNOCHAL FEVER—Acon.; Bapt.; Bell.

TRAUMATIC FEVER—Acon.; *Arn.*; Ars.; Cinch.; Lach. See Injuries (Generalities).

TYPHUS FEVER—Acet. ac.; Agar.; *Ail.*; Apis; *Ars.*; Arum; *Bapt.*; *Bell.*; Calc. c.; *Camph.*; Chin. s.; Cinch.; Crot.; Helleb.; *Hyos.*; Kreos.; *Lach.*; Merc. i. r.; Merc. s.; Merc. v.; Mur. ac.; Nit. ac.; Op.; Phos. ac.; Phos.; Pyr.; *Rhus t.*; Stram.; Ver. a.

Cellulitis, adenitis (salivary)—Bell.; Chin. s.; *Merc. i. r.*

Nervous symptoms—Agar.; Bell.; *Hyos.*; Lach.; Op.; Phos. ac.; Phos.; *Stram.*

Toxemia—Ars.; *Mur. ac.*; Pyr.; Rhus t. See Typhoid.

URETHRAL FEVER—Acon.; Ars.; Chin. ars.; Cinch.; *Gels.*; Hep.; Lach.; Phos.; Rhus t.; Sil.

WORM FEVER—Bell.; *Cina*; *Merc. s.*; Santon.; Sil.; Spig.; Stann.

YELLOW FEVER—*Acon.*; Ant. t.; Apis; Arg. n.; *Ars.*; Bell.; *Bry.*; Cadm. s.; Camph.; Canth.; Carb. ac.; Carbo v.; Chin. s.; Cinch.; Coff.; Crot. casc.; Crot.; Cupr.; Gels.; Guaco; *Hyos.*; Ipec.; *Lach.*; Merc.; Op.; *Phos.*; Plumb.; Sab.; Sul. ac.; Tereb.; Ver. a.

NERVOUS SYSTEM

BRAIN: EPILEPSY—(grand mal): *Absinth.;* Æth.; *Agar.;* Am. br.; Amyl; *Arg. n.;* Art. v.; Ars.; Aster.; Atrop.; Aur. br.; Avena; *Bell.;* Bor. Bufo; *Calc. ars.; Calc. c.;* Calc. p.; Camph.; Can. ind.; *Caust.;* Cic. mac.; *Cic.;* Cim.; Cocc.; Con.; Cupr. ac.; *Cupr. m.;* Ferr. cy.; Ferr. p.; Gels.; Glon.; Hep.; *Hydroc. ac.; Hyos.; Ign.;* Illic.; Indigo; Irid.; *Kali br.;* Kali cy.; Kali m.; Kali p.; *Lach.;* Mag. c.; Mag. p.; Meli.; Methyl. bl.; Nit. ac.; *Nux v.; Œnanthe;* Op.; Œstrus; Passifl.; Phos.; Picrot.; Plumb. m.; Psor.; *Salam.;* Santor.; Sec.; *Sil., Solan. c.;* Spiræa; *Stram.;* Strych.; *Sul.;* Sumb.; Tar. h.; Tub.; Val.; *Verb.;* Viscum; Zinc. cy.; Zinc. v.; Zizia.

CAUSE—CONCOMITANTS—Aura absent: Zinc. v.

Aura absent; several fits, close together—Art. v.

Aura begins, as painful spot, between shoulders, or dizziness, flashes of heat, from abdomen to head—Indigo.

Aura begins, as sensation of mouse running up limb; heat from stomach; visual or aural disturbance—*Bell.;* Calc. c.; Sul.

Aura begins, in brain, as a wavy sensation—Cim.

Aura begins, in knees, ascends to hypogastrium—Cupr. m.

Aura begins, in left arm—Sil.

Aura begins, in solar plexus—Bufo; Calc. c.; Nux v.; Sil.

Aura begins, in stomach or genitals—Bufo.

Aura begins, in upper or lower limbs—Lyc.

Aura descends—Calc. c.

Aura felt, in heart region—Calc. ars.

During full moon; nocturnal—Calc. c.

During new moon; nocturnal—Caust.; Cupr. m.; Kali br.; Sil.

During sleep—Bufo; Cupr.; Lach.; Op.; Sil.

Followed by deep sleep—Æth.; Hyos.; Kali br.; Lach.; *Op.*

Followed by hiccough—Cic.

Followed by nausea, vomiting—Bell.

Followed by prostration—Æth.; *Chin. ars.;* Cic.; Hydroc. ac.; Sec.; Sil.; Strych.; Sul.

Followed by rage, automatic impulse—Op.

Followed by restlessness—Cupr. m.

Followed by tumor—Arg. n.; Cic.

From eruptions, suppressed—Agar.; Calc. c.; Cupr. m.; Psor.; *Sul.*

From fright, emotional causes—*Arg. n.;* Art. v.; Bufo; Calc. c.; Cham.; Hyos.; Ign.; Sil.; Stram.

From hysteria—Asaf.; Cocc.; Cupr. m.; Hyos.; *Ign.;* Mosch.; Œnanthe; Solan. c.; Sumb.; Tar. h.; Zinc. v.

From injury—Con.; Cupr. m.; Meli.; Nat. s.

From jealousy—Lach.

From menstrual disturbances—Arg. n.; Bufo; Caul.; Caust.; Ced.; *Cim.;* Cupr. m.; Kali br.; *Millef.;* Œnanthe; Puls.; Solan. c.

From pregnancy—Œnanthe.

From scleroses; brain tumors—Plumb. m.
From sexual disturbances—Art. v.; *Bufo;* Calc. c.; Plat.; Stann.; **Sul.**
From syphilis, tubercular—Kali br.
From taking cold; nocturnal; worse right side—Caust.
From valvular disease—Calc. ars.
From vital drains; onanism—Lach.
From wet exposure—Cupr. m.
From worms—Cic.; Cina; Indigo; Sant.; Sil.; Stann.; Sul.; Teucr.
In children—Æth.; Art. v.; *Bell.;* Bufo; Calc. c.; Cham.; Cupr. m.; Ign.; Sil.; Sul.

Periodical seizures—Ars.; Cupr. m.
Preceded, by cold on left side of body—Sil.
Preceded, by dilated pupils—Arg. n.
Preceded, by gastric flatulency—*Arg. n.;* Nux v.; Psor.; Sul.
Preceded, by irritability, rambling—Bufo.
Preceded, by malaise—Cic.
Preceded, by memory, confused—Lach.
Preceded, by palpitation, vertigo—Lach.
Preceded, by sudden cry—Cupr. m.; Hydroc. ac.
Preceded, by tremblings, twitchings—Absinth.; Aster.
Preceded, by vesicular eruption—Cic.
Recent cases—*Bell.;* Caust.; Cupr. m.; *Hydroc. ac.; Ign.;* Op.; Plumb. m.; Stram.
Recurrent, several times daily—Art. v.; Cic.
Status epilepticus—Acon.; Æth.; *Bell.;* Cocc.; Œnanthe; Plumb.; Zinc. m.
With consciousness—Ign.
With face red, thumbs clenched, jaws locked, foam at mouth, eyes turned downwards, pupils fixed, dilated, pulse small, quick, hard—Æth.
With paralysis following—*Caust.;* Plumb. m.; Sec.
With swelling of stomach, screaming, unconsciousness, trismus, distorted limbs; frequent during night; recurrent tendency—Cic.
With vertigo (epileptic)—Arg. n.; Bell.; Calc. c.; Caust.; Cocc.; Cupr.; Hydroc. ac.; Nit. ac.; Op.; Sil.; Stram.

PARALYSIS—**Remedies in general:** Absinth.; *Acon.;* Agar.; Alum.; Angust.; Aragal.; Arg. iod.; *Arg. n.;* Ars. iod.; Asaf.; Astrag.; Aur.; Bar. ac.; Bar. c.; Bar. m.; *Bell.;* Calc. caust.; Calend.; Can. ind.; Carbon. oxy.; Carbon. s.; *Caust.;* Chin. s.; Cic.; *Cocc.;* Colch.; Con.; *Cupr. m.; Dulc.;* Gels.; Graph.; Grind.; *Guaco;* Helod.; Hydroc. ac.; Hyos.; *Hyper.;* Ign.; Iris fl.; Kali br.; *Kali c.;* Kali iod.; Kali p.; Lach.; Latrod. has.; Lol. tem.; Merc. c.; Nat. m.; Nux v.; *Oleand.;* Op.; Ox. ac.; Oxytr.; *Phos.;* Physal.; Physost.; Picr. ac.; Plat.; Plectranth.; Plumb. ac.; *Plumb. iod.;* Plumb. m.; *Rhus t.;* Stann.; Staph.; Sec.; Strych. ferr. cit.; Sul.; Tab.; Thall.; Ver. a.; Xanth.; Zinc. m.; Zinc. p.

TYPE—**Agitans:**—*Agar.;* Ars.; *Aur. sul.;* Avena; Bufo; *Camph. monobr.;* Can. ind.; Cocaine; Cocc.; Con.; *Dub.;* Gels.; Helod.; *Hyos.; Hyosc. hydrobr.;* Kali br.; Lathyr.; Lolium; Mag. p.; Mang. ac.; Merc. s.; *Merc.;* Nicotine; Phos.; Physos.; *Plumb.;* Scutel.; Tab.; Tar. h.; Zinc cy.; Zinc. vicr.

NERVOUS SYSTEM

Ascending spinal—Alum.; Bar. ac.; *Con.;* Gels.; Lathyr.; Led.; *Ox. ac.;* Phos.; Picr. ac.; Sec. See Spine.

Bulbar—Guaco; Mang. ox.; Plumb. m.

General of insane—Ant. c.; Ars.; Aur.; Bell.; *Can. ind.;* Caust.; Hyos.; Kali br.; Kali iod.; Merc. c.; Nat. iod.; Nux v.; Op.; *Phos.;* Physost.; Plumb.; Stram.; Sul.; Ver. a.

Gradually appearing—Caust.

HEMIPLEGIA—Ambra; *Arn.;* Ars.; *Aur. m.;* Bapt.; *Bar c.;* Bothrops; Carbon. s.; *Caust.;* Chenop.; *Cocc.;* Cur.; Elaps; Hydroc. ac.; Irid.; *Lach.;* Nux v.; *Oleand.;* Phos.; Physost.; Picr. ac.; *Rhus t.;* Sec.; Stann.; Strych.; Ver. v.; Vipera; Xanth.

Hemiplegia, left—Ambra; *Arn.;* Bapt.; Bell.; Cocc.; Cupr. ars.; *Lach.;* Lyc.; Physost.; Ver. v.; Xanth.

Hemiplegia, right—Bell.; *Caust ,* Chenop.; Cur.; Elaps; Irid.

Hysterical—Acon.; Arg. n.; Asaf.; Cocc.; *Ign.;* Phos.; *Tar. h.*

Infantile (poliomyelitis anterior)—*Acon.;* Æth.; Bell.; *Calc. c.; Caust.,* Chrom. s.; *Gels.;* Lathyrus; Nux v.; Phos.; *Plumb. m.;* Rhus t.; Sec.; Sul. See Spine.

Labio-glosso-pharyngeal—Anac.; Bar. c.; *Bell.;* Caust.; Cocc.; Con.; Gels.; Mang. binox.; Nux v.; Oleand.; *Plumb.*

Landry's paralysis—Aconitin.; Con.; Lyssin.

Lead—*Alumen;* Caust.; Cupr.; Kali icd.; Nux v.; Op.; Plumb.; Sul. ac.

LOCALIZED, in ankles, in afternoon—Cham.

Localized, in arms, hands—Cupr. m.; Thyr.

Localized, in bladder—Caust.; Nux v.

Localized, in chest—Gels.

Localized, in eye muscles—Caust.; Con.; *Gels.;* Phos.; Physost.; Rhus t.

Localized, in face (Bell's palsy)—Acon.; *Am. phos.;* Bar. c.; Bell.; Caust.; Cur.; Gels.; Graph.; *Kali chlor.;* Nat. m.; Rhus t.; Solan. ves.; *Zinc. picr.*

Localized, in feet at night—Cham.

Localized, in forearm (wrist drop)—Cur.; Ferr. ac.; Plumb. ac.; Plumb. m.; Ruta Sil.

Localized, in motor nerves—Cur.; Cystisin; Gels.; *Ox. ac.;* Phos.; Physost.; Xanth.

Localized, in neck—Cocc.

Localized, in sensory nerves—*Cocaine;* Laburn.; Plat.

Localized, in sphincters—Ars.; *Caust.;* Gels.; Naja; Nux v.; Phos.; Physost.

Localized, in throat, vocal cords—Bell.; Bothrops; Canth.; *Caust.;* Cocaine; Cocc.; *Gels.;* Kali p.; Ox. ac.; Plumb.

PARAPLEGIA—Acon.; Alum.; Anhal.; *Arg. n.;* Arn.; Ars.; *Bell.;* Caul.; *Caust.;* Cocc.; Con.; *Cupr. m.;* Cur.; Dulc.; Formica; Geis.; *Hyper.;* Kali iod.; *Kali tart.;* Kal.; Lach.; *Lathyr.;* Latrod. has.; Mang. ac.; Merc. c.; Nux v.; Ox. ac.; Phos.; Physost.; Picr. ac.; *Plumb. ac.;* Rhus t.; Sec.; Strych.; Thall.; Thyr.

Paraplegia, hysterical—*Cocc.;* Con.; Cupr.; *Ign.;* Nux v.; Plumb.; *Tar. h.*

Paraplegia, spastic—Gels.; Hyper.; *Lathyr.;* Nux v.; Plectranth.; Sec. See Sclerosis (Spine).

POST-DIPHTHERITIC—*Arg. n.;* Aur. mur.; Avena; Botul.; *Caust.;* Cocc.; Con.; *Diph.; Gels.;* Kali iod.; *Lach.;* Nat. m.; Nux v.; Phos.; Phyt.; Plumb. ac.; Plumb. m.; Rhod.; Rhus t.; Sec.

Pseudo-hypertrophic—Cur.; *Phos.;* Thyr.

Rheumatic—*Caust.;* Dulc.; Lathyr.; Phos.; *Rhus t.;* Sul.

Spinal origin—Alum.; Bell.; Can. ind.; *Con.;* Irid.; *Lathyr.;* Phos.; Physost.; *Picr. ac.;* Plumb.; Xanth.

PETIT MAL—*Art. v.;* Bell.; Caust.; Phos.; *Zinc. cy.*

SLEEP—DROWSINESS: Æth.; Am. c.; Ant. c.; *Ant. t.; Apis;* Apoc.; Arn.; Aur.; *Aur. mur.;* Bapt.; Bar. mur., Can. ind.; *Carbon. ox.;* Carbon. s.; Caust.; *Cinch.; Clem.;* Coca; Cocc.; Cornus fl.; *Cycl.;* Dub.; Ferr. p.; *Gels.; Helleb.;* Helon.; Hydroc. ac.; Hyper.; *Indol;* Kali br.; Kali c.; Laburn.; Lathyrus; Linar.; Lob. purp.; *Lupul.; Morph.;* Naja; *Nux m.; Op.;* Phos. ac.; Phos.; Pyr.; Rhus t.; Rosmar.; Sarcol. ac.; *Scrophul.;* Selen.; Senec.; Sulphon.; Thea; Zinc. m.

Drowsiness, after meals—Bism.; *Cinch.;* Graph.; Kali c.; *Lyc.;* Nux m.; Nux v.; Paul.; *Phos.;* Puls.; Scrophui. See Indigestion (Stomach).

Drowsiness, during day—*Agar.;* Alum.; *Am. c.;* Anac.; *Ant. c.; Calc. c.;* Calc. p.; Can. s.; Carbo v.; *Cinch.;* Cinnab.; *Colch.;* Euphras.; Graph.; Indol; Kali c.; Lupul.; *Lyc.;* Mag. m.; Merc. c.; Merc.; *Nat. c.;* Nat. m.; Nux m.; Op.; *Phos.; Sep.;* Sil.; Spong.; Staph.; *Sul.;* Tub.

Drowsiness, during day, wakeful at P. M.—*Abies n.;* Cinnab.; Colch.; Graph.; Lach.; *Lyc.;* Merc.; Phos. ac.; Sil.; Staph.; Thea. See Insomnia.

Drowsiness, in A. M. and forenoon—Alum.; Anac.; *Am. c.;* Bism.; Carbo v.; Nat. m.; *Nux v.;* Petrol.; Zinc. m.

Drowsiness, in early evening—Calc. c.; Mang. ac.; *Nux v.;* Phos.; Puls.; Sep.; *Sul.*

Drowsiness, in evening, while sitting reading—Nux v.

Drowsiness, yet cannot sleep—Ambra; *Apis; Bell.;* Can. ind.; Caust.; *Cham.;* Coca; Coff.; Cupr. m.; Ferr. m.; *Gels.;* Lach.; Morph.; *Op.;* Sil.; Stram.

INCUBUS (nightmare)—Acon.; Am. c.; Arn.; *Aur. br.;* Bapt.; *Can. ind.;* Chloral; *Cina;* Cyprip.; Daphne; *Kali br.;* Kali p.; Op.; *Nux v.;* Nit. ac.; Pæonia; Pariet.; Phos.; Ptel.; Scutel.; Solan. n.; Sul.

INSOMNIA (sleeplessness)—Remedies in general: Absinth.; *Acon.;* Agar.; Alfal.; Alum.; Ambra; Am. c.; *Anac.;* Ant. c.; Apis; Apomorph.; Aquil.; Arn.; Arg. n.; *Ars.; Aur.;* Avena; Bept.; *Bell.;* But. ac.; Cact.; Caffeine; *Calc. c.;* Camph.; Camph. monobr.; *Can. ind.;* Caul.; *Cham.;* Chin. s.; Chloral; Chrysanth.; *Cim.; Cinch.; Coca;* Cocaine; *Cocc.;* Coff.; Col.; *Cyprip.;* Daphne; Dipod.; *Gels.; Hyos.;* Hyosc. hydrob.; *Ign.;* Iod.; *Kali br.;* Kali p.; Lecith.; Lil. t.; *Lupul.;* Lyssin; Mag. p.; Merc.; *Nux v.; Op.; Passifl.;* Phos.; Picr. ac.; *Puls.;* Selen.; *Scutel.;* Stann.; Staph.; Sulphon.; *Sul.; Sumb.;* Stram.; Tela ar.; Thea; Val.; Xanth.; Yohimb.; Zinc. p.; Zinc. v.

NERVOUS SYSTEM

CAUSES—OCCURRENCE—Abdominal disturbances:—Ant. t.; **Cupr. m.**
Aching in bones—Daphne.
Aching in legs, yet cannot keep them still—Med.
Aching in muscles, too much exhausted, tired out—Helon.
Alcoholic, drug, habits—Ars.; Avena; Can. ind.; *Cim.*; Gels.; *Hyos.*: Nux v.; Op.; Sec.; Stram.; *Sumb.*
Anxiety, driving him out of bed, aggravated after midnight—Ars.
Aortic disease—Crat.
Arterial pulsations—Acon.; *Bell.*; *Cact.*; *Glon.*; Sec.; Selen.; Sul.; **Thea.**
Banqueting, late suppers—Puls.
Bed feels too hard, cannot lie on it—Arn.; Bry.; *Pyr.*
Bed feels to hot, unable to lie on it—Op
Chest oppression—Physal.
Chronic nicotinism—Plant.
Coffee, abuse—Cham.; *Nux v.*
Coldness of body—*Acon.*; Ambra; Camph.; Carbo v.; Cistus; *Ver. a.*
Coldness of knees—Apis; *Carbo v.*
Cramps—Argen. mex.; Col.; Cupr. m.
Delirium—Acon.; *Bell.*; Cact.; Calc. c.; *Can. ind.*; Gels.; *Hyos.*; Kali br.; Phos.; *Stram.*; Ver. a. See Mind.
Dentition—Bell.; Bor.; *Cham.*; Coff.; Cyprip. See Teeth.
Menopause; women with prolapsus uteri or uterine irritation—Senec.
Mouth and throat sore—Arum; Merc.
Multiple neuritis—Con.
Weaning of child—Bell.

DREAMS—Accidents, falling from height, etc.: Arn.; Bell.; Calc. c.; *Dig.*; Lyc.; Nit. ac.; Sil.; Ver. a.
Animals, snakes—Arg. n.; Daphne; Lac c.; Op.; Ran. sc.
Anxious—Abies n.; *Acon.*; Ambra; Anac.; *Apis*; *Arg. n.*; Arn.; *Ars.*; *Bell.*; Bry.; Calc. c.; Caust.; Can. ind.; Canth.; *Cham.*; Cinch.; Euphorb.; dath.; Ferr. p.; Graph.; Ign.; Kali c.; Lyc.; Nat. m.; Nit. ac.; Nux v.; Oxytr.; Puls.; *Rhus t.*; Sec.; Sep.; *Sil.*; Staph.; *Sul.*; Zinc. m.
Business matters he forgets during day—Selen.
Confused—Alum.; Cinch.; Glon.; Helleb.; Hydroc. ac.; Phos.
Continues, after being apparently awake—Calc. c.; Cinch.; Nat. m.
Death, or dead persons—Arn.; *Ars.*; Calc. c.; Can. ind.; Crot. casc.; Crot ; Elaps; *Lach.*; Nit. ac.; Ran. sc.
Dreamful—Alum.; Brom.; Con.; Hyos.; Ign.; Lyc.; Nit. ac.; Phos.; Sep.
Drinking—Ars.; Med.; Nat. m.; Phos.
Exertion of body, toil, business—Apis; Ars.; Bapt.; *Bry.*; Nat. m.; **Nux v.**; Phos.; Puls.; *Rhus t.*; Selen.; Staph.
Fantastic, pleasant—Op.
Fires, flames, lightning—Bell.; Euphras.; Lach.; Phos.
Flying through air—Apis; *Rhus gl.*; Sticta.
Forgotten matters—Selen.
Happy dreams—Sul.
Hemorrhage—Phos.

NERVOUS SYSTEM

Horrible—Adon. v.; *Arg. n.*; *Aur.*; Bapt.; *Bell.*; *Cact.*; Calc. c.; **Can. ind.**; Castor.; *Cham.*; *Cinch.*; *Colch.*; Eupion; Graph.; *Hyos.*; **Kali br.**; Kali c.; *Lil. t.*; Lyc.; *Merc. c.*; Nux v.; Op.; Phos.; Psor.; **Puls.**; Ran. sc.; *Rhus t.*; Sec.; Sep.; Stram.; *Sul.*; Thea; *Zinc. m.*

Images bewildering, figures—Bell.; Hyos.

Lascivious—Arg. n.; Ars.; *Can. ind.*; Canth.; *Cob.*; *Diosc.*; Ham.; **Hyos.**; Ign.; Nat. m.; Nit. ac.; Op.; Phos. ac.; *Phos.*; Sil.; *Staph.*; **Thuya**; Ustil.; Ver. v. See Emissions (Male Sexual System).

Laughs, during—Alum.; Caust.; Hyos.; Lyc.

Robbers—Bell.; *Nat. m.*; Psor.; Ver. a.

Vivid—Agar.; *Arg. n.*; Brom.; *Can. ind.*; Cenchris; Cham.; Coff.; Daphne; Diosc.; Hydroc. ac.; *Hyos.*; Indol; Iod.; Mang. ac.; Nat. m.; Petrol.; Phos.; Puls.; Pyr.; *Sul.*; Tub.; Ver. v. See Anxious.

Dry mouth—Apis; Calc. c.; Caust.; Lach.; *Nux m.*; *Paris*; Puls.; Tar. h.

Emotional causes (grief, worry, anxiety, over-excitement, nervousness)—Absinth.; *Acon.*; *Alfal.*; *Ambra*; Am. val.; Aur.; Bry.; *Can. ind.*; Cham.; Chin. ars.; Chloral; *Cim.*; Coca; *Coff.*; Col.; *Gels.*; *Hyos.*; Hyosc. hydrobr.; *Ign.*; *Kali br.*; Mosch.; Nat. m.; *Nux v.*; Op.; Passifl.; Phos. ac.; Plat.; Senec.; *Sep.*; *Stram.*; Sul.; Thea; Val.; Zinc. v.

Exhaustion, debility, over-exertion of mind or body—Arn.; Ars.; Avena; Can. ind.; Chin. s.; Cnloral; *Cim.*; *Cinch.*; Coca; *Cocc.*; *Colch.*; Dipod.; *Gels.*; Hyos.; Kali br.; *Nux v.*; Passifl.; Piscidia; *Phos.*

Eyes, half open, during—Bell.; *Cham.*; Hyos.; Ipec.; *Op.*; Pod.; *Zinc. m.* See Eyes.

Every second night—Cinch.; Lach.

Fears suffering from mental and physical exhaustion on waking—Lach.; Syph.

Formication in calves and feet—Sul.

Grinding of teeth—*Bell.*; Cic.; *Cina*; Helleb.; Kali br.; *Pod.*; *Santon.*; Spig.; Zinc. m.

Heat in general—Acon.; Arn.; Bar. c.; *Bell.*; Bor.; Caust.; **Cham.**; Hep.; Kali br.; Mag. m.; Meph.; Op.; *Sanic.*; Sil.; *Sul.*

Hunger—*Abies n.*; Apium gr.; *Cina*; Ign.; Lyc.; *Psor.*; Sul.

Hyperacute senses—Asar.; *Bell.*; Calad.; Calc. br.; **Cham.**; **Cocc.**; **Coff.**; Ign.; Nux v.; *Op.*; Tar. h.; Val.; Zinc. v.

In aged—*Acon.*; Ars.; Op.; Passifl.; *Phos.*

In children—*Absinth.*; *Acon.*; Ars.; *Bell.*; Calc. br.; *Cham.*; Cina; Cyprip.; Hyos.; Kali br.; *Passifl.*; Phos.; Puls.; Sul.

Itching—Acon.; *Agar.*; Alum.; Psor.; Teucr.; Sul.; Val.

Itching of anus—*Aloe*; Alum.; Coff.; Ign.; *Indigo.*

Itching of scrotum—Urt.

Mental activity, flow of ideas—Acon.; Apium gr.; Apis; Bry.; Calc. c.; *Cinch.*; *Cocc.*; *Coff.*; Gels.; Hep.; *Hyos.*; Lyc.; Meph.; *Nux v.*; Puls.; Sep.; Ver. a.; Yohimb.

Moaning, whining, during—Ant. t.; Arn.; Ars.; Aur.; *Bapt.*; *Bell.*; Carbo v.; *Cham.*; Cic.; Cupr. ac.; *Gels.*; *Helleb.*; Hyos.; Kali br.; Lach.; Lyc.; *Mur. ac.*; Nat. m.; Nit. ac.; *Op.*; *Pod.*; Puls.; Rhus t.; Ver. a.

Mouth, open—Merc.; Rhus t.; Samb.

Nose stopped up must breathe per orem—Am. c.; Lyc.; Nux v.; Samb.

NERVOUS SYSTEM

Pains—Ars.; Can. ind.; *Cham.;* Col.; Mag. m.; Merc.; Passifl.; Puls.; Sinap. n.

Palpitation—Acon.; Alum.: Am. c.; *Cact.; Icd.;* Lil. t.; Lycop.; Rhus t.; Sep.

Picks at bed clothes, during—Op.

POSITION—Must lie in knee-chest position: Med.

Must lie on back—Am. c.; *Ars.;* Cina.

Must lie on back with thighs drawn upon abdomen, hands above head; disposition to uncover lower limbs—Plat.

Must lie on belly—Acet. ac.; Am. c.

Must lie on hands and knees—Cina.

Must lie with hands over head—Ars.; Nux v.; Plat.; Puls.; Sul.; Ver. a.

Must lie with hands under head—Acon.; Ars.; Bell.; Cinch.; Col.; Plat.

Must lie with legs apart—Cham.; Plat.

Must lie with legs crossed—Rhod.

Must lie with one leg drawn up, other stretched out—Stann.

Must move or fidget feet constantly—Zinc. m.

Must stretch violently for hours—Amyl; Plumb. m.

RESTLESSNESS, awakens frequently (catnaps)—Bar. c.; *Calc. c.;* Dig.; Ferr. m.; *Ign.;* Lyc.; Nit. ac.; Nux v.; *Phos.;* Plat.; Sarcol. ac.; *Selen.;* Sil.; Stram.; *Sul.*

Restlessness, during—Acon.; *Agar.;* Alum.; Ambra; Apis; Apoc.; Arg. n.; Arn.; *Ars.; Bapt.; Bell.;* Bry.; Calc. c.; *Can. ind.;* Castor.; Caust.; *Cham.;* Cina; *Cim.;* Cinch.; Coca; Cocaine; *Coff.;* Eup. perf.; Gels.; Glon.; Graph.; *Hyos.; Ign.; Jal.;* Kali br.; Lac d.; Lyc.; Menthol; Nit. ac.; Nux v.; Passifl.; Psor.; Ptel.; Puls.; Radium; *Rhus t.;* Ruta; Santon.; Sarcol. ac.; *Scutel.; Stram.;* Stront. c.; Sulphon.; *Sul.;* Tar. h.; Thea; Zinc. m.

Restlessness, kicks off clothes—Hep.; Op.; Sanic.; *Sul.*

Restlessness, rolling head—Apis; *Bell.;* Helleb.; *Pod.;* Zinc. m.

Sexual causes—Can. ind.; *Canth.;* Kali br.; *Raph.* See Sexual System.

Shocks, electric-like, on falling asleep—Ant. t.; *Cupr. m.;* Ign.; Ipec.

Shrieks, screams, awakens frightened—Ant. c.; Ant. t.; *Apis;* Aur.; *Bell.;* Bor.; *Bry.;* Cham.; *Cic.; Cina;* Cinch.; *Cupr. ac.;* Cyprip.; Dig.; *Helleb.; Hyos.;* Ign.; Iodof.; Kali br.; Lyc.; Nux m.; Phos.; Psor.; Puls.; Spong.; *Stram.;* Tub.; Zinc. m.

Singing, during—Bell.; Croc.; Phos. ac.

Singing on awakening—Sul.

Skin dry—Thea.

Sleepless, in evening, before midnight—*Ars.;* Lach.; *Lil. t.;* Nat. m.; Nux v.; Phos. ac.; Phos.; *Puls.; Rhus t.;* Selen.; Thuya.

Sleepless, after 2-3 A. M.—Apium gr.: Bapt.; Bellis; Bry.; *Calc. c.;* Cinch.; *Coff.;* Gels.; *Kali c.;* Kal.; Nat. c.; Nat. m.; Nit. ac.; *Nux v.; Selen.;* Sep.

Snoring, during—Cinch.; Laur.; *Op.;* Sil.; Stram.; Tub.; *Zinc. m.*

Soporous, deep, heavy sleep—Am. c.; Ant. c.; *Apis;* Arn.; Cinch.; *Cupr. m.; Helleb.;* Hyos.; Kali br.; Lact. v.; Laur.; Lonic.; Lupul.; *Morph.;* Naja; Nux m.; *Op.; Phos. ac.;* Piscidia; Pod.; Rhus t.; Sec.; *Stram.;* Sul.

Spasmodic symptoms, during (jerkings, twitchings, startings)—*Acon.*; *Æth.*; *Agar.*; Ambra; Ant. c.; *Apis*; Ars.; *Bell.*; Bor.; Brom.; Bry.; Calc. c.; Carbo v.; Castor.; Caust.; *Cham.*; *Cina*; Cinch.; *Cupr. ac.*; Daphne; Helleb.; *Hyos.*; *Ign.*; Kali c.; *Lyc.*; Morph.; Nit. ac.; Nux v.; Passifl.; Phos.; Samb.; Sil.; *Stram.*; *Sul.*; Tar. h.; Val.; *Zinc. m.*; Zizia.

Suddenly wide awake—Sul.

Suffocation, loss of breath, on falling asleep—*Am. c.*; Ars.; *Cur.*; Graph.; *Grind.*; Kali iod.; *Lach.*; Lac c.; *Merc. pr. rub.*; Morph.; Naja; Op.; *Samb.*; *Spong.*; Stront. c.; Sul.; Teucr.

Sweating, during—*Æth.*; *Calc. c.*; *Cham.*; *Cinch.*; Op.; Phos. ac.; *Psor.*; Sil.; Ver. a. See Night Sweats (Fever).

Talking, during—Bar. c.; Bell.; Bry.; Carbo v.; *Cina*; **Graph.**; *Helleb.*; Hyos.; Kali c.; Lyc.; Sep.; Sil.; Sul.; *Zinc. m.*

Tea, abuse—Camph. monobr.; Cinch.; Nux v.; Puls.

Tobacco—Gels.

Unrefreshing, awakens wretched—Alum.; *Ant. c.*; Apium gr.; *Ars.*; Brom.; Bry.; *Cinch.*; Cob.; *Con.*; Dig.; Ferr. m.; Graph.; *Hep.*; *Lach.*; Lil. t.; *Lyc.*; Mag. c.; Merc. c.; Myr.; *Nux v.*; Op.; Phos.; Ptel.; *Puls.*; Rhus t.; Sarcol. ac.; Sep.; *Sul.*; Syph.; Thuya; Thymol; Tub.; Zinc. m.

Walking, during (somnambulism)—Art. v.; *Bry.*; *Kali br.*; Pæonia; Sil. See Mind.

Yawning, stretching, limbs—Acon.; *Agar.*; *Amyl*; Ant. t.; Arn.; Asar.; Calc. c.; Carls.; Castor.; Cepa; *Chel.*; *Cina*; Cinch.; Coca; Crot.; Cupr. ac.; Elat.; Euphras.; **Gels.**; Hep.; Hydroc. ac.; *Ign.*; Kali c.; Lyc.; Mang.; Morph.; *Nat. m.*; *Nux v.*; Plumb. m.; *Rhus t.*; Sec.; *Sil.*; *Sul.*

GENERALITIES—ADYNAMIA (general weakness, debility): Abies c.; *Acet. ac.*; Adren.; *Æth.*; *Ail.*; *Alet.*; Alston.; Ambra; Am. c.; *Anac.*; *Ant. t.*; *Antipyr.*; Apis; *Arg. n.*; *Arn.*; *Ars. iod.*; *A.e.*; Asaf.; Aur.; Aur. mur.; *Avena*; *Bals. per.*; *Bapt.*; Bar. c.; Bellis; Bry.; *Calc. c.*; Calc. hypophos.; *Calc. p.*; *Camph.*; Can. s.; Canth.; Carb. ac.; Carbo v.; Caul.; *Caust.*; *Chin. ars.*; *Chin. s.*; *Cinch.*; Coca; *Cocc.*; *Colch.*; Con.; Crat.; Crot.; *Cupr. m.*; *Cur.*; *Dig.*; Dipod.; Diph.; Dulc.; Echin.; *Ferr. cit. et chin.*; *Ferr. m.*; Ferr. mur.; Ferr. p.; Ferr. picr.; *Gels.*; Helleb.; *Helon.*; Hep.; Hydr.; Hyos.; Ign.; *Iod.*; Ipec.; *Irid.*; Iris; Kali br.; *Kali c.*; Kali iod.; *Kali p.*; Lac c.; Lach.; Lact. ac.; Lil. t.; Lith. c.; Lith. chlor.; Lob. purp.; *Lyc.*; Mag. m.; Mag. p.; Meli.; Merc. c.; *Merc. cy.*; Merc. i. r.; Merc.; Murex; *Mur. ac.*; *Nat. c.*; *Nat. m.*; Nat. sal.; *Nit. ac.*; Nux v.; Op.; Ornithog.; Ox. ac.; *Phos. ac.*; *Phos.*; Physost.; Phyt.; *Picr. ac.*; Plumb. m.; *Psor.*; Rhus t.; *Ruta*; Sang.; Sarcol. ac.; Sec.; *Selen.*; Sep.; *Sil.*; Solid.; Spong.; Stann.; Stroph.; Strych.; Sulphon.; *Sul. ac.*; Sul.; *Tab.*; Tanac.; Tereb.; **Thea**; *Thuya*; Tub.; Uran. n.; Val.; *Ver. a.*; *Zinc. ars.*; Zinc. m.; *Zinc. p.*; Zinc. picr.

Adynamia, collapse—Acetan.; Acon.; *Ant. t.*; Arn.; *Ars.*; *Camph.*; Carb. ac.; *Carbo v.*; Colch.; Crat.; Crot.; Cupr. ac.; *Dig.*; Diph.; Hydroc. ac.; Laur.; Lob. infl.; Lob. purp.; Med.; Merc. cy.; *Morph.*; Mur. ac.; Nicot.; Op.; Pelias; Phos.; *Sec.*; Sul. ac.; *Tab.*; *Ver. a.*; *Zinc. m.*

Adynamia, afebrile—Ars.; Bapt.; Carbo v.; Cinch.

Adynamia, from acute diseases, mental strain—Abrot.; Alet.; *Alston.;* Anac.; Avena; *Calc. p.;* Carbo an.; *Carbo v.; Chin. ars.; Cinch.;* Coca; Cocc.; Colch.; Cupr. m.; Cur.; Dig.; Fluor. ac.; Gels.; *Helon.; Irid.;* Kali ferocy.; *Kali p.;* Lathyr.; Lob. purp.; Macroz.; Nat. sal.; Nux v.; *Phos. ac.; Phos.;* Picr. ac.; *Psor.;* Selen.; Sil.; Staph.; Strych. p.; Sul. ac.; Zinc. ars.

Adynamia, from anæsthetics; surgical shock—Acet. ac.; Hyper.

Adynamia, from depressing emotions—Calc. p.; Ign.; *Phos. ac.*

Adynamia, from diphtheria, stupor, cold limbs, low temperature, pulse rapid, weak—Diph.

Adynamia, from drugging—Carbo v.; Helon.; Nux v.

Adynamia, from excesses, vital drains—Agar.; Anac.; *Calc. p.; Carbo v.;* Caust.; Chin. s.; *Cinch.;* Corn. fl.; Cur.; Gins.; Kali c.; Nat. m.; *Phos. ac.; Phos.;* Selen.; Stroph.

Adynamia, from heat of summer—Ant. c.; *Gels.;* Lach.; *Nat. c.;* Selen.

Adynamia, from inebriety, bilious or remittent fevers—Eup. perf.

Adynamia, from injuries—*Acet. ac.;* Arn.; Calend.; Carbo an.; *Sul. ac.*

Adynamia, from jaundice—Ferr. picr.; Picr. ac.; Tarax.

Adynamia, from loss of sleep—*Cocc.;* Colch.; Nux v.

Adynamia, from menses; talking even fatigues—Alum.

Adynamia, from prolapsus, protracted illness, defective nutrition—Alet.; Helon.

Adynamia, from some deep-seated dyscrasia—Abrot.; Eup. perf.; Hydr.; Iod.; Nat. m.; Nit. ac.; *Psor.;* Sul. ac.; *Sul.;* Tub.; Zinc. m.

Adynamia, hysterical—Nat. m.

Adynamia, in aged—Bar. c.; Carbo v.; *Con.;* Cur.; Eup. perf.; Glycerin; Nit. ac.; Nux m.; *Phos.;* Selen.

Adynamia, nervous—Ambra; Anac.; **Cur.;** Gels.; Kali br.; *Phos. ac.; Phos.;* Rhus t.; Sil.; Staph.; Zinc. m.

Adynamia, with erethism—Ars.; Cinch.; Sil.

Adynamia, with frequent, faint spells during day—Murex; Nux m.; Sep.; *Sul.;* Zinc. m.

Adynamia, without erethism—Phos. ac.

Adynamia, without organic lesion or cause—Psor.

Adynamia, worse from ascending—Calc. c.; Iod.; Sarcol. ac.

Adynamia, worse from descending—Stann.

Adynamia, worse from exertion, walking—*Ars.;* Bry.; Calc. c.; Caust.; Cycl.; Ferr. m.; Lac d.; Merc. v.; Nat. c.; Nux m.; Phos. ac.; *Picr. ac.;* Sarcol. ac.; Sep.; Rhus d.; *Stann.;* Thea; Ver. a.

Adynamia, worse in A. M.—*Acal.;* Bar. m.; Bry.; Calc. c.; Con.; Corn. c.; Lac c.; Lach.; Lyc.; *Nat. m.; Nit. ac.;* Phos; Psor.; Sep.; Stann.; Sul ; Tub.

Adynamia, worse in women worn out from hard mental and physical work, or, from indolence and luxury—Helon.

ALCOHOLISM—Acon.; *Agar.;* Ant. t.; *Apoc.;* Apomorph.; Ars.; Asar.; Aur.; *Avena;* Bell.; Bism.; Calc. ars.; Calc. c.; Can. ind.; *Caps.;* Chimaph.; *Cim.; Cinch. rub.;* Cocc.; Crot.; *Cupr. ars.; Gels.;* Hydr.; *Hyos.;* Ichthy.; Kali iod.; Lach.; Led.; Lob. infl.; Lupul.; *Nux v.; Op.;* Phos.; Psor.; *Querc.; Ran. b.;* Stercul.; Stram.; Stroph.; *Strych.*

m.; *Sul. ac.*; *Sul.*; Syph.; Tub.; Zinc. m. See Chronic Gastritis (Stomach).

Alcoholism, hereditary tendency—Asar.; Psor.; Sul.; Sul. ac.; Syph.; Tub.

Alcoholism: to overcome habit—Angel.; Bufo; *Cinch. rub.*; Querc.; Stercul.; Sul. ac.; Sul.

ATHETOSES—Lathyr.; Strych.

BERI-BERI—*Elat.*; Lathyr.; Rhus t.

CHOREA (St. Vitus dance)—Absinth.; *Agar.*; Agaricin; *Arg. n.*; *Ars.*; Art. v.; Asaf.; Aster.; Avena; *Bell.*; Bufo; *Calc. c.*; Calc. p.; *Caust.*; Cham.; Chloral; Cic.; *Cim.*; *Cina*; Cocaine; *Cocc.*; Con.; Croc.; *Cupr. ac.*; *Cupr. m.*; Eup. ar.; Ferr. cy.; *Ferr. red.*; Hippom.; Hyos.; Ign.; Iod.; Kali br.; Latrod.; *Mag. p.*; *Myg.*; *Nat. m.*; Nux v.; Op.; Phos.; Physost.; Pictrox.; Psor.; Puls.; Santon.; *Scutel.*; Sep.; Solan.; *Spig.*; *Stram.*; *Strych.*; Strych. p.; Sulphon.; Sul.; *Sumb.*; Tanac.; *Tar. h.*; Thasp.; Thuya; Ver. v.; Viscum; Zinc. ars; *Zinc. br.*; Zinc. cy.; *Zinc. m.*; Zinc. v.

CAUSE—OCCURRENCE—Anemia: Ars.; Cinch.; *Ferr. red.*; Hyos.

Corybantism—Bell.; Hyos.; Stram.

Eruptions, suppressed—Zinc. m.

Fright—Calc. c.; Cim.; Cupr.; Ign.; Laur.; Nat. m.; Stram.; Tar. h.; Zinc. m.

Nervous disturbances—*Asaf.*; Bell.; *Cim.*; *Cocc.*; Croc.; Gels.; Hyos.; Ign.; Kali br.; Op.; Sticta; Stram.

Onanism—Agar.; Calc. c.; Cinch.

Pubertic—Asaf.; Caul.; *Cim.*; Ign.; Puls.

Reflex, from dentition, pregnancy—Bell.

Relief, from music, sight of bright colors—Tar. h.

Relief, from sleep—*Agar.*; Cupr. m.

Rheumatism—Caust.; *Cim.*; Spig.

Rhythmical motions—Agar.; Caust.; Cham.; Cim.; Lyc.; *Tar. h.*

Scrofulous, tubercular—Calc. c.; *Calc. p.*; Caust.; *Iod.*; Phos.; Psor.

Worms—Asaf.; Calc. c.; *Cina*; Santon.; *Spig.*

Worse, at approach of thunder storm—*Agar.*

Worse, during sleep—Tar. h.; Zizia.

Worse, face—*Caust.*; Cic.; Cupr.; Hyos.; *Myg.*; Nat. m.; Zinc. m.

Worse, from cold, noise, light, emotions—Ign.

Worse, in spasms, partial, changing constantly—Stram.

Worse, left arm, right leg—Agar.; Cim.

Worse, right arm, left leg—Tar. h.

Worse, right side, tongue affected, staccato speech—Caust.

Worse unilaterally—Calc. c.

CONVULSIONS—Remedies in general: *Absinth.*; Acon.; *Æth.*; Agar.; Alum. sil.; Antipyr.; Arg. n.; Ars.; *Art. v.*; Atrop.; *Bell.*; Camph.; Can. ind.; Canth.; Carb. ac.; Castor.; *Cham.*; Chloroform; Cic. mac.; Cic.; Cim.; *Cina*; Cocc.; Cupr. ac.; *Cupr. ars.*; *Cupr. m.*; Dulc.; Euonym.; Gels.; *Glon.*; Helleb.; *Hydroc. ac.*; Hyper.; *Hyos.*; Ign.; Illic.; Iris fl.; *Kali br.*; *Laburn.*; Laur.; Lonic.; Lyssin; *Mag. p.*; Morph.; Nat. s.; Nux v.; *Œnanthe*; Op.; Ox. ac.; Passifl.; Phos.;

NERVOUS SYSTEM

Physost.; Plat.; Plumb. chrom.; Plumb.; *Santon.; Sil.; Solan. c.;* Solan. n.; *Stram.;* Strych.; Sul.; Upas art.; *Upas t.;* Ver. a.; Ver. v.; Verbena; Zinc. m.; Zinc. oxy.; Zinc. s.

CAUSE AND TYPE—Anger affects mother's milk—Cham.; Nux v.

Apoplectic; in inebriates; hemorrhagic or broken down systems—Crot.

Carphopedal—Cupr. ac.; Ign.

Cataleptic—Cic.; *Mosch.*

Cerebral sclerosis or tumor—Plumb. m.

Children, infants, from reflex causes, dentition—Absinth.; Acon.; *Æth.;* Art. v.; *Bell.;* Calc. c.; *Camph. monobr.;* Caust.; *Cham.;* Chloral; *Cic.;* Cina; Cocc.; *Cupr. m.;* Cyprip.; Glon.; Helleb.; Hydroc. ac.; *Hyos.; Ign.; Kali br.;* Kreos.; Laur.; *Mag. p.;* Meli.; Mosch.; Nux v.; *Œnanthe;* Op.; *Santon.;* Scutel.; Stann.; Stram.; Zinc. m.; Zinc. sul. See Worms.

Clonic—Antipyr.; Apis; Bell.; Camph.; Carb. ac.; Cina; *Cupr. m.;* Gels.; Hyos.; Ign.; *Nicot.;* Plumb. m.; Upas art.

Crying; approach of strangers—Op.

Exanthemata—Acon.; *Bell.;* Glon.; Thea; Ver. v.

Exanthemata, suppressed—Apis; Ars.; *Cupr. m.;* Op.; Stram.; *Zinc. m.;* Zinc. s.

Foot sweat, suppressed—Sil.

Fright—Acon.; Cupr. m.; Hyos.; *Ign.;* Op.; Stram.

Fright, anger or emotional disturbance in nervous, plethoric persons—Kali br.

Grief, or any emotional excitement—Ign.

Hypochondriacal—Mosch.; Stann.

Hysterical—Absinth.; Asaf.; Asar.; Castor.; Caul.; Cim.; Cocc.; *Gels.;* Hydroc. ac.; *Hyos.;* Ign.; Kali p.; *Mosch.;* Nux m.; Plat.; Stann.; Tar. h.

Injury—Cic.; Hyper.

Isolated groups of muscles—Acon.; *Cic.;* Cina; Cupr.; Ign.; Nux v.; Stram.; Strych.

Labor—Acon.; Bell.; Cic.; Cupr. m.; Glon.; Hyos.; Ign.; Kali br.; Œnanthe; Stram.; Ver. v. See Female Sexual System.

Meals followed by vomiting, shrieking, spasms—Hyos.

Menses suppressed—Gels.; Millef. See Female Sexual System.

Metastases, from other organs—Apis; Cupr.; Zinc. m.

Prodromata—Acon.; Bell.; Cham.; Ipec.; Op.

Reflected light from water, mirror—Bell.; Lyssin; *Stram.*

Sleep, loss of—Cocc.

Spinal origin—Acon.; *Cic.;* Cim.; Hydroc. ac.; *Hyper.;* Ign.; Nux v.; Œnanthe; *Physost.*

Terminal stage—Op.; Plumb.; Zinc. m.

Tonic: Opisthotonos—Apis; *Cic.;* Cina; Cupr. ac.; Cupr. m.; *Hydroc. ac.; Ign.;* Ipec.; Mag. p.; Mosch., Nicot.; *Nux v.;* Physost.; Plat.; Plumb. m.; Solan. c.; Solan. n.; Stram.; *Strych.;* Upas; Ver. v.

Uremic—Carb. ac.; Cic.; Cupr. ars.; Glon.; Helleb.; Hydroc. ac.; Kali br.; Merc. c.; Œnanthe; Op.; Plumb.; Piloc.; Urt. See Urinary System.

Uterine disease—Cim.

NERVOUS SYSTEM

Vaccination—Sil.; Thuya.
Whooping cough—Cupr. m.; Kali br.
Worms—Cic.; *Cina;* Hyos.; *Indigo;* Kali br.; Sabad.; *Santon.;* Spig.; Tanac.

CONCOMITANTS—Beginning in face; unilateral; shallow breathing—Cina
Beginning in fingers, toes, radiates all over—Cupr. m.
Bladder, chest, intestines, striated muscles, cheifly involved; drowsiness, rigid limbs; sudden onset; head hot, feet cold—Bell.
Calves of legs; clenched thumbs; cyanosis—Cupr. m.
Chorea-like—Sticta.
Convulsive jerkings, of limbs and head—Bufo; Cham.; *Cic.;* Hyos.
Cyanosis—Cupr. ac.; Hydroc. ac.
Extremities cold—Bell.; Helleb.; Hydroc. ac.; *Nicot.;* Œnanthe.
Eyes half open, upturned; breathing, deep, stertorous—Op.
Eyes turned downward—Æth.
Fever; skin hot, dry; child frets, screams, gnaws its fists; twitching of single muscles—Acon.
Followed by collapse—Nicot.
Followed by deep sleep—Cupr. ac.; *Op.;* Zinc. m.
Followed by paresis—Acon.; *Elaps;* Lonic.; Plumb. m.
Followed by restlessness—Cupr. m.
No cerebral congestion—Ign.
No fever—Ign.; *Mag. p.;* Zinc. m.
Pale face; rolling eyes; gnashing teeth—Zinc. m.
Preceded, by gastro-intestinal symptoms—Æth.; Cupr. ars.
Preceded, by restlessness—Arg. n.; Hyos.
Shrieks, screams, before, and during—*Apis;* Cina; Cupr. m.; *Helleb.,* Op.
Terrible pains—Plumb. chrom.
Tremor, spasm of glottis, febrile paroxysm—Ign.
Twitchings, cramps, gastro-enteric symptoms—Nux v.
Twitchings of single muscles or groups, especially of upper body—Stram.
Twitchings over entire body—Cic.; Hyos.
Twitchings worse upper body, continue after delivery—Cic.
Violent vomiting—Æth.; Upas.
With consciousness—Cina; Nux v.; Plat.: *Stram.;* Strych.
Without consciousness—Bell.; Calc. c.; *Cic.;* Cupr. ac.; Cupr. ars.; *Cupr. m.;* Glon.; Hydroc. ac.; *Hyos.; Mosch.;* Œnanthe; *Op.;* Stram.
Worse from touch, motion, noise—Cic.; Ign.; Lyssin; Nux v.; Stram.; Strych.

DEFICIENT REACTION—Ambra; Am. c.; Calc. c.; Camph.; Caps.; *Carbo v.;* Carbon. s.; Caust.; Cic.; Cupr. m.; Helleb.; Iod.; *Laur.;* Nat. ars.; Nat. s.; *Op.; Psor.;* Radium; *Sul.; Tub.;* Val.; X-ray.; *Zinc. m.*

EXOPHTHALMIC GOITRE (Basedow's disease)—Amyl; Antipyr.; Ars.; Ars. iod.; Aur.; *Bell.;* Brom.; *Cact.;* Calc. c.; Colch.; Ephedra; Ferr. iod.; *Ferr. m.;* Ferr. p.; Fucus; *Glon.; Iod.; Lycop.;* Nat. m.; *Piloc.;* Pineal gl. ext.; Spart. s.; Spong.; *Thyr.*

MAL-DE-MER (seasickness)—Amyl; *Apomorph.;* Aqua mar.; Arn.; Cercum ox.; Chloral; *Cocc.*; Cucurb.; Glon.; Kali br.; Kali p.; Morph.; Nicot.; *Nux v.*; Petrol.; Staph.; *Tab.*; Thea; *Ther.* See Vomiting (Stomach).

MORPHINISM—Apomorph.; *Avena;* Can. ind.; Cim.; Ipec.; Lob. infl.; *Macrot.*; Nat. p.; Passifl.

MORVAN'S DISEASE—Aur.; *Aur. mur.*; Bar. mur.; Lach.; *Sec.*; Sil.; Thuya.

NERVOUS AFFECTIONS—Of cigar makers: Gels.
  Nervous affections of girls, at puberty—Caul.; *Cim.*
  Nervous affections of onanists—*Gels.*; Kali p.
  Nervous affections, from excessive delicacy and sensitiveness of the senses—Cupr.
  Nervous affections, from suppressed discharges, in the psoric—Asaf.; Merc. s.
  Nervous affections, from tobacco, in sedentary persons; dyspepsia, right prosopalgia—Sep.
  Nervous affections, from worms—*Cina;* Psor.; Sabad.

NERVOUSNESS—In general: Abies n.; Absinth.; *Acon.;* Alfal.; *Ambra;* Amyl; *Anac.;* Aquil.; Arn.; Ars.; *Asaf.;* Asar.; Avena; *Camph. mon. obr.; Cham.; Cim.; Coca;* Cocaine; *Coff.;* Cupr.; Cyprip.; Eup. ar.; *Gels.;* Glycerin, Gossyp.; Hedeoma; *Hyos.; Ign.;* Indol; *Kali br.;* Kali c.; *Kali p.; Mag. p.;* Niccol.; Nux m.; *Nux v.;* Oophor.; Op.; *Phos.;* Puls.; Santon.; Senec.; Sil.; *Stram.; Strych.;* Thea; *Ther.; Triost.; Val.;* Val. am.; Xanth.; *Zinc. m.* See Moods (Mind).
  Nervousness, hypersensitiveness—*Acon.;* Ambra; Am. val.; Angust.; Ant. c.; *Apis;* Aquil.; *Asaf.; Asar.;* Arn.; Atrop.; Aur.; *Bell.; Bor.;* Bry.; Calad.; Calc. sil.; Camph.; Can. ind.; Canth.; *Cham.;* Chin. mur.; Chrysanth.; *Cim.; Cinch.; Cocc.; Coff.; Colch.;* Con.; Cupr.; Ferr. m.; Glon.; *Hep.;* Hyper.; *Ign.;* Justicia; Kali br.; Kali c.; Kali p.; Lac c.; *Lach.;* Lyssin; Mag. p.; Med.; Morph.; Nit. ac.; Nux m.; *Nux v.;* Op.; *Phos.;* Phos. hydr.; Plat.; Puls.; Sep.; *Sil.;* Spig.; Stann.; *Staph.; Strych.; Sul.;* Tar. h.; Teucr.; *Ther.; Tub.;* Zinc. m.
  Nervousness, hypersensitiveness, to cold air, drafts—Acetan.; *Acon.;* Agar.; Allium s.; Ambra; Am. c.; Anac.; Ant. c.; Bac.; Bad.; *Bar. c.;* Bell.; Bor.; *Calc. c.; Calc. sil.;* Calend.; Camph.; *Caps.;* Carbo v.; Caust.; Cham.; *Cinch.; Cistus;* Con.; Cupr. m.; *Graph.;* Ham.; *Hep.; Kali c.;* Kali m.; Mag. m.; *Merc.; Mez.;* Nat. c.; *Nat. m.;* Nit .ac.; Nit. sp. d.; *Nux v.;* Physost.; *Psor.;* Ran. b.; Rhus t.; *Rumex;* Selen.; Sep.; *Sil.;* Strych.; Sul.; *Tub.*
  Nervousness, hypersensitive, to least pain—*Acon.;* Arn.; Aur. m.; Aur. mur.; Cact.; *Cham.; Cinch.; Coff.; Colch.;* Hep.; Hyper.; *Ign.;* Kali p.; Latrod.; Mag. p.; Med.; Meli.; Mez.; *Morph.;* Mosch.; Nit. ac.; Nux m.; *Nux v.;* Phos.; Ran. s.; Val.; Zinc. v.
  Nervousness, tremulousness, faintness—Abies c.; Ant. t.; Aquil.; *Arg. n.;* Arn.; Ars.; Asar.; *Caul.; Caust.;* Cim.; *Cinch.;* Cocc.; *Gels.;* Hyos.; Lach.; Latrod.; *Med.; Mosch.;* Murex; Nux m.; *Nux v.;* Puls.; Raph.; Sep.; Strych.; Sul.; *Sul. ac.;* Tar. h.; *Val.;* Zinc. m.

NEURASTHENIA (nervous prostration)—**Remedies in general:** Agn.; Alfal.;

Anac.; Anhal.; *Arg. n.;* Asaf.; Asar.; *Avena; Calc. c.; Calc. p.;* **Can. ind.;** *Cinch.;* Cob.; Coca; *Cocc.;* Cupr. m.; Cur.; *Fluor. ac.; Gels.;* Glycerin; Graph.; *Helon.;* Hyper.; Ign.; *Kali hypoph.; Kali p.;* Lach.; Lathyrus; *Lecith.;* Lob. purp; Mosch.; *Nat. m.; Nux v.; Onosm; Ox. ac.; Phos.;* Physost.; *Picr. ac.;* Pip. m.; Plumb.; Puls.; Sacchar. of.; Sarcol. ac.; *Scutel.; Sil.;* Stann.; Staph.; *Strych. p.;* Tar. h.; Tub.; Turnera; Verbena; Xanth.; *Zinc. m.; Zinc. p.; Zinc. picr.* See Adynamia.

Cerebral symptoms, unable to apply mind—*Anac.;* Aur.; Calc. c.; *Gels.; Kali p.;* Nux v.; *Phos. ac.;* Phos.; *Picr. ac.;* Sil.; Scutel. See Brain Fag (Mind).

From long, concentrated grief—Ign.

Gastric form—*Anac.;* Gent.; Nux v.; Strych. p.

Hypochondriacal tendency—*Aur.;* Coca; Con.; Kali br.; Nat. m.; Sul.

In females—Alet.; Aloe; Ambra; Ars.; Aur.; Bellis; Calc. c.; Cinch.; *Cocc.; Epiph.;* Ferr.; *Helon.;* Hyos.; *Ign.;* Iod.; Kali p.; *Lach.;* Lyc.; *Mag. c.;* Mag. p.; Phos. ac.; *Picr. ac.;* Puls.; *Sep.;* Sil.; Sul.; Zinc. v.

Insomnia—Ambra; Ars.; Aur.; *Cim.;* Coff.; Nux v.; Zinc. p. See Sleep.

Sexual origin—Agar.; *Agn.; Anac.;* Calad.; *Cinch.;* Coca; Gels.; Graph. Lecith.; Lyc.; Nat. m.; Nux v.; Onosm.; *Phos. ac.;* Phos.; *Picr. ac.* Plat.; *Sabal;* Selen.; Sep.; *Staph.;* Thymol; Turnera; Zinc. picr. See Female Sexual System.

NEUROSES—**Of children:** Passifl.

Neuroses of professional men—Gels.

TREMORS—**Twitchings, trembling:** Absinth.; *Agar.;* Agaricin; Anac.; *Ant. t.;* Apis; *Arg. n.;* Ars.; Bell.; Camph.; Can. ind.; *Caust.;* Cham.; Cic.; *Cim.;* Cinch.; *Cocc.;* Cod.; Ferr. p.; *Gels.;* Hep.; Hyos.; *Hyosc. hydrobr.; Ign.;* Iod.; Kali br.; Kali p.; *Lach.;* Latrod.; Lith. chlor. Lyc.; *Med.; Merc. s.;* Morph.; Mosch.; Nat. m.; *Nux v.;* Op.; Oxytr.; *Phos. ac.;* Phos.; Physost.; Plumb.; Rhus t.; Sabad.; Scutel.; Sil.; *Stram.;* Sul.; Tar. h.; Tub.; Val.; Veratrin; Ver. v.; Viscum alb.; *Zinc. m.;* Zinc. p.

Alcoholic—*Ant. t.;* Cocaine; Cocc.; *Nux v.*

Disseminated sclerosis—Acet. ac.; Ars.; *Hyos. hydrobr.*

From smoking—Kali c.; Nit. ac.; Sep.

Senile—Avena; Can. ind.; Cocaine; *Phos.*

NERVES: NEURITIS (Inflammation)—*Acon.;* Æsc.; Ananth.; Arg. n.; *Arn.; Ars.; Bell.;* Bellis; Benzin. din.; Berb. v.; *Carbon. s.; Caust.; Ced.; Cepa;* Cim.; Con.; Ferr. p.; *Gels.; Hyper.;* Merc.; Nux v.; Pareira; Phos. ac.; Phos.; *Plumb.;* Plumb. phos.; Rhus t.; Sang.; *Stann.,* Stront. c.; Strych.; *Thall.;* Urt.; Zinc. p.

TYPE—**Alcoholic:** Nux v.; Strych.

Diphtheritic—Gels.

Of anterior crural—Pareira.

Of circumflex—Sang.

Of lesser sciatic—Æsc.

Of lumbo-sacral plexus—Berb. **v.**

NERVOUS SYSTEM 947

Of upper dorsal roots—Ananth.
Injuries of nerves—Bellis; Cepa; *Hyper.*; Phos. ac.
Multiple—Bov.; Con.; Morph.; Thallium.
Retro-bulbar, with sudden loss of sight—Chin. s.
Traumatic—Arn.; Calend.; *Cepa; Hyper.*

NEURALGIA—Remedies in general: Acetan.; *Aconitin; Acon.*; Agar.; Am picr.; Am. val.; Amyl; Aran.; *Arg. n.*; *Arn.*; *Ars.*; Atrop.; *Bell.*; *Bry.*; Cajup.; *Can. ind.*; Caust.; Cepa; *Cham.*; *Chel.*; *Chin. ars.*; *Chin. s.*; *Ced.*; *Cim.*; *Cinch.*; *Coff.*; *Col.*; Commocl.; Con.; Cornu. fl.; Diosc.; *Gels.*; Glon.; *Gnaph.*; *Hyper.*; *Ign.*; Ipec.; Kali ars.; *Kali bich.*; Kali ferrocy.; Kali iod.; *Kal.*; Lach.; Mag. c.; *Mag. p.*; Menyanth.; *Mez.*; *Morph.*; Nat. m.; Niccol. s.; Nux v.; Onosm.; Ox. ac. Paris; *Phos.*; *Phyt.*; Plant.; Plat.; Prun. sp.; *Puls.*; *Ran. b.*; *Rhod.*; Sil.; *Spig.*; *Stann.*; Staph.; *Sul.*; Sumb.; Thea; Ther.; Thuya; Tub.; Val.; *Ver. a.*; *Verbasc.*; Xanth.; Zinc. p.; *Zinc. v.*

CAUSE—TYPE—Anemia: *Ars.*; Cinch.; *Ferr.*; Kali ferrocy.; Puls.
Chronic cases, or later life—*Arn.*; Kreos.; *Phos.*; Sul.; Thuya.
Climacteric—Lach.
Gout, rheumatism—Cim.; *Colch.*; Col.; Kal.; Phyt.; Ran. b.; *Rhod.*; Rhus t.; Sul.
Idiopathic cases—Acon.; Ars.
Influenza, debility—Ars.
Malaria—Aran.; *Ars.*; Ced.; *Chin. s.*; Cinch.; Menyanth.; Nat. m.; Niccol. s.; Stann.; Sul.
Recent origin, occurring in young—*Acon.*; *Bell.*; Col.; *Gels.*; Kal.; Spig.
Syphilis—*Kali iod.*; Mez.; Phyt.
Traumatic, in amputated limbs—Am. m.; *Arn.*; *Cepa; Hyper.*; Kal.; Phos. ac.; Symphyt.
Zoster, after—*Mez.*; Morph.

LOCATION—Brachial plexus, cervico-brachial: *Acon. r.*; *Bry.*; Cepa; Cham.; Coccus; Corn. fl.; Hyper.; *Kal.*; *Merc.*; *Nux v.*; Paris; *Rhus t.*; *Sul.*; Tereb.; *Ver. a.*
Cervico-occipital—Bell.; Bry.; Chin. s.; Cinch.; Nux v.; Puls.; Zinc. p.
Ciliary—*Cim.*; Gels.; Mez.; Nat. m.; *Spig.* See Ciliary Neuralgia (Eye).
Crural anterior—Am. m.; Coff.; *Col.*; Gels.; *Gnaph.*; *Limul.*; Nat. ars.; Œnanthe; Solan. lyc.; Spig.; *Staph.*; Sul.; Xanth.
Infra-orbital—*Arg. n.*; Bell.; Mag. p.; Mez.; Nux v.; Phos. See Trifacial.
Intercostal—Acon.; Aran.; Arn.; *Ars.*; Ars. iod.; *Asclep. t.*; Aster.; Bell.; Brom.; Bry.; Chel.; Cim.; Gaulth.; Mag. p.; Menthol; *Mez.*; Morph.; Nux v.; Paris; Phos.; Puls.; *Ran. b.*; Rhod.; Samb.; Zinc. m.
Lumbo-abdominal—Aran.; Bell.; Clem.; Col.; Cupr. ars.; Ham.; Mag. p.; Nux v.
Phrenic—Bell.

SCIATICA—Acetan.; *Acon.*; *Am. m.*; Apoc.; Arn.; *Ars.*; Ars. met.; Ars. s. r.; *Bell.*; Bry.; Caps.; Carbon. oxy.; Carbon. s.; *Cham.*; Cinch.; Col.; Cotyled.; Diosc.; Gaulth.; Gels.; *Gins.*; *Gnaph.*; Hymosa; Hyper.; Ign.; Indigo; Iris; Kali c.; *Kali iod.*; Kali p.; Lac c.; Lyc.; Mag. p.; Nat. s.; Nyctanth.; Nux v.; Pall.; *Phyt.*; Plumb.; Polyg.; Ran. b

Rhus t.; *Ruta;* Sal. ac.; Sep.; Staph.; Strych.; *Sul.;* Sul. rub.; Syph.; Tellur.; Tereb.; Theine; Thuya; Val.; Ver. a.; *Viscum;* Xanth.; Zinc. v.

Sciatica, acute cases—*Acon.;* Bry.; Cham.; *Col.;* Ign.

Sciatica, chronic cases—*Ars.;* Calc. c.; Kali iod.; Lyc.; Phos.; *Plumb.;* Ran. b.; *Rhus t.;* Sul.; Zinc. m.

Sciatica, in summer, croupy cough in winter—Staph.

Sciatica, rheumatic—Acon.; Bry.; *Cim.;* Guaiac.; Hymosa; Led.; *Rhus t*

Sciatica, syphilitic— *Kali iod.;* Merc. c.; Phyt.

Sciatica, uterine—Bell.; Ferr.; Graph.; Merc.; *Puls.;* Sep.; Sul.

Sciatica, vertebral origin—Lac c.; Nat. m.; Phos.; Sil.; Sul.; Tellur.

Spermatic cord—*Clem.;* Col.; Ham.; *Ol. an ;* Ox. ac.; Rhod.; Spong. See Male Sexual System.

Spine—Paris. See Spine.

Sub-orbital—Caust.; Colch.; Con.; Kali c.; Phos. See Trifacial.

Supra-orbital—Arg. n.; Asaf.; *Ced.;* Chel.; *Chin. s.;* Cim.; *Kali bich.;* Mag. p.; Morph.; *Nux v.;* Ran. b.; *Spig.;* Stann.; Theine; Tongo; Viola od. See Prosopalgia (Face).

Teeth—Kreos.; Merc.; Mez.; Plant.; Staph.; Verbasc. See Odontalgia (Teeth).

Trifacial—*Acon.;* Amyl; *Aran.; Arg. n.; Ars.;* Arundo; *Bell.;* Cact.; Ced.; Cepa; *Cham.; Chel.; Cim.;* Cinch.; Colch.; Col.; Ferr.; *Gels.;* Glon.; *Kal.;* Mag. p.; Merc.; *Mez.;* Nat. s.; *Nux v.;* Phos.; Puls.; Rhus t.; Sabal; Sang.; *Spig.;* Stann.; Thuya; Tongo; Ver. a.; *Verbasc.;* Zinc. m.; *Zinc. v.* See Prosopalgia (Face).

Ulnar—Hyper.; Kal.; Lycopers.; Oxytr.; Rhus t.

TYPE OF PAIN—Bruised: Apis; Arn.; Bellis; Corn. fl.; Phyt.; Ruta.

Burning—Acon.; Anthrac.; Apis; *Ars.;* Caps.; Cepa; Sal. ac.; Spig.

Cramp-like, constrictive—Am. m.; *Cact.;* Caul.; Cim.; *Col.;* Con.; Cupr. m.; Gnaph.; Iris; *Mag. p.;* Nux v.; *Plat.;* Plumb.; Stann.; Sul.; Thuya; *Verbasc.*

Drawing—*Cham.;* Cinch.; Col.; Phos. ac.; Phos.; *Puls.;* Spig.; *Stann.;* Sul.; Verbasc. See Tearing.

Intermittent—*Ars.;* Chin. s.; *Cinch.; Col.;* Cupr. m.; *Ign.;* Mag. p.; Nux v.; *Spig.;* Sul. See Periodical.

Lancinating, electric shock like—Acon.; *Bell.;* Cact.; Caust.; Cim.; Col.; Daphne; Gels.; Mag. c.; *Mag. p.; Nux v.;* Phyt.; Plumb.; *Strych.;* Sul. ac.; Ver. a.; *Verbasc.;* Xanth.; Zinc. p.

Localized, in spots—Ign.; Kali bich.; Lil. t.; Ox. ac.

Onset gradual, cessation gradual—Arg. n.; Plat.; *Stann.;* Sul.; Ver. a.

Onset sudden, cessation sudden—*Bell.;* Carb. ac.; Chrom. ac.; Col.; Kali bich.; *Mag. p.;* Ovig. p.; Oxytr.

Periodical—*Aran.; Ars.; Ced.;* Chin. s.; Chrom. ac.; Kali bich.; *Niccol. s.;* Nux v.; Ox. ac.; Parth.; Sal. ac.; *Spig.;* Sul.; Toxicophis; Verbasc.

Plug-like—Anac.

Severe, drives him frantic—Acon.; Arg. n.; Ars.; *Bell.; Cham.;* Carb. ac.; Cinch.; Coff.; Colch.; *Col.;* Kreos.; *Mag. p.;* Morph.; Nux v.; Ox. ac.; *Spig.;* Ver. a.

Splinter-like—Ign.; Rhus t.

Tearing, shifting, darting, shooting—Æsc.; Arg. n.; *Ars.; Bell.;* Bry.; Caust.; *Cham.;* Cinch.; *Col.;* Diosc.; Gels.; Gnaph.; Ign.; Kal.; *Mag. p.;* Mez.; Nux v.; Paraf.; Phos.; Phyt.; Puls.; Rhus t.; Ruta; Sang.; *Spig.;* Tereb.

Tearing, shooting, along tracts, of large nerves—Gels.

Tearing, shooting, darting like chain lightning, ending in sharp, vice-like grip—Cact.

Tearing, shooting, to chest, trunk—Corn. fl.

Tearing, shooting, to extremities—Col.; Gnaph.; Graph.; Kal.; Pall.

Tearing, shooting, to face, shoulder, pelvis—Arundo.

Tearing, shooting, upwards—Kal.

CONCOMITANTS—Alternates with pain elsewhere; not deeply rooted cases—Ign.

Anesthesia—*Acon.;* Ars.; Kal.

Anguish, restlessness—Acon.; Ars.

Arms feel cold, swollen, paralyzed—Ver. a.

Beginning, in pneumogastric nerve disorders—Arn.

Cardiac anxiety—Spig.

Coldness—Agar.; Ars.; *Menyanth.;* Mez.; Nat. m.; Nux v.; Plat.; Puls.; Rhus t.; Sep.; Spig.; Ver. a.

Congestive symptoms—Acon.; Bell.; Gels.

Eructations, gastric symptoms—Ver. a.; Verbasc.

Face pale, restlessness, sweat—Spig.

Face red—Acon.; *Bell.;* Cham.; Verbasc.

Fainting, sudden—Cham.; Hep.; Morph.

Heat of one part, coldness of other—Pimenta.

Hyperesthesia—*Bell.;* Coff.; Ign.; Kali iod.; **Tereb.**

Lachrymation—Chel.; Mez.; *Puls.;* Rhus t.

Mania following—Cim.

Muscular contraction, spasmodic—Am. m.; *Bell.;* Gels.; Mag. p.; *Nux v.;* Plat.; Plumb. m.; Zinc. m.

Nervous agitation—*Acon.;* Am. val.; Ars.; *Cham.; Coff.;* Gels.; *Mag. p.;* Spig.

Numbness—*Acon.;* Agar.; Caust.; *Cham.;* Col.; Glon.; *Gnaph.;* Graph.; Kal.; Lac c.; Led.; Lith. c.; Merc.; Mez.; *Plat.; Rhus t.;* Sep.; Spig.

Salivation, stiff neck—Mez.

Skin, feels pinched—Sul. ac.

Torpor—Plat.

Weakness—*Ars.;* Cinch.; Colch.; Gels.; Kal.; *Ver. a.*

MODALITIES—AGGRAVATION: Bending back—Caps.

Cold—*Ars.;* Bell.; Caps.; Cinch.; Col.; Kali bich.; *Mag. p.;* Rhus t.; Ruta.

Exertion, mental—Kal.

Jar, concussion—*Bell.;* Caps.; *Spig.;* Tellur.

Left side—Acon.; *Ars.;* Caust.; Ced.; Colch.; *Col.;* Iris; Kali bich.; Mag. c.; *Mez.;* Morph.; Nux v.; Rhus t.; *Spig.;* Sumb.

Lying down—Am. m.; Gnaph.

Lying, on affected side—Col.; Kali iod.

Midnight—Ars.; Bell.; Mez.; Sul.
Morning—Acon.; Chin. s.; Nux v.
Morning, 9 A. M.-4 P. M.—Verbasc.
Motion—Acon.; Ars.; Bell.; *Bry.*; Cinch.; Coff.; Colch.; Col.; Gnaph.; Nux v.; Phyt.; Ran. b.; *Spig.*; Verbasc.
Night—Acon.; *Ars.;* Bell.; *Cham.;* Cim.; Coff.; Ginseng; Ign.; *Kali iod.;* Mag. p.; Merc.; Mez.; Plat.; Phyt.; Puls.; *Rhus t.;* Ruta; Sal. ac.; Syph.; Tellur.
Noon (12-1)—Nat. m.; Sul.
Pressure—Ars.; Gels.; Plumb.; Verbasc.; Zinc. m.
Rest, first beginning to move—Lac c.; Rhus t.
Rest, sitting—Am. m.; Ars.; Mag. c.; *Rhus t.;* Val.
Right side—*Bell.;* Chel.; Diosc.; Gnaph.; *Kal.; Lyc.;* Mag. p.; Morph.; Puls.; Ran. b.; Sul. ac.; Tellur.
Standing, resting foot on floor—Bell.; Val.
Stooping or straightening limb after previous exertion—Spig.
Talking, sneezing, change of temperature—Verbasc.
Touch—Ars.; *Bell.;* Bry.; *Cinch.;* Col.; *Lach.;* Mag. p.; Mez.; *Nux v.;* Plumb.; Spig.
Touching or closing teeth—Verbasc.
Warmth—Cham.; Mez.; Plumb.; *Puls.;* Xanth.

AMELIORATION—Bending backward: Diosc.
Bending forward—Col.
Closing eyes—Bry.
Cold—Ars.; Puls.
Daybreak—Syph.
Flexing thigh, on abdomen—Gnaph.
Kneeling down, pressing head firmly against floor—Sang.
Lying still, rest—Am. m.; Bry.; Diosc.; Kreos.; *Mag. p.;* Nux v.
Motion, walking—Am. m.; *Ars.; Diosc.; Ign.;* Kali bich.; Kali iod.; Mag. c.; Ox. ac.; *Puls.; Rhus t.;* Sep.; Sul.; Val.
Pressure—Ars.; Bell.; *Bry.;* Coff.; *Col.; Mag. p.;* Menyanth.; *Mez.;* Nux v.; Plumb.; Spig.
Rubbing—Acon.
Sitting—Bell.; Gnaph.
Warmth—*Ars.;* Bell.; Col.; *Mag. p.;* Morph.; Nux v.; Phos.; Rhus t.

SLEEPING SICKNESS—Ars.; Atoxyl.

SPINAL CORD—Anemia: Agar.; *Plumb.;* Sec.; Strych. p.; Tar. h.
Burning—Agar.; *Alum.;* Alum. sil.; Ars.; Bell.; Gels.; *Guaco;* Kali c.; Kali ferrocy.; Kali p.; Med.; Nux v.; Phos. ac.; *Phos.;* Physost.; *Pict ac.;* Strych. p.; Sul.; *Zinc. m.*
Coldness—Cim.; Strych.
Concussion—*Arn.;* Bellis; Cic.; Con.; *Hyper.;* Physost.
Congestion—Absinth.; Acon.; Agar.; Arn.; Bell.; *Gels.;* Hyper.; *Nux v.;* Onosm.; Oxytr.; Phos.; Physost.; Sec.; Sil.; *Strych.;* Tab.; Ver. v.
DEGENERATION (Softening, sclerosis, etc.)—Alum.; Alum. sil.; Arg. n.; Aur.; *Aur. mur.;* Bar. mur.; Carbon. s.; Naja; Ox. ac.; *Phos.;* Physost.; Pier. ac.; *Plumb. iod.;* Plumb. m.; Zinc. See Locomotor Ataxia.

NERVOUS SYSTEM 951

Degeneration, lateral sclerosis—*Arg. n.;* Cupr.; Hyper.; **Lathyrus**; Plumb.

Degeneration, multiple sclerosis—*Arg. n.; Atrop.; Aur.;* Bar. c.; Bell.; Calc.; Caust.; Chel.; *Crot.;* Gels.; *Lathyr.;* Lyc.; *Nux v.;* Ox. ac.; Phos.; Physost.; Plumb.; Sil.; Strych.; Sul.; Tar. h.; Thuya.

Hemorrhage in—Acon.; Arn.; Bell.; Lach.; Nux v.; Sec.

HYPERESTHESIA—Abrot.; Acon.; Agar.; Apis; Arg. n.; *Ars.; Bell.;* Bry.; *Chin. ars.;* Chin. s.; *Cim.; Cocc.;* Crot.; *Hep.; Hyper.; Lach.; Lac c.;* Lob. infl.; *Ign.;* Med ; Menisp.; Nat. m.; *Ox. ac.;* Phos. ac.; Phos.; Physost.; Pod.; Ran. b.; Rhus t.; Sec.; Senec. jac.; *Sil.; Strych. p.;* Sul.; *Tar. h.;* Tellur.; *Ther.;* Viscum; Zinc. m.

Hyperesthesia, between vertebræ—Chin. s.; Nat. m.; Ther.

Hyperesthesia from using arms in sewing, typewriting, piano playing—Agar.; *Cim.;* Ran. b.

Hyperesthesia, middorsal—Strych. p.; Tellur.

Hyperesthesia, sacral—Lob. infl.

Hyperesthesia, sits sideways to prevent pressure on spine—Chin. s.; Ther.; Zinc. m.

Hyperesthesia, spasmodic pain in chest and cardiac region from touch—Tar. h.

Hyperesthesia, worse from least jar or noise—Ther.

INFLAMMATION (meningitis)—Acon.; *Bell.;* Bry.; Kali iod.; Merc.; Nat. s.; Ox. ac.; Ver. v. See Myelitis.

Inflammation (myelitis)—*Acon.;* Arg. n.; *Arn.; Ars.;* Bell.; Bellis; Bry.; Chel.; *Cic.;* Con.; Crot.; Dulc.; Gels.; Hyos.; Hyper.; Kali iod.; Lach.; *Lathyr.; Merc.;* Naja; Nat. s.; *Nux v.; Ox. ac.; Phos.;* Physost.; Picr. ac.; *Plumb. m.;* Rhus t.; *Sec.;* Stram.; *Strych.;* Ver. a.; Zinc. p.

Inflammation, chronic (myelitis)—*Ars.: Crot.;* Lathyr.; *Ox. ac.; Plumb. m.;* Strych.; Thallium.

Inflammation, spasmodic form—Arg. n.; Ars.; Chel.; Merc.; Ver. a.

IRRITATION—*Agar.;* Ambra; *Arg. n.;* Arn.; Bell.; *Bellis;* Chin. ars.; Chin. s.; *Cim.;* Cob.; *Cocc.;* Cupr.; Gels.; *Guaco; Hyper.; Ign.;* Kali c.; Kali p.; Naja; *Nat. m.; Nux v.;* Ox. ac.; Phos.; *Physost.,* Picr. ac.; Plat.; Puls.; Ran. b.; *Sec.;* Sep.; *Sil.;* Staph.; Strych. p.; Sul.; *Tar. h.; Tellur.;* Ther.; Tub.; *Zinc. m.;* Zinc. v. See Hyperesthesia.

Irritation, from sexual excesses—Agar.; Kali p.; Nat. m.

LOCOMOTOR ATAXIA—Agar.; *Alumen;* Alum. chlor.; *Alum.;* Am. m.; Angust.; Arag.; *Arg. n.; Ars.;* Ars. br.; *Atrop.; Aur. mur.; Bell.;* Can. ind.; Carbon. s.; Carbo v.; Caust.; Chrom s.; Condur.; *Con.;* Cur.; Dub.; *Ferr. picr.; Fluor. ac.;* Gels.; Hyos.; *Ign.;* Kali br.; *Kali iod.;* Lathyr.; Lyc.; *Mag. p.;* Merc. c.; Nat. iod.; Nit. ac.; *Nux v.;* Onosm.; *Ox. ac.;* Pedic.; *Phos.;* Phos. hydr.; *Physost.; Picr. ac.;* Picrot.; *Plumb. m.; Plumb. phos.;* Rhus t.; Ruta; Sabad.; *Sec.; Sil.;* Stram.; *Strych.;* Tar. h.; Thall.; Thiosin.; *Zinc. p.;* Zinc. s.

CONCOMITANTS—**Early stage:** Angust.; Atrop.; *Bell.;* Con.; Ign.; Nux v.; Sec.; Strych.; Tar. h.; Zinc. m.; Zinc. s.

Early and urinary symptoms—Bell.; Berb. v.; Equis.; Ferr. p. See Urinary System.

Fulgurating pains—*Acetan.*; *Æsc.*; Agar.; Alum.; *Am. m.*; Angust.; Arg. n.; *Ars.*; Ars. iod.; *Atrop.*; Bar. m.; *Bell.*; Berb. v.; Dig.; *Fluor. ac.*; Guaiac.; Hyos.; Ign.; *Kal.*; Lyc.; Merc. c.; Nit. ac.; Nux m.; *Nux v.*; *Phos.*; *Physost.*; Piloc.; Plumb. iod.; Plumb. m.; Sabad.; Sant.; Sec.; Sil.; *Stront. c.*; Strych.; Thall.; Thiosin.; Zinc. m.; Zinc. p.; Zinc. s.

Gastric symptoms—*Arg. n.*; Bell.; Carbo v.; Ign.; Lyc.; *Nux v.*; Thiosin.

Muscular weakness, anæsthesia of skin, and muscular sense—Can. ind.

Ocular symptoms—Bell.; Con.; Ferr. picr.; Phos. See Eye.

Sexual excitement—Kali br.; Picr. ac.; Phos.

Syphilitic cases—*Kali iod.*; Merc. c.; Nit. ac.; Sec.

Ulcer of heel—Sil.

Vesical and anal symptoms—Alum.; Fluor. ac.; Ign.; Nux v.; Strych.; Tar. h.; Thiosin.

PAIN IN SPINE—Abrot.; Acon.; Adon. v.; *Agar.*; *Arg. n.*; Cact.; Cim.; Gels.; *Hyper.*; Lact. v.; Lob. syph.; Menisp.; Niccol. s.; *Ox. ac.*; Paraf.; Physost.; Strych.; Sec.; Tar. h.; Ther.; *Zinc. m.* See Backache (Locomotor System).

PARESIS—Cocc.; Con.; *Irid.*; Plectranth.; Plumb. iod.; Sec.; *Strych.* See Paralysis.

TETANY—Acon.; Cocc.; Graph.; Lyc.; Merc.; Plumb.; Sec.; *Solan. n.*

TETANUS—Aconitin; *Acon.*; Amyl; Angust.; Arn.; Bell.; Calend.; Camph.; Carbon. s.; Chloral; *Cic.*; *Cocc.*; Con.; Cupr.; *Cur.*; Gels.; *Hydroc. ac.*; Hyos.; *Hyper.*; Ign.; *Ipec.*; Kali br.; Lach.; Laur.; Led.; Lyssin; Mag. p.; Morph.; Mosch.; Nicot.; *Nux v.*; Œnanthe; *Op.*; Ox. ac.; *Passifl.*; *Physost.*; Phyt.; Plat.; Scorpio; *Stram.*; *Strych.*; Tab.; Tereb.; Thebain; *Upas*; Ver. a.; Zinc. m. See Trismus (Face).

TIC CONVULSIF—Arg. n.; Hyos.; Laur.; Lyc.; Sep.; Tar. h.; Zinc.

WEAKNESS OF SPINE—*Æsc.*; Alum. sil.; Arg. n.; Bar. c.; *Calc. p.*; Cocc.; Con.; Nat. m.; Phos.; Picr. ac.; Selen.; Sil.; *Strych.*; Zinc. picr. See **Back (Locomotor System).**

GENERALITIES

ABSCESS—Acute: Acon.; *Ananth.;* Anthrac.; Apis; *Arn.;* Ars.: *Bell.;* Calc. hypoph.; *Calc. s.;* Calend.; *Carb. ac.;* Chin. s.; Cinch.; Crot.; Fluor. ac.; *Hep.;* Hippoz.; *Lach.;* Lapis alb.; Lyc.; *Merc. s.; Myrist. seq.; Nit. ac.;* Phos. ac.; Phos.; *Rhus t.; Sil.;* Sil. mar.; Syph.; *Sul.; Tar. c.;* Vespa.

About bones—Asaf.; *Aur.;* Calc. fl.; Calc. hypoph.; Calc. p.; Fluor. ac.; Mang.; *Phos.;* Puls.; *Sil.;* Symphyt.

About joints—Calc. hypoph.; Sil.

Chronic—Arn.; Calc. c.; *Calc. fl.;* Calc. iod.; Calc. p.; Carbo v.; Cham.; Cinch.; Fluor. ac.; Graph.; Hep.; *Iod.;* Iodof.; Kali iod.; Merc. i. r.; *Merc. s.;* Ol. j. as.; Phos.; *Sil.;* Sul.

Muscles, deep—Calc. c.

Psoas abscess—Sil.; Symphyt.

To abort—Apis; Bell.; Bry.; *Hep.;* Merc. s.

To hasten suppuration—Guaiac.; *Hep.;* Lach.; *Merc. s.;* Operc.; Phos.; Phyt.; *Sil.*

ACROMEGALY—Pituit. ext.; Thyr.

ADDISON'S DISEASE—*Adren.;* Ant. c.; Apomorph.; *Arg. n.; Ars.;* Ars. iod.; Bac.; Bell.; Calc. ars.; Calc. c.; Hydroc. ac.; *Iod.;* Kreos.; Nat. m.; Nit. ac.; Phos.; Sec.; *Sil.;* Spig.; Sul.; *Suprarenal ext.;* Thuya; *Tub.;* Vanad.

ANEMIA—Chlorosis: Acet. ac.; *Alet.;* Alum.; *Arg. n.; Arg. oxy.;* Arn.; *Ars.;* Aur. ars.; Bism.; Calc. ars.; *Calc. c.;* Calc. lact.; *Calc. p.;* Calop.; Carbo v.; Chin. ars.; *Chin. s.;* Cic.; *Cinch.;* Con.; Crat.; Crot.; Cupr ars.; *Cupr. m.; Cycl.;* Ferr. ac.; *Ferr. ars.;* Ferr. carb.; Ferr. et. chin.; Ferr. p.; *Ferr. iod.; Ferr. m.;* Ferr. mur.; Ferr. oxy.; *Ferr. red.;* Gossyp.; *Graph.; Helon.;* Hydr.; Iod.; *Irid.;* Kali bich.; *Kali c.;* Kali p.; Lecith.; *Lyc.; Mang. ac.;* Merc. s.; Nat. c.; *Nat. m.; Nit. ac.;* Nux v.; Petrol.; *Phos.;* Phyt.; Picr. ac.; Plat.; *Plumb. ac.; Puls.;* Rubia; Sacchar. of.; *Sec.; Sep.;* Sil.; *Strych. et ferr. cit.; Sul.;* Thyr.; Vanad.; Zinc. ars.; Zinc. mur.

From cardiac disease—Ars.; Crat.; Stroph.

From grief—Nat. m.; *Phos. ac.*

From malaria—Alston.; Ars.; *Nat. m.;* Ostrya; Robin.

From menstrual derangements—Arg. oxy.; Ars.; *Calc. c.;* Calc. p.; Crat.; *Cycl.;* Ferr.; *Graph.;* Kali c.; Mang. ac.; *Nat. m.;* Puls.; Sep.

From nutritional disturbances—Alet.; Alum.; Calc. p.; Ferr.; Helon.; Nux v.

From suboxidation—Picr. ac.

From syphilis—Calop.

From vital drains, exhausting disease—Acet. ac.; Alston.; Calc. p.; Chin. s.; *Cinch.; Ferr.;* Helon.; Kali c.; *Nat. m.;* Phos. ac.; Phos.

Hemorrhagic chlorosis—Arg. oxy.; *Ars.;* Calc. c.; Crot.; Ign.; Nat. br.

Pernicious anemia—Ars.; *Phos.;* Picr. ac.; Thyr.

954 GENERALITIES

Type, erythistic; worse in winter—Ferr. m.

ASPHYXIA—Am. c.; *Ant. t.*; *Hydroc. ac.*; Sul. hydr.; Upas.
  Asphyxia neonatorum—*Ant. t.*; Laur.

BLOOD—Disorganization: Ail.; Am. c.; *Anthrac.*; Arn.; *Ars.*; Ars. hydr.; Bapt.; Carb. ac.; *Crot.*; *Echin.*; Kreos.; *Lach.*; *Mur. ac.*; Phos.; Psor.; *Pyr.*; *Rhus t.*; Tar. c. See Pyemia.

BONES—Club-foot: Nux v.; Phos.; Strych.
  Cold feeling—Zinc. m.
  Condyles, epiphyses, swollen—Conchiolin; Rhus t.
  Condyles, sutures, affected—Calc. c.; Calc. p.
  Cranial bones, thin, soft—Calc. c.; *Calc. p.*
  Crooking—Am. c.; Calc. c.; Calc. p.; Iod.; Sil.
  Development, tardy—*Calc. c.*; Calc. fl.; *Calc. p.*; Sil.
  Enlargement (acromegaly)—Pituit. ext.; Thyr.
  Exostoses—Arg. m.; Aur.; Calc. c.; *Calc. fl.*; Fluor. ac.; Hekla; *Kali bich.*; *Kali iod.*; Lapis alb.; Malandr.; Merc. c.; *Merc. phos.*; Merc. s.; Mez.; Phos.; *Plumb. ac.*; Ruta; *Sil.*; Still.; Sul.; Zinc. m.
  Fractures, shock—Acon.; Arn.
  Fractures, slow union—*Calc. p.*; Calend.; Iod.; Mang. ac.; *Mez.*; Phos. ac.; *Ruta*; *Sil.*; *Symphyt.*; Thyr.
  Inflammation (osteitis)—Asaf.; Aur. iod.; *Aur.*; Conchiol.; Hekla; Hep.; Iod.; *Kali iod.*; *Merc. s.*; *Mez.*; *Nit. ac.*; Phos. ac.; Phos.; Staph.; Still.; Stront. c.
  Inflammation, chronic (osteitis deformans)—Aur.; Calc. p.; Hekla; Nit. ac.
  Inflammation, (osteo-myelitis)—Acon.; Chin. s.; Gun powder; Phos.

NECROSIS—Angust.; *Arg. m.*; Ars.; *Asaf.*; Aur. iod.; *Aur. m.*; Calc. c.; *Calc. fl.*; Calc. hypophos.; Calc. p.; Calc. sil.; Cinch.; Con.; *Fluor. ac.*; Graph.; Hekla; *Hep.*; Iod.; Kali bich.; Kali iod.; Lach.; Med.; *Merc. s.*; Mez.; *Nat. sil. fl.*; *Nit. ac.*; Phos. ac.; *Phos.*; Plat. mur.; *Sil.*; Staph.; Sul. ac.; Symphyt.; Syph.; Sul.; Thea; Ther.; *Tub.*; Vitrum
  Facial—Hep.; Mez.; Sil.
  Femur—Stront. c.
  Long bones—Angust.; Asaf.; *Fluor. ac.*; Mez.; Stront. c.
  Mastoid, palatine, cranial, nasal—Aur. m.
  Mastoid, temporal—Calc. fl.; Caps.
  Nasal—Aur.; Kali bich.
  Skull—Fluor. ac.
  Sternum—Con.
  Tarsus—Plat. mur.
  Tibiæ—Asaf.; Carb. ac.; Hep.; Lach.; Nit. ac.; Phos.
  Vertebræ—Calc. c.; Nat. m.; Phos. ac.; Sil.; Sticta; Syph.
  Vertebræ, inferior maxilla—Phos.

NODES—Asaf.; *Aur. mur.*; Cinnab.; Fluor. ac.; Kali bich.; Kali iod.; Merc.; Mez.; Nux v.; Phyt.; Sil.; Still. See Syphilis (Male Sexual System).

PAIN—Agar.; Angust.; *Asaf.*; *Aur. m.*; Aur. mur.; Bry.; Castor eq.; Caust.; Cinch.; Crot.; Crot. casc.; *Eup. perf.*; Euphorb.; *Fluor. ac.*; Guaiac.; Hep.; Iod.; Ipec.; *Kali bich.*; *Kali iod.*; Lyc.; Lyssin; Mang. ac.;

GENERALITIES 955

Merc. c.; Merc. s.; *Mez.*; Phos. ac.; Phos.; *Phyt.*; *Rhod.*; Rhus t.; *Ruta*; Sil.; *Staph.*; Sul.; *Symphyt.*; Syph.; Ther.; Vitrum.
Burning—Aur.; Euphorb.; Fluor. ac.; Kali iod.; Phos. ac.; Sul.
Constricting, band-like—*Apis*; Carb. ac.; Hep.; Nit. ac.; Sul.
Drawing, pressing, sensitiveness—Nit. ac.
Gnawing, digging—*Aur.*; Carb. ac.; Kali iod.; Mang. ac.; Merc.; Symphyt.
Growing—Guaiac.; Mang. ac.; Phos. ac.
In coccyx—Castor eq.
In face, feet—Aur. m.
In long bones—Cinnab.; Eup. perf.; Staph.; Stront.; Syph.
In shin bones—Agar.; Asaf.; Castor eq.; Carb. ac.; Dulc.; *Mez.*; Staph.; Still.; Syph.
In skull—Eup. perf.; Kali bich.
In vertebræ—Agar.
Influenzal—Eup. perf.
Localized in spots, worse, from weather changes—Rhod.
Nocturnal—*Asaf.*; *Aur.*; Fluor. ac.; Hep.; Iod.; *Kali iod.*; Lach.; Mang. ac.; *Merc.*; *Mez.*; Phos. ac.; Phyt.; Rhod.; Still.; Syph.
Pricking—Arn.; *Symphyt.*
Sore, bruised, aching—Cinch.; Conchiol.; Eup. perf.; Lyssin; *Phyt.*; Ruta.
Sore, bruised, as if scraped—*Ipec.*; Paris; *Phos. ac.*; Rhus t.
Sore, bruised, worse, from cold; wandering—Kali bich.
Tearing—Caust.; Colch.; Fluor. ac.; Phos. ac.
Throbbing, jerking, darting, drawing, hypersensitiveness—Asaf.
Worse, from damp weather—Merc.; Mez.; Nit. ac.; Phyt.; Rhus t.; Still.; Syph.

PERIOSTITIS—**And periosteal affections**: Apis; Aran.; *Asaf.*; *Aur. m.*; *Aur. mur.*; Calc. c.; Cinch.; Clem.; Colch.; Con.; Ferr. iod.; Graph.; *Guaiac.*; Hekla; Iod.; *Kali bich.*; *Kali iod.*; Mang. ac.; *Merc. s.*; *Mez.*; *Nit. ac.*; Phos. ac.; Phos.; *Phyt.*; Plat. mur.; Rhod.; Rhus t.; *Ruta*; Sars.; *Sil.*; Still.; Symphyt.

SOFTENING, Mollities Ossium—Calc. c.; *Calc. iod.*; Calc. p.; Guaiac.; Iod.; Merc. s.; *Phos.*

SPINAL bifida—Bry.; *Calc. p.*; Psor.; Tub.
Spinal caries (Pott's disease)—Arg. m.; Aur.; Calc. c.; Calc. iod.; *Calc. p.*; Con.; *Iod.*; Kali iod.; Merc. i. r.; *Phos. ac.*; *Phos.*; Pyr.; *Sil.*; Still.; Sul.; *Syph.*; Tub.; Vitrum.
Spinal curvature—Calc. c.; *Calc. p.*; Ferr. iod.; Phos.; *Sil.*; Sul.; Ther.
Wounds—Ruta; Symphyt.

BUBONIC PLAGUE—Anthrac.; Ant. t.; *Ars.*; Bapt.; Bell.; Bubon.; Carbo v.; Cinch.; *Crot.*; Ign.; Iod.; *Lach.*; Naja; Operc.; *Phos.*; *Pyr.*; Rhus t.; *Tar. c.*

CANCER—**Remedies in general**: Acet. ac.; Ananth.; *Ant. chlor.*; Apis; *Ars.*; Ars. br.; Ars. iod.; *Aster.*; Aur. ars.; Aur. m. n.; Bapt.; Bism.; Brom.; Calc. c.; Calc. iod.; Calc. ox.; Calend.; Carb. ac.; *Carbo an.*; Carbon. s.; Carcinos.; Choline; Cic.; Cinnam.; *Cistus*; Condur.; Con.;

Cupr. ac.; Eosin.; Euphorb.; Form. ac.; Formica; Fuligo; *Galium ap.;* Guaco; Graph.; Ham.; *Hoang n.; Hydr.;* Iod.; Kali ars.; *Kali cy.;* Kali iod.; *Kreos.;* Lach.; Lapis alb.; Lyc.; Maland.; Med.; Phos.; Phyt.; Radium; Rumex; ac.; Sang.; *Semperv. t.;* Scirrhin.; Sedum rep.; Sep.; Sil.; Symphyt.; Sul.; Taxus; *Thuya.*

Cancer, of antrum—Aur.; Symphyt.

Cancer, of bone—Aur. iod.; Phos.; Symphyt.

Cancer, of bowel, lower—Ruta.

Cancer, of breast—Ars. iod.; Bar. iod.; Brom.; Bufo; Carbo an.; Carcinos.; Condur.; *Con.;* Form. ac.; Graph.; *Hydr.;* Phyt.; *Plumb. iod.;* Nat. cacodyl.; Scirrhin. See Female Sexual System.

Cancer, of cæcum—Ornithog.

Cancer, of glandular structures—Hoang nan.

Cancer, of omentum—Lob. erin.

Cancer, of stomach—Acet. ac.; *Ars.;* Bism.; Cadm. s.; *Condur.;* Form. ac.; Hydr.; Kreos.; Ornithog.; Phos.; Sec. See Stomach.

Cancer, of uterus—*Aur. m. n.;* Carbo an.; Carcinos.; Fuligo; Hydr.; Iod.; Lapis alb.; Nat. cacodyl.; Nit. ac.; Sec. See Female Sexual System.

Cancer, to relieve pains—Alveloz.; *Apis;* Anthrac.; *Ars.;* Aster.; Bry.; *Calc. ac.;* Calc. c.; Calc. ox.; Carcinos.; Ced.; Cinnam.; Condur.; Con.; Echin.; *Euphorb.; Hydr.;* Mag. p.; Morph.; Op.; Ova t.; Phos. ac.; Sil.

CARTILAGES (perichondritis)—Inflammation: Arg. m.; Bell.; Cham.; Cim.; Oleand.; Plumb.; *Ruta.*

Cartilages, pains—Arg. m.; Ruta.

Cartilages, ulceration—Merc. c.

CELLULAR TISSUE—Indurated: *Anthrac.;* Carbo an.; Graph.; *Kali iod.;* Kreos.; Merc.; Plumb. iod.; *Rhus t.;* Sil.

CELLULITIS—Apis; Arn.; *Ars.;* Bapt.; Crot.; *Lach.;* Mang. ac.; *Merc. i. r.; Rhus t.;* Sil.; Vespa.

COMPLAINTS—ABUSE of alcoholic beverages: *Agar.;* Apomorph.; Ant.; *Ars.;* Asar.; Aur.; Calc. ars.; Carbo v.; Carbon. s.; Card. m.; Coca; Cocc.; Colch.; Eup. perf.; Hydr.; Ipec.; Lach.; Led.; *Lob. infl.;* Lyc.; Nux v.; Querc.; *Ran. b.;* Strych.; Sul. ac.; Sul.; Ver. a. See Alcoholism (Nervous System).

Abuse of aconite—Sul.

Abuse of arsenic—Carbo v.; Ferr.; Hep.; *Ipec.;* Samb.; Ver. a.

Abuse of belladonna—Hyos.; Op.

Abuse of bromide of potassium—Camph.; Helon.; Nux v.; Zinc. m.

Abuse of camphor—Canth.; Coff.; Op.

Abuse of cantharis—Apis; Camph.

Abuse of chamomilla—Cinch.; Coff.; Ign.; Nux v.; Puls.; Val.

Abuse of chloral—Can. ind.

Abuse of chlorate of potash—Hydr.

Abuse of cod liver oil—Hep.

Abuse of coffee—Cham.; Guar.; *Ign.; Nux v.*

Abuse of colchicum—Led.

Abuse of condiments—Nux v.

Abuse of digitalis—Cinch.; Nit. ac.
Abuse of drugs in general—Aloe; Hydr.; *Nux v.;* Teucr.
Abuse of ergot—Cinch.; Lach.; Nux v.; Sec.; Solan. n.
Abuse of iodides—Ars.; Bell.; *Hep.;* Hydr.; Phos.
Abuse of iron—Cinch.; *Hep.; Puls.*
Abuse of lead (plumbism)—*Alum.;* Bell.; Carbon. s.; Caust.; *Col.;* Iod.; Kali br.; *Kali iod.;* Merc.; Nux v.; *Op.;* Petrol.; Plat.; Sul. ac.
Abuse of magnesia—Nux. v.; Rheum.
Abuse of mercury—Angust.; Ant. t.; Arg. m.; Asaf.; *Aur.;* Carbo v.; Caust.; Cinch.; Clem.; Dulc.; Fluor. ac.; Guaiac.; *Hep.;* Iod.; *Kali iod.;* Lach.; Mez.; *Nit. ac.;* Op.; Plat. mur.; Phyt.; Pod.; Puls.; Rhus g.; Sars.; Sul.
Abuse of narcotics—Acet. ac.; Apomorph.; Avena; Camph.; Can. ind.; Cham.; Cim.; Ipec.; Macrot.; Mur. ac.
Abuse of nitrate of silver—Nat. m.
Abuse of phosphorus—Lach.; Nux v.
Abuse of quinine—*Ars.;* Bell.; Col.; Carbo v.; Eucal.; Ferr.; *Ipec.;* Lach.; Menyanth.; *Nat. m.;* Parth.; *Puls.;* Selen.
Abuse of salt (halophagia)—Ars.; Carbo v.; Nat. m.; *Nit. sp. d.; Phos.*
Abuse of stramonium—Acet. ac.; Nux v.; Tab.
Abuse of strychnine—Cur.; *Eucal.;* Kali br.; Physost.
Abuse of sugar—Merc. v.; Nat. p.
Abuse of sulphur—Puls.; Selen.
Abuse of tar, locally—Bov.
Abuse of tea—Abies n.; *Cinch.; Diosc.;* Ferr.; Puls.; *Selen.;* Thuya.
Abuse of tobacco—*Abies n.; Ars.;* Calad.; Calc. p.; Camph.; Chin. ars.; Cinch.; Coca; *Gels.; Ign.; Ipec.;* Kal.; Lyc.; Mur. ac.; *Nux v.;* Phos.; *Plant.;* Plumb.; *Sep.; Spig.;* Staph.; Tab.; Ver. a.
Abuse of tobacco, in boys—Arg. n.; Ars.; Ver. a.
Abuse of turpentine—Nux m.
Abuse of vegetable medicines—Camph.; *Nux v.*
Abuse of veratrum—Camph.; Coff.
Anæsthetic vapors, antidote—*Acet. ac.;* Am. caust.; Amyl; Hep.; Phos.

BITES of insects, snakes, dogs—Acet. ac.; Am. c.; Am. caust., Anthrac.; *Apis;* Arn.; *Ars.;* Bell.; Calad.; Camph.; *Ced.;* Crot.; *Echin.;* Golond.; *Grind.;* Guaco; Gymnen.; Hydroc. ac.; *Hyper.;* Kali perm.; Lach.; *Led.;* Mosch.; Pyr.; Salag.; Sisyr.; Spiræa; Trychnos.
Charcoal fumes, illuminating gas, ill effects—Acet. ac.; Am. c.; Arn.; Bell.; Bov.; Coff.; Op.

CHECKED discharges, ill effects—Abrot.; Asaf.; Aur. mur.; *Bar. c.;* Bry.; *Graph.;* Lach.; *Lob. infl.;* Med.; Merc. s.; *Psor.;* Sanic.; *Sil.;* Stram.; Sul.; Zinc. m.
Checked foot sweat, ill effects—*Bar. c.;* Cupr.; Formica; Graph.; Psor.; Sanic.; *Sil.;* Zinc. m.
Checked gonorrhœa, ill effects—Graph.; Psor.; *Med.; Thuya;* X-ray.
Checked, sweats, ill effects—*Acon.;* Bellis; Dulc.; Rhus t.

CHRONIC DISEASES, to begin treatment—Calc. c.; Calc. p.; *Nux v.;* Puls.; *Sul.*

CICATRICES, affections—Calc. fl.; *Fluor. ac.;* Hyper.; Phyt.; Sil.; *Thiosin.*
Cicatrices, freshen up, reopen—*Caust.;* Fluor. ac.; *Graph.;* Mag. pol. am.; Sil.
Cicatrices, itch—Fluor. ac.
Cicatrices, pain during change of weather—Nit. ac.
Cicatrices, turn green—Led.
Cicatrices, turn red or blue—Sul. ac.

COMPLAINTS, appear, atypically—Mosch.
Complaints, appear, diagonally, upper left, lower right side—*Agar.;* Ant. t.; Stram.
Complaints, appear, diagonally, upper right, lower left side—Ambra; Brom.; Med.; Phos.; Sul. ac.
Complaints, appear, from above downwards—Cact.; *Kal.*
Complaints, appear, from below, upwards—Led.
Complaints, appear, gradually—Calc. sil.; Cinch.; Radium; Tellur.
Complaints, appear, gradually, cease gradually—Arg. n.; *Plat.;* Stann.; Stront. c.; Syph.
Complaints, appear, gradually, cease suddenly—Ign.; *Puls.;* Sul. ac.
Complaints, appear, in small spots—Coff.; *Ign.; Kali bich.;* Lil. t.; *Ox. ac.*
Complaints, appear, suddenly, cease gradually—Puls.; Sul. ac.
Complaints, appear, suddenly, cease suddenly—*Bell.;* Cact.; Carb. ac.; Eup. perf.; Eup. purp.; Ign.; Kali bich.; Lyc.; *Mag. p.;* Nit. ac.; Oxytrop.; Petrol.; Poth.; *Strych.;* Tub.
Complaints, appear, suddenly, tension acutely increases, leaves with a snap on first motion—Puls.; Rhus t.
Complaints, fatal issue; to induce "euthanasia"—Amyl; Ant. t.; *Ars.;* Carbo v.; Lach.; Tar. h.
Complaints, from chilling—*Acon.;* Coff.; Dulc.; Nux v.; Sil.
Complaints, from exposure of feet—*Calc. c.;* Cupr. m.; Nux m.; Sil.
Complaints, from exposure, to cold dry wind—*Acon.;* Bry.; Caust.; Hep.; Rhod.
Complaints, from living in cool, damp places—Ant. t.; *Aran.;* Ars.; Ars. iod.; Calc. c.; Calc. sil.; *Dulc.;* Nat. s.; Nux m.; *Rhus t.;* Tereb.
Complaints, from overlifting—Arn.; Carbo an.; Carbo v.; Kali c.; Lyc.; *Nat. c.;* Nat. m.; Phos.; *Rhus t.;* Sep.; Sul.
Complaints, from working, in clay, cold water—Calc. c.; Mag. p.
Complaints, improve, then relapse continually—Sul.
Complaints, improve, then remain stationary—Caust.; Psor.; *Sul.*
Complaints, in extremes of life—Ant. c.; *Bar. c.;* Lyc.; Millef.; Op.; *Ver. a.*
Complaints in fleshy persons—Allium s.; Am. c.; Am. m.; Ant. c.; Aur. m.; Bar. c.; Blatta or.; Calc. ars.; *Calc. c.; Caps.;* Carbo v.; Ferr.; *Graph.;* Kali bich.; Kali br.; *Kali c.;* Lob. infl.; Op.; Phyt.; Puls.; Thuya. See Obesity.
Complaints, in old people—Agar.; Aloe; Alumen; *Alum.;* Ambra; Ant. c.; Ars.; Aurant.; Aur. m.; *Bar. c.; Bar. m.;* Caps.; *Carbo an.;* Carbo v.; Colch.; *Con.;* Crot.; Fluor. ac.; Hydr.; Iod.; Kali c.; Lyc.; Millef.; Nit. ac.; Nux m.; *Op.;* Phos.; Sec.; Sul. ac.; *Ver. a.*
Complaints, wander, or shift about, erratic, changeable—Apis; Bell.; Benz.

GENERALITIES

ac.; Berb. v.; *Dios.;* *Ign.;* *Kali bich.;* *Kali s.;* *Lac c.;* Lil. t.; **Mag. p.;** Magnolia; *Mang. ac.;* Phyt.; *Puls.;* Sanic.; Syph.; *Tub.*

Complaints, with painlessness—Op.; *Stram.*

ERUPTIONS, exanthemata, suppressed, or repercussed, ill effects—*Apis;* Ars.; Asaf.; *Bry.;* Camph.; Caust.; *Cic.;* *Cupr.;* *Helleb.;* **Mag. s.;** Op.; Psor.; Puls.; Stram.; *Sul.;* *Tub.;* X-ray; *Zinc. m.*

Foreign bodies, in larynx, trachea—Ant. t.; Ipec.; Sil.

Growth, too rapid, ill effects—*Calc. c.;* *Calc. p.;* Ferr. ac.; Irid.; Kreos.; *Phos. ac.;* *Phos.*

Mental labor, sufferings from—*Arg. n.;* *Gels.;* Graph.; Lyc.; **Nat. c.;** *Nux v.;* Phos. ac.; Sil.

Mining, ill effects—Card. m.; Nat. ars.

Mountain climbing, aviation, ill effects—Ars.; Coca.

Night watching, mental strain, ill effects—Bellis; Caps.; Caust.; *Cocc.;* Colch.; Cupr.; Dipod.; *Gels.;* *Ign.;* Lac d.; Nit. ac.; *Nux v.;* *Phos. ac.;* *Zinc. ac.* See Neurasthenia (Nervous System).

Nutritional disturbances, development tardy—Bac.; *Bar. c.;* *Calc. c.;* *Calc. p.;* Caust.; Kreos.; Lac d.; Med.; Nat. m.; Pinus sylv.; *Sil.;* Thyr.

Poison oak, and rhus poisoning—Am. c.; *Anac.;* Apis; Arn.; Astac.; Cim.; *Crot. t.;* Cyprip.; Echin.; Erech.; Euphorb. d.; Graph.; *Grind.;* Hedeoma; Hydrophyl.; *Led.;* Mez.; Plant.; Prim. ob.; Rhus d.; *Rhus t.;* *Sang.;* Sep.; Tanac.; Urt.; Vanillin; Verb.; *Xerophyl.*

PROMAINE poisoning (decayed food)—Absinth.; Acet. ac.; *Ars.;* Camph.; Carbo an.; Carbo v.; Cepa; Crot.; *Cupr. ars.;* Gunpowder; Kreos.; Pyr.; Urt.; *Ver. a.*

Ptomaine poisoning (mushrooms)—Agar.; Atrop.; *Bell.;* Camph.; Pyr.

Sewer gas, or noxious effluvia, ill effects—Anthrac.; *Bapt.;* Phyt.; Pyr.

Sun exposure, ill effects: SUNSTROKE (coup-de-soleil): Acon.; *Ant. c.;* *Bell.;* Bry.; Cact.; Camph.; *Gels.;* *Glon.;* Hydroc. ac.; Lach.; *Nat. c.;* Op.; Stram.; Usnea; *Ver. v.* See Collapse (Nervous System); Modalities.

Vaccination, ill effects—Acon.; *Ant. t.;* Apis; Bell.; Crot.; Echin.; *Malandr.;* Merc. s.; *Mez.;* Sars.; Sep.; *Sil.;* Sul.; *Thuya.*

Vital drains, ill effects—Calc. p.; *Cinch.;* Ham.; Kali c.; Kali p.; Nat. m.; *Phos. ac.;* Phos.; Psor.; Sep.; Staph.

DEGENERATION—Fatty: Ars.; Aur.; *Cupr.;* Kali c.; *Phos.;* Vanad.

DROPSY—Acetan.; *Acet. ac.;* Acon.; *Adon. v.;* Amelop.; Am. benz.; *Apis;* *Apoc.;* Arg. phos.; *Ars.;* Ars. iod.; Asclep. s.; Asclep. vinc.; Benz. ac.; *Blatta am.;* Brass.; Bry.; Cact.; Calc. ars.; Calc. c.; Caffeine; *Gahinca;* Card. m.; *Cinch.;* Cochlear.; Colch.; *Conv.;* Cop.; *Crat.;* *Dig.;* *Dulc.;* Elat.; Eup. purp.; Euphorb.; Ferr.; *Fluor. ac.;* Galium; *Helleb.;* Hep.; Iod.; Iris; Iris germ.; Jatropha; *Junip.;* Kali ac.; *Kali ars.;* Kali c.; *Kali iod.;* *Kali n.;* Lac d.; *Lach.;* Lact. v.; *Liatris;* Lyc.; Merc. d.; Nasturt.; Nit. sp. dulc.; Onisc.; *Oxydend.;* *Phaseol.;* Phos.; *Piloc.;* Prun. sp.; Psor.; Querc.; Rhus t.; *Samb. can.;* Samb.; *Scilla;* Solan. n.; Solid.; *Stroph.;* Strych. ars.; Tereb.; Teucr. sc.; **Thlaspi;** Toxicophis; Urium; Ur. ac.

From abuse of quinine—Apoc.

From alcoholism—Ars.; Fluor. ac.; Sul.

From eruption suppressed, sweat, rheumatism—Dulc.
From heart disease—*Adon. v.;* Apis; *Apoc.;* Arn.; *Ars.;* Ars. iod.; **Asclep. s.;** Aur. m.; *Cact.; Caffeine;* Collins.; *Conv.; Crat.; Dig.; Digitalin;* Iod.; Kal.; Liatris; Merc. d.; *Stroph.* See Heart.
From kidney disease—Ampel.; Ant. t.; *Apis;* Apoc.; Ars.; Asclep. s.; Aspar.; Chimaph.; *Dig.;* Digitalin; Eup. purp.; Helon.; Lac d.; Liatris; *Merc. c.;* Merc. d.; Plumb.; Tereb.; Uric. ac. See Urinary System.
From liver disease—*Apoc.;* Ars.; Asclep. s.; Aur.; Card. m.; Caenoth.; Chel.; Chimaph.; Lac d.; Liatris; *Lyc.;* Mur. ac.; Polymnia. See Liver (Abdomen).
From menstrual disorder at puberty, or menopause—Puls.
From spleen disease—Ceanoth.; Liatris; Querc.; Scilla. See Spleen (Abdomen).
From remittent fever—Helleb.
From scarlet fever—Acon.; *Apis;* Apoc.; *Ars.;* Asclep. s.; Colch.; Dig.; Dulc.; *Helleb.; Hep.;* Junip.; Lach.; Piloc.; Scilla; *Tereb.*
From suppressed exanthemata—Apis; Helleb.; Zinc. m.
From suppressed intermittents—Carbo v.; Cinch.; Ferr. m.; Helleb.; Lac d.
Dropsy, in newborn—Apis; Caffeine; Carbo v.; Dig.; Lach.
Dropsy, with diarrhœa—Acet. ac.
Dropsy, with serum oozing—Ars.; Lyc.; Rhus t.
Dropsy, with soreness in uterine region—Conv.
Dropsy, with suppressed urine, fever, debility—Helleb.
Dropsy, with thirst—*Acet. ac.;* Acon.; *Apoc.;* Ars.
Dropsy, without thirst—Apis; Helleb.

LOCATION—Abdomen—ASCITES: Acet. ac.; *Adon. v.;* Apis; *Apoc.;* Ars.; Aur. m.; Aur. m. n.; *Blatta am.;* Cahinca; Canth.; *Cinch.;* Cop.; *Dig.;* Digitalin; Fluor. ac.; *Helleb.;* Iod.; Kali c.; Lact. v.; Led.; *Lyc.;* Nat. chlor.; Oxydend.; *Prun. sp.;* Samb.; *Senec.;* Sep.; Tereb.; Uran. n.

Chest (hydrothorax)—*Apis;* Apoc.; *Ars.;* Ars. iod.; Colch.; *Dig.;* Helleb.; Kali c.; Lach.; Lact. v.; *Merc. sul.;* Scilla; *Sul.* See Chest.

Extremity, left—Cact.

General—ANASARCA:—Acetan.; Acet. ac.; Acon.; Eth.; *Apis;* Apoc.; Arn.; *Ars.;* Cahinca; *Cinch.; Conv.;* Cop.; Crat.; *Dig.;* Dulc.; Ferr. m.; *Helleb.;* Kali c.; *Liatris;* Lyc.; *Merc. c.;* Oxydend.; Picr. ac.; Prun. sp.; Tereb.; Uran. n. See Dropsy.

EFFUSION—Threatening: *Apis;* Bry.; Cic.; Cinch.; *Helleb.;* Iodof.; Op.; Tub.; *Zinc. m.*

GLANDERS—Acon.; Ars.; Chin. s.; *Crot.;* Hep.; Hippoz.; *Kali bich.;* Lach.; *Merc. s.;* Phos.; Sep.; Sil.; Thuya.

GLANDS—Abscess: Bell.; Calc. c.; Calc. iod.; Cistus; Hep.; Lapis alb.; *Merc.;* Nit. ac.; Rhus t.; *Sil*

Affections, traumatic—Aster.; Con.

Atrophy—Iod.

Induration—Alumen; Ars.; Ars. br.; *Aster.;* Aur. mur.; Bad.; *Bar. c.; Bar. iod.;* Bar. m.; Bell.; Berb. aq.; *Brom.;* Calc. c.; Calc. chlor.; *Calc. fl.; Carbo an.;* Cinch.; *Cistus;* Clem.; *Con.;* Dulc.; Graph.; Hekla;

Iod.; Kali iod.; *Lapis alb.*; Merc. i. fl.; Merc. i. r.; Operc.; Phyt.; *Rhus t.*; *Spong.*; Thyr.: Trifol. r.

Inflammation (ADENITIS)—Acute: Acon.; Ail.; Alumen; Ananth.; *Apis;* Ars. iod.; Bar. c.; Bar. iod.; *Bell.*; *Cistus;* Clem.; *Dulc.*; Graph.; *Hep.*; Iod.; *Iodof.*; *Kali iod.*; *Merc. i. r.*; *Merc. s.*; Operc.; *Phyt.*; Rhus t.; Sil.; *Sil. mar.*

Inflammation, chronic: GLANDULAR SWELLINGS—Acon. lyc.; *Ail.*; *Alnus*; Apis; Ars. br.; Ars.; *Ars. iod.*; Arum; Astacus; Aur. mur.; Bad.; *Bar. c.;* Bar. iod.; Bar. mur.; *Brom.*; *Calc. c.*; *Calc. fl.*; *Calc. iod.*; Calc. p.; Calend.; *Carbo an.*; *Cistus;* Clem.; *Con.*, Coryd.; Crot.; Dulc.; Ferr. iod.; *Filix*; Graph.; Hep.; *Iod.*; *Kali iod.*; Lach.; *Lapis alb.*; Lyc.; Med.; Merc. cy.; Merc. i. fl.; *Merc. i. r.*; Merc. s.; Nit. ac.; *Phyt.*; Psor.; Rhus t.; *Rumex*; Sal. mar.; Scirrhin.; *Scrophul.*; *Sil.*; Sil. mar.; *Spong.*; *Sul.*; Taxus; Thiosin.; Thuya; Tub.

LOCATION—OF GLANDULAR AFFECTION: Axillary: Acon. lyc.; *Aster.*; *Bar. c.*; Bell.; Calc. c.; Carbo an.; *Con.*; Elaps; Graph.; Hep.; Jugl. r.; *Lact. ac.*; Nat. s.; Nit. ac.; Phyt.; Raph.; Rhus t.; Sil.; Sul.

Bronchial—Bell.; Calc. c.; Calc. fl.; *Iod.*; Merc. c.; Tub.

Cervical—Acon. lyc.; *Am. c.*; Astac.; Bac.; *Bar. c.*; Bar. iod.; *Bell.*; *Brom.*; Calc. c.; Calc. chlor.; Calc. fl.; Calc. iod.; *Carbo an.*; Caust.; *Cistus;* Dulc.; Graph.; Hekla; *Hep.*; Iod.; Kali iod.; Kali m.; *Lapis alb.*; Mag. p.; *Merc. i. fl.*; *Merc. i. r.*; Merc.; Nit. ac.; *Rhus t.*; Rhus r.; Rhus v.; Sal. mar.; Sil.; Spong.; *Still.*; Sul.

Inguinal—Apis; Ars.; Aur.; Bac.; *Bar. c.*; Bar. m.; Bell.; *Calc. c.*; Carbo an.; Clem.; Dulc.; Graph.; Kali iod.; *Merc. i. fl.*; *Merc. s.*; *Nit. ac.*; Ocim.; Pall.; Pinus sylv.; Rhus t.; Sil.; Sul.; Xerophyl.

Mesenteric—*Ars.*; Ars. iod.; Bac.; Bar. c.; Bar. mur.; *Calc. c.*; **Calc. fl.**; *Calc. iod.*; Con.; Graph.; *Iod.*; Iodof.; Lapis alb.; Merc. c.; Mez.; Tub. See Tabes Mesenterica.

Parotid—Inflammation (Parotitis, Mumps): *Acon.*; Ail.; Am. c.; Anthrac.; Ant. t.; Aur. mur.; *Bar. c.*; Bar. m.; *Bell.*; *Brom.*; Calc. c.; Carbo an.; Cham.; Cistus; Dulc.; Euphras.; Ferr. p.; Hep.; *Kali bich.*; Kali m.; Lach.; Mag. p.; *Merc. c.*; Merc. cy.; Merc. i. fl.; Merc. i. r.; *Merc. s.*; *Phyt.*; Piloc.; *Puls.*; *Rhus t.*; *Sil.*; Sul. iod.; Trifol.; Trifol. r.

Parotitis, gangrenous—Anthrac.

Parotitis, metastases to brain—Apis; Bell.

Parotitis, metastases to mammæ ovaries—Con.; Jabor. Puls.;

Parotitis, metastases to testes—Aur.; *Clem.*; *Ham.*; *Puls.*; Rhus t.

Parotitis, persistent—Bar. ac.; Bar. c.; *Con.*; *Iod.*; Sil.

Sebaceous glands—Lyc.; Psor.; Raph.; Sil.; Sul. See Skin.

Submaxillary—Alnus; *Arum*; Asimina; *Bar. c.*; Brom.; Calc. c.; Calend.; Cham.; Cistus; Clem.; Iod.; *Kali bich.*; Kali m.; Lyc.; Mag. p.; Merc. cy.; *Merc. i. r.*; Merc. s.; Nat. m.; Petrol.; Pinus sylv.; Phyt.; *Rhus t.*; Sil.; Staph.; Sul.; Trifol.; Trifol. r.

Thyroid (Goitre, bronchocele)—Adren.; Am. c.; Am. m.; Apis; Aur. sul.; Bad.; Bar. iod.; *Bell.*; *Brom.*; Calc. c.; Calc. fl.; Calc. iod.; Caust.; Chrom. s.; Cistus; *Crot. casc.*; Ferr. m.; *Fluor. ac.*; *Fucus*; Glon.; Hep.; *Hydr.*; Hydroc. ac.; *Iod.*; *Iodothyr.*; *Iris*; Kali c.; *Kali iod.*; *Lapis* *alb.*; Mag. p.; Merc. i. fl.; *Nat. m.*; Phos.; Phyt.; Pineal gl. ext.; Puls.; Sil.; *Spong.*; Sul.; *Thyr.*

Thyroid—(EXOPHTHALMIC GOITRE—Basedow's disease)—Amyl; Ars.; Ars. iod.; Aur.; Bad.; Bar. c.; *Bell.*; Brom.; *Cact.*; *Calc. c.*; Can. ind.; Chrom. s.; Colch.; Con.; Echin.; Ephedra; Ferr. iod.; *Ferr. m.*; Ferr. p.; *Fluor. ac.*; Fucus; *Glon.*; *Iod.*; Jabor.; *Lycop.*; Nat. m.; *Piloc.*; Spart. s.; Spong.; Stram.; *Thyr.*

Paroxysm—Cact.; Dig.; Glon.; Samb.

GRANULATIONS—Exuberant: Calend.; Nit. ac.; Sab.; *Sil.*; Thuya. See Ulcers.

GREASE—In horse: Thuya.

HEMOPHILIA—Small wounds, bleed profusely, or protractedly: *Adren.*; Ail.; Ars.; Bov.; Calc. lact.; Cinch.; *Crot.*; Ferr. m.; *Ham.*; Kreos.; *Lach.*; Merc.; Millef.; *Nat. sil.*; Phos.; Sec.; Tereb.

HEMORRHAGES—Acal.; *Acet. ac.*; *Achillea*; *Acon.*; *Adren.*; Alumen; Alum.; Anthrac.; *Arn.*; Ars. hyd.; Bell.; Bothrops; *Bov.*; *Cact.*; Canth.; Carbo v.; Chin. s.; *Cinch.*; *Cinnam.*; Croc.; *Crot.*; Dig.; Elaps; Erech.; Ergotin; *Erig.*; Ferr. m.; *Ferr. p.*; Ficus; Gall. ac.; Gelatin; *Geran.*; *Ham.*; *Hydrastin*; *Ipec.*; Kali c.; Kreos.; Lach.; Meli.; Merc. cy.; *Millef.*; Mur. ac.; Nat. sil.; *Nit. ac.*; Op.; *Phos.*; Puls.; *Sab.*; Sanguis.; *Sec.*; *Sul. ac.*; Sul.; *Tereb.*; Thlaspi; Tilia; *Trill.*; Ustil.; Ver. a.; Xanth.

Hemorrhage, chronic effects—Stront. c.

Hemorrhage, from traumatism—Aran.; *Arn.*; Bov.; Euphorb. pil.; Ham.; *Millef.*; Trill.

Hemorrhage, hysterical (hemosialemesis)—Bad.; Croc.; Hyos.; Ign.; Kali iod.; Merc. s.; Sticta; Sul.

Hemorrhage, with face intensely red, preceding—Meli.

Hemorrhage, with fainting tinnitus, loss of sight, general coldness, even convulsions—*Cinch.*; Ferr. m.; Phos.

Hemorrhage, with no mental anxiety—Ham.

Hemorrhage, with putrescence; tingling in limbs; debility—Sec.

Hemorrhage, without fever or pain—Millef.

Blood, bright red—*Acon.*; Bell.; Erech.; *Erig.*; Ferr. m.; *Ferr. p.*; *Ipec.*; Led.; *Millef.*; Nit. ac.; Phos.; Phos.; Sab.; *Trill.*; Ustil.

Blood, clotted, partly fluid—Erig.; Ferr.; Plat.; Puls.; Ratanh.; *Sab.*; Ustil.

Blood, dark, clotted—Alum.; Anthrac.; Cinch.; *Croc.*; Crot.; *Elaps*; Merc. cy.; Merc.; Mur. ac.; Plat.; *Sul. ac.*; Tereb.; *Thlaspi*; Trill.

Blood, decomposes rapidly—Acet. ac.; Am. c.; Anthrac.; *Crot.*; Lach.; Tereb.

Non-coagulable; intermittent—Phos.

Non-coagulable, thin, dark—*Crot.*; Elaps; *Lach.*; *Sec.*; Sul. ac.

Thin, pale, fluid—Ferr.; Tilia.

Venous, dark, clotted—Ham.; Mangif. ind.

Vicarious—Acet. ac.; Ham.

HODGKIN'S DISEASE (pseudo-leukemia)—Acon. lyc.; Acon.; Ars.; Ars.

GENERALITIES

iod.; Bar. iod.; Calc. fl.; Ferr. picr.; *Iod.;* Kali m.; **Nat. m.; Phos.;** Scrophul.

HOOK-WORM DISEASE—Carbon. tetrachl.; Chenop.; Thymol.

INFLAMMATIONS—Abrot.; Acon.; *Agros!.;* Apis; Arn.; Ars.; *Bell.; Bry.;* Canth.; Chel.; Cinch.; *Ferr. p.;* Hep.; *Iod.;* Kali bich.; Kali c.; Kali iod.; Kali m.; Kali s.; *Nat. nit.; Spiranth.;* Sul.; *Ver. v.;* Vib. op.

Inflammation, passive—*Dig.; Gels.;* Puls.; Sul.

Inflammation, surgical—Acon.; *Anthrac.;* Arn.; Ars.; Ars. iod.; *Bell.;* Bellis; Calend.; Calc. s.; Echin.; Gun powder; *Hep.;* H*y*per.; Iod.; Merc. c.; Merc. i. r.; Myrtis. s.; *Pyr.;* Rhus t.; *Sil.* See Pyemia.

Inflammation, to favor absorption—Ant. t.; Apis; *Kali iod.;* Kali m.; Lyc.; Phos.; Sul.

INJURIES (traumatisms)—Acet. ac.; Acon.; Angust.; *Arn.; Bellis;* Bufo; *Calend.; Cic.;* Crot. t.; Euphras.; Glon.; *Ham.; Hyper.; Led.;* Mag. c.; Millef.; Nat. s.; Physost.; *Rhus t.;* Ruta; Stont. c.; Sul. ac.; Verb.

Bruises, contusions—Acet. ac.; *Arn.;* Bellis; *Con.;* Echin.; Euphras.; *Ham.; Hyper.;* Led.; *Rhus t.; Ruta;* Sul. ac.; *Symphyt.;* Verb.

Bruises, of bone—Arn.; Calc. p.; *Ruta; Symphyt.*

Bruises, of breast—Bellis; *Con.*

Bruises, of eye—Acon.; *Arn.;* Ham.; *Led.; Symphyt.*

Bruises, of parts, rich in sentient nerves—Bellis; *Hyper.*

Bruises, with persistence of ecchymosis—Arn.; Led.; *Sul. ac.*

Burns, scalds—Acet. ac.; Acon.; Arn.; *Ars.;* Calc. s.; Calend.; Camph.; *Canth.;* Carb. ac.; *Caust.;* Gaulth.; Grind.; Ham.; *Hep.; Jabor.; Kali bich.;* Kreos.; Petrol.; Rhus t.; Tereb.; *Urt.*

Burns, fail to heal, or ill effects—Carbo ac.; Caust.

Chronic effects of injuries—*Arn.;* Carbo v.; *Cic.; Con.;* Glon.; **Ham.;** Hyper.; Led.; *Nat. s.; Stront. c.*

Mental symptoms, from injuries—Cic.; *Glon.;* Hyper.; Mag. c.; *Nat. s.*

Post-operative disorders—Acet. ac.; Apis; *Arn.; Bellis;* Berb. v.; *Calend.;* Calc. fl.; Camph.; Croc.; Ferr. p.; *Hyper.;* Kali s.; Millef.; Naja; Nit. ac.; Raph.; Rhus t.; *Staph.; Stront.;* Ver. a.

Prostration, from injuries—*Acet. ac.;* Camph.; Hyper.; *Sul. ac.;* Ver. a.

Sprains, strains—Acet. ac.; *Acon.;* Agn.; *Arn.;* Bell.; *Bellis; Calc. c.;* Calc. fl.; Calend.; *Carbo an.;* Formica; *Hyper.;* Millef.; Nux v.; Rhod.; *Rhus t.; Ruta;* Stront.; *Symphyt.*

Sprains, tendency to—Nat. c.; Nat. m.; Psor.; *Sil.*

Tetanus prevented—Hyper.; Physost.

Wounds, bleed profusely—Arn.; *Crot.;* Ham.; Kreos.; *Lach.;* Millef.; *Phos. ac.*

Wounds, bleed profusely, after a fall—*Arn.;* Ham.; Millef.

Wounds, bluish, discolored—*Lach.;* Lyssin.

Wounds, bullet, from—Arn.; Calend.

Wounds, contused—*Arn.;* Ham.; Sul. ac.; Symphyt.

Wounds, dissecting, post-mortem—*Anthrac.; Apis;* Ars.; Crot.; *Echin.; Lach.; Pyr.* See Pyemia.

Wounds, incised—Arn.; Calend.; Ham.; Hyper.; Led.; *Staph.*

GENERALITIES

Wounds, involving muscles, tendons, joints—Calend.

Wounds, lacerated—Arn.; *Calend.*; Carb. ac.; Ham.; Led.; *Hyper.*; Staph.; Sul. ac.; Symphyt.

Wounds, punctured—Apis; Hyper.; *Led.*; Phaseol.

Wounds, with burning, cutting, shooting—Nat. c.

Wounds, with gangrenous tendency—Calend.; Sal. ac.; Sul. ac. See Dissecting.

LEUCOCYTHEMIA—leukemia: Aran.; *Ars.*; *Ars. iod.*; Bar. iod.; Benzol.; Bry.; Calc. c.; Ceanoth.; Chin. s.; Con.; *Ferr. picr.*; Ipec.; Merc.; *Nat. m.*; Nat. s.; Nux v.; Phos.; *Picr. ac.*; *Thuya.* See Anemia.

Leucocythemia, splenic—*Ceanoth.*; Nat. s.; Querc.; Succin.

LYMPHANGITIS—Anthrac.; *Apis*; Ars. iod.; *Bell.*; Bothrops; Bufo; Crot.; Echin.; Hippoz.; *Lach.*; Latrod. k.; Merc. i. r.; *Merc. s.*; Myg.; Pyr.; Rhus t.

MARASMUS (emaciation, atrophy, wasting)—*Abrot.*; Acet. ac.; Ant. iod.; Arg. m.; *Arg. n.*; *Ars.*; Ars. iod.; Bar. c.; *Calc. c.*; Calc. p.; Calc. sil.; Carbo an.; Carbo v.; Caust.; Cetrar.; Cinch.; Clem.; Ferr. m.; *Ferr. p.*; Fluor. ac.; Glycerin; Helon.; *Hep.*; *Hydr.*; *Iod.*; Kali iod.; Kali p.; Kreos.; Led.; *Lyc.*; Mang. ac.; *Merc. c.*; Merc. s.; Nat. c.; *Nat. m.*; *Ol. j. as.*; Op.; *Phos. ac.*; Phos.; Phyt.; *Plumb. ac.*; Plumb. iod.; *Plumb. m.*; Psor.; Ricin.; Rhus t.; *Samb.*; *Sanic.*; *Sars.*; Sec.; Selen.; *Sil.*; Stann.; Staph.; *Sul.*; *Syph.*; Tereb.; *Thuya*; *Tub.*; Uran.; Vanad.; *Ver. a.*; Zinc. m.

Affected parts, atrophy—Ars.; *Caust.*; Graph.; Led.; Selen.

Atrophy of children—*Abrot.*; Arg. n.; *Ars.*; Ars. sul.; Bac.; Bar. c.; *Calc. p.*; Calc. sil.; *Iod.*; *Nat. m.*; *Ol. j. as.*; Phos.; Pod.; Psor.; Sanic.; Sars.; *Sul.*; Thyr.; *Tub.*

Atrophy of face, hands, legs, feet, single parts—Selen.

Atrophy of legs—*Abrot.*; *Am. m.*; *Arg. n.*; Iod.; Pinus sylv.; Sanic.; Tub.

Atrophy of mesenteric glands (tabes mesenterica)—Ars.; Bapt.; Bar. c.; Calc. ars.; *Calc. c.*; Calc. chlor.; Calc. hypophos.; Calc. iod.; *Calc. p.*; Con.; Hep.; *Iod.*; Merc. c.; Plumb. ac.; Sacchar. of.; Sil.

Atrophy of neck, flabby, loose skin—Abrot.; Calc. p.; Iod.; *Nat. m.*; Sanic.; Sars.

Atrophy, from above, downwards—Lyc.; Nat. m.

Atrophy, from below upwards—Abrot.

Atrophy, neck so weak, unable to hold head up—*Abrot.*; Æth.; Calc. p.

Atrophy, progressive, muscular—Ars.; Carbon. s.; Hyper.; Kali hypoph.; Phos.; Physost.; *Plumb.*; Sec.

Atrophy, rapid—Iod.; Plumb. m.; Samb.; *Thuya*; *Tub.*

Atrophy, rapid, with cold sweat, debility—Ars.; *Tub.*; Ver. a.

Atrophy, with bulimia—*Abrot.*; Acet. ac.; Ars. iod.; Bar. c.; Calc. c.; Con.; *Iod.*; *Nat. m.*; Sanic.; Tub.; Thyr.

Atrophy, with shrivelled up look—Abrot.; *Arg. n.*; Fluor. ac.; Kreos.; Op.; Sanic.; Sars.; Sil.; *Sul.*

MUSCLES—Inflammation (myositis): *Arn.*; Bell.; *Bry.*; Hep.; Kali iod.; Merc. s.; *Mez.*; Rhus t.

Muscles, pain (myalgia)—*Acon.*; Ant. t.; *Arn.*; Ars.; Bell.; Bellis; Bry.;

GENERALITIES

Carbon. s.; Caust.; *Cim.;* Colch.; *Dulc.; Gels.;* Led.; *Marcot.;* Merc.; Morph.; Nux v.; *Ran. b.; Rham. cal.; Rhus t.; Ruta;* Sal. ac.; Stram.; *Strych.;* Val.; *Ver. a.;* Ver. v. See Rheumatism (Locomotor System).

Muscles, pain cramp-like—Ant. t.; Cholas ter.; *Cim.;* Colch.; Col.; *Cupr. m.; Mag. p.;* Nux v.; Op.; Plumb. ac.; Sec.; *Sul.;* Syph.; Ver. a.

Muscles, pain, hysterical—Ign.; Nux v.; Plumb.; Puls.

Muscles, soreness, stiffness—Angust.; *Arn.;* Bad.; *Bapt.;* Bell.; *Bellis; Bry.;* Caust.; Cic.; *Cim.;* Cupr. ac.; *Gels.;* Guaiac.; Ham.; *Helon.;* Jacar.; *Magnol.;* Merc.; Myr.; *Phyt.;* Pyr.; *Rhus t.; Ruta;* Sang.

Muscles, twitchings—Acon.; *Agar.;* Angust.; Apis; Ars.; Asaf.; Atrop.; *Bell.; Bry.;* Caust.; *Cham.; Cic.; Cim.;* Cina; *Cocc.;* Cod.; *Col.;* Croc.; *Cupr. m.;* Ferr. red.; Gels.; Helleb.; *Hyos.; Ign.;* Kali br.; Kali c.; Lupul.; Mez.; *Morph.; Myg.; Nux v.;* Op.; Phos.; Physost.; Plumb. ac.; Puls.; *Santon.;* Sec.; Spig.; *Stram.; Strych.;* Tar. h.; Ver. v.; *Zinc. m.;* Zizia.

Muscles, weakness, debility—Acet. ac.; *Alet.; Alumen;* Alum.; Am. caust.; Anhal.; *Ant. t.;* Arg. n.; Ars.; Bry.; Calc. c.; Carbo v.; Caust.; Colch.; Collin.; *Con.; Gels.; Helleb.;* Helon.; Hep.; Hydr.; Ign.; Kali c.; Kali hypophos.; *Kali p.;* Kal.; Lob. infl.; Mag. p.; Merc. v.; *Mur. ac.;* Nux v.; Onosm.; Pall.; Physal.; Physost.; *Picr. ac.;* Plumb. ac.; Rhus t.; Sabad.; *Sarcol. ac.;* Sil.; *Strych.;* **Tab.;** *Ver. a.; Ver. v.; Zinc. m.* See Adynamia (Nervous System).

MUTINISM of childhood—Agraph.

MYXEDEMA—Ars.; Prim. ob.; *Thyr.*

OBESITY (adiposis, corpulence)—*Am. br.;* Am. c.; Ant. c.; Ars.; *Cals. ars.; Calc. c.; Calop.;* Caps.; Col.; *Fucus;* Graph.; *Iodothyr.;* Kali br.; Kali c.; Lac d.; Mang. ac.; Phos.; *Phyt.;* Sabal; *Thyr.;* Tussil. fr.

Obesity, in children—*Ant. c.;* Bar. c.; *Calc. c.; Caps.;* Ferr. m.; Kali bich.; Sacchar. of.

POLYCYTHEMIA—Phos.

PROPHYLACTICS—Catheter fever: Camph. ac.

Cholera—Ars.; Cupr. ac.; Ver. a.

Diphtheria—Apis (30); Diph. (30).

Erysipelas—Graph. (30).

Hay fever—Ars.; Psor.

Hydrophobia—Bell.; Canth.; Hyos.; Stram.

Intermittent fever—Ars.; Chin. s.

Measles—*Acon.;* Ars.; Puls.

Mumps—Trifol. rep.

Pus infection—Arn.

Quinsy—Bar. c. (30).

Scarlet fever—Bell. (30); Eucal.

Variola—Ant. t.; Hydr.; Kali cy.; *Malandr.;* **Thuya;** *Vaccin.;* Variol.

Whooping cough—Dros.; Vaccin.

PYEMIA, SEPTICEMIA—*Acon.; Anthrac.;* Apium v.; *Arn.; Ars.;* Ars. iod.; Atrop.; *Bapt.;* Bell.; Bothrops; *Bry.;* Calend.; *Carb. ac.; Chin. ars.; Chin. s.;* Crot.; *Echin.;* Gun powder; Hippoz.; Hyos.; Irid.; *Lach.;* Latrod. has.; Merc. cy.; Merc. s.; Methyl. bl.; Mur. ac.; Nat.

sul. carb.; *Pyr.*; *Rhus t.*; *Sec.*; Sepsin; Sil.; Streptococcin; **Tar. c.**; Ver. a.

RACHITIS (rickets)—*Ars.*; Ars. iod.; Calc. ac.; *Calc. c.*; Calc. hypoph.; *Calc. p.*; Calc. sil.; Ferr. p.; Fluor. ac.; Hekla; Hep.; *Iod.*; Kali iod.; Mag. m.; Med.; Merc. s.; Nit. ac.; *Phos. ac.*; *Phos.*; Pinus sylv.; Sanic.; *Sil.*; Sul.; Supraren. ext.; Ther.; Thuya; Thyr.; *Tub.* See Scrofulosis.

SCROFULOSIS—*Æthiops*; Alnus; Alum.; Ars.; *Ars. iod.*; *Aurums*; Bac.; Bad.; *Barytas*; Brom.; *Calcareas*; Caps.; Carbo an.; *Caust.*; Cinnab.; Cistus; Clem.; Con.; Diph.; *Dulc.*; *Ferrums*; Fluor. ac.; *Graph.*; Helleb.; *Hep.*; Hydr.; *Iodides*; Iodof.; Kali bich.; Kali iod.; Kreos.; Lapis alb.; Lyc.; Mag. m.; *Mercuries*; Mez.; Nit. ac.; Ol. j. as.; Petrol.; Phos. ac.; Phos.; Plumb. iod.; Psor.; Ruta; Samb.; Sedum; *Sil.*; Sil. mar.; Still.; *Sul.*; Ther.; *Tub.*; Viola tr.

SCURVY (scorbutus)—Acet. ac.; *Agave*; Alnus; *Ars.*; Bov.; Carbo v.; Chin. s.; Cinch.; *Ferr. p.*; Galium ap.; Ham.; Kali chlor.; Kali p.; Kreos.; Lach.; *Merc. s.*; *Mur. ac.*; Nat. m.; Nit. ac.; Nitro. mur. ac.; Phos. ac.; *Phos.*; Rhus t.; Staph.; Sul. ac.; Sul.; Urium.

SENILE DECAY—*Agn.*; *Arg. n.*; Ars.; *Bar. c.*; Can. ind.; *Con.*; Fluor. ac.; Iod.; *Lyc.*; *Oophor.*; Phos.; Thiosin.

SENSATION, of burning—*Acon.*; *Agar.*; Agrost.; Anthrac.; *Apis*; *Ars.*; Bell.; *Calad.*; *Canth.*; *Caps.*; Carbo an.; *Caust.*; *Cepa*; Cham.; *Doryph.*; Eosin; Kreos.; Ol. an.; Phos. ac.; *Phos.*; Pip. m.; Pop. c.; Rhus t.; *Sang.*; Sec.; *Sul.*; Tar. h.

Sensation, of constriction—Alum. sil.; *Anac.*; Asar.; *Cact.*; Caps.; *Carb. ac.*; Col.; Iod.; Lach.; Mag. p.; Naja; Nat. m.; *Nit. ac.*; Plumb. m.; Sec.; *Sul.*

Sensation, of numbness—*Acon.*; *Agar.*; Alum. sil.; *Ambra*; Ars.; Bov.; Calc. p.; *Ced.*; *Cham.*; Cic.; *Cocaine*, Cod.; *Con.*; Helod.; Ign.; Irid.; Kali br.; Nux v.; *Oleand.*; Onosm.; Ox. ac.; *Phos.*; *Plat.*; Plumb.; Raph.; *Rhus t.*; Sec.; Stann.; Thallium.

Sensation, of numbness, attending pains—*Acon.*; Can. ind.; *Cham.*; Con.; *Kal.*; *Plat.*; *Rhus t.*; Stann.; Staph.

Sensation, of stitching—Acon.; *Asclep.*; *Bry.*; Kali c.; Mag. p.; Nat. s.; Nit. ac.; *Ran. b.*; Rumex; Scilla.

TUMORS—Ananth.; Aur. m. n.; *Bar. c.*; Bar. iod.; Bar. m.; Bellis; Calc. ars.; *Calc. c.*; *Calc. fl.*; Cistus; Col.; Con.; Eucal.; *Ferr. iod.*; Ferr. picr.; Form. ac.; Galium ap.; *Graph.*; Hekla; Hydr.; Kali br.; Kali iod.; Kreos.; Lach.; Lapis alb.; *Lob. erin.*; Lyc.; Malandr.; Mancin.; Med.; Merc. i. r.; Merc. per.; Nat. cacodyl.; Nat. sil.; *Phos.*; Phyt.; Plumb. iod.; Psor.; *Semperv. t.*; *Sil.*; Thiosin.; Thuya; Thyr.; Urea; Uric ac. See Cancer.

Cystic—Apis; *Bar. c.*; Calc. c.; Calc. p.; Calc. s.; *Iod.*; *Kali br.*; Platanus; Sil.; Staph. See Scalp (Head); Skin.

Bone-like, protuberances—*Calc. fl.*; *Hekla*; Lapis alb.; Malandr.; Ruta; Sil.

Enchondroma—Calc. fl.; Lapis alb.; Sil.

Epithelial—Acet. ac.; Ferr. picr. See Skin.

GENERALITIES

Epulis—Calc. c.; **Plumb. ac.;** *Thuya.*
Erectile—Lyc.; *Phos.*
Fibroid—*Calc. iod.;* Calc. s.; Chrom. s.; Graph.; Hydrast. m.; Kali iod.; Lapis alb.; Sec.; *Sil.;* Thiosin.; Thyr. See Uterus.
Fibroid, hemorrhage—*Hydrast. m.;* Lapis alb.; Sab.; Thlaspi; *Trill.;* Ustil.
Fungoid—Clem.; Mancin.; Phos.; *Thuya.*
Ganglion—Benz. ac.; Kali m.; *Ruta; Sil.*
Lipoma—*Bar. c.;* Calc. ars.; Calc. c.; Lapis alb.; Phyt.; *Thuya;* Uric ac.
Naevus on right temple, flat; in children—Fluor. ac.
Neuroma—Calend.; Cepa.
Nodulated, of tongue—Galium ap.
Papillomata—Ant. c.; Nit. ac.; Staph.; *Thuya.*
Polypi—*Calc. c.;* Cepa; *Formica;* Kali bich.; Kali s.; Lemna; Nit. ac.; *Phos.;* Psor.; Sang.; *Sang. n.;* Sil.; Teucr.; *Thuya.* See Nose, **Ear,** Uterus.
Ranula—Ambra; Thuya.
Sarcocele—Merc. i. r. See Male Sexual System.
Tumors of urinary passages—Analinum.
Vascular in urethra—Can. s.; *Eucal.*
Wen—Bar. c.; Benz. ac.; Calc. c.; Con.; Daphne; Graph.; Hep.; **Kali c.**: Mez.

MODALITIES

AGGRAVATION—Acids:—*Ant. c.;* Ant. t.; Ferr. m.; Lach.; Merc. c.; Nux v.; Phos.; *Sep.* See Stomach.

Afternoon—Æsc.; Alum.; Am. m.; Ars.; *Bell.;* Cenchris; Cocc.; Coccus; Fagop.; Kali bich.; Kali c.; Kali cy.; Kali n.; Lil. t.; Lob. infl.; *Rhus t.;* Sep.; Sil.; Still.; *Thuya;* Verbasc.; Xerophyl.; X-ray.

Afternoon, late—*Apis;* Aran.; Carbo v.; Colch.; *Col.;* Helleb.; *Lyc.;* Mag. p.; Med.; Meli.; Ol. an.; *Puls.;* Sabad.; Zinc. See Evening.

Air cold, dry—Abrot.; Acon.; Æsc.; Agar.; Alum.; *Ars.;* Asar.; Aur. m.; Bac.; Bar. c.; Bell.; *Bry.;* Calc. c.; *Camph.;* Caps.; Carbo an.; *Caust.;* Cham.; Cinch.; Cistus; Cupr. m.; Cur.; Euphorb. d.; *Hep.;* Ign.; *Kali c.;* Mag. p.; *Mez.;* Nat. c.; *Nux v.;* Plumb.; *Psor.;* Rhod.; *Rumex;* Selen.; Sep.; Sil.; *Spong.;* Tub.; Urt.; Viola od.; Viscum.

Air, open—*Acon.;* Agar.; Benz. ac.; Bry.; Cadm. s.; *Caps.;* Carbon. s.; *Cham.;* Cic.; Cocc.; Coff.; Coral.; Crot.; *Cycl.;* Epiph.; Euphras.; Ign.; Kal.; Kreos.; Linar.; Mosch.; *Nux v.;* Ran. b.; *Senega;* Solan. lyc.; Thea; X-ray. See Air, Cold.

Anger—*Bry.;* Cham.; Col.; Ign.; *Nux v.; Staph.* See Emotions (Mind).

Arms moved backward—Sanic.

Ascending stairs—Am. c.; *Ars.;* But. ac.; Cact.; *Calc. c.;* Can. s.; Cocc.; Glon.; *Kali c.;* Menyanth.; Spong.

Autumn; warm days, cold, damp nights—Merc. v.

Bathing—*Ant. c.;* Bellis; Calc. c.; Caust.; Formica; Mag. p.; Nux m.; Physost.; *Rhus t.;* Sep.; *Sul.* See Water.

Bed, turning in—*Con.;* Nux v.; Puls.

Beer—Bry.; *Kali bich.;* Nux m.

Bending double—Diosc.

Bending forward—*Bell.;* Kal.; Nux v.

Biting hard—Am. c.; *Verbasc.*

Breakfast, after—Cham.; *Nux v.;* Phos.; *Thuya;* Zinc. m. See Eating.

Breakfast, before—Croc.

Bright objects—*Bell.;* Canth.; Coccinel.; *Lyssin; Stram.*

Brushing teeth—Coccus; Staph.

Celibacy—Con.

Coffee—Aster.; Can. ind.; *Canth.;* Carbo v.; Caust.; *Cham.;* Ign.; Kali c.; *Nux v.;* Psor.; Thuya.

Coitus, after—Agar.; *Calad.;* Calc. s.; *Cinch.;* Kali c.; Nux v.; *Phos. ac.;* Phos.; *Selen.;* Sep.

Cold—Acon.; Agar.; Alumen; *Alum.;* Am. c.; Ant. c.; *Ars.;* Bad.; Bar. c.; Bell.; *Bry.;* Calc. c.; *Camph.;* Caps.; *Caust.;* Cham.; Collins.; Cocc.; Coff.; Con.; Crot. casc.; *Dulc.;* Formica; *Hep.;* Ign.; *Kali c.;* Kali p.; Kreos.; Lach.; Lob. infl.; *Mag. p.;* Merc.; *Mez.;* Mosch.; Nit. ac.; Nux m.; *Nux v.;* Ran. b.; *Rhod.;* Rhus t.; *Rumex;* Ruta; Sabad.; *Selen.; Sep.; Sil.;* Spig.; *Stram.;* Stront.; Sul. ac.; Tab.; Ver. a.; Xerophyl.

Concussion—Cic. See Jar.

Consolation—Cact.; Graph.; *Helleb.*; Ign.; Lil. t.; *Nat. m.*; Sabal; Sep.; Sil.
Contact, of clothing, about neck—Glon.; *Lach.*; Sep. See Touch.
Conversation—Ambra; Cocc.; *Phos. ac.*; *Stann.* See Talking.
Cough—Ars.; Bry.; *Cina*; Hyos.; *Phos.*; Sep.; *Tellur.* See Respiratory System.
Damp living houses—Ant. t.; *Aran.*; Ars.; *Dulc.*; *Nat. s.*; Tereb.
Dampness—Amphis; *Aran.*; *Ars. iod.*; Aster.; Bar. c.; *Calc. c.*; Calend.; Carbo v.; Chimaph.; Chin. s.; Cinch.; Colch.; Crot.; Cur.; *Dulc.*; Elat.; Euphras.; Formica; Gels.; Kali iod.; Lathyr.; Lemna; Magnol.; Meli.; Mur. ac.; *Nat. s.*; Nux m.; *Petrol.*; *Phyt.*; Radium; Rhod.; *Rhus t.*; Ruta; Sep.; Sil.; Still.; Sul.; Tub.
Dampness, cold—Am. c.; Ant. t.; Aran.; Arn.; Asclep. t.; Aster.; Bor.; *Calc. c.*; *Calc. p.*; *Dulc.*; Gels.; *Guaiac.*; Mang. ac.; *Merc.*; Nux m.; Nux v.; Physal.; *Phyt.*; *Rhus t.*; Sil.; Thuya; Urt.; Ver. a.
Dampness, warm—Bapt.; Brom.; Carbo v.; Carbon. s.; *Gels.*; Ham.; Phos.; Sep.
Dark—*Ars.*; Calc. c.; Carbo an.; Phos.; *Stram.* See Emotions (Mind).
Daylight to sunset—Med.
Defecation, after—Æsc. See Stool (Abdomen).
Dentition—Æth.; *Bell.*; Bor.; Calc. c.; Calc. p.; Cham.; *Kreos.*; Phyt.; Pod.; *Rheum*; Zinc. m. See Teeth.
Dinner, after—Ars.; *Nux v.* See Stomach.
Direction, diagonally—*Agar.*; Bothrops.
Direction, diagonally, upper left, lower right—Agar.; Ant. t.; Stram.
Direction, diagonally, upper right, lower left—Ambra; Brom.; Med.; Phos.; Sul. ac.
Direction, downward—*Bor.*; Cact.; Kal.; Lyc.; *Sanic.*
Direction, outwards—Kali c.; Sul.
Direction, upwards—Benzin.; Eup. perf.; *Led.*
Drinking, during—Bell.
Eating—Abies n.; Æsc.; Æth.; Agar.; *Aloe*; Ant. c.; *Arg. n.*; *Ars.*; Bry.; *Calc. c.*; Carbo v.; Caust.; Chionanth.; Cina; *Cinch.*; Cocc.; Col.; Con.; *Crot. t.*; Dig.; *Graph.*; Hyos.; *Ipec.*; Kali bich.; *Kali c.*; Kali p.; Kreos.; Lach.; *Lyc.*; Mag. m.; Nat. m.; Nit. ac.; *Nux v.*; Ol. an.; Petrol.; Phos.; *Puls.*; Rheum; Rumex; Samb.; *Sep.*; Sil.; *Staph.*; Strych.; Sul.; Thea; Zinc. m. See Indigestion (Stomach).
Emotional excitement—Acon.; *Ambra*; *Arg. n.*; Aur.; Cinch.; Cob.; *Coff.*; *Colch.*; Collins.; Col.; Con.; Cupr. ac.; *Gels.*; Hyos.; *Ign.*; Kali p.; Lyssin; Nit. sp. d.; *Nux v.*; Petrol.; Phos. ac.; *Phos.*; Sil.; Staph. See Mind.
Erratic, shifting, constantly changing, symptoms—Apis; Berb. v.; *Ign.*; Kali bich.; *Kali s.*; *Lac c.*; Lil. t.; *Mang. ac.*; Paraf.; Phyt.; *Puls.*; Sanic.; *Tub.*
Evening—*Acon.*; *Alfal.*; *Ambra*; Am. br.; Am. m.; Apis.; Ant. t.; Arn.; Bell.; Bry.; Cajup.; Carbo v.; Caust.; *Cepa*; Cham.; Colch.; Crot.; Cycl.; Diosc.; Euonym.; Euphras.; Ferr. p.; *Helleb.*; *Hyos.*; *Lyc.*; Kali s.; Merc. c.; *Merc.*; Mez.; Nit. ac.; *Phos.*; Plat.; Plumb.; *Puls.*; Ran. b.;

Rumex; Ruta; *Sep.;* Sil.; Stann.; Sul. ac.; *Syph.;* Tab.; Vib. op.; X-ray; Zinc. m.

Eyes, closing—*Bry.;* Sep.; Ther.

Eyes, motion of—*Bry.;* Nux v.; Spig.

Eyes, opening of—Tab.

Fasting—Croc.; Iod.

Fats—Carbo v.; *Cycl.;* Kali m.; *Puls.;* Thuya.

Feet, exposure—Con.; Cupr.; *Sil.*

Feet hanging down—Puls.

Fish—Nat. s.; Urt.

Fog—Bapt.; Gels.; Hyper. See Dampness.

Fright—*Acon.;* Gels.; *Ign.;* Op.; Ver. a.

Fruit—*Ars.;* Bry.; *Cinch.; Col.;* Ipec.; Samb.; *Ver. a.*

Gaslight—*Glon.;* Nat. c.

Grief—Aur.; Gels.; *Ign.; Phos. ac.;* Staph.; Ver. a. See Emotions (Mind).

Hair-cut—Acon.; *Bell.;* Glon.

Head, uncovering—Bell.; Sil. See Air, Cold.

High altitudes—Coca.

Hot drinks—Chionanth.; Lach.; Stann.

Inspiration—*Acon.; Bry.;* Phos. b.; Ran. b.; Spig. See Respiratory System.

Intermittently—Anac.; *Cinch.;* Strych. See Periodical.

Jar—Arn.; *Bell.;* Berb. v.; *Bry.; Cic.;* Crot.; Glon.; Ign.; Nux v.; *Spig.;* Ther.

Laughing—Arg. m.; *Dros.;* Mang. ac.; *Phos.;* Stann.; Tellur.

Laundry work—Sep.

Left side—Agar.; Arg. m.; Arg. n.; Asaf.; Aster.; *Bellis;* Ceanoth.; Chimaph.; Cim.; Colch.; Cupr. m.; Erig.; *Lach.;* Lepid.; *Lil. t.;* Ox. ac.; Pulex; Rumex; Sapon.; Sep.; Ther.; *Thuya;* Ustil.

Left side, then right side—Lac c.; *Lach.*

Light—Acon.; *Bell.;* Calc. c.; Coca; *Con.;* Colch.; Graph.; Ign.; *Lyssin;* Nux v.; *Phos.;* Spig.; *Stram.*

Liquors—*Agar.;* Ant. c.; *Can. ind.; Carbo v.;* Cim.; *Lach.;* Led.; *Nux v.;* Ran. b.; *Stram.; Sul. ac.; Zinc. m.* See Alcoholism (Nervous System).

Localized spots—Coff.; *Ign.;* Kali bich.; Lil. t.; Ox. ac.

Looking, downwards—Acon.; *Kal.;* Oleand.; *Spig.;* Sul.

Looking, intently, at objects—Cina; Croc.

Looking upwards—Benzoin; Calc. c.; *Puls.;* Sul.

Lower half of body—Bac. t.

Lying down—Ambra; Ant. t.; Arn.; *Ars.;* Arum; Aur.; *Bell.;* Can. s.; Caust.; Cenchris; *Con.;* Croc.; *Diosc.;* Dros.; Dulc.; *Glon.; Hyos.;* Iberis; Ipec.; Kreos.; *Lach.;* Lyc.; Menyanth.; Nat. m.; Nat. s.; Plat.; *Phos.; Puls.; Rhus t.; Rumex;* Ruta; Samb.; Sil.; Tarax.; *Trifol.;* X-ray.

Lying, on back—Acet. ac.; *Nux v.;* Puls.; Rhus t.

Lying, on left side—Arg. n.; *Cact.;* Calad.; Coccus; Iberis; *Kali c.;* Lyc.; Magnol.; *Phos.;* Plat.; Ptel.; Puls.; *Spig.;* Viscum.

Lying, on painful, or affected side—Acon.; Ars.; Bar. c.; Calad.; Hep.; *Iod.; Kali c.; Nux m.;* Phos.; Ruta; Sil.; Tellur.; Vib. op.

Lying, on painless side—*Bry.;* Cham.; Col.; Ptel.; *Puls.*
Lying, on right side—Can. ind.; *Mag. m.;* Merc.; *Rhus t.;* Scroph; Stann.
Lying, with head low—Ars.
Masturbation—Calc. c.; *Cinch.;* Con.; *Nux v.; Phos. ac.;* Sep.; *Staph.*
Medicines, patent, aromatic, bitter vegetable pills—Nux v.
Menses, after—Alum.; *Bor.; Graph.;* Kreos.; Lil. t.; Nat. m.; Nux v.; Sep.; *Zinc. m.*
Menses, at beginning, and close—Lach.
Menses, before—Am. c.; *Bov.; Calc. c.;* Cocc.; Con.; Cupr. m.; *Gels.; Lach.;* Lyc.; Mag. m.; *Puls.;* Sars.; *Sep.;* Ver. a.; *Zinc. m.*
Menses, during—Am. c.; Arg. n.; *Bell.;* Bov.; Cham.; *Cim.;* Con.; *Graph.;* Ham.; Hyos.; *Kali c.;* Mag. c.; *Nux v.; Puls.; Sep.;* Sil.; Sul.; Ver. a.; *Vib. op.* See Menstruation (Female Sexual System).
Mental exertion—Agar.; Aloe; Amyl; *Anac.; Arg. n.;* Aur. m.; Calc. c.; Calc. p.; *Cim.; Cocc.;* Cupr. m.; *Gels.;* Ign.; Kali p.; *Nat. c.;* Nat. m.; *Nux v.; Phos.;* Phos. ac.; *Picr. ac.;* Sabad.; Sep.; *Sil.;* Thymol. See Mind.
Midnight, after—Apis; *Ars.;* Bell.; Carbo an.; *Dros.;* Ferr. m.; *Kali c.;* Kali n.; Nit. ac.; *Nux v.;* Phos.; *Pod.;* Rhus t.; Sil.; Thuya.
Midnight, at—Aran.; *Ars.;* Mez.
Midnight, before—Arg. n.; Bron..; Carbo v.; Cham.; *Coff.;* Led.; Lyc.; *Merc.;* Mur. ac.; Nit. ac.; Phos.; *Puls.;* Ran. s.; *Rhus t.; Rumex; Spong.;* Stann.
Milk—*Æth.;* Ant. t.; Calc. c.; *Carbo v.;* Cinch.; Homar.; Mag. c.; Nit. ac.; Sep.; *Sul.*
Misdeeds of others—Colch.; *Staph.*
Moon, full—*Alum.;* Calc. c.; Graph.; Sabad.; *Sil.*
Moonlight—Ant. c.; Thuya.
Moon, new—Alum.; Caust.; Clem.; *Sil.*
Morning—*Acal.;* Alum.; Ambra; *Am. m.;* Arg. n.; Aur.; *Bry.; Calc. c.;* Can. ind.; Croc.; Crot.; Fluor. ac.; Glon.; Ign.; *Kali bich.;* Kali n.; Lac c.; *Lach.;* Lil. t.; Lith. c.; Magnol.; Med.; Myg.; *Nat. m.;* Niccol.; *Nit. ac.;* Nuph.; *Nux v.;* Onosm.; *Phos.;* Phos. ac.; *Pod.; Puls.;* Rhus t.; Rumex; Sep.; Sil.; Stellar.; Strych.; *Sul.; Verbasc.*
Morning, early (2-5 A. M.)—*Æth.; Æsc.; Aloe;* Am. c.; Bac.; Bell.; Chel.; Cina; Coccus; Cur.; *Kali bich.; Kali c.;* Kali cy.; Kali p.; Nat. s.; *Nux v.;* Ox. ac.; *Pod.;* Ptel.; Rhod.; *Rumex; Sul.;* Thuya; Tub.
Morning, (10-11 A. M.)—Gels.; *Nat. m.; Sep.;* Sul.
Mortification from an offense—*Col.;* Lyc.; Staph.
Motion—*Æsc.;* Agar.; Aloe; Am. c.; Amyl; Anhal.; Apis; *Bell.; Berb. v.;* Bism.; *But. ac.;* Cact.; Cadm. s.; *Calad.;* Calc. ars.; Camph.; Ceanoth.; *Cim.;* Cinch.; *Cocc.;* Colch.; Cupr. m.; Dig.; Equis.; Ferr. p.; *Gels.;* Gettysburg Water; Guaiac.; Helon.; *Iberis;* Ipec.; Jugl. c.; Kali m.; *Kal.;* Lac c.; *Led.;* Linar.; Lob. infl.; Mag. p.; Med.; Meli.; *Merc.; Mez.; Nat. m.;* Nat. s.; Nit. ac.; Nux m.; *Nux v.;* Onosm.; Pall.; Petrol.; *Phyt.;* Phos.; Picr. ac.; Plat.; Plumb.; Pulex; Puls. nut.; *Ran. b.;* Rheum; Ruta; *Sab.;* Sang.; Scilla; *Sec.;* Senega; Sil.; Solan. lyc.; *Spig.;* Still.; Strych.; *Sul.;* Tab.; *Tar. h.;* Thea; Thymol; Ver. a.; Viscum.
Motion, downward—*Bor.;* Gels.; Saric.

Motion, on beginning—Puls.; *Rhus t.*; Stront. c.
Mountain climbing—*Ars.*; Coca. See Ascending.
Music—*Acon.*; Ambra; Dig.; *Graph.*; *Nat. c.*; Nux v.; Pall.; Phos. ac.; Sab.; Sep.; *Thuya.*
Narcotics—Bell.; *Cham.*; *Coff.*; Lach.; *Nux v.*; Thuya.
Night—*Acon.*; Ant. t.; Arg. n.; Arn.; *Ars.*; Aster.; Bac.; Bell.; Bry.; But. ac.; Cajup.; Camph.; Caust.; Cenchris; *Cham.*; Chionanth.; Cina; Cinch.; Clem.; *Coff.*; *Colch.*; Commocl.; Con.; Crot. casc.; Cupr. m.; Cycl.; Diosc.; Dolich.; *Dulc.*; Ferr. m.; Ferr. p.; Gamb.; *Graph.*; Guaiac.; *Hep.*; Hyos.; Iod.; Iris; Kali iod.; Lach.; Lil. t.; Mag. m.; Mag. p.; Merc. c.; *Merc.*; Mez.; Nat. m.; *Nit. ac.*; Nux m.; *Phos.*; Phyt.; Plat.; Plumb.; Psor.; *Puls.*; *Rhus t.*; Rumex; Sep.; *Sil.*; Sul.; Syph.; Tellur.; Thea; Thuya; Ver. a.; Vib. op.; X-ray; *Zinc. m.* See Evening.
Noise—Acon.; Asar.; *Bell.*; Bor.; Calad.; Cham.; *Cinch.*; Cocc.; *Coff.*; Colch.; Ferr.; Glon.; *Ign.*; Lyc.; Mag. m.; Med.; Nux m.; *Nux v.*; Onosm.; Phos.; Solan. lyc.; *Spig.*; Tar. h.; *Ther.*
One half of body—*Cham.*; Ign.; Mez.; *Puls.*; Sil.; Spig.; Thuya; Val.
Overeating—Ant. c.; *Nux v.*; Puls. See Eating.
Overheating—*Acon.*; Ant. c.; *Bell.*; Brom.; *Bry.*; Calc. c.; Carbo v.; Glon.; Lyc.; Nux m.; *Nux v.*
Pastry, rich food—Carbo v.; Kali m.; *Puls.*
Peaches—Cepa; Glon.
People, presence of—Ambra.
Periodically—*Alum.*; Aran.; *Ars.*; Ars. met.; *Cact.*; Carls.; *Ced.*; Chrom. ac.; *Cinch.*; Cupr. m.; *Eup. perf.*; Ign.; Ipec.; Kali bich.; *Nat. m.*; Niccol.; Primul. ob.; Nit. ac.; Ran. s.; Sep.; Sil.; Tar. h.; *Tela ar.*; Thuya; Urt.
Periodically, every alternate day—*Alum.*; Cinch.; Fluor. ac.; Nit. ac.; Oxytrop.
Periodically, every two weeks—Niccol.
Periodically, every 2-3 weeks—Ars. met.
Periodically, every 2-4 weeks—Carls.; Ox. ac.; Sul.
Periodically, every 3 weeks—Ars.; *Mag. c.*
Periodically, every year—*Ars.*; Carbo v.; Crot.; *Lach.*; Niccol.; Sul; *Thuya*; Urt.
Periodically, 4-8 P. M.—Lyc.; Sabad.
Periodically, new and full moon—Alum.
Plants, growing near water—Nat. s.
Potatoes—Alum.
Pressure—Acon.; *Agar.*; *Apis*; Arg. m.; Bar. c.; Bor.; Calc. c.; Cenchris; Cina; Equis.; Guaiac.; *Hep.*; Iod.; Kali c.; *Lach.*; Led.; Lyc.; *Merc. c.*; Nat. s.; *Nux v.*; Onosm.; Ov. g. p.; Phyt.; Ran. b.; Sil.; *Ther.* See Touch.
Rest—Acon.; *Arn.*; *Ars.*; Asaf.; Aur.; Calc. fl.; Caps.; Commocl.; Con.; Cycl.; Dulc.; Euphorb.; *Ferr. m.*; Indigo; Iris; Kali c.; Kreos., Lith. lact.; Lyc.; Mag. c.; Menyanth.; *Merc.*; Oleand.; *Puls.*; Rhod.; *Rhus t.*; Sabad.; *Samb.*; Senega; Sep.; Stront. c.; Sul.; Tar. h.; Tarax.; Val.

Riding—Arg. m.; Berb. v.; Caust.; *Cocc.*; Lyssin; Nux m.; *Petrol.*; Sanic.; Ther.

Right side—*Agar.*; Am. c.; Anac.; Apis; Ars.; *Bell.*; Bothrops; *Bry.*; Caust.; *Chel.*; Cinnab.; Con.; Crot.; Cur.; Dolich.; Equis.; Ferr. p.; Iod.; Kali c.; Lith. c.; *Lyc.*; *Mag. p.*; Merc.; Phyt.; Pod.; Rhus t.; Sang.; Solan. lyc.; Tar. h.; Viola od.

Rising—Acon.; Am. m.; Ars.; Bell.; *Bry.*; Caps.; Carbo v.; *Cocc.*; Con.; Dig.; Ferr.; Lach.; Lyc.; *Nux v.*; Phos.; *Phyt.*; Puls.; Radium; *Rhus t.*; Sul.

Room, heated—Acon.; Alum.; Ant. c.; *Apis*; Aran. sc.; Bapt.; Brom.; Bufo; *Cepa*; Crat.; *Croc.*; Euphras.; *Glon.*; Hyper.; *Iod.*; Kali iod.; Kali s.; Lil. t.; Merc.; *Puls.*; Sab.; Vib. op. See Warmth.

Scratching—Anac.; Ars.; Caps.; *Dolich.*; Merc.; Mez.; *Puls.*; Rhus t.; Staph.; Sul.

Sea bathing—Ars.; Limulus; Mag. m.

Seashore—*Aqua m.*; Ars.; Brom.; *Nat. m.*; *Nat. s.*; Syph.

Sedentary habits—Acon.; Aloe; Am. c.; Anac.; Arg. n.; Bry.; Con.; Nux v.; Sep.

Shaving, after—Caps.; *Carbo an.*; Ox. ac.; Plumb.

Sitting—Alum.; *Bry.*; Caps.; Con.; Cycl.; Dig.; Diosc.; Dulc.; Equis.; Euphorb.; Ferr. m.; Hydrocot.; Lyc.; Indigo; Kali c.; Nat. c.; Nux v.; Phyt.; *Plat.*; Puls.; *Rhus t.*; *Sep.*; Sul.; Tarax.; Val.

Sitting, on cold steps—Chimaph.; *Nux v.*

Sleep, after—Ambra; *Apis*; Bufo; Cadm. s.; Calc. c.; *Cocc.*; Coccus; Cra.; Epiph.; Homar.; *Lach.*; Merc. c.; Morph.; *Op.*; Parth.; Picr. ac.; Rhus t.; Selen.; *Spong.*; Stram.; Sul.; Syph.; Thasp.; Tub.; Val.

Smoking—*Abies n.*; Bor.; Can. ind.; Chin. ars.; *Cic.*; Cocc.; *Gels.*; *Ign.*; Kal.; *Lact. ac.*; Lob. infl.; *Nux v.*; Puls.; Sec.; Spig.; Spong.; *Staph.*; Stellar.

Sneezing—*Ars.*; Bry.; Kali c.; Phos.; *Sul.*; Verbasc. See Jar.

Snow, melting—Calc. p.

Snow storm—Con.; Formica; Merc.; Sep.; Urt.

Solitude—*Bism.*; Kali c.; Lil. t.; Lyc.; Pall.; *Stram.* See Fears (Mind).

Soup—Alum.; Kali c. See Fats.

Spices—*Nux v.*; Phos.

Spring—Ars. br.; Aur.; Calc. p.; Cepa; Crot.; Dulc.; Gels.; Kali bich.; Lach.; *Nat. m.*; Nat. s.; Nit. sp. d.; Rhus t.; Sars.

Standing—Æsc.; Aloe; *Berb. v.*; Calc. c.; Con.; *Cycl.*; Lil. t.; Plat.; Sul.; Val.

Stimulants—Ant. c.; Cadm. s.; Chionanth.; Fluor. ac.; *Glon.*; Ign.; Lach.; Led.; Naja; *Nux v.*; Op.; *Zinc. m.*

Storm, before—*Bellis*; Meli.; *Nat. s.*; Psor.; *Rhod.*; Rhus t.

Stooping—*Æsc.*; Am. c.; Bry.; Calc. c.; Glon.; Lyssin; Merc.; Ran. b.; Spig.; *Sul.*; Val.

Straining, overlifting—Arn.; Carbo an.; *Rhus t.*; Ruta.

Stretching—Med.; Rhus t.

Sun—*Ant. c.*; Bell.; Bry.; Cact.; Fagop.; *Gels.*; *Glon.*; Lach.; Lyssin; Nat. c.; Nat. m.; Puls.; Selen. See Weather, Hot.

Sun pain—*Glon.*; Nat. m.; Sang.; Spig.; Tab.

Swallowing—Apis; *Bell.;* Brom.; Bry.; *Hep.;* Hyos.; *Lach.;* Merc. i. fl.; Merc. i. r.; *Merc.;* Nit. ac.; Stram.; Sul. See Dysphagia (Throat).

Sweating—Ant. t.; Chin. s.; *Hep.;* Merc. c.; *Merc. s.;* Nit. ac.; Op.; Phos. ac.; *Sep.;* Stram.; Ver. a.

Sweets—*Ant. c.;* *Arg. n.;* Ign.; *Lyc.;* Med.; Sang.; *Zinc. m.*

Talking—Ambra; Am. c.; Anac.; *Arg. m.;* Arum; Calc. c.; Can. s.; Chin. s.; *Cocc.;* Mag. m.; *Mang. ac.;* Nat. c.; *Nat. m.;* Phos. ac.; Rhus t.; *Selen.;* Stann.; Sul.; Verbasc.

Tea—*Abies n.;* *Cinch.;* Diosc.; Lob. infl.; Nux v.; Puls.; *Selen.;* Thuya.

Temperature, extremes of—Ant. c.; Ipec.; Lach.

Thinking of symptoms—Bar. c.; *Calc. p.;* Caust.; *Gels.;* Helon.; *Med.;* Nux v.; *Ox. ac.;* Oxytr.; Pip. m.; Sabad.; Staph.

Thunder storm, before, during—Agar.; Gels.; Med.; Meli.; *Nat. c.;* Petrol.; Phos.; Phyt.; Psor.; *Rhod.;* Sep.; Sil.

Tobacco chewing—*Ars.;* Ign.; Lyc.; Selen.; *Ver. a.*

Tobacco smoke—Acon.; Cic.; Cocc.; *Ign.;* Staph. See Smoking.

Touch—*Acon.;* Angust.; *Apis;* Arg. m.; *Arn.;* Asaf.; *Bell.;* Bor.; *Bry.;* Calc. c.; Camph.; Caps.; Carbo an.; *Cham.;* Cic.; *Cinch.;* Cocc.; Colch.; Col.; Commocl.; Cupr. ac.; *Cupr. m.;* Equis.; Euphorb. d.; Euphras.; Ferr. p.; Guaiac.; Helon.; *Hep.;* Hyos.; Ign.; *Kali c.;* *Lach.;* *Lil. t.;* Lob. infl.; Lyc.; Mag. p.; Mez.; Murex; *Nit. ac.;* *Nux v.;* Oleand.; *Ox. ac.;* Phos.; *Plumb. m.;* Puls.; *Ran. b.;* *Rhod.;* Rhus t.; Sab.; Sang.; Sep.; *Sil.;* *Spig.;* Staph.; *Strych.;* Sul.; *Tar. h.;* Tellur.; *Ther.;* Urt.; Zinc. m.

Touch of hat—Glon.

Traveling—Coca; Plat.

Twilight, to daylight—Aur.; *Merc.;* Phyt.; *Syph.*

Uncovering—Ars.; Bell.; Benz. ac.; Caps.; Dros.; Helleb.; *Hep.;* Kali bich.; *Mag. p.;* *Nux v.;* Rheum; *Rhus t.;* Rumex; *Samb.;* Sil.; Stront. c.

Vaccination, after—Sil.; Thuya.

Veal—Ipec.; *Kali n.*

Vital drains—Calc. c.; *Calc. p.;* *Carbo v.;* *Cinch.;* Con.; Kali c.; Kali p.; Nux v.; *Phos.;* Phos. ac.; Puls.; *Selen.;* Sep.; *Staph.*

Voice, using—Arg. m.; Arg. n.; Arum; Carbo v.; *Dros.;* Mang. ac.; Nux v.; *Phos.;* Selen.; *Stann.;* Wyeth.

Vomiting—Æth.; Ant. t.; *Ars.;* Cupr. m.; *Ipec.;* *Nux v.;* Puls.; Sil.

Waking—Ambra; Lach.; Nit. ac.; Nux v. See Sleep.

Warmth, heat—Acon.; Æth.; Agar.; Alum.; Ambra; Anac.; *Ant. c.;* Ant. t.; *Apis;* Arg. n.; Asaf.; Bell.; *Bry.;* Calc. c.; Camph.; *Cepa;* *Cham.;* Cinch.; Clem.; *Cammocl.;* Conv.; *Dros.;* Euphras.; Ferr. m.; Fluor. ac.; Gels.; Glon.; *Graph.;* Guaiac.; Helianth.; Hyos.; Iberis; *Iod.;* Jugl. c.; *Justicia;* Kali iod.; *Kali m.;* Lach.; *Led.;* Lyc.; Med.; *Merc.;* *Nai. c.;* Nat. m.; Nit. ac.; Nux m.; Op.; *Puls.;* Sab.; *Sec.;* Stellar.; Sul. ac.; Sul.; Tab. See Weather, Hot.

Warmth of bed—Alum.; Apis; Bellis; Calc. c.; *Cham.;* Clem.; Dros.; *Led.;* Lyc.; Mag. c.; *Merc.;* Mez.; *Puls.;* Sab.; *Sec.;* *Sul.;* Thuya; Viscum.

Washing, water—*Am. c.;* *Ant. c.;* Ars. iod.; Bar. c.; Bell.; *Calc. c.;* Canth.;

Cham.; Clem.; *Crot. casc.*; Ferr. m.; Kreos.; Lil. t.; Mag. p.; *Merc.*; Mez.; *Nat. s.*; Nit. ac.; Rhus t.; Sep.; Sil.; Spig.; *Sul.*; Urt.

Water, drinks cold—Ant. c.; Apoc.; Arg. n.; *Ars.*; Calc. c.; *Canth.*; Clem.; Cocc.; *Crot. t.*; Cycl.; Dros.; Ferr. m.; Lob. infl.; Lyc.; Nux m.; *Rhus t.*; Sabad.; Spong.; Sul.

Water, drinks warm—Ambra; Bry.; *Lach.*; Phos.; *Puls.*; Sep.; Stann.

Water, seeing or hearing—Lyssin.

Water, working—*Calc. c.*; Mag. p.

Weather changes—*Am. c.*; Bry.; Calc. c.; Calc. fl.; *Calc. p.*; Chel.; Cinch.; *Dulc.*; Mang. ac.; Mag. c.; *Merc.*; Nat. c.; Nit. ac.; *Nux m.*; Phos.; Psor.; *Ran. b.*; *Rhod.*; Rhus t.; Ruta; Sticta; Stront. c.; Sul.; Tar h. See Dampness.

Weather changes, in spring—Ant. t.; Cepa; Gels.; Kali s.; Nat. s.

Weather, dry, cold—Agar.; Alum.; Apoc.; *Asar.*; *Aur.*; *Caust.*; Dulc.; Ipec.; *Kali c.*; Kreos.; Nit. sp. d.; *Nux v.*; *Petrol.*; Rhus t.; Viscum. See Air, Cold.

Weather, hot—*Acon.*; Æth.; Aloe; Ant. c.; *Bell.*; Bor.; Bry.; Croc.; Crot.; Crot. t.; *Gels.*; *Glon.*; Kali bich.; Lach.; *Nat. c.*; *Nat. m.*; Nit. ac.; Phos.; Picr. ac.; *Pod.*; Puls.; Sab.; Selen.; Syph. See Sun.

Weather, stormy—Nux m.; *Psor.*; Ran. b.; *Rhod.*; Rhus t.

Weather, windy, dry—*Acon.*; Arum; Cham.; Cupr. m.; *Hep.*; Lyc.; Mag. c.; *Nux v.*; Phos.; Puls.; *Rhod.*

Weather, windy, moist—Cepa; Dulc.; *Euphras.*; Ipec.; *Nux m.*; Rhod.

Weeping—Cham.; *Nat. m.*; Puls.; *Sep.*; Stann.

Wet application—*Am. c.*; *Ant. c.*; Calc. c.; *Clem.*; Crot.; *Merc.*; Rhus t.; *Sul.* See Washing.

Wet exposure—Am. c.; Ant. c.; Apis; Aran.; Ars.; *Calc. c.*; Caust.; Cepa; *Dulc.*; *Elaps*; Meli.; *Merc.*; Narcissus; Nat. s.; Nux m.; *Phyt.*; Picr. ac.; Ran. b.; Rhod.; *Rhus t.*; Ruta; Sep. See Dampness.

Wet feet—Calc. c.; Cepa; Puls.; *Rhus t.*; *Sil.*

Wine—*Alum.*; Ant. c.; Arn.; *Ars.*; Benz. ac.; *Carbo v.*; Con.; Fluor. ac.; Led.; Lyc.; *Nux v.*; Op.; Ran. b.; Selen.; Sil.; *Zinc. m.*

Yawning—Cina; *Ign.*; Kreos.; *Nux v.*; Rhus t.; *Sars.*

Yearly—Lach.; Rhus r.

AMELIORATIONS—Acids: Ptel.; Sang.

Air, cool, open—*Acon.*; Æsc.; Æth.; Aloe; *Alum.*; Ambra; Am. m.; *Amyl*; Ant. c.; Ant. t.; *Apis*; *Arg. n.*; Asaf.; Bar. c.; Bry.; Bufo; Cact.; Can. ind.; *Cepa*; *Cinch.*; Clem.; Coca; Commocl.; Conv.; Crat.; Croc.; Dig.; Diosc.; Dros.; Dulc.; Euonym.; Euphras.; Gels.; *Glon.*; Graph.; Iod.; *Kali iod.*; *Kali s.*; Lil. t.; *Lyc.*; *Mag. c.*; Mag. m.; Merc. i. r.; Mez.; Mosch.; Naja; *Nat. m.*; Nat. s.; Ol an.; Phos.; *Picr. ac.*; Plat.; *Puls.*; Radium; Rhus t.; *Sabad.*; Sab.; Sec.; *Sep.*; Stellar.; Strych. p.; Sul.; *Tab.*; *Tar. h.*; Vib. op. See Warmth (Aggravation).

Air, cool, must have windows open—*Amyl*; *Arg. n.*; Bapt.; Calc. c.; *Lach.*; Med.; *Puls.*; *Sul.* See Asthma (Respiratory System).

Air, warm—Aur. m.; Calc. c.; Caust.; Led.; Mag. c.; Merc.; Petrol.; Rhus t. See Warmth.

Bathing—Acon.; Apis; Ars.; *Asar.*; *Caust.*; Euphras.; *Puls.*; Spig.

Bathing, cold—Apis; Asar.: Bufo; Meph.; Nat. m.; Sep.

Bathing, vinegar—Vespa.
Bathing, warm—Ant. c.; Bufo; Radium; *Stront.*; Thea.
Bending, double—Aloe; Cinch.; *Col.*; *Mag. p.* See Pressure.
Bending, forward—Gels.; *Kali c.*
Boring into, nose, ears—Nat. c.; Spig.
Breakfast, after—Nat. s.; Staph. See Eating.
Carrying—Ant. t.; *Cham.*
Chewing—Bry.; Cupr. ac.
Coffee—Euphras.; Fluor. ac.
Cold—Bellis; Bor.; *Bry.;* Cepa; Fagop.; Iod.; *Led.;* Lyc.; Onosm.; Op. *Phos.;* Sec.
Cold applications, washing—Alum.; *Apis;* Arg. n.; Asar.; Bell.; Ferr. p.; Kali m.; Merc.; Phos.; *Puls.;* Sab. See Bathing.
Cold water—Agar. em.; Aloe; Ambra; *Bry.;* Camph.; Can. ind.; *Caust.;* Cupr. m.; Fagop.; *Led.;* Phos.; Picr. ac.; *Puls.;* Sep.
Colors, objects, bright—*Stram.;* Tar. h.
Combing hair—Formica.
Company—Æth.; *Bism.;* Kali c.; Lil. t.; Lyc.; *Stram.*
Consolation—Puls.
Conversation—Eup. perf.
Coughing—Apis; Stann. See Respiratory System.
Covering light—Sec.
Dark—Coca; Con.; *Euphras.;* Graph.; Phos.; *Sang.*
Day, during—Kali c.; Syph. See Aggravations.
Days, alternating—Alum.
Descending—Spong.
Discharges appearances of—*Lach.;* Mosch.; Stann.; Zinc. m.
Drawing limbs up—Sep.; Sul.; Thuya.
Drinks, cold—Ambra: *Cupr. m.*
Drinks, warm—Alum.; Ars.; Chel.; *Lyc.;* Nux v.; Sabad.; *Spong.* See Warm.
Eating—Acet. ac.; *Alum.;* Ambra; *Anac.;* Brom.; Cad. m.; Caps.; *Chel.;* Cim.; Cistus; Con.; Ferr. ac.; Ferr. m.; Graph.; *Hep.;* Homar.; *Ign.;* Iod.; Kali p.; Lach.; *Lith. c.;* Nat. c.; Nat. m.; Onosm.; *Petrol.;* Phos.; Pip. nig.; *Psor.;* Rhod.; Sep.; *Spong.;* Zinc. m.
Eructations—Ant. t.; *Arg. n.;* Bry.; Carbo v.; Diosc.; *Graph.;* Ign.; Kali c.; Lyc.; Mosch.; Nux v.; Ol. an., Sang.
Evenings—Bor.; Lob. infl.; Niccol.; Nux v.; Stellar.
Excitement, pleasurable—Kali p.; Pall.
Exercise—Alumen; Brom.; Plumb. m.; *Rhus t.;* Sep. See Walking.
Expectoration—Ant. t.; Hep.; *Stann.;* Zinc. m. See Respiratory System.
Expulsion of flatus, per ano—Aloe; Arn.; Calc. p.; Corn. c.; Grat.; Hep.; Iris; Kali n.; Mez.
Fanned, being—*Arg. n.;* Carbo v.; Cinch.; Lach.; Med.
Fasting—Cham.; Con.; Nat. m.
Feet in ice water—*Led.;* Sec.
Food cold—Ambra; Bry.; Lyc.; Phos.; Sil.
Food warm—Kreos.; Lyc See Aggravations.

Forenoon, in—Lil. t.
Head bent backward—Hyper.; Senega.
Head bent forward, while lying—Col.
Head, wrapped up warm—Hep.; Psor.; Rhod.; Sil.
Head elevated—Ars.; Gels.
Heat—*Ars.;* Caps.; Gymnocl.; Xerophyl. See Warmth.
Ice, holding in mouth—Coff.
Inland, mountains—Syph.
Inspiration—Colch.; Ign.; *Spig.* See Respiratory System.
Lemonade—Cycl.
Light—Stram.
Limb hanging down—Con.
Lying down—Acon.; Anhal.; Arn.; *Bell.;* Bellis; Brom.; *Bry.;* Calad.; Calc. c.; Coff.; *Colch.;* Equis.; Ferr. m.; *Mang. ac.;* Nat. m.; Nux v.; Onosm.; *Picr. ac.;* Pulex; *Puls.;* Radium; Stann.; Strych.; Symphor.
Lying, on back with shoulders raised—Acon.; Ars.
Lying, on left side—Ign.; Mur. ac.; Nat. m.; Stann. See Aggravations.
Lying, on painful side—Ambra; Am. c.; Arn.; Bor.; *Bry.;* Calc. c.; *Col.;* Cupr. ac.; Ptel.; *Puls.;* Sul. ac. See Pressure.
Lying, on right side—Ant. t.; Nat. m.; *Phos.;* Sul.; Tab. See Aggravations.
Lying, on right side, with head high—Ars.; Cact.; *Spig.;* Spong.
Lying, on stomach—*Acet. ac.;* Am. c.; Ant. t.; *Col.;* Med.; *Pod.;* Tab.
Lying, with head high—Petrol.; Puls.; Spig.
Lying, with head low—Arn.; Spong.
Magnetized—Phos.
Menses, between—Bell.; Bov.; Elaps; Ham.; Magnol.
Menses, during—Am. c.; Cycl.; *Lach.;* Zinc. m. See Female Sexual System.
Mental occupation—Ferr. m.; Kali br.; *Helon.;* Nat. c.
Midnight, after—Lyc. See Night.
Midnight, until noon—Puls.
Mind being diverted—Calc. p.; Helon.; Ox. ac.; Pip. menth.; Tar. h.
Mornings—Apis; Jugl. c.; Still.; Xerophyl.
Motion—Abrot.; Æsc.; *Alum.;* Arn.; Ars.; Asaf.; *Aur.;* Bell.; Bellis; Brom.; *Caps.;* Cinch.; Coca; Coccus; Commocl.; Con.; *Cycl.; Diosc.; Dulc.;* Euphorb.; Ferr. m.; Fluor. ac.; Gels.; *Helon.;* Homar.; Ign.; Indigo; Iris; Kali c.; Kali iod.; Kali p.; Kreos.; Lith. c.; Lith. lact.; Lob. infl.; Lyc.; *Mag. c.;* Mag. m.; Magnol.; Menyanth.; Nat. c.; Op.; Parth.; Pip. menth.; Plat.; *Puls.;* Pyr.; Radium; Rhod.; *Rhus t.;* Ruta; Sabad.; *Samb.; Sep.;* Stellar.; Sul.; Syph.; *Val.;* Ver. a.;; Xerophyl.; Zinc. m.
Motion, slow—Agar.; Ambra; Ferr. ac.; *Ferr. m.;* Plat.; Stann.; Zinc. m.
Mouth, covered—Rumex.
Music—Tar. h.
Night—Cupr. ac.
Oil applications—Euphorb. d.
Position, change of—Apis; Caust.; *Ign.;* Nat. s.; Phos. ac.; *Rhus t.;* Val.; Zinc. m.

Position, hands and feet—Eup. perf.

Position, semi-erect—Ant. t.; Apis; Bell. See Rest.

Pressure—*Arg. n.;* Asaf.; Bor.; *Bry.;* *Caps.;* Chel.; *Cinch.;* *Col.;* Con.; Cupr. ac.; *Diosc.;* Dros.; Euonym.; Formica; Guaiac.; *Ign.;* Indigo; *Lil. t.;* Mag. m.; *Mag. p.;* Menyanth.; Nat. c.; Nat. m.; Nat. s.; Nux v.; Picr. ac.; *Plumb. m.;* Puls.; Radium; Sep.; Sil.; *Stann.;* Ver. a.

Putting feet on chair—Con.

Rest—Æsc.; Ant. c.; Bell.; *Bry.;* Cadm. s.; Can. ind.; *Colch.;* Crat.; Gettysburg Water; Gymnocl.; Kali p.; Merc. c.; Merc. v.; *Nux v.;* Phyt.; Pulex; Scilla; Staph.; Strych. p.; Vib. op.

Riding in carriage—Nit. ac.

Rising—Ambra; Am. c.; *Ars.;* Calc. c.; Lith. c.; Parth.; Samb.; Sep.

Rocking—Cina; Kali n.

Room close, in—Euphorb. d. See Warmth.

Rubbing—Anac.; Calc. c.; *Canth.;* Carb. ac.; Diosc.; Formica; Indigo; *Mag. p.;* Nat. c.; Ol. an.; Phos.; Plumb. m.; *Pod.;* Rhus t.; Sec.; *Tar. h.*

Scratching—Asaf.; *Calc. c.;* Commocl.; Cycl.; *Jugl. c.;* Mur. ac.; Nat. c.; Phos.; Sul.

Sea, at—Brom.

Seashore, at—Med.

Shaving, after—Brom.

Sipping water—Kali n.

Sitting erect—Ant. t.; Apis; Bell.

Sitting up in bed—*Kali c.;* Samb.

Sleep—Calad.; Colch.; Merc.; Myg.; *Nux v.;* Phos.; *Sang.;* Sep.

Smoking—Aran.; Tar. c.

Standing erect—Ars.; Bell.; *Diosc.;* Kali p.

Stimulants—Gels.; Glon.

Stooping—Colch.

Storm, after—Rhod.

Stretching limbs—Amyl; Plumb. m.; Rhus t.; Sec.; Teucr.

Summer, during—Alum.; Aur. m.; Calc. p.; Ferr. m.; Sil. See Warmth.

Sweat—Acon.; Ars.; Calad.; *Cham.;* Cupr. m.; Franciscea; Rhus t.; Ver. a. See Fever.

Taking hold of anything—Anac.

Thinking of symptoms—*Camph.;* Helleb.

Touch—Asaf.; Calc. c.; Cycl.; Mur. ac.; Tarax.; Thuya.

Uncovering—Apis; Camph.; Lyc.; Onosm.; Sec.; *Tab.* See Aggravations.

Urination—*Gels.;* Ign.; Phos. ac.; Sil.

Vomiting—Helianth.

Warmth, heat—*Ars.;* Aur. m.; Bad.; Bell.; Bry.; Calc. fl.; Camph.; Caust.; Cim.; *Col.; Collins.;* Coff.; Coral.; Cupr. ac.; Cycl.; *Dulc.;* Formica; *Hep.;* Ign.; Kali bich.; Kali p.; Kreos.; Lach.; Lob. infl.; Lyc.; *Mag. p.;* Nux m.; *Nux v.;* Phos. ac.; Phyt.; Psor.; Rhod.; Rhus t.; *Rumex;* Sabad.; Sep.; Sil.; Solan. lyc.; Staph.; Stram.; Sul. ac.; Thea; Ver. a.

Warmth, heat of, applications—Ars.; Bry.; Calc. fl.; *Lach.; Mag. p;* Nux m.; Radium; Rhus t.; Sep.

Warmth, of head—Bell.; Graph.; *Hep.*; *Psor.*; Sanic.; *Sil.*
Water, cold—Aloe; *Bry.*; Caust.; *Jatropha*; *Phos.*; Picr. ac.; Sep.
Water, hot—Spig.
Weather, damp, wet—Alum.; Asar.; *Caust.*; *Hep.*; Med.; Mur. ac.; Nux v.
Weather, damp, warm—Cham.; Kali c.; Sil.
Weather, dry—Am. c.; Calc. c.; Kali c.; Magnol.; Petrol.; Still. See Aggravations.
Weather, dry, warm—Alum.; *Calc. p.*; Nat. s.; Nux m.; Rhus t.; *Sul.* See Summer.
Wine—Coca.
Winter, during—Ilex.

INDEX TO REPERTORY
(Ninth Edition)

INDEX TO REPERTORY

	PAGE
Abortion	842
Abscess	953
——Retropharyngeal	762
Acidity	772
Acne	904
——Rosacea	904
Acromegaly	953
Actinomycosis	904
Addison's Disease	953
Adenitis	961
Adenoids	761
Adynamia	940
After Pains	845
Agalactea	846
Aggravations	968
Agoraphobia	691
Ague	923
Alae Nasi, Affections	734
Albuminuria	816
Alcoholism	941
Alopecia	904
Amblyopia	726
Ameliorations	975
Amenorrhoea	834
Anasarca	960
Anemia	953
——Pernicious	953
Aneurism	853
Anger, Ill Effects	690
Angina Pectoris	855
Anidrosis	905
Ankles, Weak	877
Anthrax	905
Anthropophobia	691
Antrum Affections	740
Anuria	814
Anus, Affections	788
Aortitis	853
Aphasia	698
Aphonia	897
Apthae (thrush)	750
Apoplexy	853
Appendicitis	804
Appetite Disorders	768
Arteriosclerosis	853
Arteritis	853

	PAGE
Arthritis	875
——Deformans	875
Ascarides	805
Ascites	960
Asphyxia	954
Asthenopia	727
Asthma	883
Astigmatism	727
Atheroma	853
Athetosis	942
Auricle, Affections	729
Aversions	768
Axilla, Affections	861
Azoturia	818
Backache	861
Baker's Itch (Lichen)	910
Balanitis	822
Balanopostitis	822
Barber's Itch (Sycosis)	914
Basedow's Disease	962
Bed Sores	905
Bell's Palsy	745
Beri Beri	942
Biliary Colic	800
Bilious Fever	924
Biliousness	771
Black Eye	713
Bladder, Affections	806
——Inflammation	806
——Irritable	807
——Paralysis	808
Blepharitis	720
Blepharospasm	720
Blindness (Amaurosis)	726
Blood, Disorganization	954
Bone, Affections	954
Borborygmi	774
Bowel Obstruction	802
Brachialgia	866
Bradycardia (slow pulse)	859
Brain, Concussion	700
——Congestion	700
——Inflammation	700
——Softening	700
Brainfag	689

	PAGE
Breath Offensive (Halitosis)	749
Bright's Disease	809
Bromidrosis	905
Bronchiectasis	854
Bronchitis, Acute	855
——Chronic	855
——Croupous	855
Bronchorrhoea	854
Bruises	963
Bubo	820
Bubonic Plague	955
Bulbar Paralysis	935
Bunions	873
Burns, Scalds	963
Bursitis	877
Calculi, Biliary	800
——Renal	808
Cancer	955
——Pains	956
Cancrum Oris	750
Canker Sores	750
Carbuncle	905
Cardiac Dropsy	960
——Neuroses	855
Cardialgia	771
Caries	954
Carphologia	689
Catalepsy	689
Cataract	716
Catarrh, Bladder	807
——Bronchi	855
——Larynx	896
——Nose	738
——Stomach	775
——Throat	764
——Uterus	849
Cartilages, Affections	956
Catheterism	924
Cellulitis	956
Cerebrospinal Meningitis	700
Chancre	826
Chancroid	820
Change of Life	833
Chapped Hands	866
Checked Discharges	957

	PAGE
——Eruptions	959
Cheeks, Affections	748
Cheyne-Stokes—Respiration	901
Chickenpox	927
Chilblains	905
Chilliness	919
Chloasma	905
Chlorosis	953
Cholera	790
——Infantum	790
——Morbus	790
Cholerine	790
Chordes	821
Chorea (St. Vitus Dance)	942
Choroid, Affections	716
Cicatrices	958
Ciliary Muscle, Spasm	716
——Neuralgia	716
Cirrhosis of Liver	802
Clairvoyance	689
Clergyman's Sore Throat	764
Climacteric Disorders	833
——Flushings	833
Coccygodynia	864
Colic	783
——Babies	783
——Biliary	800
——Lead	784
——Renal	808
Colitis	796
Collapse	940
Color Blindness	726
Coma	690
——Vigil	889
Comedo	905
Complaints (General)	956
Condylomata	918
Conjunctivitis	717
Constipation	790
Consumption	900
Contusions	963
Convulsions	942
——Puerperal	844
——Suppressed Eruptions	943
——Teething	943
——Uremic	943

INDEX TO REPERTORY

	PAGE
Cornea, Affections	717
Corns (Callosities)	905
Coryza	737
Cough	888
——Dry	891
——Hoarse	891
——Laryngeal	891
——Loose	891
——Nervous	891
——Phthisical	891
Cowperitis	821
Coxalgia	877
Cracked Lips	749
Cramps in Calves	870
Cretinism	689
Croup	896
——Membranous	896
Crusta Lactea	710
Cyanosis	854
Cystitis, Acute	806
——Chronic	807
Cysts	840, 914, 966
Dandruff	710
Day Blindness	726
Deafness	729
Debility	940
Decubitus (Bed Sores)	905
Delirium	689
——Tremens	689
Delusions	691
Dementia	690
Dengue	924
Dentition	758
Dermatalgia	906
Diabetes Insipidus	812
——Mellitus	819
Diaphragmitis	792
Diarrhoea, Acute	793
——Chronic	793
——Teething	794
Diphtheria	761
Diplopia	727
Dissecting Wounds	963
Dreams	937
Dropsy	959

	PAGE
Drowsiness	936
Drugs, Abuse	956
Duodenitis	799
Dysentery	799
Dysmenorrhœa	835
Dyspepsia	772
Dysphagia	762
Dyspnœa	901
——Cardiac	854
Dysuria	812
Earache (Otalgia)	732
Ecchymoses	906
Eclampsia (Convulsions)	942
——Puerperal	844
Ecthyma	906
Ectropion	720
Eczema	906
Elephantiasis	907
Emissions	824
Emphysema	898
Empyema	901
Encephalitis Lethargica	950
Endocarditis	855
Endocervicitis	847
Endometritis	849
Enteralgia	785
Enteritis, Acute	793
——Chronic	793
Entropion	720
Enuresis	806
Ephelis (Sunburn)	907
Epididymitis	828
Epilepsy (Grand Mal)	933
Epiphora	721
Epistaxis (Nose Bleed)	735
Epithelioma	907
Erotomania	698
Eructations	774
Erysipelas	907
Erythema	908
——Nodosum	908
Eustachian Deafness	730
Exophthalmic Goitre (Basedow's Disease)	944
Exostoses	954

INDEX TO REPERTORY

	PAGE
External Auditory Canal, Affections	730
Eyelids, Affections	719
Face, Eruptions	744
Fainting	859
False Labor Pains	844
Fatty Degeneration	959
Fears	690
Febricula	927
Felon (Whitlow)	918
Fever	920
Fibroid Tumors	967
Fistula, Dentalis	758
——in Ano	788
——Lachrymalis	721
Fissures	908
——Anus	788
Flatulence	774
Floating Kidney	809
Fractures	954
Freckles (Lentigo)	910
Fright, Ill Effects	690
Fungus Hematodes	908
Furuncle (Boil)	908
Gait Disorders	874
Galactorrhœa	846
Gall Stones	800
——Colic	800
Ganglion	879
Gangrene	909
Gas Fumes, Ill Effects	957
Gastralgia	777
Gastric Fever	927
——Ulcer	780
Gastritis, Acute	775
——Chronic	775
Gastro Enteritis	775
Glanders	960
Glands, Affections	960
——Swollen	961
Glaucoma	721
Gleet	821
Glossitis	755
Goitre	961

	PAGE
——Exophthalmic	962
Gonorrhœa (Specific Urethritis)	821
Gout	875
Gravel	808
Grief, Ill Effects	690
Growing Pains	864
Gum Boil	757
Gums, Affections	757
Hæmatemesis	771
Hæmaturia	816
Hæmoglobinuria	818
Hæmophilia	962
Hæmoptysis	898
Hæmorrhages	962
Hæmorrhoids	800
Hair Disorders	711
Halitosis	692
Halophagia	957
Hamstring, Contractions	875
Hay Fever	737
Headaches	706
——Anemic	702
——Chronic	702
——Congestive	702
——Nervous	702
——Sick	702
Heart, Affections	853
——Dilatation	854
——Failure	854
——Fatty Degeneration	854
——Hypertrophy	854
Heartburn (Pyrosis)	774
Hectic Fever	927
Hemicrania	703
Hemiopia	727
Hemiplegia	935
Hepatitis	803
Hernia	801
Herpes	909
——Labialis	749
——Zoster (Shingles)	909
Hiccough	771
Hip Joint Disease	877
Hives (Urticaria)	916

INDEX TO REPERTORY

	PAGE
Hoarseness	897
Hodgkin's Disease (Pseudo-leukemia)	962
Homesickness (Nostalgia)	690
Hook Worm Disease	963
Housemaid's Knee	877
Hydrarthrosis	875
Hydroa	909
Hydrocele	823
Hydrocephalus	710
Hydrophobia	691
Hydrothorax	901
Hygroma Patella	877
Hyperchlorhydria	772
Hyperidrosis	910
Hypermetropia	727
Hypertrophy of Heart	854
Hypochondriasis	691
Hysteralgia	849
Hysteria	691
Ichthyosis	910
Impacted Bowels	802
Impetigo	910
Impotence	822
Incubus (Nightmare)	936
Indigestion	772
Infantile Paralysis	935
Inflammations	963
Influenza (Grippe)	927
Inframammary Pains	832
Ingrown Toe Nail	911
Injuries	963
Insanity. (See Dementia, Mania, Melancholia.)	
Insect Bites	957
Insomnia	936
Intermittent Fever	928
Intertrigo (Chafing)	908
Intussusception	802
Iritis	721
Ischuria (Retention of Urine)	813
Jaundice	802
——Infantile	802
Jaws, Affections	745

	PAGE
Keloid	910
Keratitis	717
Kidneys, Calculi	808
——Congestion	808
——Floating	809
——Inflammation	809
Labor	844
Labrinthine, Affections	731
Lachrymal Fistula	721
——Sac, Inflammation	721
Lachrymation	721
Lactation	846
Lagophthalmos	722
Landry's Paralysis	935
Laryngismus Stridulus	897
Laryngitis, Acute	896
——Chronic	896
——Tubercular	896
Lead Colic	784
Lentigo (Freckles)	910
Leprosy	910
Leucocythemia	964
Leucoderma	910
Leucorrhœa	829
Lichen	910
Lienteria	797
Lipoma	967
Lips, Affections	749
Lithemia Lithiasis	818
Liver, Acute Yellow Atrophy	802
——Cancer	803
——Cirrhosis	802
——Congestion	803
——Fatty	803
——Hypertrophy	803
——Inflammation	803
Liver Spots (Chloasma)	905
Lochia, Disorders	845
Locomotor Ataxia	951
Low Fevers	932
Lumbago	869
Lungs, Congestion	898
——Edema	898
——Inflammation, Catarrhal	899
————Croupous	899

	PAGE		PAGE
——Paralysis	899	Muscæ Volitantes	728
Lupus	910	Mushroom Poisoning	959
Lying in Period	845	Mutinism	965
Lymphangitis	964	Myalgia	964
		Myelitis	951
Malaria	928	Myocarditis	855
Malnutrition	959	Myopia	727
Mammary Gland, Affections	831	Myositis	964
Mania	693	Myxedema	965
——a potu	689		
Marasmus	964	Nails, Affections	911
Mastitis	832	Nævus	910
Mastodynia	832	Nausea	775
Mastoid, Affections	731	Necrosis	954
Masturbation, Ill Effects	822	Nephralgia	807
Measles (Rubeola)	925	Nephritis, Acute	809
Megrim (Migraine)	702	——Chronic	809
Melancholia	693	Nephrolithiasis	808
Memory, Weak	693	Neuralgia	947
Meniere's Disease	713	——Brachial	947
Meningitis	700	——Ciliary	716
——Cerebrospinal	700	——Facial	746
——Spinal	951	——Gastric	777
——Tubercular	700	——Intercostal	947
Menopause	833	——Sciatic	947
Menorrhagia	836	——Spermatic Cord	824
Menstruation, Delayed	834	——Supraorbital	723
——Painful	835	——Uterine	849
——Profuse	836	Neurasthenia	946
——Suppressed	834	Neuritis	946
Metritis	849	Nictalopia	726
——Chronic	849	Night Sweats	923
Metrorrhagia	848	——Terrors	697
Miliaria (Prickly Heat)	910	Nipples, Affections	832
Milk Fever	845	——Ulcerated	832
——Leg	846	Nodes	826
Miscarriage, Habit	842	Nodosities, Tophi	876
——Threatened	842	Nose, External, Affections	734
Modalities	968, 975	Nostalgia	690
Mollities Ossium	955	Nymphomania	840
Moods	694		
Morning Sickness	843	Obesity	965
Morphinism	945	Odontalgia (Toothache)	759
Morvan's Disease	945	Oedema	959
Mountain Sickness	959	——Larynx	896
Mumps	961	——Lungs	898

INDEX TO REPERTORY

	PAGE
——Pedes	873
Oesophagus, Affections	761
Onychia	911
Ophthalmia	722
Optic Neuritis	723
Optical Illusions	727
Orchitis	828
Osteitis	954
Osteo-myelitis	954
Otitis Media, Acute	731
————Chronic	731
Otorrhœa	732
Ovaralgia	841
Ovarian Cyst	840
Ovaritis	840
Oxaluria	818
Oxyuris	805
Ozæna	739
Palate, Affections	751
Palpitation	856
Panaritium (Felon)	918
Pancreas, Affections	804
Pannus	725
Paralysis	934
——Acute Ascending	935
——Agitans	934
——Facial (Bell's Palsy)	935
——General of Insane	935
——Hemiplegia	935
——Hysterical	935
——Infantile (Poliomyelitis)	935
——Landry	935
——Lead	935
——Paraplegia	935
——Pneumogastric	899
——Post Diphtheritic	936
——Spinal	936
——Typists, Pianists	935
Paraplegia	935
——Spastic	936
Parotitis (Mumps)	961
Pellagra	911
Pelvic, Affections	841
——Cellulitis	841
Pemphinus	911

	PAGE
Penis, Affections	822
Pericarditis	855
Periostitis	955
Peritonitis	804
Perityphlitis	804
Pertussis (Whooping Cough)	892
Petichiae	918
Petit Mal	936
Pharyngitis, Acute	763
——Chronic	764
——Follicular	764
——Sicca	763
Phimosis, Paraphimosis	822
Phlebitis	860
Phlegmasia Alba Dolens	846
Phobias	690
Phosphaturia	818
Photophobia	725
Phthisis	900
——Laryngeal	896
Pica (Cravings)	769
Pityriasis	912
Placenta, Retained	844
Plague	955
Pleurisy	901
Pleurodynia	886
Plica Polonica	711
Pneumonia, Catarrhal	899
——Croupous	899
Poison Oak, Antidotes	959
Poliomyelitis, Anterior	935
Polychrome Spectra	727
Polypi	967
——Nasal	737
——Uterine	851
Polyuria	812
Portal Congestion	860
Post Nasal, Affections	740
——Operative Disorders	963
——Partum Hemorrhage	845
Pregnancy, Disorders	842
Priapism	821
Proctitis	789
Prolapsus Ani	789
——Uteri	847
Prophylactics	961

INDEX TO REPERTORY

	PAGE
Prosopalgia (Face Ache)	746
Prostate, Affections	823
——Hypertrophy	823
Prostatitis	823
Prurigo	912
Pruritus	912
——Ani	788
——Vulvæ	852
Psoriasis	913
Pterygium	725
Ptomaine Poisoning	959
Ptosis	719
Ptyalism (Salivation)	751
Pulmonary Oedema	898
Puerperium, Disorders (Lying in Period)	845
Pulse, Disturbances	858
Pupils, Contracted (Myosis)	725
——Dilated (Mydriasis)	725
Purpura	913
——Hemorrhagica	913
——Rheumatica	913
Pyelitis	811
Pyemia	965
Pylorus, Affections	778
Pyorrhœa Alveolaris	757
Pyrosis	774
Pyuria	818
Quinsy	766
Rachitis	966
Ranula	967
Raynaud's Disease	909
Rectal Pockets	788
Rectum, Affections	788
Reflexes, Disturbances	878
Relapsing Fever	932
Remittent Fever	932
Renal Colic	808
Retina, Affections	725
Retinitis	725
Retropharyngeal Abscess	762
Rheumatic Gout	875
Rheumatism, Acute	880
——Chronic	882

	PAGE
——Gonorrhœal	882
——Muscular	882
——Periosteal	882
Rhinitis, Acute (Cold in Head)	737
——Chronic	738
——Sicca	738
Rigid Os	844
Rigg's Disease	760
Ringworm	915
Rose Cold	737
Roseola	913
Rubella (Rotheln)	925
Rubeola (Measles)	925
Rupia	914
Salpingitis	847
Satyriasis	820
Scabies	914
Scalp, Affections	710
Scarlet Fever	926
Sciatica	947
Scleroderma	914
Sclerosis, Multiple	951
Sclerotic, Affections	726
Scrofulosis (Scrofula)	966
Scrotum, Affections	823
Scurvy (Scorbutus)	966
Sea Sickness (Mal de Mer)	944
Sebaceous Cyst	914
Seborrhœa	914
Seminal Vesiculitis	824
Senile Decay	966
Sensations	966
Septicemia	965
——Puerperal	845
Septum Ulceration	741
Sinus, Affections	740
Sleeping Sickness	950
Sleeplessness	936
Small Pox (Variola)	927
Smell, Disorders	740
Snake Poison, Antidotes	957
Sneezing	741
Somnambulism	699
Spermatic Cord, Affections	824

	PAGE
Spermatorrhœa	824
Spinal Bifida	955
——Cord, Concussion	950
——— ——Degeneration	950
——— ——Hyperesthesia	951
——— ——Inflammation	951
——— ——Irritation	951
Spleen, Affections	804
Sprains	963
Stage Fright	691
Sterility	829
Stomach, Dilatation	771
Stomatitis	750
Strabismus (Squint)	726
Strangury	814
Strophulus (Tooth Rash)	914
Stye	720
Sub-involution	846
Sudaminæ	914
Suppressed, Eruptions	959
——Menses	834
——Milk	846
Suppurations	953
Surgical Shock	941
Sweat, Disorders	922
Sycosis (Barber's Itch)	914
Syncope (Fainting)	859
Synochal Fever	932
Synovitis	875
Syphilidæ	827
Syphilis	825
——Congenital	826
Tabes Dorsalis (Locomotor Ataxia)	951
——Mesenterica	964
Tachycardia (Rapid Pulse)	858
Taenia (Tapeworm)	805
Taste, Disorders	756
Tenesmus	798
——Vesicæ	808
Teeth, Affections	758
Testalgia	828
Testes, Affections	827
Tetanus	952
Thirst	730

	PAGE
Tics	748
Tinea	915
——Versicolor	915
Tinnitus (Noises in Ears)	732
Tobacco, Abuse	957
Tongue, Affections	754
Tonsils, Deposits	766
——Hypertrophy	766
——Inflammation (Tonsilitis)	766
—— ——Phlegmonous (Quinsy)	766
Torticollis	880
Trachea, Affections	903
Trachoma (Granular Lids)	720
Traumatisms	963
Trichinæ	805
Trichophytosis (Ringworm)	915
Trismus (Lockjaw)	745
Tuberculosis	900
Tumors	966
Tympanites	786
Typhoid Fever	924
Typhus	932
Ulcer	915
Umbilicus, Affections	804
Uremia	810
Urethra, Affections	811
Urethral Caruncle	811
——Fever (Catheterism)	932
Urethritis, Specific	821
Urticaria (Hives)	916
Uterus, Affections	847
——Cancer	851
——Displacements	847
——Inflammation	849
Uvula, Affections	767
——Elongated	767
Vaccination, Ill Effects	959
Vaccinia	918
Vaginismus	851
Vaginitis	851
Valvular Diseases	860
Varicella (Chickenpox)	927
Varicocele	824

INDEX TO REPERTORY

	PAGE
Varicose Ulcers	916
——Veins	860
Variola (Small Pox)	927
Vertigo	713
Vision, Disorders	726
Vitreous Opacities	728
Vomiting	780
Vulvar Pruritus	852
Vulvitis	852
Warts	918
Waterbrash	775
Weaning Disorders	847

	PAGE
Wens	914
Whooping Cough (Pertussis)	892
Worm Fever	932
Worms	805
Wounds	963
Wrist Rheumatism	879
Writer's Cramp	879
Wry Neck	880
Yellow Fever	932
Zona Zoster	909

THERAPEUTIC INDEX

THERAPEUTIC INDEX

Any attempt to select the proper homœopathic remedy for any case except by the study of the totality of symptoms must prove futile. In order to prescribe homœopathically, the essentials for so doing must be observed,—i. e., *to let the characteristic symptoms of the individual patient, largely independent of the pathological nature of the case, be paramount in selecting the remedy.*

Such characteristics are found especially—

(1) In the location or part affected;
(2) In the sensations;
(3) In the modalities.

The study of the repertory alone will give the indicated remedy. But throughout this work are found numerous suggestions for remedies based on clinical observations or deductions from partial provings, all of which may prove most valuable additions to our Materia Medica if further verified at the bedside. As many of them have no place as yet in our published repertories, I have thought it advisable to give them a place with others in this therapeutic index, in order to bring them to the attention and further study of the physician. At best, a clinical index is but suggestive.

Abortion, threatened.—Caulophyl; Viburnum.
Abscess.—Bellad.; Merc.; *Hepar;* Silica; Ananther.
Acidity.—Calc.; *Robin.;* Sulph. ac.; Nux.
Acne.—Kal. brom.; Cimicif.; *Berb. aquif.;* Led.; Hydrocot.; Antimon.; Kali brom.
——**Rosacea.**—Oophor.; Kreos.; Sulph.; Carb. an.; Radium.
Acromegaly.—Thyroid; Chrysarob.
Actinomycosis.—Nitr. ac.; Hippoz.; Hecla.
Addison's disease.—Adrenalin; Ars.; Phos.; Calc. ars.
Adenitis.—Bell.; Merc.; Cist.; Iod.
Adenoids.—Agraphis; Calc. jod.
Adiposity.—Phytolacca; Fucus.
Adynamia.—Phos. ac.; China.
After-pains.—Caulophyl; Magnes. phos.
Agalactia.—Lactuca; Agnus; Urtica.

Ague.—Nat. mur.; China; Cedron.
Albuminuria.—Ars.; Kalmia; Merc. cor.
Alcoholism.—Quercus; Avena; Capsic; Nux.
Alopecia.—Fluor. ac.; Pix. liq.
Amenorrhoea.—Puls.; Graph.; Nat. mur.
Anasarca.—Oxydend; Elater; Liatris.
Anaemia.—Fer. cit. Chin.; Nat. m.; Calc. phos.
——**Pernicious.**—Ars.; T. N. T.
Aneurism.—Baryt.; Lycop.
Angina pectoris.—Latrodect; Cactus; Glonoin.; Bryon; Hæmatox; Oxal. ac.; Spigel.
Angioma.—Abrotan.
Ankylostomiasis.—Carduus mar.
Anorexia.—*Nux; Hydrast.; China.*
Anthrax.—*Echinacea.*
Aortitis.—*Aurum ars.*
Antrum.—Hep.; Nit. ac.; K. bich.; Euphorb.; Amyg.
Aphasia.—Bothrops; Stram.; Kal. brom.
Aphonia.—Alumen; Arg. m.; Nit. ac.; Caust.; Oxal. ac.; Spongia; Aurum.
Aphthæ.—Æthus.; *Borax;* Merc.; Nit. ac.; Kal. mur.; Hydr. mur.
Apoplexy.—Op.; Phos.; Arnica; Bellad.
Appendicitis.—Echin.; Bellad.; Laches.; Iris tenax.
Arterial tension lowered.—Gels.
Arterial tension raised.—Verat. vir.; Viscum.
Arteriosclerosis.—Am. iod.; Plumb. iod.; Polyg. avic.; Baryta; Glonoin 2x; Aurum; Carduus; Sumbul.
Arthritis.—Arbut.; Sulph.; Bry.; Elater.
Ascarides.—Abrotan.; Sabad.; Cina; Spig.
Ascites.—Acet. ac.; Apocyn.; Helleb.; Apis; Ars.; *Dig.*
Asthenopia.—Nat. mur.; Ruta; Croc.; Senega.
Asthma.—Ipec.; Ars.; Eucalypt; *Adrenalin;* Nat. sulph.
——**Cardiac.**—Conval.; Iberis; Ars. jod.
Astigmatism (myopic).—Lilium.
Atrophy.—Ol. jecor.; Iod.; Ars.
Auricular Fibrillation.—Digital.; Quinidine.
Auto-intoxication.—Skatol; Indol.; Sulph.
Azoturia.—Caust.; Senna.

Backache.—Oxal. ac.; Æsc.; Rhus; Puls.; Kal. carb.; Cimicif.; Nux; Ant. tart.; Variol.
Balonitis.—Merc.
Barber's Itch.—Sulph. iod.; Thuja.
Bed-sores.—Fluor. ac.; Arn.; Sulph. ac.
Bell's Paralysis.—Am. phos.; *Causticum;* Zinc. pic.
Beri Beri.—Elater.; Rhus; Ars.
Bilharziasis.—Antimon. tart.
Biliousness.—Yucca; Euony.; Bry.; Pod.; Merc.; Sulph.; Nux; Nyctanthes; Chelidon.
Bladder (irritable).—*Eup. purp.;* Copaiv.; Ferr.; Nux; Apis; Sarsap.
——**Hæmorrhage.**—Amygd.; Hamam.; *Nit. ac.*
Blepharitis.—Puls.; Graph.; Merc.
Blepharospasm.—Agaric.; Physost.
Blood-pressure.—High—Baryta mur.; Glonoin.; Aurum; Viscum.
Boils.—Bellis; Calc. pic.; Ferr. iod.; Ol. myr.; *Bell.;* Sil.; Hep.; Ichthyol.
Bone Affections.—Aurum; Calc. phos.; Fluor. ac.; Ruta; Mezer.; Silica; Symphyt.
Borborygmi.—Hæmatoxyl.
Bradycardia (slow pulse).—Abies nig.; *Digit.;* Kalm.; Apocn. can.
Brain, Softening.—Salamand; Phos.; Baryta.
Brain-fag.—Anhalon.; Zinc.; Phos.; Anacard.; Sil.
Bright's Disease.—Ars.; Phos. ac.; Apis; Merc. cor.; Tereb.; Kali cit.; Natrum mur.
Bromidrosis.—Silica; Calc.; Butyr. acid.
Bronchitis.—Acon.; *Bry.;* Phos.; Tart. e.; *Fer. phos.;* Sang.; Pilocarp.
——**(chronic)**—Ammoniac; Ars.; Seneg.; Sulph.; Antim. iod.
Broncho-pneumonia.—Kali bich.; Tart emet.; Tuberc.; Phos.; Squilla.
Bronchorrhœa.—Ammoniacum; Eucalyp.; *Bals. Peru;* Stan.; Bacillin.
Bulbar Paralysis.—Guaco; Plumb.; Botulin.
Bubo.—Merc.; Nit. ac.; Carb. an.; Phytol.
Burns—Cantharis; Urtica; Picric acid.

Bursæ.—Benz. ac.; Ruta; Sil.
Calculi (biliary).—China; Berberis; Chelidon.
——**(renal)**—Berberis; Pareira; Sarsap.
Cancer—(Bladder.)—Taraxac.
——**(Epithelial.)**—Acetic acid.
——**(Gastric.)**—Geranium.
——**(Rectal.)**—Ruta; Hydr.; Kal. cyan.
——**(Tongue.)**—Fuligo.
Cancer.—Semp. viv.; *Ars.*; Hyd.; Ant. chlor.; Galium.
——**Mammæ.**—Aster.; Con.; Plumb. iod.; Carcinosin.
——**Pains.**—Euphorb.
Cancrum Oris.—Secal.; Kreos.; Ars.; Baptis.
Capillary Stasis.—Capsic.; Echinac.
Carbuncles.—*Anthrac;* Ledum; Tar. cub.; *Ars.*; Lach.; Silic.
Cardiac Dropsy.—Adonis; Digit.
Cardiac Dyspnœa.—Acon. ferox.; Aspidos.
Cardialgia.—Fer. tart.
Cardio-vascular spasm.—Actæa spicata.
Caries.—Aur.; Asaf.; Sil.; Phos.
Car Sickness.—Coccul.
Caruncle, Urethral.—Thuja.
Catalepsy.—Curare; Hydroc. ac.; *Can. ind.*
Cataract.—Cineraria; *Phos.*; Platanus; Quass.; *Naphth.*; Calc. fluor.
Catarrh (chronic).—Anemopsis; Nat. sulph.; *Aur.*; *Eucaly.*; *Kal. bich.*; Puls.; Sang. nit.; Nat. carb.
Cellulitis.—Apis; Rhus; Vespa.
Cerebro-spinal Meningitis.—Cicut.; Zinc. cyan.; Cupr. acet.; Helleb.
Chancre.—Merc. bin iod.; Merc. prot.; Merc. sol.; Kali iod.
Checked Discharges.—Cupr.; Psorinum.
Cheyne-Stokes Respiration.—Grind.; Morphin.; Parthen.
Chicken-pox.—Tart. e.; Rhus; Kal. mur.
Chilblains.—Abrot.; *Agar.*; Tamus; Plantag.
Chloasma.—Sep.; Paull.
Chlorosis.—Ars.; Ferr.; Helon.; Cupr.; Puls.
Cholelithiasis.—Chionanth; Hydrast.
Cholera.—Camph.; *Verat.*; Ars.; Cupr.
Cholera Infantum.—Æthus.; Cuphea; Cal. phos.

Chordee.—Canth.; Salix; Yohimb.; Lupul.; Agave.
Chorea.—Absinth.; Agar.; Hippom.; Mygal.; Tanacet.; Tarant. hisp.; Ignat.; Zinc.; Cimicif.
Cicatrices.—Thiosin.; Graphites.
Ciliary Neuraglia.—Prunus; Spig.; Sapon.; Cinnab.
Cirrhosis of Liver.—Nasturt.; Nat. chlo.; *Merc.*
Climacteric Flushings.—Amyl nit.; *Lach.;* Sang.; Cimic.; Sep.
Coccygodynia.—Caust.; Silica.
Cold Sores.—Camphor; Dulcam.
Colic.—Cham.; Mag. phos.; Diosc.; Plumb
Colic, Renal.—Eryng; Pareira.
Colitis.—Merc. dulc.; Aloes; Allium sat.
Collapse.—Camph.; Morph.; Verat.; Ars.
Color-blindness.—Benzin.; Carb. sulph.
Coma.—Opium; Pilocarp.; Bell.
Comedones.—Abrotan.; Æthiops.; Baryta.
Condylomata.—Cinnab.; Nat. sulph.; Nit. ac.; *Thuja.*
Conjunctivitis.—Acon.; Puls.; Euphr.; Guar.
Constipation.—Opium; *Hydr.;* Iris; Verat.; Mag. mur.; Nux; Paraf.; Lac defl.; Tan. ac.; Mag. phos.; Sulph.; Alumina; Veratrum.
——**(in children)**—Æsc.; Collins.; Bry.; Alumina; Paraf.; Psorin.
Convulsions.—Hydroc. ac.; Laburn.; *Cupr.;* Cicut.; *Bell.;* Œnanth.
Corns.—Ant. curd.; Graph.; Sil.
Coryza.—Cepa; Penthor.; *Nat. mur.; Quillaya; Gels.;* Euphras.; Acon.; Ars.; Kali hyd.
Cough (dry).—Alum.; Bell.; Hyos.; Lauro.; Con.; Mentha; Rumex; Spongia; Sticta.
——**(laryngeal)**—Nit. ac.; Brom.; Caps.; Caust.; Lach.
——**(hoarse)**—Bry.; Hep.; Phos.; Samb.; Spong.; Verbasc.
——**(loose)**—Kal. sulph.; Tart. e.; Ipec.; Merc.; Puls.; Squilla; Stannum; Coccus c.
——**(phthisical)**—All. sat.; Crotal.; Phelland.; Naja.
——**(nervous)**—Ambra; Ignat; Hyos.; Kali brom.
——**(spasmodic)**—Corall.; Dros ; Mephit.; Cupr.; Mag. phos.; *Bellad.; Ipec.;* Coccus c.
Cracked Lips.—*Condur.;* Graph.; Nat. mur.

Croup.—*Acon.;* *Hep.;* Kaolin; *Spong.;* Brom.; Iod.; Kali bich.; Sang.

Cyanosis.—Tart. emet.; Carbo; Cuprum; Laches.; Laurocer.; Opium.

Cystitis.—Epigea; Saurur.; Popul.; *Canth.;* Chimaph.; Tereb.

Cysts.—Iod.; Apis.

Dandruff.—Kal. sulph.; Ars.; Lyc.; Badiaga.

Day-blindness.—Bothrops.

Deafness.—Calend.; Puls.; Hydr.; Graph.

Debility.—Chin.; Phos. ac.; Ars.; Curar; Kali phos.; Alfalfa.

——**(after gout)**—Cyprip.

Delirium.—Bell.; Hyos.; Agar.

Dentition.—Bell.; *Calc. phos.;* *Tereb.;* *Cham.*

——**(drooling)**—Trifolium; Mercur.

Diabetes.—Ars. brom.; Coca; Codein; Helleb.; Sizyg.; Phlorid.; Uran. nit.; Phosph.; Aur.

Diaphragmitis.—Cactus; Nux.

Diarrhœa.—Camph.; *Verat.;* *Ipec.;* *China;* Puls.; *Phos. ac.;* Merc.; Manzanita; Natrum sulph.; Sul.; Podophyl.

——**(chronic)**—Liatris; Chaparo; Coto; Natr. sulph.; Sulphur; Calcar.

——**(teething)**—Arundo; *Cham.;* Cal. phos.

Diphtheria.—Lach.; *Merc. cyan.;* Merc. bin iod.; Phyt.; Carb. ac.; Apis; Vinca; Nit. ac.; Echinacea.

——**(nasal)**—Am. caust.: *Kal. bich.*

Diplopia.—Bell.; Gels.; Oleand.; Hyos.

Dipsomania.—Capsicum.

Dissecting Wounds.—Crotal.; Ars.; Echinac.

Dropsy.—Apis; *Apocy. can.;* Cahinca; *Samb. can.;* Oxyd.; Helleb.; Dig.; Arsenic.

Dupuytren's Contraction.—Gels.; Thios.

Dysentery.—Asclep. t.; *Aloe;* Ipec.; *Merc. cor.;* Tromb.; Colocy.; Colchic.; Ars.; Canth.

Dysmenorrhœa.—Apiol.; Puls.; Caulop.; *Viburn.;* Mag. phos.; Aquilegia.

——**(membranous)**—Calc. ac.; Borax.

Dyspepsia.—*Nux;* Hyd.; Graph.; Petrol.; *Anacard.;* Puls.; Lycop.; Homar.; Carbo.

Dyspepsia—(Acid.)—Robinia.

——(Atonic)—Hydrastis.
——(Fermentative)—Salicyl. acid.
——(Nervous.)—Ignatia; Anacard.
Dysphagia.—Bell.; Lach.; Merc.; Cajap.; Curar.; Epilob.
Dyspnœa.—Apis; Ars.; Ipec.; Quebrach.; Spong.
Dysuria.—Tritic.; Fabian.; *Canth.;* Apis; Sarsap.; Camphor.; Bellad.

Ear-ache.—Bell.; Cham.; Mullein Oil.
Ear—(discharges).—Kal mur.
——(**very offensive**)—Elaps.
Ecchymosis.—Æthus.; *Arn.;* Rhus; Sulph. ac.
Eczema.—Arbut.; Clem.; Dulc.; *Rhus;* Sulph.; *Ars.;* Bovist.; Nat. ars.; *Anac.;* Oleand.; Petrol.; *Psorin.;* Alnus; Graphites.
Elephantiasis.—Elæis; Ars.; Hydrocot.; Lyc.
Emphysema.—Am. carb.; Ant. ars.; Lobel.
Empyemia.—Arnica.
Enteritis (acute).—Cinch.; Croton.; Podop.
——(**chronic**)—Ars.; Sulph.; Arg. nit.
Enuresis.—Benz. ac.; Caust.; Sulph.; Rhus ar.; Equiset.; Lupul.; Uran.; Physalis; Bellad.
Epididymitis.—Sabal; Puls.
Epilepsy.—Absinth.; Artem.; Sol. carol.; Fer. cyan.; Cupr.; Hyd. ac.; Sil.; Calc. ars.; *Œnanthe.*
Epistaxis.—Ambros.; Nat. nit.; *Arn.;* Ipec.; Bry.; Hamam.; Fer. phos.; *Nit. ac.;* Phosph.
Epithelioma.—Jequir.; Ars.; Thuj.; Chromic acid.
Erotomania.—Origan.; Phos.; Pic. ac.; Stram.; Plat.
Erysipelas.—Ananth.; Bell.; *Apis;* Canth.; Graph.; *Rhus;* Verat. vir.
Erythema.—Bell.; Mezer.; Antipyrin.
——**nodosum**—Apis; Rhus.
Eustachian Deafness.—Kal. sulph.; Rosa; Hydr.
Exophthalmic Goitre.—Lycopus; Pilocarp
Exostosis.—Hekla; Calc. fluor.
Exudative Pleurisy.—Abrotan.
Eyes—(Inflamed).—Acon.; Euphras.; Ruta.
——(**Detachment of retina**)—Naphthalin.

Fever.—Acon.; Agrostis; Spiranthes; *Gels.*; Bapt.; Verat. vir.; Ferr. phos.
Fibroids.—Calc. iod.
Fibroma.—Trillium; Ergot; Lapis.
Fissures.—Ledum; Graph.; Petrol.
Fistula.—Fluor. ac.; Nit. ac.; Sil.
Flatulence.—Carb.; *Asaf.*; *Nux mos.*; Mosch.; Lycop.; China; Carbol. ac.; Cajup.; Argent. nit.
Framboesia.—Jatropha; Merc. nit.
Freckles.—Badiaga; Sepia.

Gallactorrhœa.—Salvia; Calc.
Gall-stones.—China; Calc.; Berber.; Chionanth.; Calculus 8-10x trit.
Ganglion.—Ruta; Benz. ac.
Gangrene.—Euphorb.; Lach.; *Secale;* Carbo.
Gastralgia.—Bism.; Carb.; Coccul.; Nux; Cup. ars.; Petrol.; Phosph.
——**(recurring)**—Graph.
Gastric Ulcer.—Geran.; Arg. nit.; Ars.; *Atrop.;* Kal. bich.; Uran. nitr.
Gastritis.—Ars.; Nux: Oxal. ac.; Phos.; Hydr.
Gastro-enteritis.—Arg. n.; Ars.
Glanders.—Hippoz.; Merc.
Glands, Swollen.—Bell.; Merc. jod.; Phytol.; Kali hyd.; Alnus.
Gleet.—Thuja; Sepia; Santal.; Pulsat.; Abies can.
Glossitis.—Laches.; Mur. ac.; Apis.
Globus hyst.—Ignat.; Asaf.
Gonorrhœa.—Cann. sat.; Gels.; Ol. Sant.; Tussilago; Petros.; Merc.
Gout.—Amm. benz.; Lycop.; Urtica; Formica; Colchic.; Ledum; Lithium; Fraxinus.
——**(Retrocedent)**—Cajuput.
Gravel.—Hydrang.; Solidago; Lycopod.; Berberis.
Growing Pains.—Phosph. ac.; Guaiacum; Calc. phos.
Gumboil.—Bell.; Merc.; Hecla; Phosph.

Hæmatemesis.—Ipec.; Ham.; Phos.; Millefol.
Hæmaturia.—Canth.; Ham.; Tereb.; Nit. ac.

Hæmoglobinuria.—*Pic. ac.; Phos.*
Hæmophilia.—Nat. sil.; Phos.
Hæmoptysis.—Acal.; Ferr. phos.; Ipec.; Millef.; Ergot.; Eriger.; Geran.; Hydr. mur.; Allium sat.
Hæmorrhages.—Adrenalin; Hydrasing; Ipec.; Chin.; Sabina; Hamam.; Millef.; Crotal.; Trill.
——**(chronic sequelæ)**—Stront.
Hæmorrhoids.—Negundo; Scrophul.; *Aloe; Mur. ac.; Hamam.;* Fluor. ac.; *Nux;* Æs.; Collins.
Hallucinations.—Antipyr.; Stram.; Bell.
Halophagia.—Nit. sp. d.; Ars.; Phos.
Hay-fever.—Ambros.; Aral.; Cup. acet.; Napth.; Arundo; Rosa; *Sabad.;* Linum; Phleum pretense.
Headaches.—**(anæmic)**—Chin.; Ferr. phos.
——**(bursting)**—*Usnea;* Glonoin.
——**(congestive)**—Acon.; Bell.; Glon.; Lach.; Melil.; Gels.
——**(nervous)**—Cimic.; Ign.; Coff.; Guar.; Cannab.; Zinc.; Niccol.
——**(sick)**—Iris; Sang.; Nux; Chionanth.
Heart Affections.—Acon.; *Cactus; Naja; Dig.; Cræt.;* Lycop.; Spig.; Spong.; Adon.; Conval.; Phaseol.
Heartburn.—Geran.; Carbo.
Heart Failure.—Strych. sulph., 1/60-1/30 gr.; Spartein Sulph., ¼ gr.; Agaricin, 1/10 gr.; hypodermically.
Hectic Fever.—Baptis.; Ars.; Chinin. ars.
Hemicrania.—Ol. an.; Onos.; Sep.; Stann.; Coff.
Hemiplegia.—Oleand.; Coccul.; Bothrops.
Hemopia (vertical).—Titan.
Hepatitis.—Bry.; Merc.; Lach.; Natr. sulph.
Herpes—(Circinatus).—Sep.; Tellur.
Herpes Labialis.—Caps.; Nat. mur.; Rhus.
——**(preputialis)**—Hep.; Nit. ac.
——**(pudendi)**—Calad.; Nat. mur.; Nit. ac.
——**Zoster.**—Carb. oxyg.; Mentha; Ran. bulb.; Rhus.
Hiccough.—Ginseng.; Ratanh.; Nux; Sulph. ac.
Hoarseness.—Acon.; Bry.; Dros.; Carb.; Phos.; Caust.
Hodgkin's Disease.—Ars. iod.; Phos.; Iod.
Homesickness.—Caps.; Ignatia.
Hookworm.—Chenopod.; Thymol.

Housemaid's Knee.—Sticta; Slag.
Hydrocephalus.—Helleb.; Iodof.; Zinc.
Hydrocyle.—Rhodod.; Graph.; Puls.
Hydrophobia.—Xanthium; Anagallis; Canth.
Hydrothorax.—Lactuca; Ran. bulb.; Kali carb.; Merc. sulph.; Fluor. ac.; *Adonis.*
Hyperchlorhydria.—Chin. ars.; Robin.; Orexine; Arg. nit.; *Atropin;* Anacard.; Iris.
Hysteria.—Aquileg.; Castor.; Mosch.; Pothos.; Plat.; Sumb.; Valer.; Ignat.; Asaf.
Hysterical Joint.—Cotyledon.

Ichthyosis.—Ars. iod.; Syphil.
Impetigo.—Ars.; Tart. e.; Mez.
Impotence.—Agnus; Calad.; Onos.; *Phos. ac.;* Con.; Lycop.; Selen.; *Yohimbin.*
Indurations.—Carb. an.; Plumb. iod.; Alumen.
Inflammations.—Acon.; Bell.; Ferr. phos.; Sulph.
Influenza.—Eryng.; Bap.; Eucalyp.; Lobel. cerul.; *Gels.; Rhus;* Eup. perf.; Bryonia; Arsenic.
Insomnia.—*Coff.;* Cyprip.; Daph. ind.; Ignat.; Passifl.; *Aquileg.*
——**(delirium tremens)**—Sumbul.
Intermittent Fever.—Helianth.; *Chin.; Ars.;* Ipec.; *Nat. mur.;* Caps.; Tela aranea.
Iritis.—Bell.; Merc.; Clemat.; Syph.; Dubois.; Sarcolact. ac.

Jaundice.—Chionanth.; Cholest.; Bry.; Chin.; Myric.; Podop.; Mercur.; Chelid.; Kali pic.; Nat. phos.
——**(infantile)**—Lupulus; Cham.
——**(toxic)**—Trotyl.

Keloid.—Fluor. ac.
Kidneys (congestive).—Bell.; Tereb.; Canth.

Lagophthalmus.—Physos.
Laryngitis (acute).—Acon.; Hep.; Spong.; Phos.; Caust.; Arum.
Lectophobia.—Cann. sat.
Leprosy.—Elæis; Hydrocot.; Crotalus; Pyrara.
Leucocythæmia.—Ars.: Pic. ac.; Thuj.

Leucoderma.—*Ars. sul. r.*
—— **(chronic)**—Dros.; Selen.; Mang.; Argent.
Leucorrhœa.—Alum.; Calc.; Hyd.; Sulph.; Puls.; Kreos.; Sep.; Hydr.; Eucalyp.; Thuj.
—— **(in little girls)**—Calc.; Cub.; Hyp.; Asperul.
Lithiasis.—Asparag.; Lycop.; Sep.
Liver (congestion).—Berb.; Bry.; Card.; Chel.; Lept.; Merc.; Mag. mur.; Pod.; Sulph.
Liver-spots.—Nat. hyposulph.
Locomotor Ataxia.—Zinc. phos.; Plumb.; Arg. nit.; Oxal. ac.; Chromium sulph.; *Aragallis*.
Lumbago.—Guaiac.; Hyos.; *Rhus;* Tart. em.; Macrot.; Phytol.; Kali oxal.
Lungs, Congestion.—Acon.; Verat. vir.; Fer. phos.
—— **Œdema.**—Am. carb.; Tart. em.; Ars.
Lupus.—Am. ars.; Ars.; Hydrocot.; Thuja.
Lypothemia.—Ignatia; Nux mosch.

Malaria.—Alstonia; Am. pic.; Cornus.
Malnutrition.—Alfalfa; Calc. phos.
Mania.—Bell.; Hyos.; Stram.; Lach.
Marasmus.—Abrotan.; Iod.; Nat. mur.; Ars. iod.
Mastitis.—Bell.; Phytol.; Con.
Mastoid.—Caps.; Onos.; Hydr.
Measles.—Gels.; Puls.; Fer. phos.; Kal. mur.
Megrim.—Menisp.; Coff.; Sep.; Stan.
Meniere's Disease.—Carb. sulph.; Chenop.; Nat. sal.; Sal. ac.; Silica; Pilocarp. mur.
Meningitis (tubercular).—Bacil.; Cup. cyan.; Iodof.
Menorrhagia.—Chin.; Sabina; Croc.; Calc.; Plat.; Sedum; Tellur; Sanguisorba.
Menstruation.—**(cessation)**—Laches.; Puls.; Graph.; Sanguin.
—— **(delayed)**—Puls.; Calc. phos.; Cauloph.; Nat. mur.
—— **(painful)**—Bell.; Viburn. op.; Mag. phos.
—— **(profuse)**—Cham.; Ipec.; Trill.; Bellad.; Sabina.
Metritis, Chronic.—Aur. mur. nat.; Mel. c. s.; Merc.
Milk-leg.—Bufo; Ars.; Puls.; Rhus; Hamam.
Miscarriage.—**(repeated)**—Syphilin.; Bacill.
—— **(threatened)**—Sabina; Viburn. op.

Morning Sickness.—Amygdal.; Nux; Ipec.; Cucurb.; Coccul.; Apomorph.; Aletris.

Morphine Habit.—Avena.

Morvan's Disease.—Aur. mur.: Thuya.

Mountain Sickness.—Coca.

Mumps.—Bell.; Merc.; Pilocarp.; Rhus.

Muscæ Volitantes.—Caustic.; Cypriped.; China.

Mushroom Poisoning.—Absinth.

Myalgia.—Acon.; Bry.; Macrot.; Rhus.

Myelitis.—Ars.; Plumb.; Oxal. ac.; Secale; Dulc.

Myocardial Degeneration after Influenza.—Nux; Gels.

Myocarditis.—Dig.; Ars. iod.; Aur. mur.

Myositis.—Arn.; Mez.; Rhus.

Myxœdema.—Thyroid.

Nævus.—Fluor. ac.; Thuja.

Nephritis.—Meth. blue; Koch's lymph.; Berb.; Kali chlor.; Canth.; Merc. cor.; Phos.; Tereb.; Apis; Eucalyp.

Nephrolithiasis.—Pareira; Senecio aur.

Neuralgia.—Am. val.; *Acon.*; Bell.; *Spig.*; Kalm.; *Ars.*; Colocy.; Phos.; Zinc. val.

——**(lumbo-abdominal)**—Aran.

——**(periodic)**—Nic. sulph.; Ars.; Cedr.

——**(spermatic cord)**—Ol. an.; Oxal. ac.; Clemat.

Neurasthenia.—Anac.; *Zinc. pic.*; Stry. phos.; Physostig.

——**(gastric)**—Gentiana; Anacard.

Neuritis.—Stann.; Plumb.; Hyper.; Thallium; Ars.

Nictalopia.—Bell.; Helleb.

Night-sweats.—Acet. ac.; Nat. tell.; Popul.; Agaricus; Picrot.; Salvia; Pilocarp.

Nipples, Ulcerated.—Cast. eq.; Eup. ar.; Ratanh.

Nodosities of Joints.—Am. phos.

Nymphomania.—Robin.; Canth.; Hyos.; Phos.; Murex.

Obesity.—Am. brom.; Fucus; Calc.; Phyt.; Thyroid.

Oedema.—Apis; Ars.; Dig.

——**(of lungs)**—Tart. emet.

——**(pedum)**—Prunus.

Œsophagus.—Cajup.; Condur.; Bapt.

Onychia.—Silica; Psorin.

Orchitis.—Puls.; Bell.; Rhodod.; Spong.; Aur.
Osteitis.—Conchiolin.
Osteomalacia.—Phosph. ac.
Otitis Media (chronic).—Chenopod.; Cap.; Bell.; Merc.; Puls.; Calc.
Otorrhœa.—Kino; Merc.; *Calc.; Puls.;* Sulph.; Hydr.; Tellur.
Ovaralgia.—Zinc. val.; Apis; Lach.
Ovarian Cyst.—Oophor.; K. brom.; Apis.
Ovaritis.—Apis; Laches; Platina; Colocyn.; Sepia; Xanthox.
Oxaluria.—Senna; Nit. mur. ac.
Ozæna.—Alum.; Hippoz.; Aur.; Nit. ac.; Merc.; Hydr.; *Cadmium;* Sulph.

Panaritium.—Am. carb.; Fluor. ac.; Sil.
Pancreatic Troubles.—*Iris.*
Paralysis Agitans.—Aur. sul.; Hyos. hydrob.; Merc.
Paralysis.—(post-diphtheritic)—Gels.; Coccul.; Lach.; Aur. mur.; Arg. nit.
Paraplegia.—*Mang. ox.;* Kal. tart.; Lathyr.; Thall.; Hyper.; Anhalon.
Paresis.—Æsc. glab.; Badiag.
——(pneumo-gastric)—Grind.
——(respiratory)—Lobel. purp.
——(senile)—Aur. iod.; Phos.
——(spinal)—Irid.
——(typewriter's)—Stann.
Pellagra.—Bovista.
Pemphigus.—Caltha; Mancin.; Ran. scel.
Pericarditis.—Ant.; Ars.; Bry.; Colch.; Spig.; Dig.
Periostitis.—Asaf.; Aur.; K. bich.; Merc.; Phos.; Mez.; Sil.; Apis.
Peritonitis.—Apis; Bell.; Bry.; Colocy.; Merc. cor.; Sinapis; Sang. nit.; Wyeth.
Pharyngitis, follicular.—Æsc. hip.; Hydr.; Sang.; Wyethia.
——(sicca)—Dubois.
Phimosis.—Merc.; Guaiac.
Phlebitis.—Hamam.; Puls.
Phthisis.—Acalyph.; Gall. ac.; **Nat. cacod.**; Polyg. avic.; Silphium; Calc. ars.; Kreos.

──(laryngeal)—Dros.; Stan.; Selen.; Nat. selen.
Plague.—Ignatia; Operculina.
Pleurisy.—Acon.; *Bry.;* Squill.; Asclep.; Kal. c.
──(effusion stage)—Apis; *Canth.;* Ars.; Sulph.
Pleurodynia.—Bry.; Cimic.; Ran. bulb.
Plica Polonica.—Vinca; Lycop.
Pneumonia.—Bry.; Phos.; Sang.; Iod.; Chelid.; Lyc.; Pneumo-coccin.
Poison-oak.—Anac.; Xerophyl.; Grind.; Cyprip.; Rhus; Croton.; Graph.; Erecht.
Poliomyelitis.—Lathyrus; *Bungaris;* Kali phos.
Polychrome Spectra.—Anhalon.
Polypi.—Phos.; Calc.; Sang.; Thuj.
──(nasal)—Lemna; *Calc.; Teuc.*
Polyuria.—Arg.; *Phos. ac.;* Murex; Squill.; Uran.; Rhus aromat.
Porrigo capitis.—Calc. mur.
Portal congestion.—Æscul glabra.
Priapism.—Pic. ac.; Canth.
Proctitis.—Ant. crud.; Collins.; Aloe; Podop.
Prosopalgia.—Cactus; Verbas.; Kalmia; Puls.
Prostatic Hypertrophy.—Fer. pic.; Thuj.
Prostatitis.—Merc. dulc.; Sabal.; Pic. ac.; *Thuj.;* Tritic.; Staph.
Pruritus.—Antipyr.; Carbol. ac.; Dolich.; Fagop.; Sulph.; Rhus; Pulex.; Radium.
Psilosis.—Fragaria.
Psoriasis.—Kal. ars.; K. brom.; Thyroid.; *Ars.;* Graph.; *Borax;* Sulph.; Emetin ½ gr.
Pterygium.—Zinc.; Ratanh.; Sulph.
Ptomaine Poisoning.—Ars.; Kreos.; Pyrog.
Ptyalism.—Merc.; Iris; Iod.; Trifol.
Purpura.—Crotal.; Phosp.; Ars.; Hamam.; Naja.
Pyæmia.—Ars. jod.; Chinin.; Lach.; Pyrogen.
Pyelitis.—Merc. cor.; Hep.; Tereb.; Cup. ars.; Epigea; Juniperus.
Pyorrhœa.—Emetin.; Staphis.; Plantago.
Pyrosis.—Gallic ac.; Bismuth.; Caps.

Rachitis.—Calc.; Iris; Phos.; Sil.
Ranula.—Thuja; Calc.; Fluor. ac.
Raynaud's Disease.—Ars.; Secale; Cactus tincture.
Rectal Pockets.—Polygon.
Respiration (Cheyne-Stokes).—Antipyr.
Rheumatism.—Colch.; Propyl.; Acon.; *Bry.*; Dulc.; Merc.; Rhus; Cimic.
——**(chronic)**—Stellar.; Ol. jecor.; *Sulph.*; Viscum.
——**(gonorrhœal)**—Irisin; Sarsap.; Thuja.
Rhinitis (atrophic).—Lemna.
Riggs' Disease.—Calc. renal.
Ringworm.—Sepia; Tellur.; Ars.; Bacillin.

Scarlatina.—Bell.; Rhus; Stram.
——**(malignant)**—Am. carb.; Mur. ac.; Lach.; Ailanth.; Crotal.; Baptis.; Nit. ac.
Sciatica.—Cotyled.; Viscum; *Colocy.;* Rhus; *Gnaph.*
Sclerosis, multiple.—Aur. mur.
Sclerotic Degeneration.—Baryt. m.; Plumb.; Aur. mur.
Scrofula.—Æthiops; Fer. iod.; Cistus; Merc.; Calc.; Sulph.; Therid.
Scurvy.—Acet. ac.; Agave; Phos.; Merc.
Seasickness.—Apomorph.; Petrol.; *Coccul.;* Nux; Tabac.
Seborrhœa.—Heracleum.; Ars.; Graph.; Vinca; Nat mur.
Senile Decay.—Oophor.; Baryta.
Sepsis.—Crotal.; Bapt.; Echin.; Ars.; Lach.
Sleeping Sickness.—Nux mosch.; Opium; Gelsem.; *Atoxyl.*
Sleeplessness.—Tela aran.; *Coff.;* Ign.; Cimicif.; Gels.; Opium (high); Daphne; Hyos. hydrob.
Snake-poison Antidotes.—Golond.; Cedr.; Gymne.; Sisyr.; Guaco; Salag.
Somnambulism.—Kali phos.; Kali brom.
Spermatorrhœa.—Salix; Chin.; Phos. ac.; Staphys.
Spleen Affections.—Ceanoth.; Quercus; Helianth.; Nat. m.; Polymnia.
Sterility.—Agnus; Nat. m.; Borax.
Stomach Dilatation.—Hydr. mur.
Stomatitis.—Borax; Arg. nit.; Kal. mur.; *Nit. ac.*
Subinvolution.—Fraxin.; Aur. mur. nat.; Epipheg.
Sycosis.—Asterias; Thuja; Natr. sulph.; Aur. mur.

Synovitis.—Apis; Bry.; Calc. fluor.
Syphilides.—Ars. s. fl.; K. hyd.; Nit. ac.
Syphilis.—Calotropis; Coryd.; Plat. mur.; Merc.; K. hyd.; Aurum.
——**(latent)**—Ars. met.; Syphil.
——**(nodes)**—Coryd.; Stilling.; K. hyd.

Tachycardia.—*Abies nig.*; Agnus.
Tape-worm.—Filix; Cina; Ioduretted Pot. iod.
Tetanus.—Strych.; Upas; Passif.; Physos.
Thrombosis.—Borthrops.; Lach.
Tinnitus.—Antipyr.; Cannab. ind.; Carb. sulph.; Sal. ac.
Tobacco-craving.—Daph. ind.
Tonsillitis.—Am. mur.; Guaiac.; Baryta. ac.; Bell.; Merc.; Phyt.
Toothache.—Plantago; Mag. carb.; Bell.; Chamom.
Torticollis.—Lachnant.
Traumatism.—Arnica; Bellis.
Trismus.—Linum.
Tuberculosis.—Ars. jod.; Phelland.; Tuberculin.; Calcar.
Tumors.—Calc. fluor.; Conium; Baryta mur.; Thuja; Merc. iod. rub.; Hydrast.; Phytol.; Plumb. jod.
Tympanitis.—Lycop.; Tereb.; Asaf.; Erigeron.
Typhoid.—Bapt.; Mur. ac.; Ars.; Phos. ac.; Bry.
——**(diarrhœa)**—Epilob.

Ulcers.—Nit. ac.; Sil.; Ars.; Comocl.; Kal. hyd.; Lach.; Pæon.; Calend.
Uræmia.—Am. carb.; Cup. ars.; *Morph.*
Urethral Caruncle.—Cann. sat.; *Eucalyp.*
Urethritis.—Acon.; Apis; *Canth.*
——**(in children)**—Doryph.
Uric Acid Diathesis.—Hedeom.; Ocim.
Urticaria.—Ant. c.; Antipyr.; Apis; Astac.; Bombyx; Copaiv.; Fragar.; Nat. mur.
Uterine Displacement.—Abies can.; Eupion; Heliot.; Sep.; Puls.; Fraxin.; Fer. iod.
——**(induration)**—Aur. mur.; Kalmia.
——**(tumors)**—*Aur. m. nat.*

Vaginismus.—Cactus; Plumb.; Bellad.
Varicose Veins.—Calc. fluor.; Hamam.; Puls.
Variola.—Ant. tart.; Saracen.
——**(hæmorrhage)**—Crotal.; Phos.; Ars.
Vascular Tension.—Acon.; Bell.; Ver. v.
——**(with arterial lesion)**—Adrenal.; Baryt. mur.; Tabac.; Plumbum.
——**(rapid reducers)**—Glon.; Amyl.; Nat. nit.; Trinitin.
Vertigo.—Gels.; *Granat.*; Phos.; Coccul.; Con.
Venous Stasis.—*Æsc. hip.*

Warts.—Ant. c.; Caust.; Nit. ac.; *Thuj.*; Salicy. acid.
Wens.—Thuja; Benz. acid.; Bacillin.
Whooping-cough.—Castan.; *Dros.;* Cupr.; Mag. ph.; Pertuss.
Worms.—Calc.; Cina; Santon.; Spigel.; Teuc.; Naphth.
Wrist Rheumatism.—Actea spic.; Viol. od.
Writers' Cramp.—Arg. m.; Sulph. ac.
Weil's Disease.—Chelid.; Phosph.

Yellow Fever.—Cadmium; Ars.; Crotal.

LIST OF REMEDIES
COMMON NAMES

LIST OF REMEDIES
COMMON NAMES

	PAGE
Acetate of barium	106
Acetic acid	9
Acorn spirit dist.	542
Adder	676
Allspice	539
Alum of chrome	380
Alum root	435
Amber	618
Ambergris	37
American arum	141
American aspen	529
American coffee tree	317
American holly	344
American spikenard	68
Ammonia water	43
Amniotic fluid	328
Animal charcoal	168
Animal oil	431
Anise	344
Anthracite	55
Ants	292
Apple of Sodom	598
Aqua marina	462
Arbor vitae	643
Argilla	34
Arrow poison	248
Arsenic stibiatum	82
Arsenic trioxide	79
Arsenious acid	79
Arsenite of antimony	55
Ash (mountain)	465, 532
Ash (white)	295
Ashwathya	288
Asparagus	93
Balm of Gilead	529
Ballwood	316
Balsam apple	445
Balsam copaiva	234
Balsam Peru	103
Baneberry	11
Barberry	119
Barium chloride	109
Basket grass flower	680
Bayberry	451

	PAGE
Bean	503
Bearberry	663
Bear grass	683
Bear's foot	184
Beaver	180
Bedbug	203
Bee	61
Beechdrop	267
Beech nuts	267
Beechwood kreosote	382
Beet-root	122
Benzoic acid	117
Benzol	116
Betelnut	70
Bethroot	652
Betony	122
Bibernell	262
Bird cherry	532
Bisulphide carbon	175
Bitter almond	47
Bitter broom	498
Bitter cucumber	227
Bitter orange	213
Bitter sweet	260
Blackberry	189
Black garden radish	547
Blackhaw	673
Black lead	309
Black nightshade	597
Black snake root	203
Black spruce	2
Black sulphide of antimony	55
Black sulphur mercury	20
Black thorn	532
Black willow	566
Blazing star	323
Bloodroot	569
Blue bell	24
Blue cohosh	181
Blue eyed grass	308
Blue flag	355
Blue gum tree	270
Blue vervain	672
Boldo	468
Boracic acid	124

LIST OF REMEDIES—COMMON NAMES

	PAGE
Borate of sodium	126
Borax	125
Boro-glyceride	125
Box elder	17
Brazilian alfavaca	549
Brazilian burdock	163
Brazilian caroba	356
Brazilian cress	399
Brazilian snakeroot	75
Brazilian uctba	452
Broad-leaf dock	559
Bromide of arsenic	83
Bromine	130
Broom	599
Buckbean	430
Buckthorn	549
Buckwheat	281
Buchu	105
Bug agaric	19
Bugle weed	413
Burdock	394
Burning bush	273
Burr flower	280
Bush master	387
Butterbur	659
Buttercup	545
Butter nut	358
Butter of antimony	57
Button bush	210
Button snake root	269
Buttonwood	522
Cadmic sulphate	139
Calabar bean	512
Calcium sulphide	327
California clover	26
California coffee tree	548
California laurel	489
California lilac	184
California poison oak	555
California poppy	270
Calomel	270
Cancer nosode	232
Candy tuft	340
Cane-sugar	564
Caper spurge	276

	PAGE
Carbamide	661
Carbonate of baryta	106
Carbonate of lime	144
Carbonous oxide	175
Carburetted hydrogen	174
Carcinoma	179
Caroba	356
Cascara	178
Cashew nut	50
Castor oil	556
Caterpillar	94
Catnip	180
Cat's milk	386
Cat tail flag	244, 353
Cat thyme	638
Cayenne pepper	166
Cedar	360
Celandine	189
Celery	64
Centaury	160
Century plant	23
Centipede	493
Cevadilla	560
Chaste tree	23
Chestnut leaves	179
Cherry laurel	396
Chickpea	394
Chickweed	609
Chili bark	542
China clay	382
Cinnamon	211
Chinese sumach	25
Chloral hydrate	197
Chlorine	199
Chloroform	198
Christmas berry tea	345
Chrysophanic acid	201
Cloves	103
Clover	427
Club moss	409
Coal naphtha	116
Cobra	453
Cochineal	220
Cockle	336
Cockle burr	324
Cockroach	123

LIST OF REMEDIES—COMMON NAMES

	PAGE
Coffee	222
Coffee tree	317
Cod liver oil	482
Colic root	400
Colorado potato bug	258
Columbine	67
Common rush	360
Comfrey	627
Condor	229
Cone flower	263
Cooties	534
Copper	246
Copper head	185
Coral snake	264
Corkwood elm	259
Corn cockle	395, 580
Corn silk	611
Corn smutt	662
Corrosive sublimate	436
Cotton plant	308
Couch grass	654
Cowhage	257
Cowslip	157, 530
Cows milk	386
Crab apple	465
Crab's eye vine	358
Cranberry	673
Cranesbill	303
Crawfish	94
Crawley root	236
Cream	386
Cress	399
Crown glass	594
Cuban spider	632
Cutweed	307
Curds	386
Cystogen	291
Cuttlefish juice	586
Culver's root	400
Daffodil	455
Daisy	115
Damiana	659
Dandelion	633
Darnel	407
Deadly nightshade	110
Death cup	22
Digallic acid	632
Diphtheritic virus	257
Dipple's oil	481
Dita bark	82
Dogbane	65
Dog mercury	481
Dog's milk	385
Dogwood	236
Dogwood (white)	680
Dover's powder	488
Dwarf bean	503
Duckweed	399
Dusty miller	210
Dyer's weed	378
Egg shells	491
Egg vaccine	491
Eel serum	589
Elder	66, 568
Enlexing	629
Epsom salt	418
Ergot	578
European snake-root	90
Eyebright	279
False cromwell	484
Farcine	329
Fever root	653
Figwort	577
Fire weed	268
Flax	405
Flea	535
Fleabane	260
Flint	590
Fluoride of lime	149
Fluor spar	149
Fly acarus	655
Fly woodbine	408
Fluxweed	244
Forget-me-not	451
Fool's parsley	17
Formaldehyde	291
Fowler's solution	361
Foxglove	252
Fringetree	196

LIST OF REMEDIES—COMMON NAMES

	PAGE
Gallic acid	632
Gall stones	282
Garden nasturtium	118
Garden spurge	353
Garlic	29
Gentian	302
German chamomile	187
Gila monster	322
Ginger	687
Glauber's salt	466
Glycerin	306
Goa powder	201
Goatbush	189
Goat's rue	296
Gold	96
Goldenrod	598
Golden seal	332
Golden sulph. antimony	58
Gonorrhœal virus	424
Goose grass	297
Gopher plant	276
Grape fruit	213
Green dragon	87
Green lizard	323
Grease	421, 667
Grey spider	70
Ground ivy	320
Gummi gutti	298
Gunpowder	375
Hagenia	382
Haircap moss	331
Hard hack	602
Hashish	160
Hawthorn	237
Head-louse	534
Hedge hyssop	312
Hemlock	230
Hemlock spruce	1
Hellebore (American)	669
Hellebore (white)	667
Hemp	162
Hemp weed	314
Henbane	336
Herring brine	531
Hoarhound	334

	PAGE
Holly	344
Hogweed	328
Honey-bee	61
Honey with salt	427
Honeysuckle	408
Hops	408
Horse chestnut	15
Horse foot	402
Horse nettle	598
Horse radish	221
Horse thumbnail	180
Household herb	52
Houseleek	581, 582
Huckleberries	664
Hydrate of ammonia	43
Hydrobromic acid	132
Iceland moss	611
Ikshugandha	651
Indian arnica	78
Indian cockle	218
Indian hemp	65
Indian liquorice	358
Indian nettle	4
Indian pennywort	334
Indian tobacco	405
Iodide of arsenic	84
Iodide of baryta	109
Iron	283
Ironwood	491
Ivy	678
Jack-in-pulpit	87
Jambol	629
Japanese belladonna	338
Jellyfish	426
Jerusalem oak	191
Juniper	360
Kelp	296
Kermes mineral	58
King crab	402
Kissing bug	396
Knitbone	627
Knot grass	528
Knotted figwort	577

LIST OF REMEDIES—COMMON NAMES

	PAGE
Kola nut	609
Kombe seed	615
Krait	454
Labaraque's solution	458
Lady bug	217
Lady slipper	251
Lady's tresses	602
Lampblack	172
Laudanum	488
Lava	320
Lead	524
Leatherwood	443
Leech	563
Leopard's bane	76
Lesser periwinkle	674
Lettuce (acrid)	392
Lettuce (white)	392
Lily of valley	232
Lime water	147
Linden	649
Liverwort	328
Lizard	320
Lizard (green)	323
Lizard's tail	576
Loadstone	283
Lobster	330
Loco weed (purple)	95, 498
Loco weed (white)	67
Locust	557
Logwood	317
Louse	534
Lucerne	26
Lung wort	610
Madar bark	157
Madder	567
Magenta	296
Magendi's solution	488
Male fern	289
Mandrake	114
Manganese (colloidal)	423
Manganeel apple	421
Mango tree	424
Manzanita	333
Margosa	100

	PAGE
Marking nut	48
Marigold	156
Marine plasma	462
Marsh buttercup	546
Marsh mallow	93
Marsh tea	397
May apple	526
Mescal button	51
Meadow parsnip	639
Meadow saffron	224
Medical Lake salt	596
Mercuric sulphide	210
Metallic arsenic	85
Mirbane	117
Mistletoe	677
Moccasin snake	128
Monkshood	7
Moonseed	428
Morning glory	121
Mother-of-pearl	153, 320
Mother wort	437
Mountain ash	532
Mountain grape	119
Mountain laurel	380
Mug wort	86
Mullein	671
Mullet fish (red)	435
Mushroom	19
Musk	447
Musk root	626
Mustard	595
Mustard (black)	595
Myrtle	452
Nasturtium	118
New Jersey tea	184
New So. Wales black spider	395
New Zealand spider	396
Nickel	468
Nightblooming cereus	137
Night shade	110
Nipple wort	274
Nishope	485
Nitrate of silver	72
Nitro-glycerin	304
Nutmeg	473

LIST OF REMEDIES—COMMON NAMES

	PAGE
Oats	100
Ohio buckeye	17
One berry	497
Onion	27
Orange	213
Orange spider	640
Orpiment	86
Orris root	355
Ovarian extract	485
Ox-eye daisy	567
Oxgall	282
Pansy	875
Panax	304
Papal-cross spider	69
Paracoto bark	244
Paregoric	488
Parsley	503
Parsnip	498
Parsnip (meadow)	639
Partridge berry	444
Passion flower	499
Pawpaw (American)	93
Peach bark	47
Pennyroyal	319
Pennywort	237
Peony	494
Pepper (black)	520
Pepper (cayenne)	166
Peppermint	428
Peruvian balsam	103
Peruvian bark	207
Petroleum ether	117
Pheasant's eye	12
Phenazone	60
Phenol	173
Phosphate of lime	152
Pichi	281
Pine tar	521
Pine agaric	528
Pinkroot	600
Pippsissewa	193
Pitcher plant	575
Pituitary gland	520
Plant lice	192
Plantain	521

	PAGE
Plaster of Paris	154
Pleurisy root	92
Poison elder	556
Poison hemlock	230
Poison ivy	552
Poison nut	475
Poison oak	555
Poison weed	678
Poke root	514
Pomgranate	309
Pond lily	473
Pool root	572
Poor man's mercury	344
Poppy	486
Potato	598
Prickly pear	488
Prickly ash	679
Prickly poppy	70
Primrose	506, 531
Prussic acid	335
Puff adder	186
Puffball	128
Puka	130
Pumpkin seed	244
Purging nut	357
Purple fish	448
Pussy willow	566
Queen of meadow	275
Queen root	611
Quicksilver	432
Quince	210
Rabid dog saliva	335
Radish	574
Ragweed	38
Rag wort	583
Rape seed	580
Rattlesnake	240
Rattlesnake bean	185
Rattlesnake root	392
Rattlesnake weed	67
Red alder	30
Red cedar	369
Red clover	651
Red coral	235

LIST OF REMEDIES—COMMON NAMES

	PAGE
Red gum	272
Red mullet fish	435
Red onion	27
Red starfish	94
Reed	88
Reindeer flower	546
Rest harrow	637
Rhubarb	549
Rockoil	500
Rock rose	211
Roman chamomile	53
Rose	558
Rose apple	272
Rose laurel	480
Rosin weed	594
Rosin wood	313
Rue bitterwort	559
Rush	360
Sacred bark	178
Sad tree	479
Saffron	238
Sage	567
Sal ammoniac	44
Salicylic acid	565
Saliva rabid dog	335
Salt	459
Saltpetre	374
Sandal	483
Sanguinarine nitrate	571
Sanicula springs	571
Savine	563
Saw palmetto	562
Scabies vesicle	533
Scabwort	347
Scallop	68
Scarlet pimpernel	50
Scotch pine	519
Scouring rush	267
Sea kelp	296
Sea onion	604
Sea salt	462
Sea sand	594
Selenium	581
Selenium (colloidal)	582
Self-heal	527

	PAGE
Sensitive plant	555
Seven barks	321, 331
Sepsin	540
Sheele's green	245
Sheep sorrel	559
Shepherd's purse	642
Shrub yellow root	121
Shucks	611
Silicate of lime	154
Silkweed	91
Silver	71
Singhee	360
Skimmed milk	387
Skull cap	577
Skunk	430
Skunk cabbage	530
Slag	548
Smallpox virus	666
Smartweed	528
Smilax	575
Smooth sumach	552
Snail	444
Snake head	192
Snake lizard	390
Snake moss	308
Snake root	76
Snake root (European)	90
Snakewort	584
Snap dragon	403
Snowberry	626
Snow drop	297
Snow on mountain	278
Snow rose	321, 550
Soapbark	548
Soap root	573
Socotrine aloes	30
Soot	296
Sorrel acid	491
Sorrel tree	493
South American palm	334
Southern wood	2
Sowbread	249
Spanish fly	163
Spanish spider	663
Spearmint	429
Spice wood	7

LIST OF REMEDIES—COMMON NAMES

	PAGE
Spider	395
Spider (black)	395
Spider (Cuban)	454, 632
Spider (New Zealand)	396
Spider (Papal cross)	69
Spider (Spanish)	633
Spider web	69
Spindle tree	273
Spirit weed	390
Spring mushroom	22
Sponge	603
Sponge (fresh water)	102
Sponge nettle	357
Sprudel springs	178
Spurge laurel	251
Spurge olive	442
Squirting cucumber	266
Star of Bethlehem	489
St. John's wort	338
St. Ignatia's bean	342
St. Mary's thistle	176
Star grass	26
Staves acre	607
Stingfish	128
Stinging nettle	661
Stinkasand	89
Stone crop	500
Stone root	226
Storksbill	303
Strawberry	295
Strawberry tree	70
Succinic acid	618
Sugar	564
Sulphate of lime	154
Sulphuric acid	624
Sulphurous acid	625
Sumach	551
Sumach (Chinese)	25
Sundew	258
Sunflower	322
Supra-renal	13
Surucucu	444
Swallow-wort	92
Swamp milk-weed	92
Swamp walnut	236
Sweetbark	179
Sweet marjoram	489
Sweet spirits of nitre	472
Sweet vernal grass	89
Sweet water lily	473
Sycamore buttonwood	522
Syphilitic virus	627
Tamalpais lily	680
Tanin	632
Tansy	631
Tar camphor	454
Tartar emetic	58
Tartaric acid	634
Tartrate antimony and potash	58
Tea	640
Teamster's tea	412
Testicular extract	485
Thorn apple	612
Thoroughwort	274
Thumb-nail of horse	180
Thyme	647
Thyme-camphor	646
Thyroid	647
Tiger lily	400
Timothy grass	558
Tin	605
Toad	135
Toad flax	403
Toad stool	19
Tobacco	629
Tomato	596
Trailing arbutus	267
Tree moss	662
Tropical bind-weed	330
Tuberculous lung	101
Turkey pea	237
Turpentine	636
Turpethum	441
Unicorn root	323
Upas	135
Vanilla	666
Vegetable charcoal	170
Violet	674

LIST OF REMEDIES—COMMON NAMES

	PAGE
Viper	127
Viper (German)	676
Virgin bower	213
Virginia creeper	46
Virginia snake-root	76
Virginia stone crop	500
Virgin vine	497
Wahoo	273
Wall flower	415
Walnut	359
Wasp	672
Water ash	535
Water avens	331
Water dropwort	479, 504
Water hemlock	201
Water lily	473
Watermelon seed	244, 576
White agaric	124
White beth root	652
White dogwood	680
White hellebore	667
White nettle	393
Wild cherry	532
Wild elder	66
Wild ginger	91
Wild ginseng	304
Wild hops	132
Wild indigo	103
Wild primrose	530
Wild thyme	647
Wild yam	255
Willow	566
Willow herb	435
Wind flower	536
Winter cherry	511
Wintergreen	298
Witch hazel	318
Wolf's bane	11
Wolf's lung	468
Woodbine	555
Wood louse	484
Wood marsh	572
Wood sage	638
Wood sorrel	583
Wood spurge	278
Wood strawberry	295
Wood tar	286
Worm moss	207
Worm seed	205
Worm wood	4
Yarrow	444
Yeast	650
Yellow dock	558
Yellow jasmine	299
Yellow pond lily	473
Yellow sulphide of arsenic	86
Yellow viper	127
Yerba buena	443
Yerba santa	269
Yew	635

LIST OF REMEDIES
PHARMACEUTICAL
AND
LATIN NAMES

LIST OF REMEDIES
PHARMACEUTICAL AND LATIN NAMES

	PAGE
Abies Canadensis	1
Abies nigra	2
Abrotanum	2
Absinthium	4
Acalypha	4
Acanthia	203
Acarus	655
Acetanilid	5
Acetic acid	6
Achyranthes	11
Aconitum cammarum	11
Aconitum ferox	11
Aconitum lycoton	11
Aconitum napellus	7
Aconitine	11
Actæa racemosa	203
Actæa spicata	11
Adonis vernalis	12
Adonidin	13
Adrenalin	13
Æsculus glabra	17
Æsculus hippocast.	15
Æthiops antimon.	17
Æthiops merc.	17
Æthusa cynapium	17
Agaricin	124
Agaricus emeticus	23
Agaricus muscarius	19
Agaricus phalloides	22
Agave	23
Agnus castus	23
Agraphis	24
Agrimonia	324
Agropyrum	654
Agrostema	395
Agrostis	11
Ailanthus	25
Alcohol sulphuris	175
Aletris farinosa	26
Alfalfa	26
Alkekengi	511
Allium cepa	27
Allium sativum	29

	PAGE
Alnus	30
Aloe socotrina	30
Alstonia constricta	32
Althæa	93
Alumen	32
Alumina	34
Alumin. acet.	36
Alumin. chlor.	36
Alumin. oxide	34
Alumin. silic.	36, 382
Alum. sil. sulph.	548
Amanita (agaricus)	19
Amanita phalloides	22
Amanita vernus	22
Ambra grisea	37
Ambrosia	38
Ammoniacum	39
Ammonium acet.	7
Ammonium benzoicum	39
Ammonium brom.	40
Ammonium carb.	40
Ammonium causticum	43
Ammonium formald.	291
Ammonium hydrate	43
Ammonium iod.	43
Ammonium mur.	44
Ammonium phosp.	46
Ammonium picricum	46
Ammonium tart.	43
Ammon. valer.	46
Ammon. vanad.	665
Ampelopsis quin.	46
Ampelopsis trifol.	555
Amphisbœna	390
Amygdala amara	47
Amygdalus Persica	47
Amyl nitrite	47
Anacardium occid.	50
Anacardium orientale	48
Anagallis	50
Anagyris	539
Anabolinum	51
Anatherum	51

LIST OF REMEDIES—LATIN NAMES

	PAGE
Ancistrodon	185
Andira araroba	201
Andromeda	493
Androsace lactea	166
Anemopsis	52
Angelica	542
Angophora	272
Anguillar ichthy. serum	589
Angustura	52
Anilinum	53
Anisum stellatum	344
Anthemis	53
Anthracinum	54
Anthrakokali	55
Anthoxantum	89
Antiarus tox	660
Antifebrinum	5
Antimonium arsenicum	55
Antimonium chlorid.	57
Antimonium crudum	55
Antimonium jodatum	57
Antimonium sulph.	58
Antimonium tart.	58
Antipyrine	60
Aphis	192
Apiol	503
Apis mellifica	61
Apium graveolens	64
Apium virus	64
Apocynum andros	65
Apocynum cannab.	65
Apomorphia	66
Aqua calcarea	147
Aqua marina	462
Aqua regia	472
Aqua sanicula	571
Aquilegia	67
Aragallus	67
Aralia hispida	66
Aralia quinquefol	304
Aralia racemosa	68
Aranea diadema	69
Aranea scinencia	70
Arbrus precatorius	358
Arbutin	664
Arbutus	70

	PAGE
Arctosphylos	664
Arctium lappa	394
Areca	70
Argemone	70
Argentum cyan.	75
Argentum jod.	75
Argentum met.	71
Argentum nitric.	72
Argentum oxyd.	75
Argentum phos.	75
Aristolochia mil.	75, 205
Aristolochia serp.	76
Armoracia sat.	221
Arnica montana	76
Arsenicum album	79
Arsenicum brom.	83
Arsenicum hydrog.	83
Arsenicum jodatum	84
Arsenicum met.	85
Arsenicum stibiat.	82
Arsenicum sulph. flav.	86
Arsynal	458
Artanthe	384
Artemisia abrotanum	2
Artemisia absinthium	4
Artemisia maritima	592
Artemisia vulgaris	86
Arum dracontium	87
Arum Italicum	87
Arum mac.	87
Arum triphyllum	87
Arundo	88
Arundo donax	594
Asafœtida	89
Asagræa	560
Asarum can.	91
Asarum Europ.	90
Asclepias incarn.	92
Asclepias syriaca	91
Asclepias tuberosa	92
Asclepias vincetox	90
Asimina	93
Asparagus	93
Asperula	588
Aspidium	289
Aspidosperma	94

LIST OF REMEDIES—LATIN NAMES

Name	PAGE
Astacus fluv.	94
Asterias rubens	94
Astragalus	95
Athamanta	19
Atoxyl	82
Atropin	114
Atriplex	539
Aurantium	213
Aurum arsenic	98
Aurum brom.	98
Aurum jodat.	99
Aurum met.	96
Aurum mur.	98
Aurum mur. kal.	99
Aurum mur. nat.	99
Aurum sulph.	99
Avena sativa	100
Aviare	657
Azadirachta	100
Bacillinum	101
Bacillinum testium	102
Badiaga	102
Baja	196
Balsam Peru	103
Balsam tolu	103
Baptisia confusa	105
Baptisia tinctoria	103
Barosma	105
Baryta acet.	106
Baryta carb.	106
Baryta jod.	109
Baryta mur.	109
Basaka	360
Belladonna	110
Bellis perennis	115
Benzinum	116
Benzin. dinitric	117
Benzin. nit.	117
Benzoic acid.	117
Benzoin oder	7
Benzol	116
Berberis aquifolium	119
Berberis vulgaris	119
Beta vulg.	122
Betainum hydrochlor	122
Betonica	122
Bismuthum	122
Bixa	519
Blatta Americana	123
Blatta orientalis	123
Boldoa	191
Boletus laricis	124
Boletus luridus	124
Boletus satanus	124
Bolus alba	382
Bombyx	94
Boracic. acid.	124
Borax	125
Bothrops	127
Botulinum	128
Bougmancia	610
Bovista	128
Bracnyglottis	130
Branca	328
Brassica napus	580
Brassica nigra	595
Brayera	382
Bromium	130
Brucea	53
Bryonia	132
Buchu	105
Bufo	125
Bungarus	242
Bursa pastoris	642
Butyric acid	136
Cacodyl. soda	151
Cactus grandiflorus	137
Cadmium brom.	140
Cadmium iodat.	140
Cadmium oxide	140
Cadmium sulph.	139
Cæsium	493
Caffein	223
Cahinca	140
Cajuputum	141
Caladium	141
Calcarea acetica	142
Calcarea arsenica	143
Calcarea bromata	143
Calcarea calcinata	143

LIST OF REMEDIES—LATIN NAMES

	PAGE
Calcarea carbonica	144
Calcarea caustica	148
Calcarea fluorica	149
Calcarea hypophos.	153
Calcarea jodata	151
Calcarea lactic	148
Calcarea lacto-phos.	148
Calcarea muriatica	148
Calcarea ostrearum	144
Calcarea ovorum	148, 491
Calcarea oxalica	142
Calcarea phosphorica	152
Calcarea picrata	148
Calcarea renalis	153
Calcarea silicata	154
Calcarea silica fluor	393
Calcarea sulphurica	154
Calcarea sulph. stib	151
Calculus	282
Calendula	156
Calotropis	157
Caltha palustris	157
Camphora	158
Camphora monobrom.	160
Camphoric acid.	159
Cancer astacus	94
Canchalagua	160
Cannabis Indica	160
Cannabis sativa	162
Cantharidin	166
Cantharis	163
Capparis	435
Capsella	642
Capsicum	166
Carbamide	661
Carbo animalis	168
Carbo vegetabilis	170
Carbolic. acid.	173
Carboneum	172
Carbon. hydrog.	174
Carbon. oxygenisatum	175
Carbon. sulphuratum	175
Carbon. tetrachol.	169, 646
Carcinosin	179
Carduus benedictus	177
Carduus marianus	176

	PAGE
Carissa schim.	259
Carlsbad	178
Cascara sagrada	178
Cascarilla	179
Cassia acutif.	585
Castanea vesica	179
Castor equi.	180
Castoreum	180
Catalpa	94
Cataria	180
Caulophyllum	181
Causticum	181
Ceanothus Amer.	184
Ceanothus thrysif	184
Cedron	185
Cenchris	185
Centaurea	168
Cepa	27
Cephalanthus	210
Cerefolius	493
Cerium oxalicum	187
Cereus Bonplandii	186
Cereus serpentinus	186
Cetraria	610
Cephalantus	210
Cetonia	114
Chaulmoogra	519
Chamomilla	187
Chaparro	189
Cheiranthus	153, 415
Chelidonin	191
Chelidonium	189
Chelone	192
Chenopodium	191, 675
Chenopod. aphis	192
Chenopod. vulvar.	531
Chimaphila maculata	194
Chimaphila umbel.	193
China off.	207
Chininum arsenicosum	194
Chininum muriaticum	195
Chininum salicylicum	196
Chininum sulphuricum	195
Chiococca	140
Chionanthus	196
Chloralum	197

LIST OF REMEDIES—LATIN NAMES

	PAGE
Chloroform	198
Chlorum	199
Cholas terrapina	248, 557
Cholesterinum	199
Choline	634
Chopcheenee	372
Chromic acid.	200
Chromium sulph.	200
Chrysanthemum	567
Chrysarobinum	201
Cicera arist.	493
Cicuta virosa	201
Cicuta maculata	203
Cimex	203
Cimicifuga	203
Cina	205
Cinchona	207
Cineraria	210
Cinnabaris	210
Cinnamonum	211
Cistus	211
Citric acid.	213
Citrus decumana	213
Citrus limonum	213
Citrus vulgaris	213
Clematis erecta	213
Clematic vitalba	214
Clotho arictans	186
Cobaltum	215
Coca	215
Coeainum	216
Coccinella	217
Cocculus	218
Coccus cacti	220
Cochlearia	221
Codeinum	221
Coffea cruda	222
Coffea tosta	223
Colchicum	224
Colchicin	225
Collinsonia	226
Colocynthis	227
Colostrum	387
Comocladia	229
Conchiolin	153
Condurango	229

	PAGE
Conium	230
Convallaria	232
Convolvulus	121
Copaiva	234
Coqueluchin	500
Corallium	235
Coralorhiza	236
Cornus alternifolia	236
Cornus circinata	236
Cornus florida	236
Corydalis	237
Coto	244
Cotyledon	237
Coumarin	650
Cratægus	237
Crocus sativa	238
Crotalus cascavella	242
Crotalus horridus	240
Croton tiglium	242
Cubeba	243
Cucurbita	244
Cucurbita citrellus	244
Culex	302
Cuphea	244
Cupressus austral	645
Cupressus Lawson	645
Cuprum aceticum	245
Cuprum arsenitum	245
Cuprum cyanatum	248
Cuprum metallicum	246
Cuprum oxyd	248
Cuprum sulphuricum	248
Curare	248
Cuscus	51
Cusparia	52
Cyclamen	249
Cydonia	210
Cymarin	65
Cynanchum	92
Cypripedium	251
Cysticin	249, 385
Cystisus laburnum	385
Cystisus scopar	599
Damiana	659
Daphne Indica	251

LIST OF REMEDIES—LATIN NAMES

	PAGE
Datura arborea	610
Derris pin	205
Diadema	69
Dicentra	237
Dictamnus	589
Digitalis	252
Digitoxinum	254
Dioscorea	255
Diosma	256
Diphtherinum	257
Diphtherotoxin	257
Dipodium	228
Diptrix	650
Dirca palustris	443
Ditain	32
Dolichos	257
Dorema	39
Doryphora	258
Drosera	258
Duboisia	259
Duboisin sulph.	260
Dulcamara	260
Echinacea	263
Eel serum	254
Egg vaccine	491
Elæis	334
Elaps corallinus	264
Elaterium	266
Electricitas	682
Electron	618
Elemuy	191
Emetine	353
Enlexing	629
Eosin	266
Ephedra	413
Epigea	267
Epilobium	435
Epiphegus	267
Equisetum	267
Eranthis hymnalis	11
Erechtites	268
Ergot	578
Ergotin	580
Erigeron	268
Eriodictyon	269

	PAGE
Erodium	303
Eryngium	269
Erythræ chiron	160
Erythrinus	435
Erythroxylon	215
Eschscholtzia	270
Eserine	513
Escoba amargo	498
Ether	19
Eucalyptol	272
Eucalyptus	270
Eucalypt. rostr.	265
Eucalyptus tereticoris	272
Eugenia jambos	272
Eugenia cheken	272
Euonymin	273
Euonymus atrop	273
Euonymus Europa	273
Eupatorium aromat	274
Eupatorium perfol.	274
Eupatorium purpur.	275
Euphorbia amygdal	278
Euphorbia corollata	278
Euphorbia hypericif.	353
Euphorbia lathyris	276
Euphorbia marg	278
Euphorbia pilulifera	278
Euphorbia polycarpa	308
Euphorbia prost.	308
Euphorbia resinifera	277
Euphorbium	277
Euphrasia	279
Eupion	280
Fabiana	281
Fagopyrum	281
Fagus	267
Fel tauri	282
Ferrum aceticum	285
Ferrum arsenicum	285
Ferrum bromatum	285
Ferrum citric	194
Ferrum cyanatum	285
Ferrum iodatum	282
Ferrum magneticum	283
Ferrum metallicum	283

LIST OF REMEDIES—LATIN NAMES

	PAGE
Ferrum muriaticum	285
Ferrum pernitricum	286
Ferrum phosphoricum	286
Ferrum picricum	288
Ferrum protoxal	286
Ferrum pyrophos	288
Ferrum sulphuricum	286
Ferrum tartaricum	286
Ferula glauca	489
Ferula sumbul	626
Ficus Indica	488
Ficus relig.	288
Ficus venosa	444
Filix mas	289
Fluoric acid	289
Fluoroform	259
Formalin	291
Formic acid	292
Formica rufa	292
Fragaria	295
Franciscea	295
Frangula	549
Fraxinus	295
Fucus	296
Fuligo ligni	296
Fushina	166, 296
Gadus morrhua	483
Gaertner	534
Galanthus niv.	297
Galega	296
Galipea	52
Galium	297
Gallic acid	297
Gambogia	298
Garcinia morella	298
Gaultheria	298
Gelatin	353
Gelsemium	299
Genista	378
Gentiana cruciata	302
Gentiana lutea	302
Gentiana quinquef	302
Gettysburg water	303
Geranin	303
Geranium	303

	PAGE
Geum	331
Ginseng	304
Glanderine	329
Glechoma hed.	320
Glonoine	304
Glycerinum	306
Gnaphalium	307
Golondrina	308
Gossypium	308
Granatum	309
Graphites	309
Gratiola	312
Grindelia	313
Guaco	314
Guaiacol	316, 384
Guaiacum	315
Guano	174
Guao	229
Guarana	499
Guarea	366
Guipsine	678
Gummi gutti	298
Gunpowder	375
Gymnenma	308
Gymnocladus	217
Hæmatoxylon	317
Hagenia Abys.	382
Hamamelis	318
Hedeoma	319
Hedera	304
Hedera helix	320
Hedysarum	163
Hekla lava	320
Helianthus	327
Heliotropium	459
Helix tosta	444
Helleborus fœtidus	322
Helleborus niger	321
Helleborus orientalis	322
Helmintochortos	207
Heloderma	322
Helonias	323
Henchera	485
Hepar sulphuris	326
Hepatica	328

LIST OF REMEDIES—LATIN NAMES

	PAGE
Heracleum	328
Hippomanes	328
Hippozæninum	329
Hippuric acid	329
Hoang-nan	330
Hoitzia	114
Homarus	330
Humea elegans	531
Humulus lupulus	408
Hura	331
Hydrangea	331
Hydrargyrum	432
Hydrastinum mur.	333
Hydrastis	332
Hydrast. sulph.	333
Hydrobromic acid	132
Hydrocotyle	334
Hydrocyanic acid	335
Hydrophobinum	335
Hydrophyllum	280
Hydropiper	528
Hyoscyamus	336
Hyoscin hydrobrom	338
Hypericum	338
Iberis	340
Ichthyolum	341, 589
Ichthyotoxin	254
Ictodes	530
Ignatia	342
Ikshugandha	651
Ilex aquif.	344
Ilex cassine	345
Illecebrum	135
Illicium	344
Indigo	346
Indium	346
Indol	346
Ingluvin	187
Insulin	629
Inula	347
Iodoformum	348
Iodothyrine	648
Iodum	349
Ioduretted potass. jod.	351
Ipecacuanha	352

	PAGE
Ipomœa	121
Iridium	854
Iridium chlor.	854
Iris factissima	355
Iris florentina	355
Iris germanica	355
Iris minor	355
Iris tenax	855
Iris versicolor	855
Isotonic plasma	462
Jaborandi	517
Jacaranda caroba	356
Jacaranda gualandai	356
Jacea (Viola tricolor)	675
Jalapa	357
Jambosa	272
Jatropha curcas	357
Jatropha urens	357
Jequiritol	358
Jequirity	358
Jonosia	358
Juglandin	359
Juglans cinerea	358
Juglans regia	359
Juncus effusus	360
Juniperus communis	360
Juniperus Virginianus	360
Justicia	360
Kalagua	657
Kali aceticum	369
Kali arsen.	361
Kali bichromicum	361
Kali bromatum	364
Kali carbonicum	366
Kali chloricum	369
Kali citricum	369
Kali cyanatum	370
Kali ferrocynatum	369
Kali hydroiodicum	370
Kali hypophos	378
Kali muriaticum	373
Kali nitricum	374
Kali oxalicum	369
Kali permanganum	376

LIST OF REMEDIES—LATIN NAMES

	PAGE
Kali phosphoricum	377
Kali picricum	369
Kali picro-nitricum	369
Kali salicylicum	369
Kali silicum	379
Kali sulphuratum	379
Kali sulphuricum	379
Kali sulph. chrom.	380
Kali tartaricum	369
Kali telluricum	369
Kalmia	380
Kaolinum	382
Kava-kava	519
Kino	265
Koch's lymph	657
Kola	609
Kousso	382
Krameria	357
Kreosotum	382
Laburnum	385
Lac caninum	385
Lac defloratum	387
Lac felinum	385
Lac vaccinum	386
Lac vacc. coagulatum	386
Lac. vacc. floc.	386
Lacerta	323
Lachesis	387
Lachesis lanceolat	127
Lachnantes	390
Lactic acid.	391
Lactuca virosa	392
Laffa acutang	159
Laminum	393
Lapathum	559
Lapis albus	393
Lapis renalis	177
Lappa	394
Lapsana com.	274
Lathyrus	394
Latrodectus hasselti	395
Latrodectus kalipo	396
Latrodectus mactans	395
Laurocerasus	396
Lava scoriæ	320

	PAGE
Lecithin	397
Ledum	397
Lemna minor	399
Leonurus	437
Lepidium	399
Leptandra	400
Leptilon	268
Levico	82, 101
Liatris spic.	400
Lignum vitæ	315
Lillium tigrinum	400
Limulus	402
Linaria	403
Linum	403
Lippia Mexicana	354
Lithinum benzoicum	405
Lithium brom.	405
Lithium carbonicum	403
Lithium lacticum	405
Lithium chlor	405
Lobelia acetum	406
Lobelia card.	407
Lobelia cerufla	406
Lobelia erinus	228, 406
Lobelia inflata	405
Lobelia purpurescens	407
Lobelia syphilitica	406
Lolium temulentum	407
Lonicera	408
Lonicera periclymenum	408
Luminal	198
Lupulin	408
Lupulus	408
Lycopersicum	596
Lycopodium	409
Lycopus	413
Lyssin	385
Lysimachia	658
Macrotin	205
Macrotys racemosa	203
Macrozamia	195, 378
Macuna	548
Madura alb.	331
Magnesia carbonica	414
Magnesia muriatica	415

	PAGE
Magnesia phosphorica	417
Magnesia sulphurica	418
Magnet artif.	623
Magnet. p. ambo.	682
Magnet. pol. Arctio.	623, 682
Magnet. pol. Austral.	623, 682
Magnolia	420
Mahonia	119
Malandrinum	421, 667
Malaria officinalis	467
Mallein	329
Manaca (Francisces)	295
Mancinella	421
Mandragora	114
Manganum aceticum	422
Manganum (Colloidal)	423
Manganum mur	423
Manganum ox.	423
Manganum sul.	423
Mangifera	151, 424
Manzanita	333
Mapato	547
Marrubium	334
Marum verum	638
Matico	384
Medicago	384
Medorrhinum	424
Medusa	426
Mel cum sale.	427
Melilotus	427
Melilotus alba	428
Menispermum	428
Mentha piperita	428
Mentha puleg.	429
Mentha virid.	429
Menthol	429
Menyanthes	430
Mephitis	430
Mercurialis perennis	431
Mercurius acetic	435
Mercurius auratus	435
Mercurius biniod	440
Mercurius bromatus	435
Mercurius corrosiv.	436
Mercurius cum kali	435
Mercurius cyanatus	438

	PAGE
Mercurius dulcis	439
Mercurius iod. flav.	440
Mercurius iodatus rub.	440
Mercurius nitrosus	435
Mercurius phosphor.	435
Mercurius præcip. rub.	435
Mercurius protoiod	440
Mercurius sol. Hahn. (Indications same as Mercurius vivus).	
Mercurius sub. corros.	436
Mercurius sulphuricus	441
Mercurius sulph. rub.	210
Mercurius tannicus	435
Mercurius vivus	432
Methylene blue	441
Methylium salicyl.	299
Mezereum	442
Micania guacho	308
Micromeria	443
Mikania	314
Millefolium	444
Millepedes	484
Mimosa	555
Mirbane	117
Mitchella	444
Momordica bals.	445
Momordica charant.	243
Monsonia	437
Morphinum	445
Moschus	447
Muco-toxin	329
Mucuna	257
Mullein oil	671
Murex	448
Muriatic acid	449
Muscarin	22
Mygale	450
Myosotis	451
Myrmexine	292
Myrica	451
Myristica	452
Myroxylon pereirae	103
Myrtus checkan	452
Myrtus communis	452

LIST OF REMEDIES—LATIN NAMES

	PAGE
Nabalus	392
Naja tripudians	453
Naphthaline	454
Narcissus	455
Nasturtium	416
Natrum arsenicum	456
Natrum cacodyl.	458
Natrum carbonicum	456
Natrum chloratum	458
Natrum choleinicum	468
Natrum hyposulph.	468
Natrum iodatum	468
Natrum lacticum	464
Natrum muriaticum	459
Natrum nitricum	463
Natrum nitrosum	464
Natrum phosphoricum	463
Natrum salicylicum	465
Natrum selenicum	462
Natrum silico-fluor.	464
Natrum silicum	462
Natrum succinate	467
Natrum sulpho-carbol.	464
Natrum sulphuricum	466
Natrum sulphurosum	464
Natrum taurochol	191
Natrum telluricum	464
Nectandra amar	506
Negundium	17
Nepeta	585
Nerium odorum	480
Neurin	634
Niccolum met.	468
Niccolum sulph.	469
Nicotinum	631
Nitric acid	469
Nitri spiritus dulcis.	472
Nitro-muriatic acid	472
Nitrum	374
Nuphar luteum	473
Nux mochata	473
Nux vomica	475
Nyctanthes	275, 479
Nymphæa	473
Ocimum canum	479

	PAGE
Œnanthe	479
Oenothera	195, 506, 530
Œstrus cameli	346
Oleander	480
Oleum animale	481
Oleum cajaput	141
Oleum caryophyllum	103
Oleum jecoris	482
Oleum myristica	474
Oleum santali	483
Oleum succinum	38
Oleum wittnebianum	141
Oniscus asellus	484
Ononis spinosa	637
Onosmodium	484
Oophorinum	485
Operculina	485
Opii et ipecac	488
Opium	486
Opuntia	488
Orchitinum	485
Oreodaphne	489
Orexine tann.	557
Origanum	489
Ornithogalum	474, 489
Orobanche	267
Orpiment	86
Osmium	490
Ostrya	491
Ouabain	259
Ova tosta	491
Ovi gall. pellicula	491
Oxalic acid	491
Oxalis	583
Oxydendron	493
Oxytropis	493
Ozonum	589
Pæonia	494
Pakur	444
Palladium	495
Pambotano	196
Panacea arv.	344
Panax	304
Pancreatinum	356
Papaver somnif.	486

	PAGE
Paraffine	496
Pareira brava	497
Parietaria	497
Paris quadrifolia	497
Parthenium	498
Passiflora	499
Pastinaca	498
Paullinia	499
Paghala malli	479
Pecten	68
Pedicularis	580
Pediculus	534
Pelius	676
Pelletierine	309
Penthorum	500
Pepsinum	356
Periploca graeca	92
Petiveria	395
Petroleum	500
Petroselinum	503
Pertussin	179, 500
Peumus boldus	468
Phaseolus	503
Phellandrium	504
Phenazone	60
Phenol	173
Phleum	558
Phloridzin	661
Phosphoric acid	504
Phosphorus	507
Phosphorus hydrogen	511
Phosphor. pentachl.	510
Physalis	511
Physostigma	512
Phytolacca	514
Phytolacca berry	516
Pichi	281
Picric acid	516
Picrotoxin	219
Pilocarp. mur.	518
Pilocarpus	517
Pimenta	539
Pimpinella	262
Pinus canadensis	1
Pinus Lambertina	519
Pinus sylvestris	519

	PAGE
Piper augustifolia	384
Piperizine	513
Piper methysticum	519
Piper nigrum	520
Piscidia	680
Pituitrin	520
Pix liquida	521
Planifolia	666
Plantago	521
Plantanus	522
Platina metallicum	522
Platina muriaticum	523
Platina mur. nat.	523
Plectranthus	526
Plumbago	309, 412
Plumbum aceticum	526
Plumbum chromicum	526
Plumbum iodatum	526
Plumbum metallicum	524
Plumbum phosph.	526
Plumeria cell.	308
Pneumo coccin	511
Pneumo toxin	511
Pneumus Boldo	468
Podophyllum	526
Pollatin	562
Polygonum aviculære	528
Polygonum persicaria	528
Polygonum punctatum	528
Polygonum sagit.	528
Polymnia	184
Polyporus off.	124
Polyporus pin.	528
Polytrichum junip	331, 654
Populus candicans	529
Populus tremuloides	529
Potass xantate	176
Pothos fœtidus	530
Prenanthes serp.	392
Primula farinosa	530
Primula obconia	531
Primula veris	530
Propylamin	531
Protargol	75
Prunella	527
Prunus padus	532

LIST OF REMEDIES—LATIN NAMES

	PAGE
Prunus spinosa	532
Prunus Virginiana	532
Psoralea	278
Psorinum	533
Ptelea	535
Pulex irritans	535
Pulmo vulpis	465
Pulsatilla Nuttaliana	539
Pulsatilla nigricans	436
Pyrara	623
Pyrogenium	540
Pyrus	465, 532
Quassia	541
Quebracho	94
Quercus gland. spiritus.	542
Quillaya	542
Quinidin	209
Rademacher's liquor	686
Radium	542
Rana bufo	135
Ranunculus acris	545
Rananculus bulbosus	545
Ranunculus flammula	546
Ranunculus glacialis	546
Ranunculus repens	546
Ranunculus sceleratus	546
Raphanus	547
Ratanhia	547
Resorcin	557
Rhamnus Calif.	548
Rhamnus cath.	549
Rhamnus pursh.	178
Rheum	549
Rhodallin	641
Rhodium	550
Rhododendron	550
Rhus aromatica	551
Rhus diversiloba	555
Rhus glabra	552
Rhus radicans	555
Rhus toxicodendron	552
Rhus venenata	556
Ricinus communis	556
Robinia	557

	PAGE
Rosa damascena	558
Rosmarinus	564
Rubia tinctor	567
Rubus vill.	189
Rudbeckia	263
Rumex aceto	559
Rumex crispus	558
Rumex obtus	559
Ruta graveolens	559
Sabadilla	560
Sabal serrulata	562
Sabina	563
Saccharin	565
Saccharum lactis	565
Saccharomyces	650
Saccharum officinalis	564
Salaginella	308
Salamandra	136
Salicylicum acidum	565
Salix nigra	566
Sal marinum	462
Salol	566
Salufer	464
Salvia officinalis	567
Salvia sclerata	567
Sambucus Canadensis	568
Sambucus nigra	568
Sanguinaria	569
Sanguinaria nitrica	571
Sanguinaria tartar	571
Sanguisorba off.	114, 564
Sanguinsuga	564, 653
Sanicula	510
Sanicula aqua	571
Santalum	234
Santoninum	572
Saponaria	573
Saponin	574
Saraca Indica	539
Sarco lactic acid	574
Sarracenia	575
Sarsaparilla	575
Saururus	576
Saw palmetto	562
Scirrhinum	232

LIST OF REMEDIES—LATIN NAMES

	PAGE
Scolopendra	493
Scoparium	599
Scopola	338
Scopolam. hydrobrom.	338
Scorpio	672
Scrophularia	577
Scutellaria	577
Secale cornutum	578
Sedum acre	581
Sedum alpestra	581
Sedum repens	581
Sedum telephicum	581
Selaginella	308
Selenicereus	137
Selenium	581
Sempervivum tector	582
Senecio	583
Senecio jacobœa	584
Senega	584
Senna	585
Sepia	586
Sepsin	541
Serpentaria per. (Aristolochia)	76
Serum anguillæ	589
Serratula	400
Silica marina	594
Silicea	590
Silica fluor. calcar.	393
Sil. sul. calc. alum.	548
Silphion cyrenaicum	594
Silphium	594
Simaba	214
Simaruba ferr.	185
Sinapis alba	595
Sinapis nigra	595
Sisyrinchium	308
Skatol	595
Skookum-chuck	596
Slag	548
Soda cacodyl.	151
Soda taurocholate	199
Sodii bicarbonas	458
Sodium chloroaurate	99
Solanum aceticum	598
Solanum Carolinese	598

	PAGE
Solanum lycopersicum	596
Solanum mammosum	598
Solanum nigrum	597
Solanum oleraceum	598
Solanum pseudocaps	598
Solanum tuberosum	598
Solanum tuber. ægro.	598
Solanum vesicarum	511, 598
Solidago	598
Spartein sulph.	599
Spartium scoparium	599
Sphingurus	645
Spigelia	600
Spigel. mar.	602
Spiræa	602
Spiranthes	602
Spirit aetheris comp.	198
Spirit. gland. quercus.	542
Spiritus glycer. nit.	304
Spongia tosta	603
Squilla	69.
Stannum iodatum	606
Stannum metallicum	605
Staphylocin	541
Staphysagria	607
Stellaria	609
Sterculia	609
Sticta pulmonaria	610
Stigmata maydis	611
Stillingia	611
Stovain	217
Stramonium	612
Streptoccocin	541
Strontia brom.	614
Strontia carb.	613
Strontia iodatum	614
Strontia nit.	614
Strophanthus	615
Strychninum	616
Strychnin. ars.	617
Strych. et. fer. cit.	617
Strychnin. nit.	617
Strychnin. phos.	618
Strychnin. sulph.	617
Strychnin. valerian	617
Strychnos gaulth	330

LIST OF REMEDIES—LATIN NAMES

	PAGE
Strychnos tiente	659
Succinic acid	618
Succinum	618
Sucrose	564
Sulfonal	619
Sulphur	620
Sulphur hydrogen	623
Sulphur iodatum	623
Sulphur terebinthin	622
Sulphuric acid	624
Sulphurous acid	625
Sumbul	626
Supra-renal extract	13
Symphoricarpus	626
Symphytum	627
Syphilinum	627
Syzygium	629
Tabacum	629
Tamus	22
Tanacetum	631
Tannic acid	623, 632
Taraxacum	633
Tarentula Cubensis	632
Tarentula Hispania	633
Tartar emetic	58
Tartaric acid	634
Taxus baccata	635
Tela aranea	69
Tellurium	635
Terebene	637
Terebinthina	636
Terpin hydrate	455
Testa præparata	148, 491
Tetradymite	636
Teucrium marum	638
Teucrium scorodonia	638
Thallium	639
Thaspium	639
Thea	640
Thebainum	513
Theridion	640
Thiosinaminum	291, 641
Thlaspi bursa	642
Thuja	643

	PAGE
Thymol	646
Thymus	647
Thymus gland	648
Thyroidine	647
Tilia Europœa	649
Tinctura acris	181
Tinospora	184
Titanium	649
T. N. T.	117, 653
Tongo	650
Torula	650
Toxicophis	128
Trachinus	128
Tradescantia	654
Triatema	396
Tribulus	651
Trifolium pratense	651
Trifolium repens	652
Trillium cernum	652
Trillium pendulum	652
Trimethylamin	531
Trinitrophenol	516
Trinitrotoluene	117, 653
Trional	619
Triosteum perfol	653
Triticum	654
Trombidium	655
Tropæolum	118
Trotyl. (T. N. T.)	117
Trychnos gaultheriana	334
Trychosanthes	669
Tuberculinum	655
Turnera	659
Turpenthum minerale	441
Tussilago farfara	659
Tussilago fragrans	659
Tussilago petasites	659
Typha latif.	244, 353
Ucuba (Brazilian)	452
Ulmus	675
Upas antiaris	660
Upas tiente	659
Uranium nitricum	660
Urea	661
Uric. acid	661

Urinum	661
Urotropin	292
Urtica	661
Usnea	662
Ustilago	662
Uva ursi	663
Vaccinium myrtyllus	664
Vaccinum	664
Valeriana	664
Vanadium	665
Vanilla	666
Variolinum	666
Veratrina	669
Veratrinum	669
Veratrum album	667
Veratrum viride	669
Verbascum	671
Verbena	672
Veronal	198
Vesicaria	166
Vespa crabro	672
Viburnum opulus	673
Viburnum prunifol	673
Vinca minor	674
Vincetoxinum	92
Viola odorata	674
Viola tricolor	675
Vipera	676
Viscum album	677
Vitex trif.	78
Vitrum	594
Woorari	243
Wyethia	678

Xanthium	336
Xanthorrhœa	121
Xanthorrhiza	121
Xanthoxylum	679
Xerophyllum	680
Xiphosura	402
X-Ray	681
Yerba buena	443
Yerba mansa	52
Yerba santa	269
Yatren	351
Yohimbinum	682
Yucca filamentosa	683
Zea	611
Zea Italica	663
Zincum	683
Zincum aceticum	686
Zincum ars.	686
Zincum bromatum	686
Zincum arsen	686
Zincum carb.	686
Zincum cyanatum	686
Zincum metallicum	683
Zincum muriaticum	686
Zincum oxydatum	686
Zincum phosphoricum	686
Zincum picricum	687
Zincum sulphuricum	686
Zincum valerian	687
Zingiber	687
Zizia aurea (Thaspium)	639

50 Homoeopathic Indian Drugs

ABROMA AUGUSTA
(Olat Kambal)

Olat Kambal, Devil's Cotton, Olak Tambol.

First Prover : Dr. D.N. Ray.
N.O. : Sterculiaceae.
(N.O. : Natural Order).

Clinical : Albuminuria ; sleeplessness ; amenorrhoea ; carbuncle ; diabetes mellitus and insipidus ; debility ; dysmenorrhoea ; weakness of brain.

Mind : Irritable ; excitable mood ; illhumour ; forgetfulness ; absent minded ; depression ; morose ; anxious ; unable to moody.

Head : Empty feeling ; rolling of the head and vertigo ; heaviness and discomfort, much giddiness.

Eyes : Weakness of vision ; puffiness of the lids ; heaviness ; eyes easily tired; inclination to drop eyes closed; pain and watering of the eyes; conjunctiva becomes pale.

Ears : Shortness of hearing ; buzzing in the ears ; discharge from the ears.

Nose : Sneezing several times ; watering ; dryness of the nose with desire to rub.

Face : Pale, yellow, wrinkled, old looking ; itching eruption on the face with burning sensation ; furuncles of the face.

Throat : Dry; burning sensation; painful; difficulty in swallowing solids but drinking relieves throat symptom temporarily.

Mouth : Almost constant dryness of the mouth ; drinks large quantities of cold water at a time yet dryness persists ; dry and clean tongue ; indistinct speech ; lips dry and bluish.

Appetite : Unnatural appetite, can eat short after a good meal.

Stomach : Hungry feeling with faint feeling; desire for all kinds of food; a feeling of emptiness in the stomach.

ABROMA AUGUSTA

Abdomen : Flatulence with distension of abdoman.

Stool : Constipation brownish, black, knotty, hard ; lumpy stool with much straining.

Urinary Symptoms : Profuse urination day and night, frequent urination; dryness of the mouth and great thirst; desire to drink after urination which relieves thirst ; urination to lead exhaustion; fishy odour of the urine; slight sediment; diabetes mellitus ; nocturnal enuresis; burning in urethra; white ulcers in the mouth of prepuce caused by excessive passage of sugar in the urine ; inability to retain urine.

Heart : Weakness of the heart ; palpitation worse on movement; faint-feeling.

Respiratory Symptoms : Cough with purulent expectoration; pain in the chest ; lumpy sputum white or yellowish in colour, worse in cold air, agg. in the evening and night ; during coughing patient presses the chest.

Skin : Dry skin, scratching ; burning ; small boils in summer, carbuncles, etc.

Neck, Back, Limbs : Dull pain in the back extremities ; emaciation and weakness of the limbs ; pain in the kidney region.

Male Sexual Symptoms : Absence of sexual desire, inability to coition, becomes exhausted after coition ; swelling and hanging of the testis.

Female Sexual Symptoms : Irregular catamenia ; blood is dark, clotted, profuse or scanty and pale amenorrhoea or dysmenorrhoea ; leucorrhoea profuse, white, thin, watery; chlororis ; colicky pain in the lower abdomen 2-3 days before menses ; hysteria associated with menstrual disorders.

Sleep : Drowsiness ; insomnia, prostration and aversion to do any labour ; unrefreshed sleep, sleeps better in the early part of the morning.

Fever : Dry heat over the whole body ; great thirst.

Potency of Choice : Mother-tincture, 2x, 3x.

ABROMA RADIX
(Olat Kambal Root)

Olat Kambal Mul., Devil's Cotton.

First Prover : Dr. D.N. Ray.
N.O. : Sterculiaceae.

Clinical : Female disorders.

Mind : Mental and other symptoms also tally with the symptoms of Abroma-augusta.

Female Sexual Symptoms : Irregular menstrual disorder; dysmenorrhoea; menstrual flow may be copious or scanty; leucorrhoea.

Potency of Choice : Mother-tincture, 2x, 3x.

ACALYPHA INDICA
(Muktajhuri or Muktabarshi)

Aritta Manjarie, Khokali, Indian Acalypha, Kup paimeni, Harita Manjiri, Vahchni Kanto, Indra Maris.

First Prover : Dr. M.L. Sircar.
N.O. : Euphorbiaceae.

Clinical : Cough; diarrhoea; flatulence; haemoptysis.

Respiratory Symptoms : Violent, dry cough followed by bloody expectoration; pure blood comes in the morning and dark lumps of clotted blood in the evening; cough becomes violent at night; constant and severe pain is felt in the chest.

Abdominal Symptoms : Burning is felt in the intestine and stomach; spluttering diarrhoea with forcible expulsion of noisy flatus; gripping pain in the abdomen, tenesmus; rectal haemorrhage, worse in the evening.

Skin : Jaundice; circumscribed furuncle-like swelling; itching etc.

Potency of Choice : Mother-tincture, 3x, 6x, are generally used.

ACHYRANTHES ASPERA
(Apamarga)

Apang, Latjira, Aghada, Kutri, Na-yurivt, Apa-kharevazhun.

First Prover : Dr. S.K. Ghosh.
N.O. : Amaranthaceae.

Clinical : Astringent ; diarrhoea ; diuretic ; dysentery ; menorrhagia ; bad effects of dog and snake bites.

Abdominal Symptoms : Acute diarrhoea and cholera ; watery stool ; yellowish and mixed with flakes of mucus profuse in quantity ; excessive thirst ; pain in the stomach ; nausea and vomiting.

Skin : Boils, carbuncles ; foul swelling, poisonous ulcers etc. ; red spot in the skin, burning pain all over the body.

Pulse : Thready pulse.

Potency of Choice : Mother-tincture, 3x, 3, 6.

AEGLE-MARMELOS AND AEGLE-FOLIA
(Bel Fruit)

Sriphala, Bilwa, Bengal-quince, Bilinu-phal, Vilwa-pazhan, Bilwa-pandu.

First Prover : Dr. P.P. Biswas.
N.O. : Rutaceae.

Clinical : Bleeding piles ; diarrhoea ; dysentery ; fever with dropsy ; impotency.

Mind : Commits mistakes in spelling.

Head : Headache appears 4-8 p.m. ; heat in the vertex appears in the evening which is better by eating.

Face : Flushes of heat from face and eye and ear too, which disappears after eating.

Respiratory Symptoms : Catarrh ; bronchitis ; pneumonia ; cough.

Dropsy : Dropsy of any part of the body ; upper part of the eyelid swollen ; dropsical swelling due to heart diseases. Excellent medicine in beri-beri.

Pulse : Full, strong and irregular, which is a characteristic.

G-I Symptoms : Indigestion ; abdominal colic ; piles ; constipation. There is no desire for food ; anorexia; waterbrash from the mouth ; disorder of stomach ; flatulence ; wind comes out with loud noise, worse in the afternoon ; amoetic and bacillary dysentery.

Urinary Symptoms : Urine decreases considerably ; patient feels slight pain in the back and lumbar region, which is worse in the afternoon.

Male Sexual Symptom : Sexual impotency.

Skin : Itching ; ringworm.

Fever : Used in influenza when the fever is continued type; chronic fever associated with hepatic and splenic disorders.

Potency of Choice : Mother-tincture, 3x, 6, 30, 200.

ANDERSONIA OR AMOORA ROHITAKA
(Rohitaka)

Royna, Rohera, Rohido, Harinhara, Pitaraj.

First Prover : Dr. P.P. Biswas.
N.O. : Mediaceae.

Clinical : Chronic fever ; general debility ; enlarged glands ; liver and spleen disorders; leucorrhoea.

Mind : Memory becomes dull and disordered; mistakes in spelling, place, etc. ; can't fix mind in any subject ; easily angered.

Head : Heat in the vertex ; giddiness ; pain in the temples associated with heat which is relieved by cold air and cold application.

Face : Flushes of heat in the face ; burning sensation in the face including eyes.

Mouth : Insipid taste in the mouth ; bad and bitter taste in the morning.

Abdomen : Burning sensation in the stomach ; enlargement of the liver and spleen ; nausea and vomiting.

Fever : Feverish with headache ; aching pains ; burning of hands and feet.

Pulse : Full and slightly rapid.

Potency of Choice : 3x, 6x, 30 etc.

ANDROGRAPHIS PANICULATA
(Kalmegh)

Mahateekta, Kiryat, Kirata, The Great Bhunimba.

First Prover : Dr. P.P. Biswas.
N.O. : Acanthaceae.

Kalpanath, Kiryato, Olen-
kirayet, Nalavemu, Nilavambu,
Nilavoepu, The Great King of
Bitters etc.

Clinical : First stage of cold and cough ; convalescence after prolonged fever ; general debility ; infantile liver ; jaundice.

Mind : Despondency ; no desire to do any work or talk ; restless ; easily angered.

Head : Giddiness ; heaviness and throbbing pain in the occiput.

Eyes : Redness of the eyes, yellowish tinge in the eyes.

Nose : Watery discharge from the nose with occasional sneezing.

Mouth : Bitter taste in the mouth with dryness and burning in throat and white coating of the tongue.

Abdomen : Burning in chest ; heaviness of abdomen without any hungry feeling ; enlarged liver ; infantile jaundice.

Stool : Alternate diarrhoea and constipation ; frequent urging for stool without evacuation ; black, hard stool ; yellowish loose stool.

Urine : High-coloured urine ; thick and yellow in colour.

Fever : Fever with chilliness and heat all over the body ; there is headache with thirst ; burning all-over the body relieved by cold air water ; fever comes at 11 A.M. again at 7-8 P.M. ; intermittent or remittent fever ; disinclined to move during fever.

Potency of Choice : Mother-tincture, 3x, 6x, 30.

ATISTA INDICA OR GLYCOSMIS PENTAPHYLLA
(Ash-sheora)

Bannimbu, Vanamenibuka, Keimira.

First Pover : Dr. Kati Kumar Bhattacharyya.
N.O. : Rutaceae.

Clinical : Bilary colic ; diarrhoea ; flatulence.
Mind : Weak memory ; indifferent mood ; vigourless.

Head : Vertigo in the morning ; gnawing pain in one temple at a time.

Eye : Photophobia ; on opening the eyes light trembles before him for a few seconds, oblige him to shut his eyes ; trembling of light before eyes, after sleep.

Ear : Unusually increased hearing, humming sound in the ear.

Nose : Nose-bleed ; dry coryza.

Teeth : Bleeding gums ; dull pain at the root of the teeth.

Dryness : Unquenchable thirst during hot stage.

Tongue : Constant spitting in the morning with occasional belching of salty water ; sour water-brush.

Throat : Inflammation of the tonsils persist few weeks after fever.

Stomach : Canine hunger ; aversion to liquid foods and strong desire for lime-juice ; throbbing at the pit of the stomach, heaviness in the stomach ; flatulence temporarily relieved by eructations ; indigestion due to worms ; frequent eructation after a meal; heartburnt 3-4 hours after food.

Abdomen : Colicky pain round the naval makes the patient senseless ; tenesmus and drawing pain in the renal region.

Heart and Pulse : Palpitation during fever ; pulse full, hard, quick during fever but very weak and slow after remission of fever.

Stool : Constipation and watery diarrhoea during the whole period of fever : pale earthly stool ; bloody mucous stool with or without force.

Male Sexual Symptoms : No sexual desire ; erection at night without any cause ; peculiar electric-like throbbing in urethra for few seconds.

Limbs : Weakness and heaviness in the limbs ; legs 'go to sleep'; cramping while getting straight.

Fever : Chill without thirst, heat with intense thirst, fever comes at 5–10 A.M. and subsides at 3–4 A.M., every alternate day appearance of fever.

Potency of Choice : Mother-tincture, 2x, 3x, 6 etc.

ATISTA RADIX
(Root of Ash-sheora)

Bannimbu, Vanamenibuka.   N.O. :   Rutaceae.

Clinical : Dysentery ; worm-complaints.

Stool Symptoms : It is more powerful than Atista-indica used in dysentery both amoebic and bacillary ; patient passes only blood along with intense naval pain ; dysentery appearing in autumn ; also used for worm complaints ; flatulence and biliary colic.

Potency of Choice : Mother-tincture, 3x, 12, 30.

AZADIRACHTA INDICA OR MELIA AZADIRACHTA
(Nim)

Nimba, Margosa tree, Vembaka, Bal-nimb, Vembu, Vepa, The Neem, Nim.

First Prover : Dr. P.C. Mazumder.

N.O. : Meliaceae.

Clinical : Oezena ; pemphigus ; scabies.

Mind : Depressed ; forgetful, mistakes in writing and spelling ; forgets the names of very familiar persons, or what has been done previous day.

Head : Giddiness ; esp. at 10 A.M., worse when rising from sitting posture; throbbing headache; esp., right sided; worse in the open air, agg. by stooping ; scalp is painful and sensitive to touch, even hair is painful.

Eyes : Eyes are red, congested, burning, dull and heavy; pressive pain in right eye-ball.

Ears : Buzzing in the ears like tickling with a feather, worse on opening the mouth.

Nose : Watery discharge from the nose.

Mouth : Putrid taste in the mouth ; no thirst but mouth is clammy and bitter ; tongue is painful ; burning, felt as scalded ; papillae seems enlarged and prominent ; saliva tastes salty ; difficulty in deglutition, esp. water and meat ; very much thirsty, sp. at long intervals or sometimes thirstless.

Throat: Left sided sore throat.

Abdomen: Great uneasiness in abdomen with flatulence passing offensive flatus ; twisting pain in the epigastrium ; clutching pain in the umbilical region obliging to bend forward ; heart-burn and water-brush.

Stool: Insufficient stool ; small, hard and knotty when constipated but natural stools are copious, soft and semi-solid ; burning in bowels.

Genital System (Male): Great excitement of sexual organ in male ; urine scanty ; high coloured urine, scalding, strong odour.

Respiratory Organs: Very troublesome cough after bathing at 1 P.M. ; sputa is white, thick and in small lumps, expelled with much difficulty

Extremities: Numbness of the limbs ; burning of the soles and hands; rheumatic pains in the lower extremities.

Sleep and Dreams: Sleeplessness and tossing in bed ; dreams of quarrels, beating etc. in the latter part of the night.

Skin: Itching without eruption.

Fever: Fever with chill or without chill from 4-30 P.M. and abates from 7-30 P.M. ; gnawing heat with burning of various parts of the body, copious sweat, esp. on forehead, neck, upper part of the body ; no sweat in the lower parts of the body.

Potency of Choice: 6, 30, 200.

BLATTA ORIENTALIS
(Arsula or Telapoka)

Indian cockroach.   First Prover : Pt. Iswar Chandra
N.O. : Vidyasagar Orthoptera.

Clinical: Asthma ; bronchitis ; cough ; dyspnoea etc.

Respiratory System: It is an excellent remedy for asthma ; in acute cases it acts better in low potencies but in chronic cases it needs higher potencies ; patient gets aggravated in rainy weather ; asthma associated with bronchitis, cough, dyspnoea, phthis, pus-like mucous and threatened suffocation.

Potency of Choice: Mother-tincture, 3x, 6x.

BLUMEA ODORATA
(Kuksima)

Kukundar, Kukurmota. N.O : Compositae.

Clinical : Cough; fever; haemorrhage; hoarseness.

Haemorrhage : It has got reputation in bleeding piles; in diarrhoea or dysentery associated with blood; excellent results in miscarriage where haemorrhage is profuse; in bloody leucorrhoea and menorrhagia it exerts powerful influence to arrest bleeding.

Fever : In tertian fever.

Cough : It is a very good medicine to control cough-hoarseness due to cough ; trumpet-like sound or barking-like sound associated with cough.

Potency of Choice : Mother tincture, 2x, 3x.

BOERHAAVIA DIFFUSA
(Punarnava)

Sothaghuni, Sant, Ghetuli, Itsit, Mukukrattai.

First Prover : S.C. Ghosh.
N.O : Nyctagineae

Clinical : Asthma; beri-beri; high blood pressure; dropsy; jaundice; gonorrhoea; heart troubles; bites of venomous animals etc.

Head : Terrible; bursting; right sided headache better by cold application ; giddiness.

Cough : Coryza with dry cough and thick white expectoration.

Heart : Frequent palpitation and intermittent throbbing pain in cardiac region.

Liver : Slight pain in the hepatic region was felt on touch or pressure and better by hard pressure ; cirrhosis of liver.

Swelling : Swelling of eyelids; hands; abdomen; legs and feet.

Urinary Organs : Scanty, high coloured urine; strangury.

Pain : Rheumatic pains all over the body.

Potency of Choice : Mother tincture.

BRAHMI

Clinical : Impaired memory; whooping cough. It is mostly used as a tonic for absent-mindedness and short of memory. It is also used for whooping cough.

Potency of Choice : Mother-tincture.

CAESALPINIA BONDUCELLA
(Nata)

Kuberakshi, Nata-karanja, Sugar-ghota, Fevernut, Physicnut, Bonducnut, Devil's testicle, Kazhar-shikkay.

First Prover : K.K. Bhattacharjee.
N.O. : Leguminosae.

Clinical : Fever, headache etc.

Mind : Metal depression; lack of enthusiasm.

Head : Terrible headache; better by wrapping, by pressure.

Eyes : Terrible pain as if burn before and during invasion of fever, relieved by cold applications.

Tongue : Slight white coating on the tongue ; bloodless white moist tongue ; thirst for cold water.

Abdomen and Stomach : Gurgling in lower abdomen; enlargement of liver and spleen, which is painful to touch; desire for boiled rice, meat or other hard substance ; aversion to liquid food.

Stool : Hard, saffron-coloured or liquid and yellow coloured stool.

Fever : Regular; fever with chill and shivering on one day and on the other day it appears with slight chill; fever comes at 8-10 A.M. or 2-4 P.M. In intermittent fever there is no thirst when fever comes at after noon; again in morning fever there is thirst in hot stage. Flushed face ; hot breath ; hurried respiration. After the remission of fever patient feels extremely weak, disinclined to do any work even to talk; with closed eyes, likes to sleep.

Skin : Dry, dirty, small eruption like mosquito bites.

Back : Drawing pain in back after cold bath.

Potency of Choice : Mother-tincture, 2x, 3x.

CALOTROPIS GIGANTEA
(Akanda)

Arka, Mandara, Gigantic Swallow-woop. First Prover: E.B. Evatts.
Ekke, Jellude, Badabadam,   N.O. : Asclepiadeae.
Mudar.

Clinical : Asthma; ascites; cough; catarrh; chronic rheumatism; diarrhoea; dysentery; elephantisis; pneumonic tuberclosis; poisonous snake-bite; leprosy; intestinal worms; skin-disease; syphilis.

Mind : Depressed; tired-feeling; restless.

Head : Dizziness; dull occipital headache from 11 A.M. ; head hot; throbbing painful, confusion; faint and giddiness with inclination to vomit.

Face : Face hot, cheeks burns like fire; lips and throat dry.

Mouth : Foul breath; pains on moving jaws; soreness of mouth.

Stomach : Constant eructations.

Urinary Organs : Frequent urination ; urine dark red ; strong smell.

Respiratory Organs : Oppression of chest, short breath.

Pulse : Quick.

Upper Limbs : Cramping pain in the centre of right palm when grasping anything, lasting for many days. Pain in the wrist joint, agg. on movement.

Lower Limbs : Slight pain inside the right thigh just below the groin, sore, swollen, painful on every step; intermittent cramping pain in left foot, compels to move always in bed; pain agg. at rest, so severe as to bring pain to eyes, pain relieved after taking coffee.

Fever : Frequent chill passing up through the spine; head hot, body cold; cheeks burn like fire, chill returned towards bedtime even when close to fire; fits of perspiration alternate with chills.

Potency of Choice : Mother-tincture, 2x, 3x, 6.

CALOTROPIS LACTUM
(Glue of Calotropis)

Akanda, Madar, Gigantic
Swallow-woop, Arka.   N.O. : Asclepiadeae.

It is prepared from milk juice or glue of Calotropis gigantea and usually the cases which are not benefited by the employment of Calotropis gigantea yields to the therapeutic properties of Calotropis lactum. Purging; vomiting; toothache; enlargement of spleen; diseases of the eye and skin are successfully treated by this drug.

Potency of Choice : 3x, 6x.

CARICA PAPAYA
(Penpay)

Popaiya, Papend, Aranda, Kharguza, Popayi, Boppaiya, Papaya, Kappalam, Pappayam, Paputn, Melonenbum.

First Prover: D.N. Ray.
N.O. : Passifloreae.

- **Clinical** : Abortion; dyspepsia; conjunctivitis; enlarged liver; spleen; uterine disorders.
- **Gastro - Intestinal Symptoms** : Enlarged liver and spleen with fever. In dyspepsia; weak digestion, undigested stool in small quantities for many times a day; white coated tongue; intolerance of milk. It promotes digestion, esp. of those whose stomach can't tolerate meat or milk.
- **Eye** : Yellow discolouration of conjunctiva.
- **Female Sexual System** : It aids menstrual discharge; helps uterine contraction and induces abortion when locally applied to the mouth of the uterus.

Potency of Choice : Mother-tincture, 1x, 3x (trit.).

CEPHALANDRA INDICA
(Telakucha)

Bimba, Kanduri, Ki-bill, Korai, Kabare-hindi.

First Prover : S.C. Ghosh.
N.O. : Cucurbitaeae.

- **Clinical** : Diabetes mellitus and insipidus; skin affections; jaundice; dropsy etc.
- **Mind** : Morose, fretful; disinclined to do any work, gloomy ; memory partially gone; oversensitiveness (mentally and physically).
- **Head** : Giddiness worse after urination ; weakness.
- **Eyes** : Burning of eyes.

Face : Burning of face.

Mouth : Dryness of mouth with great thirst for large quantity of water at a time.

Throat : Dryness of throat.

Appetite : Loss of appetite.

Abodmen : Flatulency.

Urine : Profuse urination; weakness and exhaustion after urination; sugar in the urine; diabetes mellitus.

Stool : Greenish mucous; tinged with blood and pain before and during stool.

Burning : All over the body.

Pulse : Weak and intermittent.

Potency of Choice : Mother tincture, 1x, 3x.

CLERODENDRON INFORTUNATUM
(Bhat)

Bhanta, Ghantakarna, Bhandira, Kari.   N.O. : Leguminosae.

Clinical : Gastric trouble.

Gastro-Intestinal Symptoms : Diarrboea associated with nausea; colic due to worm affections; stools are liquid, deep yellow, frothy ; nausea is a prominent symptom, associated with watering in mouth-ptyalism.

Fever : Fever with enlargement of liver and spleen fever comes in the afternoon; burning sensation is felt in the eyes and face.

Potency of Choice : Mother tincture, 3x, 6, 30.

COLEUS AROMATICUS
(Pashanbhed'

Himsagar, Patharkuchi, Pather-chue.

Clinical : Gonorrhoea; urinary trouble.

Genito Urinary System : Strangury, suppression of urine; gonorrhoea, with burning sensation during and after urination; cystitis, vesical catarrh.

Potency of Choice : Mother-tincture, 2x.

CYNODON DACTYLON
(Durba)

Hurialea-grass, granthi,
Doorve, Garike, Arugu, Talla.   N.O. : Graminae.

Clinical : Haemorrhage; dysentery; dropsy; leucorrhoea.

Haemorrhage : Either haematemesis ; epistaxis ; haemoptysis ; bleeding due to cut or wounds, bleeding piles; cynodon is effacious.

Urinary and G.U. System : Retention or suppression of urine ; vesical calculus ; secondary syphilis.

Eye : Catarrhal ophthalmia.

Stomach and Abdomen Symptoms : Chronic diarrhoea; anasarca ; bilious vomiting.

Potency of Choice : Mother tincture, 3x.

DESMODIUM GANGETICUM
(Shalpani)

Sarivan, Shalaparni, Gitanaram. First Prover : Dr. A.C. Bhaduri.
N.O. : Leguminosae.

Clinical : Fever; headache; meningitis, etc.

Head : Cerebro-spinal meningitis; headache associated with a sensation as if all sides of the head are bound with a tape.

Pain : Neuralgia pain all over the body, could not sit straight on account of spinal pain; burning sensation in hands and feet and flushes of heat from the face.

Sensorium : Sleeplessness, comatose sleep.

Fever : Intermittent or remittent fever with sleeplessness and drowsiness ; fever comes at 7 A.M. with slight chill, lasting for 2-3 hours ; burning sensation and hot flushes from the face ; remission of fever with perspiration.

Potency of Choice : Mother tincture, 3x, 6x, 30.

EMBELIA RIBES
(Biranga)

Baberang, Vidanga,   First Prover: Babu Sris Chandra Ghosh.
Baburung, Karkannic,   N.O. : Myrsineae.
Vaynvilamgan.

Clinical: Children's remedy; worm killer; besides this diarrhoea; pyspepsia and flatulence owing to worms.

Mind: Morose; irritable, fretful; ill-humoured; restless.

Nose: Itching sensation, priks his nose.

Mouth: Dry tongue; grinding of the teeth.

Stomach: Flatulency, diarrhoea, dyspepsia, terrible nausea; great hungry soon after a meal.

Rectum: Itching in rectum; undigested stool with worms.

Urine: Pungent, blood-coloured.

Sleep: Shriek out during sleep, distrubed sleep.

Fever: Fever comes in the morning, ranging 101-103° F.
  Note: Also called as 'Krimigna' which literally means killer of worms.

Potency of Choice: Mother-tincture, 3x, 6, 30.

FICUS RELIGIOSA
(Ashwattha)

Pippala, Pipal, Sacred-Fig,   First Prover: Dr. S.C. Ghosh.
Arshemaram, Aveyal, Jeri.   N.O.: Moraceae.

Clinical: Haemorrhage-arrester; bleeding piles; epistaxis; dysentary mixed with blood; haemoptysis; haematemesis; haematuria; menorrhagia; metrorrhagia etc.

Mind: Unwilling to move, sad, melancholic; very much sensitive to noise.

Head: Nausea; vertigo; burning in vertex; vertigo with slight headache.

Mouth: White tongue with profuse saliva.

Nose: Epistaxis.

Stomach: Vomiting of bright red blood; great repugnance to all foods; sick-feeling in the stomach.

Respiration: Difficulty in breathing; cough; haemoptysis.

Stool: Blood dysentery.

Urinary Organs: Frequent micturition; blood in the urine.

Female Sexual Organs: Menorrhagia; bearing down pain in the lower abdomen.

Potency of Choice: Mother tincture, 3x. 6, 30.

FICUS INDICA OR BENGALENSIS
(Bot)

Bor, Banyan tree, Vata, Bar, Mari.

N.O. : Urticaecae.

Clinical : It possesses greater anti-haemorrhagic properties than Ficus religiosa. Haemorrhage from throat or mouth due to any cause when the colour of blood is pure red; haemorrhage before any evacuation ; bloody leucorrhoea etc.

Haemorrhage : Anti-haemorrhagic property ; successfully arrests haemorrhage from piles, mouth or throat ; or in chronic blood dysentery ; haemorrhage during menses or before any evacuation or bloody leucorrhoea.

Urinary : Gonorrhoea and diabetes associated with burning sensation during urination ; haematuria.

Generals : Nervous debility due to seminal loss ; copious haemorrhage etc.

GENTIANA CHIRATA OR SWERTIA CHIRATA
(Chirata)

Nela-verum, Kirata-tikla, Chitrata.

First Prover : Dr. Kali Kumar Bhattacharjee.

N.O. : Gentianaceae.

Clinical : Anti-pyretic or febrifuge (fever-killer) ; well indicated in dyspepsia ; hyperacidity ; functional inactivity of liver ; flatulence ; anorexia ; worm troubles etc. Popular remedy for chronic fevers.

Mind : Dullness of mind, desire to lie down.

Head : Coldness of head ; dull pain of temples; gradually extends in the whole head.

Nose and Eyes : Burning sensation felt in the eyes and flushes of heat from the nostril.

Ear : Hissing sound in the ear.

Mouth : Bad taste in the mouth in the morning and foul smell.

Tongue : Yellowish coated tongue ; heaviness ; difficulty in speech.

Throat : Pain is felt in the throat, better by hot drinks ; dry hacking cough.

Abdomen : Flatulency ; pain with enlarged liver and spleen, esp. right-sided renal pain ; desire for butter and meat.

Urinary Organs : Red-coloured urine; burning while urinating.

Male Sexual System : Weakness of sexual power ; slight discharge of semen.

Extremities : Aching pain in the extremities; weakness in legs; difficulty in walking.

Fever : Coldness lasts long with nausea and bile vomiting ; hot stage lasts for 3 to 4 hours, then sweating stage appears; desire for hot water after the cold stage.

Potency of Choice : Mother tincture, 3x, 6.

GYMNEMA SYLVESTRE
(Mesharingi or Gurmar)

Mesha-stringa (Ram's horn).   First Prover : Lt. Col. R.N. Chopra.

Chhota—dudhilata, Shirn-kuranja, Kavali.   N.O. : Asclepiadceae.

Clinical : 'Sugar-killer'—excellent medicine for diabetes mellitus, also effacious in poisonous snake-bites.

Urinary : Profuse urination loaded with sugar. After passage of wine patient exclaims, 'this passing of urine in large quantities has made me very weak'. Colour : white ; Quantity : copious ; Specific gravity : high.

Skin : Burning all over the body ; diabetic carbuncle.

Tongue : Great thirst.

Sexual System : Weakness of sexual power.

Potency of Choice : Mother tincture, 3x, 6.

HOLARRHENA ANTIDYSENTERICA OR WRIGHTIA TINCTO
(Kurchi)

Kutaji, Kaluoga, Indrayava, Indrajaverw, Pandrakura, Kurchi-conessi, Telli-cherry bark.

First Prover : Dr. Mahendra Lal Sircar.

N.O. : Apocynaceae.

Clinical : Acute and chronic dysentery ; fever etc., anti-pyretic and anti-dysenteric.

Gastro-Intestinal Symptoms : Dysentery associated with weakness; emaciation; loss of appetite; colicky pain around the navel ; more mucous but blood is less.

Potency of Choice : Mother tincture, 3x, 6x.

HYDROCOTYLE ASIATICA
(Thankuni)

Indian Pennywort, Kurivana, Valla-rai.

First Prover : Dr. Boiien.
N.O. : Umbelliferae.

Clinical : Excellent medicine in jaundice ; leprosy ; skin diseases ; syphilis ; gonorrhoea ; dropsy ; leucorrhoea ; elephantiasis. It is a diuretic, aperient and tonic ; effacious in nervous debility and seminal weakness.

Mind : Gloomy; misanthropy; desire for solitude; indifference; loquacity ; weakness of memory.

Head Vertigo with torpor; neuralgic pain in external frontal nerve ; occiput acutely sensitive.

Note—'Sushruta' has found it useful in increasing memory.

Stomach : Anorexia, then strong appetite ; aversion to tobacco smoking.

Rectum : Burning and itching in anus; weight in rectum.

Urinary Organs : Frequent desire to urinate ; urine becomes brown on standing; turbid with sediment.

Male Sexual System : Drawing pain in spermatic cords ; impotency ; indifference to intercourse.

Female Sexual Organs : Leucorrhoea ; heaviness in uterus; vulva, vagina and cervix are red, severe labor-like pain in uterus.

Respiratory Organs : Dryness of larynx; weak voice; talking makes fatigue ; difficult to expectorate the bronchial mucous ; shortness of breath.

Heart and Pulse : Constriction of heart ; cardiac spasm ; irreugular beating of heart; pulse strong and full, regular.

Skin : Circular spots with raised scaly edges ; miliary eruptions on neck, back, chest ; itching at the tip of the nose; thickening of the epidermoid layer and exfoliation of scales ; syphilitic affections ; stomatitis, either apthous or syphilitic.

Fever : Shivering in afternoon ; hands and feet cold, ameliorated by rubbing and becomes cold on ceasation of rubbing.

Potency of Choice : Mother-tincture, 3x, 6x.

HYGROPHILIA SPHINOSA
(Kule Khara)

Ikshugandha, Kokilaksha,
Talmakhana, Gokshura,　　　　N.O. : Acanthaceae.
Tolimkhana, Nirguviveru,
Gokhulajanum.

Clinical : Anasarca and dropsy ; gonorrhoea ; insomnia ; impotency ; rheumatism ; leucorrhoea ; various skin troubles ; urinary troubles and calculus ; hepatic obstrution with dropsy and anasarca.

Skin : Skin troubles worse from heat and better from cold.

Fever : Malaria associated with urticaria. With the rise of temperature there is intense itching which is relieved by cold application ; fever appears in the morning without chill or thirst.

Potency of Choice : Mother tincture, 3x, 6x, 30.

JANOSIA OR JONOSIA ASOKA OR SARACA INDICA
(The Asoka Tree)

Asoka, Kankeli, Asok,　　　　First Prover : Dr. D.N. Roy.
Ashopalava.　　　　　　　　　N.O. : Leguminosae.

Clinical : Various uterine disorders ; astringent menstrual troubles chiefly in menorrhagia.

Mind : Good-natured ; affectionate ; easily weeping; excitable and fatigued, does not like to do any work ; absent minded ; slow to understand ; hysterical ; impatient ; satisfied with small things ; distrubed sleep, insomnia ; dreams of travelling or of fear.

Head : Stupefying or congestive headache; headache better by free menstrual flow; periodical headache better by bathing; heaviness of head ; vertigo.

Eyes : Conjunctiva becomes red with burning and itching ; lachyrymation ; photophobia ; styes on the upper eyelids ; short sighted : tired feeling in the eyes with least exertion.

Nose : Profuse watering of the nose, sneezing; soreness of the nortrils ; obstruction of the nose ; anosmia ; epistaxis.

Ears : Pain in the ears ; hardness of hearing after severe cold.

Face : Pale face ; alternately heat and red ; pimple on face.

Mouth : Dryness with excessive thirst, drinks large quantity of water at a time; thickly white or brown coated tongue; bleeding gums ; toothache

Throat : Redness of throat with sore feeling ; easily takes cold ; cough.

Appetite : Desire for sweet, sour things ; disinclined to milk.

Stomach : Excessive nausea, sometimes with bile-vomiting ; pain in epigastrium ; colicky pain ; no desire for food; eats little.

Abdomen : Hard, distended abdomen with passage of foul smelling air up and down; worse in the evening.

Stool : Obstinate constipation ; passes stool on every third or fourth day ; pain before stool ; soreness in anus ; blind or bleeding piles with itching and smarting ; large, hard stool covered with mucus.

Urinary Organs : Frequent, bloody, scanty and involuntary m cturition at night; tenderness in bladder and pain in lion.

Male Sexual Organs : Swollen testicle ; drawing pain in the spermatic cord : itching in the scrotum ; seminal discharge with or without dreams.

Female Sexual Organs : Headache due to suppression of menses ; delayed or irregular menses ; menstrual discharge is scanty, pale, watery; foul smelling, blackish, amenorrhoea at puberty with headache; palpitation; hysteria with loss of appetite.

Constipation : Better by commencement of free flow ; menorrhagia; metrorrhagia; leucorrhoea from delayed menses or in the place of menses ; infantile leucorrhoea, small girl becomes emaciated inspite of regular nourishment ; menstrual colic ; headache due to scanty flow of menses with severe pain in all over the lower part of the abdomen.

Respiratory Organs : Hurried respiration ; difficulty in breathing when walking and worse in the afternoon, evening; hacking cough.

Heart : Pain over pre-cardium; palpitation of heart, worse on movement, walking or bending forward ; tight feeling across the chest ; pulse full ; hard, quick.

Pain : Pain in back and sacrum, radiated towards abdomen and thighs.

Limbs : Weak feeling in limbs ; pain in small joints ; shifting pain ; numbness of the limbs.

Fever : Chill without thirst ; dry heat with restlessness ; red cheeks; flushed face; running of the nose.

Potency of Choice : Mother tincture, 2x, 3x.

JUSTICIA ADHATODA
(Vasaka)

Baidyamata, Arusha,
Adhatodai, Malabar-nut.

First Prover : Dr. S.C. Ghosh.
N.O. : Acanthaceae.

Clinical : Excellent in all sorts of cough and cold. It is proclaimed that no death can take place from cough of any kind, if Vasaka can display its healing properties.

Mind : Low spirited; over-sensitive to external impression; anxious ; no desire to talk.

Head : Burning sensation over the forehead ; heaviness and fullness of head ; hot sensation; pulsation in both sides of the head.

Face : Pale, blue ring around the eyes.

Mouth : Dry tongue with excessive thirst for cold water.

Stool : Obstinate constipation.

Respiratory Symptoms : Constrictive pain in the lungs ; tightness across the chest ; whole body tremble while coughing with haerrptysis after severe dyspnoea and shortness of breathing ; expectoration is yellowish, dry, rusty ; patient gets worse while lying on the left side ; dry cough from sternal region; hoarseness; cough with sneezing; asthmatic attacks ; patient can't endure a close warm room ; whooping cough.

Fever : Chilly every evening with night sweats, also useful in consumption and other lung affections, attended with cough and hectic fever.

Potency of Choice : 3x, 6x, 30.

JUSTICIA RUBRUM
(Rakta Vasaka)

Justicia rubrum is highly efficacious where Justicia adhatoda is used but failed and there is more bloody expectoration or blood vomiting (as in tuberculosis). It is a grand remedy in haemoptysis also.

Potency of Choice : Mother-tincture, 3x, 6.

LEUCAS ASPERA
(Drona)

Dronapushpi, Dandakalasa,
Guldera, Kulannaphul, Kumki.   N.O. : Labiatae.

Clinical : Intermittent fever ; asthma ; cough ; dysentery ; jaundice; enlargement of liver and spleen ; bite of venomenous animals; skin troubles etc.

Snake Bite : In case of snake bites : Mother-tincture is to be applied both externally and internally : 10 - 15 drops per dose, every 15 – 20 minutes interval, until the patient feels better. In case of scorpion bites also its action is noticed udoubtedly—the burning pains disappears within very short period.

Potency of Choice : Møther tincture, 2x, 3x.

LUFFA AMARA
(Titpolla)

Dhamarjab, Titpolla.   First Prover : Dr. S.C. Ghosh.
                       N.O.   : Cucurbitaceae.

Clinical : Enlarged spleen ; fever ; hepatic congestion. It is also used as a tonic.

Mind : Anxious.

Mouth : Dry with excessive thirst, bitter taste in the mouth.

Stool and Vomiting : Passes loose stool, rice watery avery at fifteen minutes interval ; vomitus is watery or bile, sometimes mucous appeared every half an hour, sometime purging and vomiting simultaneously.

Sensation : Burning sensation all over the body, sometimes with chilliness.

Pulse : Feeble, weak pulse.

Body : Cold with perspiration.

Potency of Choice : Mother tincture, 3x, 6x.

LUFFA BINDAL
(Ghosalata)

Debdali, Koshataki.   N.O. : Cucurbitaceae.

Clinical : Chronic malarial fever ; gall-stone colic ; dropsy ; acute and chronic nasal catarrh ; enlarged liver and spleen. It controls piles successfully. (Some authors also recommend its use externally over the piles.)

Suitability : Those who are very susceptible to cold or

changes of weather or those who are attacked with catarrh off and on, are specially benefited by this drug.

Potency of Choice : Mother tincture, 3x, 6.

MENISPERNUM
(Rakta Kanthalia)

Clinical : Menorrhagia.

Mind : Despondent.

Head : Giddiness of the head and ringing in the ears.

Haemorrhage : Copious bleeding during menses ; patient becomes extremely weak due to excessive bleeding ; blood oozes out of the uterus and the haemorrhage gets worse from or during movement ; colour of blood is bright red and it is clotted ; copious, bleeding ; pain in lower abdomen ; excessive haemorrhage after delivery.

Potency of Choice : Mother tincture, 3x, 6x.

NYCTANTHES ARBORTRISTIS
(Shephalika)

Siuli, Harsinghar.　　　　First Prover : Dr. S.C. Ghosh.
　　　　　　　　　　　　N.O. : Oleaceae.

Clinical : Remittent fever; rheumation ; sciatica ; constipation ; headache.

Mind : Anxious; restless.

Head : Dull headache; giddiness.

Mouth : Thickly coated tongue with white or yellowish fur.

Stomach : Burning sensation in stomach better by cold applications ; profuse bilious vomiting with nausea.

Abdomen : Tenderness in liver, sensitive ; stitches in liver.

Stool : Constipated, bilious stools accompanied by nausea.

Urine : High coloured urine.

Fever : Insatiable thirst exists before and during chill and heat ; nausea may or may not be present ; drinking causes vomiting.

Potency of Choice : Mother-tincture.

OCIMUM CARYOPHYLLATUM
(Dulal Tulasi)

Clinical : Spermatorrhoea ; gonorrhoea ; haematuria ; blood dysentery.

Urinary Organs : Frequent micturition; extreme burning during urination, passage of pus with urine ; haematuria. Has decided action upon the kidney, bladder and urethra. In gonorrhoea in the first stage when there is excessive burning during urination which is mixed with pus.

Potency of Choice : Mother tincture, 3x, 6x.

OCIMUM SANCTUM
(Tulasi)

Vishnupriya, Tulasi,
Divya, Bharati, Krishna-mul,
Kala Tulasi, Shiva Tulasi,
Holy Basil.

First Prover : Dr. Mure
N.O. : Labiatae.

Clinical : Asthma ; catarrh ; cold ; cough ; fever : Dr. Mure reports specific for the worm affections.

Mind : Forgetful, lack of concentration ; disturbed child cries peevish, does not like to lie on bed ; prostration, drowsiness ; falls asleep while answering.

Head : Headache heavy, throbbing pain, as if nails were driven into it, relieved by pressure ; giddiness worse while walking, better by wrapping up the head ; heat on vertex better by pouring cold water over there and fanning.

Eyes : Pain, redness ; lachrymation of eyes due to nasal catarrh; ophthalmia, mist before the eyes when fixing them on something.

Ears : Noise in the ears ; loud sound appears to be very painful. Watery discharge from the ear ; offensive pus from the ear ; shortness of hearing ; hot flushes in the ear.

Nose : Nasal catarrh associated with sneezing ; white or yellow discharge from the nose ; nostrils ulcerated ; epistaxis.

Face and Mouth : Face pale or red ; lips are bright red ; watery salivation ; putrid and bitter taste in the mouth ; aphthae in mouth ; tongue is bright red or sides are red but middle portion is deeply coated ; lips dry and black, as if burnt.

Throat : Pain in the throat with difficulty in deglutition. Pain while coughing, hoarseness.

Chest : Chest pain while coughing; sneezing ; can't lie quiet in bed in asthma ; pain in the middle of the sternum.

Stomach and Abdomen : Flatulency ; eructation ; hiccough ; gurgling sound in the abdomen ; want of appetite, heaviness in abdomen, no relief after stool ; gripping pain in liver or spleen.

Fever : Excellent remedy in influenza and fevers associated with cough; acute pains in the body; bone-pains; soreness of the muscles and terrible headache ; typhoid fever with chilliness ; burning sensation all over the body; delirium; drowsiness and comatose condition.

Stool : Copious, offensive, mucous or bloody, yellow or greenish ; involuntary during high fever ; diarrhoea in rainy season or autumn.

Urine : Involuntary urination of children, burning while urinating, frequent desire to urinate.

Female Discharges : Offensive lochia lasts for a long period ; profuse bloody discharge after delivery ; leucorrhoea.

Potency of Choice : Mother-tincture, 3x.

OLDENLANDIA HERBACEA
(Khetpapra)

Kshetra-parpata, Daman papar, First Prover : Dr. P.P. Biswas.
Vero-nela Vemu, Poriengo,   N.O : Rubiaceae.
Kazuri, Two flowered Indian Madder.

Clinical : Low form of fevers, gastric troubles ; nervous depressions ; jaundice etc.

Fever : Rise of temperature in early morning with chill, thirst, headache, burning sensation all over the body. Intensity of fever graudally lessens. Fevers either remittent, or intermittent coming with bilious symptoms. Fever appears with greater intensity one day and on the next day it is of a milder character.

Gastro-Intenstinal Symptoms : Bilious vomiting; bilious loose stool.

Potency of Choice : Mother tincture, 3x, 6x, 30.

RAUWOLFIA SERPENTINA
(Chandra)

Sarpagandha, Chandrika,
Chandra, Chotachand,
Dhanmarna, Dhanbarua,
Covannamilpori, Patalagandhi.

N.O. : Apocynaceae.

Clinical : High blood pressure; irritative condition of central nervous system ; insanity ; violent maniacal symptoms. Fever during puerperium. In high blood-pressure without marked atheromatous changes in the vessels. It is also acts as a sedative.

Potency of Choice : Mother tincture.

SOLANUM XANTHOCARPUM
(Kantikari)

Kantikari, Nidigdhika,
Katele, Bhuringni, Warumlea, Kandan-
kattiri, Pinna-mulaka.

N.O : Solanaceae.

Clinical : Excellent remedy for hoarseness with cough ; catarrhal fever ; chest pain ; respiratory diseases with aphonia, broncho-pneumonia ; retention of urine. It is also a bronchitis sovereign remedy in asthma. It is also a sure preventive against small-pox.

Respiratory Symptoms : Hoarseness with cough ; bronchitis ; pneumonia ; broncho-pneumonia ; asthma etc.

Fever : Fever with thirst ; aversion to food ; burning sensation and pain over whole body.

Urinary Organs : Stricture, retention or suppression of urine and stone.

Potency of Choice : Mother tincture, 2x, 3x.

SYZYGIUM JAMBOLANUM OR EUGENIA JAMBOLANA
(Kala Jam)

Nilaphala, Jaman, Jambudo,
Nacraedu, Nagum, Navil, Naval,   N.O. : Myrtaceae.
Naeralu, Sittalchini, Jambul,
Black plum.

Clinical : Diabetes, mellitus and insipidus ; prickly heat ; pimples ; itch ; emaciation ; weakness.

Urine : Diabetes and insipidus ; much thirst with profuse flow of wine in every two hours. No other remedy causes in so marked degree the diminution and disappearance of sugar in the urine.

Skin : Prickly heat in upper part of the body ; small red pimples, which itched violently ; old ulcers of the skin ; diabetic ulceration ; old ulcers of skin, probably of a diabetic foundation.

Potency of Choice : Mother tincture, 2x, 3x.

TERMINALIA ARJUNA
(Arjuna)

Vellaimarudamarum,   First prover : Dr. S.C. Ghosh.
Shardul, Sajadan.   N.O. : Combrataceae.

Clinical : Diseases of the heart, both organic and functional ; angina pectoris ; suffocation ; vertigo. In fractures, pain all over the body owing to a fall and all sorts of ecchymosis the action of this drug in such cases is supreme. In spermatorrhoea and in gonorrhoea it is also effacious.

Mind : Nervous.

Head : Giddiness.

Ear : Ringing in the ear.

Mouth : Bitter taste in the mouth.

Urine : Scanty urine.

Heart : Population, angina pectoris, weakness and pain in the heart.

Potency of Choice : Mother tincture, 3x.

TERMINALIA CHEBULA
(Haritaki)

Abhaya, Pathya, Har, Harara, Harrar, Hirda, Harda, Kadakai, Kadut-key (tree), Kadut-kaypinji (fruit). Karaka, Kurka (tree).

First Prover : Dr. B. Dutta.
N.O : Combrataceae.

Clinical : Bleeding piles; diarrhoea ; chronic dysentery ; constipation; colic (biliary) ; headache ; vertigo ; dropsy and in some skin diseases it is found to be effacious.

Mind : Indifferent, easily indisposed with constant yawning.

Head : Vertigo remains whole day and night aggravated by 'hot sun's rays' ; agg. from motion, hard pressure. ameliorated by cold bathing, in the evening, from dry cold air, sleep, eating.

Mouth : Profuse salivation with intense thirst for cold water ; sensation of dryness in upper jaw ; gums swollen and hard; foul breath ; foetid eructation.

Tongue : Flabby, dry, brown coating on the tip of the tongue ; sore and raw tongue.

Stomach : Sensation of fullness in stomach.

Pain : Intense pain in loin, aggravated on sitting, better by lying down on bed or sleeping ; pain in the back of the neck ; pressive pain in right chest or heart.

Stool : Frequent desire for stool but passes only small quantity with great force or nothing comes out ; sweat during stool ; pressive pain ; itching and sensation of fullness in the rectum. In diarrhoea ; small quantity of faeces mixed mucous. flatulance associated with burning in the stomach. In constipations hard small stool.

Urine : Scanty urine, frequency of urination increases at night.

Extremities : Muscular pain in deltoid muscles; itching better by scratching

Pulse : Quick, irregular, hard or weak sometimes.

TINOSPORA CORDIFOLIA
(Gulancha)

Ninjara, Guluchee, Guruchi,   N.O. : Menispermaceae.
Gilo, Gularich, Gulwali,
Gharol, Gula-veli, Shindil,
Kodi, Tippa-tige, Guluchi ;
Amritvel, Heart-leaved, Moon-seed.

Respiration : Hot, deep breathing.
Potency of Choice : Mother tincture, 3x, 6x, 30.

Clinical : Seminal debility ; fevers, esp. in intermittent fevers; jaundice ; splenic affections ; leprosy ; leucorrhoea ; rheumatism; skin diseases; secondary syphilis, genito-urinary troubles such as gonorrhoea, dysurea, etc.

Fever : Acute or chronic malarial fever ; temperature rises in the afternoon with chill and shievering, bilious vomiting with thirst and headache. Chronic slow fever with history of gonorrhoea and weakness due to seminal loss. Bad effect of quinine which causes continuation of fever with burning in hands face ; jaundice, etc.

Urine : Frequent passage of small quantity of urine with burning while urinating ; urine mixed with pus.

Heart : Excessive palpitation of heart.

Potency of Choice : Mother tincture, 2x, 3x, 6x,

TRICHOSANTHES DIO1
(Patal)

Patola, Parver, Palwal,   First Prover : **Dr. P.P. Biswas.**
Kombu-pudalai, Kammu-potla,   N.O. Cucurbitaceae.
Wild snakegourd.

Clinical : Chronic malarial fever, kala-azar ; nausea and vomiting.

Mind : Despondent.

Head : Vertigo while lying in bed, terrible headache during fever.

Eyes : Yellow colour, dilated pupil.

Mouth : Thirst ; with dryness of throat ; slimy salivation ; bad taste ; constant water-brush from the mouth ; bitter taste in the mouth.

Throat : Sore throat.

Vomiting, Eructation and Hiccough : Nausea and water-brush along with distension of abdomen. Vomitus is stringy mucus, may be streaked with blood. Eructation and vomiting after drinking water.

Hunger : Extreme hunger, must eat something in the morning, great desire for cold things.

Burning : Burning sensation in the whole body, associated with thirst.

Abdomen : Empty feeling in abdomen, uneasiness in the abdomen, hot feeling in abdomen at 11 A.M. Owing to enlargement of liver and spleen, pain is felt, which is worse from sneezing, coughing, motion, etc.

Stool : Copious, greenish-yellow, liquid, mixed with bile and mucous : bloody stool, become exhausted owing to frequent passage of stool ; smarting pain in anus.

Urinary Organs : Scanty, red urine, retention of urine along with purging and vomiting.

Lower Extremities : Swelling of the lower extremities.

Fever : Comes at 11 A.M.—12 noon with chilliness ; during fever burning sensation of the whole body ; with the rise of temperature associated with headache, thirst etc. Acute fever associated with vomiting, nausea, water brash ; intensity of fever rises next day. Used in all kinds of fever with predominance of bilious symptoms. Headache, waterbrash and nausea are the keynote symptoms of its administration. In chronic fever there is enlargement of liver and spleen.

Potency of Choice : Mother tincture, 3x, 6x, 30.

VERNONIA ANTHELMINTICA
(Somaraja)

Vakuehi, Somraja, Bakchi,   N.O : Comporitae.
Kali-jiri, Kadvo-jiri,
Kattu-shiragam, Adavi-jilakara.

Clinical : It has a remarkable anti-helminthic property and however it is distinctly effective in thread-worm infections. It is also useful in the trouble arises in consequence with worm troubles ; nocturnal enuresis, grinding of the teeth at night etc.

Potency of Choice ; Mother tincture, 3x.

Relationship of Remedies and Sides of the Body

RELATIONSHIP OF REMEDIES AND SIDES OF THE BODY

R. Gibson Miller

B. JAIN PUBLISHERS (P) LTD.
USA — EUROPE — INDIA

RELATIONSHIP OF REMEDIES WITH DURATION OF ACTION
(R. Gibson Miller)

1 Remedy	2 Complements	3 Remedies that Follow Well	4 Inimicals	5 Antidotes	6 Duration
Ac. acet	China.	—	Borax, Caust. Nux. Ran-b. Sars.	Acon. Natr-m. Nux. Sep. Tabac.	14-20 d.
Ac. fluor	Sil. Coca	Graph. Ac. nitric.	—	Sil.	30 d.
Ac. lactic.	—	Psor.	Coff.	Bry.	—
Ac. mur.	—	Calc. Kali-c. Nux. Puls. Sep. Sulph. Sil.	—	Bry. Camph.	35 d.
Ac. nitric.	Ars. Calad.	Arn. Arum-t. Bell. Calc. Carb-v. Kali-c. Kreos. Merc. Phos. Puls. Sil. Sulph. Sep. Thuja.	Lach. after Calc.	Acon. Calc. Hep. Con. Merc. Mez. Sulph.	40-60 d.
Ac. phos.	—	Ars. Bell. Chin. Caust. Ferr. Ac. fluor. Lyc. Nux. Puls. Rhus. Selen. Sep. Sulph. Verat.	—	Camph. Coff. Staph.	40 d.
Ac. sulph.	Puls.	Arn. Calc. Con. Lyc. Plat. Sep. Sulph.	—	Puls.	30-40 d.

RELATIONSHIP OF REMEDIES

1 Remedy	2 Complements	3 Remedies that Follow Well	4 Inimicals	5 Antidotes	6 Duration
Acon.	Arn. Coff. Sulph.	Abrot. Arn. Ars. Bell. Bry. Cact. Calc. Cocc. Canth. Coff. Hep. Ipec. Kali-bro. Merc. Puls. Rhus. Sep. Spig. Spong. Sulph. Sil.	—	Ac. acet. Bell. Berb. Coff. Nux. Paris. Sulph. Vinum.	
Aesc-H.	—	—	—	Nux.	30 d.
Aeth.	Calc.	—	—	Veget. Acids.	20-30 d.
Agar.	—	Bell. Calc. Cupr. Merc. Op. Puls. Rhus. Sil. Tuberc.	—	Calc. Puls. Rhus. Vinum	40 d.
Agnus	—	Ars. Bry. Calad. Ign. Lyc. Puls. Selen. Sulph.	—	Camph. Nux.	8-14 d.
Allium cepa	Phos. Puls. Sars. Thuj.	Calc. Sil.	All-s. Aloe Scilla	Arn. Cham. Nux. Thuj. Verat.	1 d.
All-s.	Ars.	—	Aloe All-c. Scilla	Lyc.	—
Aloe	Sulph.	Kali-b. Sep. Sulph. Ac. sul.	All-s.	Camph. Lyc. Nux. Sulph.	30-40 d.
Alum.	Bry. Ferr.	Arg-m. Bry.	—	Bry. Camph. Cham. Ipec.	40-60 d.
Alumen	—	—	—	Cham. Nux. Ipec. Sulph.	Long- acting.

RELATIONSHIP OF REMEDIES

1 Remedy	2 Complements	3 Remedies that Follow Well	4 Inimicals	5 Antidotes	6 Duration
Ambra	—	Lyc. Puls. Sep. Sulph.	—	Camph. Coff. Nux. Puls. Staph.	40 d.
Amm-carb.	—	Bell. Bry. Lyc. Puls. Phos. Rhus. Sep. Sulph. Verat.	Lach.	Arn. Camph. Hep.	40 d.
Am-mur.	—	Ant-c. Coff. Merc. Nux. Phos. Puls Rhus. Sanic.	—	Coff. Hep. Nux	20-30 d.
Anac.	—	Lyc. Puls. Plat.	—	Clem. Crot-t. Coff Juglans Ran-b. Rhus.	30-40 d.
Angust.	—	Bell. Ign. Lyc. Sep.	—	Coff.	20-30 d.
Ant-crud.	Scilla	Calc. Lach. Merc. Puls. Sep. Sulph.	—	Calc. Hep. Merc.	40 d.
Ant-tart.	Ipec.	Bar-c. Cina. Camph. Ipec. Puls. Sep. Sulph. Tereb. Carbo-v.	—	Asaf. Chin. Cocc. Ipec. Laur. Op. Puls. Rhus. Sep.	20-30 d.
Apis	Natr-m.	Arn. Ars. Graph. Iod. Lyc. Puls. Nat-m. Stram. Sulph.	Rhus.	Ac. carbol. Ac. lact. Canth. Ipec. Lach. Led. Natr-m. Plant.	
Arg-met.	—	Calc. Puls. Sep.	—	Merc. Puls.	30 d.

RELATIONSHIP OF REMEDIES

1 Remedy	2 Complements	3 Remedies that Follow Well	4 Inimicals	5 Antidotes	6 Duration
Arg-nit.	—	Bry. Calc. Kali-c. Lyc. Merc. Puls. Sep. Spig. Spong. Sil. Verat.		Ars. Calc. Lyc. Natr-m. Merc. Phos. Puls. Rhus. Sep. Sil. Sulph.	30 d.
Arnica	Acon. Ip-c. Verat. Hyper. Rhus.	Acon. Ars. Bell. Ac. sul. Bry. Bar-m. Berb. Cact. Calc. Chin. Cham. Calend. Con. Curare. Hep. Ipec. Nux. Phos. Led. Puls. Psor. Rhus Ruta. Sulph. Verat.	—	Acon. Ars. Camph. Chin. Ign. Ipec.	6-10 d.
Arsen.	All-s. Carb-v. Natr-s. Phos. Pyrog. Thuja	Aran. Arn. Apis. Bell. Ac. fluor. Bar-c. Cact. Calc-ph. Chsm. Chin. Cic. Ferr. Hep. Iod. Ipec. Kali-b. Lach. Lyc. Merc. Ntr-s. Nux. Phos. Ran-sc. Sulph. Thuja. Verat.	—	Chin. Sul. Camph. Carb-c. Chin. Euph. Ferr. Graph. Hep. Iod. Ipec. Kali-b. Merc. Nux. Nux-m. Op. Samb. Sulph. Tabac. Verat.	60-90 d.
Arum-t.	—	Euphm.	Calad.	Ac. acet. Bell. Ac. lact. Puls.	1-2 d.
Asaf.	—	Chin. Merc. Puls.	—	Caust. Camph. Chin. Merc. Puls. Valer.	20-40 d.
Asar.	—	Ac. sul. Bism. Caust. Puls. Sil.	—	Ac. acet. Camph.	8-14 d.
Asclep-t.	—	—	—	—	40-60 d.

RELATIONSHIP OF REMEDIES

1 Remedy	2 Complements	3 Remedies that Follow Well	4 Inimicals	5 Antidotes	6 Duration
Aster-r.	—	—	Coff. Nux.	Plb. Zinc	—
Aur-m-n.	—	—	Coff.	—	—
Aurum	—	Ac-nitric. Acon. Bell. Calc. Chin. Lyc. Merc. Puls. Rhus. Sep. Sulph. Syph.	—	Bell. Chin. Cocc. Coff. Cupr. Merc. Puls. Spig. Sol-n.	50-60 d.
Badiaga	od. Merc. Sulph.	Lach.	—	—	—
Baptisia	—	Ac. nitric. Tereb. Crotal. Ham. Pyrog.	—	—	6-8 d.
Bar-c.	Dulc.	Ant-t. Con. Chin. Lyc. Merc. Ac. nit. Psor. Puls. Rhus. Sep. Sulph. Tuberc.	after Calc.	Ant-t. Bell. Camph. Dulc. Zinc.	40 d.
Bellad.	Calc.	Ac. mur. Acon. Ars. Cact. Calc. Cham. Carb-v. Chin. Con. Curare. Hep. Hyos. Lach. Merc. Mosch. Merc-i-r. Nux. Puls. Rhus. Sep. Sil. Stram. Sulph. Seneg. Valer. Verat.	Ac. acet. Dulc.	Acon. Camph. Coff. Hep. Hyo. Merc. Op. Puls. Sabad. Vinum.	1-7 d.
Berb.	—	—	—	Camph. Bell.	20-30 d.
Bism.	—	Bell. Calc. Puls. Sep	—	Coff. Calc. Caps. Nux.	20-50 d.
Borax	—	Ars. Bry. Calc. Lyc. Nux. Phos. Sil.	Ac. acet. Vinum	Cham. Coff.	30 d.

RELATIONSHIP OF REMEDIES

1 Remedy	2 Complements	3 Remedies that Follow Well	4 Inimicals	5 Antidotes	6 Duration
Bovista	—	Alum. Calc. Rhus. Sep. Verat.	Coff.	Camph.	7-14 d.
Brom.	—	Arg-n. Kali-c.	—	Am-c. Camph. Mgn-c. Op.	20-30 d.
Bryonia	Alum. Rhus.	Ac. mur. Alum. Ara. Abrot. Ant-t. Bell. Berb. Cact. Carb-v. Dulc. Hyos. Kali-c. Nux. Phos. Puls. Rhus. Sil. Sabad. Squil. Sulph.	—	Ac. mur. Acon. Alum. Camph. Cham. Chel. Clem. Coff. Ign. Nux. Puls. Rhus. Seneg.	7-21 d.
Cactus	—	Dig. Eupat. Lach. Nux. Sulph.	—	Acon. Camph. Chin.	7-10 d.
Cadmium	—	Bell. Carb-v. Lobel.	—	—	—
Calad.	Ac. nitric.	Acon. Canth. Caust. Puls. Sep. Selen.	Arum-t.	Camph. Caps. Carb-v. Ign. Hyos. Merc.	30-40 d.
Calc-ars.	—	Con. Glon. Op. Puls.	—	Carb-v. Glon. Puls.	—
Calc-c.	Bell. Rhus.	Ac. nitric. Aran. Agar. Bell. Borax. Bism. Dulc. Graph. Ipec. Kali-b. Lyc. Ntr-c. Nux. Phos. Puls. Plat. Pod. Rhus. Sil. Sep. Sars. Therid. Tuberculin.	Ac. nitric. Bar-c. and Sulph. do not follow. After Kali-b. and Ac. nitric.	Ac. nitric. Bry. Camph. Chin. Ipec. Nit-sp-d. Nux. Sep. Sulph.	60 d.
Calc-fluor.	—	Ac. phos. Calc-ph. Ntr-m. Sil.	—	—	—

RELATIONSHIP OF REMEDIES

1 Remedy	2 Complements	3 Remedies that Follow Well	4 Inimicals	5 Antidotes	6 Duration
Calc-phos.	Ruta Sulph. Zinc.	Rhus. Sulph. Iod. Psor. Sanic.	—	—	60 d.
Calend.	Hep.	Ac. nitric. Arn. Ars. Bry. Phos. Rhus.	Camph.	Arn.	—
Camphor.	Canth.	Ars. Ant-t. Bell. Cocc. Nux. Rhus. Verat.	After Kali-n.	Canth. Dulc. Nit-s-d. Op. Phos.	1 d.
Cann-sat.	—	Bell. Hyos. Lyc. Nux. Op. Puls. Rhus: Verat.	—	Camph. Merc.	1-10 d.
Canth.	Camph.	Bell. Kali-Iod. Merc. Phos. Puls. Sep. Sulph.	Coff.	Acon. Apis. Camph. Kali-n. Laur. Puls. Rheum.	30-40 d.
Caps.	—	Bell. Cina. Lyc. Puls. Sil.	—	Ac. sul. Calad. Camph. Chin. Cina.	7 d.
Carb-an.	Calc-ph.	Ac. nitric. Ars. Bell. Bry. (Carb-v.) Phos. Puls. Sep. Sil. Sulph. Verat.	Csrb-v.?	Ars. Camph. Nux. Vinum	60 d.
Carb-veg.	Dros. Kali-c. Phos.	Ac. phos. Ars. Acon. Chin. Dros. Kali-c. Lyc. Nux. Puls. Scp. Sulph. Verat.	Carb-an. ? Kreos. does not follow.	Ars. Camph. Coff. Lach. Nits-d.	60 d.
Caulop.	—	—	Coff.	—	—

RELATIONSHIP OF REMEDIES

1 Remedy	2 Complements	3 Remedies that Follow Well	4 Inimicals	5 Antidotes	6 Duration
Caust.	Petros. Coloc. Carb-v.	Ant-t. Arum-t. Coloc. Calc. Guaia. Kali-i. Lyc. Nux. Puls. Rhus. Ruta. Sep. Sil. Stann. Sulph.	Ac. acet. Cotf Phos.	Asaf Coloc. Dulc. Guaia. Nux	50 d.
Cepa (see Allium c.)	—	—	—	—	—
Cham.	Bell Mgn-c.	Acon. Arn. Bell. Bry. Cact. Calc. Cocc. Form. Merc. Nux. Puls. Rhus Sep. Sil. Sulph.	Zinc.	Acon. Alum. Borax. Camph. Chin. Cocc. Coff. Coloc. Con. Ign. Nux. Puls. Valer.	20-30 d.
Chelid.	—	Acon. Ars. Bry. Cor-r. Ipec. Led. Lyc. Nux. Sep. Spig. Sulph.	—	Acon. Cham. Coff. Acids. Vinum	7-14 d.
China	Ferr.	Ac. acet. Ac. phos. Ars. Arn. Asaf Bell. Calc. Carb-v. Calc-ph. Ferr. Lach. Merc. Puls. Phos. Sulph. Verat.	After Dig. and Selen.	Aranea. Arn. Apis. Ars. Asaf. Bell. Bry. Carb-v. Carb-an. Calc. Caps. Caust. Cedr. Cina. Eupat. Ferr. Ipec. Lach. Led. Lyc. Meny. Merc. Ntr-c. Ntr-m. Nux. Puls. Rhus. Sep. Sulph. Verat.	14-21 d.
Cicuta	—	Bell, Hep, Puls, Rhus. Op. Sep.	—	Arn. Coff. Op. Tabac.	35-40 d.
Cimicif.	—	—	—	Acon. Bspt.	8-12 d.

RELATIONSHIP OF REMEDIES

1 Remedy	2 Complements	3 Remedies that Follow Well	4 Inimicals	5 Antidotes	6 Duration
Cina	—	Calc. Chin. Ign. Nux. Plat. Puls. Rhus. Sil. Stann.	—	Arn. Camph. Chin. Caps. Pip-n.	14-20 d.
Cistus	—	Bell. Carb-v. Mgn-c. Phos.	Coff.	Sep. Rhus.	—
Clemat.	—	Calc. Rhus. Sep. Sil. Sulph.	—	Bry. Camph. Cham. Anac. Crot-t. Rhus. Ran-b.	14-20 d.
Cobalt.	—	—	—	—	30 d.
Coccul.	—	Ars. Bell. Hep. Ign. Lyc. Nux. Rhus. Puls. Sulph.	Coff.	Camph. Cham. Cupr. Ign. Nux.	30 d.
Coffea	Acon.	Ac. fluor. Acon. Aur. Bell. Lyc. Nux. Op. Sulph.	Canth. Caust. Cocc. Ign.	Ac. acet. Acon. Cham. Chin. Grat. Merc. Nux. Puls. Sulph.	1- 7 d.
Colch.	—	Carb-v. Merc. Nux. Puls. Sep. Rhus	—	Bell. Camph. Cocc. Led. Nux. Puls. Spig.	14-20 d.
Collins.	—	Aloe. Aesc-h. Con.	—	Nux.	30 d.
Coloc.	—	Bell. Bry. Caust. Cham. Merc. Nux. Puls. Spig. Staph.	—	Camph. Caust. Cham. Coff. Op. Staph.	1-7 d.
Conium	Bar-m.	Arn. Ars. Bell. Calc. Calc-ars. Cic. Dros.	—	Ac. nitric. Coff. Dulc.	30-50 d.

RELATIONSHIP OF REMEDIES

1 Remedy	2 Complements	3 Remedies that Follow Well	4 Inimicals	5 Antidotes	6 Duration
		Lyc. Nux. Psor. Phos. Puls. Rhus Stram. Sulph.		Nit-s-d.	
Cor-r.	—	Sulph.	—	Merc. Calc.	—
Crocus	—	Chin. Nux. Puls. Sulph.	—	Acon. Bell. Op.	8 d.
Crot-h.	—	—	—	Lach.	30 d.
Crot. tig.	—	Rhus	—	Anac. Ant-t. Clem. Rhus Ran-b.	30 d.
Cuprum	Calc.	Ars. Apis, Bell. Calc. Caust. Cic. Hyo. Kali-n. Puls. Stram. Verat. Zinc.	—	Bell. Camph. Cic. Chin. Cocc. Con. Dulc. Hep. Ipec. Merc. Nux Puls. Verat.	40-50 d.
Cycl.	—	Phos. Puls. Rhus. Sep. Sulph.	—	Camph. Coff. Puls.	14-20 d.
Digit.	—	Ac. acet. Bell. Bry. Cham. Lyc. Nux. Op. Phos. Puls. Sep. Sulph. Verat.	Nit-s-d. Chin.	Ac. nitric. Apis. Camph. Calc. (Colch.) Nux. Op.	40-50 d.
Dios.	—	—	—	—	1-7 d.
Dros.	Nux.	Calc. Cina. Con. Puls. Sulph. Verat.	—	Camph.	20-30 d.
Dulc.	Bar-c. Calc. Kali-s. Sulph.	Calc. Lyc. Rhus. Sep. Bell.	Ac. acet. Bell. Lach.	Camph. Cupr. Ip. Kali-c. Merc.	30 d.

RELATIONSHIP OF REMEDIES

1 Remedy	2 Complements	3 Remedies that Follow Well	4 Inimicals	5 Antidotes	6 Duration
Eupat. Perf.	—	Natr-m. Sep. Tubercul.	—	—	1- 7 d.
Euphorb	—	Ferr. Lach. Puls. Sep. Sulph.	—	Ac. acet. Camph.	50 d.
Euphras.	—	Acon. Alum. Calc. Con. Lyc. Merc. Nux. Phos. Puls. Rhus. Sil. Sulph.	—	Caust. Camph. Puls.	7 d.
Ferr.	Alum. Chin. Ham.	Acon. Arn. Bell. Chin. Con. Lyc. Merc. Phos. Puls. Verat.	Ac. acet.	Ars. Arn. Bell. Chin. Hep. Ipec. Puls. Sulph. Verat.	50 d.
Fluor-ac. (see Ac. Fluor.)					
Gamb.		—	—	Camph. Coff. Coloc. Ksli-c. Op.	1-7 d.
Gelsem.	—	Bapt. Cact. Ipec.	—	Atrop. Chin. Coff. Dig.	30 d.
Glon.	—	—	—	Acon. Camph. Coff. Nux.	1 d.
Graph.	Araen. Caust. Ferr. Hep. Lyc.	Euphm. Ntr-s. Sil.	—	Acon. Ars. Nux.	40-50 d.
Guaiac.	—	Calc. Merc.	—	Nux.	40 d.
Hamam.	Ferr.	Arn.	—	—	—
Helleb.	—	Bell. Bry. Chin. Lyc. Nux. Phos. Puls. Sulph. Zinc.	—	Camph. Chin.	20-30 d.

RELATIONSHIP OF REMEDIES

1 Remedy	2 Complements	3 Remedies that Follow Well	4 Inimicals	5 Antidotes	6 Duration
Hepar	Calend.	Ac. nitric. Abrot. Acon. Arum-t. Hell. Bry. Calend. Iod. Lach. Merc. Nux. Rhus. Sep. Spong. Sil. Sulph.	—	Ac. acet. Ars. Bell. Cham. Sil.	40-50 d.
Hyosc.	—	Bell. Puls. Stram. Verat.		Ac. acet. Ac. citric. Bell. Chin. Stram.	6-14 d.
Hyper.	—	—		Arsen. Cham. Sulph.	1-7 d
Ignatia	Ntr-m.	Al-ph. Ars. Bell. Calc. Chin. Cocc. Lyc. Puls. Rhus Sep. Sil. Sulph.	Coff. Nux. Tabac.	Ac. acet. Arn. Cocc. Cham. Puls.	9 d.
Iod.	Bad. Lyc.	Acon. Arg-n. Calc. Calc-ph. Kali-b. Lyc. Merc. Phos. Puls.	—	Ant-t. Apis. Ars. Acon. Bell. Camph. Chin. Chin-s. Coff. Ferr. Graph. Grat. Hep. Op. Phos. Spong. Sulph. Thuja.	30-40 d.
Ipec.	Ant-t. Arn. Cupr.	Aranea Ant-cr. Ant-t. Apis Arn. Ars. Bell. Bry. Cact. Cadm. Calc. Cham. Chin. Cupr. Ign. Nux. Pod. Phos.	—	Arn. Ars. Chin. Nux. Tabac.	7-10 d.

RELATIONSHIP OF REMEDIES

1 Remedy	2 Complements	3 Remedies that Follow Well	4 Inimicals	5 Antidotes	6 Duration
		Puls. Rheum. Sep. Sulph. Tabac. Verat.			
Kali-bi.	Ars.	Ant-t. Berb. Puls.	Does not follow Calc.	Ars. Lach. Puls.	30 d.
Kali. brom.	—	Cact.	—	Camph. Helon. Nux. Zinc.	—
Kali. carb.	Carb-v. Nux.	Ac. fluor. Ac. nitric. Ars. Carb-v. Lyc. Phos. Puls. Sep. Sulph.		Camph. Helon. Coff. Nit-s-d. Dulc.	40-50 d.
Kali-iod.	—	—	—	Am-m. Ars. Chin. Merc. Rhus. Sulph. Valer.	20-30 d.
Kali-nit.	—	Bell. Calc. Puls. Rhus. Sep. Sulph.	Camph. Does not follow	Nit-s-d.	30-40 d.
Kali-sulph.	—	Ac. acet. Ars. Calc. Hep. Kali-c. Puls. Rhus. Sep. Sil. Sulph.	—	—	—
Kalmia	Ac. benz.	Calc. Lith. Lyc. Ntr-m. Puls. Spig.	—	Acon. Bell. Spig.	7-14 d.
Kreos.	—	Ac. nitric. Ars. Bell. Calc. Kali-c. Lyc. Nux. Rhus. Sep. Sulph.	After Carb-v.	Acon. Nux	15-20 d.

RELATIONSHIP OF REMEDIES

1 Remedy	2 Complements	3 Remedies that Follow Well	4 Inimicals	5 Antidotes	6 Duration
Lach.	Ac. nitric. Hep. Lyc.	Acon. Ars. Alum. Bell. Brom. Carb-v. Caust. Con. Cact. Calc. Cic. Chin. Euphm. Hep. Hyos. Kali-b. Lac-c. Lyc. Merc. Merc-i-fl. Nux. Ntr-m. Oleand. Phos. Puls. Rhus. Sil. Sulph Tarent.	Ac. acet. Ac. carbol. Ac. nitric Dulc. Am-c. Psor.	Ac. nitric. Ac. phos. Alum. Ars. Bell. Calc. Cham. Cocc. Carb-v. Coff. Hep. Led. Merc. Nux. Op.	30-40 d.
Lactic-ac. (see Ac. lactic.)					
Laur.		Bell. Carb-v. Phos. Puls. Verat.	—	Camph. Coff. Ipec. Op. Nux-m.	4-8 d.
Ledum	—	Ac. Sulph. Acon. Bell. Bry. Chel. Nux. Puls. Rhus. Sulph.	Chin.	Camph.	30 d.
Lil-tig.	—	—	—	Helon. Nux. Puls. Plat.	14-20 d.
Lycop.	Iod. Lach. Puls.	Anac. Bell. Bry. Carb-v. Colch. Dulc. Graph. Hyos. Kali-c. Lach. Led. Nux. Phos. Puls. Stram. Sep. Sil. Therid. Verat.	After Sulph. except in cycle of Sulph. Calc. Lyc. Sulph. etc. Coff.	Acon. Camph. Caust. Cham. Graph. Puls.	40-50 d.
Magn-carb.	Cham.	Caust. Phos. Puls. Sep. Sulph.	—	Ars. Cham. Merc. Nux Puls. Rheum	40-50 d.
Magn-mur.	—	Bell. Lyc. Ntr-m. Nux. Puls. Sep.	—	Ars. Camph. Cham. Nux	40-50 d.

RELATIONSHIP OF REMEDIES

1 Remedy	2 Complements	3 Remedies that Follow Well	4 Inimicals	5 Antidotes	6 Duration
Manc.	—	—	—	—	30-40 d.
Mangan.	—	Puls. Rhus. Sulph.	—	Coff. Camph.	40 d.
Medorrh.	—	Sulph. Thuja	—	Ipec.	—
Menyanth.	—	Caps. Lyc. Puls. Rhus.	—	Camph.	14-20 d.
Meph.	—	—	—	—	1 d.
Merc.	Bad.	Ac. mur. Ac. nitric. Ars. Asaf. Bell. Calc. Calc-ph. Carb-v. Chin. Dulc. Guaiac. Hep. Iod. Lach. Lyc. Phos. Puls. Rhus. Sep. Sulph. Thuja	Ac. acet. Sil. disagrees before or after potentized Mercury, but antidotes the crude substance.	Ac. nitric. Ars. Aur. Aranea. Asaf. Bell. Bry. Calad. Carb-v. Calc. Chin. Cupr. Con. Cor-r. Clem. Dphn. Dulc. Ferr. Guaia. Hep. Iod. Kali-i. Kali-chl. Kali-b. Lach. Mez. Nux-m. Op. Pod. Phyt. Rata. Sars. Staph. Sep. Still. Spig. Sulph. Stram. Valer.	30-60 d.
Mezer.	—	Calc. Caust. Ign. Lyc. Merc. Nux Phos. Puls.	—	Acon. Bry. Calc. Kali j. Merc. Nux. Acids.	30-60 d.
Millef.	—	—	Coff.	Arum-m.	1-3 d.
Mosch.	—	—	—	Camph. Coff.	1 d.
Mur-ac. (see Ac. mur.)					

RELATIONSHIP OF REMEDIES

1 Remedy	2 Complements	3 Remedies that Follow Well	4 Inimicals	5 Antidotes	6 Duration
Ntr-carb.	—	Ac. nitric. Calc. Nux Puls. Sepia Sulph. Selen.	—	Camph. Nit-s-d.	30 d.
Ntr-mur.	Apis Ign. Sep.	Apis. Bry. Calc. Hep. Kali-c. Puls. Rhug Sep. Sulph. Thuja	—	Ars. Phos. Nit-s-d. Sepia. Nux.	40-50 d.
Ntr-sul.	Ars. Thuja	Bell. Thuja	—	—	30-40 d.
Nitric-ac. (see Ac. nitric.)					
Nux-mos.	—	Ant-t. Lyc. Nux Puls. Rhus. Stram.	—	Camph. Gels. Laur. Nux. Op. Valer. Zinc.	60 d.
Nux vom.	Sulph. Kali-c. Sepia	Ac. phos. Aranea. Aesc. Ars. Act-sp. Bell. Bry. Cact. Carb-v. Calc. Cocc. Colch. Cobalt. Hyos. Lyc. Phos. Puls. Rhus Sep. Sulph.	Ac. acet. Ign. Zinc.	Acon. Ars. Bell. Camph. Cham. Cocc. Coff. Euphm. Op. Puls. Thuja	1-7 d.
Oleander	—	Con. Lyc. Ntr-m. Puts. Rhus. Sep. Spig.	—	Camph. Sulph.	20-30 d.
Opium	—	Acon. Ant-t. Bell Bry. Hyos. Nux-m. Nux. Samb.	—	Ac. acet. Ac. mur. Bell. Cham. Cic. Coff Cupr. Gels. Ipec. Merc. Nux Puls. Ver. Zinc.	7 d.

RELATIONSHIP OF REMEDIES

1 Remedy	2 Complements	3 Remedies that Follow Well	4 Inimicals	5 Antidotes	6 Duration
Paris	—	Calc. Led. Lyc. Nux. Puls. Phos. Rhus. Sep. Sulph.	Fer. ph.	Coff.	2-4 d.
Pallad.	Plat.	—	—	Chin. Bell. Glon.	—
Petrol.	—	Ac. nitric. Bry. Calc. Lyc. Nux. Puls. Sep. Sil. Sulph.	—	Cocc. Nux.	40-50 d.
Phos-ac. see Ac. phos.)					
Phosph.	Ars. All-c. Carb-veg.	Ars. Bell. Bry. Carb-v. Chin. Calc. Kali-c. Lyc. Nux. Puls. Rhus. Sep. Sil. Sulph.	Caust.	Coff. Calc. Mez. Nux. Sep. Tereb.	40 d.
Plat.	—	Anac. Arg-m. Bell. Ign. Lyc. Puls. Rhus. Sep. Verat.	—	Bell. Nit-s-d. Puls.	35-40 d.
Plumb.	—	Ars. Bell. Lyc. Merc. Phos. Puls. Sil. Sulph.		Ac. sul. Alum. Alumen. Ant-cr. Ars. Bell. Cocc Caust. Hep. Hyos. Kali-bro. Kreos. Nux. Nux-m. Op. Petr. Plat. Stram. Zinc.	20-30 d.

RELATIONSHIP OF REMEDIES

1 Remedy	2 Complements	3 Remedies that Follow Well	4 Inimicals	5 Antidotes	6 Duration
Pod.	(Sulph.)	—		Ac. lact. Coloc. Lept. Nux.	30 d.
Psor.	Sulph. Tubercul.	Alum. Borax. Bar-c. Carb-v. Chin. Sulph.	Sep.?	Coff.	30-40 d.
Pulsat.	Ac-sul. Lyc. All-c. Sil. Kali-s. Stann. Kali-m. (Tubercul.)	Ac. nitric. Anac. Ant. Ant-t. Asaf. Ars. Bell. Bry. Calc. Euphm. Graph. Ign. Kali-s. Kali-m. Lyc. Nux. Phos. Rhus. Sep. Sil. Sulph.	—	Asaf. Coff. Cham. Ign. Nux. Stann.	40 d.
Ran-b.	—	Bry. Ign. Kali-c. Nux. Rhus. Sep. Sabad.	Ac. acet. Staph. Sulph. Vinum	Anac. Clem. Bry. Camph. Crot-t. Puls. Rhus	30-40 d.
Ran-sc.		Bell. Lach. Phos. Puls. Rhus. Sil.	—	Camph.	30-40 d.
Rheum	Mgn.c.	Bell. Puls. Rhus. Sulph.	—	Camph. Cham. Coloc. Merc. Nux. Puls.	2-3 d.
Rhod	—	Arn. Ars. Calc. Con. Lyc. Merc. Nux. Puls. Sep. Sil. Sulph.	—	Bry. Camph. Clem. Rhus.	35-40 d.
Rhus.	Bry. Calc.	Ac. mur. Ac. phos. Ars. Aran. Arn. Bell. Bry. Herb. Cact. Calc. Calc-ph.	Apis disagrees, but Phos. follows well.	Anac. Acon. Am-c. Bell. Bry. Camph. Coff. Clem. Crot-t. Graph.	1-7 d.

RELATIONSHIP OF REMEDIES

1 Remedy	2 Complements	3 Remedies that Follow Well	4 Inimicals	5 Antidotes	6 Duration
		Cham. Con. Graph. Hyos. Lach. Merc. Nux. Puls. Phos. Sep. Sulph.	(Kent).	Guaiac. Grindel. Lach. Ran-b. Sulph. Sep.	
Ruta	Calc-ph.	Ac. phos. Ac. sulph. Calc. Caust. Lyc. Puls. Sep. Sulph.	—	Camph.	30 d.
Rumex	—	Calc.	—	Bell. Camph. Con. Hyos. Lach. Phos.	—
Sabad.	Sepia	Ars. Bell. Merc. Nux. Puls.	—	Con. Puls.	20-30 d.
Sabina	Thuja	Ars. Bell. Puls. Rhus. Spong. Sulph.	—	Puls.	20-30 d.
Sambuc.	—	Ars. Bell. Con. Dros. Nux. Phos. Rhus. Sep.	—	Ars. Camph.	1 d.
Sarsap	All-c. Merc. Sepia	All-c. Bell. Hep. Merc. Phos. Rhus Sep. Sulph.	Ac. acet.	Bell. Merc. Sepia	35 d.
Secale	—	Acon. Ars. Bell. Chin. Merc. Puls.	—	Camph. Op.	20-30 d.
Selen.	—	Calc. Merc. Nux. Sep.	Chin. Vinum	Ign. Puls.	40 d.
Senega	—	Arum-t. Calc. Lyc. Phos. Sulph.	—	Arn. Bell. Bry. Camph.	30 d.

RELATIONSHIP OF REMEDIES

1 Remedy	2 Complements	3 Remedies that Follow Well	4 Inimicals	5 Antidotes	6 Duration
Sepia	Nux Natr-m. Sabad.	Bell. Calc. Con. Carb-v. Dulc. Euphm. Graph. Lyc. Ntr-c. Nux. Petr. Puls. Sars. Sil. Sulph. Rhus. Tarant.	Bry. Lach.	Acon. Ant-cr. Ant-t. Sulph. Nit-s-d. Veget. Acids.	40-50 d.
Silicea	Ac. fluor. Calc. Puls. Thuja Sanic.	Ac. fluor. Aran. Ars. Asaf. Bell. Calc. Clem. Graph. Hep. Lach. Lyc. Nux. Phos. Puls. Rhus. Sep. Sulph. Tubercul. Thuja	Merc.	Ac. fluor. Camph. Hep.	40-60 d.
Spigel.	—	Arn. Ars. Bell. Calc. Cimic. Dig. Iris. Kali-c. Kalm. Nux. Puls. Rhus. Sep. Sulph. Zinc.	—	Aur. Camph. Cocc. Puls.	20-30 d.
Stront.	—	Bell. Caust. Kali-c. Puls. Rhus. Sep. Sulph.	—	Camph.	40 d.
Spongia	—	Ac. fluor. Brom. Bry. Con. Carb-v. Hep. Kali-bro. Nux. Phos. Puls.	—	Camph.	20-30 d.
Squil.	—	Ars. Bar-c. Ign. Nux. Rhus. Sil.	All-s.	Camph.	14-20 d.
Stann.	Puls.	Calc. Kali-c. Nux. Phos. Puls. Rhus. Sulph.	—	Puls.	35 d.

RELATIONSHIP OF REMEDIES

1 Remedy	2 Complements	3 Remedies that Follow Well	4 Inimicals	5 Antidotes	6 Duration
Staph.	Caust. Coloc.	Ac. fluor. Calc. Caust. Coloc. Kali-c. Ign. Lyc. Nux. Puls. Rhus. Sulph. Selen.	Ran-b.	Ambra. Camph.	20-30 d.
Stram.	—	Acon. Bell. Bry. Cupr. Hyos. Nux.	Coff.	Ac. acet. Bell. Hyos. Nux Op. Puls. Tabac.	—
Sulph.	Acon. Ars. Aloe. Bad. Nux. Psor	Ac. Nitric. Aesc-h. Acon. Alum. Apis. Ars. Bell. Bry. Bar-c. Berb. Borax. Calc. Carb-v. Euphm. Graph. Guaiac. Kali-c. Merc. Nux. Phos. Puls. Pod. Rhus. Sars. Sep. Samb.	Sulph. follows Lyc. but Lyc. does not fotlow Sulph. (Kent.) Ran-b.	Acon. Camph. Ars. Cham. Chin. Con. Caust. Nux. Merc. Puls. Rhus. Sep. Sil.	40-60 d.
Sul-ac. (see Ac. sulph.)					
Tabac.	—	Carb-v	—	Ac. acet. Ars. Clem. Cocc. Ign. Ipec Lyc. Phos. Nux Puls. Sep. Verat. Staph.	—
Tarax.	—	Ars. Asaf. Bell. Chin. Lyc. Rhus. Staph. Sulph.	—	Camph.	14-21 d.
Tellur.	—	—	—	Nux.	30-40 d.
Therid	—	—	—	Acon. Mosch. Graph.	30 d.
Teucrium	—	Chin. Puls. Sil.	—	Camph.	14-21 d.

RELATIONSHIP OF REMEDIES

1 Remedy	2 Complements	3 Remedies that Follow Well	4 Inimicals	5 Antidotes	6 Duration
Thuja	Ars. Ntr-s. Sabina Sil. Medor.	Ac. nitric. Asaf. Calc. Ign. Kali-c. Lyc. Merc. Puls. Sabin. Sil. Sulph.	—	Camph. Cham. Cocc. Merc. Puls. Sulph. Staph.	60 d.
Tubercul.	Psor. Hydras. Sulph. Bell. Calc.	Calc-ph. Calc. Sil. Bar-c.	—	—	—
Valer.	—	Puls. Phosp.	—	Bell. Coff. Camph. Puls. Merc.	8-10 d.
Verbasc.	—	Bell. Chin. Lyc. Puls. Stram. Sulph. Sep. Rhus.	—	Camph.	8-10 d.
Verat.	Arn.	Acon. Ars. Arn. Arg-n. Bell. Carb-v. Chin. Cupr. Cham. Dulc. Ipec. Puls. Rhus. Sep. Samb. Sulph.	—	Acon. Ars. Camph. Chin. Coff.	20-30 d.
Viol-od.	—	Bell. Cina. Cor-r. Nux. Puls.	—	Camph.	2-4 d.
Viol-tr.	—	Puls. Rhus. Sep. Staph.	—	Camph. Merc. Puls. Rhus.	8-14 d.
Vespa.	—	—	Arg-n.	Ac. acet. Apis	—
Zinc.	—	Hep. Ign. Puls. Sep. Sulph.	Cham. Nux. Vinum	Camph. Hep. Ign.	30-40 d.

THE SIDES OF THE BODY AND DRUG AFFINITIES
(From Boenninghausen's *Lesser Writings*)

Most drugs having manifested their action more or less on either side of the body, both during the proving and during their use in disease, the great question is, on which side this action was more particularly manifest. This distinction as well as the degrees of this action seemed to me best indicated by different print. The same plan was pursued in my repertories of the anti-psoric and non-anti-psoric drugs, and the public seemed to be pleased with it. For the benefit of those who do not possess these repertories which are partly out of the market or have been replaced by the later works of Jahr, Mueller, Possart, and others, I will state that I used four different kinds of type.

1. COMMON TYPE, like: Agar., Alum., Ang., Ant. tart., Aur., etc., this kind of type indicates the lowest degree of action.
2. BOLD TYPE, such as: **Acon. Amm., Anac.,** etc.; this kind of print indicates: the next higher degree of action.
3. ITALICS, such as: *Ambr., Amm. mur., Ant. crud.,* etc.; this kind of print indicates the third degree, which is pretty thoroughly verified and confirmed by experience; and lastly
4. BOLD TYPE WITH ASTERISK, such as: ***Brom., *Sep.,** etc.; this is the highest and most distinguished degree.

It seems impossible that, in such an arrangement as this, incorrect statements should have occurred; on the other hand, finding a remedy is facilitated by the alphabetical order which has uniformly been observed.

In the second part of this work, the drug affinities, the remedies which belong to the lowest degree, have been omitted for the purpose of avoiding all unnecessary crowding of mere names which would simply tend to embarrass the reader; the other three degrees have been distinguished by the same varieties of print as in the first part. This second part contains the result of the examination to which I have subjected, for a number of years past, my former labors in reference to the same subject, and which has convinced me that an excessive number of remedies rendered their proper application in disease so much more difficult.

In conclusion I need scarcely remark that both parts of this little work, should only be looked upon and used as means of *facilitating the selection* of the proper remedy, and that the homoeopathic law *similia similibus* should always remain the supreme guide in the treatment of disease whenever the characteristic symptoms of the drug are indicated with sufficient clearness to enable us to decide that the spirit of the remedy which we select, is in harmony with the character of the disease.

THE SIDES OF THE BODY

INTERNAL HEAD

LEFT SIDE

Acon., Agar. Alum., *Ambr.,* **Amm.,** A. mur., **Anac.,** Ang. *Ant. crud.,* Ant. tart., *Ap., Arg., Arn.,* **Ars.,** *Asaf., Asar., Aur.,* Bar., Bell., Bism., Bor., *Bov.,* ***Brom., Bry.,** Calad., *Calc.,* Camph., Cann., Canth., *Caps.,* **C. an.,** C. veg., **Caust.,** *Cham.,* Chel., **Chin.,** *Cic., Cina.,* **Clem.,** Cocc., Coff., **Colch.,** *Coloc.,* Con., **Creos.,** *Croc.,* **Cupr.,** *Cycl., Dig.,* Dros., **Dulc.,** *Euph.,* Euphr., Ferr., Fluor., *Graph., Guaj.,* Hell., Hep., Hyosc., Ignat., *Jod.,* **Ipec.,** Kali, *Lach.,* **Laur.,** Led., Lyc., **M. arct.,** *M. austr., Magn.,* **Mang.,** Mar., **Men.,** *Merc.,* Mezer., Millef., Mosch., **M. ac.,** Natr., N. mur., **Nitr.,** *N. ac., N. mosch.,* **N. vom.,** *Oleand.,* Op., *Par.,* **Petr., Posph., Ph-ac.,** *Plat.,* Plumb., *Psor.,* **Puls.,** R. bulb., R. Scel., Rheum, *Rhod.,* **Rhus.,** Ruta, Sabad., **Sabin.,** *Samb.,* **Sarsap.,** Scill., S. corn., *Selen.,* Seneg., ***Sep.,** Sil., *Spig.,* **Spong., Stann., Staph.,** Stram., Stront., *Sulph.,* **S. ac., Tar.,** Thuj., Valer., **Veratr.,** Verb., V. od., Viol. tric., Vit., Zinc.

RIGHT SIDE

Acon., **Agar.,** *Alum.,* Ambr., Amm., A. mur., Anac., Ang., Ars., Ant. crud., Ant. tart., **Ap.,** Arg., **Arn.,** Ars., **Asaf.,** Asar., Aur., Bar., ***Bell.,** *Bism., Bor.,* Bov., Brom., *Bry.,* **Calad., *Calc.,** Camph., **Cann.,** *Canth.,* **Caps.,** C. an., ***C. Veg.,** *Caust.,* **Cham.,** *Chel.,* Chin., Cic., *Cina,* Clem., Cocc., Coff., **Colch.,** Coloc., Con., Creos., Croc., Cupr., Cycl., Dig., **Dros.,** *Dulc.,* Euph., Euphr., Ferr., *Fluor.,* **Graph.,** Guaj., **Hell.,** *Hep.,* **Hyos., *Ignat.,** Jod., Kali, **Lach.,** Laur., Led., *Lyc.,* M. arct., M. austr., **Mago.,** Mang., *Mar.,* Men., Merc., Mezer., **Millef.,** *Mosch.,* M. ac., Natr., N. mur., Nitr., N. ac., **N. mosch.,** *N. vom.,* **Oleand.,** Op., Par., Petr., **Phosph., Phosph. ac., Plat., Plumb.,** Psor., **Puls.,** *R. bulb.,* **R. scel.,** Rheum, Rhod., *Rhus,* Ruta, ***Sabad.,** *Sabin.,* Samb., Sarsap., Scill., S. corn., Selen., Seneg., **Sep., *Sil., Spig.,** Spong., Stann., **Staph., Stram., Stront., Sulph.,** *S. ac.,* Tar., *Thuj., Valer.,* Veratr., *Verb.,* Viol. od., Viol. tric., **Vit., Zinc.**

EARS

Acon., Agar., Alum., **Ammon.,** Anac., **Ang., Ant. crud., Ant. tart.,** Arg., *Ars., Asar.,* Aur., **Bar.,** Bell., **Bor.,** Calc., Caps., **C. an., C. veg.,** Caust., Cham., *Chel.,* Chin., ***Clem.,** Cocc., **Coloc.,** *Dig., Dulc.,* **Euph.,** *Graph.,* **Hep.,** Jod., Kali, Laur., **Lyc., Magn.,** M. mur., Mang., Men., *Merc.,* Millef., **M. ac.,** *Natr., N. mur.,* Nitr., N. ac., **Oleand., Petr., Phosph., Ph-ac., Plat., Rhod.,** Rhus., ***Ruta, Seneg., Sep., Sil., Spig.,** Staph., Stront., **Sulph., *Tar., Thuj., Verb.,** V. tric., Zinc.

Agar., Alum., *Ambr.,* Amm., **A. mur.,** Anac., Ang., **Aur., Bell.,** Bor., **Brom.,** *Bry.,* ***Calc., *Canth.,** Caps., C. an., C. veg., Caust., *Chel.,* Chin., Clem., Coloc., ***Con., Creos.,** Dig., *Dros.,* Graph., **Guaj.,** Hep., **Jod.,** *Kali,* Laur., **Led., Lyc.,** M. mur., **Mang.,** *Men.,* Merc., ***Mezer.,** M. ac., **Natr.,** N. mur., **Nitr.,** *N. ac.,* Petr., Phosph., Ph. ac., Plat., Psor., *Puls.,* R. bulb., **R. scel.,** Rhod., *Rhus.,* **Sabad.,** Sarsap., Sep., *Sil.,* Spig., **Spong.,** Stann., *Staph., Stront.,* Thuj., **Veratr.,** V. tric., **Vit., Zinc.**

THE SIDES OF THE BODY

EYES

LEFT SIDE

Acon., **Agar.,** Alum., Ambr., Amm., A. mur., Anac., **A. cr.,** A. tart., Ap., **Arn.,** *Ars., Asaf., Asar.,* **Aur.,** Bar., ***Bell., Bor.,*** Bov., Brom., *Bry.,* Calad., **Calc.,** Camph., Canth., Caps., C. an., C. veg., **Caust.,** *Chel., Chin.,* Cina, **Clem.,** Colch., **Con., Croc., Dros.,** Euph., **Euphr.,** Ferr., **Fluor.,** Hell., ***Hep.,*** Ignat., Jod., Kali, *Laur.,* **Lyc., M. arct.,** *M. austr.,* **Magn.,** Mar., **Men., Merc.,** Mezer., *Millef.,* M. ac., **N. mur.,** Nitr., **N. ac.,** *N. vom.,* **Oleand., Op.,** Par., Petr., **Phosph., Ph. ac.,** Plat., *Plumb.,* **Psor., Puls.,** R. bulb., R. scel., **Rheum.,** Rhod., **Rhus, Ruta,** Sabad., **Sabin.,** Sarsap., *Scill.,* **Selen.,** Seneg., *Sep.,* **Sil.,** *Spig.,* ***Spong.,*** **Stann.,** Staph., Stram., **Stront., *Sulph.,*** S. ac., *Tar., Thuj.,* Valer., Veratr., **V. od., V. tr.,** Zinc.

RIGHT SIDE

Acon., Agar., **Alum.,** Ambr., *Amm.,* A. mur., Anac., **Ang.,** A. cr., **A. tart.,** Ap., **Arn., Ars., Asaf.,** Asar., Aur., **Bar., Bell., Bism.,** Bor., **Bov., Brom.,** Bry., Calad., ***Calc.,*** *Camph.,* ***Cann.,*** *Canth.,* Caps., C. an., *C. veg.,* **Caust., Cham.,** Chel., Chin., *Cic.,* Cina, *Clem.,* Coff., Colch., ***Coloc.,*** *Con.,* **Creos.** Croc., **Cycl.,** *Dig.,* Dros., **Euph.,** Euphr., **Ferr.,** *Fluor.,* **Graph., Guaj., Hep., Hyosc., Ignat.,** Jod., *Kali,* Laur., **Led., *Lyc.,* M. art.,** M. austr., **M. mur.,** *Mang.,* **Mar.,** *Merc.,* Millef., **M. ac.,** *Natr.,* ***N. mur.,*** *Nitr.,* ***N. ac.,*** **N. mosch.,** N. vom., Oleand., *Par.,* ***Petr.,*** Phosph., Ph. ac., ***Plat.,*** *Plumb.,* **Psor., Puls., R. bulb.,** *R. scel.,* Rheum., *Rhod.,* ***Rhus,*** Ruta, Sabad., Sarsap., Scill., Selen., ***Seneg.,*** **Sep., *Sil.,* Spig.,** Spong., Stann., *Staph.,* Stram., **Sulph.,** S. ac., Tar., Thuj., **Valer.,** Veratr., V. tr., **Vit.,** Zinc.

EARS

Acon., Agar., Alum., **Ambr.,** *Amm.,* A. mur., ***Anac.,*** Ang., A. cr., *Ap.,* Arg., *Arn.,* **Ars., *Asaf,*** Asar., *Aur.,* Bar., Bell., **Bism., *Bor.,*** Brom., *Bry.,* Calad., **Calc.,** *Camph.,* Cann., Canth., **Caps.,** C. an., **C. veg., Caust.,** Chel., Chin., Cic., Clem., Colch., Con., **Creos.,** Croc., Cupr., Cycl., Dig., Dros., *Dulc.,* Euph., Euphr., Ferr., Fluor., ***Graph., *Guaj.,*** Hep., ***Ignat.,*** Jod., Kali, Lach., *Laur.,* Lyc., Mang., Mar., Men., *Merc.,* Mezer., *Millef.,* **M. ac.,** Natr., N. mur., Nitr., **N. ac.,** N. mosch., ***Oleand.,*** Par., Petr., **Phosph.,** Ph. ac., Plat., Plumb., *Psor.,* **Puls.,** R. bulb., R. scel., Rheum., **Rhod., Rhus,** Sabad., **Sabin.,** Sarsap., Scill., Selen., Seneg., **Sep.,** Sil., **Spig.,** Spong., **Stann.,** Staph., **Sulph.,** Tar., Thuj., Valer., Veratr., *Verb.,* ***Viol. od.,*** Viol. tric., Vit., Zinc.

Acon., *Agar., Alum.,* Ambr., Amm., A. mur., Anac., Ang., *A. crud.,* Ap., Arg., Arn., Ars., Asaf., **Asar., Bar., *Bell.,*** Bor., *Bov.,* Brom., Bry., **Calad.,** *Calc.,* **Cann.,** Canth., C. an., C. veg., **Caust., Cham.,** Chel., Chin., Cic., Clem., **Cocc., Colch.,** Coloc., **Con.,** Creos., Croc., **Cupr., Cycl.,** Dig., Dros., Dulc., Euph., Euphr., Ferr., ***Fluor.,*** Graph., **Hell.,** *Hep.,* **Hyosc., *Jod.,*** *Ipec.,* *Kali,* **Lach.,** Laur., **Led.,** *Lyc.,* **M. arct., Magn., M. mur.,** Mang., Mar., Men., Merc., Mezer., Millef., M. ac., Natr., N. mur., *Nitr., N. ac.,* **N. mosch.,** ***N. vom.,*** Par., **Petr.,** Phosph., **Ph. ac., *Plat.,*** Plumb., Psor., *Puls.,* **R. bulb.,** *R. scel.,* Rheum, Rhod. *Rhus.,* Ruta, Sabad., Sabin., **Samb.,** *Sarsap.,* Spill., Selen., Seneg., Sep., *Sil.,* Spig., ***Spong.,*** Stann., Staph., Sulph., S. ac., Tar., *Thuj.,* Valer., **Veratr.,** Verb., Zinc.

1103

THE SIDES OF THE BODY

NOSE

LEFT SIDE

Agar., *Amm.,* **A. mur.,** Anac., **A. cr., Ap.,** Ars., **Asar.,** *Aur., Bell., Bor., Bov.,* Brom., **Bry., Calc.,** Canth., **Caps.,** C. an., ***C. veg.,** *Caust.,* Chel., **Chin.,** *Cina,* Cocc., *Coff., Coloc.,* Dros., **Dulc.,** Fluor., Graph., **Hell.,** Hep., Kali., Laur., Lyc., M. arct., **Magn., M. mur.,** Mar., *Merc.,* ***N. mur.,** N. ac., *N. mosch.,* **N. vom., Oleand.,** Petr., **Phosph.,** *Plat.,* Psor., Puls., ***Rhod., Rhus,** Sabin., **Sarsap.,** ***Sep.,** *Sil.,* **Spong.,** Stann., **Staph., Sulph.,** Tar., **Thuj.,** V. tr., Zinc.

RIGHT SIDE

Acon., **Alum., Ambr.,** Amm., A. mur., Anac., A. crud., **Asaf., Aur.,** *Brom., Bry.,* **Calad.,** *Calc.,* **Canth.,** C. an., C. veg., Caust., *Chel.,* **Cic.,** Cocc., **Colch.,** ***Con.,** *Croc.,* Dros., *Fluor., Graph.,* Hep., *Jod., Kali,* Laur., Lyc., **M. arct., Mang.,** *Mar.,* Merc., **Natr.,** N. mur., **Nitr.,** *N. ac.,* **N. vom.,** Petr., *Phosph., ph-ac.,* Plat., *Psor.,* Puls., *R. bulb.,* **R. scel.,** *Rhus,* Sabin., Sarsap., Sep., *Sil.,* ***Spig.,** Stann., *Sulph.,* S. ac., Tar., *Thuj.,* **Veratr., V. od.,** V. tr., **Vit.,** Zinc.

FACE

Acon., Alum., **Amm.,** Anac., **A. cr.,** A. tart., **Ap.,** Arg., **Arn.,** Ars., *Asaf.,* **Asar.,** Aur., **Bar., Bell., Bor., Bov.,** *Brom.,* Bry., **Calc.,** *Cann.,* **Canth., Caps.,** *C. an.,* **C. veg., Caust.,** Cham., Chel., Chin., Cic., **Cina,** *Clem.,* Cocc., **Coff.,** Colch., *Coloc.,* **Con.,** Creos., **Cupr.,** Dig., Dros., **Dulc., Euph., Euphr.,** Fluor., Graph., Guaj., **Hell.,** Hep., *Hyosc.,* **Ignat.,** Jod., Kali, **Lach.,** Laur., **Led.,** Lyc., ***M. arct.,** Magn., M. mur., Mang., Mar., Men., **Merc., Mezer.,** Millef., Mosch., *M. ac.,* Natr., **N. mur.,** Nitr., N. ac., N. mosch., N. vom., *Oleand.,* Par., Petr., Phosph., **Ph. ac., Plat.,** Plumb., Psor., **Puls.,** R. bulb., *Rhod.,* **Rhus, Ruta, Sabad., Sabin., Samb., Seneg.,** Sep., Sil., Spig., *Spong.,* Stann., Staph., Stram., Stront., **Sulph.,** S. ac., Tar., **Thuj.,** valer., **Veratr., Verb., V. od.,** *V. tr.,* Zinc.

Acon., **Agar., Alum.,** Amm., *A. mur.,* **Anac.,** A. cr., A. tart., Ap, **Arg.,** Arn., *Ars.,* Asaf., Asar., *Aur.,* **Bar., *Bell., Bism.,** Bor., Brom., *Bry.,* ***Calc.,** Cann., ***Canth., Caps.,** C. an., C. veg., *Caust.,* Cham., **Chel.,** Chin., Cina, *Cocc.,* **Colch.,** Coloc., **Con.,** Creos., Cupr., **Cycl.,** Dig., **Dros., Dulc.,** Euph., *Fluor.,* **Graph.,** Guaj., *Hep.,* Hyos., Jod., **Kali, Lach.,** Laur., Led., ***Lyc.,** M. arct., **Magn.,** M. mur., **Mang., Mar., Men.,** *Merc.,* **Mezer.,** Millef., **Mosch.,** *Natr.,* N. mur., **Nitr.,** *N. ac.,* **N. mosch., *N. vom.,** Oleand., Par., Petr., *Phosph.,* Ph. ac., Plat., **Plumb.,** *Psor.,* **Puls.,** R. bulb., R. scel., **Rheum.,** *Rhus.,* Sabad., Sabin., **Sarsap., Sep.,** *Sil., Spig.,* Spong., Stann., *Staph.,* Stram., Stront., **Sulph.,** S. ac., **Tar., Thuj., Valer.,** Veratr., **Verb.,** *Vit.* Zinc.

TEETH

Acon., *Agar.,* **Alum.,** Ambr., **Amm., A. mur.,** Anac., *Ap., Arn.,* **Asaf., Asar., Aur.,** *Bar.,* Bell., *Bor.,* **Brom., Bry., Calc.,** Canth., **C. ar., C. veg., *Caust., *Cham., Chel.,** *Chin.,* ***Clem., Colch., Con., Creos.,**

Agar., Alum., **Ambr., Amm.,** Anac., *Ang.,* Ap., **Aur., Bav., *Bell., Bov.,** Brom., *Bry.,* Calc., **Camph., Cann.,** Canth., C. an., C. veg., **Caust., Chin., Coff.,** Colch., **Coloc.,** Con., *Creos.,* ***Fluor., Graph.,** *Hell.,* Jod.,

THE SIDES OF THE BODY

LEFT SIDE

Croc., Cycl., Euph., Fluor., Graph., *Guaj.*, Hyosc., Jod., Kali., *Laur.*, Led., Lyc., *M. arct.*, Mar., *Merc.*, *Mezer., Millef., N. mur., Nitr., *N. mosch.*, N. vom., Oleand., *Phosph.*, Puls., R. scel., Rheum., *Rhod.*, Rhus., Sabad., Sabin., Samb., Selen., Seneg., *Sep., *Sil., Spig.,* Spong., *Staph., Stront., Sulph., *Thuj., Veratr., Verb., *Zinc.*

RIGHT SIDE

Kali., Lach., Laur., Lyc., *Magn.*, Mang., Mar., Merc., Mezer., Natr., N. mur., N. ac., *N. vom.*, Oleand., *Petr.*, Ph. ac., *Psor.*, Puls., *R. bulb.*, R. scel., Rhod., Rhus, Ruta, *Sabad.*, Sarsap., Sep., Sil., Spig., Spong., *Staph., Stront., Sulph:, *Tar., Thuj.*, Valer., *Verb.*, Vit., Zinc.

MOUTH AND FAUCES

Acon., Alum., Ang., A. crud., A. tart., Ap., Aur.. Bar., *Bell., Bov., Calc., C. an., C. veg., *Caust.,* Colch., Creos., Croc., Cupr., Dros., Euph., Fluor., *Graph.,* Hep., Jod., *Kali,* Lach., Lyc., M. austr., Mar., Men., Mezer., Millef., N. mur., N. ac., N. mosch., *N. vom.,* Oleand., Phosph., Ph-ac., Plat., Psor., *puls.,* Rhod., *Rhus,* Sabad., Sabin., *Seneg.,* *Sep., Sil., Spig., *Sulph.,* Tar., Thuj., Veratr., *Zinc.*

Alum., *Amm.,* A. crud., Ars., Aur., Bov., Brom., Calc., *C. veg.,* Caust., Chin., Coloc., Creos., *Dros., Fluor.,* Graph., Jod., Lach., M. arct., Mar., *Merc., Millef., N. mur., N. ac., N. vom., Petr., Plat., Plumb., Psor., R. bulb., Rhus, Sabad., Sep., Sil., Spig., Stann., Sulph., Thuj., Zinc.

HYPOCHONDRIA

Acon., Agar., Alum., Amm., A. *mur.*, Anac., *A. crud:,* Ap., Arg., *Arn., Ars.,* *Asaf., *Asar.,* Aur., Bell., *Bor.,* Brom., Bry., Calad., Calc., *Cann.,* C. an., *C. veg.,* Caust:, *Cham.,* Chel., *Chin.,* Cocc., Coff., Con., Creos., Cupr., Dig., Dulc., *Euph.,* Ferr., *Fluor., Graph., Hep., *Ignat., Jod., Ipec., Kali., Laur., Lyc., Mang., Mar., Merc., *Mezer.,* Millef., Mosch., *M. ac.,* Natr., N. mur., Nitr., *N. Ac., N. vom., Oleand., Par., Petr., Phosph., Ph-ac., Plat., Plumb., Puls., *Psor.,* R. bulb., R. Scel., *Rheum.,* Rhod., Rhus, Ruta., Sabad., Sarsap. Scill., S. corn., Seneg., *Sep.,* Sil., Spig., Stann., Staph., *Sulph., S. ac., Valer., *Verb.,* V. tric., *Vit.,* Zinc.

*Acon., Agar., *Alum., Ambr.,* *Amm., A. mur., *Anac.,* Ang., A. crud., Ap., Arn., Ars., Asaf., *Bar., *Bell., Bor., *Bry., Calad., *Calc., Canth.,* C. an., C. veg., Caust., Chel., Chin., Clem., *Cocc., Colch., Con., Creos., *Dig.,* Dulc., Ferr., Fluor., Graph., Hep., Hyosc., Ignat., Jod., *Kali, *Lach.,* Laur., Led., *Lyc., M. arct., M. austr., *M. mur., Mang., Mar., *Merc.,* Millef., Mosch., Natr., *N. mur.,* N. ac., N. mosch., *N. vom., Par., *Petr.,* Phosph., Ph. ac., Plat., Plumb., Psor., Puls., R. bulb., R. Scel., Rhod., Rhus., Ruta, *Sabad.,* Sabin., *S. corn.,* Selen., Sep., Sil., Spig., Stann. Staph., Sulph., S. ac., *Valer.,* veratr., Verb., Vit., Zinc.

THE SIDES OF THE BODY

ABDOMEN

LEFT SIDE

Acon., Agar., **Alum.**, Ambr., *Amm.*, *A. mur.*, Anac., Ang., A. crud., *A. tart.*, Ap., Arg., Arn., Ars., *****Asaf.**, **Asar.**, **Aur.**, Bar., **Bell.**, Bov., **Brom.**, *Bry.*, Calc., Camph., **Cann.**, Canth., **Caps.**, C. Veg., Caust., *Cham.*, Chel., **Chin.**, *Cina*, Cocc., Colch., Coloc., **Con.**, **Creos.**, Croc., *Cupr.*, **Dig.**, *****Dulc.**, Euph., *****Fluor.**, *****Graph.**, *Guaj.*, *****Hep.**, Ignat., **Jod.**, *Kali.*, Laur., **Led.**, *Lyc.*, **M. arct.**, M. austr., M. mur., **Mang.**, Mar., **Men.**, Merc., **Mezer.**, *Millef.*, **M. ac.**, Natr., *N. mur.*, N. ac., N. mosch., **N. vom.**, **Oleand.**, Op., *Par.*, Petr., **Ph. ac.**, Plat., *****Plumb.**, **Psor.**, *Puls.*, R. bulb., *****Rheum.**, Rhod., Rhus., **Ruta**, **Sabad.**, Sabin., **Samb.**, *Sarsap.*, Scill., **Selen.**, Sep., Sil., *Spig.* **Spong.**, Stann., **Staph.**, *****Sulph.**, **S. ac.**, *****Tar.**, Thuj., *Valer.*, **Verb.**, V. tric., Vit., Zinc.

RIGHT SIDE

Agar., *Ambr.*, A. mur., Anac., **Ang., A. crud.**, Ap., Arg., **Arn.**, *****Ars.**, psaf., Aur., *Bar.*, Bell., **Bism.**, **Bry.**, **Calad.**, Calc., Csmph., Cann., *Canth.*, *C. an.*, *C. Veg.*, *Caust.*, Chel., Chin., **Cic.**, **Clem.**, Cocc., **Colch.**, *Coloc.*, Con., Creos., **Croc.**, Cupr., **Cycl.**, Dig., **Dros.**, Dulc., Fluor., Graph., Guaj., *Ignat.*, Jod., **Ipec.**, Kali., *Lach.*, Laur., *Lyc.*, M. austr., **M. mur., Mar.**, Men., **Merc.**, Mezer., Millef., **Mosch.**, Nstr., N. mur., *Nitr.*, N. ac., N. mosch., **N. vom.**, Oleand., Petr., **Phosph.**, Ph. ac., **Plat.**, Plumb., Psor., Puls., R. bulb. **R. scel.**, Rhod., *Rhus.*, Sabad., **Sabin.**, Samb., Scill., *Seneg.*, Sep., Sil., Spig., Spong., **Stann.**, **Stront.**, Sulph., Tar., *Thuj.*, Verb., **V. tric.**, Vit., Zinc.

ABDOMINAL RINGS

Agar., **Alum.**, **Ambr.**, *Amm.*, A. mur., **A. crud.**, *Ap.*, **Arg.**, Arn., **Asar.**, Aur., Bell., Calc., Camph., **Cann.**, Canth., C. an., **Chel.**, Cocc., **Dig.**, *Dulc.*, *****Euph.**, Fluor., Graph., *Ignat.*, Kali., Laur., .Lyc., **M. arct.**, **M. austr.**, *****Magn.**, **M. mur.**, **Merc.**, *N. ac.*, N. mosch., **N. vom.**, **Par.**, **Phosph.**, Rhod., Rhus., **Sabad.**, Sabin., Sarsap., **Sep.**, Sil., **Spig.**, Spong., **Stann.**, **Staph.**, *Sulph.*, **S. ac.**, **Tar.**, **Veratr.**, V. tr., Vit., Zinc.

Alum., Amm., *A. mur.*, **Ap., Ars.**, *Aur.*, **Bell., Bor.**, *****Calc.**, Camph., Cann., Canth., C. an., *C. veg.*, **Cic., Clem., Cocc.**, *Coloc.*, **Con.**, Dig., **Dros.**, Dulc., Fluor., Graph., **Hell., Jod., Ipec.**, *****Kali**, *****Lach.**, *Laur.*, *****Lyc.**, **Mang., Mar.**, *Merc., Mezer.*, *****N. vom.**, **Op.**, *Petr.*, **Ph.ac.**, **Psor.**, *****Puls.**, **R. bulb.**, *****Rhod.**, *****Rhus.**, **Ruta**, **Sabin.**, Sarsap., *Seneg.*, **Sep.**, *Sil.*, Spig., Spong., Stann., *Staph.*, **Stront.**, Sulph., *****S. ac.**, *****Thuj.**, *Valer.*, *Veratr.*, Vit., Zinc.

SEXUAL ORGANS

Agar., Alum., Ambr., **A. mur.**, *Ang.*, **A. cr.**, *Ap.*, **Arg., Am., Bar.**, *Brom.*, **Bry.**, Calc., **Cann., Chin.**, **Clem.**, **Colch., Con., Euph.**, *Fluor.*, **Graph.**, *Kali.*, Lyc., M. arct., *Magn.*, Mar., Men., **Merc.**, Mezer., **Natr.**, *N. ac.*,

Acon., Alum., **Ap.**, *Arn.*, Aur., **Bism.**, *****Calc.**, **Cann.**, **Canth.**, *****Caust.**, *Clem.*, **Coff.**, *Coloc.*, Con., **Croc.**, *Graph.*, *****Hep.**, *Jod.*, *Lach.*, *Lyc.*, M. arct., Mar., *Men.*, *Merc.*, Mezer., **M. ac.**, N. ac., *****N. vom.**, Petr., Puls.,

THE SIDES OF THE BODY

LEFT SIDE

Petr., *Ph. ac.,* **Plumb., Puls.,** *Rhod.* **Rhus. Sabad.,** Selen., **Sep.,** Sil., Spig., Staph., Tar., **Thuj., *Zinc.**

RIGHT SIDE

Rhod., *Sabin.,* **S. corn.,** Selen., *Sil., Spig.,* *****Spong.,** Staph., **Sulph., *S. ac.,** Tar., *Valer.,* **Veratr.,** *Zinc.*

NECK AND NAPE OF THE NECK

Alum., Amm., Anac., Ang., A. cr., **A. tart., Ag., Arg.,** Asaf., Aur., *Bell., Bism.,* Bry., **Calc., Camph., Canth., Caps.,** C. veg., *****Caust., Chel., Chin., Cina,** Cocc., *Colch., Coloc., Con.,* **Cupr., Dulc., *Fluor.,** Guaj., *Hep.,* Jod., *Kali., Lach., Laur.,* **Led., Lyc., M. austr.,** *****Mar., Men., Merc.,** *Mezer.,* **Natr., N. mur., Nitr., *N. ac.,** *N. vom.,* Oleand., **Petr.,** Ph. ac., **Plat., Plumb., Puls.,** Rhod., Sabin., **Sarsap.,** *Seneg., Sil.,* **Spig.,** *Spong.,* Staph., **Sulph.,** *S. ac.,* Thuj., Vit., Zinc.

Acon., Alum., **A. mur., Anac.,** Ang., *****Ap., A. crud.,** Arg., **Arn.,** Ars., *****Asaf.,** *Asar.,* Aur., **Bar.,** Bell., **Bor., Bov., Brom., Bry., *Calc., Canth., C. an., C. veg.,** Caust., **Cic.,** Cocc., Colch., **Coloc., Croc., Cycl.,** Fluor., *Guaj.,* **Hyosc., Ignat.,** Kali, Lach., Laur., *Lyc.,* Mar., Merc., Mezer., **Mosch., N. vom.,** *Oleand.,* **Par.,** ph. ac., **Psor.,** Rhod., **Rhus.,** *Sabin.,* **Scil.,** Selen., **Sep., Sil.,** Spig., **Spong., Staph.,** Stram., *****Sulph., S. ac.,** *Tar., Thuj.,* **Veratr., V. tr.,** Vit., Zinc.

CHEST

Acon., **Agar.,** Alum., Ambr., **Amm., *A. mur., Anac.,** Ang., **A. cr.,** *A. tart., Ap.,* Arg., Arn., **Asaf.,** Asar., **Aur., Bar., Bell., Bism.,** Bor., **Bov.,** Brom., **Bry., Calad., Calc., Camph.,** *Cann.,* **Canth., Caps., C. an.,** *C. veg., Caust., Cham.,* **Chel.,** *Chin.,* **Cina,** Clem., *Cocc.,* Colch., Coloc., **Con.,** *Creos.,* **Croc., Cupr., Cycl.,** Dig., **Dros.,** *Dulc.,* *****Euph., *Fluor.,** Graph., *Guaj.,* **Hep.,** Hyosc., *Ignat.,* *****Kali,** Lach., *****Laur.,** Led., *****Lyc.,** Mag., *M. arct., M. austr.,* **Magn.,** *Mang.,* Mar., *Men., Merc.,* Mezer., Millef, **Mosch.,** M. ac., **Natr.,** *N. mur.,* **Nitr., *N. ac.,** N. mosch., *****N. Vom.,** *Oleand.,* Par., Petr., *Phosph., Ph. ac.,* **Plat., Plumb.,** Psor., **Puls.,** *R. bulb.,* R. scel., **Rheum.,** *Rhod.,* *****Rhus,** *Ruta,* Sabad., *Sabin.,* Sarsap., **Scill.,** *****Seneg., Sil.,** *Spig., Spong.,* **Stann.,** *****Staph.,** Stront., *****Sulph.,** *S. ac,* **Tar.,** *Thuj., Valer.,* **Veratr., Verb.,** *V. tr.,* Vit., Zinc.

Acon., Agar., **Alum.,** Ambr., *Amm.,* A. mur., Anac., Ang., A. cr., A. tart., **Arg.,** *****Arn., Ars.,** *Asaf.,* Asar., *Aur.,* Bar., *****Bell.,** Bism., *Bor.,* Bov., *Bron.,* **Bry.,** Calad., **Calc.,** Camph., **Cann.,** *Canth.,* Caps., *****C. an., C. veg.,** Caust., **Cham.,** Chel., *Chin.,* Cic., Cina, Clem., **Cocc., Colch., *Coloc.,** Con., Creos., Croc., Cupr., Cycl., *Dig.,* Dros., **Dulc.,** Euph., Fluor., **Graph.,** *Hep., Hyos.,* Ignat., *****Jod., Ipec.,** Kali., *****Lach.,** Laur., **Led.,** *Mgs.,* **M. arct.,** M. austr., *M. mur.,* Mang., **Mar.,** Men., **Merc.,** Mezer., Millef., M. ac., Natr., **N. mur.,** Nitr., **N. ac.,** N. mosch., **N. vom.,** Oleand., *Op.,* **Par.,** Petr., **Phosph., Ph. ac.,** Plat., Plumb., **Psor., *Puls., R. bulb., R. scel.,** Rheum., **Rhus, Ruta, Sabad.,** Sabin., Sarsap., *Scill.,* Seneg., **Sep., *Sil., Spig.,** Spong., Stann., Staph., Stront., **Sulph.,** S. ac, *Tar.,* Thuj., Valer., *Veratr.,* **V. tric., Vit.,** Zinc.

THE SIDES OF THE BODY

BACK

LEFT SIDE

Acon., Agar., Alum., Ambr., **Amm.**, A. mur., Anac., Ang., A. cr., A. tart., Ap., Arg., **Ars., Asaf.,** Aur., Bar., *Bell., Bism., Bry., Calc., Cann., Canth., C. an., **C. Veg.,** Caust., Chel., Chin., Cina, **Cocc.,** Colch., **Coloc.,** Con., **Creos., Croc., Cupr., Dig.,** *Dros., **Dulc.,** Euph., **Ferr., Fluor.,** Graph., Guaj., **Hell.,** Hep., Ignat., Jod., **Kali.,** Laur., **Led., Lyc., Mgs., M. austr.,** Mang., Mar., Men., Merc., Mezer., **Millef., Mosch.,** M. ac., **N. mur., Nitr.,** N. ac., N. vom., Oleand. Par., Petr., Phosph., **Ph-ac.,** Plat., Plumb., **Psor., Puls.,** R. scel., **Rhod., Rhus.,** Ruta, Sabad., Sabin., Sarsap., *Scill., Seneg., Sep., *Sil., **Spig.,** Spong., Stann., **Staph., Stront.,** Sulph., S. ac., Tar., **Thuj.,** Valer., Veratr., Verb., V. tric., Vit., Zinc.

RIGHT SIDE

Acon., Agar., Alum., Ambr., Amm., **A. mur.,** Anac., Ang., **A. cr., A. tart.,** Ap., **Arg.,** Arn., **Ars.,** Asaf., **Asar., Aur.,** Bar., Bell., **Bor., Brom.,** *Calc., Cann., Canth., C. an., C. veg., **Caust.,** Chel., Chin., *Cic., Cina, Cocc., **Colch.,** Coloc., Con., Cupr., Dig., Dros., Dulc., Euph., *Fluor., Guaj., Hep., **Jod., Kali.,** Laur., Lyc., M. arct., M. austr., Mar., Men., Merc., Mezer., Millef., Mur. ac., N. mur., N. ac., N. vom., Oleand., Petr., Phosph., Plat., *Plumb., R. bulb., R. scel., Rhod., Rhus., Ruta, **Sabad.,** Samb., Sarsap., **Sep., Sil.,** Spig., Spong., Stann., Staph., **Sulph.,** S. ac., Tar., Thuj., Verb., V. tric., Vit., *Zinc.

UPPER EXTREMITIES

Acon., Agar., Alum., Ambr., Amm., A. mur., *Anac., Ang., A. crud., **A. tart.,** Ap., Arg., *Arn., **Ars., Asaf.,** Asar., Aur., Bar., **Bell.,** Bism., Bor., Bov., **Brom., Bry., Calad., Calc., Camph., Cann.,** Canth., Caps., C. an., **C. veg.,** Caust., Cham., Chel., **Chin., Cic., Cina.,** Clem., **Cocc., Coff.,** Colch., Coloc., **Con.,** Creos., **Croc.,** Cupr., **Cycl.,** Dig., Dros., Dulc., Euph., **Euphr.,** Ferr., Fluor., Graph., Guaj., Hell., Hep., **Hyosc., Ignat., Jod., Ipec., *Kali., Lach., Led.,** Lyc., Mgs., M. arct., *M. austr., Magr., M. mur., Mang., Mar., **Men., Merc.,** Mezer., Millef., **Mosch., M. ac.,** Natr., **N. mur., Nitr.,** N. ac., **N. mosch., N. vom.,** Oleand., **Op.,** Par., Petr., Phosph., Ph. ac., Plat., Plumb., **Psor., Puls.,** R. bulb., R. scel., Rheum, Rhod., *Rhus., Ruta, Sabad., *Sabin., Samb., Sarsap., *Scill., S. corn., Selen.,

Acon., Agar., Alum., Ambr., Amm., **A. mur.,** Anac., Ang., A. crud., A. tart., **Ap.,** Arg., Arn., Ars., Asaf., Asar., Aur., Bar., *Bell., *Bism., Bor., Bov., Brom., *Bry., Calad., *Calc., Camph., Cann., Canth., Caps., C. an., **C. Veg.,** *Caust., Cham., Chel., Chin., Cic., Cina, Clem., Cocc., Coff., Colch., *Coloc., Con., Creos., Croc., Cupr., Cycl., **Dig., Dros., Dulc.,** Euph., Euphr., **Ferr.,** Fluor., *Graph., Guaj., Hell., Hep., Hyosc., Ignat., Jod., **Ipec.,** Kali, Lach., Laur., Led., **Lyc., Mgs.,** M. arct., M. austr., **Magn.,** M. mur., Mang., Mar., Men., Merc., Mezer., Millef., Mosch., M. ac., Natr., N. mur., Nitr., N. ac., N. mosch., N. vom., Oleand., Op., Par., **Petr.,** *Phosph., **Ph. ac.,** Plat., Plumb., Psor., **Puls.,** R. bulb., R. scel., **Rheum.,** *Rhod., Rhus., Ruta, Sabad., Sabin., Samb., Sarsap., Scill., S. corn., Selen., Seneg., *Sep.,

1108

THE SIDES OF THE BODY

LEFT SIDE

Seneg., **Sep.**, **Sil.**, Spig., Spong., ***Stann.**, **Staph.**, **Stram.**, **Stront.**, ***Sulph.**, S. ac., *Tar.*, **Thuj.**, *Valer.*, **Veratr.**, *Verb.*, Viol. od., *V. tric.*, Vit., **Zinc.**

RIGHT SIDE

*Sil., Spig., Spong., Stann., **Staph.**, Stram., Stront., **Sulph.**, *S. ac.*, Tar., **Thuj.**, Valer., Veratr., Verb., **Viol. od.**, V. tr., **Vit.**, **Zinc.**
Acon., *Agar.*, Alum., ***Ambr.**, **Amm.**, A.

LOWER EXTREMITIES

mur., **Anac.**, Ang., A. crud., *A. tart.*, *Ap.*, *Arg.*, **Arn.**, **Ars.**, ***Asaf.**, **Asar.**, *Aur.*, *Bar.*, **Bell.**, Bism., **Bor.**, **Bov.**, Brom., **Bry.**, *Calad.*, ***Calc.**, Camph., Cann., Canth., Caps., C. an., C. veg., *Caust.*, Cham., **Chel.**, Chin., *Cic.*, ***Cina.**, **Clem.**, **Cocc.**, Colf., Colch., **Coloc.**, **Con.**, *Creos.*, *Croc.*, Cupr., Cycl., **Dig.**, Dros., **Dulc.**, **Euph.**, **Euphr.**, ***Ferr.**, **Fluor.**, **Graph.**, **Guaj.**, *Hell.*, ***Hep.**, *Hyosc.*, **Ignat.**, *Jod.*, Ipec., Kali, **La'ch.**, Laur., **Led.**, ***Lyc.**, **Mgs.**, M. arct., *M. austr.*, *Magn.*, M. mur., Mang., **Mar.**, *Men.*, *Merc.*, *Mezer.*, Millef., **Mosch.**, M. ac., Natr., N. mur., Nitr., ***N. ac.**, N. mosch., **N. vom.**, Oleand., Op., Par., **Petr.**, **Phosph.**, Ph. ac., **Plat.**, Plumb., **Psor.**, **Puls.**, **R. bulb.**, R. scel., *Rheum.*, Rhod., ***Rhus**, *Ruta,* Sabad., *Sabin.*, Samb., Sarsap., Scill., S. Corn., *Selen.*, **Seneg.**, **Sep.**, ***Sil.**, Spig., Spong., **Stann.**, Staph., Stram., **Stront.**, ***Sulph.**, *S. ac.*, Tar., Thuj., **Valer.**, **Verat.**, Verb., V. od., V. tr., **Vit.**, *Zinc.*

Acon., Agar., **Alum.**, Ambr., Amm., A. mur., Anac., **Ang.**, A. crud., A. tart., **Ap.**, **Arg.**, *Arn.*, ***Ars.**, Asaf., Asar., *Aur.*, Bar., ***Bell.**, Bism., Bor., Bov., **Brom.**, ***Bry.**, Calad., **Calc.**, **Camph.**, Cann., *Canth.*, Caps., **C. an.**, **C. veg.**, **Caust.**, Cham., Chel., **Chin.**, Cic., Cina., Clem., *Cocc.*, *Coff.*, Colch., ***Coloc.**, *Con.*, Creos., Croc., **Cupr.**, Cycl., Dig., **Dros.**, Dulc., Euph., Ferr., *Fluor.*, ***Graph.**, **Guaj.**, Hell., **Hep.**, Hyosc., **Ignat.**, Jod., Ipec., Kali, ***Lach.**, *Laur.*, **Led.**, **Lyc.**, Mgs., M. arct.; M. austr., *Magn.*, M. mur., Mang., **Mar.**, **Men.**, **Merc.**, **Mezer.**, **Millef.**, Mosch., M. ac., **Natr.**, **N. mur.**, Nitr., **N. ac.**, *N. mosch.*, ***N. vom.**, **Oleand.**, Op., *Par.*, Petr., ***Phosph.**, *Ph. ac.*, Plat., Plumb., **Psor.*, **Puls.*, R. bulb., *R. scel.*, Rheum., ***Rhod.**, **Rhus**, Ruta, *Sabad.*, *Sabin.*, *Samb.*, ***Sarsap.**, Scill., ***S. Corn.**, Selen., Seneg., ***Sep.**, **Sil.**, Spig., **Spong.**, St:nn., *Staph.*, **Stram.**, Stront., **Sulph.**, S. ac., *Tar.*, *Thuj.*, Valer., *Veratr.*, *Verb.*, V. od., *V. tr.*, Vit., **Zinc.**

GENERAL SYMPTOMS

Acon., **Agar.**, Alum., Ambr., Amm., A. mur., *Anac.*, Ang., *A. crud.*, *A. tart.*, ***Ap.**, **Arg.**, **Arn.**, Ars., ***Asaf**, ***Asar.**, Aur., **Bar.**, Bell., Bism., Bor., **Bov.**, *Brom.*, Bry., Calad., Calc., Camph., Cann., Canth., ***Caps.**, C. an., C. veg., Caust., *Cham.*, Chel., *Chin.*, Cic., ***Cina.**, **Clem.**, Cocc., Coff., Colch., Coloc., Con., *Creos.*, ***Croc.**, **Cupr.**, Cycl., **Dig.**,

Acon., Agar., **Alum.**, Ambr., Amm., A. mur., Anac., **Ang.**, A. cr., A. tart., Ap.; Arg., Arn., Ars., Asaf., Asar., **Aur.**, Bar., ***Bell.**, *Bism.*, Bor., Bov., Brom., *Bry.*, Calad., ***Calc.**, Camph., **Cann.**, ***Canth.**, Caps., C. an., C. veg., **Caust.**, Cham., Chel., Chin., Cic., Cina, Clem., **Cocc.**, Coff., *Colch.*, ***Coloc.**, *Con.*, Creos., Croc., Cupr., Cycl., Dig., **Dros.**, Dulc.,

THE SIDES OF THE BODY

LEFT SIDE

Dros., *Dulc.,* ***Euph.,** *Euphr.,* Ferr., Fluor., Graph., *Guaj.,* Hell., Hep., Hyosc., **Ignat.,** Ipec., Kali., Lach., Laur., Led., Lyc., Mgs., *M. arct.,* ***M. austr., Magn.,** M. mur., Mang., Mar., Men., Merc., **Mezer., Millef.,** Mosch., *M. ac.,* Natr., N. mur., Nitr., **N. ac.,** N. mosch., N. vom., ***Oleand.,** Op., *Par.,* Petr., Phosph., Ph. ac., Plat., Plumb., Psor., Puls., R. bulb., R. scel., *Rheum.,* Rhod., Rhus., *Ruta,* Sabad., *Sabin.,* Samb., Sarsap., ***Scill.,** S. corn., ***Selen.,** Seneg., Sep., Sil., *Spig.,* Spong., ***Stann.,** Staph., **Stram.,** Stront., ***Sulph.,** S. ac., **Tar., Thuj., Valer.,** Veratr., **Verb.,** *V. odor., v. tric.,* **Vit., Zinc.**

RIGHT SIDE

Euph., Euphr., Ferr., **Fluor.,** Graph., Guaj., Hell., Hep., Hyosc., Ignat., *Jod., Ipec.,* Kali., ***Lach.,** Laur., Led., ***Lyc., Mgs.,** M. arct., M. austr., Magn., *M. mur., Mang., Mar.,* Men., Merc., Mezer., Millef., **Mosch., M. ac.,** *Natr.,* N. mur., **Nitr.,** N. ac., *N. mosch.,* ***N. vom.,** Oleand., **Op.,** Par., *Petr.,* **Phosph.,** Ph. ac., Plat., **Plumb.,** Psor., *Puls.,* R. bulb., ***R. scel.,** Rheum., Rhod., *Rhus.,* Ruta, *Sabad.,* Sabin., Samb., ***Sarsap.,** Scill., ***S. corn.,** Selen., Seneg., Sep., *Sil.,* Spig., Spong., Stann., *Staph.,* Stram., **Stront.,** Sulph., **S. ac.,** Tar., Thuj., Valer., **Veratr.,** Verb., Viol. od., Viol. tric., *Vit.,* Zinc.

GENERAL SYMPTOMS

LEFT UPPER SIDE
RIGHT LOWER SIDE

Alum., Anac., Arn., Ars., **Bar., Bell., Brom.,** Camph., Caps., *C. an.,* Cham., **Chin., Coff., Con.,** Cycl., Euphr., *Fluor.,* Hep., *Kali.,* Lach., Laur., Led., M. arct., M. austr., M. mur., **Mar.,** Men., **Merc.,** Millef., M. ac., N. mur., Nitr., N. ac., **N. mosch.,** N. vom., **Oleand.,** Op., **Par., Ph. ac.,** *Puls.,* R. scel., Rhod., *Rhus.* Sabad., **Sabin.,** Samb., **Sarsap.,** *Scill.,* **S. corn., Seneg.,** Spong., *Stann.,* **Staph.,** Stram., **Sulph., *Tar.,** *Thuj.,* Valer., Veratr., Verb., V. tric.

LEFT LOWER SIDE
RIGHT UPPER SIDE

Acon., Agar., *Ambr., Amm., A. mur., Ang., A. crud., A. tart., **Arg.,** Asar., **Bism.,** *Bor., Bov.,* Bry., Calad., *Calc.,* Cann., C. veg., *Caust.,* Chel., Cic., **Cina,** Colch., **Coloc.,** Croc., Cupr., **Dig.,** Dulc., Euph., **Euphr.,** *Ferr.,* Graph., Hell., Hyosc., Ignat., Jod., Ipec., *Lyc.,* Mgs., Magn., Mang., Mezer., **M. ac.,** Natr., **N. vom., *Phosph.,** Plat., **Plumb.,** R. bulb., **Rheum, Rhus,** Ruta, Selen., *Sil.,* Spig., ***S. ac.,** V. od., Vit.

FEBRILE SYMPTOMS

Agar., Ambr., **A. crud.,** Arn., **Bar.,** Caust., Cham., *Chin.,* Dig., **Lyc., Par.,** *Plat.,* Puls., ***Rhus,** Ruta, Spig., ***Stann.,** Sulph., **Thuj., Verb., Vit.**

Ambr., *Bell.,* **Bry., Caust.,** Chin., Cocc., **Fluor.,** Nat., *N. vom.,* ***Phosph., *Puls.,** *R. bulb.,* **Sabin.,** Spig., Verb.

DRUG AFFINITIES

ACON.	— *Arn., Ars.,* ***Bell., *Bry., *Canth., *Cham.,** *Coff,* **Croc., Dulc., Graph.,** *Lyc.,* ***Merc.,** *Millef., N. vom., Op., Phosph., Ph. ac., Puls.,* ***Rhus, Ruta, *Sep.,** *Sulph., Valer.,* **Veratr.**
AGAR.	— *Bell.,* ***Calc.,** *Cocc.,* **Coff., *Lyc.,** *N. ac.,* ***N. vom.,** *Petr., Phosph., Puls., Sep.,* ***Sil.,** *Sulph.*
ALUM.	— ***Bry.,** *Calc., Cham.,* **Ignat.,** *Ipec.,* **Lach.,** *Lyc., N. mur.,* **Phosph., Plumb.,** *Puls.,* **Veratr.**
AMBR.	— *Bell., Calc., Lyc., N. vom., Puls.,* **Staph.,** *Sulph.*
AMM.	— *Brom., Calc.,* **Fluor.,** *Hep., Phosph., S corn.*
A. MUR.	— *Ars.,* **N. vom.,** *Puls., Rhus.*
ANAC.	— **Calc.,** *Coff., Con., N. mur.*
ANG.	— **Bry., Calc., Lyc.,** *Rhus.,* **Verb.**
A. CRUD.	— *Ars.,* **Bism., Brom., *Hep., Ipec., *Merc., Puls.,** *Sep.,* ***Sulph.**
A. TART.	— ***Bell.,** *Chin., Cocc.,* **Con.,** *Ipec., Op., Puls., Sep.*
APIS M.	— ***Ars.,** *Bell., Canth., Chin.,* **Ferr., Graph.,** *Hep.,* **Jod., Kali, Lach.,** *Lyc., Merc., Millef.,* ***Puls.,** *Sep., Sulph.*
ARG.	— **Merc.**
ARN.	— *Acon., Arn.,* **Bry., Cann., Caps.,** *Chin.,* ***Cic.,** *Ferr., Ignat.,* ***Ipec.,** *Merc.,* **Millef.,** *Puls.,* **Rhus, Sabin., Samb.,** *Scill., Seneg., Veratr.,* ***Zinc.**
ARS.	— **Acon., A. mar.,** *Ant. cr, Arn.,* ***Ap.,** *Bar.,* **Brom.,** *Bry.,* **Calc.,** *C. veg.,* ***Cham., *Chin.,** *Coff., Dig.,* **Colch., Dulc., Eupb., *Ferr.,** *Graph.,* ***Hep.,** *Ignat.,* ***Jod., *Ipec., Kali,** *Lach.,* ***Lyc., Mang., *Merc., Mosch., M. ac.,** *N. mur.,* **N. vom.,** *Petr., Phosph., Ph. ac.,* **Plumb., R. Scel.,** *Samb., Scill., S. corn., Sep., Sill,* **Stam.,** *Staph.,* ***Sulph., S. ac.,** *Veratr.*
ASAF.	— **Aur.,** *Caust.,* ***Chin., Men., *Merc.,** *N. ac., Ph. ac.,* **Plat.,** *Puls., Sep.*
ASAR.	— *Cupr., N. vom., Phosph.*
AUR.	— **Asaf, Calc., Coff.,** *Merc., N. vom., Puls.,* **Phosph.**
BAR.	— *Ars.,* **Calc., N. vom., Sep., Zinc.**
BELL.	— ***Acon.,** *Agar., Ambr., A. tart., Ap., Bry.,* ***Calc., Cann., Canth., Caust.,** *Cham., Chin.,* **Cic., Cina,** *Coff., Colch., Coloc., Croc., Cupr.,* **Dig.,** *Graph.,* **Hell., *Hep., Hyosc.,** *Jod.,* ***Lach.,** *Merc.,* ***Mosch.,** *N. ac.,* ***N. vom.,** *Op., Ph-ac.,* **Plat.,** *Plumb.,* **Puls.,** *Rheum., Rhus., Sarsap., Seneg.,* ***Sep., Sil.,** *Stram.,* **Sulph.,** *Valer.*
BISM.	— **A. crud., *Calc.,** *Cocc.,* **Ignat.,** *Spig.,* **Staph.**
BOR.	— *Bry., Calc., Cham.,* **Coff.,** *Sil., Sulph.*
BOV.	— **N. ac.,** *Selen.,* **Sil.**
BROM.	— ***Amm., A. crud., Ars., Camph., Coff.,** *Hep.,* **Jod., Magn., N. Mur., Op.,**

DRUG AFFINITIES

	Phosph., *Spong.*
BRY.	— *****Acon., *Alum., Ang.,** *Ars.,* **Bell., Bor., Calc.,** *C. veg.,* **Caust.,** *Chin., Clem.,* **Coloc.,** *Dulc.,* **Guaj.,** *Jod.,* Ipec., *Kali, Led., Lyc., Mezer.,* **Millef., Phosph., *Puls.,** *R. bulb.,* *****Rhod., *Rhus.,** Scill., Seneg., **Sep.,** Veratr.
CALAD	— *Canth.,* *****Caps.,** *Ignat.,* **N. vom.**
CALC.	— *****Agar., Alum.,** *Ambr. Amm.,* **Anac., Ang., Ars., Aur., Bar., *Bell., *Bism.,** *Bor.,* **Bry.,** *Cann.,* Caust., **Chel.,** *Chin.,* **Cocc., Cupr.,** *Fluor.,* **Graph.,** *Ignat.,* **Jod., *Ipec.,** *Kali,* *****Lyc.,** *M. mur.,* **Men., Merc., *Natr.,** Nitr., *****N. ac., *N. Vom.,** *Petr.,* **Phosph.,** *Ph. ac.,* *****Puls.,** *Rhus.,* Sabin., *****Sarsap.,** *Selen., Sep.,* *****Sil., *Sulph.,** Caust., Veratr., Vit.
CAMPH.	— **Brom.,** *Canth.,* *****Op., Verat.**
CANN.	— **Arn.,** *Bell.,* **Calc., Canth.,** Coloc., *Euph.,* Men., **N. mur.,** *N. ac.,* **Puls.,** *Thuj.*
CANTH.	— *****Acon.,** *Ap.,* Bell, **Calad.,** *Camph.,* **Cann.,** *Laur.,* *****Lyc., *Puls.**
CAPS	— **Arn., *Calad.,** Cham., **Chin.,*Cina,**Ignat., **N. vom.,** Puls.
C. AN.	— **C. veg.,** Rhod., *****Thuj.**
C. VEG.	— *Ars.,* **Bry., C. an., *Chin.,** *Dulc., Ferr,. Ignat.,* **Ipec.,** *Kali, Lach.,* *****Merc.,** *N. mur.,* **N. ac.,** *N. vom.,* **Op.,** *Petr.,* **Puls., Rhod.,** *Sep., Sulph.,* Veratr.
CAUST.	— *Asaf.,* **Bell.,** *Bry.* **Calc., Cocc.,** *Clem.,* **Coloc., Creos., Cupr., Graph., Hep.,** *Ignat.,* *****Lach.,** Lyc., *****Natr.,** *N. vom.,* **Phosph.,** *Plat.,* **Puls., Rhod., Rhus., *Sep.,** Sil., *****Sulph.**
CHAM.	— *****Acon., Alum.,** *Ars.,* **Bell., Bor., Caps.,** *Chin., Cina,* *****Cocc., Coff.,** **Coloc., *Hep., *Ignat.,** Ipec., Lyc., **Magn., *N. vom.,** Petr., *****Puls.,** *Rheum.,* **Rhus., Stram.,** *Sulph., Valer.*
CHEL.	— **Calc., Lyc., Puls., Sulph.**
CHIN.	— **Amm.,** *A. tart., Ap.,* *****Arn., *Ars., *Asaf., *Bell.,** *Bry.,* **Calc., Caps.,** *****C. veg.,** *Cham., Cupr., Cycl., Dig.,* *****Ferr., Fluor.,** *Hell., Jod.,* *****Ipec., *Lach., *Merc.,** **Millef.,** *N. mur.,* **N. vom., Phosph.,** *Ph. ac.,* **Plumb., *Puls.,** *Samb., Sep., Stann., Sulph.,* **S. ac., *Veratr.**
CIC.	— *****Arn.,** **Bell.,** *Dulc.,* **Lyc., Merc., Op., Rhus., Stram., Veratr.**
CINA.	— **Bell., *Camps.,** *Chin.,* **Dros., Hyosc., Merc., Phosph., Veratr.**
CLEM.	— *Bry.,* **Graph.,** *Merc.,* *****Rhod.,** *Rhus.*
COCC.	— **Agar.,** *A. tart., Bism.,* **Calc., Caust.,** *****Cham.,** *Cupr.,* *****Ignat., *Ipec.,** *Kali,* **Mosch., N. mosch.,** *N. vom.,* **Oleand.**
COFF.	— Acon., **Agar., Anac., Ars., Aur.,** *Bell.* **Bor., Brom., Caps.,** *Cham.,* *****Coloc., Con.,** *Ignat.,* **Magn., Mar., Merc., Mosch.,** *N. vom.,* **Op., Puls. Sulph.,** *Valer., Veratr.*
COLCH.	— **Ars.,** *Bell., Fluor.,* **Merc.,** *N. vom., Op.,* **Puls.**

DRUG AFFINITIES

COLOC.	— *Bell.*, **Bry.**, **Cann.**, *Caust.*, **Cham.**, *****Coff.**, **Magn.**, *Rheum.*, *S. corn.*, *****Staph.**
CON.	— *Anac.*, **A. tart.**, *Coff*, **Cupr.**, **Cycl.**, **Dig.**, **Dulc.**, *****Lach.**, *Lyc.*, *N. ac.*, **N. vom.**, *Puls.*, **Vit.**
CREOS.	— **Caust.**, *N. mur.*, *****N. Vom.**, *Sep.*, *Sulph.*
CROC.	— **Acon.**, **Bell.**, *Op.*, **Plat.**
CUPR.	— **Bell.**, **Calc.**, *Caust. Chin.*, **Cocc.**, **Con.**, *Dulc.*, *****Hep.**, *Hyosc.*, *Ignat.*, **Ipec.**, *Lyc.*, **Merc.**, *N. vom.*, *Op.*, **Ph. ac.**, *****Puls.**, *Sep.*, **Sil.**, **Sulph.**, *****Veratr.**
CYCL.	— **Con.**, *Puls.*
DIG.	— *Ars.*, **Bell.**, **Chin.**, **Con.**, **Merc.**, *N. vom.*, *Op.*, **Phosph.**, **Ph. ac.**, *Plat.*, *Puls.*, **Spig.**, **S. ac.**
DROS.	— **Cina**, **Hep.**, **Ipec.**, *N. vom.*, **Sep.**, *Spong.*, *Veratr.*
DULC.	— **Acon.**, **Ars.**, **Bry.**, *Cic.*, **Con.**, **Cupr.**, **Led.**, **Merc.**, *N. vom.*, **Ph. ac.**, **Puls.**, *Rhus.*, **Sep.**, **Sulph.**
EUPH.	— **Ars.**, **Lyc.**, **Merc.**, *Mezer.*, **Puls.**, **Rhus.**, **Sep.**, *Zinc.*
EUPHR.	— *Cann.*, *Hep.*, *N. vom.*, **Spig.**
FERR.	— **Ap.**, *Arn.*, *****Ars.**, *C. veg.*, **Chin.**, *****Hep.**, *Ipec.*, **Puls.**, **Sulph.**, **S. ac.**, *Veratr.*
FLUOR.	— **Amm.**, *Calc.*, **Chin.**, *Colch.* *****Graph.**, *****N. ac.**, *Sil.*
GRAPH.	— **Acon.**, **Ap.**, *Ars.*, **Bell.**, **Calc.**, *Caust.*, *****Fluor.**, **Guaj.**, *Kali*, *Lyc.*, **Magn.**, *****Natr.**, *N. ac.*, *N. vom.*, *Phosph.*, *****Puls.**, *Sep.*, **Sil.**, **Sulph.**, *Thuj.*, **Vit.**
GUAJ.	— **Bry.**, **Graph.**, **Merc.**
HELL.	— **Bell.**, *Chin.*, **Phosph.**
HEP.	— *Amm.*, *****A. Crud.**, **Ap.**, *****Ars.**, *****Bell.**, **Brom.**, **Caust.**, *****Cham.**, *****Cupr.**, **Dros.**, *Euphr.*, *****Ferr.**, **Ignat.**, *****Jod.**, *****Lach.**, **Lyc.**, *****Merc.**, *N. ac.*, *Rhus.*, *Sep.*, *****Sil.**, *****Spong.**, **Sulph.**, *Thuj.*, *****Zinc.**
HYOSC.	— *****Bell.**, *Cina. Cupr., Op., Ph. ac., Plumb.*, *****Stram.**, *Valer.*, *Veratr.*
IGNAT.	— **Alum.**, *Arn.*, *Ars.*, *Bism.*, **Calad.**, **Calc.**, **Caps.**, *C. veg.*, *Caust.*, *****Cham.**, **Cocc.**, *Coff.* **Cupr.**, **Hep.**, **Ipec.**, **Lyc.**, **Mar.**, *Mgs.*, *M. arct.*, *M. austr.*, *N. vom.*, **Ph. ac.**, *Plat.*, **Puls.**, **Ruta.** *Selen.*, **Stram.**, **Valer.**, *****Zinc.**
JOD.	— **Ap.**, *****Ars.**, *Bell.*, **Brom.**, **Bry.**, **Calc.**, **Chin.**, *****Hep.**, **Kali**, **Lyc.**, **Merc.**, *Par.*, *Phosph.* **Sil.**, *Spong.*, **Sulph.**
IPEC.	— **Alum.**, **A. crud.**, *****A. tart.**, *****Arn.**, *****Ars.**, **Bry.**, *****Calc.**, **C. Veg.**, **Cham.**, **Chin.**, **Cocc.**, **Cupr.**, **Dros.**, **Ferr.**, **Ignat.**, *Laur.*, *Nitr.*, *****N. vom.**, **Op.**, **Phosph.**, **Puls.**, **S. ac.**, *Veratr.*
KALI.	— **Ap.**, *Ars.*, **Bry.**, **Calc.**, **C. Veg.**, **Cocc.**, **Laur.**, *Lyc.*, **Magn.**, *Natr.*, *N. mur.*, *****N. ac.**, **N. vom.**, *Phosph.*, *****Puls.**, **Sil.**
LACH.	— **Alum.**, **Ap.**, *Ars.*, *****Bell.**, *C. veg.*, *****Caust.**, **Chin.**, *****Con.**, *****Hep.**, *****Lyc.**, *****Merc.**, *N. vom.*, *Ph. ac.*, *****Plat.**, *****Puls.**, *Stann.*, **Zinc.**
LAUR.	— *Canth.*, *Ipec.*, **Kali**, **Merc.**, *Spig.*

DRUG AFFINITIES

LED. — *Bry.,* **Dulc., Lyc., Puls.**

LYC. — **Acon., Agar., Alum., Ambr., Ang., Ap., *Ars.,** *Bry.,* ***Calc., *Canth., Caust., *Cham., Chel., Chin., Cic.,** *Con.,* **Cupr., Euph.,** *Graph.,* **Hep., Ignat., Jod.,** *Kali.,* ***Lach., Led., M. mur.,** *Mang.,* **Merc.,** *M. ac.,* ***Natr., N. ac., *N. vom.,** *Petr.,* **Phosph., Ph. ac., *Puls.,** *Rhus.,* **Sep., Sil., Vit.**

MGS — *Ignat.,* **Zinc.**

M. ARCT. — **Bell.,** *Ignat., M. austr.,* **Puls., Zinc.**

M. AUSTR. — *Ignat. M. arct., N. vom.,* **Zinc.**

MAGN. — **Ars., Brom.,** *Cham.,* **Coff.,** *Coloc.,* **Graph.,** *Kali.,* **M. mur.,** *N. vom.,* **Puls.,** *Rheum.*

M. MUR. — *Calc.,* **Lyc., Magn., N. Vom., *Sep., Sulph.**

MANG. — **Bry.,** *Lyc.,* **Puls.**

MAR. — **Coff., Ignat.**

MEN. — **Asaf., Calc., Cann., Plat., Sep.**

MERC. — **Acon., *A. Crud., Ap., Arg., Arn., Ars., *Asaf., Aur., *Bell., Bry.,** *Calc.,* ***C. veg., *Chin., Cic., Cina., Clem., Coff., Colch., Cupr., Dig.,** *Dulc.,* ***Euph., Guaj., *Hep., Jod., *Lach., Laur., Lyc., Mezer., *N. ac., N. vom., *Op., Ph. ac., Plat.,** *Puls.,* **Rheum., Rhod., Rhus.,** *Sarsap.,* **Selen., Sep.,** *Sil.,* **Spig., *Staph., *Sulph.,** *Thuj.,* **Valer.,** *Veratr.,* **Vit.,** *Zinc.*

MEZER. — **Bry., Euph.,** *Merc.* **M. ac.,** *N. ac., Rhus.,* **Sil., Verb.**

MILLEF. — **Acon., Ap., Arn., *Bry., Chin., *N. vom., *Puls.,** *Scill.*

MOSCH. — ***Bell., Cocc., Coff., N. vom., Op., Phosph.**

M. AC. — *Ars.,* ***Bry.,** *Lyc.,* **M. ac.**

NATR. — ***Calc., Caust.,** *Graph.,* **Kali, *Lyc.,** *N. mur.* ***Puls., Sep., Sil., Spig., Sulph.**

N. MUR. — **Alum., Anac.,** *Ars.,* **Brom., Cann.,** *C. veg., Chin., Creos.,* **Kali,** *Natr.,* **N. vom.,** *Petr.,* ***Puls.,** *Ruta,* **Spig., Vit.**

NITR. — **Calc.,** *Ipec.*

N. AC. — **Agar.,** *Asaf.,* **Bell.,** *Bov.,* ***Calc.,** *Cann., C veg., Con., Fluor.,* **Graph., *Hep., *Kali, Lyc., *Merc., Mezer., *Petr.,** *Puls., Rhus.,* ***Sep., Sulph.,** *Thuj.*

N. MOSCH. — **Cocc., Ignat., N. vom., Sep.**

N. VOM. — **Acon., *Agar.,** *Ambr.,* **A. mur., *Ars., Asar., Aur., Bar., *Bell., Calad., *Calc., Caps.,** *C. veg., Caust.,* ***Cham., Chin.,** *Cocc., Coff, Colch., Con.,* ***Creos.,** *Cupr., Dig.,* **Dros.,** *Dulc., Euphr. Graph.,* **Guaj., Ignat., *Ipec., Kali,** *Lach.,* ***Lyc., M. austr., Magn., Merc., *Millef., Mosch., M. ac., N. mur., *Op., Par., *Petr., *Phosph., Plumb.,** *Puls., Rheum.,* ***Rhus.,** *Selen.,* **Sep., Sil.,** *Stram.,* **Sulph.,** *valer.*

1114

DRUG AFFINITIES

OLEAND.	— **Cocc.**, *Vit.*
OP.	— *Acon., A. tart.,* ***Bell., Brom., Camph.,** C. veg., *Cic., Coff.,* **Colch.,** *Croc., Cupr., Dig.,* Hyosc., *Ipec.,* ***Merc., Mosch.,** *N. vom.,* **Phosph., Ph. ac., *Plumb., Stram.**
PAR.	— *Jod.,* N. vom., **Phosph.**
PETR.	— **Agar.,** *Ars.,* **Calc.,** C. veg., **Cham.,** *Lyc.,* N. mur., *N. ac.,* ***N. vom., Phosph., Puls.,** *Sil.,* **Sulph.,** *Thuj.*
PHOSPH.	— **Acon., Agar., Alum.,** *Amm. Ars.,* **Aur., Brom.,** *Calc., Caust.,* **Chin., Cina., Dig.,** *Graph.,* **Hell.,** *Jod.,* **Ipec.,** *Kali,* **Lyc., Mosch., *N. vom., Op., Par., Petr., *Puls., S. corn., Sep., Sil., Stront., Veratr., Verb.**
PH. AC.	— **Acon.,** *Ars., Asaf.,* **Bell., Calc.,** *Chin.,* **Cupr.,** *Dig.,* **Dulc.,** *Hyosc.,* **Ignat.,** *Lach., Lyc.,* **Merc., Op.,** *Rheum,* **Rhus.,** *Staph.,* **Veratr.,** Zinc.
PLAT.	— **Asaf, Bell.,** *Caust.,* **Croc.,** *Dig., Ignat.,* ***Lach., Men., Merc., *Plumb., *Puls.,** *Sabad.,* **Sabin., Stront., Vit.**
PLUMB.	— *Alum., Ars., Bell.,* **Chin.,** *Hyosc.,* **N. mur.,** *N. vom.,* ***Op., *Plat.,** *Stram.,* **Sulph.,** *S. ac.*
PULS.	— **Acon.,** *Agar., Alum., Ambr.,* **A. mur., A. crud.,** *A. tart., Ap., Arn., Asaf., Aur.,* ***Bell., *Bry., Calc., Cann., *Canth., Caps.,** C. veg., *Caust.,* ***Cham., Chel.,** *Chin., Coff., Colch., Con.,* ***Cupr.,** *Cycl., Dig.,* **Dulc., Euph., Ferr., *Graph., Ignat., Ipec., *Kali, *Lach., Led., *Lyc., M. arct., Magn., Mang., Merc., *Millef., *Natr., *N. mur., *N. ac.,** *N. vom.,* **Petr., Phosph., *Plat.,** *R. bulb.,* **Rheum.,** *Rhus., Sabad.* ***Sep.,** *Sil.* **Spig., *Stann.,** *Sulph.,* ***S. ac., Valer., Verb., Vit.**
R. BULB.	— *Bry., Puls.,* **Staph., Sulph., Verb.**
R. SCEL.	— **Ars., Puls., Veratr.**
RHEUM.	— *Bell., Cham., Coloc.,* **Magn.,** *Merc.,* ***N. vom.,** *Ph. ac.,* **Puls.**
RHOD.	— **Bry., Calc.,** C. an., C. veg., *Caust.,* ***Clem., Merc.,** N. vom., ***Rhus,** Sep.
RHUS.	— **Acon., A. mur.,** *Ang.,* **Arn., *Ars.,** *Bell.,* ***Bry.,** *Calc., Caust.,* **Cham.,** Cic., *Clem., Coff.,* **Dulc., Euph.,** *Hep., Lyc.,* **Merc.,** *Mezer.,* N. ar., ***N. vom., Phosph., Ph. ac.,** *Puls.,* ***Rhod., Samb., *Sep., Sil.,** *Sulph.,* **Veratr.**
RUTA.	— **Ignat.,** *N. mur.*
SABAD.	— **Plat.,** *Puls.*
SABIN.	— **Arn., Calc., Plat.**
SAMB.	— **Arn.,** *Ars.,* **Chin., Rhus.**
SARSAP.	— **Bell., *Calc.,** *Merc.,* **Sulph.**
SCILL.	— *Arn., Ars.,* **Bry., Millef.**
S. CORN.	— **Amm.,** *Ars., Bell., Coloc.,* **Phosph., Veratr.**

DRUG AFFINITIES

SELEN. — *Alum., *Bry., Bov., Calc., Ignat., **Merc.**, *N. vom., Puls., Sep., **Sulph.**, **Thuj.**

SENEG. — Arn., Bell., Bry., **Stann.**

SEP. — *Acon., Agar., A. crud., A. tart., Ap., Ars., Asaf., Bar., *Bell., Bry., Calc., C. veg., *Caust., *Chin., Clem., Creos., **Cupr.**, Dros., Dulc., Euph., Graph., Hep., Lyc., *M. mur., Men., **Merc.**, Natr., *N. ac., N. vom., Phosph., *Puls., *Rhod., **Rhus.**, Selen., *Sil., *Sulph., Veratr., Vit.

SIL. — Agar., Ars., **Bell.**, Bor., *Calc., Caust., **Cupr.**, Fluor., **Graph.**, *Hep., Jod., Kali, Lyc., Merc., Mezer., Natr., N. vom., Petr., Phosph., Puls., **Rhus.**, *Sep., Staph., **Sulph.**

SPIG. — Bism., Dig., Euph., Laur., Merc., Natr., N. mur., Puls., Veratr.

SPONG. — Brom., Dros., *Hep., **Jod.**

STANN. — **Ars.**, **Chin.**, Lach., *Puls., Seneg., Sulph., Valer.

STAPH. — Ars., Bism., *Coloc., Merc., Ph. ac., R. bulb., Sil., Sulph., Thuj.

STRAM. — **Bell.**, **Cham.**, Cic., Hell., *Hyosc., Ignat., N. vom., Op., Plumb., Veratr.

STRONT. — Phosph., Plat., Sulph.

SULPH. — Acon., Ambr., A. crud., Ap., *Ars., Bell., Bor., *Calc., C. veg., *Caust., Cham., Chel., Chin., Coff., Creos., Dulc., Ferr. Graph., Hep., Jod., *Merc., N. ac., N. vom., Petr., *Puls., R. bulb., **Rhus.**, Sarsap., Selen., *Sep., Sil., **Stann.**, Staph., Stront., Thuj., Valer., **Vit.**

S. AC. — Ars., Chin., Dig., Ferr., Ipec., Plumb., *Puls.

TAR. — **Con.**, **Kali**, Puls., Valer.

THUJ. — Cann., *C. an., Hep., Graph., Merc., N. ac., Petr., **Puls.**, Selen., **Staph.**, Sulph.

VALER. — **Acon.**, Bell., Cham., Coff., Hyos., **Ignat.**, **Merc.**, N. vom., **Puls.**, **Stann.**, Sulph.

VERATR. — Acon., **Alum.**, Arn., Ars., Bry., Calc., Camph., C. Veg., *Chin., Cic., Cina, Coff., *Cupr., Dros., Ferr., Hyos., Ipec., Merc., Phosph., Ph. ac., S. corn., Sep., Spig., Stram.

VERB. — Ang., Mezer., Phosph., Puls., R. bulb.

VIOL. OD. — N. vom., Phosph.

VIOL. TR. — Bar., N. ac., Rhus.

VIT. — Calc., Con., Graph., Lyc., Merc., N. vom., Oleand., Puls., Rhod., Sep., Sulph.

ZINC. — *Arn., *Bar., C. veg., Euph., *Hep., *Ignat., Lach., Mgs., M. arct., M. austr., *Merc., Ph. ac.

ESSENTIALS
OF
RARE AND UNCOMMON
REMEDIES

Otherwise referred to in 'Relationship' of the Remedies dealt with in the 'Pocket Manual'

(reproduced from 'Regionals of Boericke' 1991 Edition)

ACONITUM CAMMARUM (in 'relationship' of **Aconite nap.**)
Headache with vertigo and tinnitus, Cataleptic Symptoms Formication of tongue, lips and face.

ACONITUM FEROX (in 'relationship' of **Aconite nap.**)
—Indian Aconite—Rather more violent in action than **Acon. nap.** It is more diuretic and less antipyretic. It has proved valuable in *Cardiac dyspnoea* and acute gout. *Dyspnoea. Must it up. Rapid respiration.* Anxiety, with suffocation from feeling of paralysis in respiratory muscles. Cheynes stokes Breathing.

ACONITUM LYCOTONUM (in 'relationship' of **Aconite nap.**)
—Great yellow woflbane—swelling of gland; Hodgkins disease. Diarrhoea after eating pork. Itching of nose, eyes, anus and vulva. Skin of nose cracked; taste of blood.

ACONITUM LYCOTONUM (in 'relationship' of **Baryta iod.**)
Swelling of cervical, axillary and mammary glands.

ACONITUM LYCOTONUM (in 'relationship' of **Calc. iod.**)
Swelling of glands, Hodgkin's disease.

ESSENTIALS OF RARE AND UNCOMMON REMEDIES

AGARIC EMETIC (in 'relationship' of **Veratalli.**)
Vertigo, longing for ice-cold water; burning pains in stomach.

AGARIC PHALLOIDES (in 'relationship' of **Verat alb.**)
Cholera, cramps in stomach, cold extremities, urine suppressed.

AGARIMONIA (in 'relationship' of **Helonias.**)
—Cocklaburr—painful kidneys, impaired digestion and menstrual difficulties; Bron-chorrhoea and catarrh of bladder cough with profuse expectoration attended with expulsion of urine. Tincture 1-10 gtt.

AGARIMONIA (in 'relationship' of **Solidago virga**)
Pain in the region of kidney.

AGROSTEMA (in 'relationship' of **Secale cor.**)
—Corn cockle—active constituent is *Saponis* which causes violent sneezing and sharp burning taste; burning in stomach, extends to oesophagus, neck and breast; vertigo, headache, difficult-locomotion, burning sensation.

AGROSTIS (in 'relationship' of **Aconite nap.**)
Acts like Aconite in fever and inflammations.

ALSTONIA CONSTRICTA (in 'relationship' of **Alstonia scholaris**)
A bitter bark or native **quinine** of Australia.

ALTHEA (in 'relationship' of **Asparagus off.**)
—Marsh mallow—contains asparagin, irritable bladder. Throat and bronchi.

ALUMINIUM ACETATE (in 'relationship' of **Alumina**)
—Solution—Externally a lotion for putrid wounds and skin affections. Arrests haemorrhage from inertia of uterus. Parenchymatous haemorrhage from various organs 2-3% solution. Haemorrhage following tonsillectomy is controlled by rinsing out naso-pharynx with a 10% solution.

ALUMINIUM CHLORIDUM (in 'relationship' of **Alumina**)
Pains of locomotor ataxia. Lower trits in water.

ACONITINE (in 'relationship' of **Aconite nap.**)

Heavy feeling as of lead, pain in supraorbital nerve, ice-cold sensation creeps up; hydrophobia symptoms. Tinnitus aurium—3x. Tingling sensation.

ACHYRATHES (in 'relationship' of **Aconite nap.**)

—a Maxican drug—very similar to **Acon.** in fevers, but of larger range, being also adapted to typhoidal states and intermittents. Muscular rheumatism. A great diaphoretic—use 6x.

ADONIDIN (in 'relationship' of **Adonis vernalis**)

A cardia tonic and diuretic. Quarter grain daily, or two to five grains of first decimal trit, increases arterial pressure and prolongs the diastole, favouring emptying engorged veins. Is an excellent substitute for **Digitalis** and is not cumulative in action.

AESCULUS GLABRA (in 'relationship' of **Aesculus hipp**)

—Ohio—Buckeye— Proctitis. Very painful, dark purple external haemorrhoids, with constipation and vertigo and portal congestion. Speech thick, tickling in throat, impaired vision, paresis.

AESTRUS CAMELI (in 'relationship' of **Indigo**)

An Indian medicine for epilepsy.

AETHOLPS ANTIMONALIS (in 'relationship' of **Aethiops merc.**)

—Hydrargyrum stibiato sulfuratum—often more effective than **Aethiops marc.** in scrofulous eruptions, glandular swelling, otorrhoea and *scrofulous eye affections,* corneal ulcers 3rd trit.

AGARIC EMET. (in 'relationship' of **Agaricus musc**)

Severe vertigo; all symptoms *better, cold water; longing for ice-water;* gastritis cold sweat, vomiting, sensation as if stomach was suspended on a string.

AGARICIN (in 'relationship' of **Boletus laricis**)

—An active constituent of Polyporus officinate—phthisical and other enervating night-sweats 1-4 to 1-2 gr. doses; also in chorea in dilatation of heart with pulmonary emphysema, fatty degeneration, profuse persperation and erythema.

ESSENTIALS OF RARE AND UNCOMMON REMEDIES

AMANITA PHALLOIDES (in 'relationship' of **Agari. musc**)

—Death Cup or Deadly Agaric— The poison is a toxalbumin resembling the poison in the rattle snake and the poison excreted by the cholera and diphtheria germs. It acts on the red blood corpuscles, dissolving them so that blood escapes into the alimentary canal and the whole system is drained. The amount of this toxic principle is small, even handling of specimen and breathing of spores affects some people unpleasantly. The poison is slow in development. Even 12 to 20 hours after taking it the patient feels all right, but vertigo, violent choleric symptoms with rapid loss of strength with death. The second and third day, preceded by stupor and spasms. Fatty degeneration of liver, heart, and kidneys, haemorrhages in lungs, pleura and skin (Dr. J. Schier). Vomiting and purging. Continuous urging to stool, but *no gastric, abdominal or rectal pain*. Intense thirst for cold water, dry skin. Lethargic but mentally clear. *Sharp changes* from rapid to slow and from slow to rapid breathing, extreme collapse, suppressed urine, but not cold extemities or cramps.

AMANITA VERNUS (in 'relationship' of **Agariam musc**)

—A spring mushroom. A variety of Agaricus.

AMANITA VERNUS (in 'relationship' of **Agaricus musc.**)

—**Spring mushroom—a variety of** *Agar Phalloids—Death cup-active principle in Phallin, active like Muscarine.*

AMBER (in 'relationship' of **Ambra grisea**)

—Succinum. q.v. Moschus frequently follows advantageously.

AMMON ACET. (in 'relationship' of **Acetic acid**)

Profuse saccharine urine, patient is bathed in sweat.

AMMONIUM FORMAL. (in 'relationship' of **Formaliss**)

Cystogen—Prevents decomposition of urine in the bladder, kidneys and ureters. Turbid urine rendered clear and non-irrigating; phosphatic deposits dissolved, and growth of pyogenic bacteria arrested. Five to seven grains, two to four times daily, dissolved in hot water, after meals.

AMMONIUM TART. (in 'relationship' of **Amon. Jodat**)

By hacking cough after every cold.

ESSENTIALS OF RARE AND UNCOMMON REMEDIES

AMMONIUM VALER (in 'relationship' of **Valeriana**)
Neuralgia, gastric disturbance ; and great nervous agitation. Insomnia especially during pregnancy and menopause.

AMMON VALERIAN (in 'relationship' of **Zinc met.**)
Violent neuralgia with great nervous agitation.

AMPELOPSIS TRIFOLA (in 'relationship' of **Rhus tox**)
—Three leaf woodbine—Toxic dermatitis due to vegetable poisons-30 and 200. Very similar to Rhus poisoning. Desensitizing against Ivy poisoning by use of ascending doses of the tincture by mouth or by hypodermic injections is commended by old school authorities. But is not as effective as the homoeopathic remedies.

AMPHISBAENA (in 'relationship' of **Hekla lava**)
—Snail like lizard—has a great affinity for jaw bones, worse by air and dampness.

AMPHISBAENA (in 'relationship' of **Lachesis**)
—Snake lizard—right jaw swollen and painful, lancinating pains ; headaches. Eruptions of vesicles and pimples.

AMPHISBAENA (in 'relationship' of **Phos**)
Right jaw swollen and painful.

AMYGDALUS AMARA (in 'relationship' of **Amygd. persica**)
—Bitter Almond—Pains through tonsils, throat dark, difficult swallowing, vomiting, cough with sore chest.

ANAGYRIS (in 'relationship' of **Pulsatilla**)
Headache, amenorrhoea.

ANACARDIUM OCCI. (in 'relationship' of **Anancard.**)
Cashew nut-erysipelas vesicular, facial eruption.

ANACARD OCCI. (in 'relationship' of **Anacard ori.**)
—Cashew nut—erysipelas vesicular facial eruptions, anaesthetic variety of leprosy; warts. Corns, ulcers, cracking of the skin on soles of feet.

ANDROSACE LACTEA (in 'relationship' of **Cantharis**)
Urinary troubles diuretic; dropsy.

POCKET MANUAL OF MATERIA MEDICA: BOERICKE

ANGELICA (in 'relationship' of **Quercus gland, spirit**) 52

Produces disgust for liquor, also for atony of different organs, dyspepsia, nervous headache etc. Chronic bronchitis to increase expectoration-Tincture 5 drops 3 times a day.

ANGELICA (in 'relationship' of **Quercus Ps.S.**)

Produces disgust for liquor (in tincture five drops three times daily), also for atony of different organs, dyspepsia, nervous headache etc.; chronic bronchitis to increase expectoration.

ANGOPHORA (in 'relationship' of **Eucalyp. glob.**)

—Red Gum—Dysentery, pains, tenesmus; better lying flat on face.

ANTHOXANTUM (in 'relationship' of **Arundo**)

—Sweet vernal grass—A popular medicine for hay-fever and coryza.

ANTIARUS TOX (in 'relationship' of **Upas tiente**)

A deadly poison to the muscular system. It suspends both voluntary muscular action and that of the heart without causing convulsions Used in Java as an arrow poison (Merrell).

ANTIARUS TOXICARID (in 'relationship' of **Upas tiente**) 617

—Upas antiaris—a deadly posion to the muscular system. It suspends both voluntary muscular action and that of arrow poison (Merrel). Differs in producing *clonic spasms*, violent vomiting, diarrhoea, great prostration.

ANTIM. CHLORIDUM (in 'relationship' of **Antim crud.**)

—Butter of Antimony—A remedy for cancer. Mucous membranes destroyed. Abrasions. Skin cold and clammy. Great prostration of strength 3rd trit.

ANTIMONIUM JODAT (in 'relationship' of **Antim crud.**)

Uterine hyperplasia; humid asthma. Pneumonia and bronchitis; loss of strength and appetite, yellowish skin, sweaty, dull and drowsy.

In sub-acute and chronic colds in chest which have extended downwards from head and have fastened themselves upon the bronchial tubes in the form of hard croupy cough with a decided wheeze and inability to raise the sputum, especially in the aged and weak patients (Bacmeister). Stage of resolution of pneumonia slow and delayed.

AQUA CALCAREA (in 'relationship' of **Calc. carb.**) 191
—Lime water—½ teaspoonful in milk as injection for oxyuria vermicularis.

AQUA MARINA (in 'relationship' of **Natr. mur.**)
—Isotonic plasma—Marine plasma is a sea water taken some miles from shore and some depth below surface, filtered and diluted with twice as much pure fresh water. It acts primarily on the blood, as in intoxications, scrofulous conditions, enteritis. It disintoxicates in cancer (administered subcutaneously in the treatment of diseases of skin, kidney and intestines, gastro-enteritis and tuberculosis).
Scrofulous affections of children-Lympth adenitis. Lupus, eczema, varicose ulcers. A great *"blood purifier and vitalizer"*. Potentized sea water in weakness, lack of reaction; symptoms worse seaside. Goitre.

APIOL (in 'relationship' of **Petroselinum**)
—An active principle of Parsley—Dysmenorrhoea.

APIUM VIRUS (in 'relationship' of **Apis mell.**)
Auto—toxaemia with pus products.

ARALIA HISPIDA (in 'relationship' of **Apocy. cann.**) 122
—Wild Elder—a valuable diuretic, useful in dropsy of the cavities, either due to hepatic or renal disease with constipation. Urinary disorders, especially with dropsy. *Scudder* advises doses of five to thirty drops in sweetened cream of tartar, solution.

ARBUTIN (in 'relationship' of **Uva ursi**) 620
A crystaleized glucoside of uva; found also in Kalmia, Gaultheria and other genera of the family of *Eriaceae,* given in doses of 3 to 8 grain with sugar three times a day used as an urinary antiseptic and diuretic.

ARETOSPHYLOS MANZA. (in 'relationship' of **Uva ursi**)
Acts on renal and reproductive organs. Gonorrhoea, vesical catarrh, diabetes, menorrhagia. Tincture of leaves.

ARGENTUM CYAN. (in 'relationship' of **Argn. nit.**) 129
Angina pectoris, asthma, spasm of oesophgus.

ESSENTIALS OF RARE AND UNCOMMON REMEDIES

ARGENTUM IODAT. (in relationship of **Argen. nit.**)
Throat disosders, hoarseness, glands affected.

ARGENTUM OXYD. (in 'relationship' of **Argen. nit.**)
Chlorosis with menorrhagia and diarrhoea.

ARGENTUM PHOSPH. (in 'relationship' of **Argen. nit.**)
An excellent diuretic in dropsy.

ARGOTIN (in 'relationship' of **Secale cor.**)
Beginning arterio sclerosis progressing rather rapidly. Increased blood pressure: 2x trit. Edema, gangrene and purpura haemorrhagica; when **Secale** fails.

ARISTO. SERPEN. (in 'relationship' of **Aristo. mil.**) 12y
Virginia Snake Root—Symptoms of intestinal tract; colliquative diarrhoea, meteorism. Flatulent dyspepsia. Brain congestion. Distention and cutting pains in abdomen. Symptoms like those of poison-oak.

ARSENIC STIBIA. (in 'relationship' of **Arsenic Album**)
Chest inflammation of children, oppression, hurried respiration, crepitant rales.

ARS. SULPH. RUB. (in 'relationship' of **Ars. sulph. flav.**)
Influenza with intense catarrhal symptoms, great prostration and high temperature, purulent discharges, psoriasis, *Acne and sciatica.* Chilly even before fire. Itching in various parts. Pellagra.

ARSYNAL (in 'relationship' of **Natr. carb.**)
—Disodium methylarsenate— Introduced by M.A. Gautier for phthisis in the second stage 4 to 6 centigrammes per day for one week followed by a week's intermission. But much smaller doses, i.e. 1x to 3x are followed by improvement, lessened fever, night sweat and haemoptysis ceasing.

ARUM ITALICUM (in 'relationship' of **Arum dracon.**)
—Brain fag with headache in occipital region.

ARUM MACULATUM (in 'relationship' of **Arum dracon.**)
Inflammation and ulceration of mucous membranes. Nasal irritation with polypus.

POCKET MANUAL OF MATERIA MEDICA: BOERICKE

ESSENTIALS OF RARE AND UNCOMMON REMEDIES

ARUNDO DONAX (in 'relationship' of **Silicea**)

Acts on excretory and generative organs, suppuration, especially chronic, and where the ulceration is fistulous, especially long bones. Itching eruptions on chest, upper extremities and behind ears.

ASARUM CANADENSA (in 'relationship' of **Asarum Europ**)

—Wild Ginger—Colds followed by amenorrhoea and gastro-enteritis. Suppressed colds.

ASCLEPIA NCAR. (in 'relationship' of **Asclep. tuber.**)

—Swamp Milk Weed—Chronic gastric catarrh and leucorrhoea. Dropsy with dyspnoea.

ASCLEPIAS VINCETOXICUM (in 'relationship' of **Asclepias Syri.**)

Swallow—wart.

ASPERULA (in 'relationship' of **Sepia**)

—Nacent oxygen—Distilled water charged with the gas—leucorrhoea of young girls and uterine catarrh.

ASPIDIUM ALHAMANT. (in 'relationship' of **Filex mas.**)

—Panna—Removes tape worm; 3 doses, 2 grammes each, all in half hour, fasting in a glass of milk.

ATHAMANTHA (in 'relationship' of **Aethusa cyn.**)

Confused head, vertigo better lying down, bitter taste and saliva. Hands and feet icy cold.

ATOXYL. (in 'relationship' of **Arsenic Album**)

—Sodium arseniate—sleeping sickness; commencing optic atrophy. use in 3x.

ATRIPLEX (in 'relationship' of **Pulsatilla**)

Uterine symptoms, amenorrhoea; hysteria; coldness between shoulders, dislike of warm food. Craves strange food, palpitation, sleeplessness.

ATRPIA (in 'relationship' of **Belladonna**)

Alkaloid of **Bellad**. Cover more the neurotic sphere of Balladonna action. *Great dryness of throat*, almost impossible to swallow. Chronic stomach affections, with great pain and vomiting of all food. Peritonitis. All kinds of illusion of sight. Everything appears large. (Platina opposite) *Hypochlorhydria*, pyrosis. Motes over everything. On reading *words run together;* double vision, all *objects seem to be elongated*. Eustachian tube and tympanic congestion. Affinity for the pancreas. Hyperacidity of stomach. Paroxyms of gastric pain, ovarian neuralgia.

AURANTIUM (in 'relationship' of Citrus vulg.)

—Orange—Neuralgic and skin symptoms. Itching, redness and swelling of hands. Diseases of the aged with coldness and chilliness. Boiled dried *orange peel* excites the intestines in a manner similar to other forms of cellulose or agar. There is an increased flow of bile which continues for hours. It unites both a cholagogue action with a mechanical stimulus to peristalsis.

AURUM ARSENIC (in 'relationship' of Aurum met.)

Chronic aortitis; lupus, phthisis, in syphilitic, headache; also in anaemia and chlorosis. It causes rapid increase of appetite.

AURUM BROM. (in 'relationship' of Aurum met.)

Headache with neurasthenia, megrin, night terrors, valvular disease.

AURUM CANADENSA (in 'relationship' of Asarum Euro.)

—Wild Ginger—Colds followed by amenorrhoea and gastro-enteritis, suppressed colds.

AURUM IOD. (in 'relationship' of Aurum met.)

Chronic pericarditis, valvular diseases, arterio-sclerosis, ozaena, lupus, osteitis, ovarian cysts, myomata uteri are pathological lesions, that offer favourable ground for the action of this powerful drug. Senile paresis.

AURUM MUR. (in 'relationship' of Aurum met.)

Burning yellow acrid leucorrhoea; heart symptoms, glandular affections. Warts on tongue and genitals; sclerotic and exudative degeneration of the nervous system. Multiple sclerosis. Morvan's disease, 2nd. trit.

Aur. mur, is a sycotic remedy, causing suppressed discharges to reappear. Valuable in climacteric haemorrhages from the womb. Diseases of frontal sinus. Stitching pain in left side of forehead.

ESSENTIALS OF RARE AND UNCOMMON REMEDIES

Weariness, aversion to all work. Drawing feeling in stomcah. cancer, tongue as hard as leather; induration after glossitis.

AURUM MUR. KALI. (in 'relationship' of **Aurum met.**)
Double chloride of Potassium and gold—uterine induration and haemorrhage.

AURUM MUR. (in 'relationship' of **Aurum met.**) 149
Paralysis agitans; constant nodding of the head; affections of mammae. Swelling, pain, cracked nipples with lancinating pains.

AVIARE (in 'relationship' of **Tuberculinum**) 597
Tuberculin from birds—Acts on the apices of the lungs; has proved an excellent remedy in influenzal bronchitis symptoms similar to tuberculosis; relieves the debility, diminishes the cough, improves the appetite and braces up the whole organism; acute broncho-pulmonary diseases of children, itching of the palms and ears, *cough* acute inflammatory, irritating, incessant and tickling; loss of strength and appetite.

BACILLIN TESTICUM (in 'relationship' of **Bacillinum**)
Acts especially on lower half of the body.

BAJA (in 'relationship' of **Chin. Sulph.**) 232
—An East India drug—said to be almost infallible in intermittent fever; quartan type; pulsating, headache injected eyes, flushed face. Liver and spleen enlarged. Oedema.

BALSAMUM TELU. (in 'relationship' of **Balsam peru.**)
Balsam of Myroxylon toluifera—Chronic bronchitis with profuse expectoration.

BAPTISIA CONFUSIA (in 'relationship' of **Baptisia**)
Pain in right jaw and oppression in left-hypochondrium, producing dyspnoea and necessity to assume erect position.

BENZIN (in 'relationship' of **Benzenum**)
—Petroleum ether—not as pure a compound as B ..zene (Benzol). It is the same but with a mixture of hydrocarbons. It seems to exercise a special influence on the nervous system and on the blood Oxyhaemoglobenaemia. Physical weakness, cramps. exaggeration of

12 ESSENTIALS OF RARE AND UNCOMMON REMEDIES

knee jerks, nausea, vomiting, dizziness, *heaviness* and coldness of limbs. Tremor of eyelids and tongue.

BENZIN DINITRICUM (in 'relationship' of **Benzenum**) 164

D.N.B.—The most obvious results of poisoning by skin absorption are changes in the red blood corpuscles and liver degeneration in amblyopia, colour-blindness, retinitis. Field of vision contracted and black urine.

BENZOIN (in 'relationship' of **Acetic acid**)
—spice wood—for night sweats.

BETAINUM HYDRO. (in 'relationship' of **Beta. vulg.**)
Obtained from the Beet root itself seems to be the best adapted to phthisical patients. Children yield very quickly to the action of the remedy. 2x trit.

BIXA ORELLANA (in 'relationship' of **Piper methy.**)
South American plant related to Chaulmoogra, recommended for leprosy, eczema and elephantiasis.

BOLDO (in 'relationship' of **Chelidonium majus**) 228
—Bolda fragrans—Bladder atony; cholecystitis and biliary calculus. Bitter taste, no appetite; constipation, hypochondriasis languor, congestion of liver; burning weight in liver and stomach. Painful hepatic diseases. Disturbed liver following malaria.

BOLETUS LURIDUS (in 'relationship' of **Boletus laricis**) 171
Violent pain in epigastrium, urticaria tuberosa.

BOLETUS SATNUS (in 'relationship' of **Boletus laricis**)
Dysentery, vomiting, great debility cold extremities, spasm of face and extremities.

BOMBYX (in 'relationship' of **Astagus fluvia**)
—Caterpillar—Itching of whole body. (Urticaria).

BOUGMANCIA CANDIDA (in 'relationship' of **Sticta**) 575
Cannot concentrate thoughts; brain floats in thousands of problems and grand ideas. Floating sensation as if ideas were floating out side of brain. Headache, heartburn. Burning sensation around cardiac end of

stomach, extending to oesophagus with sense of constriction. Heat and fullness over liver region.

BRASSICA NAPUS (in 'relationship' of **Secale cor.**)
—Red seed—Dropsical swellings, scorbutic mouth, voracious appetite, tympanitis; Drooping of nails, gangrene.

BRUCEA (in 'relationship' of **Angustura vera**)
—Bark of Nux vomica or Angustura falsa—Tetanic spasms with undisturbed consciousness, worse noise, liquids, paralyzed lower extremities, worse least touch, *cries for fear of being touched.* Painful jerking of legs; cramp-like pain in knees; rigid and lame limbs of paralysis. For pain in passing of calculus.

BUNGARUS FASCIATUS (in 'relationship' of **Naja tripud.**)
Banded Krait—This venom produces a condition like an acute polio—encephalitis and myelitis, both symptomatically and histologically.

BUNGARUS KRAIT (in 'relationship' of **Crotalus hord**)
Poliomyelitis.

CACODYLATE OF SODA (in 'relationship' of **Calc. fluor.**) 193
Tumors.

CADMIUM BROM (in 'relationship' of **Cadmium sulph.**)
Pain and burning in stomach, and vomiting.

CADMIUM JODAT (in 'relationship' of **Cadmium sulph.**)
Itching of anus and rectum felt during the day only; constipation, frequent desire, tenesmus, abdomen bloated.

CAESIUM (in 'relationship' of **Oxalic acid**)
Pain in lumbar region and tesicle. Headahce, darting through temples. Diarrhoea and colic; languor.

CAFFEIN (in 'relationship' of **Coffea cruda**) 257
A crystalline alkaloid—is a direct heart stimulant and diuretic. Dropsy depending on cardiac insufficiency. Myocardial degeneration Cardiac insufficiency in pneumonia and other infectious diseases. Raises the blood presure, increases pulse rate and stimulates the heart muscle; hence, a support in extreme feebleness or threatened failure

POCKET MANUAL OF MATERIA MEDICA: BOERICKE

Stimulates the respiratory centre, nerve centres and *increases diuresis*. One of the best stimulants of the vaso-motor centres. Acute pulmonary edema. Brachialgia and other neuralgias characterized by *nocturnal exacerbations*. Jousset uses equal parts of caffein and sachar lac. 3 grains taken in divided doses every other day. Hypodermically. 1/4 grain. Excruciating facial neuralgia from decayed teeth.

CALCAREA BROM (in 'relationship' of Calc. carb.) 191

Removes inflammatory products from uterus; children of lax fiber, nervous and irritable, with gastric and cerebral irritation. *Tendency to brain disease.* Insomnia and cerebral congestion. 1x. trit.

CALCAREA CALCINATA (in 'relationship' of Calc. carb.)

—Calcined oyster-shell— A remedy for warts. Use 3d trit.

CALCAREA CAUST. (in 'relationship' of Calc. carb.)

—Slaked lime—pain in back, heels, jaws and malar bones, also symptoms of influenza.

CALCAREA HYPOPHOS. (in 'relationship' of Calc. phos)

It is to be preferred when it seems necessary to furnish the organism with liberal doses of phosphorus in consequence of continued abscesses having reduced the vitality. Give first and second decimal trits.

Loss of appetite, rapid debility, night sweats; Acne pustulosa. Pallor of skin, habitually *cold extremities*. Phthisis, diarrhoea and cough; acute pains in chest. Mesenteric tuberculosis. Bleeding from lungs; angina pectoris; asthma; affections of arteries. Veins stand out like whipcords. Attacks of pain occurring two hours after meals (relieved by a cup of milk or light food.)

CALCAREA LACTIC (in 'relationship' of Calc. carb.)

Anaemias, haemophilia, urticaria, where the coagulability of the blood is diminished; nervous headache with oedema of eyelids, lips or hands; 15 grain three times a day, but low potencies often equally effective.

CALCAREA OXALICA (in 'relationship' of Calcarea acet.)

Excruciating pains of open cancer.

ESSENTIALS OF RARE AND UNCOMMON REMEDIES 15

CALCAREA RENALIS (in 'relationship' of **Calc. phos.**)
—Lapis renalis—Arthritic.

CALC. LACTO-PHOS. (in 'relationship' of **Calc. carb.**)
5 grain 5 times a day in cyclic vomiting and migraine.

CALCAREA MUR. (in 'relationship' of **Calc. carb.**)
—Calcium chloratum—Rademacher's Liquor-Boils. *Porrigo Capitis. Vomiting of all food and drink*, with gastric pain. Impetigo, glandular swellings, angioneurotic oedema. Pleurisy with effusion. Eczema in infants. 1 part to 2 of distilled water, of which take 15 drops in half a cup of water, five times daily.

CALCAREA PICRATA (in 'relationship' of **Calc. carb.**) 191
Peri-follicular inflammation; a remedy of prime importance *in recurring or chronic boils*, particularly when located on parts thinly covered with muscle tissue, as on shin bones, coccyx, *auditory canal*, dry, scurfy accumulation and exfoliation of epithelial scales, etc. styes, phlyctenules. Use 3x trit.

CALCAREA PIC (in 'relationship' of **Picricum acid**)
Boils in and around ears.

CALCAREA RENALIS (in 'relationship' of **Calc. phos.**) 196
Lapis renalis—Arthritic nodosities. Rigg's disease; lessens tendency to accumulation of tartar on teeth; gravel and renal calculi.

CALC. SULPH-STIBIATA (in 'relationship' of **Calc. fluor.**)
Acts as an haemostatic and absorptive in uterine myoma.

CALCULOBILI (in 'relationship' of **Fel. tauri**)
Triturate Gall Stones—Gall stones 10-12x.

CAMPHOR MONO-BROM. (in 'relationship' of **Chin. sulph.**)
Intensifies the action of **Quinine** and renders it more permanent.

CAMPHORIC ACID (in 'relationship' of **Camphora**)
A prophylactic against catheter fever; cystitis, 15 grains three times a day; also for prevention of night sweats.

CANTHARIDIN (in 'relationship' of **Cantharis**)
Glomerular nephritis. The immediate pharmacologial action of

Cantharidin is irritability of the capillaries, rendering the passage of nutritive fluids through them less difficult. This is most marked in the capillaries of the kidneys. The increase of blood sugar coincident with the glomular nephritis appears to be a valuable observation.

CAPPARIS CORIACCEA (in 'relationship' of **Mercurius**)
Polyuria, glandular affections, mucous diarrhoea with tenesmus and mucous discharges; ptyalism, dysphagia; wasting of body and much debility; cholera infantum.

CARBON TETRA. (in 'relationship' of **Carbo. anii.**)
Causes fatty liver.

CARBON TETRA. (in 'relationship' of **Thymol**)
A vermifuge and vermicide of great potency, and has shown itself to be the best vermifuge for the treatment of hookworm in a country where the disease predominates. It is non-toxic and palatable. A single dose of 3c.c. (Dr. Lambert, Suva Fiji and Dr. W.G. Smilie and S.B. Parsosa of Sao Paulo Brazil.)

CARBONEUM (in 'relationship' of **Carbo veg.**)
Lampblack—Spasms commencing in tongue, down trachea and extremities. Tingling sensation.

CARDUUS BENEDICTUS (in 'relationship' of **Card. mari**)
Strong action on eyes, and sensation of contraction in many parts. Stomach symptoms similar.

CASCARA SAGRADA (in 'relationship' of **Rhamnus calif**)
Palliative in constipation, as an intestinal tonic, and dyspepsia dependent thereon 10-15 drops of tincture.

CATALPA (in 'relationship' of **Aspidosperma**)
Difficult respiration.

CEANOTHUS TRYSIFLO. (in 'relationship' of **Ceanothus**) 222
California Lilac—Pharyngitis, tonsillitis, nasal catarrh, diphtheria Tincture internally as a gargle.

CENTAUREA (in 'relationship' of **Capsicum**)
Surging of blood, homesickness and intermittent fever.

ESSENTIALS OF RARE AND UNCOMMON REMEDIES

CEPHALANTHUS (in 'relationship' of **Cinchona off.**)
—Button Bush—Intermittent fever, sore throat, rheumatic symptoms, vivid dreams.

CEREFOLIUS (in 'relationship' of **Oxydendron**) 481
Dropsy, Bright's disease, cystitis.

CEREUS SERAN. (in 'relationship' of **Cereus bomplandi**)
Very irritable with tendency to swear; wild anger and low morals Disturbance in speech; in writing leaves off the last-syllable. Paralyzed feeling. Pains in heart, and dwindling of sexual organs. Emissions followed by pain in testicles.

CETONIA (in 'relationship' of **Belladonna**) 162
Useful in epilepsy and hydrophobia (A.E. Lavine).

CETRARIA (in 'relationship' of **Sticta**) 575
—Iceland Moss—Chronic diarrhoea, phthisis, bloody expectoration. Is used as a decoction and boiled with milk as an expectorant and nutrient in bronchorrhoea catarrh etc.

CHAULMOOGRA (in 'relationship' of **Piper methysticum**)
Taraklogenos—The oil and its derivatives are to a certain extent effective in the treatment of *leprosy,* especially in early cases.

CHEIRANTHUS (in 'relationship' of **Calc. phos**)
Effects of cutting wisdom teeth.

CHEIRANTHUS (in 'relationship' of **Mag. carb.**) 416
—Wall flower—Deafness, Otorrhoea, nose stopped up at night *from irritation of cutting wisdom-teeth.*

CHELIDONIN (in 'relationship' of **Chelidonium majus.**)
Spasms of smooth muscles everywhere, instestinal colic, uterine colic, bronchial spasm, tachycardia etc.

CHENOPOD. VULV. (in 'relationship' of **Propylamin**)
The plant has an odour of decaying fish and contains a large amount of Propylamine. Weakness in lumbar and dorsal region.

CHIMAPHILA MACU. (in 'relationship' of **Chima. umbel.**)
Intense gnawing hanger; burning fever, sensation of swelling in arm

pits.

CHININUM MUR. (in 'relationship' of **Chin. ars.**)

In severe neuralgic pains around eyes, with chills; exaggerated sensitiveness to alcohol and tobacco; prostration and restlessness.

CHININUM SALICYL (in 'relationship' of **Chin sulph.**)

Deafness, tinnitus, and Meniere's disease.

CHOLAS TERRAPINA (in 'relationship' of **Cupr. met.**)

Cramps in calves and feet; rheumatism, with cramplike pains.

CHOLINE (in 'relationship' of **Taraxacum**)

A constitution of Taraxacum root, has given encouraging results in the treatment of cancer. Choline is closely related to *Neurin,* it is the "Cancronie" of Prof. Adamkiewiez (E. Schlegel).

CHOLOS TERRA. (in 'relationship' of **Ricinus Common.**)

Cramps of muscles.

CHOLOS TERRAPINA (in 'relationship' of **Verat alb.**) 624

Cramps in calves.

CHOPHEENEE (in 'relationship' of **Kali hydriod.**) 381

A Hindu remedy for syphilitic eruptions, ulceration and bone pains; use tincture.

CHROMIUM SULPH. (in 'relationship' of **Crom. acid**)

Locomotor ataxia, goitre, *prostatic hypertrophy.* Herpes preputials. Wry neck. Also exophthalmic, inhibits the vagus, relieving tachycardia. Act like a nerve tonic where there is lack of nervous tone. Fibroid tumors. Infantile paralysis.

Adult dose 3 to 5 grains after meals at bedtime.

CHRYSANTHE. LEUCAN. (in 'relationship' of **Salvia offi.**)

—Ox-eye Daisy—Has specific action on Sudoriparous glands. Quietens nervous system like *Cypripedium.* Right sided tearing pains in bones of jaw and temple. Pain in teeth and gums, worse touch, better warmth. Irritable and tearful. Here use 12x. *Insommia and night-sweats.* For colliquative sweating and hyperaesthesia of nervous system, material doses of tincture.

ESSENTIALS OF RARE AND UNCOMMON REMEDIES

CHRYSAROBIN (in 'relationship' of **Carbolic acid**) 213

Locally in ringworms of the scalp 5-10 percent in glycerine and alcohol. Equal parts.

CICER ARIETINUM (in 'relationship' of **Oxalicum acid**)

—Chick-pea—Lithiasis, Jaundice, liver affections; diuretic.

CICUTA MACULATA (in 'relationship' of **Cicuta virosa**)

Water Hemlock—Effects very similar; the most prominent symptom being: Falls unconscious, tetanic or clonic convulsions. Body covered with sweat. Consider in epilepsy and tetanus. Tincture and lower potencies.

CITRIC ACID (in 'relationship' of **Citrus vulg.**)

Useful in *scurvy* and chronic rheumatism and haemorrhages. All forms of *dropsy* are benefited with **Citric acid** and lemon juice, tablespoonful every 3-4 hours.

Pains from cancer of tongue. Used as local application and mouthwash, one dram to 8 ozs. of water. For cancer pains generally, often effective.

CITRUS DECUMANA (in 'relationship' of **Citrus vulg.**) 246

—Grape fruit—Tinnitus, *head noises* and singing in ears. Sensation of pressure in the temporal region.

CITRUS LIMONUM (in 'relationship' of **Citrus vulg.**) 246

Scorbutus, sore throat and cancer pains; checks excessive menstruation.

CLEMATIS VITALBA (in 'relationship' of **Clematis erecta**)

Varicose and other ulcers.

CLOTHO ARICLANS (in 'relationship' of **Cenchris contor.**)

—Puff Adder—Should have a great sphere of usefulness in many conditions where excessive swelling is a leading feature.

CODEIN (in 'relationship' of **Opium**)

Dry, teasing, incessant cough; twitching of muscles especially those of eyelids.

COFFEA TOSTA (in 'relationship' of **Coffea cruda**) 254

Roasting develops certain vitamin-like substances (P.T. Matter).

CROTALUS CASC. (in 'relationship' of **Crotalus hord.**)
Thoughts and dreams of death. Paralysis of articulation, embarrassed stertorous breathing and semi-consciousness. A magnetic is produced; cutting sensation all around the eyeball.

CROTALUS CASC. (in 'relationship' of **Lachesis**)
Often completes curative work of Lachesis.

CUCURBITA CITRELLS (in 'relationship' of **Sarsa.**)
—Watermelon. Infusion of the seeds act promptly in painful urination with constriction and backache, relieves pain and stimulates flow.

CULEX (in 'relationship' of **Gelsemium**)
Vertigo on blowing nose with fulness of the ears.

COUMARIN (in 'relationship' of **Tongo**) 608
A constituent of Anthoxanthum, Asperula and Tongo-to be compared in hay-fever.

CUPRESSUS AUSTRALIS (in 'relationship' of **Thuja**)
Sharp, prickling pain, general feeling of warmth, rheumatism and gonorrhoea.

CUPRESSUS LAWSONIA. (in 'relationship' of **Thuja**)
Terrible pains in stomach. Acts like Thuja.

CUPRUM CYAN. (in 'relationship' of **Cupr. met.**)
Meningitis basilaria.

CUPRUM OXY. NIG. (in 'relationship' of **Cupr. met.**) 274
All kinds of worms including tape worm and trichinosis according to Zopfy's 60 years experience.

CUPRUM SULPH. (in 'relationship' of **Cupr. met.**) 274
Burning at vertex. Incessant smasmodic cough: worse at night; tongue and lips bluish. Locally in 1 per cent solution for inoperable sarcoma.

CYDONIA VULGARIS (in 'relationship' of **Cinchona off.**)
—Quincy—supposed to be of use to strengthen the sexual organs and stoh. stomach.

CYSTISIN (in 'relationship' of **Curare**) 275
Motor paralysis.

Pigeons which have developed "deficiency", neuritis and paralysis on diet of polished rice lost their disabilities on the addition of 8cc to a 5% infusion of coffee to their food-unroasted coffee was useless.

COLCHICINE (in 'relationship' of **Colchicum**)
Intestinal catarrh with shreddy membranes; convulsive jerkings of right hand; rheumatic fever, gout, endo and pericarditis, pleurisy, arthritis deformans in early stages, *intense pain of rheumatism,* 3x trit.

COLLOIDA MANGANESE (in 'relationship' of **Mang. acet.**)
Boils and other staphylococcal infections.

COLOSTRUM (in 'relationship' of **Lac. deflo.**)
Diarrhoea in infants, whole body smells sour.

CORNUS ALTERIFOLIA (in 'relationship' of **Cornus Circinata**) 265
—Swamp Walnut— Weak and tired disturbed sleep, fever, restlessness, eczema, *skin cracked;* chest feels cold, as if full of ice.

CORNUS FLORIDA (in 'relationship' of **Cornus Circinata**) 265
Chronic malaria; indigestion and distressing acid hertburn; general debility from loss of fluids and night sweats; neuralgic pains in arms, chest, and trunk, and sensation as if broken in two, intermittent fever, with drowsiness; feels cold, but is warm to touch; great exhaustion in intervals; general clammy sweat. Chill is preceded by drowsiness, heat is associated with drowsiness. Headache after quinine.

CORYDALIS (in 'relationship' of **Stillingia**)
Syphilitic nodes.

COTO (in 'relationship' of **Cuphea.**)
Para Coto Bark—Intestinal catarrh, chronic, copious, exhausting diarrhoea and dysentery; Colliquitive sweats of phithisis and chronic diarrhoea.

CONVOLVULUS DUAR TINUS (in 'relationship' of **Berle. vulg.**)
—Morning Glory—Pain in left lumbar muscles on stooping. Kidney disorders with pain in back. Much abdominal flatulence. Aching in top of right shoulder renal colic; aching in small of back and extremities.

CYMARIN (in 'relationship' of **Apocynum cann.**)
—Active principle of **Apocyn.** lowers pulse rate and increases blood-pressure.

CYNANCHUM (in 'relationship' of **Asclep. syriaca**)
A gastro-intestinal irritant, producing vomiting and purging-useful in dropsy diabetis, great thirst, profuse urination.

DERRIS PINNATA (in 'relationship' of **Cimicifuga race.**) 239
Neuralgic headache of rheumatic origin.

DERRIS PINATA (in 'relationship' of **Kalmia lati.**) 288
Neuralgic headache of rheumatic origin.

DICTAMUS (in 'relationship' of **Sepia**)
—Burning Bush—Soothes labour pains; metrorrhagia, leucorrhoea, and constipation also somnambulism.

DIGITOXINUM (in 'relationship' of **Digit**)
—Digitalis dissolved in chloroform with a very marked yellow vision and distressing nausea, aggravated by *Champagne and aerated waters*.

DIPHTHEROTOXIN (in 'relationship' of **Caust.**) 222
Follows Caust. in chronic bronchitis.

DIPHTHEROTOXIN (in 'relationship' of **Dephtherinum**) 283
—Cahis—chronic bronchitis with rales, *Cartier* suggests it in the vagoparalytic forms of Bronchitis of the aged or in toxic bronchitis after grip.

DIPODIUM PUNCT. (in 'relationship' of **Colocynthis**) 258
Writhing. Twisting like a dying snake. Intractable insomnia.

DIRCA PALUSTRIS (in 'relationship' of **Mezereum**) 438
—Leather wood—A gastro-intestinal irritant inducing salivation, emesis and purgation; cerebral hyperaemia; neuralgic pains, with depression, palpitation, and dyspnoea.

DITAIN (in 'relationship' of **Alstonia scholasis**) 93
—Active principle—is anti-periodic like **quinine,** but without dyspepsia and debility.

ESSENTIALS OF RARE AND UNCOMMON REMEDIES

DUBOISON SULPHATE (in 'relationship' of **Dubosia**) 285

Hystero-epilepsy. Motor restlessness of insane. Has been used as a substitute for Atropia in doses of 1.20 of a grain hypodermically. 1-100 gr. sedative in mania. 2-4 milligrams a day.

ELAEIS (in 'relationship' of **Hydrocotyle**)

—South American Palm—Scleroderma, elephantiasis, leprosy, skin thickened, itching and hardened. Anaesthesia.

ELECTRICITAS (in 'relationship' of **X-ray**)

—Sugar of milk saturated with the current—Anxiety, nervous tremors, restlessness, palpitation, headache. Dreads approach of thunder-storms, heaviness of limbs.

EEL SERUM (in 'relationship' of **Digit**)

Experiments show great analogy between the serum and the venom of Vipera. Indicated whenever the systole of the heart is insufficient, decompensated valvular disease, irregular pulse due to fibrillation of the auricle. Assytole, feeble, frequent, irregular pulse, dyspnoea and scanty urine. Liver enlarged, dyspnoea, albuminuria. No. oedema.

EEL SERUM (in 'relationship' of **Vipera**)

Heart and kidney disease. Failure of compensation and impending asystole.

ELEMUY GAUTERIA (in 'relationship' of **Chelid. majus**) 228

Stones in kidney and bladder; grain doses of powdered bark in water or 5 drops of tincture. Pellagra.

EMETINE (in 'relationship' of **Ipecac**) 364

A principle alkaloid of Ipecac. A powerful amebicide, but is not a bactericide. Specific for amaebiasis, of remarkable value in treatment of amaebic dysentery; also as a remedy in Pyorrhoea 1/2 gr. daily for three days, then less. Emetin 1/2 gr. hypodermically, in Psoriasis. Emetin hydrocin 2x, diarrhoea with colicky, abdominal pains and nausea. **Emetin** for endamoebic dysentery. In Physiological doses must be carefully watched. May produce hepatization of lungs, rapid heart action, tendency for the head to fall forward and lobar pneumonia.

ESSENTIALS OF RARE AND UNCOMMON REMEDIES

EPHEDRA (in 'relationship' of **Lycopus. verg.**) 415

—Teamaster's Tea—Exophthalmic goitre; eyes feel pushed out with *tumultous* action of heart.

EPILOBIUM (in 'relationship' of **Arsenic album.**)

Intractable diarrhoea of typhoid.

EPSOM SALT (in 'relationship' of **Baryta carb.**)

An antidote for poisonous doses.

ERATHIS HYMNALIS (in 'relationship' of **Aconite nap.**)

—Winter Aconite—acts on solar plexus and works upwards causing dyspnoea. Pain in occiput and neck.

ERGOTIN (in 'relationship' of **Secale cor.**)

Beginning ateriosclerosis progressing rather rapidly. Increased blood pressure: 2x trit. Oedema, gangrene and purpura haemorrhagia; when secale, though indicated fails.

ERODIUM (in 'relationship' of **Geranium macu**)

Hemlock—Stork's bill. p. popular haemostatic in Russia, and especially used for metrorrhagia and menorrhagia.

ERYTHRINUS (in 'relationship' of **Mercurius**)

South American Red Mulltet Fish—In pityriasis rubra and syphilis; red rash on chest.

ESCHSCHOLTZIA (in 'relationship' of **Opium**)

—California Poppy—a harmless soporific.

ESERINE (in 'relationship' of **Physostigma**) 497

—The alkaloid of Physostigma—slows action of heart and increases arterial tension; in ciliary spasm and spasmodic *astigmatism* due to irregular action of ciliary muscles; blepharo-spasm; *pupils contracted*. Twitching of lids, soreness of eyeballs, blurring of vision *after using eyes*. Pains around eyes and head. Used locally to contract the pupil. *Eserine* contracts the pupils dilated by *Atropin*, but not those dilated by *Gelsemium*. Internally 6x.

ESERIN SALICYLATE (in 'relationship' of **Physostigma**)

Post-operative intestinal paralysis; meteorism. Hypodermically

ESSENTIALS OF RARE AND UNCOMMON REMEDIES 25

ETHER (in 'relationship' of **Chloroformum**) 234
Post-operative Bronchitis. (Prof. Bier)

EUCALYPTOL (in 'relationship' of **Eucalyp. glob.**) 294
Depresses temperature of healthy body more than *Quinine;* acts on kidneys like Terebinthina.

EUCALYPTUS, OIL OF (in 'relationship' of **Eucalyp. globe.**) 294
Produces remarkable bodily exhaustion, no desire for any motion; unable to do any real mental work, study etc. The volatile oil possesses in common with other terpenes, the property of converting water, in presence of air and sunlight, into hydrogen peroxide, or to convert oxygen into ozone, which is the explanation usually given of its deodorizing and antiseptic properties (Merrel). Locally, in catarrhal affections, especially when of a suppurating or putrid nature.

EUCALYPTUS ROSTRA. (in 'relationship' of **Elaps coral**)
Offensive dark discharge from right ear.

EUCALYPTUS TERET. (in 'relationship' of **Eucalyp. globe.**) 294
Menstrual cough and *prostration.*

EUGENIA CHEKUN (in 'relationship' of **Eugenia jambos**)
Chronic bronchitis.

EUONYMIN (in 'relationship' of **Euonymus atro**)
Albuminuria—1x trit.

EUONYMUS (in 'relationship' of **Euonymus atro**)
—Spindle-tree—Liver disorders, biliousness, lumbago, gastric derangements with albuminuria. Cutting pains in malar bones, tongue, penis up to bladder.

EUPHORBIA AMYGDAL. (in relationship' of **Euphorbium**) 299
—Wood Spurge—pain in antrum, illusion of smell, odor of mice. Sense of taste blunted. Diarrhoea, stools difficult, with painful, anal spasm.

EUPHORBIA COROL. (in 'relationship' of **Euphorbium**)
—Large Flowering Spurge—a diaphoretic expectorant and

POCKET MANUAL OF MATERIA MEDICA: BOERICKE

cathartic of the old school in gastro-enteric disturbances, with deathly nausea. Vomiting of food, water and mucus, and copious evacuations. Attacks recur after short intermissions. Feeling of clawing in stomach; cold sweat.

EUPHORBIA HYPERICI. (in 'relationship' of **Ipecac.**)

—Garden spurge—Very similar to **Ipecac.** Irritation of the respiratory and gastro-intestinal tracts and female organs.

EUPHORBIA MARGI. (in 'relationship' of **Euphorbium**)

—Snow on the mountain—Honey from the flowers is poisonous, detected by the hot, acrid taste. The milky juice produces skin symptoms like *Rhus.*.

EUPHORBIA PROSTA. (in 'relationship' of **Goldonrina**)

Used by Indian as an infallible remedy against bites of poisonous insects and snakes, especially the rattle-snake.

EUPHORBIA PILUL. (in 'relationship' of **Euphorbium**)

Pillbearing spurge—Humid asthma, Cardiac dyspnoea, hay-fever and bronchitis. Urethritis, with intense pain on urinating, and much urging. Acrid leucorrhoea, worse least movment. Haemorrhages from sunstroke and traumatism.

FAGUS (in 'relationship' of **Epiphagus**)

—Beech-nuts—headache and salvation; swelling of mouth; dread of water.

FABIANA (in 'relationship' of **Pareira brava**)

—Pichi—Dysuria; post-gonorrhoeal complications, gravel; vesical catarrh.

FERRUM ACETICUM (in 'relationship' of **Ferrum met.**)

Alkaline urine in acute diseases. Pain in right deltoid. Epistaxis; especially adapted to thin; pale, weak children who grow rapidly and are easily exhausted; *varices of the feat*; copious expectoration of greenish pus, asthma; worse, sitting still and lying, phthisis, constant cough, vomiting of food after eating haemoptysis.

FERRUM ARSENICUM (in 'relationship' of **Ferrum met.**)

Enlarged liver and spleen, with fever; undigested stool; albuminuria

ESSENTIALS OF RARE AND UNCOMMON REMEDIES

simple and pernicious anaemia and chlorosis. Skin dry. Eczema, psoriasis, impetigo. Use 3x trituration.

FERRUM BROMATUM (in 'relationship' of **Ferrum met.**)

Sticky, excoriating leucorrhoea; uterus heavy and prolapsed, scalp feels numb.

FERRUM CITRICUM (in 'relationship' of **Chin. ars.**)

In nephritis with great anaemia; acid dyspepsia in chloros's Morbus maculosus werlhoffii.

FARRUM CYANATUM (in 'relationship' of **Ferrum met.**)

Neuroses with irritable weakness and hypersensitiveness, especially of a periodical character; *epilepsy;* cardialgia, with nausea, flatulence, constipation, alternating with diarrhoea; chorea.

FERRUM CYANATUM (in 'relationship' of **Silicea**)

Epilepsy, neuroses, with irritable weakness and hyper-sensitiveness, especially of a periodical character.

FERRUM MURIATICUM (in 'relationship' of **Ferrum met.**)

Arrested menstruation, tendency to seminal emissions or copious urination at puberty; very dark, watery stools; diphtheria; phlegmonous erysipelas; pyelitis; heaemoptysis of dark, clotty blood; dyspareunia; pain in *right shoulder*, right elbow, and marked tendency to cramps and round red spots on cheeks; bright crystals in urine. Anaemia 3x after meals. Tincture 1-5 drops 3 times daily for chronic interstitial nephritis.

FERRUM PIC (in 'relationship' of **Picricum acid**) 500

Buzzing in ear, deafness, chronic gout; epistaxis; Prostatic troubles.

FERRUM PROTOX. (in 'relationship' of **Ferrum met.**)

Anaemia. Use 1x trit.

FERRUM PYROPHOS (in 'relationship' of **Ferrum phos.**)

Congestion of brain and headache following great loss of blood; tarsal cysts.

FERRUM SULPH (in 'relationship' of **Ferrum met.**)

Watery and painless stools; menorrhagia, pressing, throbbing between periods with rush of blood to head. Basedow's disease. Erethism—Pain in gall-bladder; toothache; acidity; eructation of food in mouthfuls.

FERRUM TART. (in 'relationship' of **Ferrum met.**)
Cardialgia; heat at cardiac orifice of stomach.

FERULA GLAUCA (in 'relationship' of **Origanum**) 478
Violent sexual excitement in women; icy coldness in occiput.

FICUS CARICA (in 'relationship' of **Sempervi. tect.**)
—Fig—The milky juice of the freshly broken stalk applied to warts; causes their disappearance.

FICUS VENOSA (in 'relationship' of **Millefolium**)
—Pakur—Haemorrhage from bowels and lungs.

FLUOROFORM (in 'relationship' of **Drosera**)
Paroxysms, considered specific for whooping-couph. 2 per cent watery solution, 2-4 drops.

FORMIC ACID (in 'relationship' of **Formica rufa**)
Chronic myalgia. Muscular pains and soreness. Gout and articular rheumatism, which appear suddenly. Pain usually worse on right side, motion and beter from pressure. *Failing vision.* Increases muscular strength and resistance to fatigue. Feels stronger and more 'fit' in products of disassimilation, particularly urea. *Tremor.* Tuberculosis, products of disassimilation, particularly area. *Tremor.* Tuberculosis, chronic nephritis and carcinoma, lupus etc. have been treated successfully with injections of Formic acid of a dilution corresponding to the 3rd and 4th centesimal. In prescribing it for varicose veins, polypi, catarrh, *Dr. J.H. Clarke* orders an ounce or two of a solution of *Formic acid* in the proportion of one part of the acid to eleven of distilled water. Of this solution one teaspoonsful is taken in a tablespoonful of water after food once or twice daily. Pain in aponeurosis and muscles of head, neck and shoulders before a snowstorm. *Rhus, Dulca, Urtica* and *Juniperus* contain *Formic acid. Wood alcohol*, when taken as a constituent of a beverage so common in these prohibition days, is not eliminated easily and is slowly converted into *Formic acid*, attacking the brain and causes death or blindness. Dr. Sylwestrowicz of Hering Research

Laboratory of Hahnemann College, Philadelphia contributes his experience with **Formic Acid**, as follows: "The best field for the formic acid treatment are cases of atypical gout. Under this classification are to be mentioned disturbances in the muscles such as myositis, periostitic processes of the bones in form of doughy swelling, changes of the fascias such as Dupuytren's contraction, skin troubles such as chronic eczema, psoriasis and loss of hair, kidney disturbances such as subacute and chronic nephritis. In these cases *Formic acid* in 12x and 30x, hypodermically 1 cc. is indicated at intervals of 2-4 weeks. Eight till twelve days after the first injection an aggravation is often noticed.

In acute rheumatic fever and acute gonorrhoeic arthritis *Formic acid* 6x, every six days 1 cc., sometimes 12x in sensitive patients shows often splendid results abolishing the pains and preventing reoccurrence.

Chronic arthritis needs a special discussion. Clinical experiments of the Hering Research Laboratory of the Hahnemann Medical College of Philadelphia on a great number of cases of arthritis with *Formic acid* showed that it preferably acts on the ligaments, capsula and bursa of the joints. Such kind of cases respond very readily to treatment.

The prognosis depends to a large extent upon the etiology of the case. The most satisfactory cases are chronic arthritis in connection with gouty diathesis. Chronic arthritis following an attack of acute rheumatic fever shows also remarkable results although often pains of neuralgic character persisting in certain spots are very stubborn. Finally chronic arthritis of traumatic nature can be cured by *Formic acid*. In the latter case *Formic acid* 6x showed quicker and better results than 12x or 30x whichare indicated in the previous cases. In general the disappearance of the stiffiness of the joint is the first sign of improvement. Then the pain and swelling cease gradually in 1-6 months time.

The prognosis of the formic acid treatment is not so favourable in chronic arthritis in which deformans processes have already taken place on the articular surfaces. Such processes in the beginning can be checked completely, advanced cases frequently show an improvement. But there is always the possibility that this improvement is only temporary. This is particularly to be expected in the cases of the so-called arthritis deformans in which even the inflammations on the ligaments and capsula are of a very progressive character."

Dose—Sixth to thirtieth attenuation.

FORMIC ACID (in 'relationship' of Tuberculinum)

Tuberculosis, chronic nephritis, malignant tumors; pulmonary tuberculosis, not in third stage, however; lupus; carcinoma of breast and stomach; Dr. Krull uses injections of solution corresponding to the 3rd centesimal potency; these must not be repeated before six months.

FRANGULA RHAMNUS (in 'relationship' of Rhamnus calif)

—Eurpean Buckthorn—a rheumatic remedy for abdominal symptoms, colic diarrhoea; haemorrhoids especially chronic.

FRANXINUS EXCELSIOR (in 'relationship' of Franxi. Ameri)

—European Ash—*Gout;* rheumatism Infusion of ash-leaves. Rademacher.

GADUS MORRHUA (in 'relationship' of Oleum jeco asel.) 473

—Cod—frequent breathing; with flapping of alae nasi; rush of blood to chest; pain in lungs and cough; dry heat in palms.

GAERTNER (in 'relationship' of Psorinum)

Pessimistic, lack of confidence, subjective troublesome eye symptoms, fear of heights. Urticaria, use 30th and 200th (Wheeler).

GELATIN (in 'relationship' of Ipecac)

Has a marked effect on coagulability of blood. Hypodermically, or if by mouth a 10 per cent jelly, about 4 oz., 3 times a day.

GALEGA (in 'relationship' of Franxinus Ameri)

—Goat's Rue—Backache; debility; anaemia and impaired nutrition. Increases the quantity and quality of the milk in nursin women, also the appetite.

GENISTA (in 'relationship' of Kali phos.)

—Dyer's Weed—contains scopolamin; frontal headache and vertigo, worse motion, better open air and eating. Dry throat, awakes with waterbrash. Itching eruption on elbows, knees and ankles. Promotes diuresis in dropsical conditions.

ESSENTIALS OF RARE AND UNCOMMON REMEDIES

GENTIANA CRUCIATA (in 'relationship' of **Gentiana lutea**)

Throat symptoms in addition to similar stomach symptoms, dysphagia, vertigo with headache; pressing inward sensation in eyes, constricted throat and head and abdomen. Distention, fulness and tightness in abdomen. Creeping over body as from fleas.

GENTIANA QUIN. FLORA (in 'relationship' of **Gentina lutea**) 321

Intermittent fever, dyspepsia, cholera infantum, weakness.

GERANIN (in 'relationship' of **Geranium macu.**) 322

Constant hawking and spitting in elderly people.

GEUM (in 'relationship' of **Hydrangea**) 345

—Water Avens—Severe jerking pains from deep in the abdomen to end of urethra; affections of bladder, with pains in penis; worse, eating; relaxed mucous membranes, with excessive and depraved secretions; imperfect digestion and assimilation.

GLACHOMA (in 'relationship' of **Paeonia**)

—Ground Ivy—Rectal symptoms.

GLACHOMA HEDERACCA (in 'relationship' of **Hedeoma**)

—Grand Ivy—Haemorrhoids with rectal irritation and bleeding. Diarrhoea. Anus feels raw and sore. Cough with laryngeal and tracheal irritation. Glandula sub-mentalis inflamed.

GUAIACOL (in 'relationship' of **Guaiacum**)

Locally in gonorrhoeal epididymitis 2 parts to 30 parts of vaseline.

GUAIACOL (in 'relationship' of **Kreosotum**)

A principle constituent of Kreosote and similar in action. Used in pulmonary tuberculosis—Dose 1 to 5 drops.

GUALANDAI (in 'relationship' of **Jacaranda**)

In syphilitic symptoms, especially of eye and throat. Chancroids; *atonic ulcers*. Dark, painless diarrhoea.

GUANO (in 'relationship' of **Carboic acid**)

Violent headache as from a band around head. Itching of nostrils, back, thighs, genitals, and symptoms like hay-fever.

ESSENTIALS OF RARE AND UNCOMMON REMEDIES

GUIPSINE (in 'relationship' of **Viscum album**)
—An active principle—exalts the hypotensive properties of Viscum.

GUNPOWDER, BLACK (in 'relationship' of **Silicea**)
Abscesses, boils, carbuncles, limb purple 3x.

HEDERA (in 'relationship' of **Ginseng.**)
—Ivy—mental depression and skin irritation antidoted by Gunpowder.

HEDERA HELIX (in 'relationship' of **Hedeoma**)
—Common Ivy—Delirium and chronic convulsions, chronic hydrocephalus, Rhinorrhoea, cerebro-spinalis. Cataract. Acts on blood vessels and menorrhagia.

HEDERA MELIX (in 'relationship' of **Viscum album**)
—Ivy-Intercranial pressure.

HEDYSARUM (in 'relationship' of **Cannabis sat**)
—Brazilian Burdock—Gonorrhoea and inflammation of penis.

HELLOTROPEUM (in 'relationship' of **'Natr. chlor.**)
Uterine displacement, with active bearing-down sensation and loss of voice; membranous dysmenorrhoea.

HELIX TOSTA (in 'relationship' of **Millefolium**) 439
—Snail—Haemoptysis, diseases of chest, consumption.

HELLEBOR FAETIDUS (in 'relationship' of **Helleborus**) 337
— Polymnia-Bear's foot—Acts especially on spleen (Ceanothus) also rectum and sciatic nerve, splenic pains extend to scapula, neck, head, worse left side and evening, chronic ague cake, hypertrophied uterus; glandular enlargement; hair and nails fall of; skin peeling.

HELLEBOR ORIENTALIS (in 'relationship' of **Helleborus**)
Salivation.

HELMINTOCHORTOS (in 'relationship' of **Cina**) 241
—Worm-moss—Acts very powerfully on intestinal worms, especially the lumbricoid.

HENCHERA (in 'relationship' of **Mercurius**)

—Alum root—Gastro-enteritis, nausea, vomiting of bile and frothy muscus; stools watery, profuse, slimy, tenesmus, never get done feeling. Dose 2 to 10 drops of tincture.

HOITZIA (in 'relationship' of **Belladonna**)

A Mexican drug similar in action to *Bellad.* Useful in fever, scarlatinal eruptions, measles, urticaria etc. High temperature with eruptive fever. Dry mouth and throat, red face, injected eyes, delirium.

HUMEA ELEGANS (in 'relationship' of **Primula ob.**)

Similar skin symptoms.

HYDRASTINUM MUR. (in 'relationship' of **Hydrastis**)

—Muriate of Hydrastis—Locally in aphthous sore mouth, ulcers, ulcerated sore throat, ozaena, etc. Internally, 3rd dec. trit. It is a uterine haemostatic and vaso-contractor; metrorrhagia, especially from fibroid tumors; haemorrhages; *in dilatation of the stomach* and chronic digestive disorders.

HYDRASTIN SULPH (in 'relationship' of **Hydrastis**)

Haemorrhages of bowels in Typhoid.1x.

HYDROBROMIC ACID (in 'relationship' of **Bromum**) 17t

Throat dry and puckering; constriction in pharynx and chest; waves of heat over face and neck; pulsating tinnitus with great nervous irritability (Houghton); vertigo, palpitation; arms heavy; seemed as if parts did not belong to him. Seems to have a specific effect on the inferior cervical ganglion, increasing the tonic action of the sympathetic, thus promoting vaso-constriction. Relieves headache, tinnitus and vertigo, especialy in vasomotor stomach disturbance. 20 drops.

HYDROPHYLLUM (in 'relationship' of **Euphrasia**) 301

—Burr-flower—Catarrhal inflammation of eyes; hot lachrymation with itching, swollen lids, dull headache; also for effects of Poison-Oak.

HYOSC. HYDROBROM (in 'relationship' of **Hyoscyamus**)

—Scopolamine hydrobromide—Paralysis agitans; *tremors of disseminated sclerosis*. Sleeplessness and nervous agitation. Dry cough in phthisis. Similar in its effects to alcohol, both recent and remote. Corresponds to the effects of strong poisons introduced into or generated within the body. Symptoms of uraemia and acute nervous exhaustion. A remedy for shock 3rd and 4rth dec. trituration. In physiological dosage (1-200 gr.) mania and chorea; Insomnia.

IKSHUGANDHA (in 'relationship' of **Caladium seg.**)
Sexual weakness, emissions, prostatic enlargement.

ILEX CASSINE (in 'relationship' of **Ilex aqui.**)
—Chrismas berry Tea—Excellent diuretic and substitute for tea.

ILEX PARAGUAYENSIS (in 'relationship' of **Ilex aqui.**)
—Yerba Mate—Persistent epigastric pain; sense of dryness of mouth and pharynx, anorexia pyrosis, nervous depression, neurasthenia. Somnolence; incapacity for work, diminution of urinary secretion, headache and pruritus. Hemicrania. Renal colic. Is said to be of use as a prophylactic against sunstroke, being a safe stimulant to the circulation, to diaphoresis and diuresis.

ILEX VOMITORIA (in 'relationship' of **Ilex aqui.**)
—Yaupon— Emetic properties—Possesses also tonic and digestive qualities, free from sleepless effects. Has an active principle said to act as a powerful diuretic-employed in nephritis and gout.

ILLECEBRUM (in 'relationship' of **Bryonia**)
A Mexican drug—Fever with catarrhal symptoms, gastric and typhoid fever symptoms.

INGLUVIN (in 'relationship' of **Ceruim oxalicum**)
—Made from gizzard of a fowl—Vomiting of pregnancy; gastric neurasthenia. Infantile vomiting and diarrhoea. 3x trit.

INSULIN (in 'relationship' of **Syzygium**) 589
An aqueous solution of an active principle from pancreas which affects sugar metabolism. If administered at suitable intervals in

diabetes meleitus, the blood sugar is maintained at a normal level and the urine remains free of sugar. Overdosage is followed by weakness and fatigue tremulousness and profuse sweating.

IODOTHYRINE (in 'relationship' of **Thyroidinum**)

The active principle isolated from thyroid gland, a substance rich in **Iodine** and nitrogen, affects metabolism, reducing weight, may produce glycosuria. Use cautiously in obesity, for a fatty heart may not be able to maintain the accelerated rhythm. Milk contains the internal secretion of the thyroid.

IRIDIUM CHLORIDE (in 'relationship' of **Iridium**)

Produces salivation and stiffness of jaws followed by head and nervous symptoms. Congestion of nares and bronchi. Dragging pain in lower back. Headache worse right side, heavy feeling as of liquid lead.

IRIS FLORENTINA (in 'relationship' of **Iris versi.**)
—Orris root—Delirium, convulsions, and paralysis.

IRIS GERMANICA (in 'relationship' of **Iris versi.**) 365
—Blue Garden Iris—dropsy and freckles.

IRIS FACTISSIMA (in 'relationship' of **Iris versi.**)
Headache and hernia.

IRIS TENAY (in 'relationship' of **Iris versi.**) 365
—Iris minor—dry mouth; deathly sensation at point of stomach, *pain in ileo-caecal region;* appendicitis. Pain from adhesions after.

JATROPHA URENS (in 'relationship' of **Jatropha**)
—Sponge nettle—Oedema and cardiac paresis.

JEQUIRITOL (in 'relationship' of **Jequirity**)

In cases of trachoma and pannus to engraft a new purulent inflammation. The proteid poisons contained in **Jaquirity** seeds are almost identical in their pathological and toxic properties with the similar principles found in snake venom.

JUGLANDIN (in 'relationship' of **Juglan cin.**)
Duodenal catarrh, bilious diarrhoea.

JUNIPERUS VIRGINI. (in 'relationship' of **Juniper. com.**)

ESSENTIALS OF RARE AND UNCOMMON REMEDIES

Red Cedar—Violent tenesmus vesical. Persistent dragging in back; hyperaemia of the kidneys; pyelitis and cystitis: dropsy of the aged with suppressed urine. Dysuria, burning, cutting pain in urethra when urinating. Constant urging, appoplexs, convulsions, strangury, uterine haemorrhage.

KALAGUA (in 'relationship' of **Tuberculinum**)
Garlicky odour of all secretions and breath.

KALI ACETICUM (in 'relationship' of **Kali carb.**)
Diabetes, diarrhoea, dropsy, alkaline urine, very much increased in quantity.

KALI CITRICUM (in 'relationship' of **Kali carb.**)
Bright's disease—1 gr to wine-glass of water.

KALI FERROCYANATUM (in 'relationship' of **Kali carb.**)
—Prussian blue—Physical and mental prostration following infection. Inability to sustained routine work. Neuralgic affections depending on impoverished blood and exhausted nerve centres, bearing down sensations and gastric sinking; profuse pus like leucorrhoea and passive haemorrhage—6x.

KALI HYPOPHIS (in 'relationship' of **Kali phos.**)
Debility—with wasting of muscular tissue. Phosphoturia with general anaemia or leucocythemia. Effects of excessive tea drinking. Chronic bronchitis where the expectoration is *thick* and *fetid,* sometimes *scanty* and *tough.* Dose—5 grain of crude to 3x.

KALI OXALICUM (in 'relationship' of **Kali carb.**)
Lumbago, convulsions.

KALI PICRICUM (in 'relationship' of **Kali carb.**) 378
Jaundice, violent eructations.

KALI PICRO-NITRICUM (in 'relationship' of **Kali Carle**)
Jaundice and violent eructations, also see Kali picricum.

KALI SALICYLICUM (in 'relationship' of **Kali carb.**)
Vomiting especially of pregnancy; arterio-sclerosis, with chronic rheumatism.

POCKET MANUAL OF MATERIA MEDICA: BOERICKE

ESSENTIALS OF RARE AND UNCOMMON REMEDIES

KALI SILICUM (in 'relationship' of **Kali carb.**)
Gouty nodosities.

KALI SULPH CHROMICO (in 'relationship' of **Kali sulph**)
—Alum of chrom— 3x. Produces in the nasal passages very fine threads from the septum to external wall.

KALI TELLURICUM (in 'relationship' of **Kali carb.**)
Garlicky odor of breath, salivation, swollen tongue

KERMES MINERAL (in 'relationship' of **Antim crud.**)
—Stibiat sulph rub—Bronchitis.

KINO (in 'relationship' of **Elaps coral.**) 289
—from Pterocarpus—Haemoptysis and haemorrhage from intestines.

KINO (in 'relationship' of **Kali mur.**) 352
Otorrhoea with stitches in right ear.

KOCH'S LYMPH (in 'relationship' of **Tuberculimum**)
Acute and chronic parenchymatous nephritis; produces, pneumonia, broncho-pneumonia, and congestion of the lungs in tuberculous patients, and is a remarkably efficacious remedy in lobular pneumonia—(broncho-pneumonia).

LAC FELINUM (in 'relationship' of **Lac cann.**)
—Cat's milk—Ciliary neuralgia, eye symptoms, photophobia; asthenopia; dysmenorrhoea.

LAC VACCINUM (in 'relationship' of **Lac. cann.**)
—Cow's milk—headache, rheumatic pains, constipation.

LAC VACCINUM COAGULATUM (in 'relationship' of **Lac. cann.**)
—Curds—Nausea of pregnancy.

LACERIA (in 'relationship' of **Heloderma**)
—Green Lizard—Skin eruptions. Vesicle under tongue. Increased mental acumen. Difficult swallowing. Constant accumulation of saliva in the mouth. *Nausea;* violent pressure in stomach.

LAC VACCINI FLOC (in 'relationship' of **Lac. Can.**)
—Cream—diphtheria, leucorrhoea, menorrhagia, dysphagia.

LACTIS VACCINI FLOC (in 'relationship' of **Lac. cann.**)

—Cream—Diphtheria, leucorrhoea, menorrhagia, dysphagia.

LATRODEC. HASSEL. (in 'relationship' of **Latro. mac.**)

—New South Wales Black Spider—Long lasting effects seem to indicate it in a 'chronic' blood poisoning. Arrests intense pain in pyaemias. Great oedema in neighbourhood of wound; paralysis of limbs, with great wasting of muscles. Violent, darting, burning pains, preceding paralysis; vertigo, tendency to fall forward. Septicaemic conditions; constant delusion of *flying*. Loss of memory roaring noises.

LATRODEC. KALIPO (in 'relationship' of **Latro. mac.**)

—New Zealand Spider—Lymphangitis and nervous twitchings, scarlet burning eruptions.

LAFFA ACUTANGULA (in 'relationship' of **Camphora**) 201

Whole body ice-cold, with a restlessness and anxiety, burning thirst.

LAPSANA COMMUNIS (in 'relationship' of **Eupat. aroma.**)

—Nipple wort—useful in sore nipples and piles.

LAPATHUM (in 'relationship' of **Rumex crisps.**)

—Broad leaf dock—nosebleed and headache following pain in kidney; leucorrhoea.

LAPATHUM (in 'relationship' of **Sepia**)

Leucorrhoea with constriction and expulsive effort through womb and pain in kidneys.

LEONURUS (in 'relationship' of **Merc cor.**)

—Mother wort—Influences pelvic organs; allays spasm and nervous irritability, promotes secretion and reduces febrile excitment. Valuable in suppressed menses and *lochia,* dysentery; vomiting, frightful pains in abdomen, violent thirst. Tongue dry and cracked.

LEVICO (in 'relationship' of **Bacillinum**)

5 to 10 drops, follows as an intercurrent where much debility is present. (Burnett).

LEVICO WATER (in 'relationship' of **Arsenic album**)

Contains Ars., Iron and Copper—Chronic and dyscratic skin

ESSENTIALS OF RARE AND UNCOMMON REMEDIES

diseases, chorea minor and spasms in scrofulous and anaemic children. Favours assimilation and increases nutrition. Debility and skin diseases, especially after the use of higher potencies where progress seems suspended—10 drops in warm water 3 times a day after meals (Burnett).

LIPPA MEXICANA (in 'relationship' of **Ipecac**)

Persistent, dry, hard, bronchial cough-asthma and chronic bronchitis.

LITHIUM BENZOICUM (in 'relationship' of **Lithium carb.**)

Deep-seated pains in loins; in small of back; uneasiness in bladder. Cystic irritation. Gallstones. Frequent desire. Diminishing uric-acid deposit.

LITHUM BROMATUM (in 'relationship' of **Lithium carb.**)

Cerebral congestion, threatened apoplexy, insomnia and epilepsy.

LINUM CATHARTI. (in 'relationship' of **Linum. usitat.**) 406

—Purging flax—Similar respiratory symptoms, but also colic and diarrhoea.

LITHIUM CHLOR. (in 'relationship' of **Lithium carb.**)

Symptoms of cinchonism, viz.; Dizzy head, full, *blurring of vision*. Ringing in ears; marked tremors; *general weakness;* marked muscular and general prostration; no gastro-intestinal effects. Nose sore, heartburn, pain in teeth.

LITHIUM LACTICUM (in 'relationship' of **Lithium carb.**) 407

Rheumatism of shoulder, and small joints relieved by moving about, worse resting.

LOBELIA CARDINALIS (in 'relationship' of **Lobelia purp.**) 409

Debility, especially of lower extremities; oppressed breathing, pleurisy, *sticking pain* in chest on taking a long breath. Pain in left lung, intermitting pricking during the day.

LOBELIA CERULEA (in 'relationship' of **Lobelia infla**) 409

Or SYPHILITIA—gives a perfect picture of sneezing influenza, involving the posterior nares, palate, and fauces. Very depressed. Pain in the forehead over eyes; pain and gas in bowels, followed by copious watery stools with tenesmus and soreness of anus. Pain in knees. Prickling in soles. *Great oppression in lower part of chest.* Dry hacking cough. Breathing difficult. Dull aching pain over root of nose. Eustachian catarrh. Pain in posterior part of spleen.

LOBELIA ERINUS (in 'relationship' of **Lobelia infla.**)

Malignant growth, extremely rapid development; colloid cancer of the omentum; Cork-screw-like pains in abdomen, great dryness of skin, nasal and buccal mucous membranes; distaste for brandy; dry eczematous patches covering points of first fingers. Malignant disease of the face Epithelioma.

LOBELIA ERINUS (in 'relationship' of **Colocynthis**)

Violent cork—Screw like pains in abdomen.

LOBELIA ERINUS (in 'relationship' of **Lobelia infla.**)

Malignant growths, extremely rapid development; colloid cancer of the omentum, cork-screw like pains in abdomen; great dryness of skin, nasal and buccal mucous membranes; distaste for brandy; dry, eczematous patches covering points of first fingers. Malignant disease of the face Epithelioma.

LOBELIA PURPURA. (in 'relationship' of **Natr. salicy.**)

Drowsiness, dizzyness, headache between eyebrows; cannot keep eyes open; tongue white-feels paralyzed as also do the heart and lungs; intense prostration of all vital forces; deadly chill, without shivering useful for the low nervous prostration of grippe.

LOBELIA SYPHILITICA (in 'relationship' of **Lobel. infla.**)

Or CERULEA—Gives a perfect picture of sneezing influenza, involving the posterior nares, palate, and fauces. Very depressed pain in forehead over eyes; pain and gas in bowels, followed by copious watery stools with tenesmus and soreness of anus. Pain in knees. Pricking in soles. *Great oppression in lower part of chest,* as if air could not reach there. *Pain in chest under short ribs of left side.* Dry hacking cough. Breathing difficult. Dull aching pain over root of nose. Eustachian catarrh. Pain in posterior part of spleen.

LONICERA PERICYL. (in 'relationship' of **Lomicera xylos**)

—Honey suckle—irritability of temper, with violent outburst [Crocus].

ESSENTIALS OF RARE AND UNCOMMON REMEDIES 41

LUMINAL (in 'relationship' of **Chloralum**)
Sleeplessness with skin symptoms in migraine; lethargy like epidemic encephalitis.

MACROTIN (in 'relationship' of **Cimicifuga race.**)
Especially for lumbago.

MACROZAMIA SPIRALIS (in 'relationship' of **Chin. ars.**)
Extreme debility after illness; collapse.

MACROZAMIA SPIRALIS (in 'relationship' of **Kali phos.**)
Extreme debility after severe illness; colapse. Wearness from no assignable cause, no pains. Boring pain at vertex, vomiting and retching all night; impossible to open eyes, giddiness and cold.

MACUNA PRURENS (in 'relationship' of **Ratanhia**)
—Doticose—Piles with burning; haemorrhoidal diathesis.

MADUR ALBUM (in 'relationship' of **Hura Brazi**)
Calotropis—Leprosy; livid and gangrenous tubercles; thickening of the skin.

MAGNES ARTIFICIALIS (in 'relationship' of **Sulphur**)
Great hunger in evening, profuse sweat on face, bruised pain in joints, rectal constriction after stool.

MAGNETIS POLI AMBO (in 'relationship' of **X-ray**)
—The Magnet—Sugar of milk or distilled water exposed to influence of entire mass Burning lancinations throughout the body; pains as if broken in joints, when cartilages of two bones touch; shooting and jerkings; headache as if a nail were driven in; tendency of old wounds to bleed afresh.

MAGNETIS POLUS ARCTI. (in 'relationship' of **Sulphur**)
Anxious, *coldness of eyes as if a piece of ice lay in orbit,* increased flow of saliva, constipation, sopor, trembling, abdominal flatulence.

MAGNETIS POLUS ARCTI. (in 'relationship' of **X-ray**)
—North pole of the magnet—Disturbed sleep, somnambulism, cracking in cervical vertebrae, sensation of coldness; toothache.

MAGNETIS POLUS AUSTR. (in 'relationship' of **Sulphur**)
Dryness of lids, easy dislocation of ankle, ingrowing toe-nails, aching in patella, shooting in soles.

MAGNETIS POLUS AUSTRA. (in 'relationship' of **X-ray**)
—South pole of the magnet—Severe pain in inner side of nail of the big toe, *ingrowing toe*-nail, easy dislocation of joints of foot; feet are painful when letting them hang down.

MALÁRIA OFFICINALIS (in 'relationship' of **Natr sulph.**)
—Decomposed vegetable matter—has evident power to cause the disappearance of the plasmodium of malaria. Malarial cachexia. General sense of weariness. Spleen affections. Malaria and rheumatism. Functional hepatic disease—6th potency and higher.

MANDRAGORA (in 'relationship' of **Belladonna**)
—Mandrake—An ancient narcotic with restless excitability and bodily weakness. Desire for sleep. Has antiperiodic properties like **China** and **Aranea**. Useful in epilepsy and hydrophobia.

MANDRAGORA (in 'relationship' of **Podophyllum**)
—also called Mandrake—must not be confounded with Podoph. Great desire for sleep; exaggeration of sounds and enlarged vision. Bowels inactive; stools large, white and hard.

MANGANUM MUR (in 'relationship' of **Mang. acet.**) 422
Painful ankles, bone pains.

MANGANUM OXYDAT (in 'relationship' of **Mang. acet.**)
Pain in tibia, dysmenorrhoea, colic, and diarrhoea. Easily fatigued and heated; sleepy. Stolid, mask-like faciеas; low monotonous voice "Economical Speech". Muscular twitching, cramps in calves; stiff leg muscles; occasional uncontrollable laughter. Peculiar slapping gait. Symptoms Similar to paralysis-agitans, progressive lenticular degenerations and pseudo sclerosis. Workers in Manganum binoxide are frequently affected with bulbar paralysis. Use 3x.

MANGANUM SULPH. (in 'relationship' of **Mang acet**)
Liver affections, excess of bile; a powerful intestinal stimulant.

ESSENTIALS OF RARE AND UNCOMMON REMEDIES

MANGIFERA INDICA (in 'relationship' of **Calc. fluor**)
Varicose veins.

MANZANITA (in 'relationship' of **Hydrastis**)
Diarrhoea, gonorrhoea gleet, leucorrhoea, catarrhal conditions.

MARRUBIUM (in 'relationship' of **Hydrastis**)
—Hoarhound—a stimulant to mucous membranes; especially laryngeal and bronchial, chronic bronchitis, dyspnoea, and hepatic disorders; colds and cough.

MATICO (in 'relationship' of **Kreosotum**)
—Artanthe or Piper augus tifolia—Gonorrhoea, haemorrhage from lungs; Catarrhal conditions of genito-urinary organs and gastro-intestinal tract. Topically a haemostatic. Difficult dry, deep, winter cough-Use Tincture.

MELIOTUS ALBA (in 'relationship' of **Melilotus**)
—White Clover—Practically the same action Haemorrhages, congestive headaches, engorged blood vessels, sparsms.

MENTHA PULEGIUM (in 'relationship' of **Mentha pip.**)
—European pennyroyal—pain in bones of forehead and extremities.

MENTHA VIRDIS (in 'relationship' of **Mentha pip.**)
—Spearmint—Scanty urine with frequent desire.

MERCUR. ACET (in 'relationship' of **Mercurius**)
Congestion with stiffness, dryness and heat of parts affected. Eyes inflamed, burn and itch. Lack of moisture. Throat dry, talking difficult. Pressure in lower sternum; Chancre in urethra; tinia capitis favosa margin of ulcers painful.

MERCUR. ACET (in 'relationship' of **Merc sulph.**)
Cutting in urethra when last drop is flowing out.

MERCUR. AURATUS (in 'relationship' of **Mercurius**)
Psoriasis and syphilitic catarrh; brain tumors; caries of nose and bones; ozaena; swelling of testicles.

MERCUR. BROMATUS (in 'relationship' of **Mercurius**) 432
Secondary syphilitic skin affection.

POCKET MANUAL OF MATERIA MEDICA: BOERICKE

MERCUR. NITROSUS (in 'relationship' of **Mercurius**) 432
—Nitrate of Mercury—Especially in pustular conjunctivitis and keratitis; gonorrhoea and mucous patches, with *sticking pains*; syphilides.

MERCUR. PHOSPHORI. (in 'relationship' of **Mercurius**)
Nervous diseases from Syphilis; exostoses.

MERCUR. PRAECUPITA. (in 'relationship' of **Mercurius**)
Suffocative attacks at night on lying down *while on the point of falling asleep*, obliged to jump up suddenly which relieves, gonorrhoea; *urethra felt as a hard string;* chancroid; phagedenic ulcer and bubo; pemphigus, mucous patches. eczema with rhagades and fissures, barber's itch; blepharitis, internally and externally; deaden heaviness in occiput, with otorrhoea.

MERCUR. TANNICUS (in 'relationship' of **Mercurius**)
Syphilides in patients with gastro-intestinal diseases, or if very sensitive to ordinary mercurial preparations.

METHYLIUM SALICYLI. (in 'relationship' of **Gaultheria**)
—An artificial gaultheria oil for rheumatism, especially when the salicylates cannot be used. Pruritus and epididymitis locally. After **Cantharis** in burns.

MICANIA GUACHO (in 'relationship' of **Golondrina**.)
A Brazilian snake cure.

MIMOSA (in 'relationship' of **Rhus tox**.) 531
—Sensitive Plant—rheumatism. Knee stiff, lancinating pains in back and limbs. Swelling of ankle. Legs tremble.

MIRBANE (in 'relationship' of **Benzeum**)
Dark, black blood, coagulates with difficulty, venous hyperaemia of the brain and general venous engorgement. Burning taste in mouth. Blue lips, tongue, skin, nails and conjunctiva. Cold skin, pulse small, weak, breathing slow and irregular, unconsciousness, symptoms of apoplectic coma. *Rolling of eyes balls in their vertical axis; pupils dilated.* Nystagmus. Respiration very slow, difficult sighing.

MOMORDICA CHARANTIA (in 'relationship' of **Croton tig**)
—Hairy momordica—has marked drastic properties, producing colic,

ESSENTIALS OF RARE AND UNCOMMON REMEDIES — 45

nausea, vomiting, cholera-like symptoms, abdomen seems full of fluid discharged explosively, thin, watery, yellow, great thirst.

MOMORDI. CHARANTIA (in 'relationship' of **Momord. Bals.**)

—Indian Variety—More severe symptom-intestines full of yellow watery fluid, discharged explosively-cramps, thirst, prostration, choleraic symptoms similar to Croton and Elaterium etc.

MONSONIA (in 'relationship' of **Merc cor.**)

—An American plant belonging to the geraneaceae used for dysentery in material doses.

MUCO-TOXIN (in 'relationship' of **Hippozaenium**)

Cahis' preparation with the micro coccus catarrhales. Freedlander's Bacillus of Pneumonia and the micrococcus tatragenius for acute and chronic mucus, catarrhs in children and old people.

MUCUNA URENS (in 'relationship' of **Sedum acre.**)

Haemorrhoidal diathesis and diseases depending thereon.

MULLEIN OIL (in 'relationship' of **Verbascum**)

Locally for earache and dry, scaly condition of meatus. Also for teasing cough at night or lying down. Internally, tincture and lower potencies. Enuresis, five drop doses night and morning.

MUSCARINE (in 'relationship' of **Agaricus musc.**)

—The alkaloid of **Agaricus**— has much power over secretions, increasing lachrymal, salivary, hepatic etc., but diminishing renal; probably neurotic in origin, stimulating the terminal fibres of the secretory nerves of all these structures, hence *salivation, lachrymation and excessive perspiration.* **Atropin** exactly opposes **Muscarine.** Resembles **Pilocarpin** in action.

MUSTARD OIL (in 'relationship' of **Sinapis nig.**)

By inhalation acts on the sensory nerve ending of the trigeminal. Relieves pain in middle ear disorder and in painful condition of nose, nasal cavities, and tonsils.

MYRTUS CHEKAN (in 'relationship' of **Eugenia jambob.**)

Chronic bronchitis.

POCKET MANUAL OF MATERIA MEDICA: BOERICKE

MYRTUS CHEKON (in 'relationship' of **Stannum**)

Chronic bronchitis, cough of phthisis, emphysema, with gastric catarrhal complications and thick, yellow, difficult sputum. Old persons with weakened power of expectoration.

NABALUS (in 'relationship' of **Lactuca vrosa**.)

—Prenanthes serpentaria—Rattle snake root—while Lettuce, similar to Lacluca. Chronic diarrhoea, worse after eating, nights and towards morning. Pain in abdomen and rectum; emaciation. Dyspepsia, with acid burning eructation. *Craving for acid food.* Leucorrhoea with throbbing in uterus.

NARCISSUS POETICUS (in 'relationship' of **Verat alb**.)

Gastro-enteriti. with much griping and cutting pain in bowels. Fainting, trembling, cold limbs, small and irregular pulse.

NASTURTIUM AQUA. (in 'relationship' of **Mag. mur**.)

—Water-cress—useful in scorbutic affections and constipation, related to strictures of urinary apparatus; supposed to be aphrodisiacal in its action. Is also antidotal to *tobacco* narcosis and sedative in neurotic affections, neurasthenia, hysteria. Cirrhosis of liver and dropsy.

NATRUM CACODYL (in 'relationship' of **Natr. carb**.)

Foul breath and mouth with bad odour. Dry dermatitis of the skin of abdomen. Maglignant growth (In phthisis 5 centigram), hypodermically daily. Increases number of red blood corpuscles to double.

NATRUM CHOLEIN. (in 'relationship' of **Natr. sulph**.)

—Fel Tauri Depuratum—Constipation; chronic gastric and intestinal catarrh; Cirrhotic liver, diabetes, *nape of neck pains; tendency to sleep after eating,* much flatus; ascites.

NATRUM HYPOSUL. (in 'relationship' of **Natr. sulph**)

Liver spots locally and internally.

NATRUM IODAT (in 'relationship' of **Natr. sulph**.)

Incipient rheumatic endocarditis; Chronic bronchitis, rheumatism and tertiary syphilis. Chronic catarrhal affections, arteriosclerosis. Has various symptoms, as *angina pectoris*, vertigo, dyspnoea becomes less marked after continued use— 5-10grs. 3 times a day.

ESSENTIALS OF RARE AND UNCOMMON REMEDIES

NATRUM LACTIC (in 'relationship' of **Natr. phos.**) 455
Rheumatism and gout, gouty concretions; rheumatism with diabetes.

NATRUM NITROSUM (in 'relationship' of **Natr. phos.**) 455
Angina pectoris. Cyanosis, fainting, copious liquid stools at night throbbing and fullness; faintness, nervous pain in head, nausea, eructations, blue lips.

NATRUM SELEN (in 'relationship' of **Natr. phos.**) 455
Chronic laryngitis and laryngeal phthisis; hoarseness of singers, expectorate small lumps of mucus with frequent clearing of throat.

NATRUM SELENICUM (in 'relationship' of **Natr. mur.**)
Laryngeal phthisis with expectoration of small lumps of bloody mucus and slight hoarseness.

NATRUM SILICOFLUOR. (in 'relationship' of **Natr. phos.**)
—Salufer—a cancer remedy, tumors, bone affections, caries, lupus, and ethmoidits. Must be used carefully.

NATRUM SILICUM (in 'relationship' of **Natr. mur.**)
Haemophilia, Scrofulous bone affections; given intravenously every 3 days for *senile pruritus*.

NATRUM SILICUM (in 'relationship' of **Silicea**)
Tumors, haemophilia, arthritis; 3 drops dose thrice a day in milk.

NATR. SUL.-CARBOL (in 'relationship' of **Natr. phos.**)
Pyaemia; purulent pleurisy, 3 to 5 grains every three hours.

NATRUM SULPH. (in 'relationship' of **Natr. phos.**)
Diarrhoea with yeasty stool.

NATRUM SUCCINATE (in 'relationship' of **Natr. sulph.**)
Catarrhal jaundice, every 3 hours.

NATRUM TELL. (in 'relationship' of **Natr. phos.**)
Breath has odour of garlic; night sweats of phthisis.

NECTRANDA AMARA (in 'relationship' of **Phos. acid**)
Watery diarrhoea, dry tongue, colic, bluish ring around sunken eyes, restless sleep.

NYMPHEA ODORATA (in 'relationship' of **Nuphar luti**)
—Sweet Water Lily—early morning diarrhoea, acrid leucorrhoea, offensive ulcers; bronchorrhoea; ulcerative sore throat.

OLEUM, CARYOPH. (in 'relationship' of **Balsam paru.**)
—Oil of Cloves—in *profuse* septic expectoration. 3-5 drops in milk or capsules.

NEGUND. AMERI. (in 'relationship' of **Aesculus hipp.**)
—Box elder—Engorgement of rectum and piles with great pain, ten-drop doses of tincture every two hours.

NEPETA CATARIA (in 'relationship' of **Senega**)
—Catnip—to break up a cold; infantile colic; hysteria.

NERIUM ODORUM (in 'relationship' of **Digit.**) 280
Resembles in heart effects, but also has an action like **strychnia** on spinal cord. Spasms appear more in upper part of body. Palpitation; strengthens weak heart. Lock-jaw.

NICOTINUM (in 'relationship' of **Tabacum**)
Alternate tonic and clonic spasms, followed by general relaxation and trembling; nausea, cold sweat, and speedy collapse; head drawn back, contraction of eyelids and masseter muscles; muscles of neck and back rigid; hissing respiration from spasm of laryngeal and bronchial muscles.

OENOTHERA (in 'relationship' of **Chin ars.**)
Effortless diarrhoea with nervous exhaustion, incipient hydrocephaloid.

OENOTHERA BIENNIS (in 'relationship' of **Phos. acid**) 492
—Everything primrose—Effortless diarrhoea with nervous exhaustion. Incipient hydrocephaloid. Whooping-cough and spasmodic asthma.

OESTRUS CAMELI (in 'relationship' of **Indigo**)
An Indian medicine for epilepsy.

OLIUM MYRISTICA (in 'relationship' of **Nux mosch.**)
—Oil of Nutmeg—as a remedy for boils, felons, poisonous ulcers, it has been used in the 2x potency.

OLEUM SUCCINUM (in 'relationship' of **Ambra grisea**)
Hiccough.

ESSENTIALS OF RARE AND UNCOMMON REMEDIES 49

ONONIC SPINOSA (in 'relationship' of **Terebinthina**)

—Harrow—Diuretic, Lithontriptic. Chronic nephritis; diuretic effects like *Juniper;* Calculus nosebleed, worse washing face.

ORCHITINUM (in 'relationship' of **Ophorinum**)

—Testicular Extract—Sexual weakness after ovariotomy; senile decay.

OREXINE TANNATE (in 'relationship' of **Robinia**)

Hyperchlorhydria; deficient acid and slow digestion; 14 hourly doses.

OUABAIN (in 'relationship' of **Drosera**) 284

—from leaves of Carissa schimperi—Arrow poison. Respiratory spasm-Whooping cough is cut short in first stage and reduced in frequency of attacks and hastens convalescence.

OVA TOSTA (in 'relationship' of **Calc. carb.**)

—Toasted egg shells—*backache and leucorrhoea.* Feeling as if back were broken in two; tired feeling. Also effective in controlling suffering from cancer.

OXALIS ACET. (in 'relationship' of **Sempervi. tect.**)

—Wood Sorrel—The inspissated juice used as a cautery to remove cancerous growths of the lips.

OZONUM (in 'relationship' of **Sepia**)

Sacral pains, tied feeling through pelvic viscera and perineum.

PAMBOTANO (in 'relationship' of **Chin. sulph.**) 232

—Mexican remedy for intermittent and tropical fevers.

PANACEA AROENSIS (in 'relationship' of **Ignatia**) 356

—Poor man's Mercury—Sensitiveness over gastric region with hunger but an aversion to food.

PANCREATINUM (in 'relationship' of **Iris versi.**)

A combination of several enzymes—Indicated in intestinal indigestion; pain an hour or more after eating. Lienteric diarrhoea. 3-5 grains, better not given during the active period of stomachic digestion.

ESSENTIALS OF RARE AND UNCOMMON REMEDIES

PARIETARIA (in 'relationship' of **Pareira brava**) 34

Renal calculi; nightmare, patient dreaming of being buried alive.

PASTINACA (in 'relationship' of **Paris quad.**) 485

—Parsnip—Loquacity; delirium tremens; illusions of vision; intolerance of milk; Roots used dietically, cooked in water or as broth or as salad for consumption and "kidney stones".

PECTEN (in 'relationship' of **Aralia racemosa**)

—Scallop—Humid asthma. Quick, laboured breathing. Constriction of chest, especially right side. Asthma preceded by coryza and burning in throat and chest. Attack ends with copious expectoration of tough, frothy mucus. Worse at night.

PEDICULARIS CAN. (in 'relationship' of **Secale cor.**)

Symptoms of locomotor ataxia; spinal irritation.

PEDICULUS (in 'relationship' of **Psorinum**)

—Head louse—Psoric manifestations in children. Eruption on dorsum of hands, feet, neck. Prurigo; pellagra. unusual aptitude for study and work. Pediculus (Cooties) transmit typhus and trech fever.

PELIUS BERUS (in 'relationship' of **Vipera.**)

—Adder—Prostration and fainting, faltermg pulse, skin yellow, pain about navel. Swelling of arm, tongue, right eye; giddiness, nervousness, faintness, sickness, compression of chest could not breath properly or take a deep breath; aching and stiffness of limbs, joints stiff, collapsed feeling, great thirst.

PELLETIERNE (in 'relationship' of **Granatum**)

—One of its constituents—an anthelminitic, especially for tapeworm.

PEPSINUM (in 'relationship' of **Iris. versi.**)

Imperfect digestion with pain in gastric region. Marasmus of children who are fed on artificial foods. Diarrhoea due to indigestion. 3-4 grains. Diseases of pancreas, gout, diabetes.

PERIPLOCA GRAECA (in 'relationship' of **Ascelp. tuber**)

—One of the Asclepiades—Cardiac tonic, acts on circulation and respiratory centre, accelerating respiration in a ratio disproportionate to pulse.

PEUMUS BOLDUS (in 'relationship' of **Nat. sulph**)

—Boldo—atomic states of stomach and intestinal canal; liver states following malaria. Burning weight in region of liver and stomach, bitter taste, languor; abscess of liver; asthma, bronchitis, cattarrh, oedema of lung.

PHELEUM PRATENSE (in 'relationship' of **Sabadilla**)

—Timothy—Hay fever—Potentized-12-specific for many cases and evidently acts in a desensitizing manner (Rabe).

PEHLEUM PRATENSE (in 'relationship' of **Rosa damas**) 533

—Timothy grass—Hey fever with asthma; watery coryza, itching of nose and eyes, frequent sneezing, dyspnoea. Use 6-30 potency Rabe.

PHIORIDZIN (in 'relationship' of **Uranium nit.**)

A glucosidal principle obtained from the bark of the root of the apple and other fruit trees. Produces diabetes and fatty degeneration of the liver, intermittent fever. Daily doses, 15 grains. Phlorizin causes glycosuria. No Hypergalycemia results. It compels the secretory epithelium of the kidney to break down serum albumin into sugar. There is no increase in blood sugar.

PHOSPH HYDROGENATUS (in 'relationship' of **Phos.**)

Crumbling teeth; hyperaesthesia; locomotor ataxia.

PHOSPH. PENTACHLORIDE (in 'relationship' of **Phos.**)

Great soreness of mucous membrane of eyes and nose; throat and chest sore.

PHYTOLACCA BERRY (in 'relationship' of **Phytolacca**)

Sore throats and in the treatment of obesity.

PICROTOZIN (in 'relationship' of **Cocculus**)

—alkaloid of Cocculus—Epilepsy, hernia, locomotor ataxia, night-sweats.

PILOCARPIN MUR. (in 'relationship' of **Pilocarpul micro.**)

Meniere's disease, rapidly progresive phthisis, with free haemorrhages, profuse sweating-2x trit.

ESSENTIALS OF RARE AND UNCOMMON REMEDIES

PIMENTA (in 'relationship' of **Pulsatilla**)
—Allspice—one sided neuralgias, parts of body hot and cold.

PIMPINELLS (in 'relationship' of **Dulcamara**)
—Bibernell—Respiratory mucous membrane sensitive to draughts, pain and coldness in occiput and nape. Whole body weak; heavy head and drowsiness; lumbago and stiff neck; pain from nape to shoulder; Chilliness.

PINUS LAMBERTINA (in 'relationship' of **Pinus sylvest**)
Sugar Pine—Constipation, amenorrhoea, abortion. Pinus lambertina sap is a decided carthartic. Delayed and painful menstruation.

PIPERAZINUM (in 'relationship' of **Physostigma**)
Uric acid conditions. Pruritus Gout and urinary calculi. *Constant backache.* Skin dry, urine scanty. Rheumatic urethritis. Give one grain daily in carbonated water. First and second decimal trituration three times a day.

PISCIDIA (in 'relationship' of **Xanthoxylum**)
White dogwood—a nerve sedative. *Insomnia due* to worry, nervous excitement, spasmodic coughs; pains of irregular menstruation; regulates the flow. Neuralgic and spasmodic effections. Use tincture in rather material doses.

PITUITRIN (in 'relationship' of **Secale cor.**)
Dilated os, little pain, no progress. Dose 1/2 cc, repeat in half hour, if necessary. Hypodermically contra indicated in 1st. stage of labour, Valvular lesions or deformed pelvis.

PLATINUM MURIATICUM (in 'relationship' of **Platina**)
Achieves beneficial result after Iodide of Potash fails to cure in syphilitic affection; violent occipital headaches, dysphagia, and syphilitic throat and bone affections; caries of bones of feet.

PLATINA MUR. NAT (in 'relationship' of **Platina**) 505
Polyuria and salivation.

PLECTRANTHUS (in 'relationship' of **Plumb. met.**) 507
Paralysis, spastic, spinal form.

PLUMBAGO (in 'relationship' of **Rhus. tox.**)
Eczema of vulva.

PLUMBAGO LITTORALIS (in 'relationship' of **Lyco.**)
A Brazilian plant—Costive with red urine, pain in **kidneys** and joints and body; generally milky saliva, ulcerated mouth.

PLUMBUM ACET. (in 'relationship' of **Plum. met.**)
Painful cramps in paralyzed limbs, severe pain and muscular cramps in gastric ulcer; locally as an application (**non-homoeopathic**) in moist eczema, and to dry up secretions from mucous surface. Care must be used, as sufficient lead can be absorbed to produce lead poison, one to two drams of the *liquor plumbi subacetatis* to the ounce of water; also in pruritus pudendi equal parts of the *liquor plumbs and glycerin.*

PLUMB. CHROMICUM (in 'relationship' of **Plumb. met.**)
Convulsions with terrible pains; pupils greatly dilated; retracted abdomen.

PLUMBUM IOD (in 'relationship' of **Baryta mur.**)
Compare in sclerotic degeneration especially of spinal cord, liver, and heart also **Plumbum met.** and **Aurum mur.** Which will often accomplish more in Sclerotic and exudative degeneration than other remedies. Multiple Sclerosis, fulgurating pains, tremors. Morvan's disease, hypertrophy of fingers.

PLUMBUM IOD (in 'relationship' of **Merc. iod. flav.**)
Mammary tumors.

PLMB. IODAT (in 'relationship' of **Plum. met.**)
Has been used empirically in various forms of paralysis, sclerotic degenerations, especially of spinal cord, atrophies, arterio-sclerosis, pellagra. Indurations of mammary glands, *especailly when a tendency to become inflamed appears; sore and painful.* Induration of great hardness and associated pains of Tabes.

PLUMS. PHOSPH. (in 'relationship' of **Plumb. met.**)
Loss of sexual power; *locomotor ataxia.*

PLUMERIA CELLINUS (in 'relationship' of **Golondrina**) 326
Tincture internally and locally every 15 minutes for snake poisoning.

ESSENTIALS OF RARE AND UNCOMMON REMEDIES

PNEUMOCOCIN (in 'relationship' of **Phosphorus**)
Pneumonia and paralytic phenomena; pleuritic pain and pain in ilio-caecal region [Cartier].

PNEUMOTOXIN (in 'relationship' of **Phosphorus**)
Cahis taken from the Diplococcus lanceolatus of Fraenkel. Pneumonia, pleurisy and other respiratory disorders.

POLYCTRICHUM (in 'relationship' of **Hydrangea**)
—Haircap moss—according to Dr. A.M. Cushing in mother tincture or infusion for enlarged prostate-prostatitis.

POLYGONUM AVI. (in 'relationship' of **Polygo. punct.**)
—Knotgrass— in material doses of tincture, found useful in phthisis pulmonalis and intermittent fever, and especially in *arterio-sclerosis*.

POLYGONUM AVI. (in 'relationship' of **Sulphiums**)
Phthisis. Given in material doses of mother ticture.

POLYGONUM PERSI. (in 'relationship' of **Polygo. punct.**)
Reneal colic and calculi, gangrene.

POLYGONUM SAGI. (in 'relationship' of **Polygo. punct.**)
—Arrow—leaved tear thumb—2x for *pains of nephritic colic*; supparative nephritis lancinating pains along spine; itching of had palate; burning inner side of right foot and ankle. (C.M. Boger)

POLYMANIA UVEDALIA (in 'relationship' of **Ceanothus**)
—Bearsfoot—acute splenitis with tenderness over left hypochondriac region, spleen enlarged, ague cake. Vascular atony tissues sodde , falbby and non-elastic. Enlarged glands, influences all ductless glands.

POLYTRICHUM JUNIPER. (in 'relationship' of **Triticum.**)
—Ground Moss—Painful urination of old people; dropsy, urinary obstruction and suppression.

POPULUS TREMUL (in 'relationship' of **Sabal serru.**)
Prostatic enlargement with cystitis.

POTASS XANTATE (in 'relationship' of **Carbon. sulph**) 215
Similar in action. Acts on cortical substance; loss of memory, marked blood degeneration; impotence and senility.

PRIMULA FARINOSA (in 'relationship' of **Primula veris.**)
—the Wild Prim Rose—Dermatitis, especially on index fingers and thumb.

PROTARGOL (in 'relationship' of **Argen nit.**) 129
Gonorrhoea after acute stage 2 per cent. solution; syphilitic mucous patches, chancres and chancroids, 10 per cent. solution applied twice a day; ophthalmia neonatorum, 2 drops of 10 percent solution.

PRUNELLA (in 'relationship' of **Podophyl.**)
—Self heal—Colitis.

PRUNUS PODUS (in 'relationship' of **Prunus spin.**)
—Bird cherry—Sore throat, pressure behind sternum and sticking pain in rectum.

PRUNUS VIRGINIANA (in 'relationship' of **Prunus spin.**) 512
—Wild cherry=*Heart tonic* relieves the flagging and distended ventricle; irritable heart; dilatation of right heart; *cough worse at night—on lying down*; weak digestion especially in elderly people; chronic bronchitis; increases muscular tone.

PSORALEA (in 'relationship' of **Euphorbium**) 299
A Columbean plant—Pains of cancer, ulcers. Leucorrhoea fetid. Pruritus uterine tumors.

PULMO VULPIS (in 'relationship' of **Nat. sulph**)
—Wolf's lung—persistent shortness of breath causing a paroxysm of asthma on the slightest motion. Strong, sonorous bubbling rales. 1x trit.

PULS. NUITALIANA (in 'relationship' of **Pulsatilla**)
Identical effects.

PYRARARA (in 'relationship' of **Sulphur**) 584
—a fish caught in the Amazon, clinically used for various skin affections. Lepra, tuberculosis, syphilides, varicosities, etc.

PYRUS (in 'relationship' of **Prunus spin.**) 512
—Mountain Ash—irritation of eyes; constriction around waist; spasmodic pains in uterus, bladder, heart, cold water sensation in

stomach, coldness extends up oesophagus; neuralgic and gouty pains.

PYRUS MALUS (in 'relationship' of **Natr. salicy.**)
—Crab apple tree—Labyrinthine vertigo.

QUEBRACHO (in 'relationship' of **Aconite nap.**)
Cardiac dyspnoea.

QUINIDIN (in 'relationship' of **Cinchona off.**)
Paroxysmal tachycardia and *auriculae fibrillation*. Heart is slowed, and the auriculo-ventricular conduction time is lengthened. Dose ½ gram t.i.d.

QUINIDIN (in 'relationship' of **Digit.**)
—Isomeric methoxyl compound—Restores normal rhythm in auricular fibrillation, often supplements the action of Digitalis. Two doses of 3 grains each, three hours apart—if no symptoms of cinchonism develop, 4 doses 6 grs. each daily (C. Harlan Wells). Paroxysmal tachycardia. Establishes normal heart rhythm at least temporarily, less in valvular lesions.

RADEMACHER'S SOLUTION (in 'relationship' of **Zinc met.**)
638

Five drops three times a day in water, for those who are compelled to work, on an insufficient amount of sleep.

RANUNCULUS ACRIS (in 'relationship' of **Ranun bulb.**)
Pain in Lumbar muscles and joints by bending and burning in body.

RANUNCULUS FLAM. (in 'relationship' of **Ranun bulb.**)
Ulceration; gangrene of arm

RANUNCULUS GLACI. (in 'relationship' of **Ranun. bulb.**)
—Reindeer flower Carlina—Pulmonary affections; broncho—pneumonical influenza—enormous weight in head with vertigo and sensation of impending apoplexy; night sweats—more on thighs.

RANUNCULUS REPENS (in 'relationship' of **Ranun. bulb.**)
Crawling sensation in forehead and scalp in evening in bed.

RESORCIN (in 'relationship' of **Ricinus commun.**)
Summer complaints with vomiting; destroys organic germs of

putrefaction.

RHAMNUS FRANGU. (in 'relationship' of **Rhamn. calif.**) 526
—European Buckthorn—a rheumatic remedy. Abdominal symptoms, colic, diarrhoea; haemorrhoids, especially chronic.

RHUS DIVERSILOBA (in 'relationship' of **Rhus tox.**)
—California Poison Oak— antidote to Rhus; violent skin symptoms, with frightful itching; much swelling of face, hands and genitals; skin very sensitive; eczema and erysipelas, great nervous weakness, tired from least effort; goes to sleep from sheer exhaustion.

RHUS RADICANS (in 'relationship' of **Rhus tox**)
—Almost identical action—Burning in tongue; tip feels sore, pains are often semilateral and in various parts, often remote and successive. Many symptoms are better after a storm has thoroughly set in especially after an electric storm. Has pronounced yearly aggravation (Lachesis). **Rhus radicans** has headache in occiput, even pain in nape of neck and from there pains draw over the head forwards.

ROSMARINUS (in 'relationship' of **Sabina**)
Menses too early, violent pains followed by uterine haemorrhage. Head heavy, *drowsy*. Chilly with icy coldness of lower extremities without thirst, followed by heat. Memory deficient.

RUBIA TINCTORUM (in 'relationship' of **Saliva offi.**)
—Madder—A remedy for the spleen. (Ceanothus.) Chlorosis and amenorrhoea; tuberculosis. Anaemia; undernourished conditions: splenic anaemia. Dose, 10 drops of tincture.

RUBUS VILLOSUS (in 'relationship' of **Chamomilla**)
—Blackberry—Diarrhoea of infancy; stools watery and clay coloured.

RUMEX ACETOSA (in 'relationship' of **Rumex crisp.**)
Sheep sorrel—gathered in June and dried, used locally for Epithelioma of face. (*Cowperthwaite*). Dry, unremitting short cough and violent pains in the bowels; uvula elongated; inflammation of oesophagus; also cancer.

RUMEX OBTUSIFOLIUS (in 'relationship' of **Rumex crisp.**)

—Lapathum—Broad-leaf dock for nosebleed and headache following, pain in kidney; leucorrhoea.

SACCHARUM LACTIS (in 'relationship' of **Sacch offi.**)

—Sugar of milk—lactose—Diuresis; amblyopia; *cold pains*, as if produced by fine, icy cold needle with tingling, as if frost bitten; great physical exhaustion. *Sugar of milk* in large doses to develop the Bacillus acidophilus to correct putrefactive intestinal conditions and also constipation.

SALAMAND. (in 'relationship' of **Bufo**)

Epilepsy and softening of brain.

SAL MARINUM (in 'relationship' of **Natr. mur.**)

—Sea salt—Indicated in chronic enlargement of glands, especially cervical. Suppurating glands. It appears likely to become a most useful remedy as an auxiliary, if not a principal, in the treatment of diseases in patients of a strumous diathesis. Also useful in constipation.

SALOL (in 'relationship' of **Salicylic acid**) 539

Rheumatic pains in joints, with soreness and stiffness, headache over eyes; urine violent smelling.

SALUFER (in 'relationship' of **Natrum Phos.**)

A cancer remedy; tumors, bone affections, caries, lupous, ethmoidits. Must be used carefully.

SALVIA SCLERATA (in 'relationship' of **Salvia offi.**)

Tonic, influence on nervous system; dose, teaspoonful to one pint hot water, as inhalent for sponging.

SAMBUCUS CAN. (in 'relationship' of **Samb. nig.**) 541

Great value in dropsies, large doses required, fluid extract ¼ to 1 teaspoonful three times daily.

SANGUIN. TART. (in 'relationship' of **Sanguin nit.**)

Exophthalmos; *mydriasis*; dim vision.

SANGUISORBA (in 'relationship' of **Sabina**) 538

Venous congestion and passive haemorrhages; varices of lower extremities; dysentery. *Long lasting profuse menses* with congestion to head and limbs in sensitive, irritable patients. *Climacteric* haemorrhages. Use 2x attenuation.

SANGUISORBA OFF. (in 'relationship' of **Belladonna**)

Profuse, long-lasting menses, especially in nervous patients with congestive symptoms to head and limbs. Passive haemorrhage at climacteric. Chronic motritis. Haemorrhage from lungs. Varices and ulcers. Use 2x-3x.

SANGUINSUGA (in 'relationship' of **Phos.**) 495
—Leech—*Persistent haemorrhage;* effects of use of leeches.

SANGIUSUGA (in 'relationship' of **Sabina**)
—The leech—Haemorrhages, especially bleeding from anus-use 6x.

SANGUISUGA (in 'relationship' of **Trillium pend.**)
—The leech—Haemorrhages; bleeding from anus.

SANTALUM (in 'relationship' of **Copaiva**) 263
Aching in kidney.

SAURURUS (in 'relationship' of **Sarsa.**)
—Lizard's tail—Irritation of kidneys, bladder, prostate and urinary passages. Painful and difficult micturition; cystitis with strangury.

SAXONITE (in 'relationship' of **Skookum chuck**)
Appears to have remarkable cleansing, deodorizing and soothing properties for the skin (Cowperthwaite). Eczema, scalds, burns, sores and haemorrhoids.

SCIRRIHNUM (in 'relationship' of **Conium**)
—Cancer nosode—Cancerous diathesis; enlarged glands; cancer of breast; worms.

SCOLOPENDRA (in 'relationship' of **Oxylic acid**)
—Centipede—Terrible pain in back and loins, extending down limbs, return periodically, commencing in head, to toes. Angina pectoris. Inflammation, pain and gangrene. Pustules and abscesses.

SCORPIO (in 'relationship' of **Vespa crabro.**)
Salvation; strabismus; tetanus.

60

SCOPOLA (in 'relationship' of **Hyoscyamus**)

—Japanese Belladonna—chemically identical with Hyoscine. Joyous delirium, ticking of lips and smacking of mouth; sleepless, tries to get out of bed; sees cats, picks imaginary hairs, warms hands before imaginary fire, etc.

SEDUM ACRE (in 'relationship' of **Plantina**)

Sexual irritability, relieves irritation of nerve centres and gives rest.

SEDUM REPENS (in 'relationship' of **Sedum acre**) 551

—Sedum alpestre—Cancer, specific action on abdominal organs; pain loss of strength.

SEDUM TELEPHIUM (in 'relationship' of **Sedum acre**) 551

Uterine haemorrhages, also of bowels and rectum, *menorrhagia*, especially at climacteric.

SELAGINELLA (in 'relationship' of **Golondrina**)

Macerate in milk, locally and internally for bites of snakes and spiders.

SENECIO JACOBAEA (in 'relationship' of **Senecio aur.**)

Cerebro-spinal irritation, rigid muscles, chiefly of neck and shoulder; also in cancer.

SEPIN (in 'relationship' of **Pyrogenium.**) 519

—A toxin of Proteus vulgaris, prepared by Dr. Shedd, same symptoms as **Pyrogen.** of which it is the main constituent.

SHUCKS (in 'relationship' of **Stigmata maydis.**)

As a decoction used for chronic malaria, teaspoonful doses freely. (Dr. E.C. Lowe, England)

SILICA MARINA (in 'relationship' of **Silicea**)

—sea-sand—*Inflamed glands* and commencing suppuration. Constipation. 3x trit. for some time.

SILPHION CYREN. (in 'relationship' of **Silphium**)

Phthisis pulmonum. with incessant cough, profuse night sweats, emaciation etc.

SINAPIE ALBA (in 'relationship' of **Sinapis nig.**)

—White Mustard—throat symptoms marked, *especially pressure and burning, with obstruction in oesophagus;* sensation of lump in oesophagus behind the Manubrium sterni and with much eructation; similar symptoms in rectum.

SISYRINCHIUM (in 'relationship' of **Golondrina**) 326

—Blue eyed grass—10 to 15 drop doses of tincture for rattle snake bite.

SLAG (in 'relationship' of **Ratanhia**)

—Blast Iron Furnace Cinder—Anal itching, piles and constipation; housemaid knee; abdominal flatulence, distention and lumbago.

SLAG SILICA (in 'relationship' of **Alumina**) 96

—Sulphocalcite of Alumina—anal itching, piles, constipation, flatulent distention, 3x.

SODII BICARBONAS (in 'relationship' of **Natr. carb.**) 450

Vomiting of pregnancy with acetonuria, 30 grains in water spread over twenty-four hours.

SOLANUM ACET. (in 'relationship' of **Solanum nig.**) 564

Threatening paralysis of the lungs. in the course of bronchitis in the aged and children. Must cough a long time before able to raise expectoration.

SOLANUM CAROLIN. (in 'relationship' of **Solanum nig.**)

—Horse-nettle—Convulsions and epilepsy; 20 to 40 drop doses; of great value in grand-mal of idiopathic type where the disease has begun beyond age of childhood, hysterio-epilepsy, also in whooping cough.

SOLANUM MAMM. (in 'relationship' of **Solanum nig.**)

—Apple of Sodom—Pain in left hip joint.

SOLANUM OLERA. (in 'relationship' of **Solanum nig.**)

Swelling of mammary glands, with profuse secretion of Milk.

SOLANUM PSEUDO. (in 'relationship' of **Solanum nig.**)

Acute pain in lower abdomen.

SOLANUM TUBERO. (in 'relationship' of **Solanum nig.**)

Cramps in calves and contractions of fingers; spitting through closed teeth.

SOLANUM TUBEROSUM (in 'relationship' of **Solan. nig.**)

—Potato berries—Cramps in the calves of legs and fingers.

SOLANUM TUB., AEGRO. (in 'relationship' of **Solan. nig.**)

—Diseased potato—Prolapse of the rectum, patulous anus, offensive breath and odour of body; tumors of rectum look like decayed potato; dreams of pools of blood.

SOLANUM VESICARIUM (in 'relationship' of **Solanum nig.**) 564

Recommended in facial paralysis.

SPIGELIA MARYLANDICA (in 'relationship' of **Spigelia**) 568

Maniacal excitement, paroxysmal laughing and crying, loud, disconnected talking, vertigo, dilated pupils, Congestions.

SPHIGURUS (in 'relationship' of **Thuja**)

Falling out of hair from beard; pain in jaw joint and zygoma.

SPHINGURUS (in 'relationship' of **Verbascum**)

Pain in zygoma.

SPIRITUS RETH. COMP. (in 'relationship' of **Chloroform**)

—Hoffman's Anodyne—Flatulence, Angina pectoris, 5 drops to 1 dram in water.

SQUILL. CONVOLVULUS (in 'relationship' of **Ipecac.**)

Colic and diarrhoea.

STANNUM 10 D. 3X. (in 'relationship' of **Stannum**) 572

Valuable in chronic chest diseases, characterized by plastic tissue changes. Persistent inclination to cough, excited by tickling dry spot in the throat, apparently at root of tongue. Dryness of throat. Trachial and bronchial irritation of smokers. Pulmonary symptoms; cough, loud, hollow, ending with expectoration. State of purulent infiltration. *Advanced* phthisis sometimes when *Stannum iod* has not taken effect, an additional dose of Iodine in milk caused the drug to have its usual beneficial effect (Stonham.)

STANNUM OID (in 'relationship' of **Stannum**) 572

Valuable in chronic chest disease characterized by plastic tissue changes. Persistent inclination to cough, excited by itching dry spot in the throat, apparently at root of tongue. Dryness of throat, Trachial and bronchial irritation of smokers. Pulmonry symptoms; cough, loud, hollow, ending with expectoration. [Phellandrium] State of purulent infiltration. *Advanced* phthisis. Sometime when stann. Iod has not taken effect, and additional dose of Iodein in milk caused the drug to have its usual benificial effect.

STAPHYLOCCIN (in 'relationship' of **Pyrogenium**)

Where the staphylococcus is the chief bacterial factor, as acne, abscess, furuncle; empyema endocarditis.

STREPTOCCIN (in 'relationship' of **Pyrogenium**)

Anti-febrile action; septic symptoms in infectious diseases. Rapid in its action, especially in effect on temperature.

STOVAIN (in 'relationship' of **Cocaina**)

An analgesic, a vasomotor dilator. Antidote to disagreeable effects occasionally resulting from injection of cocaina into skin or gums, drop doses of nitro-glycer 1% solution.

STREPTOCCIN (in 'relationship' of **Pyrogenium**)

Anti-febrile action; septic symptoms in infectious diseases. Rapid in its action, especially in its effects on temperature.

STRONTIUM BROM. (in 'relationship' of **Strontia**)

Often gives excellent results where a bromide is indicated. Vomiting of pregnancy. Nervous dyspepsia. It is anti-fermentative and neutralizes excessive acidity.

STRONTIA JODAT. (in 'relationship' of **Strontia**)

Arterio-sclerosis.

STRONTIA NUT. (in 'relationship' of **Strontia**)

Morbid cravings; headache and eczema behind ears.

STRYCHNINUM ARS. (in 'relationship' of **Strychninum**)

Paresis in the aged, relaxed musculature Prostration. Psoriasis; chronic diarrhoea with paralytic symptoms; compensatory hypertrophy or neart with beginning fatty degeneration; marked dyspnoea when lying down; oedema of lower extremities, urine scanty, high specific gravity, heavily loaded with glucose. Diabetes 6x trit.

STRYCHN. et FERR.CIT. (in 'relationship' of Strychninum)

Chlorotic and paralytic conditions; dyspepsia, with vomiting of ingesta; 2x and 3x trit.

STRYCHNINUM NIT. (in 'relationship' of Strychninum) 580

Removes craving for alcohol. 2x and 3x. use for two weeks.

STRYCHNINUM SULPH. (in 'relationship' of Strychninum) 580

Gastric atony.

STRYCHN. VALER. (in 'relationship' of Strychninum)

Exhaustion of brain-power; women of high nervous erethism. 2x. trit.

SUCCINIC ACID. (in 'relationship' of Succinum)

Hay-fever. Paroxysmal sneezing, dropping of watery mucus from nostrils; asthma. Inflammation through respiratory tract; causing asthma, chest pains etc. itching of eyelids and canthi and nose worse drafts. Use 6 to 80th potency.

SULPHUR HYDROGEN. (in 'relationship' of Sulphur) 584

Delirium, mania, asphyxia.

SULPHUR TERBINTH. (in 'relationship' of Sulphur)

Chronic rheumatic arthritis; chorea.

TAMUS. (in relationship' of Agaricus musc.) 85

Chilblains and freckles.

TANNIC ACID (in 'relationship' of Sulphur)

Nasal haemorrhages, elongated uvula; gargle; constipation.

TAUROCHOLATE SODA (in 'relationship' of Cholest.)

Dr. I.P. Tessier, in an interesting study of the action of bile and its salts, in hepatic affections, analyzes a number of experiments by leading authorities, with the object of determining this action, and concludes that the Taurocholate of soda homoeopathically has a useful remedy against certain forms of hypoglobular anaemia The claim that its pathogenesis and toxicology clearly indicate its value, and that it should also serve us as a remedy in cases of hypertrophy of the spleen and ganglia. He calls our attention to the fact that it produces dyspnoea, the cheyne—stokes rhythm, actue pulmonary oedema, and intense exaggeration of the cardiac-pulsations. offering a good field for clinical studies and experimentation of great interest which may give fruitful and important results.

TELA ARANEARUM (in 'relationship' of **Aranea diadema**)

—Spider's web—Cardiac sleeplessness, increased muscular energy. Excitement and nervous agitation in febrile state. Dry asthma, harassing coughs; periodic headaches with *extreme nervous erethism. Obstinate intermittents.* Acts immediately on arterial system, pulse full, strong, compressible. Lowers pulse rate frequency. Marked periodical diseases, hectic, broken down patients symptoms come on *suddenly* with cool *clammy* skin. Numbness of hands and legs when at rest. *Continued chilliness.*

TELA ARANEARUM (in 'relationship' of **Taraxacum**)

Nervous asthma and sleeplessness.

TEREBENE (in 'relationship' of **Terebinthina**)

Chronic bronchitis and winter coughs; subacute stages of inflammation of respiratory tract loosens secretion, relieves tightened feeling, makes expectoration easy. Neurotic cough. Huskiness of public speakers, and singers. Cystitis when urine is alkaline and offensive. 1x.

TERPIN HYDRAT (in 'relationship' of **Naphthaline**)

Whooping-cough, hay asthma and bronchial affections. 1-2 grain doses.

TETRODYMITE (in 'relationship' of **Tellurium**)

Crystals from Georgia and North Carolina containing Bismuth, Tellurium, and Sulphur: Coccygodynia, ulceration of nails, pains in hands, in small spots, ankles, heels, and tendo-Achilles.

TEUCRIUM SCOR. (in 'relationship' of **Teuc. marum**)

—Woodsage-Tuberculosis with muco-purulent expectoration; dropsy; orchitis and *tuberculous epidymitis;* especially in young, thin individuals with tuberculosis of lungs, glands, bones and uro-genitals. 3x.

THYMOL (in 'relationship' of **Phos.**)

Typical sexual neurasthenia; irritable stomach; aching throughout lumbar region; worse mental and physical exertion.

THYMUS GLAD EXT. (in 'relationship' of **Thyroid.**)

Arthritis deformans; metabolic osteoarthritis, 5 grain tablet 3 times daily. High potencies very efficient in exophthalmic goitre.

TINOSPORA CORDIFOLIA (in 'relationship' of **Ceanothus**)

A Hindoo medicine for chronic cases of fever with enlarged spleen.

TOSTA PRAEP. (in 'relationship' of **Ovigalli pell**)

—Roasted egg shells—Calcarea ovorum—Leucorrhoea and backache. A feeling as if the spine were broken and wired or tied together with a string. Pain of cancer warts. *Also Egg Vaccine for asthma.* Much interest is shown in Dr. Fritz Talbot's method to ease one form of asthma in children by use of egg vaccine Asthma due to susceptibility of the proteid substance in eggs can be cured by immunizing against egg poison by repeated doses of egg white. After the skin has been cleaned with soap and alcohol the egg-white is rubbed into a slight scratch.

TOXICOPHIS (in 'relationship' of **Bothrops lanci.**)

—Moccasion snake—pain and fever recur annually, after bite from this snake, and sometimes changes location with disappearance of first symptoms. An annual dryness of skin follows the bite. Oedematous swellings and periodical neuralgia. Pain travels from one part to another. Other snake poisons notably **Lachesis.**

TRACHINUS (in 'relationship' of **Bothrops lanci.**)

—Stingfish—intolerable pains, swellings, acute blood poisoning, gangrene.

TRADESCANTIA (in 'relationship' of **Triticum**)

Haemorrhage from ear and upper air passages; painful urination, urethral discharge; scrotum inflamed.

TRIATEMA (in 'relationship' of **Lactrodectone mac.**)

—Kissing bug—Sweating with violent itching of fingers and toes.

ESSENTIALS OF RARE AND UNCOMMON REMEDIES

Smothering sensation and difficult breathing succeeded by fainting and rapid pulse.

TRIFOLIUM REPENS (in 'relationship' of **Trifol. prat.**)

—White clover—Prophylactic against mumps, feeling of congestion in salivary glands, pain and hardening, especially submaxillary; worse, lying down. Mouth filled with watery saliva, *worse lying down*. Taste of blood in mouth and throat. Sensation as if heart would stop, with great fear, better sitting up or moving about; worse when alone, with cold sweat on face.

TRILLIUM ERUNUM (in 'relationship' of **Trillium pend.**)

Eye symptoms everything looks bluish; greasy feeling in mouth.

TRIONAL (in 'relationship' of **Sulfonal**)

Insomnia associated with physical excitement; vertigo, loss of equilibrium, ataxia, nausea, vomiting, diarrhoea, stertorous breathing, cyanosis, tinnitus, hallucinations.

TRYCHOSATHES (in 'relationship' of **Verat. alb.**)

Diarrhoea, pain in liver, dizziness after every stool.

TRYCHNOS GAUL. (in 'relationship' of **Hyderoc.**)

Bites of serpents, ulcers and cutaneous affections generally.

TUSSILAGO FAR. (in 'relationship' of **Tussilago pet.**)

Cough and as an intercurrent remedy in phthisis pulmonalis.

TUSSILAGO FRAG. (in 'relationship' of **Tussilago pet.**)

Pylorus pain, plethora and corpulency.

TYPHA LATIFOLIA (in 'relationship' of **Cuphea**)

—Cat tail flag—Diarrhoea, dysentery, summer complaints of children. Tincture and first attenuation.

TYPHA LATIFOLIA (in 'relationship' of **Ipecac**)

—Cat tail flag—Dysentery, diarrhoea and other summer complaints.

ULMUS (in 'relationship' of **Viola od.**)

Formication in feet, numb, creeping pains in legs and feet; rheumatic pains above wrists; numbness, tingling, and full soreness where gastrocnemius gives off its tendon.

UPAS ANTIARIS (in 'relationship' of Upas tients)

—resinous exudation of *Antiarus toxicaria*. A deadly poison to the muscular system. It suspends both voluntary muscular action and that of the heart without causing convulsions, used in lava as an arrow poison (Merrell). Differs in producing *clonic spasms*, violent vomiting, diarrhoea, great prostration.

URIC ACID (in 'relationship' of Urea)

Gout, gouty eczema, rheumatism, lipoma.

URINUM (in 'relationship' of Urea)

Acne, boils, scurvy, dropsy.

UROTROPIN (in 'relationship' of Formalin)

A diuretic and solvent of uric acid concretions; relieves cystitis associated with putrefaction. Three to five grain well-diluted. When administered invariably appears in the cerebro-spinal fluid and therefore advised in threatened meningeal infection.

VACCINUM MYRTILLUS (in 'relationship' of Uva ursi.)

—Huckleberries—Dysentery; typhoid, keeps intestines aseptic and prevents absorption and reinfection.

VERATRINA (in 'relationship' of Sabadilla) 536

An alkaloid of Sabad. and Verat., locally in neuralgias, and for removal of dropsy. Give 5 grains to 2 drams. Lanolin rubbed on inside of thighs, causes diuresis.

VERATRINE (in 'relationship' of Verat alb.)

Increased vascular tension. It relaxes it and stimulates the elimination of toxins by skin, kidneys and liver.

VERATRINUM (in 'relationship' of Verat alb.)

—An alkaloid from seeds of Sabadilla—electric pains, electric shocks in muscles, fibrillary twitchings.

VERONAL (in 'relationship' of Chloralum)

—A dangerous drug, made by the action of alcohol upon urea and contains the same radical that alcohol does. Makes a man just as drunk as pure alcohol. Staggers, cannot stand up—Confluent reddish spots;

dermatitis, itching of glans and prepuce; circumscribed dermatitis patch on first metacarpal phalangeal joint.

VESICARIA (in 'relationship' of **Cantharis**)

Urinary and kidney remedy. Smarting, burning sensation along urethra and in bladder with frequent desire to void urine often with strangury. Cystitis irritable bladder. 5-10 drops of tincture.

VIBURNUM PRUNI. (in 'relationship' of **Veburnum opu.**)

—Black Haw—habitual miscarriage; *after pains*; cancer of the tongue; obstinate hiccough; supposed to be a uterine tonic. Morning sickness, menstrual irregularities of sterile females with uterine displacements.

VITEX TRIFOLIO (in 'relationship' of **Arnica mont.**)

—Indian Arnica—sprains and pains. Headache in temples, pain in joints; pain in abdomen; pain in testicles.

VITRUM (in 'relationship' of **Silicia**)

—Crown glass—Potts' disease, after silica, necrosis, discharge thin, watery, fetid. Much pain, fine grinding and grating like grit.

XANTATE (in 'relationship' of **Carboneum sulph.**)

Similar in action. Acts on cortical substance; loss of memory, marked blood degeneration; impotence and senility

XANTHORRHIZA API. (in 'relationship' of **Berberis vulg.**)

—Shrub yellow Root—contain Berberine. Dilatation of stomach and intestine, atony, enlarged spleen.

XANTHORRHOEA ARBO. (in 'relationship' of **Berberis vulg.**)

Severe pain in Kidney, cystitis and gravel. Pain from ureter to bladder and testicles. Pain in small of back returns from least chill or damp.

XANTHIUM SPINOSUM (in 'relationship' of **Hydrophob.**)

—Cockle—said to be specific for hydrophobia and is recommended for chronic cystitis in women.

ZEA ITALICA (in 'relationship' of **Ustilago maydis**)

Possesses curative properties in skin diseases, particularly in psoriasis and eczema rubrum. Mania after bathing. Impulse to suicide particularly by drowning. Easily angered. Appetite increased, voraceous, alternating with disgust for food. Pyrosis, nausea, vomiting, better drinking wine.

ZINCUM ACETICUM (in 'relationship' of Zinc. met.)

Effects of night watching and erysipelas, brain feels sore. Rademacher's solution, five-drop doses three times a day in water, for those who are compelled to work, on an insufficient amount of sleep.

ZINCUM ARS. (in 'relationship' of Zinc. met.)

Chorea, anaemia, *profound exhaustion* on slight exertion. Depression and marked involvement of lower extremities.

ZINCUM BROMATUM (in 'relationship' of Zinc. met.)

Dentition, chorea, hydrocephalus.

ZINCUM CARB. (in 'relationship' of Zinc. met.)

Post-gonorrhoeal throat affections, tonsils swollen, bluish superficial spots.

ZINCUM CYANATUM (in 'relationship' of Zinc. met.)

Meningitis and cerebro-spinal meningitis, paralysis agitans, chorea and hysteria.

ZINCUM MURIAL (in 'relationship' of Zinc. met.)

Disposition to pick the bed clothes; sense of smell and taste perverted; bluish green tint of skin; cold and sweaty.

ZINCUM OXYDATUM (in 'relationship' of Zinc. met.)

Nausea and sore taste. Sudden vomiting in children. Vomiting of bile and dirrhoea. Flatulent abdomen. Watery stool with tenesmus. Debility after grip. Fiery red face, *great drowsiness* with dreams like unrefreshed sleep. Similar to effects of night watching. Mental and physical exertion (Rademacher).

ZINCUM PHOS. (in 'relationship' of Zinc. met.)

Herpes zoster 1x.

ZINCUM PHOS. (in 'relationship' of Zinc. met.)

Neuralgia of head and face; lightning-like pains in locomotor ataxia, brain-fag nervousness and vertigo, sexual excitement and sleeplessness.

ESSENTIALS OF RARE AND UNCOMMON REMEDIES

ZINC. PIC. (in 'relationship' of **Picricum acid**)
Facial palsy and paralysis agitans.

ZINCUM PICRICUM (in 'relationship' of **Zinc. met.**) 638
Facial paralysis; brain fag; Headache in Bright's disease; seminal emissions; loss of memory and energy. Oxide of zinc is used locally as an astringent and stimulant application to unhealthy ulcers, fissures, intertigo, burns, etc.

ZINCUM SULPH. (in 'relationship' of **Zinc. met.**)
Not repeated frequently (high potency) will clear up opacities of Cornea (Mc Ferland) corneitis; granular lids; tongue paralyzed; cramps in arms and legs, trembling and convulsions. Hypochondriasis due to masturbation, nervous headache.